www.wadsworth.com

wadsworth.com is the World Wide Web site for Wadsworth Publishing Company and is your direct source to dozens of online resources.

At *wadsworth.com* you can find out about supplements, demonstration software, and student resources. You can also send e-mail to many of our authors and preview new publications and exciting new technologies.

wadsworth.com
Changing the way the world learns®

An Invitation to Health

Ninth Edition

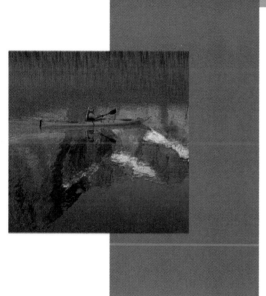

Dianne Hales

Wadsworth Publishing Company
I T P® **An International Thomson Publishing Company**

Australia • Canada • Mexico • Singapore • Spain • United Kingdom • United States

Publisher: *Peter Marshall*
Development Editor: *Barbara Yien*
Editorial Assistant: *Keynia Johnson*
Marketing Manager: *Joanne Terhaar*
Marketing Assistant: *Colleen Delgado*
Project Editor: *Sandra Craig*
Print Buyer: *Barbara Britton*
Permissions Editor: *Robert Kauser*
Production: *The Book Company*

Text and Cover Designer: *Delgado Design*
Photo Researcher: *Myrna Engler*
Copy Editor: *Jane Townsend*
Illustrators: *Impact Publications; Precision Graphics*
Cover Photograph: *Waterfowl Lake, Banff National Park, Alberta.*
James Kay Photography
Compositor: *Parkwood Composition Service*
Printer: *Von Hoffmann Press*

Printed in the United States of America
1   2   3   4   5   6   7   04   03   02   01   00

ExamView[R] and *ExamView Pro*[R] are trademarks of FSCreations, Inc. Windows is a registered trademark of the Microsoft Corporation used herein under license. Macintosh and Power Macintosh are registered trademarks of Apple Computer, Inc. Used herein under license.

Library of Congress Cataloging-in-Publication Data
Hales, Dianne R., 1950–
    An invitation to health / Dianne Hales.--9th ed.
        p. cm.
    Includes bibliographical references and index.
    ISBN 0-534-57753-9
    1. Health. 2. Self-care, Health. I. Title.

RA776.H148 2001
613--dc21
                            00-036512

Wadsworth/Thomson Learning
10 Davis Drive
Belmont, CA 94002-3098
USA

For more information about our products, contact us:
Thomson Learning Academic Resource Center
1-800-423-0563
http://www.wadsworth.com

International Headquarters
Thomson Learning
International Division
290 Harbor Drive, 2nd Floor
Stamford, CT 06902-7477
USA

UK/Europe/Middle East/South Africa
Thomson Learning
Berkshire House
168-173 High Holborn
London WC1V 7AA
United Kingdom

Asia
Thomson Learning
60 Albert Street, #15-01
Albert Complex
Singapore 189969

Canada
Nelson Thomson Learning
1120 Birchmount Road
Toronto, Ontario M1K 5G4
Canada

To my husband, Bob, and my daughter, Julia, who make every day an invitation to joy.

Preface

To the Student

An Invitation to Health is an invitation to you. What you learn in this course will have a direct impact on how you'll look, feel, and act—now and for decades to come.

Perhaps you are in good health and think that you know all that you need to know about how to take care of yourself. If so, take a minute and ask yourself some questions:

- How well do you understand yourself? Are you able to cope with emotional upsets and crises? Do you often feel stressed out?

- How nutritiously do you eat? Are you always going on—and off—diets? Do you exercise regularly?

- How solid and supportive are your relationships with others? Are you conscientious about birth control and safer-sex practices?

- Do you get drunk or high occasionally? Do you smoke?

- Are you a savvy health-care consumer? Do you know how to evaluate medical products and health professionals?

- How much do you know about complementary and alternative medicine?

- If you needed health care, do you know where you'd turn or how you'd pay? What do you know about your risk for infectious diseases, heart problems, cancer, or other serious illnesses?

- Have you taken steps to insure your personal safety at home, on campus, or on the streets?

- What are you doing today to prevent physical, psychological, social, and environmental problems in the future?

As you consider these questions, chances are there are some aspects of health you've never considered before—and others you feel you don't have to worry about for years. Yet the choices you make and the actions you take now will have a dramatic impact on your future.

Your health is your personal responsibility. Over time, your priorities and needs will inevitably change, but the connections between various dimensions of your well-being will remain the same: The state of your mind will affect the state of your body, and vice versa. The values that guide you through today can keep you mentally, physically, and spiritually healthy throughout your lifetime. Your ability to cope with stress will influence your decisions about alcohol and drug use. Your commitment to honest, respectful relationships will affect the nature of your sexual involvements. Your eating and exercise habits will determine whether you develop a host of medical problems.

An Invitation to Health, Ninth Edition, is packed with information, advice, recommendations, and research, and provides the first step in taking full charge of your own well-being. An important theme of this book is prevention. Ultimately, the power of prevention belongs to you—and it's a lot easier than you might think. You might simply add a walk or workout to your daily routine. You might snack on fruit instead of high-fat foods. You might cut back on alcohol. You might buckle your seatbelt whenever you get in a car. These things may not seem like a big deal now, yet they may well make a crucial difference in determining how active and fulfilling the rest of your life will be.

This textbook is an invitation—an invitation to health in its broadest sense, to personal fulfillment, to life itself. Its pages provide the practical tools you need to work toward achieving your full potential. I hope that you keep this book and use it often as your personal health manual. I also hope that you accept this invitation in another sense—that you live what you learn and make the most of your life—now and through all the years and adventures the future may bring you.

May you live long and well,

Dianne Hales

To the Instructor

*A*n *Invitation to Health,* Ninth Edition, introduces students to a way of thinking about their health and their future that is informed by the most current research available. The text outlines the keys to preventing the major killers of Americans—heart disease, cancer, and accidents—and to preparing for a life of health in the fullest sense of the word. **Health** is defined in the broadest possible way—not as an entity in itself, but as a process of discovering, using, and protecting all the resources within the individual, family, community, and environment. It is a subject that encompasses mind, body, and spirit, and the ninth edition brings this vision fully to life by providing students with the information and inspiration they need to make healthful decisions and changes.

Overview of the Ninth Edition

The ninth edition includes a wealth of new research, references, and features. Yet my essential themes will be familiar to those who have used previous editions of this text: I continue to place a strong emphasis on personal responsibility, a commitment to prevention, practical applications of knowledge, and a focus on behavioral change.

The ninth edition is organized into six sections, with a total of 20 chapters. In response to the high interest that has developed in consumer health, alternative medicine, and violence prevention, I have added two new chapters to this edition with expanded coverage of these topics: Chapter 11, "Consumerism, Self-Care, and Complementary/Alternative Medicine," and Chapter 18, "Staying Safe: Preventing Injury, Violence, and Victimization."

Three new features to this edition—*The X & Y Files, FAQs* (Frequently Asked Questions), and *Consumer Health Watch*— reflect my commitment to engaging students in their study of health in ways that make the content as relevant to their lives as possible. *The X & Y Files* brings students cutting-edge research on gender differences in various aspects of health. Guaranteed to spark spirited classroom discussions, *The X & Y Files* reports research on how men and women tend to differ in important ways that relate to health, such as in their susceptibilities to certain diseases, their vulnerabilities to stress, and their ways of communicating with others. Meanwhile, *FAQs* grab students' interest by presenting them with commonly asked questions at the beginning of each chapter, along with page references directing them to where the answer is found within the text. Finally, *Consumer Health Watch* focuses on topics like evaluating health information on the Internet, selecting a therapist, choosing a personal trainer, and evaluating complementary/alternative treatments—providing guidelines for how to be a smart and savvy health consumer. These, along with highly praised retained features like *Campus Focus, Pulsepoints, Self-Surveys, Strategies for Change, Strategies for Prevention,* and *Health Online,* are described in more detail in the "Features" section in this preface.

Another change to this edition is that coverage of topics related to health and aging are now integrated into chapters throughout the text in a new feature called *Across the Lifespan,* instead of appearing in a separate chapter. This allows you to cover topics related to health and aging *throughout* the course term, rather than in just one chapter or week during the course term. In addition, topics related to race, ethnicity, and other forms of diversity are now fully integrated into each chapter instead of in a separate boxed format, which

has allowed me to include more health-relevant data on diverse populations than ever before. (See page xxxii for an index of health topics that pertain to specific racial and ethnic groups.)

Because the field of health science is so broad and changes so rapidly, keeping up with the most recent developments is critical. This ninth edition incorporates *the most current research* you will find in a college health textbook—some of which was added as this book was going to press! You will find several hundred 1999 citations, the majority of which are from primary sources, including professional books; medical, health, and mental health journals, health education periodicals; scientific meetings; federal agencies; publications from research laboratories and universities; and personal interviews with specialists in a number of fields. In addition, this textbook offers your students access to *InfoTrac College Edition,* an online library of literally hundreds of academic journals and popular periodicals. With a simple key word search, your students can find reliable information on any health topic, in a database that is updated daily and available to them 24 hours a day—a powerful way to stay abreast of up-to-the-minute health research and information. See the "Ancillary Package" section of this preface for more information on *InfoTrac* and other supplements available with this textbook.

The following is a chapter-by-chapter listing of just some of the key topics I've added, expanded, or revised for the ninth edition.

Chapter 1: An Invitation to Health for the Twenty-First Century

- Expanded discussion of spiritual health and its relationship to longevity
- A progress report on Healthy People 2000 and the goals of Healthy People 2010
- A report on health progress around the world
- New data on minority populations in the United States
- New data from a government survey on risky behavior among today's youths
- New discussion of gender differences in life expectancy and susceptibility to disease

Chapter 2: Personal Stress Management

- An expanded definition of "stress" that differentiates acute, episodic, and chronic stress
- A new section on the effects of stress on the body, covering how stress hormones work and their relationship to cardiovascular (and other) diseases

- New research on the link between stress and the common cold
- New section on anger management and conflict resolution
- Expanded discussion of strategies for coping with stress
- New strategies for improving time management
- Research on people who have thrived in the face of adversity
- New discussion of gender differences in stress levels reported by college-age men and women

Chapter 3: Feeling Good

- A new section on "positive psychology," an approach to mental health that emphasizes building personal strengths rather than simply treating weaknesses
- A new section on health and "spiritual intelligence"
- A new section on "positive self-talk"
- Recent research on the links between happiness and factors like prosperity, marital status, and disability
- New research on how certain foods may influence our moods
- New research on how the Internet may be contributing to depression and loneliness

Chapter 4: Caring for the Mind

- New information on the mental health of college students
- Expanded discussion of antidepressants
- Expanded discussion of attention deficit hyperactivity disorder (ADHD)
- Expanded discussion of the costs of mental illness to our society
- New information on mind-mood products like St. John's Wort, valerian, kava, and gingko biloba
- A new *Across the Lifespan* section on how a person's psychological health early in life may affect his or her well-being later on
- Discussion of hormone replacement therapy as a treatment for Alzheimer's

Chapter 5: The Joy of Fitness

- The latest findings on the exercise habits of Americans
- Expanded discussion of muscular fitness and body composition
- New section on how much exercise is needed for optimal health

- New section on exercise motivation
- New section on how to design an aerobic workout
- Expanded discussion of performance-enhancing drugs and supplements, including androstendione, creatine, GBL, and energy bars
- New discussion of how to evaluate fitness products and programs
- New discussion of gender differences in athletic abilities

Chapter 6: Nutrition for Life

- New data on the eating habits of Americans
- Expanded discussion of carbohydrates, dietary fiber, fats, and cholesterol
- New tables on the functions, deficiency symptoms, and toxicity symptoms of key vitamins
- Expanded discussion of antioxidants and phytochemicals
- Expanded discussion of the safety and effectiveness of dietary supplements
- New research on eggs and heart health
- New information on lactose intolerance
- A new section on dietary reference intakes (DRIs), recommended daily allowances, and daily values
- A new section on what terms like *fat-free, lean, lite* and *low-calorie* really mean
- A new section on Mediterranean diets
- Expanded discussion of food poisoning

Chapter 7: Eating Patterns and Problems

- Expanded discussion of body mass index (BMI)
- New research on unhealthy eating behavior and obesity in children and adolescents
- Expanded discussion of the causes and victims of anorexia and bulimia
- Updated government guidelines on obesity
- New information on FDA-approved weight loss drugs like Meridia and Xenical
- New discussion of the gap between real and "ideal" body images among both men and women

Chapter 8: Communication and Relationships

- New section on the science behind attraction
- New research on oxytocin

- New research on breakups
- Updated data on the percentage of young adults living at home
- Updated data on the marital status of Americans
- Updated data on the percentage of interracial couples in the United States
- New research on cohabitation and marriage
- New data on the structure of American families
- New data on the percentage of mothers who work
- New discussion of changing marital roles
- New data on single fathers
- New discussion of gender differences in communication

Chapter 9: Personal Sexuality

- New cross-cultural research on girls' responses to menarche
- New research on menopause and hormone replacement therapy
- Expanded discussion of circumcision
- New data on the sexual activity of adolescents, college students, and middle-aged and older Americans
- New research on the existence/nonexistence of a "homosexuality gene"
- Expanded discussion of abstinence
- New data on college students' attitudes toward sex
- Expanded discussion of Viagra and its effects
- New discussion of the usage of X-rated Internet sites

Chapter 10: Reproductive Choices

- Expanded discussion of unintended pregnancies
- Updated information on selecting birth control methods
- New research on whether oral contraceptives reduce the risk of some diseases while increasing the risk of others
- Updated information on the contraceptive sponge
- New discussion of contraceptives around the world
- New data on the effectiveness of "morning after" pills
- Expanded discussion of abortion, including a cross-cultural comparison of abortion rates around the world
- New research on the psychological effects of abortion
- New discussion on women who decide to remain childfree

Chapter 11: Consumerism, Complementary/Alternative Medicine, and the Health-Care System

- New information on home health tests
- New discussion on evaluating online medical advice
- Expanded discussion of dental health, including new research linking dental health to longevity
- Expanded coverage about how to effectively communicate with your doctor
- New coverage of elective treatments like laser vision surgery and cosmetic surgery
- Expanded coverage of complementary and alternative medicine, including why people seek alternative therapies, what these therapies are, what research has shown about their effectiveness, and how to evaluate them
- New information on herbal remedies
- Expanded discussion of managed care, including coverage of a "patient's bill of rights" and comparison of care quality in HMOs versus traditional fee-for-service practices

Chapter 12: Defending Yourself from Infectious Diseases

- New research on immunity and stress
- New research on immunotherapy
- New research on how to treat the common cold
- New information on vaccines for flu prevention and Lyme disease
- Expanded discussion of hepatitis B, hepatitis C, and chlamydia
- Expanded discussion of sexually transmitted diseases among those under 25
- Fully updated coverage of AIDS, including current statistics on people living with HIV, current rate of new infections, expanded discussion of HIV testing, and current AIDS treatments

Chapter 13: Keeping Your Heart Healthy

- Fully updated statistics on heart disease
- New discussion of the heart benefits of physical activity and good nutrition
- Expanded discussion of factors related to heart disease risk, including psychological and social factors, homocysteine, bacterial infection, and cocaine use

- Expanded discussion of how to lower cholesterol
- Updated coverage of arrythmias and mitral valve prolapse

Chapter 14: Lowering Your Risk of Cancer and Other Major Diseases

- Fully updated statistics on cancer
- Expanded coverage of how cancer develops
- New discussion of how cancer has affected minority populations
- New research on how nutrition may affect cancer risk
- Expanded discussion of chemoprevention, including tamoxifen and finasteride
- Completely revised and updated coverage of breast, cervical, and prostate cancer
- New research on cancer treatments and survivorship

Chapter 15: Drug Use, Misuse, and Abuse

- Updated statistics on drug use in America
- New tables on common over-the-counter medications, as well as commonly abused legal and illegal drugs
- New section on the selling of prescription drugs online
- New discussion of gender differences in drug use
- Updated section on drug use on college campuses
- New research on marijuana as a medical treatment and on "marijuana withdrawal syndrome"
- Expanded discussion of GHB ("blue nitro" or "the date rape drug")

Chapter 16: Alcohol Use, Misuse, and Abuse

- Updated statistics on alcohol use in America
- Updated discussion of binge drinking and underage drinking
- Updated discussion of drinking on college campuses
- New section on drinking among minority populations
- New research on the effectiveness of legal age limit laws
- New section on treating alcohol problems in the elderly

Chapter 17: Tobacco Use, Misuse and Abuse

- Updated statistics on tobacco use in America

- Updated coverage of smoking among minority populations, women, and campus populations
- New section on bidis (skinny, flavored cigarettes that are popular among young people)
- Updated section on cigar use
- New section on lifelong risks to smokers' children
- Updated coverage of strategies for quitting, including discussion of buproprion (Zyban)

Chapter 18: Staying Safe: Preventing Injury, Violence, and Victimization

- Expanded discussion of safety on the road, including road rage, driver safety, the dangers of cell phones, and cycling safely
- Updated coverage of computer safety, including prevention of repetitive motion injury and vision problems
- New discussion of violence in America, hate crimes, and use of guns and firearms
- New statistics on crime victims by age, race, and gender
- Updated coverage of sexual harassment on campus

Chapter 19: When Life Ends

- New cross-cultural discussion on finding meaning in death
- New coverage of pain relief for the terminally ill

Chapter 20: Working Toward a Healthy Environment

- Updated coverage of the state of the environment today, including new discussions of environmental health threats, multiple chemical sensitivity (MCS), and pollution-induced health problems
- New statistics on the growth of the global population
- Expanded coverage of global warming and ozone pollution
- New research on the health risks of electric and magnetic fields around power lines

Hales Health Almanac

- Complete updating of "Your Health Directory," including several organizations' web sites

Features and Pedagogy

FAQ—Frequently Asked Questions, new to this edition, are found at the beginning of each chapter, immediately engaging students with commonly asked questions such as "Should I take vitamin supplements?" "What can help me relax?" "How can I reduce my cancer risk?" "Is it possible to overdose on caffeine?" Page references are included after each question, and each corresponding heading is marked with an icon, signaling that this is where the answer can be found.

The X & Y Files, new to this edition, are found throughout the text and present what scientific research has revealed about health-related differences between men and women. Much of this research is truly groundbreaking, since until very recently, most studies—since proven erroneous—were conducted on male subjects only (the assumption being that women were essentially smaller versions of men). Among the topics covered: differences in susceptibility to heart attacks, cancer, liver failure, autoimmune disorders, and other diseases; differences in stress vulnerabilities; differences in athletic capabilities; differences in communication styles; differences in vulnerability to alcoholism and drug use; and more.

Campus Focus, one of the text's most popular features, uses pie charts and bar graphs to present eye-catching data on college populations that relate to nearly every chapter topic in the text. Topics include student stress levels, mental health, fitness activity, prevalence of eating disorders, sexual activity, drug and alcohol use, and more. Campus data have been completely updated for this edition.

Health Online presents more engaging and reliable Internet resources than you will find in any other college textbook on the market. Appearing in every chapter, it includes a list of web sites relevant to chapter topics (along with descriptions of each); a "Campus Chat" discussion question that students can answer online on the web site accompanying this text at **http://health.wadsworth.com** (where they can compare their answers with those of other students nationwide); and a suggested reading from the InfoTrac online library—a terrific way to have students research topics on the Internet from *trusted and credible* sources. Moreover, students can go to **http://health.wadsworth.com** to find link updates, over 500 additional health-related links (researched by a health professor), and additional suggested readings on InfoTrac, complete with review/discussion questions.

Pulsepoints is a popular feature that appears in every chapter, offering a snappy list of relevant, practical health tips. Examples include "Top Ten Stress Busters" (Ch. 2), "The Top Ten Ways to Cut Fat" (Ch. 6), and "Ten Characteristics of a Good Relationship" (Ch. 8).

Self-Surveys appear in every chapter and allow students to assess themselves on topics like "Rate Your Diet" (Ch. 6), "Which Contraceptive is Right For You?" (Ch. 10), and "Are You Doing Your Part for the Planet?" (Ch. 20).

Strategies for Change appear throughout the text and provide practical, checklist-format behavioral change strategies for achieving better health.

Strategies for Prevention appear throughout the text and provide effective, checklist-format strategies for preventing health problems and reducing health risks.

Consumer Health Watch, new to this edition, focuses on consumer-related health topics and provides guidelines for being a savvy and informed health consumer. Topics include selecting a therapist, evaluating mind-mood medications like St. John's Wort, selecting a personal trainer, evaluating weight-loss diets, online dating, bogus HIV tests, evaluating alternative treatments, and more.

Across the Lifespan, new to this edition, appears throughout the text and focuses on health issues as they relate to aging, as well as on how health changes now can result in benefits later in life.

The Wellness Inventory is a self-inventory that precedes Chapter 1. It allows students to assess how their lifestyles rate in various areas of wellness, providing a useful springboard for deciding which areas they would like to pay special attention to and improve.

Hales Health Almanac appears at the end of the text and includes resources related to finding health information on the Internet; what to do in an emergency; a consumer's guide to medical tests; tables for counting calories and fat in specific foods; and a comprehensive health directory of contact information for various health organizations.

In addition:

• *Learning Objectives* open each chapter and outline the most essential information on which students should focus while reading.

• *Key Terms* are boldfaced when they first appear in the chapter and are listed at the end of each chapter with page references. They are also defined in the Glossary at the end of the book.

- *Making This Chapter Work for You* appears at the end of each chapter, providing a bulleted summary of key points covered in the chapter.
- *Critical Thinking Questions* are included at the end of each chapter and ask the students to consider some applications of the chapter's coverage, or weigh in on a health-related controversy.
- *CNN Video Discussion Questions* are included at the end of each chapter. These are designed to work in conjunction with the video of CNN health clips that has been developed with this edition. The CNN health video is complimentary with adoption of this textbook.

Ancillary Package

An extraordinary package of support materials is available for instructors and students using this textbook:

Instructors Guide—Contains chapter outlines, learning objectives, discussion questions, a video list, and more. Also includes a section for Canadian instructors.

Test Bank—Completely revised for this edition, the Test Bank contains hundreds of multiple-choice, fill-in-the-blank, and essay questions.

ExamView^R Computerized Test Bank—Deliver and customize tests in minutes with this easy-to-use assessment and tutorial system. *ExamView^R* guides you step-by-step through the process of creating print or online tests, and allows you to see the test you are creating on the screen exactly as it will print or display online. With ExamView's complete word processing capabilities, you can also enter an unlimited number of new questions or edit existing questions.

Full-Color Transparency Acetates—More than 100 transparency acetates are available with this text, consisting of text art as well as supplementary outlines.

PowerPoint Presentations—More than 100 power-point slides are available, consisting of text art as well as supplementary outlines.

HealthLink Presentation CD-ROM—*HealthLink* is the perfect software tool to help you present dynamic lectures! It contains art, photos, and other resources designed to spark classroom discussion and enhance presentations. *HealthLink* may be used with PowerPoint or other electronic lecture programs, and may also be used on the web.

Study Guide—Contains learning objectives, key terms, review questions, practice test questions, and more.

Web Tutor—This web-based learning tool helps professors take the personal health course beyond classroom boundaries to an anywhere, anytime environment. Students have access to study tools that correspond chapter by chapter and topic by topic with the book, including flashcards, practice quizzes, and online tutorials. Professors can use *Web Tutor* to provide virtual office hours, post syllabi, set up threaded discussions, and track student progress on the practice quizzes. *Web Tutor* is easily customizable to specific course needs. *Available on Web CT or Blackboard.*

Profile Plus Software—The most comprehensive software package available with any health textbook, *Profile Plus* allows students to generate personalized fitness and wellness profiles, conduct self-assessments, analyze their diets, tailor exercise prescriptions to their individual needs, keep an exercise log, and much more!

Diet Analysis Plus Software—*Diet Analysis Plus* software allows students to determine the best ways to adjust their food intake and better meet their nutritional needs. Students create their own personalized profile based on height, weight, age, sex, and activity level, and input the type and serving size of foods they consume each day for up to seven days. The program then calculates Recommended Nutrient Intakes and Allowances (RDAs/RDIs), goal percentages, and actual percentages of the essential nutrients, vitamins, and minerals consumed based on the student's personal profile. The software includes the newest Dietary Reference Intakes.

The U.C. Berkeley Wellness Newsletter—This respected newsletter imparts up-to-date consumer information related to health and wellness. Typical topics include the benefits of soy, butter vs. margarine, reducing risks for heart disease, and so on.

CNN Health Video—Launch your lectures with riveting footage from CNN, the world's leading 24-hour global news television network. The *CNN Today: Health* video allows you to integrate the newsgathering and programming power of CNN into the classroom to show students the relevance of course topics to their everyday lives. Organized by topics introduced in the text, the clips are presented in short 2-to-5 minute segments, and a new video is available each year.

Wadsworth Video Library for Health—A comprehensive library of videos is available for adopters of this textbook. Contact your local Wadsworth/Thomson Learning representative for more information.

InfoTrac College Edition—The latest news and research articles online—updated daily and spanning four years! Choose to package *InfoTrac College Edition* with this text and you and your students will have four months of free access to an easy-to-use online database of reliable, full-length articles (not abstracts) from hundreds of top academic journals and popular sources. Ideal for launching lectures, igniting discussions, and opening whole new worlds of information and research for students.

Web Site—You will find both student and instructor resources for this text (including self-quizzes and web links for students and downloadable manuals and PowerPoint presentations for instructors), at **http://health.wadsworth.com**

Personal Daily Log—Contains an exercise pyramid, a "How Long Will You Live?" chart based on lifestyle choices, study and exercise tips, time management strategies, goal-setting worksheets, cardiorespiratory exercise record forms, strength training record form, a daily nutrition diary, and more.

Wellness Worksheets—Contains detachable wellness worksheets, a complete wellness inventory, and self-surveys.

Health Explorer: Internet Resources—A handy full-color trifold brochure containing dozens of useful health and wellness Internet links.

To Order

To adopt *An Invitation to Health*, or to receive additional review copies of this book, contact your local ITP/Thomson Learning representative. You may also send your request on department letterhead to:

Wadsworth Publishing Company
Health Marketing Manager
10 Davis Dr.
Belmont, CA 94002

Or, send in your request via our website at **http://www.wadsworth.com**

Acknowledgments

I am deeply indebted to the many instructors and students, reviewers, editors, and others without whom this book would never have enjoyed so many years of success.

For the ninth edition, I was fortunate to work with a great team at Wadsworth. Peter Marshall and Barbara Yien both provided editorial expertise and invaluable input to improve the manuscript and keep the ninth edition on track. Sandra Craig and Dusty Friedman and The Book Company deserve tremendous credit for coordinating the many pieces that go into a four-color textbook and for producing a beautiful book on a demanding schedule. I appreciate the talents of Jane Townsend for her meticulous copyedit of the manuscript, Delgado Design for working up the wonderful cover, and Bob Kauser for his work on the permissions for this edition. Jean Thompson has done a wonderful job preparing promotional materials for the ninth edition, and Joanne Terhaar is directing an exceptional marketing effort. Thanks also to Keynia Johnson and Michelle Eng for their assistance on this project.

Finally, let me express my thanks to the reviewers whose input has been so valuable through these many editions. For the ninth edition, I thank the following for their helpful assistance:

Ghulam Aasef, Kaskaskia College
Andrea Abercrombie, Clemson University
Judy Baker, East Carolina University
Betsy Bergen, Kansas State University
Nancy Bessette, Saddleback College
Patti Cost, Weber State University
Maxine Davis, Eastern Washington University
Robert Dollinger, Florida International University
Mary Gress, Lorain County Community College

Ron Heinrichs, Central Missouri State University
Kim Hyatt, Weber State University
Dee Jacobsen, Southeastern Louisiana University
John Janowiak, Appalachian State University
Peggy Jarnigan, Rollins College
David Langford, University of Maryland, Baltimore County
Norbert Lindskog, Harold Washington College
Rick Madson, Palm Beach Community College

Ashok Malik, College of San Mateo
Miguel Perez, University of North Texas
Pamela Pinahs-Schultz, Carroll College

Andrew Shim, Southwestern College
Steve Singleton, Wayne State University

For their help as reviewers or focus group participants from previous editions, I want to thank the following:

Marcia Ball, James Madison University
Rick Barnes, East Carolina University
Lois Beach, SUNY-Plattsburg
David Black, Purdue University
Jill M. Black, Cleveland State University
Cynthia Pike Blocksom, Cincinnati Health Department
James Brik, Willamette University
Mitchell Brodsky, York College
Jodi Broodkins-Fisher, University of Utah
James G. Bryant, Jr., Western Carolina University
Marsha Campos, Modesto Junior College
James Lester Carter, Montana State University
Lori Dewald, Shippensburg University
Julie Dietz, Eastern Illinois University
Gary English, Ithaca College
Michael Felts, East Carolina University
Kathie C. Garbe, Kennesaw State College
Gail Gates, Oklahoma State University
Dawn Graff-Haight, Portland State University
Carolyn Gray, New Mexico State University
Janet Grochowski, University of St. Thomas
Stephen Haynie, College of William and Mary
Michael Hoadley, University of South Dakota
Linda L. Howard, Idaho State University
Jim Johnson, Northwest Missouri State University
Chester S. Jones, University of Arkansas
Herb Jones, Ball State University
Jane Jones, University of Wisconsin, Stevens Point
Lorraine J. Jones, Muncie, Indiana
Becky Kennedy-Koch, Ohio State University
Mark J. Kittleson, Southern Illinois University
Darlene Kluka, University of Central Oklahoma
Debra A. Krummel, West Virginia University
Roland Lamarine, California State University, Chico
Beth Lanning, Baylor University
Loretta Liptak, Youngstown State University
S. Jack Loughton, Weber State University
Michele P. Mannion, Temple University
Esther Moe, Oregon Health Sciences University
Anne O'Donnell, Santa Rosa Junior College
Randy M. Page, University of Idaho

Carolyn P. Parks, University of North Carolina
Anthony V. Parrillo, East Carolina University
Janet Reis, University of Illinois at Urbana-Champaign
Steven Sansone, Chemeketa Community College
Larry Smith, Scottsdale Community College
Carl A. Stockton, Radford University
Linda Stonecipher, Western Oregon State College
Emogene Johnson Vaughn, Norfolk State University
David M. White, East Carolina University
Sabina White, University of California—Santa Barbara
Robert Wilson, University of Minnesota
Roy Wohl, Washburn University
Martin L. Wood, Ball State University

Please R.S.V.P.

This book is an invitation to good health in its broadest sense—to personal fulfillment, to life itself. Its pages provide the practical tools students need to achieve their full potential. I also hope that your students accept this invitation in another sense: that they live what they learn and make the most of their health and of their lives.

I also have another invitation for you—a request to tell us what you think. *An Invitation to Health* was created for your students and for you. I would like to know what I'm doing right, what could be done better, and what I might include or drop in future editions. Your opinions and ideas matter a great deal to me, and I look forward to hearing from you.

Dianne Hales
c/o Wadsworth Publishing Company
10 Davis Dr.
Belmont, CA 94002

You may also contact the editor at **http://health.wadsworth.com** with your comments.

About the Author

Dianne Hales, one of the most widely published and honored health journalists in the country, is a contributing editor for *Parade, Ladies Home Journal,* and

Working Mother and has written more than 1,000 articles for national publications. Her trade books include *Just Like a Woman: How Gender Science Is Redefining What Makes Us Female* and the award-winning compendium of mental health information, *Caring for the Mind: The Comprehensive Guide to Mental Health.* Dianne Hales is one of the few journalists to be honored with national awards for excellence in magazine writing by both the American Psychiatric Association and the American Psychological Association. She also has won the "EMMA" (Exceptional Media Merit Award) for health reporting from the National Women's Political Caucus and Radcliffe College, and numerous writing awards from various organizations, including the Arthritis Foundation, California Psychiatric Society, CHAAD, Council for the Advancement of Scientific Education, National Easter Seal Society, and the New York City Public Library.

Brief Contents

Contents

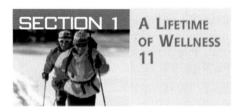

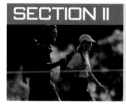

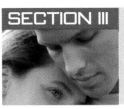

SECTION III RESPONSIBLE SEXUALITY 219

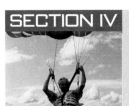

SECTION IV PERSONAL HEALTH RISKS 333

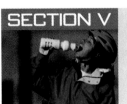

SECTION V AVOIDING HEALTH RISKS 441

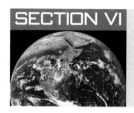

SECTION VI HEALTH IN CONTEXT 561

FEATURES

Pulsepoints

Self-Survey

The X & Y Files

Campus Focus

FEATURES, CONTINUED

Consumer Health Watch

Integrated Coverage of Race and Ethnicity relating to

An Invitation to Health

What Is Wellness?*

by John W. Travis, M.D.

Most of us think in terms of illness, and assume that the absence of illness indicates wellness. There are actually many degrees of wellness, just as there are many degrees of illness. The Wellness Inventory is designed to stir up your thinking about many areas of wellness.

While people often lack physical symptoms, they may still be bored, depressed, tense, anxious, or generally unhappy with their lives. Such emotional states often set the stage for physical and mental disease. Even cancer may be brought on through the lowering of the body's resistance from excessive stress. These same emotional states can also lead to abuse of the body through smoking, overdrinking, and overeating. Such behaviors are usually substitutes for other, more basic human needs such as recognition from others, a more stimulating environment, caring and affection from friends, and greater self-acceptance.

Wellness is not a static state. High-level wellness involves giving good care to your physical self, using your mind constructively, expressing your emotions effectively, being creatively involved with those around you, and being concerned about your physical, psychological and spiritual environments.

Instructions:

Set aside a half hour for yourself in a quiet place where you will not be disturbed while taking the Inventory. Record your responses to each statement in the columns to the right where:

2 = Yes, usually
1 = Sometimes, maybe
0 = No, rarely

Select the answer that best indicates how true the statement is for you presently.

After you have responded to all the appropriate statements in each section, compute your average score for that section and transfer it to the corresponding box provided around the Wellness Inventory Wheel on page 3. Your completed Wheel will give you a clear presentation of the balance you have given to the many dimensions of your life.

You will find some of the statements are really two in one. We do this to show an important relationship between the two parts—usually an awareness of an issue, combined with an action based on that awareness. Mentally average your score for the two parts of the question.

Each statement describes what we believe to be a wellness attribute. Because much wellness information is subjective and "unprovable" by current scientific methods, you

*Abridged from the Wellness Index in *The Wellness Workbook*, Travis & Ryan, Ten Speed Press, 1988. Used with the permission of John Travis.

(and possibly other authorities as well), may not agree with our conclusions. Many of the statements have further explanation in a footnote (noted with an asterisk). We ask only that you keep an open mind until you have studied available information, then decide.

This questionnaire was designed to educate more than to test. All statements are worded so that you can easily tell what we think are wellness attributes (which also makes it easy to "cheat" on your score). This means there can be no trick questions to test your honesty or consistency—the higher your score, the greater you believe your wellness to be. Full responsibility is placed on you to answer each statement as honestly as possible. It's not your score but what you learn about yourself that is most important.

If you decide that a statement does not apply to you, or you don't want to answer it, you can skip it and not be penalized in your score.

Transfer your average score from each section to the corresponding box around the Wheel. Then graph your score by drawing a curved line between the "spokes" that define each segment. (Use the scale provided—beginning at the center with 0.0 and reaching 2.0 at the circumference.) Last, fill in the corresponding amount of each wedge-shaped segment, using different colors if possible.

Conclusions

When you have completed the Wellness Inventory, study your wheel's shape and balance. How smoothly would it roll? What does it tell you? Are there any surprises in it? How does it feel to you? What don't you like about it? What do you like about it?

We recommend that you use colored pens to go back over the questions, noting the ones on which your scores were low and choosing some areas on which you are interested in working. It is easy to overwhelm yourself by taking on too many areas at once. Ignore, for now, those of lower priority to you. Remember, if you don't enjoy at least some aspects of the changes you are making, they probably won't last.

Sample Questions

	Yes, usually 2	Sometimes, maybe 1	No, rarely 0
1. I am an adventurous thinker.	✔		
2. I have no expectations, yet look to the future optimistically.		✔	
3. I am a nonsmoker.	✔		
4. I love long, hot baths.			✔

Total points for this section = **5**   **4** + **1** + **0**

Divided by **4** (number of statements answered) = **1.3** Average score for this section.

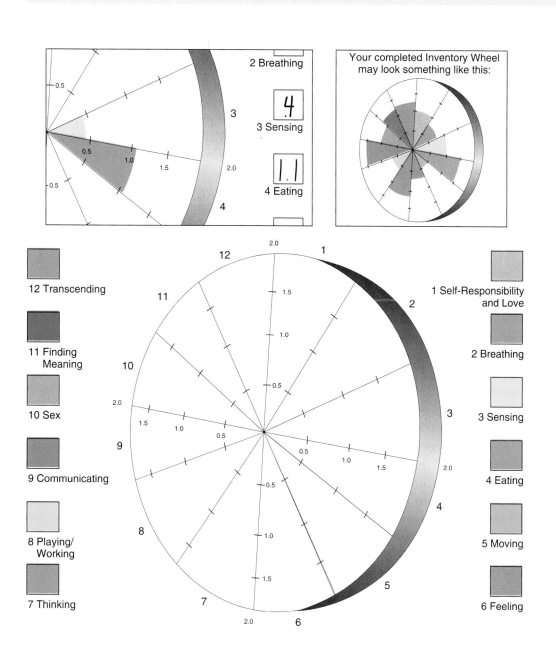

2 Breathing

3   Sensing .4

4 Eating 1.1

Your completed Inventory Wheel may look something like this:

12 Transcending

11 Finding Meaning

10 Sex

9 Communicating

8 Playing/ Working

7 Thinking

1 Self-Responsibility and Love

2 Breathing

3 Sensing

4 Eating

5 Moving

6 Feeling

Section 1 Wellness, Self-Responsibility and Love

	Yes, usually	Sometimes, maybe	No, rarely
	2	1	0
1. I believe how I live my life is an important factor in determining my state of health, and I live it in a manner consistent with that belief.	2		
2. I vote regularly.[1]	2		
3. I feel financially secure.		1	
4. I conserve materials/energy at home and at work.[2]	2		
5. I protect my living area from fire and safety hazards.			0
6. I use dental floss and a soft toothbrush daily.	2		
7. I am a nonsmoker.	2		
8. I am always sober when driving or operating dangerous machinery.	2		
9. I wear a safety belt when I ride in a vehicle.	2		
10. I understand the difference between blaming myself for a problem and simply taking responsibility (ability to respond) for that problem.	2		

Total points for this section = ☐ 17 ☐   _____ + _____ + _____

Divided by _____ (number of statements answered) = 1.7 Average score for this section.
(Transfer to the Wellness Inventory Wheel on **p. 3**)

Section 2 Wellness and Breathing

	Yes, usually	Sometimes, maybe	No, rarely
	2	1	0
1. I stop during the day to become aware of the way I am breathing.			0
2. I meditate or relax myself for at least 15 to 20 minutes each day.			0
3. I can easily touch my hands to my toes when standing with knees straight.[3]	2		
4. In temperatures over 70° F (21° C), my fingers feel warm when I touch my lips.[4]		1	
5. My nails are healthy and I do not bite or pick at them.	2		
6. I enjoy my work and do not find it overly stressful.		1	
7. My personal relationships are satisfying.	2	1	
8. I take time out for deep breathing several times a day.		1	
9. I have plenty of energy.		0	
10. I am at peace with myself.		1	

Total points for this section = ☐   _____ + _____ + _____

Divided by _____ (number of statements answered) = 1.1 Average score for this section.
(Transfer to the Wellness Inventory Wheel on **p. 3**)

---

[1] Voting is a simple measure of your willingness to participate in the social system, which ultimately impacts your state of health.
[2] Besides recycling glass, paper, aluminum, and other recyclables, if you purchase products that are reusable rather than disposable, and are packaged with a minimum of material, you will reduce the drain of resources and the toxic load on the environment caused by the disposal of wastes.
[3] A lack of spinal flexibility is usually a symptom of chronic muscle tension as well as indicative of a poor balance of physical activities.
[4] If your hand temperature is below 85° F (30° C) in a warm room, you're cutting off circulation to your hands via an overactive sympathetic nervous system. You can learn to warm your hands with biofeedback and to thereby better relax.

Section 3   Wellness and Sensing

	Yes, usually	Sometimes, maybe	No, rarely
	2	1	0
1. My place of work has mostly natural lighting or full-spectrum fluorescent lighting.[5]	2	___	___
2. I avoid extremely noisy areas or wear protective ear covers.[6]	2	___	___
3. I take long walks, hikes, or other outings to actively explore my surroundings.	___	1	___
4. I give myself presents, treats, or nurture myself in other ways.	2	___	___
5. I enjoy getting, and can acknowledge, compliments and recognition from others.	2	___	___
6. It is easy for me to give sincere compliments and recognition to other people.	2	___	___
7. At times I like to be alone.	___	1	___
8. I enjoy touching or hugging other people.[7]	2	___	___
9. I enjoy being touched or hugged by others.[8]	2	___	___
10. I get and enjoy backrubs or massages.	2	___	___

Total points for this section = ☐   ___ + ___ + ___

Divided by _____ (number of statements answered) = ____ Average score for this section.
(Transfer to the Wellness Inventory Wheel on **p. 3**)

Section 4   Wellness and Eating

	Yes, usually	Sometimes, maybe	No, rarely
	2	1	0
1. I am aware of the difference between refined carbohydrates and complex carbohydrates and eat a majority of the latter.[9]	___	___	0
2. I think my diet is well balanced and wholesome.	___	1	___
3. I drink fewer than five alcoholic drinks per week.	2	___	___
4. I drink fewer than two cups of coffee or black (nonherbal) tea per day.[10]	2	___	___
5. I drink fewer than five soft drinks per week.[11]	2	___	___
6. I add little or no salt to my food.[12]	___	1	___
7. I read the labels for the ingredients of all processed foods I buy and I inquire as to the level of toxic chemicals used in production of fresh foods—choosing the purest available to me.	___	1	___
8. I eat at least two raw fruits or vegetables each day.	___	1	___
9. I have a good appetite and am within 15% of my ideal weight.	___	1	___
10. I can tell the difference between "stomach hunger" and "mouth hunger," and I don't stuff myself when I am experiencing only "mouth hunger."[13]	2	___	___

Total points for this section = ☐   ___ + ___ + ___

Divided by _____ (number of statements answered) = 1.3 Average score for this section.
(Transfer to the Wellness Inventory Wheel on **p. 3**)

---

[5] Full-spectrum light, like sunlight, contains many different wavelengths. Most eyeglasses, and the glass windows in your home or car, block the "near" ultraviolet light needed by your body. Special bulbs and lenses are available.

[6] Loud noises that leave your ears ringing cause irreversible and cumulative nerve damage over time. Ear plugs/muffs, obtained in sporting goods stores, should be worn around power saws, heavy equipment, and rock concerts!

[7,8] Long recognized by hospitals as therapeutic, touch can be a powerful preventative as well.

[9] Refined carbohydrates (white flour, sugar, white rice, alcohol, and others) are burned up by the body very quickly and contain no minerals or vitamins. Complex carbohydrates (fruits and vegetables) burn evenly and provide the bulk of dietary nutrients.

[10] Coffee and nonherbal teas contain stimulants that, when overused, abuse your body's adrenal glands.

[11] Besides caffeine, the empty calories in these chemical brews may cause a sugar "crash" shortly after drinking. Artificially sweetened ones may be worse. Consider the other nutrients you won't be getting, and the prices!

[12] In addition to having a presumed connection with high blood pressure, the salting of foods during cooking draws out minerals, which are lost when the water is poured off.

[13] Stomach hunger is a signal that your body needs food. Mouth hunger is a signal that it needs something else (attention/acknowledgement), which you are not getting, so it asks for food, a readily available "substitute."

Section 5 · Wellness and Moving

	Yes, usually	Sometimes, maybe	No, rarely
	2	1	0
1. I climb stairs rather than ride elevators.[14]	2		
2. My daily activities include moderate physical effort.[15]	2		
3. My daily activities include vigorous physical effort.[16]		1	
4. I run at least 1 mile three times a week (or equivalent aerobic exercise).[17]			0
5. I run at least 3 miles three times a week (or equivalent aerobic exercise).			0
6. I do some form of stretching/limbering exercise for 10 to 20 minutes at least three times per week.[18]			0
7. I do some form of stretching/limbering exercise for 10 to 20 minutes at least six times per week.			0
8. I enjoy exploring new and effective ways of caring for myself through the movement of my body.	2		
9. I enjoy stretching, moving, and exerting my body.	2		
10. I am aware of and respond to messages from my body about its needs for movement.	2		

Total points for this section = ☐   _____ + _____ + _____

Divided by _____ (number of statements answered) = _1,_ Average score for this section.
(Transfer to the Wellness Inventory Wheel on **p. 3**)

Section 6 · Wellness and Feeling

	Yes, usually	Sometimes, maybe	No, rarely
	2	1	0
1. I am able to feel and express my anger in ways that solve problems, rather than swallow anger or store it up.[19]	2		
2. I allow myself to experience a full range of emotions and find constructive ways to express them.	2		
3. I am able to say "no" to people without feeling guilty.		1	
4. I laugh often and easily.		1	
5. I feel OK about crying and allow myself to do so when appropriate.[20]	2		
6. I listen to and consider others' criticisms of me rather than react defensively.		1	
7. I have at least five close friends.	2	1	
8. I like myself and look forward to the rest of my life.	2		
9. I easily express concern, love and warmth to those I care about.	2		
10. I can ask for help when needed.		1	

Total points for this section = ☐   _____ + _____ + _____

Divided by _____ (number of statements answered) = _____ Average score for this section.
(Transfer to the Wellness Inventory Wheel on **p. 3**)

---

[14] If a long elevator ride is necessary, try getting off five flights below your destination. Urge building managers to keep stair doors unlocked.
[15] Moderate = rearing young children, gardening, scrubbing floors, brisk walking, and so on.
[16] Vigorous = heavy construction work, farming, moving heavy objects by hand, and so on.
[17] An aerobic exercise (like running) should keep your heart rate at about 60% of its maximum (120–150 bpm) for 12–20 minutes. Brisk walking for 20 minutes every day can produce effects similar to aerobic exercise.
[18] The stretching of muscles is important for maintaining maximum flexibility of joints and ligaments. It feels good, too.
[19] Learning to take charge of your emotions and using them to solve problems can prevent disease, improve communications, and increase your self-awareness. Suppressing emotions or using them to manipulate others is destructive to all.
[20] Crying over a loss relieves the body of pent-up feelings. In our culture males often have a difficult time allowing themselves to cry, while females may have learned to cry when angry, using tears as a means of manipulation.

Section 7 Wellness and Thinking

	Yes, usually	Sometimes, maybe	No, rarely
	2	1	0
1. I am in charge of the subject matter and the emotional content of my thoughts, and am satisfied with what I choose to think about.[21]		1	
2. I am aware that I make judgments wherein I think I am "right" and others are "wrong."[22]	2		
3. It is easy for me to concentrate.	2		
4. I am conscious of changes (such as breathing pattern, muscle tension, skin moisture, and so on) in my body in response to certain thoughts.[23]		1	
5. I notice my perceptions of the world are colored by my thoughts at the time.[24]	2		
6. I am aware that my thoughts are influenced by my environment.	2		
7. I use my thoughts and attitudes to make my reality more life-affirming.[25]		1	
8. Rather than worry about a problem when I can do nothing about it, I temporarily shelve it and get on with the matters at hand.	2		
9. I approach life with the attitude that no problem is too big to confront, and some mysteries aren't meant to be solved.		1	
10. I use my creative powers in many aspects of my life.	2		

Total points for this section = ☐   _____ + _____ + _____

Divided by _____ **(number of statements answered) =** 16 **Average score for this section.**
(Transfer to the Wellness Inventory Wheel on **p. 3**)

Section 8 Wellness and Playing/Working

	Yes, usually	Sometimes, maybe	No, rarely
	2	1	0
1. I enjoy expressing myself through art, dance, music, drama, sports, or other activities, and make time to do so.	2		
2. I regularly exercise my creativity "muscles."	2		
3. I enjoy spending time without planned or structured activities and make the effort to do so.	2		
4. I can make much of my work into play.	2		
5. At times I allow myself to do nothing.[26]	2	1	
6. At times I can sleep late without feeling guilty.		1	
7. The work I do is rewarding to me.	2		
8. I am proud of my accomplishments.	2		
9. I am playful and the people around me support my playfulness.		1	
10. I have at least one activity, hobby, or sport that I enjoy regularly but do not feel compelled to do.	2		

Total points for this section = ☐   _____ + _____ + _____

Divided by _____ **(number of statements answered) =** 1.7 **Average score for this section.**
(Transfer to the Wellness Inventory Wheel on **p. 3**)

---

[21] When you are unconscious of the content of your thoughts, they are more likely to control you. Observing them objectively develops self-awareness and strengthens your ability to take charge.

[22] Rather than trying to completely stop yourself from judging, you can observe your judgments as efforts by your ego to avoid getting on with life and hiding behind "right/wrong" game playing.

[23] Both biofeedback and the field of psycho-neuro-immunology have shown the connections between the mind, nervous system and body. The more you become consciously aware of that connection, the greater responsibility you can take for your health.

[24] Being aware of your internal distortion of perceptions can allow you to step back and reassess a situation more objectively.

[25] Honesty, tempered with care and concern, clears out many negative thoughts that can clutter up your mind, thus making your reality more fun. "Positive thinking" without honesty and truthfulness can backfire by suppressing valid concerns that must be addressed.

[26] Doing "nothing" can give us access to the more creative and nonverbal aspects of our being, so from another perspective, doing nothing becomes doing much more.

Section 9 — Wellness and Communicating

	Yes, usually	Sometimes, maybe	No, rarely
	2	1	0
1. In conversation I can introduce a difficult topic and stay with it until I've gotten a satisfactory response from the other person.		1	
2. I enjoy silence.	2		
3. I am truthful and caring in my communications with others.	2		
4. I assert myself (in a nonattacking manner) in an effort to be heard, rather than be passively resentful of others with whom I don't agree.[27]		1	
5. I readily acknowledge my mistakes, apologizing for them if appropriate.	2	1	
6. I am aware of my negative judgments of others and accept them as simply judgments—not necessarily truth.[28]	2		
7. I am a good listener.	2		
8. I am able to listen to people without interrupting them or finishing their sentences for them.	2		
9. I can let go of my mental "labels" (for example, this is good, that is wrong) and judgmental attitudes about events in my life and see them in light of what they offer me.	2		
10. I am aware when I play psychological "games" with those around me and work to be truthful and direct in my communications.[29]		1	

Total points for this section = ☐ _____ + _____ + _____

Divided by _____ **(number of statements answered) =** _____ **Average score for this section.**
(Transfer to the Wellness Inventory Wheel on **p. 3**)

Section 10 — Wellness and Sex

	Yes, usually	Sometimes, maybe	No, rarely
	2	1	0
1. I feel comfortable touching and exploring my body.	2		
2. I think it's OK to masturbate if one chooses to do so.		1	
3. My sexual education is adequate.	2		
4. I feel good about the degree of closeness I have with men.	2		
5. I feel good about the degree of closeness I have with women.	2		
6. I am content with my level of sexual activity.[30]	2		
7. I fully experience the many stages of lovemaking rather than focus only on orgasm.[31]	2		
8. I desire to grow closer to some other people.	2		
9. I am aware of the difference between needing someone and loving someone.	2		
10. I am able to love others without dominating or being dominated by them.	2		

Total points for this section = ☐ _____ + _____ + _____

Divided by _____ **(number of statements answered) =** 1.9 **Average score for this section.**
(Transfer to the Wellness Inventory Wheel on **p. 3**)

[27] Attacking others rarely accomplishes your goals in the long run. Persisting in your convictions without using force is more effective and usually solves the problem without creating new ones.
[28] It is important to recognize that our internal judgments of others are based on personal biases that often have little objective basis.
[29] Psychological games, defined by Eric Berne in *Games People Play,* are complex unconscious manipulations that result in the players getting negative attention and feeling bad about themselves.
[30] Including the choice to have no sexual activity.
[31] A common problem for many people is an overemphasis on performance and orgasm, rather than on enjoying a close sensual feeling with their partner whether or not they experience orgasm.

Section 11 Wellness and Finding Meaning

	Yes, usually	Sometimes, maybe	No, rarely
	2	1	0
1. I believe my life has direction and meaning.	2		
2. My life is exciting and challenging.	2		
3. I have goals in my life.	2		
4. I am achieving my goals.		1	
5. I look forward to the future as an opportunity for further growth.	-	1	
6. I am able to talk about the death of someone close to me.	2		
7. I am able to talk about my own death with family and friends.	2		
8. I am prepared for my death.			0
9. I see my death as a step in my evolution.[32]			0
10. My daily life is a source of pleasure to me.		1	

Total points for this section = ☐ _____ + _____ + _____

Divided by _____ (number of statements answered) = _____ Average score for this section.
(Transfer to the Wellness Inventory Wheel on **p. 3**)

This portion of the Inventory goes beyond the scope of most generally accepted "scientific" principles and expresses the values and beliefs of the authors. It is intended to stimulate interest in these areas. If you have strong beliefs to the contrary, you can skip the questions or make up your own.

Section 12 Wellness and Transcending

	Yes, usually	Sometimes, maybe	No, rarely
	2	1	0
1. I perceive problems as opportunities for growth.	2		
2. I experience synchronistic events in my life (frequent "coincidences" seeming to have no cause-effect relationship).[33]	2		
3. I believe there are dimensions of reality beyond verbal description or human comprehension.	2		
4. At times I experience confusion and paradox in my search for understanding of the dimensions referred to above.	2		
5. The concept of god has personal definition and meaning to me.	2		
6. I experience a sense of wonder when I contemplate the universe.	2		
7. I have abundant expectancy rather than specific expectations.		1	
8. I allow others their beliefs without pressuring them to accept mine.	2		
9. I use the messages interpreted from my dreams.		1	
10. I enjoy practicing a spiritual discipline or allowing time to sense the presence of a greater force in guiding my passage through life.	2		

Total points for this section = ☐ _____ + _____ + _____

Divided by _____ (number of statements answered) = 1.4 Average score for this section.
(Transfer to the Wellness Inventory Wheel on **p. 3**)

---

[32] Seeing your death as a stage of growth and preparing yourself consciously is an important part of finding meaning in your life.
[33] Modern physics reveals that the idea of cause and effect may be as limited as Newton's theory of a mechanical universe. It suggests that we must expand our view to see that everything in the universe is connected to everything else. (Synchronicity describes that experience.)

1

A Lifetime of Wellness

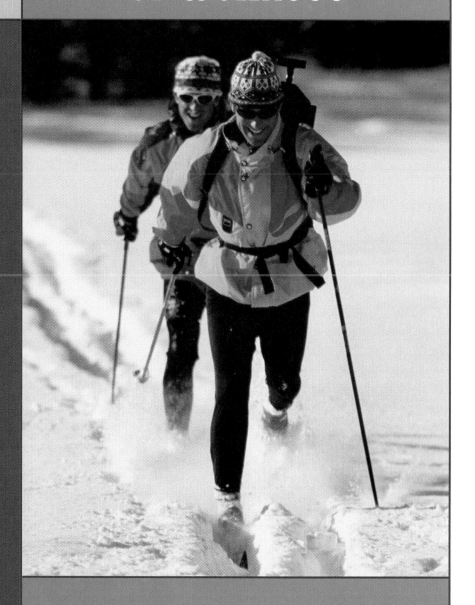

ealth may be a science; living is an art. The principles that can help you understand the science and practice the art are simple and timeless and form the basic premise of this book: You have more control over your life and well-being than does anything or anyone else. Through the decisions you make and the habits you develop, you can influence how well—and perhaps how long—you will live. This section defines the dimensions of health and provides the information you need to take charge of your well-being now and in the years to come.

1

An Invitation to Health for the Twenty-First Century

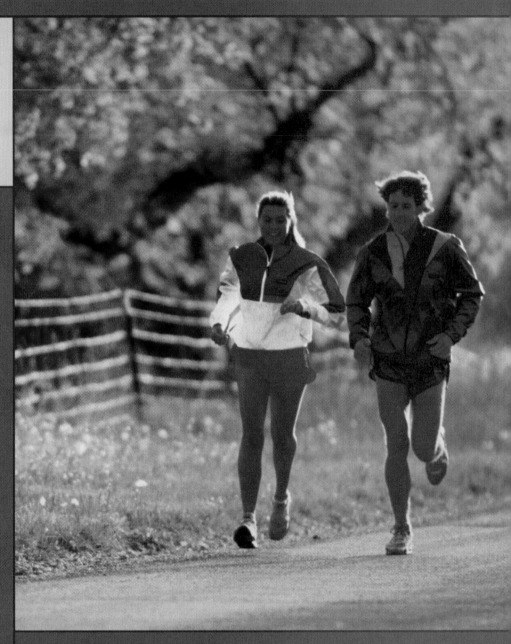

After studying the material in this chapter, you should be able to:

- **Identify** and **explain** the dimensions of health and how they relate to total wellness.
- **Explain** the principles and goals of prevention, and **differentiate** prevention from protection.
- **Explain** the principles of health promotion.
- **Discuss** the relationship between culture, economics, and health care.
- **Describe** the factors that influence the development of health behavior.
- **Create** a complete plan to change or develop a health behavior.
- **Describe** the Healthy People 2000 and Healthy People 2010 initiatives.

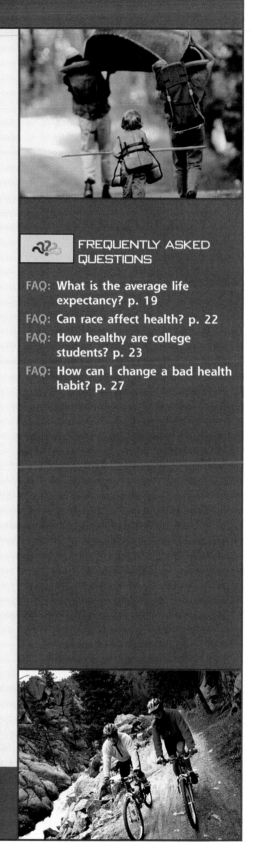

"How are you?" You may hear that question dozens of times each day.

"Fine," you answer, without thinking. But how often do you ask yourself how you *really* are? How do you feel about yourself and your life? Are you under pressure to get good grades? Are you eating well and exercising regularly? Do you have close friends with whom to share your triumphs and traumas? If you choose to be sexually active, what do you do to prevent unwanted pregnancy or sexually transmitted illnesses? Do you smoke or use drugs? How much do you drink? Are you taking steps to prevent major illnesses? Do you get regular health checkups? Are you aware of safety and environmental threats to your health? How are you going to make the most of your life? What do you hope to accomplish before you die?

This book asks these questions and many more. It is a book about you: your mind and your body, your spirit and your social ties, your needs and your wants, your past and your potential. It's about exploring options; about discovering possibilities; about what makes you unique and what makes your life worthwhile.

This is also a book about living in a human body, thinking with a human mind, responding to a world of ideas and experiences with a human spirit. You are the owner of an incredible machine, the most complex and sophisticated on earth. The human body is remarkably robust, resilient, and superbly equipped to deal with the challenges of daily living. Even processes we sometimes think of as malfunctions—a cough, a runny nose, diarrhea—can be indications of the body's capacity to heal itself.

While the body has its limits, there's no reason to tiptoe cautiously through life. We are designed to move, to think, to act—to stretch ourselves in every way. Muscles lose their tone if unexercised. Minds stagnate if we don't open them to new ideas and perspectives. If we don't make the most of what we are, we risk never discovering what we might become.

Health involves more than physical well-being. It is a state of body, mind, and spirit that must be viewed within the context of community, society, and environment. By providing the information and understanding you need to take care of your own health, *An Invitation to Health* can help you live more fully, more happily, and more healthfully. It also goes beyond the basics of health maintenance. Its primary themes— prevention of health problems, protection from health threats, and promotion of the health of others— can establish the basis for good health now and in the future.

The invitation to health that we extend to every reader is one offer you literally cannot afford to refuse: The quality of your life depends on it. ❖

FREQUENTLY ASKED QUESTIONS

FAQ: **What is the average life expectancy? p. 19**

FAQ: **Can race affect health? p. 22**

FAQ: **How healthy are college students? p. 23**

FAQ: **How can I change a bad health habit? p. 27**

The Dimensions of Health

By simplest definition, **health** means being sound in body, mind, and spirit. The World Health Organization defines health as "not merely the absence of disease or infirmity," but "a state of complete physical, mental, and social well-being."[1] Health is the process of discovering, using, and protecting all the resources within our bodies, minds, spirits, families, communities, and environment.

Health has many components: physical, psychological, spiritual, social, intellectual, and environmental. This book takes a *holistic* approach, one that looks at health and the individual as a whole, rather than part by part. Your own definition of health may include different elements, but chances are that you and your classmates would agree that it includes at least some of the following:

- A positive, optimistic outlook.
- A sense of control over stress and worries; time to relax.
- Energy and vitality; freedom from pain or serious illness.
- Supportive friends and family, and a nurturing intimate relationship with someone you love.
- A personally satisfying job.
- A clean environment.

Increasingly, Americans are striving to achieve the state of optimal health known as **wellness**. Wellness has been defined as purposeful, enjoyable living or, more specifically, a deliberate lifestyle choice characterized by personal responsibility and optimal enhancement of physical, mental, and spiritual health. Wellness means more than not being sick; it means taking steps to prevent illness and to lead a richer, more balanced, and more satisfying life. (See Pulsepoints: "Ten Simple Changes to Improve Your Health".)

While physical well-being is essential to health, the term *wellness,* as used by health professionals, has a broader meaning. To understand how the concepts of wellness and health fit together, think of an automobile transmission: Having a disease (illness) is like being in reverse; absence of disease (health) puts you in neutral; but positive health changes (wellness) push you into drive—forward motion. When your entire lifestyle is based on health-enhancing behaviors, you're in high gear and going at top speed—and you've achieved total wellness.

In wellness, health, and sickness, there's considerable overlap in the functions of the mind, body, and spirit. As scientists have shown again and again in recent decades, psychological factors play a major role in enhancing physical well-being and preventing illness, but they can also trigger, worsen, or prolong physical symptoms. "The mind clearly can have a profound effect on every aspect of physiologic functioning," says James Gordon, M.D., Director of the Center for Mind-Body Studies in Washington, DC. "Individuals who are chronically pessimistic, angry, anxious or depressed are clearly more susceptible to stress and illness, including heart disease and cancer."[2] Similarly, almost every medical illness affects people psychologically as well as physically. For example, depression is common among individuals who suffer kidney failure or neurologic disorders, such as Parkinson's disease. Understanding the various dimensions of health can help you appreciate these complex interactions.

Physical Health

The various states of good and ill physical health can be viewed as points on a continuum (see Figure 1-1). At one end is early and needless death; at the other is optimal wellness, in which you feel and perform at your very best. In the middle, individuals are neither sick enough to need medical attention nor well enough to live each day with zest and vigor. For the sake of optimal physical health, we must take positive steps away from illness and toward well-being. We must feed our bodies nutritiously, exercise them regularly, avoid harmful behaviors and substances, watch out for early signs of sickness, and protect ourselves from accidents.

Psychological Health

Like physical well-being, psychological health is more than the absence of problems or illness. Psychological

■ Figure 1-1 The wellness-illness continuum.

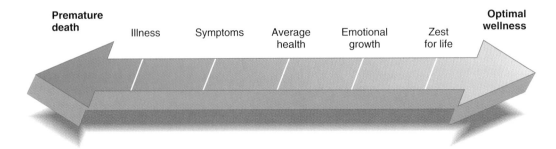

Premature death — Illness — Symptoms — Average health — Emotional growth — Zest for life — Optimal wellness

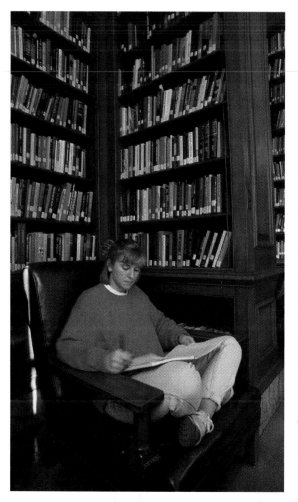
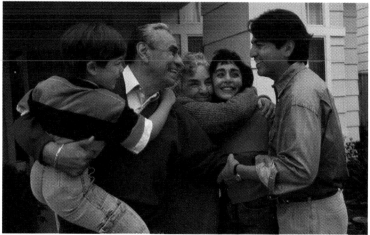
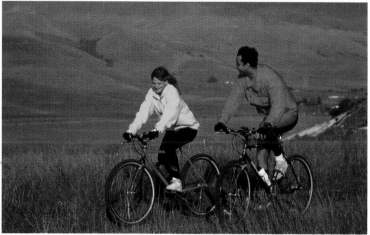

Health is the process of discovering, using, and protecting all the resources within our bodies, minds, spirits, families, communities, and environment.

PULSE points

Ten Simple Changes to Improve Your Health

1. **Use seat belts.** In the last decade seat belts have saved more than 40,000 lives and prevented millions of injuries.

2. **Eat an extra fruit or vegetable every day.** Adding more fruit and vegetables to your diet can improve your digestion and lower your risk of several cancers.

3. **Get enough sleep.** A good night's rest provides the energy you need to make it through the following day.

4. **Take regular stress breaks.** A few quiet minutes spent stretching, looking out the window, or simply letting yourself unwind are good for body and soul.

5. **Lose a pound.** If you're overweight, you may not think a pound will make a difference, but it's a step in the right direction.

6. **If you're a woman, examine your breasts regularly.** Get in the habit of performing a breast self-examination every month after your period (when breasts are least swollen or tender).

7. **If you're a man, examine your testicles regularly.** These simple self-exams can spot the early signs of cancer when they're most likely to be cured.

8. **Get physical.** Just a little exercise will do some good. A regular workout schedule will be good for your heart, lungs, muscles, bones—even your mood.

9. **Drink more water.** Eight glasses a day are what you need to replenish lost fluids, prevent constipation, and keep your digestive system working efficiently.

10. **Do a good deed.** Caring for others is a wonderful way to care for your own soul and connect with others.

health refers to both our emotional and mental states—that is, to our feelings and our thoughts. It involves awareness and acceptance of a wide range of feelings in oneself and others, the ability to express emotions, to function independently, and to cope with the challenges of daily stressors. (Chapter 3 provides more information on psychological health.)

Spiritual Health

Being *spiritual* doesn't mean belonging to a formal religion. Its essential component is a belief in some meaning or order in the universe, a higher power that gives greater significance to individual life. Spiritually healthy individuals identify their own basic purpose in life; learn how to experience love, joy, peace, and fulfillment; and help themselves and others achieve their full potential. They concern themselves with "giving, forgiving, and attending to others' needs before one's own," says psychiatrist Roger Smith, M.D., of Michigan State University. Smith notes that spiritual development "produces a new meaning in one's life through a connectedness to something greater and mysterious."[3]

Americans tend to be both spiritual and religious. According to the most recent in a series of national Gallup polls conducted over the last 60-plus years, 90 percent of Americans believe in God—an all-time high. Most Americans also say that prayer is an important part of their lives, that they believe that miracles are performed by a divine power, and that they are sometimes conscious of the presence of God. Faced with physical or psychological difficulties, most Americans turn to prayer, reading the Bible, or meditation as a way of coping.

In a national poll of 1,000 Americans, 79 percent said they believe that spiritual faith can help people recover from disease; 63 percent believe physicians should talk to patients about spiritual faith. In a survey of Americans' use of complementary/alternative medicine (discussed in Chapter 11), 25 percent said they used prayer as a medical therapy.[4]

Doctors share such beliefs: About one-third of America's medical schools now offer courses on spirituality and healing. And a growing number of doctors, while not endorsing any one approach to religion, are encouraging patients to cultivate a spiritual commitment—for the sake of their mortal bodies as well as their immortal souls.

Increasingly, health professionals have recognized the power and potential of spirituality. For 30 years, Herbert Benson, M.D., head of the Mind/Body Medical Institute at Harvard Medical School, has conducted rigorous experiments to document the influence of the spirit on health. His conclusion: The combination of relaxation and behavioral methods, such as prayer and meditation, with standard surgical and medical treatments can help relieve a host of medical problems, including chronic pain, arthritis, insomnia, and premenstrual symptoms.

Recent research also has found that "intrinsic religiosity" played a role in speeding recovery from depression and in preventing depression in hospitalized patients.[5]

Spiritual health may affect longevity. In a study of a national sample of 21,000 U. S. adults, those who attended religious services more than once a week lived an average of 7 years longer than others. African Americans who did so added 14 years to their life spans.[6]

"Religion is very, very good for you," says psychiatrist David B. Larson, M.D., president of the National Institute for Healthcare Research. In an extensive review of the medical literature, he found not only that faith, belief, and religious commitment are positive influences on physical and mental health, but also that a lack of religious practice constitutes a clear and consistent health risk factor.

"Deeply religious people of all faiths appear to benefit in five major areas," reports Dale Matthews of Georgetown School of Medicine, who reviewed more than 300 studies on healing and religion. These are: less substance abuse; lower rates of depression and anxiety, especially among women; enhanced quality of life; quicker recovery from injury or illness; and longer life expectancy. Four in five studies that looked at religion and survival found that people who went to church regularly, prayed frequently, or found religion important lived longer than those who didn't.

Social Health

Social health refers to the ability to interact effectively with other people and the social environment, to develop satisfying interpersonal relationships, and to fulfill social roles. It involves participating in and contributing to your community, living in harmony with fellow human beings, developing positive interdependent relationships with others (discussed in Chapter 8), and practicing healthy sexual behaviors (discussed in Chapters 9 and 10).

As a growing number of research studies show, social isolation increases the risk of sickness and mortality. In a landmark study of 4,725 men and women in Alameda County, California, death rates were twice as high for "loners" as for those with strong social ties. In other studies, social isolation greatly increased the risk of dying of a heart attack. In one study of 1,368 patients undergoing cardiac catheterization (a diagnostic test), those who were unmarried or did not have a close confidant were more than three times as likely to die as those with spouses or a close friend.[7] Heart attack patients have a better chance of long-term survival if

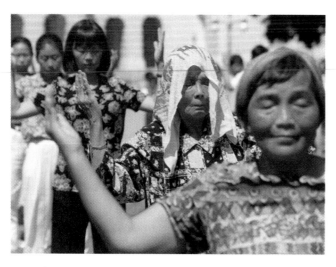

You influence your health by the choices you make about your body, your mind, and your place in the world. Take care of your health—your physical, psychological, spiritual, social, intellectual, and environmental well-being—because it can determine what you'll accomplish and become in your life.

they believe they have adequate help in performing daily tasks from family and friends.[8] Social contacts can even help ward off the common cold. In a study of 276 healthy volunteers, those with many diverse social connections (with spouses, friends, families, colleagues, and social group members) were less likely to develop colds when exposed to a virus than those who had the fewest such social ties.[9]

Health educators are placing greater emphasis on social health in its broadest sense as they expand the traditional individualistic concept of health to include the complex interrelationships between one person's health and the health of the community and environment. This change in perspective has given rise to a new emphasis on **health promotion,** which enhances health by building knowledge and skills among individuals and modifying their environment to foster healthier lifestyles.

Intellectual Health

The brain is the only organ capable of self-awareness. Every day you use your mind to gather, process, and act on information; to think through your values; to make decisions, set goals, and figure out how to handle a problem or challenge. Intellectual health refers to your ability to think and learn from life experience, your openness to new ideas, and your capacity to question and evaluate information. Throughout your life, you'll use your critical thinking skills, including your ability to evaluate health information to safeguard your well-being.

Another important component of intellectual well-being is "emotional intelligence," which is discussed in Chapter 3.

Environmental Health

You live in a physical and social setting that can affect every aspect of your health. Environmental health refers to the impact that your world has on your well-being. It means protecting yourself from dangers in the air, water, and soil, and in products you use—and also working to preserve the environment itself. (Chapter 20 offers a thorough discussion of environmental health.)

Health for the New Millennium

 ## What Is the Average Life Expectancy?

A hundred years ago, the average American could expect to live for only about 50 years. Infectious diseases, such as smallpox and tuberculosis, claimed tens of thousands of lives, particularly among the young and the poor. A high percentage of women died during childbirth or shortly afterward. By 1900, the average American woman could expect to live to an age of 50.9 years, compared with 47.9 years for a man. By 1950, women's projected life span had grown to 71.1 years and men's to 65.6. (As shown in The X & Y Files: "How Sex Differences Affect Health," this is only one of many gender-specific aspects of health.)

We have come a very long way. According to the Department of Health and Human Services, life expectancy has reached an all-time high: 76.5 years. The projected life spans of both white and black males are longer than ever: 73.8 years and 66.1 years, respectively. An estimated 15 percent decline in infant mortality rates stems from a decline in Sudden Infant Death Syndrome (SIDS), discussed in Chapter 10.

At the turn of the last century, 30.4 percent of all deaths were among children younger than age 5, and pneumonia, tuberculosis, and diarrhea were leading causes of death. Today heart disease and cancer—primarily diseases of the elderly—account for the majority of deaths. There are many reasons for this progress, including improvements in sanitation, water quality, and hygiene and the discovery of antibiotics. However, infectious disease remains a potential threat. The rise of the human immunodeficiency virus (HIV), which has infected over 33 million people worldwide and killed almost 14 million, demonstrates how unpredictable diseases can be. Other unanticipated threats include the

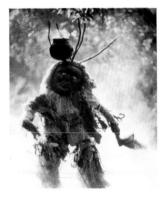

African Spirituality Dance is an essential ritual in many healing traditions of Africa. Constant rhythmic movements induce an ecstatic state that stimulates and ultimately relaxes the mind and body by shifting the focus from the self.

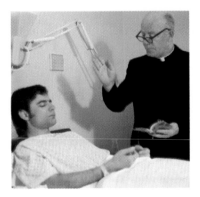

Catholicism During the sacrament of anointing of the sick, the seriously ill are anointed with oil that has been blessed by a bishop. As the oil is massaged into the forehead, the laying on of hands helps soothe and calm the patient.

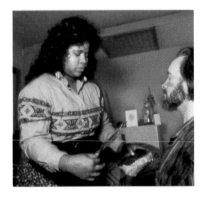

Native American Healing Each religion has its own healing rituals. Members of the Dakota/Lakota tribe, for example, conduct sweat ceremonies to heal the sick. Friends and family gather in a sweat lodge with the patient (or on her behalf) to sing and pray. It's believed that sweating heals the spirit and helps rid the body of illness.

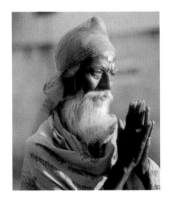

Hinduism Many followers fast regularly to cleanse their bodies of impurities. A person might also fast on behalf of a relative, hoping to please a god who can bestow health.

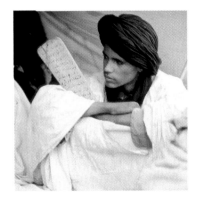

Islam When a Muslim becomes sick, loved ones read specific verses from the Koran to encourage her to be patient with her suffering.

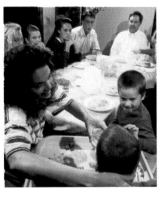

Mormonism The Mormon Word of Wisdom, a health code written in 1830, closely resembles today's nutrition guidelines, suggesting that meat be eaten sparingly and that fruits, vegetables, and grains be the foundation of the diet.

A sample of religious healing rituals. The world's religions have developed practices to promote the physical health of their followers. *Source:* Elizabeth Shaw, "Faith and Healing," *American Health*, November 1997.

resurgence of tuberculosis and the emergence of microorganisms that are resistant to available drugs.[10]

Homicide and suicide have declined as causes of death for the total population, but among young persons 15 to 24 years of age, they remain, respectively, the second and third leading causes of death. Accidents are the number-one cause of death in this age group.

Healthy People 2000

The Healthy People 2000 initiative, a nationwide program involving more than 350 organizations, achieved or made substantial progress toward achieving more than half of its health objectives during the 1990s. Areas that were successfully targeted include nutrition, maternal and child health, heart disease, mental health, control of outbreaks of waterborne diseases and food-borne infections, and reductions in oral and breast cancer deaths. Some objectives, such as a reduction in infant mortality, were only a fraction away from being met. Substantial progress also was made in child immunizations, increased breast-feeding, regular dental visits, mammography screening, and consumption of five fruits and vegetables a day.[11]

However, there was little improvement, or even movement in the wrong direction, for a fifth of the Healthy People 2000 objectives, such as reducing the number of overweight individuals in the country and increasing physical activity. A prime example of failure was the objectives related to diabetes, where incidence, prevalence, complications, and mortality all rose. Six percent of the objectives showed mixed results, 3 percent had no change from the baseline figure, and 11 percent of the objectives lacked sufficient data to assess progress.

Here is a summary of the progress made in meeting the Healthy People 2000 objectives:

- **Infants and Children:** Infant mortality declined steadily throughout the 1990s and the death rate for children 1 to 14 years of age dropped by 26 percent to surpass the objective. There was substantial progress in reducing drowning and motor vehicle crash deaths and in meeting the target for fire-related deaths. When comparing the overall mortality rates for infants and children from the inception of the Healthy People initiative in 1979 to the year 2000, there was a drop of 50 percent for infants and 40 percent for children.

- **Adolescents and young adults:** For those 15 to 24 years of age, death rates declined substantially to meet the target of 85 deaths per 100,000. Since the inception of the Healthy People initiative, the mortality rate for adolescents and young adults has dropped 26 percent. Alcohol-related motor vehicle crash deaths and suicides declined among this group, and students are now less likely to engage in such risky behaviors as fighting and weapon-carrying. On the other hand, after declining somewhat, heavy drinking remains a problem.

- **Adults:** Since the beginning of the initiative in 1979, the mortality rate has dropped 31 percent for adults between the ages of 25 and 64. Cancer death rates fell even lower than the year 2000 target, due largely to a drop in breast cancer and colorectal cancer death rates as well as a slowing of the rise in lung cancer death rates.

- **Older Adults:** Life expectancy rates rose, reflecting the continuing decline in deaths from heart disease and stroke. However, as Americans live longer, more people over 70 years of age are having difficulty performing critical functions, such as dressing, bathing, and getting out of bed. Although the decrease in the suicide rate for white males—the group at greatest risk—met the year 2000 target, rates for deaths resulting from falls and motor vehicle crashes have increased over the last decade.

Healthy People 2010

Healthy People 2010: Healthy People in Healthy Communities builds on initiatives pursued over the past two decades and presents an action agenda for the first decade of the twenty-first century. The year 2010 objectives were formulated by an alliance of 350 national organizations and 300 state health, mental health, substance abuse, and environmental agencies. To date, 47 states, the District of Columbia, and Guam have developed their own Healthy People plans for the new century.

The goals of Healthy People 2010 are increasing years of healthy life and eliminating health disparities. In addition, policy-makers have suggested four enabling goals: promoting healthy behaviors, protecting health, achieving access to quality health care, and strengthening community prevention. New areas of focus include the needs of the disabled, people with low incomes, and the chronically ill.[12]

Global Health

There were dramatic gains in life expectancy around the world in the twentieth century. For example, the average man's life span increased from 29 to 72 years in Chile and from 49 to 75 in England. Women almost everywhere live longer than men; the gender gap doubled from three to six years over the course of the last century. However, in some countries, such as the former Soviet Union, life expectancy for both sexes is falling, and in nations such as Uganda, Zambia, and the Central African Republic, life expectancy is under 50 years of age.

More than 1 billion people around the world entered the twenty-first century without modern medical care, according to the World Health Organization (WHO). Its top goals for the twenty-first century are fighting malaria and tobacco-related diseases, and combatting poverty through better health care. Another target is noncommunicable diseases, which are becoming more of a problem in both developed and developing countries.[13]

Without question, illness causes a great deal of suffering throughout the world—yet much of it can be prevented. The single most common underlying cause of

---

How Sex Differences Affect Health

The most important variable in human health may be gender. Nothing—not race, income, education, or lifestyle—has a greater impact on how our bodies function, how long we live, and the symptoms, course, and treatment of the diseases that strike us.

This realization is both new and revolutionary. For centuries, scientists based biological theories solely on a male model and viewed women as shorter, smaller, and rounder versions of men. Even modern medicine is based on the assumption that, except for their reproductive organs, both sexes are biologically interchangeable. We now know that this simply isn't so.

As "The X & Y Files" features throughout the book show, virtually every part and organ system of the body differs in men and women (see Figure 1–2). A man's core body temperature runs lower than a woman's; his heart beats at a slower rate. A woman takes 9 breaths a minute; a man averages 12. Her blood carries higher levels of protective immunoglobulin; his has more oxygen-rich hemoglobin. Her ears are more sensitive to sound; his eyes are more sensitive to light. Male brains are 10 percent larger, but certain areas in female brains contain more neurons.

Sex differences persist in sickness as well as in health. Before age 50, men are more prone to lethal diseases, including heart attacks, cancer, and liver failure. Women show greater vulnerability to chronic but non-life-threatening problems such as arthritis and autoimmune disorders. Women are twice as likely to suffer depression; men have a fivefold greater rate of alcoholism. Women outlive men by more than six years, yet they're more prone to age-related problems, such as osteoporosis and Alzheimer's disease. Health behaviors—patterns of drinking, smoking, or using seat belts—also are different in men and women. (We'll discuss these issues in later chapters.)

Even when the same disease strikes a man and a woman, it often follows a different course in each. Heart disease generally develops a decade later in women than in men, but women suffer more severe first heart attacks and are less likely to survive them. Women develop more cases of melanoma, but men are at higher risk of dying of this deadly skin cancer. Diabetes doubles the risk of heart disease in men, but increases it three- to sixfold in women. After surgery, a woman wakens from anesthesia in an average of 7 minutes, compared with slightly more than 11 minutes for a man.

The recognition of these sex differences has provided a new perspective that is transforming medical research and practice. A new science called gender-specific medicine is replacing "good-enough," one-size-fits-all health care with new definitions of what is normal in both men and women, more complex concepts of disease, more precise diagnostic tests, and more effective treatments.

---

their symptoms isn't a pathogen (disease-causing microorganism) but poverty. One-fifth of the world's 5.6 billion people live under conditions that provide little or no resources for preventing or treating illness. More than half cannot get essential medications; about a third of the world's children do not get enough to eat.[14]

Diversity and Health

We live in the most diverse nation on earth, and in one that is becoming increasingly diverse. During the 1990s, the Hispanic and Asian populations of the United States surged, growing by 35 and 40 percent, respectively. The number of African Americans grew by almost 13 percent.[15]

For society, this variety can be both enriching and divisive. Tolerance and acceptance of others have always been part of the American creed. By working together, Americans have created a country that remains a symbol of opportunity around the world. Yet members of different ethnic groups still have to struggle against discrimination. Today, in this country's third century, all Americans still aren't equal in every way, including their health and health care. Poverty remains the single greatest barrier to better health for minorities in the United States. Without adequate insurance or ability to pay, many cannot afford the tests and treatments that could prevent illness or overcome it at the earliest possible stages. Some groups, particularly African Americans, also rate the health services in their communities as lower than those available to white Americans and have more negative opinions of the health care they receive.

Race may also affect the doctor-patient relationship. African-American patients rate their doctor visits as significantly "less participatory" than do whites, according to a Johns Hopkins study. Both African-American and white patients rated their visits with

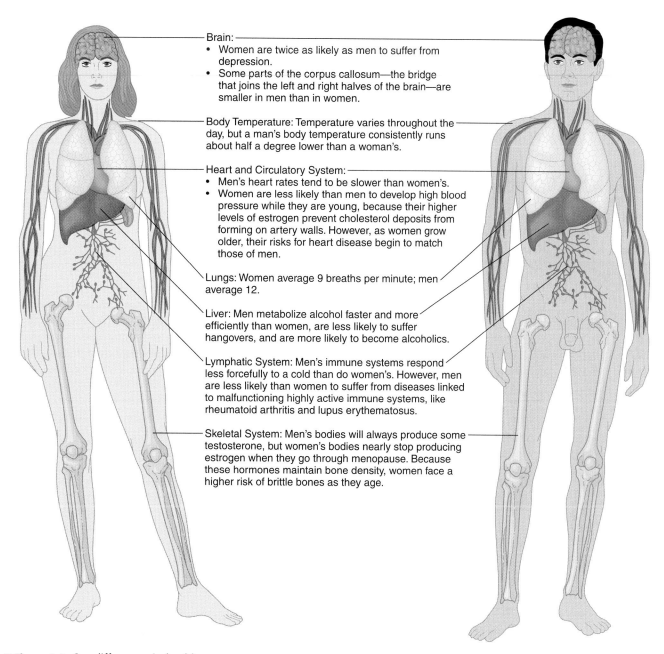

Brain:
- Women are twice as likely as men to suffer from depression.
- Some parts of the corpus callosum—the bridge that joins the left and right halves of the brain—are smaller in men than in women.

Body Temperature: Temperature varies throughout the day, but a man's body temperature consistently runs about half a degree lower than a woman's.

Heart and Circulatory System:
- Men's heart rates tend to be slower than women's.
- Women are less likely than men to develop high blood pressure while they are young, because their higher levels of estrogen prevent cholesterol deposits from forming on artery walls. However, as women grow older, their risks for heart disease begin to match those of men.

Lungs: Women average 9 breaths per minute; men average 12.

Liver: Men metabolize alcohol faster and more efficiently than women, are less likely to suffer hangovers, and are more likely to become alcoholics.

Lymphatic System: Men's immune systems respond less forcefully to a cold than do women's. However, men are less likely than women to suffer from diseases linked to malfunctioning highly active immune systems, like rheumatoid arthritis and lupus erythematosus.

Skeletal System: Men's bodies will always produce some testosterone, but women's bodies nearly stop producing estrogen when they go through menopause. Because these hormones maintain bone density, women face a higher risk of brittle bones as they age.

■ **Figure 1-2** Sex differences in health.

same-race physicians as significantly more participatory than with different-race doctors. And patients of female physicians rated their visits as more participatory than patients of male physicians.[16]

The growing influence of diverse racial and ethnic groups on our culture will affect national health priorities for many decades. As medical scientists are learning, there are clear differences with regard to disease and disability among different peoples. However, as public health experts explore the links between race, culture,

and health, they are moving beyond any narrow definition of "minority" to the broader concept of "underserved," a group made up of many cultures that also includes the homeless, rural Americans, and women. Special problems also exist for illegal Americans, who often live in extreme poverty; perform difficult, hazardous jobs; and have little or no access to health services. Even when they desperately need medical care, they may be so fearful of deportation that they do not seek help.

Diversity poses special challenges in health care. In some cultures, physicians are seen as less effective than other healers, who are believed to cure illness caused by bad karma or evil spirits. Language difficulties can create communication barriers. In addition, American physicians, trained to believe that high-tech medicine is best, may not understand or appreciate traditional healing practices. In many communities, innovative programs have begun to educate patients from other cultures about the American health-care system, as well as to educate American health-care providers about the beliefs and health practices of their diverse patients. The Institute of Medicine is urging more research on cancer in poor people and minorities.[17]

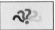 ## Can Race Affect Health?

Different racial and ethnic groups often face different health risks. Consider the following statistics:

- The infant mortality rate for African-American babies remains higher than that for white babies.

- Life expectancy for African Americans, though increasing, is 6.5 years lower than that for whites.[18]

- African Americans have higher rates of high blood pressure (hypertension), develop this problem earlier in life, suffer more severe hypertension, and have higher rates of strokes and hypertension-related deaths than whites. Cardiovascular risk is higher in minority than white youth.[19]

- African Americans have higher rates of glaucoma, systemic lupus erythematosus, liver disease, and kidney failure than whites.

- The death rate for heart disease among middle-aged black women is 150 percent higher than among white women the same age; among those with diabetes, their death rate is 134 percent higher than white female diabetics.

- Cardiologists are 60 percent less likely to refer a black woman for cardiac catheterization (a test of the heart's blood vessels) than a white woman of the same age.[20]

- Among young African-American women, breast cancer is a special threat. Of all black women diagnosed with breast cancer, 37 percent are younger than 50—compared with 22 percent of white women. Older black and Latino women have fewer mammograms than their white counterparts.[21]

- Native Americans have the highest rates of diabetes in the world. Among the Pima Indians, half of all adults have diabetes.

- Southeast Asian men have a higher incidence of lung and liver cancer than the population as a whole.

- Native Hawaiian women have a higher rate of breast cancer than women from other racial and ethnic groups.

- Native Americans, including those indigenous to Alaska, are more likely to die young, primarily as the result of accidental injuries, cirrhosis of the liver, homicide, suicide, pneumonia, and the complications of diabetes than the population as a whole.[22]

Are these increased susceptibilities the result of racial or ethnic background, the stress of living with discrimination, an unhealthy lifestyle, lack of access to health services, or poverty? It is hard to say precisely. Certainly, poverty presents the greatest barrier to making healthy lifestyle choices, seeking preventive care, and getting timely and effective treatment.

Genetic and environmental factors also may play a role. Take, for example, the high rates of diabetes among the Pima Indians. Until 50 years ago, these Native Americans were not notably obese or prone to diabetes. However, after World War II, the tribe started trading handmade baskets for lard and flour. Their lifestyle became more sedentary, and their diet, higher in fats. In addition, as researchers have since discovered, many Pima Indians have an inherited resistance to insulin that increases their susceptibility to diabetes. The combination of a hereditary predisposition and environmental factors may explain why the Pimas now have epidemic levels of diabetes.

Other groups have other vulnerabilities. Caucasians, for instance, are prone to osteoporosis (progressive weakening of bone tissue); cystic fibrosis; skin cancer; and phenylketonuria (PKU), a metabolic disorder that can lead to mental retardation. Women with Chinese or Latino backgrounds face a significantly greater risk of developing diabetes during pregnancy than African Americans or whites. Asians and Asian Americans metabolize some medications faster than whites and thus require much smaller doses. Latinos have higher rates of death from diabetes and infectious and parasitic diseases than African Americans or whites.

Health-care providers often fail to recognize such factors, in part because the discussion of ethnicity in health is politically controversial. Some fear that it could lead to misconceptions about genetic superiority or inferiority. Yet recognition of different health needs and risks is the first step toward overcoming the health problems of many Americans.

Closing the Minority Health Gap

In the words of a National Institutes of Health (NIH) report, minorities have carried "an unequal burden with respect to disease and disability, resulting in a lower life expectancy." Each year minorities in the United States—

African Americans, Latinos, Asian Americans, Pacific Islanders, Native Americans, and other groups—experience as many as 75,000 more deaths than they would if they lived under the same health conditions as the white population.

But race itself isn't the primary reason for the health problems faced by minorities in the United States. Poverty is. One in three Hispanics under age 65 has no health insurance.[23] Without adequate insurance or ability to pay, many cannot make the lifestyle choices or afford the tests and treatments that could prevent illness or overcome it at the earliest possible stages. According to public health experts, low income may account for one-third of the racial differences in death rates for middle-aged African-American adults. High blood pressure, high cholesterol, obesity, diabetes, and smoking are responsible for another third. The final third has been blamed on "unexplained factors," which may well include poor access to health care and the stress of living in a society in which skin color remains a major barrier to equality. Language, too, is a barrier. Spanish-speaking patients, for instance, have very few Hispanic health-care providers to turn to since only 3 percent of physicians in the U. S. are Hispanic.[24]

NIH has established an Office of Research on Minority Health (ORMH) with the goal of "closing the gap that currently exists between the health of minorities and the majority population." Since 1992, ORMH has provided funds for research and prevention efforts aimed at improving minority health. Some focus on prenatal care to improve survival rates. Others are educating minority youths about HIV infection and AIDS.

 ## How Healthy Are College Students?

As one of the nation's 12 million full- or part-time college students, you belong to one of the most diverse groups in America. (See Campus Focus: "A Profile of the Class of 2002.") A quarter of all 18- to 24-year-olds in the United States—some 7.1 million in all—are enrolled at one of the nation's 3,600 colleges and universities. Some of you are reentry students, back on campus for the second time; half of all college dropouts return to school within 15 years. Within the next few years, older students—most working full-time—will make up the majority of college enrollments.

As shown in the Campus Focus features throughout this book, college students often engage in behaviors that put them at risk for serious health problems. Half exercise less than five hours a week; about one in three gets less than two hours of exercise a week.[25] In one survey of community college students, 30 percent reported having had five or more sexual partners. A similar percentage of students have been tested for HIV, while one in four did not know if their partner had ever had an AIDS test.[26] Almost 80 percent have tried cigarettes, while 22 percent of men and 28 percent of women have smoked regularly.[27] Almost one in five—18 percent—of college students describe themselves as frequent binge drinkers.[28] One in four college men and one in five college women don't use seat belts regularly.[29]

These statistics reveal a gap between what students know they should be doing to ensure good health and what they actually do. And college may be an ideal time to make permanent, life-enhancing changes.

Just by educating yourself, you're likely to improve your health—now and in the future. Many risk factors for disease—including high blood pressure, elevated cholesterol, and cigarette smoking—decline steadily as education increases, regardless of how much money people make. Education may be good for the body as well as the mind by influencing lifestyle behaviors, problem-solving abilities, and values. People who earn college degrees gain positive attitudes about the benefits of healthy living, learn how to gain access to preventive health services, join peer groups that promote healthy behavior, and develop higher self-esteem and greater control over their lives.[30]

Becoming All You Can Be

By taking the Wellness Inventory ("What Is Wellness?") that precedes this chapter, you can get a snapshot of the current state of your overall health and wellness. You also can get a sense of the aspects of your life that could use some attention and improvement. As the Consumer Health Watch box "Health in a Bottle?" points out, there are no easy answers or quick solutions. Use this course as an opportunity to zero in on at least one less-than-healthful behavior and improve it. The following sections discuss some of the processes you'll have to go through in order to make a successful change for the better.

Understanding Health Behavior

Behaviors that affect your health include exercising regularly, eating a balanced, nutritious diet, seeking care for symptoms, and taking necessary steps to overcome illness, and restore well-being. If there is one health behavior that you would like to improve, you have to realize that change isn't easy. Between 40 and 80 percent of those people who try to kick bad health habits lapse back into their unhealthy ways within six weeks. To

Campus Focus

A Profile of the Class of 2002

Racial background*	
White/Caucasian	82.5%
African American/Black	9.4%
Mexican American/Chicano/Puerto Rican/other Latino	4.5%
Asian American/Asian	4.0%
American Indian	2.1%
Hours per week spent on homework	
None	2.8
Less than one	12.6
1 to 2	22.3
3 to 5	29.4
6 to 10	18.9
11 to 15	8.1
16 to 20	3.5
More than 20	2.4
Hours per week spent on prayer or meditation	
None	34.8
Less than one	32.4
1 to 2	20.5
3 to 5	7.4
6 to 10	2.7
11 to 15	.9
16 to 20	.4
More than 20	.9
Objectives considered very important by more than half of students	
Be very well off financially	74%
Raise a family	73%
Become authority in my own field	60.2%
Help others in difficulty	59.9%
More than half of students agree strongly or somewhat that:	
Men are not entitled to sex on a date	87.4%
The federal government should do more to control handguns	82.5%
Employers should be able to require drug tests	78.5%
Our society shows too much concern for criminals	72.5%
Our society should prohibit racist/sexist speech	61.8%
The wealthy should pay more taxes	58.7%
Abortion should be legal	50.9%

Source: Sax, Linda, et al. *The American Freshman: National Norms for Fall 1998.* Los Angeles: Higher Education Research Institute, UCLA, 1998.

*Some respondents checked more than one category.

make lasting beneficial changes, you have to understand the three types of influences that shape behavior: predisposing, enabling, and reinforcing factors (Figure 1-3).

Predisposing Factors

Predisposing factors include knowledge, attitudes, beliefs, values, and perceptions. Unfortunately, knowledge isn't enough to cause most people to change their behavior; for example, people fully aware of the grim consequences of smoking often continue to puff away. Nor is attitude—one's likes and dislikes—sufficient; an individual may dislike the smell and taste of cigarettes but continue to smoke regardless.

Beliefs are more powerful than knowledge and attitudes, and researchers report that people are most

Consumer Health Watch

Health in a Bottle?

Almost every week you're likely to come across a commercial or an ad for a new health product that promises better sleep, more energy, clearer skin, firmer muscles, lower weight, brighter moods, longer life—or all of these combined. As the Consumer Health Watch features throughout this book point out, you can't believe every promise you read or hear. Here are some general guidelines to keep in mind the next time you come across a health claim:

- If it sounds too good to be true, it probably is. If a magic pill could really trim off excess pounds or banish wrinkles, the world would be filled with thin people with unlined skin. Look around, and you'll realize that's not the case.

- Look for objective evaluations. If you're watching an infomercial for a treatment or technique, you can be sure that the enthusiastic endorsements have been skillfully scripted and rehearsed. Even ads that claim to be presenting the science behind a new "breakthrough" are really sales pitches in disguise.

- Consider the sources. Research findings from carefully controlled scientific studies are reviewed by leading experts in the field and published in scholarly journals. The fact that someone has conducted a study doesn't mean it was a valid scientific investigation.

- Check credentials. Anyone can claim to be a "scientist" or a "health expert." Find out if advocates of any type of therapy have legitimate degrees from recognized institutions and are fully licensed in their fields.

- Do your own research. Check with your doctor or with the student health center. Go to the library or do some online research to gather as much information as you can.

---

likely to change health behavior if they hold three beliefs.

- *Susceptibility.* They acknowledge that they are at risk for the negative consequences of their behavior.

- *Severity.* They believe that they may pay a very high price if they don't make a change.

- *Benefits.* They believe that the proposed change will be advantageous to their health.

There can be a gap between stated and actual beliefs, however. Young adults may say they recognize the very real dangers of casual, careless sex in this day and age. Yet, rather than act in accordance with these statements, they may impulsively engage in unprotected sex with individuals whose health status and histories they do not know. The reason: Like young people everywhere and in every time, they feel they are invulnerable, that nothing bad can or will happen to them, that if there were a real danger, they would somehow know it. Often it's not until something happens—a former lover may admit to having a sexually transmitted disease (STD), or there may be a pregnancy scare—that their behaviors become consistent with their stated beliefs.

The value or importance we give to health also plays a major role in changing behavior. Many people aren't concerned about their health just for the sake of being healthy. Usually they want to look or feel better, be more productive or competitive, or behave more independently. They're more likely to change, and to stick with a change, if they can see that the health benefits also enhance other important aspects of their lives.

Perceptions are the way we see things from our unique perspective; they vary greatly with age. As a student, you may not think that living a few hours longer is a significant gain; as you grow older, however, you may prize every additional second.

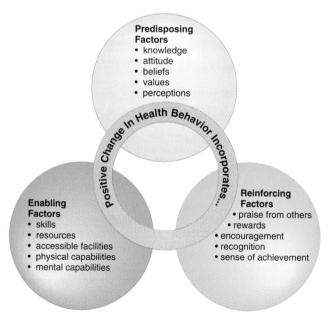

■ Figure 1-3 Factors that shape positive behavior.

Enabling Factors

Enabling factors include skills, resources, accessible facilities, and physical and mental capacities. Before you initiate a change, assess the means available to reach your goal. No matter how motivated you are, you'll become frustrated if you keep encountering obstacles. That's why breaking a task or goal down into step-by-step strategies is so important in behavioral change.

Reinforcing Factors

Reinforcing factors may be praise from family and friends, rewards from teachers or parents, or encouragement and recognition for meeting a goal. Although these help a great deal in the short run, lasting change depends not on external rewards, but on an internal commitment and sense of achievement. To make a difference, reinforcement must come from within.

A decision to change a health behavior should stem from a permanent, personal goal, not from a desire to please or impress someone else. If you lose weight for the homecoming dance, you're almost sure to regain pounds afterward. But if you shed extra pounds because you want to feel better about yourself or get into shape, you're far more likely to keep the weight off.

Strategies *for* Change

Setting Realistic Goals

Here's a framework for setting goals and objectives, the crucial preliminary step for making changes:

✔ Determine your goal or objective. Define it in words and on paper. Then test your definition against your own value system. Can you attain your goal and still be the person you want to be?

✔ Think in terms of evolution, not revolution. Revolutionary changes only inspire counterrevolutions. If you want to change the way you eat, start by changing just one meal a week.

✔ Identify your resources. Do you have the knowledge, skills, finances, time—whatever it takes? Find out from others who know. Be sure you're ready for the next step.

✔ Systematically analyze barriers. How can missing resources be acquired? Identify and select alternative plans. List solutions for any obstacles you foresee.

✔ Choose a plan. Think it through, step by step, trying to anticipate what might go wrong and why.

Making Decisions

Every day you make decisions that have immediate and long-term effects on your health. You decide what to eat, whether to drink or smoke, when to exercise, and how to cope with a sudden crisis. Beyond these daily matters, you decide when to see a doctor, what kind of doctor, and with what sense of urgency. You decide what to tell your doctor and whether to follow the advice given, whether to keep up your immunizations, whether to have a prescription filled and comply with the medication instructions, and whether to seek further help or a second opinion. The entire process of maintaining or restoring health depends on your decisions; it cannot start or continue without them.

The small decisions of everyday life—what to eat, where to go, when to study—are straightforward choices. Larger decisions—which major to choose, what to do about a dead-end relationship, how to handle an awkward work situation—are more challenging. However, if you think of decision making as a process, you can break down even the most difficult choices into manageable steps:

- *Set priorities.* Rather than getting bogged down in details, step back and look at the big picture. What matters most to you? What would you like to accomplish in the next week, month, year? Look at the decision you're about to make in the context of your values and goals (both discussed in Chapter 3).

- *Inform yourself.* The more you know—about a person, a position, a place, a project—the better you'll be able to evaluate it. Gathering information may involve formal research, such as an online or library search for relevant data, or informal conversations with teachers, counselors, family members, or friends.

- *Consider all your options.* Most complex decisions don't involve simple either-or alternatives. List as many options as you can think of, along with the advantages and disadvantages of each.

- *Tune in to your gut feelings.* After you've gotten the facts and analyzed them, listen to your intuition. While it's not infallible, your "sixth sense" can provide valuable feedback. If something just doesn't feel right, try to figure out why. Are there any fears you haven't dealt with? Do you have doubts about taking a certain path?

- *Consider a "worst-case" scenario.* When you've pretty much come to a final decision, imagine what will happen if everything goes wrong—the workload becomes overwhelming, your partner betrays your trust, your expectations turn out to be unrealistic. If you can live with the worst consequences of a decision, you're probably making the right choice.

How Can I Change a Bad Health Habit?

Change is never easy—even if it's done for the best possible reasons. When you decide to change a behavior, you have to give up something familiar and easy for something new and challenging. Change always involves risk—and the prospect of rewards.

Researchers have identified various approaches that people use in making beneficial changes. In the "moral" model, you take responsibility for a problem (such as smoking) and its solution; success depends on adequate motivation, while failure is seen as a sign of character weakness. In the "enlightenment" model, you submit to strict discipline in order to correct a problem; this is the approach used in Alcoholics Anonymous. The "behavioral" model involves rewarding yourself when you make positive changes. The "medical" model sees the behavior as caused by forces beyond your control (a genetic predisposition to being overweight, for example) and employs an expert to provide advice or treatment. For many people, the most effective approach is the "compensatory" model, which doesn't assign blame but puts responsibility on individuals to acquire whatever skills or power they need to overcome their problems.

Before they reach the stage where they can and do take action to change, most people go through a process comparable to religious conversion. First, they reach a level of accumulated unhappiness that makes them ready for change. Then they have a moment of truth that makes them want to change. One pregnant woman, for instance, felt her unborn baby quiver when she drank a beer and swore never to drink again. As people change their behavior, they change their lifestyles and identities as well. Ex-smokers, for instance, may start an aggressive exercise program, make new friends at the track or gym, and participate in new types of activities, like racquetball games or fun runs.

Social and cultural **norms**—behaviors that are expected, accepted, or supported by a group—can make change much harder if they're constantly working against a person's best intentions. You may resolve to eat less, for instance, yet your mother may keep offering you homemade fudge and brownies because your family's norm is to show love by making and offering delicious treats. Or you might decide to drink less, yet your friends' norm may be to equate drinking with having a good time.

If you're aware of the norms that influence your behavior, you can devise strategies either to change them (by encouraging your friends to dance more and drink less at parties, for example) or adapt to them (having just a bite of your mother's sweets). Another option is to develop relationships with people who share your goals and whose norms can reinforce your behavior.

Successful Change

Awareness of a negative behavior is always the first step toward changing it. Once you identify what you'd like to change, keep a diary for one or two weeks, noting what you do, when, where, and what you're feeling at the time. If you'd like, enlist the help of friends or family to call attention to your behavior. Sometimes self-observation in itself proves therapeutic: Just the act of keeping a diary can be enough to help you lose weight or kick the smoking habit.

Once you've identified the situations, moods, thoughts, or people that act as cues for a behavior, identify the most powerful ones and develop a plan to avoid them. For instance, if you snack continuously when studying in your room, try working in the library, where food is forbidden.

Planning ahead is a crucial part of successful change. If you can't avoid certain situations, anticipate how you might cope with the temptation to return to your old behavior. Develop alternatives. Visualize yourself walking past the desserts in the cafeteria or chewing gum instead of lighting a cigarette.

Some people find it helpful to sign a "contract," a written agreement in which they make a commitment to change, with their partner, parent, or health educator. Spelling out what they intend to do, and why, underscores the seriousness of what they're trying to accomplish (see Figure 1-4).

Above all else, change depends on the belief that you can and will succeed. In his research on **self-efficacy,** psychologist Albert Bandura of Stanford University found that the individuals most likely to reach a goal are those who believe they can. The more strongly they feel that they can and will change their behavior, the more energy and persistence they put into making the change. Other researchers have linked positive health change with optimism. Individuals who see themselves as optimists may underestimate their susceptibility to problems, such as hypertension, because they always expect things to turn out well. Individuals who perceive themselves as susceptible—that is, who anticipate potentially negative consequences—may be more cautious.[31]

Another crucial factor is **locus of control.** If you believe that your actions will make a difference in your health, your locus of control is internal. If you believe that external forces or factors play a greater role, your locus of control is external. Individuals with an external locus of control for health are less likely to seek preventive health care, are less optimistic about early treatment, rate their own health as poorer, and spend more time in bed because of illness than those with an internal locus of control.[32]

My Contract For Change

Date: _____

Personal Goal: _____

_____

Motivating Factors: _____

_____

Change(s) I Promise to Make to Reach This Goal:

_____

Plan for Making This Change: _____

_____

Start Date: _____

Assessment Plan: _____

_____

_____

_____

If I Need Help: _____

_____

Target Date for Reaching Goal: _____

Reward for Achieving Goal: _____

Penalty for Failing to Achieve Goal: _____

_____

Signed: _____

Witnessed By: _____

■ Figure 1-4 A sample health-change contract.

Reinforcements—either positive (a reward) or negative (a punishment)—also can play a role. If you decide to set up a regular exercise program, for instance, you might reward yourself with a new sweat suit if you stick to it for three months or you might punish yourself for skipping a day by doing ten minutes of exercises the following day.

Your **self-talk**—the messages you send yourself—also can play a role. In recent decades, mental health professionals have recognized the conscious use of positive self-talk as a powerful force for changing the way individuals think, feel, and behave. (Chapter 3 discusses self-talk as a principle of cognitive therapy.) "We have a choice about how we think," explains psychologist Martin Seligman, Ph.D., author of *Learned Optimism*. As he notes, by learning to challenge automatic negative thoughts that enter our brains and asserting our own statements of self-worth, we can transform ourselves into optimists who see what's right rather than pessimists forever focusing on what's wrong. "Optimism is a learned set of skills," Seligman contends. "Once learned, these skills persist because they feel so good to use. And reality is usually on our side."[33]

Strategies *for* Change

How to Make a Change

✓ Get support from friends, but don't expect them to supply all the reinforcement you need. You may join a group of overweight individuals and rely on their encouragement to stick to your diet. That's a great way to get going; but in the long run, your own commitment to losing weight has got to be strong enough to help you keep eating right and light.

✓ Focus on the immediate rewards of your new behavior. You may stop smoking so that you'll live longer, but take note of every other benefit it brings you—more stamina, less coughing, more spending money, no more stale tobacco taste in your mouth.

✓ To boost your self-confidence, remind yourself of past successes you've had in making changes. Give yourself pep talks, commending yourself on how well you've done so far and how well you'll continue to do.

✓ Reward yourself regularly. Plan a pleasant reward as an incentive for every week you stick to your new behavior—sleeping in on a Saturday morning, going out with some friends, or spending a sunny afternoon outdoors. Small, regular rewards are more effective in keeping up motivation than one big reward that won't come for many months.

✓ Expect and accept some relapses. The greatest rate of relapse occurs in the first few weeks after making a behavior change. During this critical time, get as much support as you can. In addition, work hard on self-motivation, reminding yourself daily of what you have to gain by sticking with your new health habit.

A New Era in Health Education

In the past, health education focused on individual change. Today many educators are using a new framework in which behavior change occurs within the context of the entire environment of a person's life. The primary themes that bring together personal health, social context, and a community focus are prevention, protection, and promotion.

The Power of Prevention

No medical treatment, however successful or sophisticated, can compare with the power of **prevention**. Two out of every three deaths and one in three hospitalizations in the United States could be prevented by changes in six main risk factors: tobacco use, alcohol abuse, accidents, high blood pressure, obesity, and gaps in screening and primary health care. Preventive efforts have already proved helpful in increasing physical activity, quitting smoking, reducing dietary fat, preventing STDs and unwanted pregnancy, reducing intolerance and violence, and avoiding alcohol and drug abuse.

Prevention can take many forms. Primary or "before-the-fact" prevention efforts might seek to reduce stressors and increase support in order to prevent problems in healthy people. Consumer education, for instance, provides guidance about how to change our lifestyle—the way we care for the basic needs of body and mind—to prevent problems and enhance well-being. Other preventive programs identify people at risk and "empower" them with information and support so they can avoid potential problems. Prevention efforts may target an entire community and try to educate all of its members about the dangers of alcohol abuse, for instance, or environmental hazards, or they may zero in on a particular group (for instance, seminars on safer sex practice offered to teens) or an individual (one-on-one counseling about substance abuse).

In the past, physicians did not routinely incorporate prevention into their professional practices. Instead, consumers played the role of Humpty-Dumpty: As long as they sat quietly on the wall, they were ignored. When they fell, the medical equivalents of all the king's horses and all the king's men came running to put them back together again. Often, however, even the best these professionals could provide was still too little, too late.

But times have changed. Medical schools are providing more training in preventive care. A growing number of studies have demonstrated that prevention saves not only money, but also productivity, health, and lives. As many as 50 percent to 80 percent of the deaths caused by cardiovascular disease, strokes, and cancer could be avoided or delayed by preventive measures. Eliminating smoking could prevent more than 300,000 deaths each year, for instance, while changes in diet could prevent 35 percent of unnecessary deaths from heart disease.[34]

The Potential of Protection

There is a great deal of overlap between prevention and **protection**. Some people might think of immunizations (discussed in Chapter 12) as a way of preventing illness; others see them as a form of protection against dangerous diseases. In many ways, protection picks up where prevention leaves off. You can prevent STDs or unwanted pregnancy by abstaining from sex. But if you decide to engage in potentially risky sexual activities, you can protect yourself by means of condoms and spermicides (discussed in Chapter 10). Similarly, you can prevent many automobile accidents by not driving when road conditions are hazardous. But if you do have to drive, you can protect yourself by wearing a seatbelt and using defensive driving techniques (discussed in Chapter 18).

The very concept of protection implies some degree of risk—immediate and direct (for instance, the risk of intentional injury from an assailant or unintentional harm from a fire) or long-term and indirect (such as the risk of heart disease and cancer as a result of smoking). In order to know how best to protect yourself, you have to be able to assess risks realistically.

Hereditary Risks

In all, more than 4,000 diseases have been traced to flaws in the basic genetic blueprints for life. "With the exception of walking across the street and being hit by a car, all disease may be genetic," says geneticist Reed Pyeritz, M.D., of Johns Hopkins School of Medicine in Baltimore. "In addition to the classical genetic disorders, most of the common diseases that get us later in life—like atherosclerosis and cancer—involve a genetic predisposition.[35]

Each individual carries about 20 abnormal genes, including 7 or 8 deadly ones. Most are hidden, but in combination with other genes or in certain environmental conditions, they can become dangerous. According to the American Society of Human Genetics, about 5 percent of adults under age 25 have a genetically linked disease; among adults over 25, 60 percent develop a genetically influenced disorder.

In addition to rare genetic syndromes, hereditary diseases include common problems such as certain types of cataracts, glaucoma, gall bladder disease, hypertension, nearsightedness, ulcers, and dyslexia. "The general perception is that all hereditary diseases are unalterable and deadly, but that's not the case," observes Pyeritz. "The vast majority don't necessarily shorten life, although they can cause pain and suffering."

Most adult-onset illnesses, such as cancer, heart disease, and alcoholism, are caused by the interaction of multiple genes and environmental factors. Other disorders can be traced to a single gene. If the gene is stronger, or dominant (as is the case for Huntington's chorea, a progressive, incurable brain disorder), each child of a carrier faces a 50 percent risk of inheriting the disease. If the gene is weaker, or recessive (as in cystic fibrosis, a disorder of the mucous and sweat glands), each child faces a 25 percent chance of having the disease and a 50 percent chance of becoming a carrier. If the X gene contributed by the mother—which joins with a Y gene from the father to create a boy or an X gene from the father to create a girl—has the harmful trait (as in hemophilia), each son has a 50 percent risk of inheriting the disorder; each daughter has a 50 percent risk of being a carrier.

In the future, millions of Americans may be able to undergo tests to find out if they have genes that increase their risk of cancer, heart disease, alcoholism, and other common problems. But how many will want to know their possible fate? "That may depend on the type of problem," says geneticist Helga Toriello, M.D., of the American Society of Human Genetics. "Knowledge can be frightening when little, if anything, can be done to alter the course of a disease. But in most cases, forewarned is forearmed."[36]

Yet genetic testing may never be able to tell individuals all they want to know. "A test can tell you only whether you have a gene or a predisposition for a disorder," says geneticist Pyeritz. "It doesn't tell you when you might develop the disease, how it might affect you, whether your symptoms will be mild or severe or what the course of the illness will be." In addition, he notes, "testing is a double-edged sword. Consumers aren't the only ones eager to find out about inherited risks. Insurance companies and employers also want to know who may be vulnerable. Testing could lead to genetic discrimination."

Testing also may provide false reassurance. "If you discover that you don't have the gene that's been linked to alcoholism, does that give you permission to drink as much as you want?" asks Toriello, pointing out that among 70 people in a recent study, 28 percent of those *without* the gene became alcohol-dependent and 23 percent of those with the gene did not.

Given the complexities and varied implications of learning about genetic risks, how much would you want to know? The answer is always profoundly personal. Knowledge can give you the power to prevent some problems or to seek early treatment for others. Yet it also can be a burden. As one woman at risk for a potentially fatal genetic disorder puts it, "You have to decide which is worse: the awful uncertainty of not knowing or the possibility of finding out that your worst fears will come true."

Assessing Risks

At this point in time, you cannot change your genes—or the risks they carry. This isn't true of all health risks. The risk of head injury is very real every single time you get on your mountain bike; however, it diminishes greatly when you put on a helmet. Today's young people face a host of risks, from the danger of being the victim of violence to the hazards of self-destructive behaviors like drinking and drugs. The CDC's Youth Risk Behavior Surveys show a decline in some risky

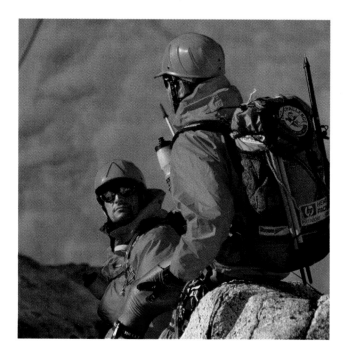

Wearing a helmet is a health choice that diminishes your risk of serious injury.

behaviors, such as carrying a weapon and not wearing a bicycle helmet, but an increase in others, including cigarette smoking and marijuana use.[37]

At any age, the greatest health threats stem from high-risk behaviors—smoking, excessive drinking, not getting enough exercise, eating too many high-fat foods, and not getting regular medical checkups, to name just a few. That's why changing unhealthy habits is the best way to reduce risks and prevent health problems.

Environmental health risks are the stuff newspaper headlines are made of (see Chapter 20). Every year brings calls of alarm about a new hazard to health: electromagnetic radiation, fluoride in drinking water, hair dyes, silicone implants, radon, lead. Often the public response is panic. Consumers picket and protest. Individuals arrange for elaborate testing. Yet how do we know whether or not alleged health risks are acceptable? Some key factors to consider:

- *Possible benefits.* Advantages or payoffs—such as the high salary paid for working with toxic chemicals or radioactive materials—may make some risks seem worthwhile.

- *Whether the risk is voluntary.* All of us tend to accept risks that we freely choose to take, such as playing a sport that could lead to injuries, as opposed to risks imposed on us, such as pollution from a nearby factory.

- *Is it fair?* The risk of skin cancer, which is increasing because of ozone depletion (see Chapter 20), affects us all. We may worry about it and take action to protect ourselves and our planet, but we don't resent it the way we resent living with the risk of violent crime because the only housing we can afford is in a high-crime area.

- *Are there alternatives?* As consumers, we may become upset about cancer-causing pesticides or food additives when we learn about safer chemicals or methods of preservation.

- *"Framing."* Our thinking about risks often depends on how they're presented or framed—for instance, if we're told that a new drug may kill 1 out of every 100 people, instead of that it may save the lives of 99 percent of those who use it.

The Promise of Promotion

If the best defense is a good offense, health **promotion** represents the ultimate form of prevention and protection. The World Health Organization defines health promotion as the process of enabling people to improve and increase control over their health. Other health specialists define it as "a science and an art devoted to helping people achieve a state of optimal health."

Education about health choices is a major aspect of health promotion.

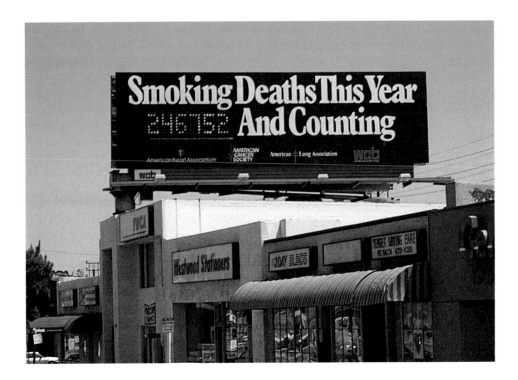

Health promotion programs emphasize health-enhancing behaviors, such as exercising regularly; eating nutritious foods; managing stress well; avoiding tobacco, excess alcohol, and drugs; forming fulfilling relationships with friends; living in a community with clean air; and having purpose in life. They may focus on risk avoidance, such as staying out of the sun at midday, and risk reduction, such as using sunscreen.

One of the best examples of how effective health promotion can be is the dramatic reduction in smoking among young African Americans. In the past, black male teenagers started smoking earlier and in much greater numbers than white adolescents. But the African-American community began to send messages to its youth. Some people whitewashed billboards advertising cigarettes. Black musicians, athletes, and celebrities stopped using cigarettes in a public, glamorized way. Most powerful of all were the messages sent from teen to teen: that smoking was a bad, uncool habit that exploited the African-American community. As discussed in Chapter 17, African-American adolescents now smoke much less than white teens.

Peer counseling—support offered by one student to another—has proven effective in many areas, from awareness of the dangers of casual, unprotected sex to education about what constitutes sexual harassment and coercion. However, often it's not enough to provide information and focus on an individual's responsibility to practice safer sex, eat less fat, exercise regularly, or stop a dangerous behavior. The reality is that all health decisions are made within the complex context of culture and community.

Increasingly, health educators are realizing that overemphasizing individual responsibility sets people up to fail and, with repeated failures, to blame themselves, even in circumstances beyond their control. A college student, for instance, may decide to eat more nutritiously. However, if the only available choices are high-fat foods in vending machines and campus cafeterias, all the good intentions and willpower in the world won't lead to success.

Many health promotion efforts look beyond the campus to make the same opportunities for nutritious food, leisure, exercise, and support open to others. To develop social responsibility in students, they encourage volunteering at community centers, homeless shelters, nursing homes, environmental agencies, and advocacy groups. Their goal is to help students define health, not only in terms of their own behaviors and well-being, but also in terms of what they can do to reach out and help others in the broader community make healthier choices and changes.

Across the Lifespan: Longer, Healthier Lives

Americans are living longer, including the most senior of our citizens. According to the U. S. Census Bureau, the ranks of centenarians nearly doubled during the 1990s, from about 37,000 at the start of the decade to more than an estimated 70,000 in 1999. Analysts at the Census Bureau

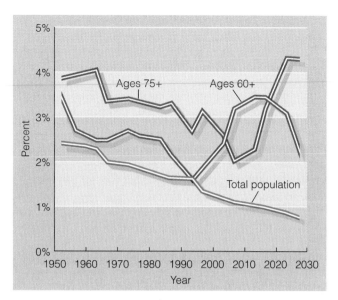

■ **Figure 1-5** Average annual percent growth of total population and older population in America.

Source: National Institute on Aging.

predict that this per-decade doubling trend may continue, with the centenarian population possibly reaching 834,000 by the middle of the twenty-first century.[38]

Four of every five centenarians are women. Approximately 78 percent of today's centenarians are white, a proportion expected to decrease to about 55 percent by 2050 as more members of different minorities extend their life spans. The nation's centenarians are concentrated on both U. S. coasts, with about 10 percent of the total number living in California and 8 percent making their homes in New York. Internationally, the U. S. may have the highest proportion of centenarians among people age 85 and older. There are approximately 120 centenarians per 10,000 people age 85 and older in the U. S.[39]

Across the Lifespan: Longer Healthspans

Americans aren't just living longer; they're staying healthy longer, increasing their "health spans" along with their life spans. The proportion of older Americans with disabilities that interfere with everyday tasks and independent living has been declining since 1982. "There are 1.5 million fewer disabled people today than there would have been if the rate hadn't dropped so dramatically," says Richard Hodes, M.D., director of the National Institute on Aging. "Now we're looking for clues so we can understand why this happened and make sure that the trend continues."[40]

Genes, as studies of identical twins have revealed, influence only about 30 percent of the rate and ways in which we age. "The rest is up to us," says Michael Roizen, M.D., of the University of Chicago, author of *RealAge,* who notes that it's

possible to become healthier, fitter, and biologically younger with time. "With relatively simple changes, someone whose chronological age is 69 can have a physiological age of 45. And the most amazing thing is that it's never too late to live younger—until one foot is 6 feet under."[41]

Staying Strong

For years, experts assumed that older meant weaker. Landmark research with frail nursing home residents in their eighties and nineties showed this isn't so. After just eight to ten weeks of strength training, even the oldest seniors increased muscle and bone, speeded up their metabolic rate, improved sleep and mobility, boosted their spirits, and gained in self-confidence. Other studies have found that exercise programs can increase lung capacity, double leg strength, decrease the risk of disability, and improve ability to walk distances, climb stairs, stoop, crouch, kneel, and carry objects.[42]

"Muscles are a big key to staying healthy longer," says Miriam Nelson, Ph.D., associate chief of the U.S.D.A. Human Physiology Laboratory at Tufts University, who explains that muscle loss starts early and proceeds silently for decades. "We start losing a third to a half pound of muscle in our mid-thirties, so by the time we reach ninety we have only half the muscle mass we did as young adults. But to be independent and healthy into advanced age, you need to be strong."

Regular resistance training—lifting hand-held weights or working on weight machines for at least ten minutes three times a week—can maintain muscle mass, prevent bone loss, and help control weight. "Exercise can make a 70-year-old person as strong and as fit as a 40-year-old," says Nelson. "And it can keep a 90-year-old mobile and independent."[43]

Thinking Young

The healthiest seniors are "engaged" in life, resilient, optimistic, productive, and socially involved, observe John Rowe, M.D., and Robert Kahn, Ph.D., of the MacArthur Foundation Research Network on Successful Aging, authors of *Successful Aging.*[44] While they are not immune to life's slings and arrows, successful agers bounce back after a setback and have a "can-do" attitude about the challenges they face. They also tend to be lifelong learners who may take up entirely new hobbies late in life—pursuits that stimulate production of more connections between neurons and may slow aging within the brain.

Just as with muscles, the best advice for keeping your brain healthy as you age is "use it or lose it." Some memory losses among healthy older people are normal, but these are reversible with training in simple methods, such as word associations, that improve recall. NIA has launched a study of Vitamin E and an experimental medication, Aricept (donepezil), as potential treatments for age-related mild cognitive impairment.

Protecting Health

Also important for a healthy old age is keeping up with immunizations against diseases, such as influenza and pneumococcal pneumonia, that take a greater toll on the elderly. For women at risk of osteoporosis, new options, including "designer estrogens" like raloxifene, can preserve their bones' health. A healthy diet, chock full of fruits and vegetables, also can contribute to a healthy old age, in part because they contain antioxidants that may ward off many age-related problems. (See Chapter 6.) Thirty minutes of moderate physi-

cal activity a day (whether it's walking, gardening, or vacuuming) can make a big difference in keeping arteries young. Other simple changes, like daily relaxation, also can help. "Most people don't realize that something as simple as flossing their teeth affects arterial health," says Roizen, who explains that the same bacteria that cause periodontal disease can trigger inflammation and constriction of the arteries. (See Chapter 11.)

"There isn't a single magic bullet that can stop the clock," says Roizen. "Instead there are lots of little things that you can do to get biologically younger. But the real pay-off of making these changes isn't the heart attack you prevent thirty years down the road. It's feeling younger and healthier right now."[45]

health **/ ONLINE**

National Center for Health Statistics
http://www.cdc.gov/nchswww/
From this site, you can read about what progress has been made toward the Healthy People project objectives, access fact sheets on a comprehensive list of topics via the "Fastats" feature, download publications, and more.

Mayo Clinic Health Oasis
http://mayohealth.org
This award-winning site provides reliable, expert advice on treating illnesses and disease prevention. It includes special centers for cancer, heart health, nutrition, men's health, and women's health topics. It also includes many online health-related assessments.

Healthfinder
http://www.healthfinder.gov/
This general health resources site features information on hot topics in health, health-in-the-media, prevention and self-care, accessing medical libraries and online journals, and more.

Please note that links are subject to change. If you find a broken link, use a search engine like http://www.yahoo.com *and search for the web site by typing in key words.*

 Campus Chat: From what sources do you receive most of your health information? (For example, personal physician, the web, newspapers, and so on.) Share your thoughts on our online discussion forum at http://health.wadsworth.com

Find It On InfoTrac: You can find additional readings related to health via InfoTrac College Edition, an online library of more than 900 journals and publications. Follow the instructions for accessing InfoTrac that came packaged with your textbook; then search for articles using a key word search.

• **Suggested article:** "Healthy People 2010: National Health Objectives for the United States," by Ronald M. Davis. *British Medical Journal*, Nov. 28, 1998, Vol. 317, p. 513.

  (1) Outline the history of the formation of national health objectives for the United States.
  (2) What are the significant differences between the "Healthy People 2010" document and the original "Healthy People 2000" objectives?

For additional links, resources, and suggested readings on InfoTrac, visit our Health & Wellness Resource Center at http://health.wadsworth.com

Making This Book Work for You

Taking Charge of Your Future

Through every chapter of this book, you'll recognize some familiar themes, messages that apply to every aspect of your health. Among the most important are the following:

- You're not simply a creature of mind, body, or spirit, but of all three. Physical, psychological, spiritual, social, intellectual, and environmental factors are interrelated in complex and crucial ways that affect your health.

- Prevention has the power to enhance the quality and duration of your life. Rather than waiting for bad health habits to take their toll, you can delay or eliminate many problems by adopting healthful behaviors now.

- Positive lifestyle changes—the basics of health promotion—enhance your health and enrich your well-being.

- You can take charge of your health and prevent illness by changing your health behaviors. The keys to success are motivation, accurate information, workable strategies, and a belief in your ability to change.

- You are not alone. Your ties to the people around you and to the environment in which you live give richness and meaning to your life.

- You face undeniable risks in life, but you can do a great deal to avoid or minimize their impact on your well-being.

To help safeguard your health, you need to understand basic theories about human health and life and to have up-to-date information about health practices. With the aid of your health instructors, *An Invitation to Health* can provide the basic knowledge and skills you need for a lifetime of well-being. But knowledge isn't enough; action is the key. The habits you form now, the decisions you make, and the ways in which you live day by day will all shape your health and your future.

This book can give you the understanding you'll need to make good decisions and establish a healthy lifestyle, but you can't simply read and study health the way you study French or chemistry—you must decide to live it.

This is our invitation to you.

 Longer Life Expectancies. What factors are contributing to longer life expectancies?

Key Terms

The terms listed here are used within the chapter. Page numbers are included for each term. A definition of each term is given in the Glossary pages at the end of this book.

health 14	promotion 31	self-talk 29
locus of control 27	protection 30	wellness 14
norms 27	reinforcements 29	
prevention 29	self-efficacy 27	

Critical Thinking Questions

1. What is the definition of health according to the text-book? Does your personal definition differ from this, and if so, in what ways? How would you have defined health before reading this chapter?

2. Where do you lie on the wellness-illness continuum? What variables might affect your place on the scale? What do you consider your optimum state of health to be?

3. In what ways would you like to change your present lifestyle? What steps could you take to make those changes?

References

1. "Constitution of the World Health Organization." *Chronicle of the World Health Organization.* Geneva, Switzerland: WHO, 1947.

2. Gordon, James. Personal interview.

3. Cunningham, Alastair. "Pies, Levels and Languages: Why the Contribution of Mind to Health Has Been Underestimated." *Advances: The Journal of Mind-Body Health,* Vol. 11, No. 2, Spring 1995.

4. Sloan, R. P., et al., "Religion, Spirituality, and Medicine." *Lancet,* Vol. 353, No. 9153, February 20, 1999.

5. Koenig, Harold. "How Does Religious Faith Contribute to Recovery from Depression?" *Harvard Mental Health Letter,* Vol. 15, No. 8, February 1999.

6. McInerney, John. "Risk of Earlier Death Cut by Going to Religious Services." National Institute of Health press release, July 1, 1999. Hummer, R. A., et al. "Religious Involvement and U. S. Adult Mortality," *Demography,* Vol. 36, No. 2, 1999.

7. "Health: That's What Friend & Family Are For." *Facts of Life: An Issue Briefing for Health Reporters from the Center for Advancement of Health,* Vol. 2, No. 6, November–December 1997.

8. Woloshin, S., et al. "Perceived Adequacy of Tangible Social Support and Health Outcomes in Patients with Coronary Artery Disease." *Journal of General Internal Medicine,* October 1997.

9. Cohen, Sheldon, et al. "Social Ties and Susceptibility to the Common Cold." *Journal of the American Medical Association,* June 25, 1997.

10. "New Report Documents Improvement in Americans' Health." CDC / NCHS Press Office, June 10, 1999.

11. Shalala, Donna. "Healthy People 2000 Review, 1998–1999." Washington, D.C.: Department of Health and Human Services, 1999. Web site: http://www.cdc.gov/nchswww

12. Healthy People 2010 Fact Sheet: *Healthy People in Healthy Communities.* Healthy People 2010 is available on the Internet at web.health.gov.healthypeople

13. *The World Health Report 1999: Making a Difference.* Geneva: World Health Organization, 1999.

14. Ibid.

15. U. S. Census Bureau.

16. Cooper-Patrick, Lisa. " Race, Gender, and Partnership in the Patient-Physician Relationship." *JAMA,* August 11, 1999.

17. Campbell, Paulette Walker. "Lawmakers Push NIH to Focus Research on Minority Populations and Cancer." *Chronicle of Higher Education,* Vol. 45, No. 26, March 5, 1999.

18. National Center for Health Statistics.

19. Araujo, David. "Cardiovascular Disease Risk Higher in Minority Youth." *Physician and Sportsmedicine,* Vol. 27, No. 7, July, 1999.

20. "Health Care: It's Better if You're White." *The Economist,* Vol. 350, No. 81, February 27, 1999.

21. Ibid.

22. Department of Health and Human Services.

23. Vitucci, Jeff. "The State of Hispanic Health." *Hispanic Business,* Vol. 21, No. 6, June 1999.

24. Marwick, Charles. "Growing Hispanic Association Serves Increasing Population." *JAMA,* May 12, 1999.

25. Sax, Linda, et al. *The American Freshman: National Norms for Fall 1998.* Los Angeles: Higher Education Research Institute, UCLA, 1998.

26. Shapiro, Johanna, et al. "Sexual Behavior and AIDS-Related Knowledge Among Community College Students in Orange County, California." *Journal of Community Health,* Vol. 24, Issue 1, February 1999.

27. Moskal, Patsy, et al. "Examining the Use of Tobacco on College Campuses." *Journal of American College Health,* Vol. 47, No. 6, May 1999.

28. Wechsler, Henry, et al. "College Alcohol Use: A Full or Empty Glass?" *Journal of American College Health,* Vol. 47, No. 6, May 1999.

29. Clark, Mary Jo, et al. "The Effects of an Intervention Campaign to Enhance Seat Belt Use on Campus." *Journal of American College Health,* Vol. 47, No. 6, May 1999.

30. Georgiou, Constance, et al. "Among Young Adults, College Students and Graduates Practiced More Healthful Habits and Made More Healthful Food Choices Than Did Nonstudents." *Journal of the American Dietetic Association,* Vol. 97, No. 7, July 1997.

31. O'Brien, William, et al. "Predicting Health Behaviors Using Measures of Optimism and Perceived Risk." *Health Values,* Vol. 19. No. 1, January–February 1995.

32. Chen, William. "Enhancement of Health Locus of Control Through Biofeedback Training." *Perceptual and Motor Skills,* Vol. 80, No. 2, April 1995.

33. Steenbarger, Brett, et al. "Prevention in College Health: Counseling Perspectives." *Journal of American College Health,* Vol. 43, January 1995.

34. Jones, Laurie. "Does Prevention Save Money?"*American Medical News,* January 9, 1995. Knapp, Jane. "A Call to Action: Institute of Medicine Report on Emergency Medical Services for Children." *Pediatrics,* Vol. 98, No. 2, July 10, 1995.

35. Pyeritz, Reed. Personal interview.

36. Toriello, Helga. Personal interview.

37. "Fact Sheet: Youth Risk Behavior Trends." CDC.

38. Cahan, Vicky. "New Census Report Shows Exponential Growth in Number of Centenarians." News release, U. S. Census Bureau, June 16, 1999.

39. Perls, Thomas, and Margery Hutter Silver. *Living to 100.* New York: Basic Books, 1999.

40. Hodes, Richard. Personal interview.

41. Roizen, Michael. *RealAge.* New York: Random House, 1999.

42. Nelson, Miriam. Personal interview.

43. Markides, Kyriakos. "Growing Younger by Keeping Up Regular Physical Activity." *Behavioral Medicine,* February 1999.

44. Rowe, John. Personal interview.

45. Roizen, Michael. Personal interview.

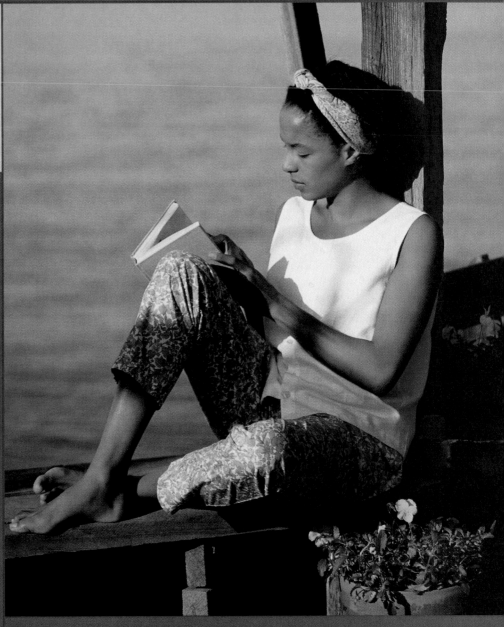

CHAPTER

2

Personal Stress Management

After studying the material in this chapter, you should be able to:

- **Define** stress and stressors and **use** the general adaptation syndrome to explain how stress relates to health.

- **Explain** the biology of stress and its relationship to heart disease, high blood pressure, the immune system, and digestive disorders.

- **List** some personal causes of stress, especially those experienced by students, and **discuss** how their effects can be prevented or minimized.

- **List** the major social stressors and **explain** how these can cause stress.

- **Describe** the symptoms of stress-related adjustment disorders.

- **Explain** how you can improve your resistance to stress, and **describe** some techniques to help manage stress.

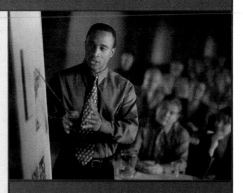

ou know about stress. You live with it every day: the stress of passing exams, preparing for a career, meeting people, facing new experiences. Everyone, regardless of age, gender, race or income, has to deal with stress—as an individual and as a member of society.

Yet stress in itself isn't necessarily bad. An individual's response to stress, not the stressful situation itself, is what matters most. Stress always involves an interaction between a life situation and a person's ability to cope. Perhaps one of the best ways to think of it is captured by the Chinese word for crisis, which consists of two characters—one means danger; the other, opportunity. Stress involves both.

By learning to anticipate stressful events, to manage day-to-day stress, and to prevent stress overload, you can find alternatives to running endlessly on a treadmill of alarm, panic, and exhaustion. The stress-management skills in this chapter provide a good start. As you organize your time, release tension, and build up internal resources, you will begin to experience the sense of control and confidence that makes stress a challenge rather than an ordeal. ❖

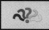 **FREQUENTLY ASKED QUESTIONS**

FAQ: **Can stress affect the heart? p. 42**

FAQ: **Can stress affect the immune system? p. 43**

FAQ: **How should I deal with anger? p. 50**

FAQ: **What can help me relax? p. 57**

FAQ: **How can I better manage my time? p. 58**

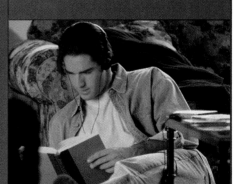

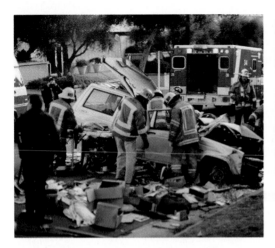 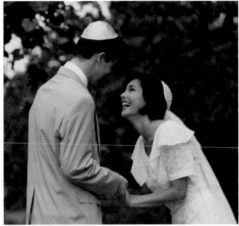

Types of stressors. An automobile accident is an example of an acute stressor. Getting married is an example of a positive stressor.

What Is Stress?

People use the word *stress* in different ways: as an external force that causes a person to become tense or upset, as the internal state of arousal, and as the physical response of the body to various demands. Dr. Hans Selye, a pioneer in studying physiological responses to challenge, defined **stress** as "the nonspecific response of the body to any demand made upon it." In other words, the body reacts to **stressors**—the things that upset or excite us—in the same way, regardless of whether they are positive or negative.

Stress can be acute, episodic, or chronic, depending on the nature of the stressors or external events that cause the stress response. Acute or short-term stressors, which can range from a pop quiz to a bomb threat in a crowded stadium, trigger a brief but intense response to a specific incident. Episodic stressors like monthly bills or quarterly exams cause regular but intermittent elevations in stress levels. Chronic stressors include everything from rush-hour traffic to a learning disability to living with an alcoholic parent or spouse.

Not all stressors are negative. Some of life's happiest moments—births, reunions, weddings—are enormously stressful. We weep with the stress of frustration or loss; we weep, too, with the stress of love and joy. Selye coined the term **eustress** for positive stress in our lives (*eu* is a Greek prefix meaning "good"). Eustress challenges us to grow, adapt, and find creative solutions in our lives. **Distress** refers to the negative effects of stress that can deplete or even destroy life energy. Ideally, the level of stress in our lives should be just high enough to motivate us to satisfy our needs and not so high that it interferes with our ability to reach our fullest potential.

What Causes Stress?

There are many biological theories of stress. The best known may be the **general adaptation syndrome (GAS),** developed by Hans Selye, who postulated that our bodies constantly strive to maintain a stable and consistent physiological state. This is called **homeostasis.** Stressors, whether in the form of physical illness or a demanding job, disturb this state and trigger a nonspecific physiological response. The body attempts to restore homeostasis by means of an **adaptive response. Allostasis** describes the body's ability to adapt to constantly changing environments.

Selye's general adaptation syndrome (GAS), which describes the body's response to a stressor—whether threatening or exhilarating—consists of three distinct stages:

1. *Alarm.* When a stressor first occurs, the body responds with changes that temporarily lower resistance. Levels of certain hormones may rise; blood pressure may increase (see Figure 2-1). The body quickly makes internal adjustments so it can cope with the stressor and return to normal activity.

2. *Resistance.* If the stressor continues, the body mobilizes its internal resources to try to sustain homeostasis. For example, if a loved one is seriously hurt in an accident, we initially respond intensely and feel great anxiety. During the subsequent stressful period of recuperation, we struggle to carry on as normally as possible, but this requires considerable effort.

3. *Exhaustion.* If the stress continues long enough, we cannot keep up our normal functioning. Even a small amount of additional stress at this point can cause a breakdown.

Another theory—the cognitive-transactional model of stress, developed by Richard Lazarus—looks at the relation between stress and health. As he sees it, stress can have a powerful impact on health. Conversely, health can affect a person's resistance or coping ability. Stress, according to Lazarus, is "neither an environmental stimulus, a characteristic of the person, nor a response, but a relationship between demands and the power to deal with them without unreasonable or destructive costs."[1] Thus, an event may be seen as stressful by one person but not by another, or it may seem stressful on one occasion but not on another. For instance, one student may think of speaking in front of the class as extremely stressful, while another relishes the chance to do so—except on days when he's not well-prepared. At any age, some of us are more vulnerable to life changes and crises than are others. The stress of growing up in families troubled by alcoholism, drug dependence, or physical, sexual, or psychological abuse may have a lifelong impact—particularly if these problems are not recognized and dealt with. Other early experiences, positive and negative, also can affect our attitude toward stress—and our resilience to it. Our general outlook on life, whether we're optimistic or pessimistic, can determine whether we expect the worst and feel stressed or anticipate a challenge and feel confident. The when, where, what, how, and why of stressors also affect our reactions. The number and frequency of changes in our lives, along with the time and setting in which they occur, have a great impact on how we'll respond.

Our level of ongoing stress affects our ability to respond to a new day's stressors. Each of us has a breaking point for dealing with stress. A series of too-intense pressures or too-rapid changes can push us closer and closer to that point. That's why it's important to anticipate potential stressors and plan how to deal with them.

Stress experts Thomas Holmes, M.D., and Richard Rahe, M.D., devised a scale to evaluate individual levels of stress and potential for coping, based on *life-change units* that estimate each change's impact. The death of a partner or parent ranks high on the list, but even changing apartments is considered a stressor. People who accumulate more than 300 life-change units in a year are more likely to suffer serious health problems. Scores on the scale, however, represent "potential stress"; the actual impact of the life change depends on the individual's response. (See Self-Survey: "Student Stress Scale," on page 47.)

In ongoing research, Holmes has evaluated variations in life events among many groups, including college students, medical students, football players, pregnant women, alcoholics, and heroin addicts. Heroin addicts and alcoholics have the highest totals of life-change units, followed by college students. In general, younger people experience more life changes than do older people; factors such as gender, education, and social class also have a strong impact.[2] Marriage seems to promote greater stability and fewer changes.

If you score high on the Student Stress Scale, think about the reasons your life has been in such turmoil. Are there any steps you could take to make your life more stable? Of course, some changes, such as your parents' divorce or a friend's accident, may be beyond your control. Even then, you can respond in ways that may protect you from disease.

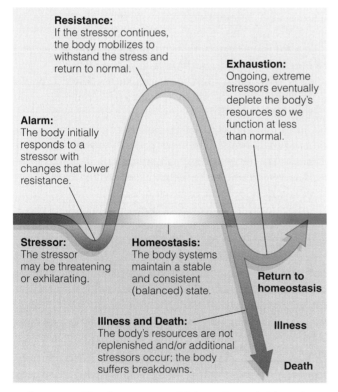

Resistance:
If the stressor continues, the body mobilizes to withstand the stress and return to normal.

Exhaustion:
Ongoing, extreme stressors eventually deplete the body's resources so we function at less than normal.

Alarm:
The body initially responds to a stressor with changes that lower resistance.

Stressor:
The stressor may be threatening or exhilarating.

Homeostasis:
The body systems maintain a stable and consistent (balanced) state.

Return to homeostasis

Illness and Death:
The body's resources are not replenished and/or additional stressors occur; the body suffers breakdowns.

Illness

Death

■ **Figure 2-1** The three stages of Selye's General Adaptation Syndrome (GAS): alarm, resistance, exhaustion.

Effects of Stress on the Body

Stress triggers complex changes in the body's endocrine, or hormone-secreting, system. A new scientific field, **psychoneuroimmunology,** has been exploring these intricate interconnections. When you confront a stressor, the adrenal glands, two triangle-shaped glands that sit atop the kidneys, respond by producing hormones, including catecholamines, cortisol (hydrocortisone), and epinephrine (adrenaline), that speed up heart rate and blood pressure and prepare the body to deal with the threat. This "fight-or-flight" response prepares you for quick action: Your heart works harder to pump more blood to your legs and arms. Your muscles tense, your breathing quickens, and your brain becomes extra alert. And because they're nonessential in a crisis, your digestive and immune systems practically shut down.

Yet stress isn't always harmful. "In spite of their bad reputation, stress hormones have a protective as well as a damaging effect on the body," observes neuroscientist Bruce McEwen. "Whether the good or bad side of stress hormone action predominates depends on the time course of the hormonal stress response, as well as the body's exposure to stress hormones."[3]

Unlike many other molecules in the body (such as the neurotransmitters that transmit messages in the brain), most stress hormones are water-insoluble, which means that they persist in the bloodstream for greater lengths of time. The effects of neurotransmitters disappear within seconds or milliseconds; stress hormones persist in the blood for hours.[4] Cortisol remains elevated for the longest period and has the most important long-term effects on our health.[5]

One effect of cortisol and the other stress hormones, for example, is to speed the conversion of proteins and fats into carbohydrates, the body's basic fuel, so we have the energy to fight or flee from a threat. Another effect is to increase appetite and food-seeking behavior. "This serves us well after running two miles," McEwen observes, "but it is not beneficial when we grab a bag of potato chips while cramming for an exam." Chronically elevated stress hormones can increase levels of insulin and, in sedentary individuals, increase body fat. They also contribute to the formation of atherosclerotic plaque in the coronary arteries.

In the brain, stress hormones linked to powerful emotions may help create long-lasting memories, such as where we were when we heard of Princess Diana's death, or the sequence of events leading up to a marriage proposal. But very prolonged or severe stress can damage the brain's ability to remember and can actually cause brain cells, or neurons, to atrophy and die.

As Figure 2-2 illustrates, persistent or repeated increases in the stress hormones can be hazardous throughout the body. Catecholamines cause a rise in blood pressure and heart rate, make breathing short and shallow, and increase the potential for blood clotting, upping the risk for stroke and heart attack. Cortisol increases glucose production in the liver, causes renal hypertension (which also raises blood pressure), and suppresses the immune system. Chronically elevated stress hormones raise the baseline anxiety level, making it harder to cope with daily annoyances.[6]

Hundreds of studies over the last 20 years have shown that stress contributes to approximately 80 percent of all major illnesses: cardiovascular disease, cancer, endocrine and metabolic disease, skin rashes, ulcers, ulcerative colitis, emotional disorders, musculoskeletal disease, infectious ailments, premenstrual syndrome (PMS), uterine fibroid cysts, and breast cysts. The New York-based American Institute of Stress reports that as many as 75 to 90 percent of visits to physicians are related to stress.[7]

The first signs of stress include muscle tightness, tension headaches, backaches, upset stomach, and sleep disruptions (caused by stress-altered brain-wave activity). Some people feel fatigued, their hearts may race or beat faster than usual at rest, and they may feel tense all the time, easily frustrated and often irritable. Others feel sad; lose their energy, appetite, or sex drive; and develop psychological problems, including depression, anxiety, and panic attacks (discussed in Chapter 4). Stress can lead to self-destructive behaviors, such as drinking, drug use, and reckless driving. Some people see such acts as offering an escape from the pressure they feel. Unfortunately, they end up adding to their stress load.

Can Stress Affect the Heart?

In the 1970s, cardiologists Meyer Friedman, M.D., and Ray Rosenman, M.D., suggested that excess stress may be the most important factor in the development of heart disease. They compared their patients to individuals of the same age with healthy hearts and developed two general categories: Type A and Type B.

Hardworking, aggressive, and competitive, Type A's never have time for all they want to accomplish, even though they usually try to do several tasks at once. Type B's are more relaxed, though not necessarily less ambitious or successful. (Of course, people who are extremely Type B may never accomplish anything.) Type-A behavior has been found to be the major contributing factor in the early development of heart disease.

The degree of danger associated with Type-A behavior remains controversial. According to a 22-year followup study of 3,000 middle-aged men by researchers at the University of California, Berkeley, both smoking and high blood pressure proved to be much greater threats than Type-A behavior with respect to heart attack risk. Of all the personality traits linked with Type-A behavior, the one that has emerged as most sinister is chronic hostility or cynicism. People who are always mistrustful, angry, and suspicious are twice as likely to suffer blockages of their coronary arteries.

"If you're racing around because you're a go-getter—you're enthusiastic, you're positive—the evidence is that it doesn't hurt you," says behavioral medicine specialist Redford Williams, M.D., of Duke

■ Figure 2-2 The effects of stress on the body.

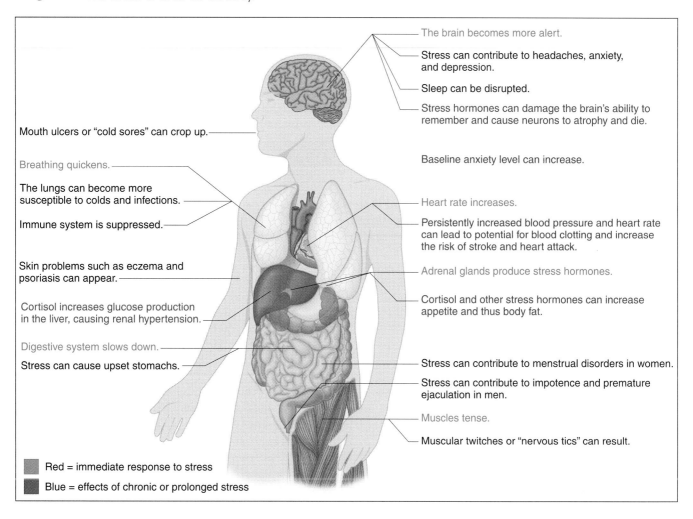

The brain becomes more alert.

Stress can contribute to headaches, anxiety, and depression.

Sleep can be disrupted.

Stress hormones can damage the brain's ability to remember and cause neurons to atrophy and die.

Baseline anxiety level can increase.

Mouth ulcers or "cold sores" can crop up.

Breathing quickens.

The lungs can become more susceptible to colds and infections.

Immune system is suppressed.

Skin problems such as eczema and psoriasis can appear.

Cortisol increases glucose production in the liver, causing renal hypertension.

Digestive system slows down.

Stress can cause upset stomachs.

Heart rate increases.

Persistently increased blood pressure and heart rate can lead to potential for blood clotting and increase the risk of stroke and heart attack.

Adrenal glands produce stress hormones.

Cortisol and other stress hormones can increase appetite and thus body fat.

Stress can contribute to menstrual disorders in women.

Stress can contribute to impotence and premature ejaculation in men.

Muscles tense.

Muscular twitches or "nervous tics" can result.

Red = immediate response to stress

Blue = effects of chronic or prolonged stress

University. On the other hand, hostile Type A's react to anger with an excessive surge of adrenaline. In Williams' studies, they also were more overweight, consumed more alcohol, smoked more cigarettes, and drank more caffeine. "Our findings suggest that hostile Type A's autonomic nervous system is balanced differently," he says.[8]

 ## Can Stress Affect the Immune System?

The powerful chemicals triggered by stress dampen or suppress the immune system—the network of organs, tissues, and white blood cells that defend against disease. Impaired immunity makes the body more susceptible to many diseases, including infections (from the common cold to tuberculosis) and disorders of the immune system itself.

As psychoneuroimmunology research has shown, traumatic stress, such as losing a loved one through death or divorce, can impair immunity for as long as a year. Even minor hassles take a toll. Under exam stress, students experience a dip in immune function and a higher rate of infections. Ohio State University researchers found a significant drop in the immune cells that normally ward off infection and cancer in medical students during exam periods.[9]

Scientists have identified what may be an important biological link between stress and the common cold: interleukin-6, a chemical pathway used by the immune system. In a 1999 study, researchers at the Children's Hospital of Pittsburgh measured the levels of 55 volunteers before infecting them with an influenza virus. While all developed flu symptoms, the concentration of IL-6, as measured from nasal secretions, was higher in those reporting greater psychological stress before being infected.[10]

Certain uplifts, including humor and altruism, may buffer the harmful effects of stress. In studies of college students, watching videotapes of comedians bolstered immune function. Altruism may be good for the body as well as the soul. Students who provided services to others or who watched a tape of Mother Teresa caring for the poor showed a temporary boost in immunity.[11]

Writing about stressful events also can improve the health of people suffering from immune disorders such as chronic asthma or rheumatoid arthritis. In one rigorously conducted study, volunteers who wrote about "the most stressful event they had ever undergone" for 20 minutes on three consecutive days showed significant improvements compared with those who spent the same amount of time writing about neutral topics. It is not known why writing about traumatic experiences can relieve immune system disorders, but the researchers theorize that it may help patients make sense of what had happened to them and come to terms with its impact.[12]

Stress and the Digestive System

Do you ever get butterflies in your stomach before giving a speech in class or before a big game? The digestive system is, as one psychologist quips, "an important stop on the tension trail." To avoid problems, pay attention to how you eat: Eating on the run, gulping food, or overeating result in poorly chewed foods, an overworked stomach, and increased abdominal pressure. The combination of poor eating habits and stress can add up to real pain in the stomach.

However, stress isn't the culprit in one common digestive problem: ulcers. As noted in Chapter 14, researchers have pinpointed a bacterium, *H. pylori,* as the cause of most peptic ulcers. Treatment with appropriate antibiotics can relieve the painful symptoms.

Good nutrition can help soothe a stressed-out stomach. Complex carbohydrates are an ideal antistress food because they boost the brain's level of the mood-enhancing chemical serotonin, says Judith Wurtman, Ph.D., a research scientist at the Massachusetts Institute of Technology. Good sources include broccoli, leafy greens, potatoes, corn, cabbage, spinach, whole-grain breads and pastas, muffins, crackers, and cereals.[13] Leafy vegetables, whole grains, nuts and seeds also are rich in other important nutrients, including magnesium and vitamin C.

Some simple strategies can help you avoid stress-related stomachaches. Many people experience dry mouth or sweat more under stress. By drinking plenty of water, you replenish lost fluids and prevent dehydration. Fiber-rich foods counteract common stress-related problems, such as cramps and constipation. It's also important not to skip meals. If you do, you're more likely to feel fatigued and irritable.

Be wary of overeating under stress. Some people eat more simply because they scarf down meals too quickly. Others reach for snacks to calm their nerves or comfort themselves. Watch out for caffeine. Coffee, tea, and cola drinks can make your strained nerves jangle even more. Also avoid sugary snacks. They'll send your blood sugar levels on a roller coaster ride—up one minute, down the next.

Other Stress Symptoms

Stress can affect any organ system in the body, causing painful symptoms or a flare-up of chronic conditions such as asthma. By interfering with our alertness and ability to concentrate, stress also increases the risk of accidents at home, at work, and on the road.

Headaches are one of the most common stress-related conditions. The most common type, tension headache, is caused by involuntary contractions of the scalp, head, and neck muscles. **Migraine headache** is the result of constriction (narrowing), then dilation (widening) of blood vessels within the brain; chemicals leak through the vessel walls, inflame nearby tissues, and send pain signals to the brain. Surveys of college women show that Type-A behavior can trigger both types of headache.

Stress also can be a culprit. The best strategy is preventive: doing a "relaxercise" a day, such as progressive relaxation or biofeedback, described in this chapter. Breathing and relaxation techniques, usually coupled with medication, also can relieve headaches after they strike.[14]

Stress also is closely linked to skin conditions. If you break out the week before an exam, you know first-hand that skin can be extremely sensitive to stress. Among the other skin conditions worsened by stress are acne, psoriasis, herpes, hives, and eczema. With acne, increased touching of the face, perhaps while cramming for a test, may be partly responsible. Other factors, such as temperature, humidity, and cosmetics and toiletries, may also play a role.

Stress and the Student

You've probably heard that these are the best years of your life, but being a student—full-time or part-time, in your late teens, early twenties, or later in life—can be extremely stressful. You may feel pressure to perform well to qualify for a good job or graduate school. To meet steep tuition payments, you may have to juggle part-time work and coursework. You may feel stressed about choosing a major, getting along with a difficult roommate, passing a particularly hard course, or living up to your parents' and teachers' expectations. If you're an older student, you may have children, housework, and homework to balance. Your days may seem so busy and your life so full that you worry about coming apart at the seams. One thing is for certain: You're not alone. (See Campus Focus: "Stress and the Class of 2002.")

Stress levels among college students rose steadily throughout the 1990s, especially among women. (See the X & Y Files: "Which Sex Is More Stressed?") In a poll of more than 300 campus counseling centers, their directors reported that increasing numbers of students were seeking help because they felt anxious, depressed, and unsure about their academic and personal lives. About 82 percent of the counselors reported an increase in hospitalizations for psychological problems, and 87

percent noted an increased severity in the students' problems.[15]

According to surveys of students at colleges and universities around the country and the world, stress levels are consistently high and stressors are remarkably similar.[16] Among the most common are:

- Test pressures.
- Financial problems.
- Frustrations, such as delays in reaching goals.
- Problems in friendships and dating relationships.
- Daily hassles.
- Academic failure.
- Pressures as a result of competition, deadlines, and the like.
- Changes, which may be unpleasant, disruptive, or too frequent.
- Losses, whether caused by the breakup of a relationship or the death of a loved one.

The X&Y Files — Which Sex Is More Stressed?

Women, who make up 56 percent of today's college students, also shoulder the majority of the stress load. In a nationwide survey of students in the class of 2002, freshmen women were five times as likely to be anxious as men. More than a third—38 percent, compared with just 19 percent of men—described themselves as "overwhelmed by all I have to do." More women than men reported feeling depressed, insecure about their physical and mental health, and worried about paying for college. More men—58.2 percent, compared with 47.5 percent of women—considered themselves above average or in the top 10 percent of people their age in terms of emotional health.

Gender differences in lifestyle may help explain why women feel so stressed. College men, the survey revealed, spend significantly more time doing things that are fun and relaxing: exercising, partying, watching TV, and playing video games. Women, on the other hand, tend to study more, do more volunteer work, and handle more household and child-care chores.

The stress gender gap, which appeared in the mid-1980s, is "one of the ironies of the women's movement," says Alexander Astin of UCLA, founder of the annual American Freshman Survey, which has tracked shifting student attitudes for 35 years. "It's an inevitable consequence of women adding more commitments and responsibilities on top of all the other things they have to cope with." He believes that college women are experi-

encing an early version of the stress that "supermoms" feel later in life when they pursue a career, care for children, and maintain a household.

Where can stressed-out college women turn for support? The best source, according to recent University of California research, is other women. In general, the social support women offer their friends and relatives seems more effective in reducing the blood pressure response to stress than that provided by men.

In a study of 109 undergraduates, men and women were asked to make a short, impromptu speech on the subject of euthanasia while wearing a blood pressure cuff. They spoke to a man or a woman who had been trained to register either positive feedback by nodding and smiling or to provide no response except for boredom. In both male and female speakers, blood pressure rose the least when a female audience member acted supportive. Blood pressure rose the most when a female listener was nonsupportive. In contrast, a supportive male listener did not have a better effect on the rise in blood pressure caused by the stress of speech-making than a nonsupportive male audience. "The smiles and nods of a woman mean something different than the smiles and nods of a man," concluded psychologist Laura Glynn, of the University of California at Irvine.

Sources: Weiss, Kenneth. "Women Feeling More Stress in College," *Los Angeles Times,* January 25, 1999. Glynn, Laura, et al. "Women's Social Support More Beneficial than Men's." *Psychosomatic Medicine*, Vol. 61, April 1999.

Campus Focus

Stress and the Class of 2002

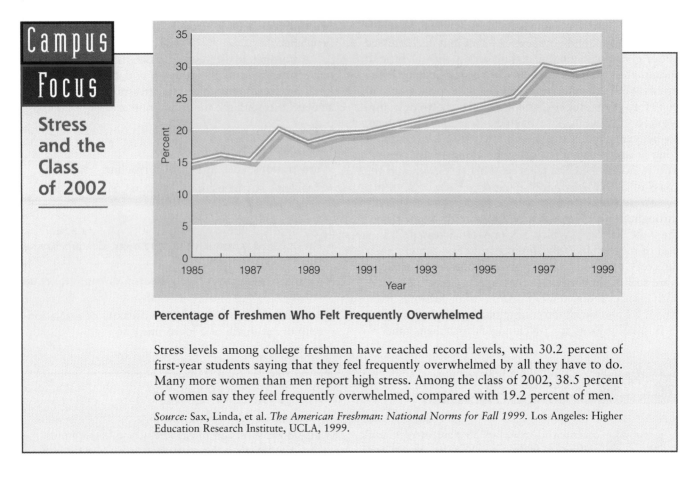

Percentage of Freshmen Who Felt Frequently Overwhelmed

Stress levels among college freshmen have reached record levels, with 30.2 percent of first-year students saying that they feel frequently overwhelmed by all they have to do. Many more women than men report high stress. Among the class of 2002, 38.5 percent of women say they feel frequently overwhelmed, compared with 19.2 percent of men.

Source: Sax, Linda, et al. *The American Freshman: National Norms for Fall 1999.* Los Angeles: Higher Education Research Institute, UCLA, 1999.

Many students bring complex psychological problems with them to campus, including learning disabilities and mood disorders like depression and anxiety. "Students arrive with the underpinnings of problems that are brought out by the stress of campus life," says

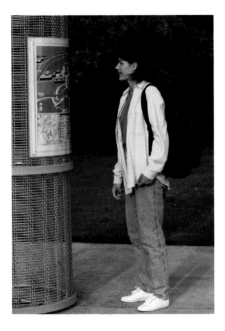

Campus life can be rather overwhelming at first, especially as a freshman with everything to learn.

one counselor. Some have grown up in broken homes and bear the scars of family troubles. Others fall into the same patterns of alcohol abuse that they observed for years in their families or suffer lingering emotional scars from childhood physical or sexual abuse.

For many students, the first year at college is the most stressful. Many have to deal with issues like sexism, racism, and financial difficulties for the first time in their lives. They may experience social discrimination in cafeterias and dorms or feel they are treated differently by professors because of their gender. Older students may feel out of place taking the same classes as 18-year-olds and fret about going into debt to pay for tuition after years of earning their own money. Students of all ages also feel intense pressure to succeed and may worry about not being able to manage their time, get good grades, or decide on a major and a career.

While the self-esteem of college freshmen typically falls, students recover their self-confidence in their second year. They become more positive, introspective, and independent and have a stronger sense of their own intellectual ability. It may well be that as students acclimate to college, they experience less stress and therefore view themselves more positively.

In some studies, certain groups of students, such as women and Asian Americans, report higher levels of

Self-*Survey* | Student Stress Scale

The Student Stress Scale, an adaptation of Holmes and Rahe's Life Events Scale for college-age adults, provides a rough indication of stress levels and possible health consequences.

In the Student Stress Scale, each event, such as beginning or ending school, is given a score that represents the amount of readjustment one has to make as a result of the change. In some studies, using similar scales, people with serious illnesses have been found to have high scores.

To determine your stress score, add up the number of points corresponding to the events you have experienced in the past 12 months.

1. Death of a close family member	100
2. Death of a close friend	73
3. Divorce of parents	65
4. Jail term	63
5. Major personal injury or illness	63
6. Marriage	58
7. Getting fired from a job	50
8. Failing an important course	47
9. Change in the health of a family member	45
10. Pregnancy	45
11. Sex problems	44
12. Serious argument with a close friend	40
13. Change in financial status	39
14. Change of academic major	39
15. Trouble with parents	39
16. New girlfriend or boyfriend	37
17. Increase in workload at school	37
18. Outstanding personal achievement	36
19. First quarter/semester in college	36
20. Change in living conditions	31
21. Serious argument with an instructor	30
22. Getting lower grades than expected	29
23. Change in sleeping habits	29
24. Change in social activities	29
25. Change in eating habits	28
26. Chronic car trouble	26
27. Change in number of family get togethers	26
28. Too many missed classes	25
29. Changing colleges	24
30. Dropping more than one class	23
31. Minor traffic violations	20
Total Stress Score _____	

Here's how to interpret your score: If your score is 300 or higher, you're at high risk for developing a health problem. If your score is between 150 and 300, you have a 50-50 chance of experiencing a serious health change within two years. If your score is below 150, you have a 1-in-3 chance of a serious health change.

Making Changes

Coping with Life Changes

If you're going through a lot of change, you can take steps to minimize harmful effects. Here are some suggestions:

- Review the Student Stress Scale often so you're familiar with different life events and the amount of stress they can cause.
- When change occurs, think about its meaning and your feelings about it.
- Try to come up with different ways of adjusting to the change.
- Don't rush into action; take time to make a careful decision.
- Pace yourself. Even if you have a lot to do, stick to a reasonable schedule that allows you some time off to relax.
- Look at each change as a part of life's natural flow, rather than as a disruption in the way things should be.

Source: Mullen, Kathleen, and Gerald Costello. *Health Awareness Through Discovery.*

stress and more intense reactions to stressors.[17] Students say they react to stress in various ways: physiologically (by sweating, stuttering, trembling, or developing physical symptoms); emotionally (by becoming anxious, fearful, angry, guilty, or depressed); behaviorally (by crying, eating, smoking, being irritable or abusive); or cognitively (by thinking about and analyzing stressful situations and strategies that might be useful in dealing with them). Social support makes a big

difference.[18] Students with a truly supportive network of friends and family available to them report greater satisfaction and less psychological distress.

Campuses are providing more "frontline services" than they have in the past, including career-guidance workshops, telephone hot lines, and special social programs for lonely, homesick freshmen. At a growing number of schools, peer mentors provide companionship and psychological support. These programs may be particularly beneficial for minorities and women, who most often feel excluded in the academic world.[19]

Strategies *for* Prevention

Reaching Out for Support

✔ If you move away from home to go to college, stay in touch with at least one friend. It's worth the effort to keep people you cherish in your life.

✔ Try different forms of "networking"—email, online, chat rooms, campus clubs, support groups.

✔ Check in with siblings. The bossy big sister and devilish little brother have done the same thing you did: They've grown up. Get to know each other as adults who share memories of the past as well as plans for the future.

✔ Make time for friends. Even half an hour for a quiet lunch or a cup of coffee with a friend can keep a relationship close.

✔ Be the kind of friend you'd like to have. If you listen when your friends need to talk, if you're considerate and caring, they will be, too.

Test Stress

For many students, midterms and final exams are the most stressful times of the year. Studies at various colleges and universities found that the incidence of colds and flu soared during finals. The reason seems to be that stress depresses the levels of the protective immune cells that ward off viruses. Students who don't come down with infections during exams often feel the impact of test stress in other ways. Many suffer headaches, upset stomachs, skin flare-ups, or insomnia.[20]

Test stress affects different people in different ways. Sometimes students become so preoccupied with the possibility of failing that they can't concentrate on studying. Others, including many of the best and brightest students, freeze up during tests and can't comprehend multiple-choice questions or write essay answers, even if they know the material.

The students most susceptible to exam stress are those who believe they'll do poorly and who see tests as extremely threatening. Unfortunately, such negative thoughts often become a self-fulfilling prophecy. As they study, these students keep wondering, "What good will studying do? I never do well on tests." As their fear increases, they try harder, pulling all-nighters. Fueled by caffeine, munching on sugary snacks, they become edgy and find it harder and harder to concentrate. By the time of the test, they're nervous wrecks, scarcely able to sit still and focus on the exam.

Can you do anything to reduce test stress and feel more in control? Absolutely. One way is to defuse stress through relaxation. In a study by researchers Janice Kiecolt-Glaser and Ron Glaser of Ohio State University, one group of students was taught relaxation techniques—such as controlled breathing, meditation, progressive relaxation, and guided imagery (visualization)—a month before finals. The more the students used these "stress busters," the higher were their levels of immune cells during the exam period. The extra payoff was that they felt calmer and in better control during their tests.[21] (See Pulsepoints: "Top Ten Stress Busters.")

Strategies *for* Prevention

Defusing Test Stress

✔ *Plan ahead.* A month before finals, map out a study schedule for each course. Set aside a small amount of time every day or every other day to review the course materials.

✔ *Be positive.* Instead of dwelling on any past failures, focus on how well you will do when you are well prepared and confident. Picture yourself taking your final exam. Imagine yourself walking into the exam room feeling confident, opening up the test booklet, and seeing questions for which you know the answers.

✔ *Take regular breaks.* Get up from your desk, breathe deeply, stretch, and visualize a pleasant scene. You'll feel more refreshed than you would if you chugged another cup of coffee.

✔ *Practice.* Some teachers are willing to give practice finals to prepare students for test situations, or you and your friends can make up tests for each other.

✔ *Talk to other students.* Chances are that many of them share your fears about test taking and may have discovered some helpful techniques of their own. Sometimes talking to your adviser or a counselor can also help.

✔ *Be satisfied with doing your best.* You can't expect to ace every test; all you can and should expect is your best effort. Once you've completed the exam, allow yourself the sweet pleasure of relief that it's over.

Minorities and Stress

Regardless of your race or ethnic background, college may bring culture shock. You may never have encountered such a degree of diversity in one setting. You probably will meet students with different values, unfamiliar

PULSE *points*

Top Ten Stress Busters

1. **Strive for balance.** Review your commitments and plans, and if necessary, scale down.
2. **Get the facts.** When faced with a change or challenge, seek accurate information, which can bring vague fears down to earth.
3. **Talk with someone you trust.** A friend or a health professional can offer valuable perspective as well as psychological support.
4. **Sweat away stress.** Even when your schedule gets jammed, carve out 20 or 30 minutes several times a week to walk, swim, bicycle, jog, or work out at the gym.
5. **Express yourself in writing.** Keeping a journal is one of the best ways to put your problems into perspective.
6. **Take care of yourself.** Get enough sleep. Eat a balanced diet. Limit your use of sugar, salt, and caffeine, which can compound stress by leading to fatigue and irritability. Watch your alcohol intake. Drinking can cut down on your ability to cope.
7. **Set priorities.** Making a list of things you need to do and ranking their importance helps direct your energies so you're more efficient and less stressed.
8. **Help others.** One of the most effective ways of dealing with stress is to find people in a worse situation and do something positive for them.
9. **Cultivate hobbies.** Pursuing a personal pleasure can distract you from the stressors in your life and help you relax.
10. **Master a form of relaxation.** Whether you choose meditation, yoga, mindfulness, or another technique, practice it regularly.

---

customs, entirely new ways of looking at the world—experiences you may find both stimulating and stressful.

If you're a minority student, you may feel a double burden. In addition to academic demands, financial worries, and the usual campus stressors, many students from racial and cultural minority groups report extra stressors that can be, as one researcher put it, "both the cause and the effect of academic difficulty."[22] Various reports have shown that African-American and non-Asian minority students at predominantly white colleges have lower grade point averages, experience higher attrition rates, and are less likely to graduate within five years or to enter graduate programs than are white students or minority students at institutions that are not predominantly white. They also experience college as more stressful and report greater feelings of not belonging.[23]

All minority students share some common stressors. In one study of minority freshmen entering a large, competitive university, Asian, Latino, Filipino, African-American, and Native-American students all felt more sensitive and vulnerable to the college social climate, to interpersonal tensions between themselves and nonminority students and faculty, to experiences of actual or perceived racism, and to racist attitudes and discrimination (discussed later in this chapter, under Societal Stressors). Despite scoring above the national average on the SAT, the minority students in this study did not feel accepted as legitimate students and sensed that others viewed them as unworthy beneficiaries of affirmative action initiatives. While most said that overt racism was rare and relatively easy to deal with, they reported subtle pressures that undermined their academic confidence and their ability to bond with the university. Balancing these stressors, however, was a strong sense of ethnic identity, which helped buffer some stressful effects.[24]

The roots of stress are complex and different for members of various minority groups. For instance,

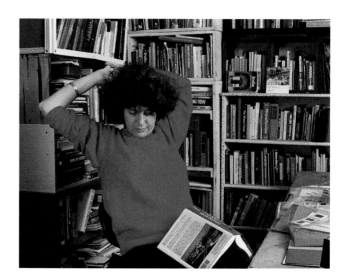

A stretch break and a few deep breaths will help make your studying more effective and will help keep your stress level down.

some African-American students tend to view white campuses as hostile, alienating, and socially isolating and to report greater estrangement from the campus community and heightened discomfort in interactions with faculty and peers.[25] Although their rates of depression are similar to those of Caucasian students, they often report higher levels of anxiety.[26] Latino students have identified three major types of stressors in their college experiences: academic (related to exam preparation and faculty interaction), social (related to ethnicity and interpersonal competence), and financial (related to their economic situation).[27]

Diversity exists within as well as among particular cultural groups, and this, too, can create stress. With more than 30 different cultures represented in the Asian-American community, for instance, there are divisions along class, ethnic, and generational lines. Some Asian students who recently immigrated to the United States report feeling ostracized by students of similar ancestry who are second- or third-generation Americans. While they take pride in being truly bicultural and bilingual, the newcomers feel ambivalent about mainstream American culture. "My parents stress the importance of traditions; my friends tell me to get with it and act like an American," says one Asian-born student who has spent five years in the United States. "I feel trapped between cultures."

Preparing for the Future

In addition to their here-and-now concerns, college students face another source of stress: concern about establishing careers after graduation. For today's students, the outlook continues to be bright. By 2005, according to the Bureau of Labor Statistics, employment will grow by 26 million jobs.[28]

More so than ever, preparation means education—and it does pay off. In the course of their careers, college graduates earn 77% more than those without degrees, reports economist John Sargent of the Bureau of Labor Statistics, who notes that "the occupations that require the most education—and, coincidentally, have the highest earnings—will be growing the fastest in the next ten years." At least a third of the fastest-growing fields, including health care and computer sciences, generally require a bachelor's degree.

Other Personal Stressors

At every stage of life, you will encounter challenges and stressors. Among the most common are those related to anger, conflict, work, and overwork.

 ## How Should I Deal with Anger?

Scientists who have studied anger observe that the two kinds of situations most likely to give rise to anger are those involving coercion and grievance. We become angry when we want someone to do what we want—whether it's to drive faster, clean up the bathroom, or pay back a loan. We also get angry when we feel mistreated, dissed, or dismissed. It's easy to blame anger on the people or situations that "caused" it. However, what we do with our anger is always our personal responsibility.[29]

Popular psychology has portrayed anger as the emotional equivalent of the steam in a pressure cooker: If it's not released, it keeps building until it explodes. "This notion has been used to justify catharsis or venting as a good way to deal with anger," says psychology professor Brad Bushman of Iowa State University. "But catharsis is worse than useless. It actually makes people more, not less aggressive."[30]

In his experiments, volunteers who'd been provoked into anger either did nothing to release their rage or pounded at a punching bag. The steamed-up sluggers became twice as aggressive. "Punching a bag or pillow to reduce anger is like using gasoline to put out a fire—it feeds the flames," says Bushman. "Letting anger out teaches people to behave aggressively. They learn to respond to frustrating situations, not by dealing with the underlying cause, but by hitting, kicking, screaming and swearing."

The consequences can be dangerous. In other research, college-age women with "Jerry-Springer-type anger" who tended to slam doors, curse, and throw things had higher cholesterol levels than those who managed to have an air-clearing discussion or to keep a lid. But locking up anger also can be hazardous to health. In a ten-year study of 200 women, University of Pittsburgh researchers analyzed personality tests of women in their forties and compared them to the thickness of their neck (carotid) arteries after menopause. (Thicker arteries increase the risk of heart attacks and strokes). Hostile women who bottled up their anger had higher heart rates, increased blood pressure, and thicker carotid arteries—and were more likely to have a heart attack by age 60.[31]

Taming a Hot Temper

"Fortunately, there are more than two solutions to the problem of anger buildup," says Bushman. "The best option is to find a way to lower the flame and reduce the heat."

- **Realize that no one else can make you mad.** A lot of angry people blame anyone and everything for their anger: the car that won't start, the kid who talks back, the driver who cuts them off. These negative thoughts are what keep your anger going. Once you come to understand that your anger is generated by how you interpret an event, you take responsibility for controlling it.

- **Use an anger mantra.** "If you get too angry too often, you have to train yourself to change the way you respond, and you do that by talking to yourself," says psychotherapist Doris Helmering, author of *Sensability: Expanding Your Sense of Awareness for a Twenty-First Century Life.* "I have my patients repeat a mantra—for instance, 'I choose not to be angry; I choose to remain in control'—3,000 times a day. That takes about an hour and 20 minutes, so I have them do it while they wash up in the morning, work out, ride to and from work. If they're skeptical, I have them try it for at least one day. They're amazed because as long as they keep at it, they don't blow up." (Eventually they can cut back to a few dozen times a day.)[32]

- **Keep an anger calendar.** Whenever you allow yourself to pout or fly into a rage, mark it with an X. "This increases your awareness and makes you account-

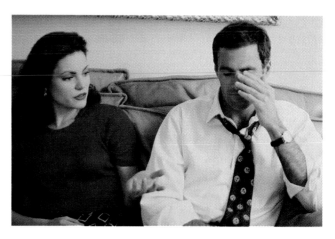

How we manage our anger has consequences on our health.

able," Helmering explains. "You can also see how many days you've made yourself and someone else miserable because of your anger."

- **Recognize your hot buttons.** Keep track of what makes you angry—ideally in writing so you can read and analyze your words and think ahead to ways you might defuse these situations.

- **If you're a hot-head, don't use words like *angry* or *furious.*** Instead, say, "I'm mildly annoyed." "No matter how loud you try to yell, 'I'm mildly annoyed,' this phrase is not going to rev up your anger," says Helmering. "But it will help you turn on your brain."

- **Avoid name-calling.** Any time you label another person—whether it's with a term as simple as "jerk" or a far more profane epithet—you put him in the category of your enemy. This makes it harder to feel any empathy, which is the best emotional antidote to anger.

- **Deal with the real issue.** "The point is not to keep saying, 'I'm so angry,' and remain actionless," says Virginia Williams, coauthor of *Life Skills.* "You want to evaluate what made you angry and move on." Even a simple assertive request or action can make a difference. (Chapter 3 discusses ways of becoming assertive.) [33]

Conflict Resolution

Disagreements are inevitable; disagreeable ways of dealing with them are not. One of the most important skills in any setting—from dormitory floor to staff meeting to corporate boardroom—is resolving conflicts. The key is to focus on the problem, not the individual. Try to put aside unconscious biases, such as assuming a person is difficult to deal with, or preconceived notions about what others really want. Rather than planning what you might say, focus your attention on what others are saying.

Among the steps that professionals recommend are the following:

Listen: In order to work through a conflict, you need to understand the other person's point of view. This demands careful listening in a quiet, private setting, away from activity and background noise. If conflict erupts in a public place, move the discussion elsewhere.

Assimilate. Rather than taking a position and focusing only on defending it, try not to shut yourself off to other possibilities. Keep open the possibility that no one party is completely right or completely wrong. In order to get a fresh perspective, consider the situation from the "third person." If you were seeing the conflict from the outside, what would you think about the information? Once you've taken in all available information, ask yourself: What do I know now about the overall situation? Has my opinion changed?

Respond. Especially if another person is responding in anger, give a calm, well-reasoned response. It will help defuse a highly emotional situation. Try to find a common goal that will benefit you both. Restate the other person's position when both of you are finished speaking so you both know you've been heard and understood.[34]

Job Stress

More so than ever, many people find that they are working more and enjoying it less. Many people, including working parents, spend 55 to 60 hours a week on the job.[35] According to sociologist John Robinson, director of the Americans' Use of Time Project at the University of Maryland, men and women between the ages 30 and 50—the peak time for parenting—have less free time than do younger or older individuals.[36] More people are caught up in an exhausting cycle of overwork, which causes stress, which makes work harder, which leads to more stress.[37]

Yet work in itself is not hazardous to health. Attitudes about work and habits related to how we work are the true threats. In fact, a job—stressful or not, enjoyable or not—can be therapeutic for survivors of heart attacks. According to a recent study sponsored by the National Institute of Mental Health, 90 percent of heart attack patients who returned to work showed decreased emotional distress—compared to increased distress among those who chose not to return to their jobs. "Even in patients who previously disliked their jobs, we found that resumption of employment substantially enhanced their psychological well-being," explains researcher Kathryn Rost of the University of Arkansas.[38]

Workaholism and Burnout

People who become obsessed by their work and careers can turn into *workaholics,* so caught up in racing toward the top that they forget what they're racing toward and why. In some cases they throw themselves into their work to mask or avoid painful feelings or difficulties in their own lives. One consequence is **burnout,** a state of physical, emotional, and mental exhaustion brought on by constant or repeated emotional pressure. Particularly in the helping professions, such as social work or nursing, men and women who've dedicated themselves to others may realize they have nothing left in themselves to give.

The early signs of burnout include exhaustion, sleep problems or nightmares, increased anxiety or nervousness, muscular tension (headaches, backaches, and the like), increased use of alcohol or medication, digestive problems, such as nausea, vomiting, or diarrhea, loss of interest in sex, frequent body aches or pain, quarrels with family or friends, negative feelings about everything, problems concentrating, job mistakes and accidents, and feelings of depression, hopelessness, and helplessness. The best way to avoid burnout is learning to cope well with smaller, day-to-day stresses. Then, tiny frustrations won't smolder into a blaze that may be impossible to put out.

Illness and Disability

Just as the mind can have profound effects on the body, the body can have an enormous impact on our emotions. Whenever we come down with the flu or pull a muscle, we feel under par. When the problem is more serious or persistent—a chronic disease like diabetes, for instance, or a lifelong hearing impairment—the emotional stress of constantly coping with it is even greater.

A common source of stress for college students is a learning disability, which may affect one of every ten Americans. Most learning-disabled have average or above-average intelligence, but they rarely live up to their ability in school. Some have only one area of difficulty, such as reading or math. Others have problems with attention, writing, communicating, reasoning, coordination, social competence, and emotional maturity—all of which may make it difficult, if not impossible, for them to find and keep jobs. Special training and a better understanding of what's wrong can make an enormous difference.

Learning disorders can be hard to recognize in adults, who often become adept at covering up or compensating for their difficulties. However, someone with a learning disability may be

- Unable to engage in a focused activity such as reading.
- Extremely distractible, forgetful, or absent-minded.
- Easily frustrated by waiting, delays, or traffic.
- Disorganized, unable to manage time efficiently and complete tasks on time.
- Hot-tempered, explosive, constantly irritated.
- Impulsive, making decisions with little reflection or information.
- Easily overwhelmed by ordinary hassles.
- Clumsy, with a poor body image and poor sense of direction.
- Emotionally immature.
- Physically restless.

Individuals with several of these characteristics should undergo diagnostic tests to evaluate their skills and abilities and to determine whether remedial training, available through state offices of vocational rehabilitation, can help.

Societal Stressors

Not all stressors are personal. Centuries ago the poet John Donne observed that no man is an island. Today, on an increasingly crowded and troubled planet, these words seem truer than ever. Problems such as discrimination and violence can no longer be viewed only as economic or political issues. Directly or indirectly, they affect the well-being of all who inhabit the earth—now and in the future. Even more mundane stressors, such as traffic, can lead to outbursts of anger that have come to be known as "road rage." (This common stress-related response is discussed in Chapter 18.)

Discrimination

Discrimination can take many forms—some as subtle as not being included in a conversation or joke, some as blatant as threats scrawled on a wall, some as violent as brutal beatings and other hate crimes. Because it can be hard to deal with individually, discrimination is a par-

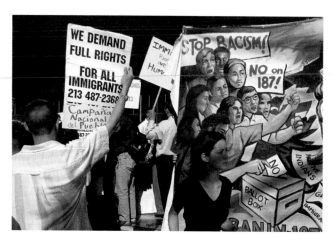

Community action can challenge the hateful assumptions that lead to discrimination, a stressor in its blatant and its subtle forms.

ticularly sinister form of stress. By banding together, however, those who experience discrimination can take action to protect themselves, challenge the ignorance and hateful assumptions that fuel bigotry, and promote a healthier environment for all.

In the last decade, there have been reports of increased intolerance among young people and greater tolerance of expressions and acts of hate on college campuses. To counteract this trend, many schools have set up programs and classes to educate students about each other's different backgrounds and to acknowledge and celebrate the richness diversity brings to campus life. Educators have called on universities to make campuses less alienating and more culturally and emotionally accessible, with programs and policies targeted not only at minority students but also at the university as a whole.

Violence

The deliberate use of physical force to abuse or injure is a leading killer of young people in the United States—and a potential source of stress in all our lives. Chances are that you or someone you know has been the victim of a violent crime, and awareness of our own vulnerability adds to the stress of daily living. The school shootings of the 1990s, particularly the massacre in Littleton, Colorado, increased the stress levels and sense of vulnerability of students of all ages across the country. The increased crime rate in inner-city communities results in stress, which leads to various health and mental problems among minority Americans. (Chapter 18 discusses violence, abuse, and other threats to personal safety.)

Strategies *for* Change

Controlling Your Own Risk for Violent Behavior

✓ When you feel angry, take a few slow, deep breaths and concentrate on your breathing.

✓ Imagine yourself at the beach, a lake, anywhere peaceful.

✓ Keep telling yourself: Calm down. I don't need to prove anything. I'm not going to let this get to me.

✓ Try to find positive or neutral explanations for what the person did to provoke you.

✓ Stop and consider the consequences. Make your goal to defeat the problem, not the other person.[39]

Coping with Stress

Although stress is a very real threat to emotional and physical well-being, its impact depends not just on what happens to you, but on how you handle it. If you tried to predict who would become ill based simply on life-change units or other stressors, you'd be correct only about 15 percent of the time.

The key to coping with stress is realizing that your *perception* and *response* to a stressor are crucial. Changing the way you interpret events or situations—a skill called *reframing*—makes all the difference. An event, such as a move to a new city, is not stressful in itself. A move becomes stressful if you see it as a traumatic upheaval rather than an exciting beginning of a new chapter in your life.

To get a sense of your own stress level, ask yourself the following questions about the preceding week of your life:

• How often have you felt out of control?

• How often have you felt confident that you'd be able to handle personal problems?

• How often have you felt things were generally going your way?

• How often have you felt that things were piling up so high you'd never be able to catch up?

Think through your answers. If the experiences of being out of control or overwhelmed outnumbered those of confidence and control, it's time to develop a stress-management plan and put it into action.

In order to achieve greater control over the stress in your life, start with some self-analysis: If you're feeling overwhelmed, ask yourself: Are you taking an extra course that's draining your last ounce of energy? Are you staying up late studying every night and missing morning classes? Are you living on black coffee and jelly doughnuts? While you may think that you don't have time to reduce the stress in your life, some simple changes can often ease the pressure you're under and help you achieve your long-term goals.

Relieving Short-Term Stress

Acute stress strikes every day: You forget your wallet. You show up late for work—again. You blow a big test. The computer crashes just as you're about to print out a term paper. Frustrated and anxious, you'd love to start the day all over again. Unfortunately, no one can undo the past. However, you can control how you react in the present. Simple exercises, like the following examples, can stop the stress buildup inside your body and help you regain a sense of calm and control. (See also Figure 2-3.)

Breathing. Deep breathing relaxes the body and quiets the mind. Draw air deeply into your lungs, allowing your chest to fill with air and your belly to rise and fall. You will feel the muscle tension and stress begin to melt away. When you're feeling extremely stressed, try this calming breath: Sit or lie with your back straight and place the tip of your tongue on the roof of your mouth behind your teeth. Exhale com-

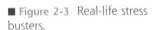

■ Figure 2-3 Real-life stress busters.

Source: Survey conducted by the University of Medicine and Dentistry of New Jersey in Newark and the Eagleton Institute in New Brunswick, N.J. Reported in *American Health,* November–December 1998.

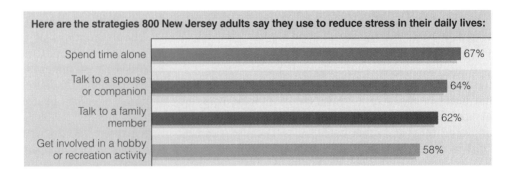

Here are the strategies 800 New Jersey adults say they use to reduce stress in their daily lives:

Spend time alone	67%
Talk to a spouse or companion	64%
Talk to a family member	62%
Get involved in a hobby or recreation activity	58%

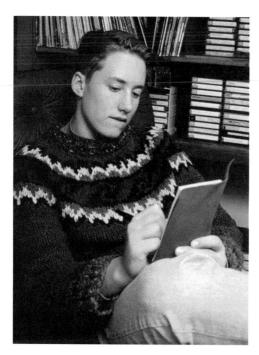

Writing in your journal about feelings and difficulties is a simple and very effective way to keep stress from building up.

pletely through the mouth, then inhale through the nose for 4 seconds. Hold the breath for 7 seconds, then exhale audibly through the mouth for 8 seconds. Repeat four times. [40]

Refocusing. Thinking about a situation you can't change or control only increases the stress you feel. Force your mind to focus on other subjects. If you're stuck in a long line, distract yourself. Check out what other people are buying or imagine what they do for a living. In the car, turn on the radio to a music station you like. Imagine that you're in a hot shower and a wave of relaxation is washing your stress down the drain.

Serenity breaks. Build moments of tranquility into your day. For instance, while waiting for your computer to warm up or a file to download, look at a photograph of someone you love or a poster of a tropical island. If none is available, close your eyes and visualize a soothing scene, such as walking in a meadow or along a beach.[41]

Stress signals. Learn to recognize the first signs that your stress load is getting out of hand: Is your back bothering you? Do you have a headache? Do you find yourself speeding or misplacing things? Whenever you spot these early warnings, force yourself to stop and say, "I'm under stress. I need to do something about it."

Reality checks. To put things into proper perspective, ask yourself: Will I remember what's made me so upset a month from now? If you had to rank this problem on a scale of 1 to 10, with worldwide catastrophe as 10, where would it rate?

Consumer Health Watch

Can Stress-Relief Products Help?

You're stressed out, and you see an ad for a product—an oil, candle, cream, satchet, herbal tea, pill, or potion—that promises to make all your cares disappear. Should you soak in an aromatic bath, have a massage, try kava-kava, squeeze foam balls? In most cases, you're probably not doing yourself much harm, but you aren't necessarily doing yourself much good either. Here are some considerations to keep in mind:

- Be wary of instant cures. Regardless of the promises on the label, it's unrealistic to expect any magic ingredient or product to make all your problems disappear.
- Focus on stress-reducing behavior, rather than a product. An aromatic candle may not bring instant serenity, but if you light a candle and meditate, you may indeed feel more at peace with yourself. Similarly, a scented pillow may not be a cure for a stress, but if it helps you get a good night's sleep, you'll cope better the following day.

- Experiment with physical ways to work out stress. Exercise is one of the best ways to lower your stress levels. Try walking, running, swimming, cycling, kick-boxing—anything physical that helps you release tension.
- Don't make matters worse by smoking (the chemicals in cigarettes increase heart rate, blood pressure, and stress hormone), consuming too much caffeine (it speeds up your system for hours), eating snacks high in sugar (it produces a quick high followed by a sudden slump), or turning to drugs or alcohol (they can only add to the stress you feel when their effects wear off.)
- Remember that stress is a matter of attitude. Remind yourself of some basic words of wisdom: Don't sweat the small stuff—and it's all small stuff.

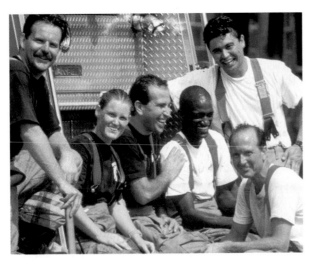

Humor is a positive coping mechanism, especially for individuals in high-stress professions.

Stress inoculation. Rehearse everyday situations that you find stressful, such as speaking in class. Think of how you might make the situation less tense, for instance, by breathing deeply before you talk or jotting down notes beforehand. Think of these small "doses" of stress as the psychological equivalent of allergy shots: They immunize you so you feel less stressed when bigger challenges come along.[42]

Rx: Laughter. Humor counters stress by focusing on comic aspects of difficult situations and may, as various studies have shown, lessen harmful effects on the immune system and overall health. However, humor may have different effects on stress in men and women. In a study of 131 undergraduates, humor buffered stress-related physical symptoms in men and women. However, it reduced stress-linked anxiety only in men. The researchers theorized that men may prefer humor as a more appropriate way of expressing emotions such as anxiety, whereas women are more likely to use self-disclosure, that is, to confide in friends.[43]

Rewriting stress scripts. Learning to identify the negative thoughts and behavior patterns that contribute to anxiety—a technique psychologists call cognitive restructuring—is another key component of stress management, says Alice Domar, author of *Healing Mind, Healthy Woman: Using the Mind-Body Connection to Manage Stress and Take Control of Your Life.* "We all have negative tapes playing in our heads," she explains. "By reprogramming them, we can improve our self-esteem and our capacity to cope with life and reduce our overall stress."[44]

Spiritual coping. Saying a prayer under stress is one of the oldest and most effective ways of calming yourself. Other forms of religious coping, such as putting trust in God and doing for others (for instance, by volunteering at a shelter for battered women,) also can provide a different perspective on daily hassles and stresses.

Sublimation. This term refers to the redirection of any drives considered unacceptable into socially acceptable channels. Outdoor activity is one of the best ways to reduce stress through sublimation. For instance, if you're furious with a friend who betrayed your trust or frustrated because your boss rejects all of your proposals, you might go for a long run or hike to sublimate your anger.[45]

Dealing with Long-Term Stress

If you're going through a transition or you're coming to terms with a setback or loss, you need time to regain a sense of perspective. Any major change, positive or negative, triggers a mixed array of feelings, and you have to sort these out by thinking through what happened, why, and where it might lead.

Journaling

One of the simplest, yet most effective, ways to work through stress is by putting your feelings into words that only you will read. The more honest and open you are as you write, the better. According to the research of psychologist James Pennebaker of the University of Texas, Austin, college students who wrote in their journals about traumatic events felt much better afterward than those who wrote about superficial topics. Recording your experiences and feelings on paper or audiotape may help decrease stress and enhance well-being.[46]

As noted earlier in this chapter, recent research has shown that writing about stressful events can actually ease the symptoms of chronic illnesses like asthma and arthritis. As psychiatrist David Spiegel, M.D., of Stanford University notes, stress affects both mind and body, and illness may trigger associations to past stressful events that were beyond individual control. Writing about traumatic experience may alter the way people think about the event, giving it order and structure and enhancing their own feelings of control.[47]

A "stress journal" can serve a similar purpose. Focus on intense emotional experiences and "autopsy" them to try to understand why they affected you the way they did. Rereading and thinking about your notes may reveal the underlying reasons for your response.

What Can Help Me Relax?

Relaxation is the physical and mental state opposite that of stress. Rather than gearing up for fight or flight, our bodies and minds grow calmer and work more smoothly. We're less likely to become frazzled and more capable of staying in control. The most effective relaxation techniques include progressive relaxation, visualization, meditation, mindfulness, and biofeedback.

Progressive relaxation works by intentionally increasing and then decreasing tension in the muscles. While sitting or lying down in a quiet, comfortable setting, you tense and release various muscles, beginning with those of the hand, for instance, and then proceeding to the arms, shoulders, neck, face, scalp, chest, stomach, buttocks, genitals, and so on, down each leg to the toes. Relaxing the muscles can quiet the mind and restore internal balance.

Visualization, or **guided imagery,** involves creating mental pictures that calm you down and focus your mind. As we note in Chapter 11, some people use this technique to promote healing when they are ill. The Glaser study showed that elderly residents of retirement homes in Ohio who learned progressive relaxation and guided imagery enhanced their immune function and reported better health than did the other residents. Visualization skills require practice and, in some cases, instruction by qualified health professionals.

Meditation has been practiced in many forms over the ages, from the yogic techniques of the Far East to the Quaker silence of more modern times. Meditation helps a person reach a state of relaxation, but with the goal of achieving inner peace and harmony. There is no one right way to meditate, and many people have discovered how to meditate on their own, without even knowing what it is they are doing. Among college students, meditation has proven especially effective in increasing relaxation. Most forms of meditation have common elements: sitting quietly for 15 to 20 minutes once or twice a day, concentrating on a word or image, and breathing slowly and rhythmically. If you wish to try meditation, it often helps to have someone guide you through your first sessions. Or try tape recording your own voice (with or without favorite music in the background) and playing it back to yourself, freeing yourself to concentrate on the goal of turning the attention within.

Mindfulness is a modern-day form of an ancient Asian technique that involves maintaining awareness in the present moment. You tune in to each part of your body, scanning from head to toe, noting the slightest sensation. You allow whatever you experience—an itch, an ache, a feeling of warmth—to enter your awareness.

Then you open yourself to focus on all the thoughts, sensations, sounds, and feelings that enter your awareness. Mindfulness keeps you in the here-and-now, thinking about what is rather than about "what if" or "if only."

Biofeedback, discussed in Chapter 11, is a method of obtaining feedback, or information, about some physiological activity occurring in the body. An electronic monitoring device attached to a person's body detects a change in an internal function and communicates it back to the person through a tone, light, or meter. By paying attention to this feedback, most people can gain some control over functions previously thought to be beyond conscious control, such as body temperature, heart rate, muscle tension, and brain waves. Biofeedback training consists of three stages:

1. Developing increased awareness of a body state or function.
2. Gaining control over it.
3. Transferring this control to everyday living without use of the electronic instrument.

The goal of biofeedback for stress reduction is a state of tranquility, usually associated with the brain's production of alpha waves (which are slower and more regular than normal waking waves). After several training sessions, most people can produce alpha waves more or less at will.

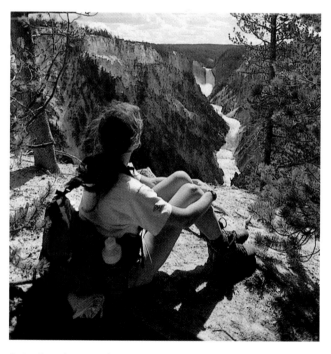

Spending time outdoors is a great way to leave behind daily tensions.

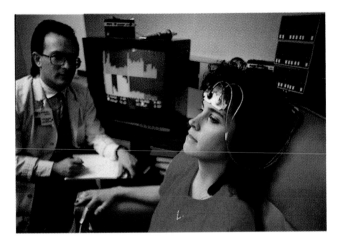

Biofeedback training uses electronic monitoring devices to teach conscious control over heart rate, body temperature, and muscle tension. Once the technique is learned, the electronic feedback is unnecessary.

Escape from the Time Trap

We live in what some sociologists call "hyperculture," a society that moves at warp speed. Information bombards us constantly. The rate of change seems to accelerate every year. The "time-saving" devices that were supposed to make life easier—pagers, cell phones, modems, faxes, palm-sized organizers, laptop computers—have simply extended the boundaries of where and how we work.[48]

As a result, more and more people are suffering from "timesickness," a nerve-racking feeling that life has become little more than an endless to-do list. [49] The best antidote is time management, and hundreds of books, seminars, and experts offer training in making the most of the hours in the day. Yet these well-intentioned methods often fail, and sooner or later most of us find ourselves caught in a time trap.

Poor Time Management

Every day you make dozens of decisions, and the choices you make about how to use your time directly affect your stress level. If you have a big test on Monday and a term paper due Tuesday, you may plan to study all weekend. Then, when you're invited to a party Saturday night, you go. Although you set the alarm for 7:00 A.M. on Sunday, you don't pull yourself out of bed until noon. By the time you start studying, it's 4:00 P.M., and anxiety is building inside you.

How can you tell if you've lost control of your time? The following are telltale symptoms of poor time management:

• Rushing.

• Chronic inability to make choices or decisions.

• Fatigue or listlessness.

• Constantly missed deadlines.

• Not enough time for rest or personal relationships.

• A sense of being overwhelmed by demands and details and having to do what you don't want to do most of the time.

One of the hard lessons of being on your own is that your choices and your actions have consequences. Stress is just one of them. But by thinking ahead, being realistic about your workload, and sticking to your plans, you can gain better control over your time and your stress levels.

 ## How Can I Better Manage My Time?

Time management involves skills that anyone can learn, but they require commitment and practice to make a difference in your life. It may help to know the techniques that other students have found most useful:

• **Schedule your time.** Use a calendar or planner. Beginning the first week of class, mark down deadlines for each assignment, paper, project, and test scheduled that semester. Develop a daily schedule, listing very specifically what you will do the next day, along with the times. Block out times for working out, eating dinner, calling home, and talking with friends as well as for studying.

• **Develop a game plan.** Allow at least two nights to study for any major exam. Set aside more time for researching and writing papers. Make sure to allow time to type and print out a paper—and to deal with emergencies like a computer breakdown. Set daily and weekly goals for every class. When working on a big project, be sure you don't neglect your other courses. Whenever possible, try to work ahead in all your classes.

• **Identify time robbers.** "If you know why or how you waste time, you can start to do something about it," says educator Beblon Parks of the Virginia Education Association. "For several days keep a log of what you do and how much time you spend doing it." You may discover that disorganization is eating away at your time or that you have a problem getting started.

(See the following section on Overcoming Procrastination.)[50]

- **Make the most of classes.** Read the assignments before class rather than waiting until just before you have a test. By reading ahead of time, you'll make it easier to understand the lectures. Go to class yourself. Your own notes will be more helpful than a friend's or those from a note-taking service. Read your lecture notes at the end of each day or at least at the end of each week.

- **Develop an efficient study style.** Some experts recommend studying for 50 minutes, then breaking for 10 minutes. Small incentives, such as allowing yourself to call or visit a friend during these 10 minutes, can provide the motivation to keep you at the books longer. When you're reading, don't just highlight passages. Instead, write notes or questions to yourself in the margins. This will help you retain more information. Even if you're racing to start a paper, take a few extra minutes to prepare a workable outline. It will be easier to structure your paper when you start writing.

- **Focus on the task at hand.** Rather than worrying about how you did on yesterday's test or how you'll ever finish next week's project, focus intently on whatever you're doing at any given moment. If your mind starts to wander, use any distraction—the sound of the phone ringing or a noise from the hall—as a reminder to stay in the moment.

- **Turn elephants into hors d'oeuvres.** "Instead of trying to eat an elephant, start by nibbling on the ears or munching on the tail," says Parks. "Cut a huge task into smaller chunks so it seems less insurmountable." For instance, break down your term paper into a series of steps, such as selecting a topic, identifying sources of research information, taking notes, developing an outline, and so on.

- **Keep your workspace in order.** Even if the rest of your room is a shambles, try to keep your desk clear. Piles of papers are distracting, and you can end up wasting lots of time looking for notes you misplaced or an article you have to read by morning. Try to spend the last ten minutes of the day getting your desk in order so you get a fresh start on the new day.

Overcoming Procrastination

Putting off until tomorrow what should be done today is a habit that creates a great deal of stress for many students. It also takes a surprising toll. In stud-

ies with students taking a health psychology course, researchers found that although procrastinating provided short-term benefits, including periods of low stress, the tendency to dawdle had long-term costs, including poorer health and lower grades. Early in the semester, the procrastinators reported less stress and fewer health problems than students who scored low on procrastination. However, by the end of the semester, procrastinators reported more health-related symptoms, more stress, and more visits to health-care professionals than nonprocrastinators. They also received significantly lower grades on term papers and exams.[51] The three most common types of procrastination are: putting off unpleasant things, putting off difficult tasks, and putting off tough decisions. Procrastinators are most likely to delay by wishing they didn't have to do what they must or by telling themselves they "just can't get started," which means they never do.

To get out of a time trap, keep track of the tasks you're most likely to put off, and try to figure out why you don't want to tackle them. Think of alternative ways to get tasks done. If you put off library readings, for instance, figure out if the problem is getting to the library or the reading itself. If it's the trip to the library, arrange to walk over with a friend whose company you enjoy.

Develop daily time-management techniques, such as a "To Do" list. Rank items according to priorities: A, B, C, and schedule your days to make sure the A's get accomplished. Try not to fixate on half-completed projects. Divide large tasks, such as a term paper, into smaller ones, and reward yourself when you complete a part.

Do what you like least first. Once you have it out of the way, you can concentrate on the tasks you do enjoy. You also should build time into your schedule for interruptions, unforeseen problems, unexpected events, and so on, so you aren't constantly racing around. Establish ground rules for meeting your own needs (including getting enough sleep and making time for friends) before saying yes to any activity. Learn to live according to a three-word motto: Just do it!

Effects of Stress on the Mind

The lifetime prevalence of major stressful events is high. In one study of 1,000 adults in four cities in the southeastern United States, 21 percent of the sample reported a traumatic event (such as a robbery, assault, or traumatic death of a loved one) during the previous year, and 69 percent reported at least one such event in their lifetime.[52] Such stressors always take a toll on an individual, and it's normal to feel sad, tense, overwhelmed, angry, or incapable of coping with the ordinary demands of daily living. Usually such feelings and behaviors subside with time. The stressful event fades into the past, and those whose lives it has touched adapt to its lasting impact. But sometimes individuals remain extremely distressed and unable to function as they once did. While the majority of individuals who survive a trauma recover, at least a quarter of such individuals later develop serious psychological symptoms.[53]

Adjustment Disorders

The term **adjustment disorder** refers to an out-of-the-ordinary response to a stressful event or situation. Any event or combination of circumstances can lead to an adjustment disorder. The stressor does not have to be extreme; even a seemingly minor event—such as learning that an ex-boyfriend or girlfriend has married—may cause great psychological pain.

Specific developmental events, such as leaving home, getting married, having a child, losing a job, or retirement, can trigger adjustment disorders. Although any one at any age can have difficulty adapting to a life crisis, most people who seek treatment for adjustment disorders are in their twenties.

The symptoms of adjustment disorders vary. After being fired, a store clerk may feel jumpy all the time, unable to sleep, irritable, and angry. A student whose boyfriend suddenly breaks up with her may find it hard to concentrate during lectures. A person identified as HIV-positive may seek out new sex partners and not use safe-sex practices.

The problem for individuals reeling from the impact of a life crisis is trying to figure out which feelings are normal and which are not. The two key signs of an adjustment disorder are distress and impairment: Individuals feel extremely upset or cannot work or relate to others the way they once did, and their symptoms persist for more than three to six months after a stressful event.[54]

There is no specific remedy for an adjustment disorder, although the goal is always the same: improving an individual's ability to adapt. Ordinarily, time helps ease the pain or difficulty of coping with a stressful situation. When the impact of a crisis is more intense, supportive counseling or brief psychotherapy (described in Chapter 4) can help an individual understand the significance of what has happened, put it into perspective, and deal with it in a healthier way.

Strategies *for* Prevention

Recognize the Warning Signals of Stress Overload

✓ Experiencing physical symptoms, including chronic fatigue, headaches, indigestion, diarrhea, and sleep problems.

✓ Having frequent illness or worrying about illness.

✓ Self-medicating, including nonprescription drugs.

✓ Having problems concentrating on studies or work.

✓ Feeling irritable, anxious, or apathetic.

✓ Working or studying longer and harder than usual.

✓ Exaggerating, to yourself and others, the importance of what you do.

✓ Becoming accident-prone.

✓ Breaking rules, whether it's a curfew at home or a speeding limit on the highway.

✓ Going to extremes, such as drinking too much, overspending, or gambling.

Posttraumatic Stress Disorder

In the past, **posttraumatic stress disorder (PTSD)** was viewed as a psychological response to out-of-the-ordinary stressors, such as captivity or combat. However, these are hardly the only experiences that can forever change the way people view themselves and their world. With the recent surge in violent crime and in natural disasters, thousands of individuals have experienced or witnessed traumatic events.[55] Children, in particular, are likely to develop PTSD symptoms when they live through a traumatic event or witness a loved one or friend being assaulted. Sometimes an entire community, such as the residents of a town hit by a devastating flood or hurricane, develops symptoms. According to recent research, almost half of car accident victims may develop PTSD. The main symptoms are re-experiencing the traumatic event, avoiding the site of the accident, refraining from driving in weather and road conditions similar to those on the day of the accident, and feeling a general increase in distress.[56]

A history of childhood sexual abuse can greatly increase the likelihood of developing PTSD.[57] An episode that repeats the abuse, such as a sexual assault or rape, can trigger an intense reaction as individuals "re-experience" the initial trauma of their youth.[58] Adolescents who are dependent on alcohol also are particularly susceptible to PTSD.[59]

In PTSD, individuals re-experience their terror and helplessness again and again in their dreams or intrusive thoughts. To avoid this psychic pain, they may try to avoid anything associated with the trauma. Some enter a state of emotional numbness and no longer can respond to people and experiences the way they once did, especially when it comes to showing tenderness or affection. Those who've been mugged or raped may be afraid to venture out by themselves.

The sooner trauma survivors receive psychological help, the better they are likely to fare. Often talking about what happened with an empathic person or someone who's shared the experience as soon as possible—preferably before going to sleep on the day of the event—can help an individual begin to deal with what has occurred. Group sessions, ideally beginning soon after the trauma, allow individuals to share views and experiences. Behavioral, cognitive, and psychodynamic therapy (described in Chapter 4) can help individuals suffering PTSD.

From Surviving to Thriving: Posttraumatic Growth

Adversity—whether in the form of a traumatic event or chronic stress—has different effects on individuals. Some people never recover and continue on a downward slide that may ultimately prove fatal. Others return, though at different rates, to their prior level of functioning. In recent years researchers have focused their attention on a particularly intriguing group: those people who not only survive stressful experiences but also thrive, that is, who actually surpass their previous level of functioning.[60]

Thriving—or, as some prefer, "posttraumatic growth"—can take many forms. A father whose child is

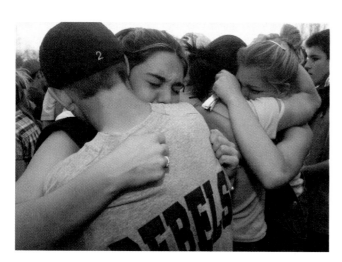

Posttraumatic stress disorder symptoms occur when we live through traumatic events. Survivors and family members can experience mild to extreme symptoms following such traumas.

kidnapped and killed may become a nationwide advocate for victims' rights. A student whose roommate dies in a car crash after a party may campaign for tougher laws against drunk driving. A couple whose premature baby spends weeks in a neonatal intensive care unit may find that their marriage has grown closer and stronger. Even though their experiences were painful, the individuals often look back at them as bringing positive changes into their lives.

Researchers have studied various factors that enable individuals to thrive in the face of adversity. These include:

- **An optimistic attitude.** Rather than reacting to a stressor simply as a threat, these men and women view stress as a challenge—one they believe they can and will overcome. Researchers have documented that individuals facing various stressors, including serious illness and bereavement, are more likely to report experiencing growth if they have high levels of hope and optimism.[61]

- **Self-efficacy.** As noted in Chapter 1, a sense of being in control of one's life can boost health, even in times of great stress.

- **Stress inoculation.** People who deal well with adversity often have had previous experiences with stress that "toughened" them in various ways, such as teaching them skills that enhanced their ability to cope and boosting their confidence in their ability to weather a rough patch.

- **Secure personal relationships.** Individuals who know they can count on the support of their loved ones are more likely to thrive.

- **Spirituality or religiousness.** Religious coping may be particularly related to growth and thriving. In particular, two types seem most beneficial: spiritually based religious coping (receiving emotional reassurance and guidance from God) and good-deeds coping (living a better, more religious life that includes altruistic acts).

Posttraumatic growth can take many forms. Some people develop new skills simply because, in order to get through the stressful experience, they had to learn something they hadn't known how to do before—dealing with health professionals, for instance, or wrangling with insurance companies or other bureaucracies. By mastering such skills, they become more fit to deal with an unpredictable world and develop new flexibility in facing the unknown.

Along with new abilities comes the psychological sense of mastery. "I survived this," an individual may say. "I'll be able to deal with other hard things in the future." Such confidence keeps people actively engaged in the effort to cope and is itself a predictor of eventual success. Stress also can make individuals more aware of the fulfilling aspects of life, and they may become more interested in spiritual pursuits. Certain kinds of stressful experiences also have social consequences. If a person experiencing a traumatic event finds that the significant others in his or her life can be counted on, the result can be a strengthening of their relationship.

Researchers are trying to determine ways in which more people can derive positive benefits from stressful experiences. One important step, they believe, is to encourage people to view a traumatic situation as an opportunity for personal growth, rather than a test of whether or not they "have what it takes" to survive. Focusing on finding meaning in their experience—what some call "cognitive coping"—can help individuals move beyond initial emotional responses such as anxiety, distress, and confusion.[62] Over time, some people may develop what may be the ultimate "gift" of a stressful experience: wisdom.[63]

Making This Chapter Work for You

Meeting the Challenge of Stress

- Stress is the physiological and psychological response to any demand placed on us, or our bodies, whether positive or negative.

- Eustress, or positive stress, challenges us to grow, adapt, and find creative solutions in our lives. Distress refers to the negative effects of stress that can deplete or even destroy life energy.

- Theories of stress include Hans Selye's general adaptation syndrome, which consists of three distinct stages: alarm, resistance, and exhaustion. The genetic-constitutional perspective looks at the role of predisposing factors, which can influence resistance and make us more or less susceptible to stress. The cognitive-transactional model of stress, developed by Richard Lazarus, looks at the interrelation between stress and health.

- Stress can contribute to heart disease, high blood pressure, immune disorders, digestive problems, and other ailments.

- Common student stressors on campus include test pressures, financial problems, personal frustrations, problems in friendships and dating relationships, daily hassles, academic failure, competitive pressure, unpleasant or disruptive changes, and personal losses. Adjusting to college life is stressful in itself.

- Minority students encounter additional stressors, including a hostile or unfriendly social climate, inter-

personal tensions between themselves and nonminority students and faculty, experiences of actual or perceived racism, and more subtle racist attitudes and discrimination.

- Jobs are a major source of stress for Americans. Two problems related to job stress are workaholism, characterized by excessive devotion to work, and burnout, a state of physical, emotional, and mental exhaustion brought on by constant or repeated emotional pressure.

- Chronic illness and disability, including learning disabilities, can be major sources of stress in an individual's life.

- Social stressors—such as discrimination and violence—also are a threat to physical and psychological well-being.

- Stress-management techniques, which include better time management, overcoming procrastination, and increased appreciation of leisure time, can help reduce distress and enhance feelings of control over daily stress.

- Techniques such as progressive relaxation, visualization, meditation, mindfulness, and biofeedback can help soothe both body and mind and reduce the harmful effects of stress.

- Stress can affect psychological well-being and cause adjustment disorders and posttraumatic stress disorder. Prompt recognition and treatment can help overcome these problems.

- Stressful experiences, though painful, can contribute to personal growth and greater resilience.

College is a perfect time to learn and practice the art of stress reduction. You can start applying the techniques and concepts outlined in this chapter immediately. You may want to begin by doing some relaxation or awareness exercises. They can give you the peace of mind you need to focus more effectively on larger issues, goals, and decisions.

You needn't see stress as a problem to solve on your own. Reach out to others. As you build friendships and intimate relationships, you may find that some irritating problems are easier to put into perspective. Don't be afraid to laugh at yourself and to look for the comic or absurd aspects of a situation. In addition, you might try some simple approaches that can help boost your stress resistance and resilience, including the following:

- *Focusing.* Take a strain inventory of your body every day to determine where things aren't feeling quite right. Ask yourself, "What's keeping me from feeling terrific today?" Focusing on problem spots, such as stomach knots or neck tightness, increases your sense of control over stress.

- *Reconstructing stressful situations.* Think about a recent episode of distress; then write down three ways it could have gone better and three ways it could have gone worse. This should help you see that the situation wasn't as disastrous as it might have been, and help you find ways to cope better in the future.

- *Self-improvement.* When your life feels out of control, turn to a new challenge. You might try volunteering at a nursing home, going for a long-distance bike trip, or learning a foreign language. As you work toward your new goal, you'll realize that you still can cope and achieve.

- *Exercise.* Regular physical activity can relieve stress, boost energy, lift mood, and keep stress under control.

If stress continues to be a problem in your life, you may be able to find help through support groups or counseling. Your school may provide counseling services or referrals to mental health professionals; ask your health instructor or the campus health department for this information. Remember that each day of distress robs you of energy, distracts you from life's pleasures, and interferes with achieving your full potential.

 Vitamin C and Stress. How can vitamin C help alleviate stress?

health / ONLINE

Stress Assess

http://wellness.uwsp.edu/Health_Service/services/stress.shtml
This online assessment from the University of Wisconsin allows you to evaluate the sources of stress in your life, identify symptoms of stress, and learn behavior modifications that can help you manage stress.

Stress Less

http://nimbus.temple.edu/~mlombard/StressLess/
This web site from Temple University provides tips for combatting student stress (such as test anxiety, financial stress, and college stress) and faculty stress (occupational stress and burnout), as well as general stress-related information.

Stress Busters

http://stressrelease.com/strssbus.html
This site focuses on managing on-the-job stress.

Please note that links are subject to change. If you find a broken link, use a search engine like http://www.yahoo.com *and search for the web site by typing in key words.*

 Campus Chat: On a scale of 1–10 (1=low, 10=high), how would you rate the level of stress in your life? What factors are causing the stress? What are some of the ways you cope with stress? Share your thoughts on our online discussion forum at **http://health.wadsworth.com**

Find It On Infotrac: You can find additional readings related to stress via InfoTrac College Edition, an online library of more than 900 journals and publications. Follow the instructions for accessing InfoTrac that came packaged with your textbook; then search for articles using a key word search.

- **Suggested article:** *7 Surefire Strategies for Stress,* by Clare Horn and Erin O'Donnell. *Natural Health,* April 1999, Vol. 29, Issue 3, p.119.

  (1) List at least five strategies for combatting stress.

  (2) What are some of the physical symptoms and long-term consequences of stress?

For additional links, resources, and suggested readings on InfoTrac, visit our Health & Wellness Resource Center at **http://health.wadsworth.com**

Key Terms

The terms listed here are used within the chapter. Page numbers are included for each term. A definition of each term is given in the Glossary pages at the end of this book.

adaptive response   40
adjustment disorder   60
allostasis   40
biofeedback   57
burnout   52
distress   40
eustress   40

general adaptation syndrome
   (GAS)   40
guided imagery   57
homeostasis   40
meditation   57
migraine headache   44
mindfulness   57

posttraumatic stress disorder
   (PTSD)   60
progressive relaxation   57
psychoneuroimmunology   41
stress   40
stressor   40
visualization   57

Critical Thinking Questions

1. Stress levels among college students have reached record highs. What reasons can you think of to account for this? Consider possible social, cultural, and economic factors that may play a role.

2. Identify three stressful situations in your life and describe how you might attempt to decrease or eliminate the stressors associated with them. Identify three examples of eustress.

3. Can you think of any ways in which your behavior or attitudes might create stress for others? What changes could you make to avoid doing so?

4. What advice might you give an incoming freshman at your school about managing stress in college? What techniques have been most helpful for you in dealing with stress?

References

1. Lazarus, R., and R. Launier, "Stress-Related Transactions Between Person and Environment." in *Perspectives in Interactional Psychology.* New York: Plenum, 1978.

2. Gadzella, Bernadette. "Student-Life Stress Inventory: Identification of and Reactions to Stressors." *Psychological Reports,* Vol. 74, No. 2, April 1994.

3. McEwen, Bruce. "Stress and Brain Development, Part 2." *Journal of the American Academy of Child and Adolescent Psychiatry,* Vol. 38, No. 1, January 1999.

4. Lombroso, Paul, and Robert Sapolsky. "Stress and Brain Development, Part 1." *Journal of the American Academy of Child and Adolescent Psychiatry,* Vol. 37, No. 12, December 1998.

5. Epel, Elissa, Bruce McEwen, and Jeannette R. Ickovics. "Embodying Psychological Thriving: Physical Thriving in Response to Stress." *Journal of Social Issues,* Vol. 54, No. 2, Summer 1998.

6. Mann, Denise. "Take It Easy: Controlling Cortisol Production Is Key to Controlling Stress." *Better Nutrition,* Vol. 61, No. 1, January 1999.

7. Langer, Stephen. "Stressless: Natural Strategies to Help You Cope." *Better Nutrition,* Vol. 60, No. 11, November 1998.

8. Williams, Redford, and Virginia Williams. *Anger Kills.* New York: Times Books, 1993.

9. Glaser, Ronald, and Janice Kiecolt-Glaser. *Handbook of Human Stress and Immunity.* San Diego: Academic Press, 1994.

10. Cohen, Sheldon, et al. "Susceptibility to the Common Cold." *Psychosomatic Medicine,* March 1999.

11. Giles, Dwight, and Janet Eyler. "The Impact of a College Community Service Laboratory on Students' Personal, Social and Cognitive Outcomes." *Journal of Adolescence,* Vol. 17, No. 4, August 1994.

12. Smyth, Joshua, et al. "Effects of Writing About Stressful Experiences on Symptom Reduction in Patients With Asthma or Rheumatoid Arthritis: A Randomized Trial." *Journal of the American Medical Association,* Vol. 281, No. 14, April 14, 1999.

13. McMahon, Ruth. "Relax!" *Vegetarian Times,* No. 255, November 1998.

14. Eller, Daryn. "Workouts That Fight Stress." *American Health,* May 1994.

15. Murray, Bridget. "College Youth Haunted by Increased Pressures." *American Psychological Monitor,* Vol. 29, No. 12, December 1998.

16. Gerdes, Eugenia, and Guo Ping. "Coping Differences Between College Women and Men in China and the United States." *Genetic, Social and General Psychology Monographs,* Vol. 120, No. 2, May 1994. Puccio, Gerard, et al. "Person-Environment Fit: Using Commensurate Scales to Predict Student Stress." *British Journal of Educational Psychology,* Vol. 63, No. 3, November 1993.

17. Demakis, George, and Dan McAdams. "Personality, Social Support, and Well-Being Among First-Year College Students." *College Health Journal,* Vol. 28, No. 2, June 1994.

18. Neville, Helen, et al. "Relations Among Racial Identity Attitudes, Perceived Stressors, and Coping Styles in African

American College Students." *Journal of Counseling and Development*, Vol. 75, No. 4, March–April 1997.

19. Murray, Bridget, "Peer Mentoring Gives Rookies 'Inside Advice.' " *American Psychological Monitor*, Vol. 29, No. 12, December 1998.

20. "College-Age Freedom Can Trigger Illness." *USA Today Magazine*, Vol. 125, No. 2610, December 1996.

21. Glaser and Kiecolt-Glaser, *Handbook of Human Stress and Immunity*. Hornig-Rohan, Mary. "Stress, Immune-Mediators, and Immune-Mediated Disease." *Advances: The Journal of Mind-Body Health*, Vol. 11, No. 2, Spring 1995.

22. Saldana, Delia. "Acculturative Stress: Minority Status and Distress." *Hispanic Journal of Behavioral Sciences*, Vol. 16, No. 2, May 1994.

23. Ibid.

24. Smedley, Brian, et al. "Minority Status Stresses and the College Adjustment of Ethnic Minority Freshmen." *Journal of Higher Education*, Vol. 64, No. 5, July–August 1993.

25. Ibid.

26. Launier, Raymond. "Stress Balance and Emotional Life Complexes in Students in a Historically African American College." *Journal of Psychology*, Vol. 131, No. 2, March 1997.

27. Solberg, V., et al. "Social Support, Stress and Hispanic College Adjustment: Test of a Diathesis Stress Model." *Hispanic Journal of Behavioral Sciences*, Vol. 16, No. 3, August 1994. Solberg, V., et al. "Development of the College Stress Inventory for Use with Hispanic Populations." *Hispanic Journal of Behavioral Sciences,* Vol. 15, No. 4, November 1993.

28. U.S. Bureau of Labor Statistics, personal inquiry.

29. Rothschild, Bertram. "A Humanistic Understanding of Anger." *Humanist*, Vol. 59, No. 1, January 1999.

30. Bushman, Brad, et al. "Catharsis, Aggression and Persuasive Influence: Self-Fulfilling or Self-Defeating Prophecies." *Journal of Personality and Social Psychology*, Vol. 76, No. 3, January 1999.

31. Matthews, Karen, et al. "Women Who Hold in Anger at Risk for Atherosclerosis." *Psychosomatic Medicine*, September–October 1998.

32. Helmering, Doris, personal interview and *Sense Ability: Expanding Your Sense of Awareness for a Twenty-First Century Life*. New York: Eagle Brook, 1999.

33. Williams, Virginia, and Redford Williams. *Life Skills*. New York: Times Books, 1999.

34. Grensing-Pophal, Lin. "Resolving Conflicts. *Nursing*, Vol. 28, No. 9, September 1998.

35. Sherwood, William. "Cat's in the Cradle," *Across the Board*, Vol. 35, Issue 10, November–December 1998.

36. John Robinson. Personal interview.

37. Kline, Marsha, and David Snow. "Effects of a Worksite Coping Skills Intervention on the Stress, Social Support and Health Outcomes of Working Mother." *Journal of Primary Prevention*, Vol. 15, No. 2, Winter 1994.

38. Rost, Kathryn, and G. Richard Smith. "Work Buffers Emotional Stress of First Heart Attack." *Archives of Internal Medicine*, February 1992.

39. Berman, Alan, et al. *Warning Signs: Are You at Risk of Violent Behavior?* Washington, D.C.: American Psychological Association, 1999.

40. Weil, Andrew. *Eight Weeks to Optimum Health*. New York: Fawcett, 1998.

41. Castleman, Michael. "37 Ways to Peace of Mind." *American Health*, April 1998.

42. Saunders, Teri, et al. "The Effect of Stress Inoculation Training on Anxiety and Performance." *Journal of Occupational Health Psychology*, Vol. 1, No. 2, pp. 170–186.

43. Abel, Millicent. "Interaction of Humor and Gender in Moderating Relationships Between Stress and Outcomes." *Journal of Psychology*, Vol. 132, No. 3, May 1998.

44. Domar, Alice. *Healing Mind, Healthy Woman: Using the Mind-Body Connection to Manage Stress and Take Control of Your Life*. New York: Delta, 1997.

45. Finnicum, Paul, and Jeffrey Zeiger. "Managing Stress Through Outdoor Recreation." *Parks & Recreation*, Vol. 33, No. 83, August 1998.

46. Pennebaker, James. "Putting Stress into Words: Health, Linguistic and Therapeutic Implications." *Behavioral Research*, Vol. 31, No. 6, 1993.

47. Spiegel, David. "Healing Words: Emotional Expression and Disease Outcome." *Journal of the American Medical Association*, Vol. 281, No. 14, April 14, 1999.

48. Bertman, Stephen. "Hyperculture Stress: How Fast Times Are Transforming America." *Vital Speeches*, Vol. 65, No. 7, January 15, 1999.

49. Japenga, Ann. "A Cure for Timesickness." *Health*, Vol. 13, No. 1, January 1999.

50. Parks, Beblon. "7 Time-Management Sanity Savers." *Instructor*, Vol. 107, No. 5, January–February 1998.

51. "Procrastinators Always Finish Last, Even in Health." *American Psychological Monitor*, Vol. 20, No. 1, January 1998.

52. Calhoun, Lawrence, and Richard Tedeschi. "Beyond Recovery from Trauma: Implications for Clinical Practice and Research." *Journal of Social Issues*, Vol. 54, No. 2, Summer 1998.

53. Spiegel, David, and Jose Maldonado. "Dissociative Disorders." *American Psychiatric Press Textbook of Psychiatry*, 3rd ed. Hales, Robert, et al. (editors). Washington, D.C.: American Psychiatric Press, 1999.

54. Hales, Dianne, and Robert E. Hales. *Caring for the Mind: The Comprehensive Guide to Mental Health*. New York: Bantam Books, 1995.

55. Breslau, Naomi, et al. "Risk Factors for PTSD-Related Traumatic Events: A Prospective Analysis." *American Journal of Psychiatry*, Vol. 152, No. 4, April 1995.

56. Blanchard, Edward, and Edward Hickling. *After the Crash: Assessment and Treatment of Motor Vehicle Accident Survivors*. Washington: APA Books, 1997.

57. Rodriguez, Ned, et al. "Posttraumatic Stress Disorder in Adult Female Survivors of Childhood Sexual Abuse: A Comparison Study." *Journal of Consulting and Clinical Psychology*, Vol. 675, No. 1, February 1997.

58. Briggs, Lynne, and Peter Joyce. "What Determines Posttraumatic Stress Disorder Symptomatology for Survivors of Childhood Sexual Abuse?" *Child Abuse and Neglect*, Vol. 21, No. 6, June 1997.

59. Deykin, E. Y., and S. L. Buka. "Prevalence and Risk Factors for Post-Traumatic Stress Disorder Among Chemically Dependent Adolescents." *American Journal of Psychiatry*, June 1997.

60. Carver, Charles. "Resilience and Thriving: Issues, Models, and Linkages." *Journal of Social Issues*, Vol. 54, No. 2, Summer 1998.

61. Park, Crystal. "Stress-Related Growth and Thriving Through Coping: The Roles of Personality and Cognitive Processes." *Journal of Social Issues*, Vol. 54, No. 2, Summer 1998.

62. Saakvitne, Karen, Howard Tennen, and Glenn Affleck. "Exploring Thriving in the Context of Clinical Trauma Theory: Constructivist Self-Development Theory." *Journal of Social Issues*, Vol. 54, No. 2, Summer 1998.

63. Massey, Sean, et al. "Qualitative Approaches to the Study of Thriving: What Can Be Learned?" *Journal of Social Issues*, Vol. 54, No. 2, Summer 1998.

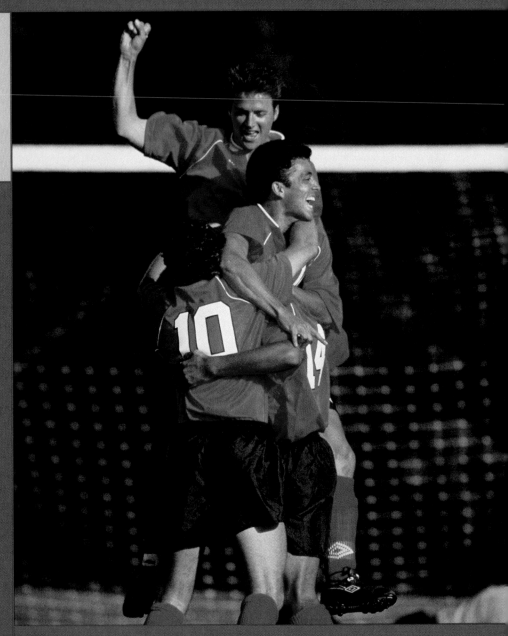

3

Feeling Good

After studying the material in this chapter, you should be able to:

- **Explain** the goal of psychological health and **list** some characteristics of psychologically healthy people.
- **Discuss** the relationship of needs, feelings, values, and goals to psychological health.
- **Define** self-esteem and **list** some strategies for boosting it, as well as some strategies for improving a negative mood.
- **Discuss** the concept of emotional intelligence.
- **List** healthy and unhealthy coping mechanisms, and **explain** ways to create more positive and effective coping mechanisms in your own life.
- **Explain** the value of sleep.

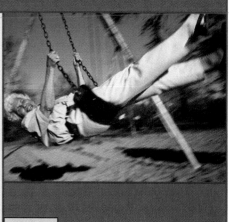

ou wake up, and the world seems new. You feel energetic, alert, eager for whatever the day will hold. You have a smile on your face and a spring in your step. The reason: You are in peak psychological health.

In every culture and country, psychologically healthy men and women generally share certain characteristics: They value themselves and strive toward happiness and fulfillment. They establish and maintain close relationships with others. They accept the limitations as well as the possibilities that life has to offer. And they feel a sense of meaning and purpose that makes the gestures of living worth the effort required.

Feeling good does not depend on money, success, recognition, or status. At any age, at any level of education and achievement, regardless of disability or disease, it is possible to find happiness and fulfillment in life. Achieving the highest possible level of psychological well-being, like achieving peak physical well-being, depends primarily on assuming responsibility for yourself. This chapter will help you accomplish this by offering insight into your needs, values, and feelings—and by providing guidance on how to manage your moods, pursue happiness, find meaning in life, and connect with others. ❖

 FREQUENTLY ASKED QUESTIONS

FAQ: **What is emotional intelligence? p. 69**

FAQ: **What is spiritual intelligence? p. 70**

FAQ: **Are there ways to boost a bad mood? p. 77**

FAQ: **What leads to happiness? p. 78**

FAQ: **How should I deal with difficult people? p. 88**

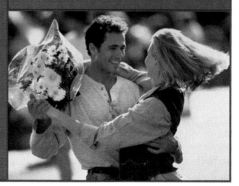

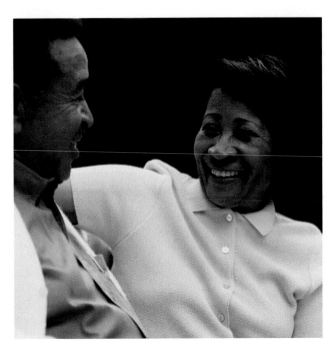

Peak psychological health. Psychologically healthy people value themselves, find meaning and purpose in life, and build close relationships with others.

What Is Psychological Health?

"A sound mind in a sound body is a short but full description of a happy state in this world," the philosopher John Locke wrote in 1693. More than 300 years later his statement still rings true. Both physical and psychological well-being are essential to total wellness. However, modern theorists have gone beyond these general requirements to analyze other components of well-being, including coping styles, goals, and adaptation to stress and change.[1]

Psychological health encompasses both our emotional and mental states—that is, our feelings and our thoughts. **Emotional health** generally refers to feelings and moods, both of which are discussed later in this chapter. Characteristics of emotionally healthy persons that psychologist Deane Shapiro identified in an analysis of major studies of emotional wellness include the following:

- Determination and effort to be healthy.
- Flexibility and adaptability to a variety of circumstances.
- Development of a sense of meaning and affirmation of life.
- An understanding that the self is not the center of the universe.

- Compassion for others.
- The ability to be unselfish in serving or relating to others.
- Increased depth and satisfaction in intimate relationships.
- A sense of control over the mind and body that enables the person to make health-enhancing choices and decisions.[2]

Mental health describes our ability to perceive reality as it is, to respond to its challenges, and to develop rational strategies for living. The mentally healthy person doesn't try to avoid conflicts and distress but can cope with life's transitions, traumas, and losses in a way that allows for emotional stability and growth. The characteristics of mental health include:

- The ability to function and carry out responsibilities.
- The ability to form relationships.
- Realistic perceptions of the motivations of others.
- Rational, logical thought processes.

There is considerable overlap between psychological and **spiritual health,** which (as defined in Chapter 1) involves our ability to identify our basic purpose in life and to experience the fulfillment of achieving our full potential. However, many people consider the two separate. "We like to think that emotional problems have to do with the family, childhood, and trauma—with personal life but not with spirituality," observes Thomas Moore, author of *Care of the Soul,* "Yet it is obvious that the soul, seat of the deepest emotions, can benefit greatly from the gifts of a vivid spiritual life and can suffer when it is deprived of them."[3]

In addition, **culture** helps to define psychological health. While, in one culture, men and women may express feelings with great intensity, shouting in joy or wailing in grief, in another culture such behavior might be considered abnormal or unhealthy. In our diverse society, many cultural influences affect Americans' sense of who they are, where they came from, and what they believe. Cultural rituals help bring people together, strengthen their bonds, reinforce the values and beliefs they share, and provide a sense of belonging, meaning, and purpose.

Strategies *for* Prevention

Tips for Psychological Fitness

✓ Recognize and express your feelings. Pent-up emotions tend to fester inside, building into anger or depression.

- ✓ Don't brood. Rather than merely mulling over a problem, try to find solutions that are positive and useful.
- ✓ Take one step at a time. As long as you're taking some action to solve a problem, you can take pride in your ability to cope.
- ✓ Get involved with others. Reach out and communicate your feelings to someone you trust, either a friend or, if necessary, a professional.

Positive Psychology

Psychology, which traditionally has focused on what goes wrong in our lives and in our minds, has turned in a new direction. Increasingly mental health professionals are concentrating on "positive psychology," an approach that emphasizes building personal strengths rather than simply treating weaknesses. One of its key beliefs is that young people who learn to be resilient and optimistic are less likely to suffer from depression and more likely to lead happier, more productive lives.[4]

The Best We Can Be

The "father" and leading proponent of positive psychology is Martin Seligman of the University of Pennsylvania, who has devoted decades to research on optimism and learned helplessness. He has called on psychologists to refocus on "the best things in life" and on positive human attributes, such as courage, love, forgiveness, and hope.[5] "The good life does not mean a Porsche, champagne, and a suntan," says Seligman, who lists such components as sanity, self-actualization, and wisdom.[6] (See Consumer Health Watch: "Choosing a Counselor.")

As he sees it, psychologists should help individuals move beyond **victimology,** which views people as passive beings who are acted upon by various forces, and which blames others for everything that goes wrong in life. "Psychology is not just the study of weakness and damage," Seligman argues, "it is also the study of strength and virtue. Treatment is not just fixing what is broken, it is nurturing what is best within ourselves."[7] The traits that may well protect us from physical and mental illness include courage, optimism, hope, interpersonal skills, a work ethic, responsibility, future-mindedness, honesty, and perseverance.[8]

What Is Emotional Intelligence?

Once a person's "IQ"—or intelligence quotient—was considered the leading determinant of achievement. However, psychologists have determined that another "way of knowing," dubbed **emotional intelligence,** may make an even greater difference in a person's personal and professional success. In his international best-seller on what some call "EQ" (for emotional quotient), psychologist Daniel Goleman identified five components of emotional intelligence: self-awareness, altruism, personal motivation, empathy, and the ability to love and be loved by friends, partners, and family

Consumer Health Watch

Choosing a Counselor

Working with a trained therapist can be a means toward greater self-understanding and personal growth. However, anyone can claim to be a counselor or psychotherapist, and you should always be sure to check the person's background and credentials. In making your final choice, here are some additional considerations to keep in mind:

- Do you feel you could work well together? Will the therapist treat you as a whole person—and focus on positive growth?
- Do you feel the therapist shows genuine concern, takes you seriously, treats you with respect, and shares or accepts your values?

- Will your therapist be supportive if you want a second opinion about a life issue or emotional problem? Will he or she work with you to evaluate others' recommendations?
- Remember that you are choosing someone in whom you may confide your most intimate secrets and fears. Of course, you want a competent therapist with the right training, knowledge, skills, and experience. But you also must choose someone you can trust.

members. People who possess high emotional intelligence are the people who truly succeed in work as well as play, building flourishing careers and lasting, meaningful relationships.[9]

Emotional intelligence isn't fixed at birth, and increasingly its precepts are being taught as part of the curriculum at primary and secondary schools. Even corporations are hiring consultants to boost employees' EQ, since it's been shown to directly affect teamwork, confidence, and productivity.[10] Emotions can be our allies, explains Dr. Jeanne Segal, helping us form loving and meaningful relationships, while making us well-rounded and profoundly sensitive beings. If repressed, they can be our enemies, oppressing us like well-armored dictators. By listening to our body's messages, we can incorporate both emotional and rational intelligence in our daily lives.[11]

In research from more than 500 companies, psychologist Goleman found that emotional intelligence is twice as important as IQ and job-specific skills in determining the success of business people. Among the emotional competencies that also can benefit students are focusing on clear, manageable goals and getting support from even a single buddy or coach.[12]

What Is Spiritual Intelligence?

Spiritual approaches to knowledge and well-being have recently become the focus of scholarly interest and research. As noted in Chapter 1, a growing number of research studies are assessing the impact of spirituality on health, and nearly 30 medical schools include courses on religion, spirituality, and health in their curricula.[13]

Mental health professionals also are recognizing the power of **spiritual intelligence**, which some define as "the capacity to sense, understand, and tap into the highest parts of ourselves, others, and the world around us." What distinguishes spiritual intelligence from spirituality is that it does not center on the worship of a God above, but on the discovery of a wisdom within. All of us are born with the potential to develop spiritual intelligence, but relatively few do. Yet its dividends are many. As one minister put it, this way of knowing provides solutions—often surprising and unexpected—to problems that had seemed insolvable.[14]

Here are some guidelines for tapping into your own spiritual intelligence:

- Build silence and solitude into your daily life. Even a few stolen moments in the early morning or evening hours can help quiet the hum of constant distractions. "There is an inner wisdom," says cardiologist Dean Ornish, "but it speaks very, very softly." He suggests ending each session with a question like "What am I not paying attention to what's important?"[15]

- Spend time in nature. There is added value in a walk on the beach, a stroll through a park, or simply looking up at the night sky—perhaps because nature helps put our mostly man-made problems into perspective.

- Keep company with the wise—either in person or through their words. Inspirational people or their writings provide both factual knowledge and insight that enables us to examine serious issues.

- Reflect on the nature of life and death. You don't need a doctorate in philosophy for this task, because the basic principles are simple: Life is precious. Life is short. Death is certain. Yet while life involves difficulties, these can be, not avoided, but transcended.

- Practice spiritual values. Spiritual intelligence is not a spectator sport. Rather than just contemplating kindness and honesty, we have to live them as best we can. One of the best places to learn and practice forgiveness is on the highway—as a much-needed antidote to road rage (discussed in Chapter 18).

- Learn to trust your spiritual intelligence. Gaining access to an inner source of wisdom is the first step; just as hard is developing the confidence to act on what we're hearing. Often it comes through "aha!" experiences, times in which we perceive the interconnectedness of seemingly random events, people, and variables in life.

Special holidays, such as Kwanzaa and Chinese New Year, bring people together in cultural celebration.

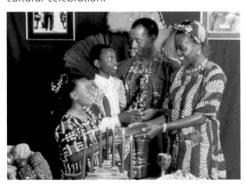

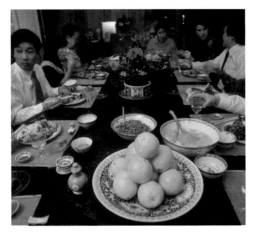

Understanding Yourself

Who are you? Probably the first answer that comes to mind is your name, because that's the way you introduce yourself to others. Of course, you are identified by numbers, too: social security, student I.D., draft regis-tration, driver's license, and credit cards. You also play many roles: To a special few, you're a son, daughter, partner, spouse, parent, or friend. To others, you're a student, voter, taxpayer, worker, colleague, or consumer. You are part of certain cultural and ethnic groups and may practice a certain religion. But when you're all alone, eye-to-eye with yourself in the mirror,

Self-*Survey* Well-Being Scale

Part I

The following questions contain statements and their opposites. Notice that the statements extend from one extreme to the other. Where would you place yourself on this scale? Place a circle on the number that is most true for you at this time. Do not put your circles between numbers.

Life Purpose and Satisfaction

1. During most of the day,
   my energy level is | very low | 1 2 3 4 5 6 7 | very high
2. As a whole, my life seems | dull | 1 2 3 4 5 6 7 | vibrant
3. My daily activities are | not a source of satisfaction | 1 2 3 4 5 6 7 | a source of satisfaction
4. I have come to expect that
   every day will be | exactly the same | 1 2 3 4 5 6 7 | new and different
5. When I think deeply
   about life | I do not feel there is any purpose to it | 1 2 3 4 5 6 7 | I feel there is a purpose to it
6. I feel that my life so far has | not been productive | 1 2 3 4 5 6 7 | been productive
7. I feel that the work* I am doing | is of no value | 1 2 3 4 5 6 7 | is of great value
8. I wish I were different
   from who I am. | agree strongly | 1 2 3 4 5 6 7 | disagree strongly
9. At this time, I have | no clearly defined goals for my life | 1 2 3 4 5 6 7 | clearly defined goals for my life
10. When sad things happen
    to me or other people | I cannot feel positive about life | 1 2 3 4 5 6 7 | I continue to feel positive about life
11. When I think about what I
    have done with my life, I feel | worthless | 1 2 3 4 5 6 7 | worthwhile
12. My present life | does not satisfy me | 1 2 3 4 5 6 7 | satisfies me
13. I feel joy in my heart. | never | 1 2 3 4 5 6 7 | all the time
14. I feel trapped by the
    circumstances of my life. | agree strongly | 1 2 3 4 5 6 7 | disagree strongly
15. When I think about my past | I feel many regrets | 1 2 3 4 5 6 7 | I feel no regrets
16. Deep inside myself | I do *not* feel loved | 1 2 3 4 5 6 7 | I feel loved
17. When I think about the
    problems that I have | I do not feel hopeful about solving them | 1 2 3 4 5 6 7 | I feel very hopeful about solving them

*The definition of work is not limited to income-producing jobs. It includes child care, housework, studies, and volunteer services.

Part II

Self-Confidence During Stress (answer according to how you feel during stressful times)

1. When there is a great deal of
   pressure being placed on me | I get tense | 1 2 3 4 5 6 7 | I remain calm

2. I react to problems and difficulties	with a great deal of frustration	1	2	3	4	5	6	7	with no frustration
3. In a difficult situation, I am confident that I will receive the help that I need.	disagree strongly	1	2	3	4	5	6	7	agree strongly
4. I experience anxiety	all the time	1	2	3	4	5	6	7	never
5. When I have made a mistake	I feel extreme dislike for myself	1	2	3	4	5	6	7	I continue to like myself
6. I find myself worrying that something bad is going to happen to me or those I love.	all the time	1	2	3	4	5	6	7	never
7. In a stressful situation	I cannot concentrate easily	1	2	3	4	5	6	7	I can concentrate easily
8. I am fearful	all the time	1	2	3	4	5	6	7	never
9. When I need to stand up for myself	I cannot do it	1	2	3	4	5	6	7	I can do it easily
10. I feel less than adequate in most situations.	agree strongly	1	2	3	4	5	6	7	disagree strongly
11. During times of stress, I feel isolated and alone.	agree strongly	1	2	3	4	5	6	7	disagree strongly
12. In really difficult situations	I feel *unable* to respond in positive ways	1	2	3	4	5	6	7	I feel able to respond in positive ways
13. When I need to relax	I experience no peace— only thoughts and worries	1	2	3	4	5	6	7	I experience a peacefulness— free of thoughts and worries
14. When I am in a frightening situation	I panic	1	2	3	4	5	6	7	I remain calm
15. I worry about the future.	all the time	1	2	3	4	5	6	7	never

Scoring

The number you circled is your score for that question. Add your scores in each of the two sections and divide each sum by the number of questions in the section.

- Life Purpose and Satisfaction: ___ ÷ 17 = ___.___
- Self-Confidence During Stress: ___ ÷ 15 = ___.___
- Combined Well-Being: (add scores for both) _____ ÷ 32 = ___.___

Each score should range between 1.00 and 7.00 and may include decimals (for example 5.15).

Interpretation:

VERY LOW: 1.00 TO 2.49
MEDIUM LOW: 2.50 TO 3.99
MEDIUM HIGH: 4.00 TO 5.49
VERY HIGH: 5.50 to 7.00

These scores reflect the strength with which you feel these positive emotions. Do they make sense to you? Review each scale and each question in each scale. Your score on each item gives you information about the emotions and areas in your life where your psychological resources are strong, as well as the areas where strength needs to be developed.

If you notice a large difference between the LPS and SCDS scores, use this information to recognize which central attitudes and aspects of your life most need strengthening. If your scores on both scales are very low, talk with a counselor or a friend about how you are feeling about yourself and your life.

Source: Copyright 1989, Dr. Jared Kass. *Inventory of Positive Psychological Attitudes.* See Credits. Reprinted by permission.[64]

who is the person you see? Who is the real you? (See Self-Survey: "Well-Being Scale.")

You may spend a lifetime searching for the answer—the most important journey you'll ever make. If you fail to find your true identity, it doesn't matter much what else you find. You can gain insight into your own personality and behavior by learning about your feelings, needs, and values.

Your Feelings

Feelings are the emotional equivalents of body temperature or blood pressure, vital signs that indicate what's going on inside us. Some feelings serve as signals leading us toward pleasure, goodness, and love and away from harm and hurt. They run the gamut from the joy of finding love, which fills us with warmth and excitement, to the cold, bleak despair of losing a cherished partner or parent.

Feelings can affect us physically as well as psychologically. Negative feelings, such as frustration and anger, can actually undermine our health, whereas love, happiness, and other positive emotions can enhance and protect our well-being. Paying attention to feelings can help us keep in tune with, and respond to, our deepest needs. (See The X & Y Files: "Which Sex Is More Emotional?")

Your Needs

Newborns are unable to survive on their own. They depend on others for the satisfaction of their physical needs for food, shelter, warmth, and protection, as well as their less tangible emotional needs. In growing to maturity, children take on more responsibility and become more independent. No one, however, becomes totally self-sufficient. As adults, we easily recognize our basic physical needs, but we often fail to acknowledge our emotional needs. Yet they, too, must be met if we are to be as fulfilled as possible.

The humanist theorist Abraham Maslow believed that human needs are the motivating factors in personality development. First, we must satisfy basic physiological needs, such as those for food, shelter, and sleep. Only then can we pursue fulfillment of our higher needs—for safety and security, love and affection, and self-esteem. Few individuals reach the state of **self-actualization,** in which one functions at the highest possible level and derives the greatest possible satisfaction from life. (See Figure 3-1.)

Your Values and Morals

Your **values** are the criteria by which you evaluate things, people, events, and yourself; they represent what's most important to you. In a world of almost dizzying complexity, values can provide guidelines for making decisions that are right for you. If understood and applied, they help give life meaning and structure.

Social psychologist Milton Rokeach distinguished between two types of values. *Instrumental* values represent ways of thinking and acting that we hold important,

---

The X&Y **Files** | **Which Sex Is More Emotional?**

Emotions know no gender. Men grieve; women rage; both sexes sigh in despair and crow with delight. Asked to record their feelings in diaries, females and males report the same beliefs about emotion and describe their experiences of emotion similarly.

Men and women may differ more in the intensity of their emotional experiences than they do in the nature of those experiences. When volunteers in a University of Illinois study logged their moods for 42 days, women reported more intense emotions of all sorts—positive and negative, pleasant and unpleasant. Men reported feeling only one emotion, anger, more frequently and fiercely.

Men also may be conditioned to hiding or downplaying emotions, and both sexes may assume that the stereotypes about women being more emotional are true. If you give women and men a questionnaire that asks them to rate themselves on various aspects of empathy, women consider themselves more empathic than men, observes psychologist Jacqueline James of the Murray Research Center at Radcliffe College. If you measure physiological repsonsiveness to another's distress or count instances of actual helping behavior during stressful situations, the sex differences disappear.

In our culture, men have traditionally been taught early on that certain feelings, like vulnerability, are not socially acceptable, observes psychologist Leslie Brody of Boston University, author of *Family, Gender and Emotion.* But as gender roles have shifted, so has emotional expression. Today men are showing a wider range of feelings—in public and private. And men who take on greater nurturing responsibilities, whether as big brothers or fathers, tend to experience and express far more of the tender emotions that men of previous generations were taught to conceal.

Yet even today men and women become emotional for different reasons. In general, relationships with friends and families and occasions such as births, reunions, separations, and deaths elicit the strongest emotional reactions in women. Men's emotions are more likely to be triggered by world events, achievements, and illnesses. Perhaps, Brody theorizes, women's traditional roles as caretakers highlight the emotional importance of family milestones, while men's long-standing roles as providers and protectors underscore the significance of events related to achievement and control.

Source: Hales, Dianne. *Just Like a Woman: How Gender Science Is Revealing What Makes Us Female.* New York: Bantam Books, 2000.

such as being loving or loyal. *Terminal* values represent goals, achievements, or ideal states that we strive toward, such as happiness.[16] Instrumental and terminal values form the basis for your attitudes and your behavior.

There can be a large discrepancy between what people say they value and what their actions indicate about their values. That's why it's important to clarify your own values, making sure you understand what you believe so that you can live in accordance with your beliefs. To do so, follow these steps:

1. Carefully consider the consequences of each choice.

2. Choose freely from among all the options.

3. Publicly affirm your values by sharing them with others.

4. Act out your values.

Values clarification is not a once-in-a-lifetime task, but an ongoing process of sorting out what matters most to you. If you believe in protecting the environment, do you shut off lights, or walk rather than drive, in order to conserve energy? Do you vote for political candidates who support environmental protection? Do you recycle newspapers, bottles, and cans? Values are more than ideals we'd like to attain; they should be reflected in the way we live day by day.

The values of society are in a state of constant change: Because of an increasing focus on individuality, organizations now place more emphasis on creativity, flexibility, and responsiveness. Because of greater value given to enriching life experiences, interest in the arts, travel, and lifelong education is growing. In health behavior, values are shifting from an emphasis on curing illness to greater commitment to promoting wellness—as seen in the decline in smoking.

The values of college students also change over the decades. In the 1960s, many young people sought to dedicate their lives to peace, saving the environment, and challenging traditional ways of doing things. By the 1980s, students tended to focus more on practical considerations and chose majors that would lead to lucrative careers. Today educators report another shift, this time toward greater concern about quality of life, community action, environmental advocacy, and helping people in need. This trend is reflected in the popularity of courses that deal with finding meaning in life.

Like our value system, our **moral** judgments—our sense of right and wrong—change throughout our life.

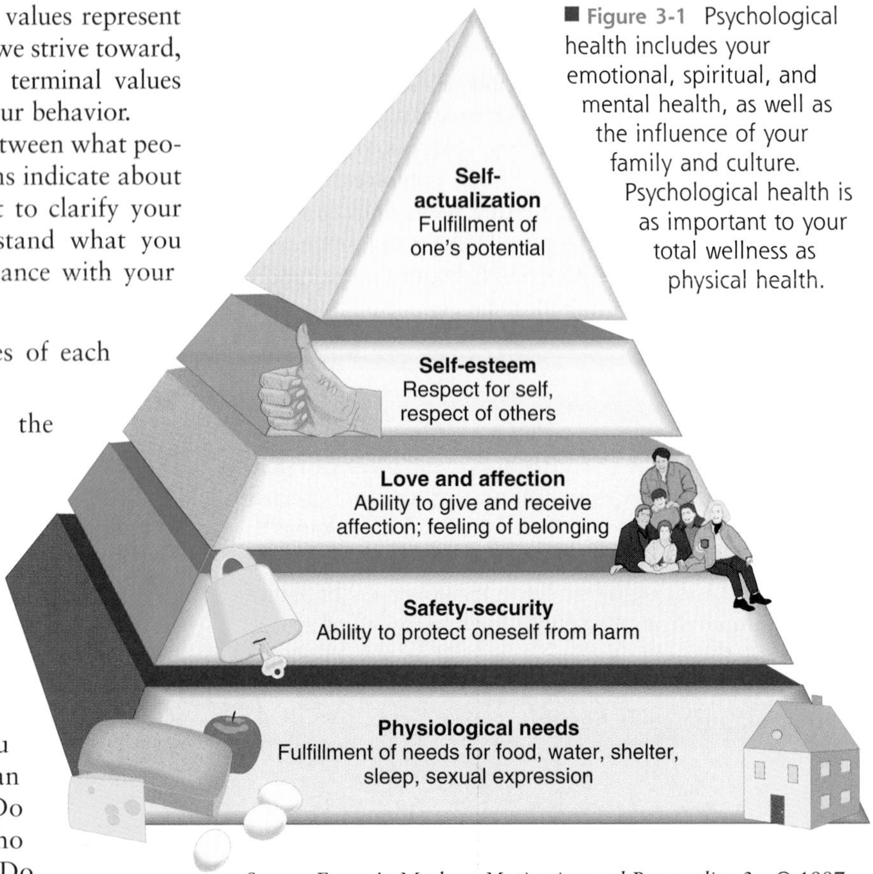

■ Figure 3-1 Psychological health includes your emotional, spiritual, and mental health, as well as the influence of your family and culture. Psychological health is as important to your total wellness as physical health.

Self-actualization
Fulfillment of one's potential

Self-esteem
Respect for self, respect of others

Love and affection
Ability to give and receive affection; feeling of belonging

Safety-security
Ability to protect oneself from harm

Physiological needs
Fulfillment of needs for food, water, shelter, sleep, sexual expression

Source: From A. Maslow, *Motivation and Personality*, 3e, © 1997. Reprinted by permission of Prentice Hall.

Strategies *for* Change

Being True to Yourself

✓ Take the tombstone test: What would you like to have written on your tombstone? In other words, how would you like to be remembered? Your honest answer should tell you, very succinctly, what you value most.

✓ Describe yourself, as you are today, in a brief sentence. Ask friends or family members for their descriptions of you. How would you have to change to become the person you want to be remembered as?

✓ Try the adjective test: Choose three adjectives that you'd like to see associated with your reputation. Then list what you've done or can do to earn such descriptions.

According to Lawrence Kohlberg's theory of moral development, we develop a sense of morality as we grow.[17] As children, we behave in certain ways because we fear punishment or expect something in return. As adolescents, we may base our judgments on peer approval above all else. At the next stage of moral development, we become more concerned about laws and authority figures, so we may work hard to please a boss or not speed to avoid getting a ticket. As our moral development continues, we make decisions based on personal honor and self-respect and on our commitment to principles of respect for others and doing the right thing. At the very highest levels, justice becomes a primary value.

Your Goals

We define ourselves not only by what we are now, but also by what we might become in the future. Career goals, in particular, have a tremendous impact. When you choose a vocation, you make a decision that affects how you spend your days, how you occupy your mind, whom you meet, and how you interact with them. College is an ideal time to think about careers, to imagine yourself in different jobs, and to prepare yourself for the type of work that most appeals to you.

The nature of students' goals often shifts during college. In a recent study of 199 undergraduates, the younger students had a greater performance orientation in their goals. This means that they pursued their goals to prove their competence to others, rather than desiring to improve their own understanding or expand their knowledge. As they progressed through college, students shifted to more of a learning orientation—that is, they sought to acquire new skills and knowledge purely for the sake of learning. They became more aware of the usefulness of knowledge and less concerned about how others saw them.[18]

Sometimes your aspirations may exceed your reach—but in stretching toward a dream, you will attain more of your potential. It is important, however, to be realistic about your abilities and opportunities. You may be the best basketball player on your block, but are you good enough to play professionally? Would it be more realistic to plan a career in coaching?

Don't underestimate your potential, but be honest. Look beyond yourself to your environment. What are the opportunities in the field that interest you most? Do you need a graduate degree? What about your financial obligations? Would you be able to get financial aid? Can you work days and study in the evenings? What about your family's involvement? Chart out a step-by-step plan to meet your goal, and remember: The first steps toward meeting any goal are the most important. If you're uncertain of which interests to pursue, look into internship programs or volunteer jobs that might

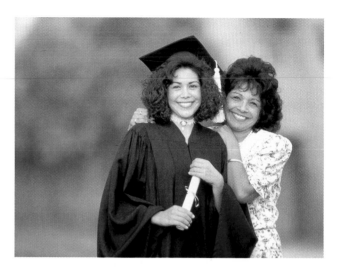

There can be great satisfaction in achieving a goal for which you worked long and hard.

give you a better sense of whether you'd be happy working in a particular field.

Boosting Self-Esteem

I am me.

In all the world there is no one else exactly like me. There are persons who have some parts like me, but no one adds up exactly like me. Therefore, everything that comes out of me is authentically mine because I alone chose it.

I own everything about me—my body, including everything it does; my mind, including all its thoughts and ideas; my eyes, including the images of all they behold; my feelings, whatever they may be—anger, joy, frustration, love, disappointment, excitement; my mouth, and all the words that come out of it, polite, sweet, or rough, correct or incorrect; my voice, loud or soft; and all my actions, whether they be to others or to myself. . . .

I own me, and therefore I can engineer me.

I am me, and I am okay.

Virginia Satir, *Peoplemaking*

After reading this declaration of **self-esteem,** think about how you feel about the person you are. Put down this book for a few minutes and draw a picture of how you see yourself. Don't worry about style or skill; simply try to capture your self-image on paper. Then analyze what you've drawn. How big is the figure you've sketched? Does it fill the page or occupy just one small corner? Is it active or still, smiling or frowning, attractive or awkward? Your drawing may hold clues to how you feel about yourself. Stop and think: What do you like about yourself? What do you dislike? What makes you unique? What gives you your greatest sense of satisfaction and pride?

Each of us wants and needs to feel significant as a human being with unique talents, abilities, and roles in life. A sense of self-esteem, of belief or pride in ourselves, gives us confidence to dare to attempt to achieve at school or work and to reach out to others to form friendships and close relationships. Self-esteem is the little voice that whispers, "You're worth it. You can do it. You're okay."

Self-esteem is based, not on external factors like wealth or beauty, but on what you believe about yourself. It's not something you're born with; self-esteem develops over time. It's also not something anyone else can give to you, although those around you can either help boost or diminish your self-esteem.

The seeds of self-esteem are planted in childhood when parents provide the assurance and appreciation youngsters need to push themselves toward new accomplishments: crawling, walking, forming words and sentences, learning control over their bladder and bowels. Two pillars of childhood self-esteem, say experts in child development, are confidence and competence. "Kids need to feel lovable and unconditionally loved to feel good about themselves," says therapist Stephanie Marston, author of *The Magic of Encouragement;* ". . . the other pillar of self-esteem is feeling capable and knowing you make a contribution to the family and later to the world."[19]

Adults, too, must consider themselves worthy of love, friendship, and success if they are to be loved, to make friends, and to achieve their goals. Low self-esteem is more common in people who have been abused as children and in those with psychiatric disorders, including depression, anxiety, alcoholism, and drug dependence. Feeling one did not receive love and encouragement as a child can also lead to poor self-esteem. Adults with poor self-esteem may unconsciously enter relationships that reinforce their self-perceptions and may prefer and even seek out people who think poorly of them.

Increasingly, educators, business managers, and health caregivers are realizing that self-esteem is critical in making teenagers less destructive, employees more productive, and welfare recipients more self-sufficient. Hundreds of schools have added self-esteem materials to their curricula, and major corporations have added self-esteem training to their employee programs. Although such efforts have their critics, programs that encourage a reality-based sense of one's worth have won respect and acceptance.

Positive Self-Talk

One of the most useful techniques for bolstering self-esteem and achieving your goals is developing the habit of positive thinking and talking. While negative obser-

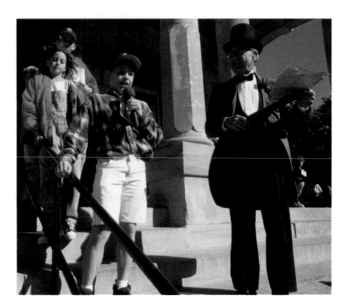

Children need opportunities to learn and succeed so that they can develop a sense of competence and self-worth.

vations, such as constant criticisms or reminders of the most minor of faults, can undermine self-image, positive affirmations—compliments, kudos, encouragements— have proven effective in enhancing self-esteem and psychological well-being. Individuals who fight off negative thoughts fare better psychologically than those who collapse when a setback occurs or who rely on others to make them feel better.

In his studies with college students, psychologist Martin Seligman has found that learning how to argue with one's negative self-evaluation can lower susceptibility to pessimism and, therefore, to depression. "It's called disputing: the act of monitoring and then arguing against the catastrophic things that you say to yourself," he says. The people most prone to pessimism tend to blame themselves for anything that goes wrong, believe that circumstances won't change, and allow the impact of a bad incident to "bleed" into every other aspect of their lives.[20]

Strategies *for* Change

How to Talk to Yourself

✓ To make sure you're sending yourself the right messages, tune into the unspoken commentary playing in your head.

✓ If you spot a self-put-down (e.g., "What a klutz!" or "I screwed up again!"), scream (silently)

"STOP!" or "DELETE!" Then give yourself a compliment to replace the criticism.

✓ If you hear your mind replaying the same negative observations again and again, try to trace them back to their source. Did they come from your parents, teachers, siblings? Say, "That's what they think, but it's not necessarily true."

✓ Make a list of the qualities you like best about yourself. Replay the list in your mind when you're feeling down about yourself.

✓ Spend more time doing those activities you know you do best. For example, if you are a good cook, prepare a meal for someone; if you are good at writing, write a letter to someone.

✓ Separate what you do, especially any mistakes you make, from who you are. Instead of saying, "I'm so stupid," tell yourself, "That wasn't the smartest move I ever made, but I'll learn from it."

Are There Ways to Boost a Bad Mood?

Feelings come and go within minutes. A **mood** is a more sustained emotional state that colors our view of the world for hours or days. According to surveys by psychologist Randy Larsen, of the University of Michigan, bad moods descend upon us an average of three out of every ten days. "A few people—about 2%—are happy just about every day," he says. "About 5% report bad moods four out of every five days."[21]

More than a dozen research laboratories are studying neurobiology and mood regulation. These scientists have found that people in various countries use many different methods to change their moods: listening to music, talking to a friend, going for a walk, keeping busy, trying to rectify a problem, eating, praying, shopping.

There are gender differences in mood management: Men typically try to distract themselves (a partially successful strategy) or use alcohol or drugs (an ineffective tactic). Women are more likely to talk to someone (which can help) or to ruminate on why they feel bad (which doesn't help).[22] Learning effective mood-boosting, mood-regulating strategies can help both men and women pull themselves up and out of an emotional slump. (See Pulsepoints: "Ten Ways to Pull Yourself Out of a Bad Mood.")

Problem-Oriented Methods

The most effective way to banish a sad or bad mood is by changing what caused it in the first place—if you can figure out what made you upset and why. "Most bad moods are caused by loss or failure in work or intimate relationships," says Larsen. "The questions to ask are: What can I do to fix the failure? What can I do to remedy the loss? Is there anything under my control that I can change? If there is, take action and solve it." Rewrite the report. Ask to take a make-up exam. Apologize to the friend whose feelings you hurt. Tell your parents you feel bad about the argument you had.

If there's nothing you can do, accept what happened and focus on doing things differently next time. "In our studies, resolving to try harder actually was as effective in improving mood as taking action in the present," says Larsen. You also can try to think about what happened in a different way and put a positive spin on it. This technique, known as *cognitive reappraisal*, or "reframing," helps you look at a setback in a new light: What lessons did it teach you? What would you have done differently? Could there be a silver lining or hidden benefit?

Emotion-Oriented Methods

If you can't identify or resolve the problem responsible for your emotional funk, the next-best solution is to concentrate on altering your negative feelings. For example, try setting a quick, achievable goal that can boost your spirits with a small success. Clean out a closet; sort through the piles of paper on your desk; write the letter to your aunt you've been putting off for weeks.

Another good option is to get moving. In studies of mood regulation, exercise consistently ranks as the single most effective strategy for banishing bad feelings. Numerous studies have confirmed that aerobic workouts, such as walking or jogging, significantly improve mood. Even nonaerobic exercise, such as weight-lifting, can boost spirits; improve sleep and appetite; reduce anxiety; irritability; and anger; and produce feelings of mastery and accomplishment.

Although it's tempting to pull away from others when you're in a slump, it's better not to withdraw. "It's never a good idea to sulk by yourself when you're feeling down," says Larsen. "Pretend to be extroverted if you have to, but do spend time with other people." As he notes, friends often can help improve your mood by giving you good feedback. But be wary of seeking out companions solely for a gripe-and-groan session. You might end up feeling worse rather than better.

Taking your mind off your troubles, rather than mulling over what's wrong, is one of the most often used mood boosters, but it's only partly successful. Simple distractions—watching television, for instance,

PULSE *points*

Ten Ways to Pull Yourself Out of a Bad Mood

1. **Accentuate the positive.** Think of the parts of your life that are going well rather than mulling over what's not.

2. **Review past successes.** Remind yourself of what you've accomplished before to motivate yourself to accomplish more in the future.

3. **Pray.** In a Gallup poll of 1007 Americans, religious practices rated as the most effective way of relieving depression.

4. **Listen to music.** While many forms of distraction help, at least temporarily, this is one of the most popular and effective mood boosters.

5. **Treat yourself.** Indulgences—big or small, expensive or not—can bring you up when you're feeling down. The reason: They make you feel special.

6. **Volunteer.** A third of Americans— some 89 million people—give of themselves through volunteer work. By doing the same, you may feel better too.

7. **Exercise.** In various studies around the world, physical exertion ranks as one of the best ways to change a bad mood, raise energy, and reduce tension.

8. **Act happy.** Putting on a happy face doesn't make problems disappear, but it does improve mood.

9. **Focus on the future.** Although you can't rewrite the past, you can learn from it. Resolve to try harder and do better the next time around.

10. **Set a limit on self-pity.** Tell yourself, "I'm going to feel sorry for myself this morning, but this afternoon, I've got to get on with my life."

or reading—work only temporarily. Activities that engage the imagination, on the other hand, seem to have more lasting effects. Listening to music, for instance, is one of the most popular and effective ways of distracting people from their troubles and changing their bad moods (see Table 3-1).

What Doesn't Work

Giving in to a bad mood and resigning yourself to feeling out of sorts practically guarantees that you won't feel better soon. Negative expectations tend to be self-fulfilling, and individuals who expect to feel bad do indeed report greater unhappiness.[23] "Venting" or "letting it all out" also does little good. "Screaming or crying only serves to reinforce a negative emotion," says Larsen. "In our studies, people who vented their emotions were more likely to remain just as upset hours afterward."

Thinking again and again about faults, failings, or misfortunes not only perpetuates a bad mood but can also contribute to depression. Individuals who ruminate in this way are less likely to engage in distracting pleasant activities—even if they believe they would enjoy them.[24] Yet, despite their low mood, they are convinced that they should perform at a high level.[25]

Turning to alcohol or drugs to escape sorrows may offer temporary relief, but once the buzz is gone, so is the good mood. And you may end up thinking even less of yourself because of your reliance on chemical crutches. Similarly, if you console yourself with ice cream, chocolate, or other tasty treats, you may be set-

ting yourself up for another slump the next time you step on the scale.

Finding Happiness

Psychologist David Myers, author of *The Pursuit of Happiness: Who Is Happy—and Why,* defines happiness as "a sense of well-being, a feeling that life as a whole is going well."[26] This state depends not on big achievements, but on little pleasures. Happiness tends to be highest when people combine frequent good experiences—the daily joys of having a caring partner, a productive job, or enjoyable hobbies—with occasional very intense pleasures, such as a special vacation or a promotion.

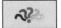 ### What Leads to Happiness?

Your happiness level may be largely genetic. In a study of sets of twins raised separately and together, psychologists concluded that, in the same way that humans have a weight set point (discussed in Chapter 7), we also have a happiness set point. Although it fluctuates somewhat, it rarely changes radically.

Happiness has a surprisingly small relationship to age, gender, or ethnicity. However, countries differ appreciably in the happiness of their people. In general, happiness is greater in more prosperous countries, but

■ Table 3-1 Mood-Boosters: What Works and What Doesn't

These are the most common ways that college students use to feel happier, release anger, or
enhance feelings of well-being. Some work better than others.

Most Effective	Partly Effective	Not Effective
Taking action to solve a problem	Socializing	"Venting"
Reappraising what happened	Distracting yourself	Blaming others
Thinking about other successes		Being alone
Rewarding yourself		Giving up
Resolving to try harder		
Making "downward" comparisons (to less fortunate individuals)		

Source: Based on research by psychologist Randy Larsen, Ph.D., of the University of Michigan.

even in the more affluent nations there seems little relationship between wealth and happiness for people who
have the basic necessities of life. In poor countries, the
rich are significantly happier than the poor. Throughout
the world, married people are happier than unmarried
individuals, and religious people are happier than those
who aren't religious.[27]

Having an unhappy childhood does not doom anyone to a lifetime of misery, but it does increase the likelihood of unhappiness in adulthood. In a study of
community college students, the vast majority reported
a happy or very happy childhood. Only 9 percent of
these students were unhappy as adults. About two-
thirds of those reporting unhappy or very unhappy
childhoods reported that they were unhappy or very
unhappy adults. The risk of having an unhappy adult-

hood was two and a half times greater for those who'd
been unhappy as children.[28]

The best predictors of happiness are the characteristics of good psychological health: high self-esteem,
optimism, extroversion, and a sense of being in control.
In addition to these four key traits, happy people are
more likely to have healthy and fit bodies; realistic goals
and expectations, supportive friendships; an intimate,
sexually warm marriage; and a faith that provides support, purpose, and acceptance.

Although research indicates no clear relationship
between wealth and happiness in developed countries,
many people still equate more money with more happiness. Yet individuals who seek nonmaterial sources of
fulfillment are far more likely to find joy, says psychologist Mihaly Csikszentmihalyi. By studying the lives of
thousands of people, he discovered that the happiest regularly experienced what he calls "flow," a state of deep
focus that occurs when individuals engage in challenging
tasks that demand intense concentration and commitment. By this definition, a challenging game of chess can
bring more happiness than a spin in a new sports car.[29]

Not even disability and illness are bars to happiness. One study of individuals who suffered accidents
resulting in quadriplegia and paraplegia found that
within six months the two groups reported nearly identical levels of happiness, despite the differences in the
severity of their injuries.[30]

Happiness is not just a state of mind but quite literally a state of brain. By means of sophisticated imaging
techniques, neuroscientists have discovered differences in
brain chemistry and activity when people are experiencing
happiness, sadness, and other moods. In both women and
men, happiness activates a specific region in the frontal
cortex (described in Chapter 4).[31]

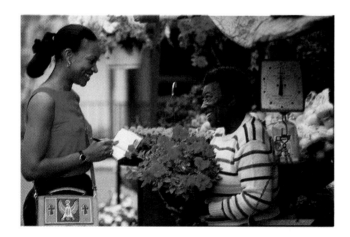

Happiness and optimism go hand in hand. Small rewards can
keep your spirits high and remind you that you are special.

Happiness affects brain functions as well as the brain itself. Studies in which individuals had to recognize or name certain words found differences in basic information processing, depending on their perceived happiness.[32] It also matters whether people link their feelings of happiness to positive or negative life events. In a study of 89 college students, the "linkers" were most likely to see their happiness as contingent on attaining important goals in life.[33]

Becoming Optimistic

The dictionary defines **optimism** as "an inclination to anticipate the best possible outcome." In *Healthy Pleasures,* Robert Ornstein and David Sobel redefine it psychologically as "the tendency to seek out, remember, and expect pleasurable experiences. It is an active priority of the person, not merely a reflex that prompts us to look on the sunny side."[34]

For various reasons—because they believe in themselves, because they trust in a higher power, because they feel lucky—optimists expect positive experiences from life. When bad things happen, they tend to see setbacks or losses as specific, temporary incidents. In their eyes, a disappointment is "one of those things" that happens every once in a while, rather than the latest in a long string of disasters. And rather than blaming themselves ("I always screw things up," pessimists might say), optimists look at all the different factors that may have caused the problem.

"What you expect is what you get," say Ornstein and Sobel, who suggest a simple test of your optimism level: Write down as many as you can of the wonderful experiences you expect to have in the future. Then describe the difficult, trying things you think might happen. How many positive experiences did you list? How many negative ones? Two years after a group of elderly men and women took this test, the optimists who had listed more positive than negative expectations reported fewer physical symptoms of ill health, fewer colds, fewer days off from work, more energy, and a greater sense of psychological well-being.

Individuals aren't born optimistic or pessimistic; in fact, researchers have documented changes over time in the ways that individuals view the world and what they expect to experience in the future. "We have a choice about how we think," asserts psychologist Martin Seligman. "We can choose to change the habits of pessimism into optimism." The key is disputing the automatic negative thoughts that flood our brains and choosing to believe in our own possibilities. "Optimism is a set of learned skills," says Seligman. "Once learned, these skills persist because they feel so good to use. And reality is usually on our side."[35]

Savoring Pleasures

"Treating yourself is one of the best ways to cheer yourself up," says psychologist Larsen of the University of Michigan. "A night out is fun in itself, but it also imparts an important message: You're worth it. As adults we all need occasional reminders that we are special and deserve some special things."

This doesn't mean you have to break the bank. When you're feeling low, even simple indulgences, like sleeping in a few extra minutes or eating your lunch out in the sun, can make you feel better. If you're feeling down, plan a reward for yourself every day, and make it a habit to include small pleasures—such as sharing a joke with a friend or taking time to watch a splendid sunset—in your daily routine.[36]

Looking on the Light Side

Humor, which enables us to express fears and negative feelings without causing distress to ourselves or others, is one of the healthiest ways of coping with life's ups and downs. Laughter stimulates the heart, alters brain wave patterns and breathing rhythms, reduces perceptions of pain, decreases stress-related hormones, and strengthens the immune system. In psychotherapy, humor helps channel negative emotions toward a positive effect.[37] Even in cases of critical or fatal illnesses, humor can help people live with greater joy until they die. It also boosts the stamina and spirits of those who care for the ill.[38]

Joking and laughing are ways of expressing honest emotions, of overcoming dread and doubt, and of connecting with others. They also can defuse rage. After all, it's almost impossible to stay angry when you're laughing. To tickle your funny bone, try keeping a file of favorite cartoons or jokes. Go to a comedy club instead of a movie. And when you see or hear something that makes you laugh out loud, don't keep it to yourself—multiply the mirth by sharing it with a friend.

Strategies *for* **Prevention**

How to Be Happy

✓ Make time for yourself. It's impossible to meet the needs of others without recognizing and fulfilling your own.

✓ Invest yourself in closeness. Give your loved ones the gift of your time and caring.

✓ Work hard at what you like. Search for challenges that satisfy your need to do something meaningful.

✔ Be upbeat. If you always look for what's wrong about yourself or your life, you'll find it—and feel even worse.

✔ Organize but stay loose. Be ready to seize an unexpected opportunity to try something different.

✔ Despite inevitable highs and lows, strive for a sense of balance.

Finding Meaning in Life

"What's it all about?" It's the question almost everyone asks sooner or later. Whether dreams come true or die, whether we achieve our goals or not, we find ourselves confronting difficult questions about the purpose of our lives. We're especially likely to ask such questions when bad things happen or when we face daunting difficulties—circumstances that are an unavoidable part of life. Many people find answers through loving relationships, spiritual development, and acts of charity and good will.

Loving and Being Loved

"One can live magnificently in this world if one knows how to work and how to love, to work for the person one loves and to love one's work," Leo Tolstoy wrote. You may not think of love as a basic need like food and rest, but it is essential for both physical and psychological well-being.

Mounting evidence suggests that people who lack love and commitment are at high risk for a host of illnesses, including infections, heart disease, and cancer. "Love and intimacy are at the root of what makes us sick and what makes us well," says cardiologist Dean Ornish, author of *Love & Survival: The Scientific Basis for the Healing Power of Intimacy*. "No other factor in medicine—not diet, not smoking, not exercise—has a greater impact."[39] (See Table 3–2, "The Price of Loneliness.")

Although being loved is enough to get us started in a healthy life, as mature individuals we need to express love as well as to receive it, to be able to form a union with another person while retaining our own identity and integrity. We evolve toward this state of loving, beginning from the infant's total self-concern and gradually learning to love others and to find fulfillment by

---

■ **Table 3-2** The Price of Loneliness: The Questions That Count

Researchers asked several groups of people questions relating to their sense of isolation. Here is what they learned about isolation as a health hazard:

Asked of women: Do you feel isolated?
Those who said yes were three and a half times as likely to die of breast, ovarian, or uterine cancer over a 17-year period.

Asked of men: Does your wife show you her love?
Men who said no suffered 50 percent more angina (chest pain) over a 5-year period than those who said yes.

Asked of male medical students: Are you close to your parents?
Those who said no were more likely to develop cancer or mental illness years later.

Asked of heart patients: Do you feel loved?
Those who felt the least loved had 50 percent more arterial damage than those who felt the most loved.

Asked of unmarried heart patients: Do you have a confidant?
Those who said no were three times as likely to die within 5 years.

Asked of heart-attack survivors: Do you live alone?
Those who said yes were more than twice as likely to die within a year.
Source: Cowley, Geoffrey. "Is Love the Best Drug?" *Newsweek*, Vol. 131, No. 11, March 16, 1998.

fulfilling the needs of others. Since relationships are so vital to our well-being, Chapter 8 is devoted to exploring our ties to friends, parents, partners, spouses, and children.

Caring for the Soul

As discussed in Chapter 1, spiritual development is part of total health. "The soul needs an intense, full-bodied spiritual life as much as and in the same way that the body needs food," observes psychologist Thomas Moore in *Care of the Soul*. "Just as the mind digests ideas and produces intelligence, the soul feeds on life and digests it, creating wisdom and character out of the fodder of experience."[40]

For years, spiritual matters were rarely recognized or discussed by mental health professionals. Until 1982, fewer than 3 percent of the articles published in leading psychiatry journals focused on spirituality or religiousity. Since then dozens of scientific studies have found that spiritual beliefs and activities—such as prayer or meditation—positively affect psychological well-being and may even speed recovery from medical illness. How? "Faith provides a support community, a sense of life's meaning, a reason to focus beyond self, and a timeless perspective on life's temporary ups and downs," observes psychologist David Meyers.

Doing Good

Altruism—helping or giving to others—enhances self-esteem, relieves physical and mental stress, and protects psychological well-being. Hans Selye, the father of stress research, described cooperation with others for the self's sake as altruistic egotism, whereby we satisfy our own needs while helping others satisfy theirs. This concept is essentially an updated version of the golden rule: Do unto others as you would have them do unto you. The important difference is that you earn your neighbor's love and help by offering them love and help.

Giving helps those who give as well as those who receive. People involved in community organizations, for instance, consistently report a surge of well-being called *helper's high*, which they describe as a unique sense of calmness, warmth, and enhanced self-worth.[41] College students who provided community service as part of a semester-long course reported changes in attitude (including a decreased tendency to blame people for their misfortunes), self-esteem (primarily a belief that they can make a difference), and behavior (a greater commitment to do more volunteer work).[42]

Many students volunteer regularly. (See Campus Focus: "Volunteerism Among Students.") The options for giving of yourself are limitless: Volunteer to serve a meal at a homeless shelter. Collect donations for a char-

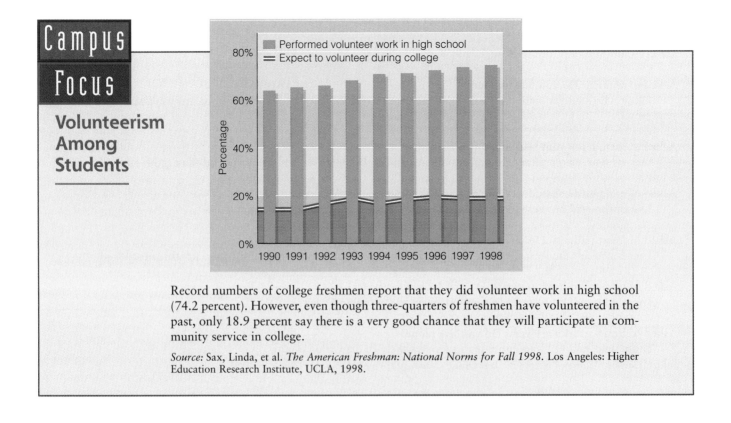

Campus Focus

Volunteerism Among Students

Record numbers of college freshmen report that they did volunteer work in high school (74.2 percent). However, even though three-quarters of freshmen have volunteered in the past, only 18.9 percent say there is a very good chance that they will participate in community service in college.

Source: Sax, Linda, et al. *The American Freshman: National Norms for Fall 1998.* Los Angeles: Higher Education Research Institute, UCLA, 1998.

ity auction. Teach in an illiteracy program. Perform the simplest act of charity: pray for others. "Whenever I hear of someone with a problem, I say three prayers for them," one woman reports; "It makes me feel better—and I hope it helps them, too."

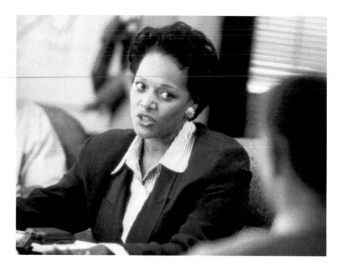

Practicing assertiveness allows you to express yourself without aggression, to communicate and accomplish your goals.

Feeling in Control

Although no one has absolute control over destiny, there is a great deal that we can do to control how we think, feel, and behave. By assessing our life situations realistically, we can make plans and preparations that allow us to make the most of our circumstances. By doing so, we gain a sense of mastery. In nationwide surveys, Americans who feel in control of their lives report greater psychological well-being than those who do not, as well as "extraordinarily positive feelings of happiness."[43]

Developing Autonomy

One goal that many people strive for is **autonomy,** or independence. Both family and society influence our ability to grow toward independence. Autonomous individuals are true to themselves. As they weigh the pros and cons of any decision, whether it's using or refusing drugs or choosing a major or career, they base their judgment on their own values, not those of others. Their ability to draw on internal resources and cope with challenges has a positive impact on both their psychological well-being and their physical health, including recovery from illness. Those who've achieved autonomy may seek the opinions of others, but they do not allow their decisions to be dictated by external influences. Because of this, it is said that their **locus of control**—that is, where they view control as originating—is *internal* (from within themselves) rather than *external* (from others).

Asserting Yourself

Being **assertive** means recognizing your feelings and making your needs and desires clear to others. Unlike aggression, a far less healthy means of expression, assertiveness usually works. You can change a situation you don't like by communicating your feelings and thoughts in nonprovocative words, by focusing on specifics, and by making sure you're talking with the person(s) who is directly responsible.

Becoming assertive isn't always easy. Many people have learned to cope by being passive and not communicating their feelings or opinions. Sooner or later they become so irritated, frustrated, or overwhelmed that they explode in an outburst—which they think of as being assertive. However, such behavior is so distasteful to them that they'd rather be passive. But assertiveness doesn't mean screaming or telling someone off. You can communicate your wishes calmly and clearly. Assertiveness is a behavior that respects your rights and the rights of other people even when you disagree.[44]

Even at its mildest, assertiveness can make you feel better about yourself and your life. The reason: When you speak up or take action, you're in the pilot seat. And that's always much less stressful than taking a back seat and trying to hang on for dear life.

Strategies *for* Change

Asserting Yourself

✔ Use "I" statements to explain your feelings. This allows you to take ownership of your opinions and feelings without putting down others for how they feel and think.

✔ Listen to and acknowledge what the other person says. After you speak, find out if the other person understands your position. Ask how he or she feels about what you've said.

✔ Be direct and specific. Describe the problem as you see it, using neutral language rather than assigning blame. Also suggest a specific solution, but make clear that you'd like the lines of communication and negotiation to remain open.

Don't think you have to be obnoxious in order to be assertive. It's most effective to state your needs and preferences without any sarcasm or hostility.

Boosting Energy

Do you drag through the day? Do you feel that you're running on empty? Sometimes the causes of fatigue are psychological, and a lack of energy can be a symptom of a mental disorder, such as depression. However, often fatigue stems from a lack of any one of three energy essentials: exercise, good nutrition, or sleep.

Exercise

While you may think that working out will wear you down, regular aerobic activities such as walking, jog-ging, cycling, or swimming in fact have the opposite effect. Daily workouts promote alertness and relax body and mind so that you sleep better and feel more ener-getic. Exercise also produces gradual psychological changes. As they condition their bodies, individuals who exercise release anger and anxiety and feel better about their bodies and lives. Seeing for themselves that they're capable of change, exercisers may feel more competent and confident about other aspects of their lives.

Almost any form of physical activity—from walking to weight-lifting—can help. (See Figure 3-2.) While even a single session does some good, a regular regimen of daily exercise is better. Individuals who regularly engage in aer-obic activity report higher energy levels, better mood, and lower likelihood of depression. (Chapter 5 provides a complete discussion of exercise and its benefits.)

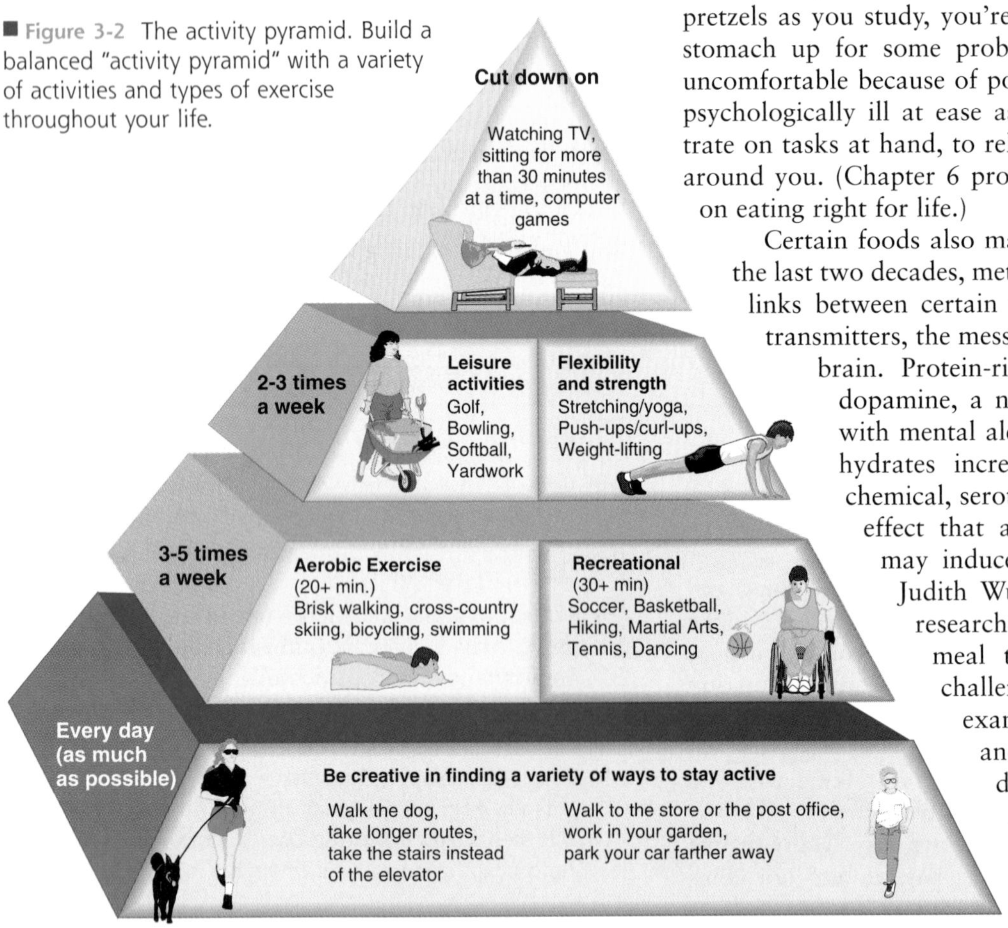

Eating Right

Both your body and mind need good nutrition to run efficiently. To keep energy levels up, try five small meals throughout the day rather than three large ones. Always start with a healthy breakfast. Take time to eat nutri-tious meals. If you wolf down a hamburger and fries in the car on your way to class, or munch on chips and pretzels as you study, you're setting yourself and your stomach up for some problems. If you're physically uncomfortable because of poor eating habits, you'll be psychologically ill at ease as well—unable to concen-trate on tasks at hand, to relax, or to enjoy the people around you. (Chapter 6 provides detailed information on eating right for life.)

Certain foods also may affect our moods. Over the last two decades, meticulous research has found links between certain types of food and neuro-transmitters, the messenger chemicals within the brain. Protein-rich foods boost levels of dopamine, a neurotransmitter associated with mental alertness and energy. Carbo-hydrates increase levels of a different chemical, serotonin, which has a calming effect that alleviates anxiety but also may induce sleepiness. According to Judith Wurtman of MIT, a leading researcher in this field, the best meal to eat before a mentally challenging event, such as a final exam, would be high in protein and low in fat and carbohy-drate (fish with a salad, for instance), while a soothing supper after a stressful day might feature carbo-hydrates, such as pasta.[45]

■ Figure 3-2 The activity pyramid. Build a balanced "activity pyramid" with a variety of activities and types of exercise throughout your life.

Cut down on
Watching TV, sitting for more than 30 minutes at a time, computer games

2-3 times a week

Leisure activities
Golf, Bowling, Softball, Yardwork

Flexibility and strength
Stretching/yoga, Push-ups/curl-ups, Weight-lifting

3-5 times a week

Aerobic Exercise
(20+ min.)
Brisk walking, cross-country skiing, bicycling, swimming

Recreational
(30+ min)
Soccer, Basketball, Hiking, Martial Arts, Tennis, Dancing

Every day (as much as possible)

Be creative in finding a variety of ways to stay active

Walk the dog, take longer routes, take the stairs instead of the elevator

Walk to the store or the post office, work in your garden, park your car farther away

Getting Enough Sleep

You stay up late cramming for a final. You drive through the night to visit a friend at another campus. You get up for an early class during the week but stay in bed until noon on weekends. And you wonder: "Why am I so tired?" The answer: You're not getting enough sleep—and you're not alone. According to the National Commission on Sleep Disorders Research, one out of every three Americans has problems sleeping. And even those who aren't having difficulty don't log as much sleep time as they'd like. Over the last century, we have cut our average nightly sleep time by more than 20 percent.[46]

Whenever we fail to get adequate sleep, we accumulate what researchers call a *sleep debt*. With each night of too little rest, our body's need for sleep grows until it becomes irresistible. "We don't tend to have a good handle on our amount of sleep debt," says psychiatrist William Dement, of Stanford University, a pioneer in sleep research. "So when we finally go bankrupt, it happens fast. People can go from feeling wide awake to falling asleep in five seconds. If you are behind the wheel of a car, you could end up dead."

While the specific amount of sleep individuals need varies from person to person, physicians have recognized "problem sleepiness" as a threat to health and safety. However, its effects are insidious, and often neither individuals nor their doctors realize that problem sleepiness is undermining emotional and physical health.[47]

One sleep disorder in particular, sleep apnea, which is characterized by breathing stoppages that disrupt restful sleep, has been linked to increased dangers during both night and day. This chronic condition can increase the risk of hypertension and other medical complications.[48] Because of daytime sleepiness, people with sleep apnea are six times more likely than others to have a traffic accident.[49] According to the Department of Transportation, each year 200,000 sleep-related accidents claim more than 5,000 lives, cause hundreds of thousands of injuries, and incur billions in indirect costs.

The only solution to sleep debt is the obvious one: paying it back. Individuals who add an hour or two to their nightly sleep time are more alert, more productive, and less likely to have accidents. And because sleepy people tend to be irritable and edgy, those who get more rest also tend to be happier, healthier, and easier to get along with.

Sleep Basics

We spend a third of our lives sleeping—more time than we spend working, loving, or playing. Although sleepers may look quiet and seem unresponsive to the world around them, their brains and bodies are going through a series of profound changes. Scientists differentiate between certain periods of the night when the eyes dart rapidly back and forth beneath closed lids, called **rapid-eye-movement (REM) sleep,** and quieter, non-REM sleep stages. Most adults spend 20 to 25 percent of the night in REM sleep, when our most vivid dreaming takes place.

Each night as you fall asleep, you go through the same sequence of sleep stages: Your body begins to slow down, and muscular tension decreases. As you enter stage 1 of non-REM sleep, your brain waves become smaller, pinched, and irregular. Mundane thoughts flit through your mind; if awakened from this twilight zone, you might deny having slept at all. As you enter stage 2, your brain waves become larger, with occasional bursts of activity. Your eyes become unresponsive, so that even if your eyelids were gently lifted, you wouldn't see. In stage 3, your brain waves are much slower and about five times larger than in stage 1. In stage 4, the most profound state of unconsciousness, your brain waves form a slow, jagged pattern; and you would be very difficult to arouse. (See Figure 3-3.)

The full journey to the depths of tranquility takes more than an hour. Then you begin your ascent—not to consciousness but to REM sleep. The muscles of your middle ear vibrate. Your brain waves resemble the patterns of waking more than of deep sleep. The muscles of your face, limbs, and trunk are slack. Your pulse and breathing quicken, and your brain temperature and blood flow increase. Your eyes dart back and forth. If wakened, you're likely to report a fantasylike dream.

Your body repeats this sequence four or five times a night. In an eight-hour night's rest, you spend two hours in REM sleep; over the course of a lifetime, you'll spend five or six years dreaming and three times that amount in the quieter stages of sleep.

How Much Sleep Is Enough?

There's no one formula for how long a good night's sleep should be. Expecting all people to need the same amount of rest would be as absurd as expecting them to eat the same amount of food every day. Normal sleep times range from five to ten hours; the average is seven and a half. About one or two people in a hundred can get by with just five hours; another small minority needs twice that amount. Each of us seems to have an innate sleep *appetite* that is as much a part of our genetic programming as hair color and skin tone.

To figure out your sleep needs, keep your wake-up time the same every morning and vary your bedtimes. Are you groggy after six hours of shut-eye? Does an extra hour give you more stamina? What about an extra two hours? Since too much sleep can make you feel sluggish, don't assume that more is always better. Listen to your body's signals, and adjust your sleep schedule to suit them.

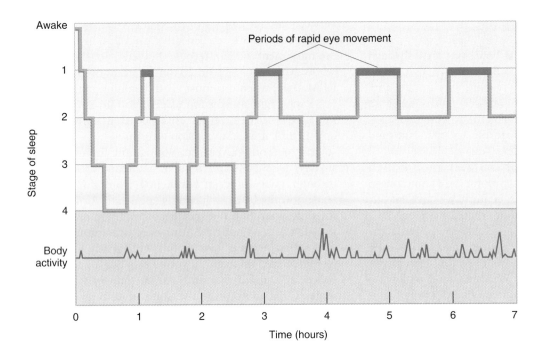

■ Figure 3-3 A sleep cycle. During the first hour or so sleep becomes deeper, then the level ascends to a period of REM sleep (indicated by thick bars). The sleep cycle is repeated, with some variations, throughout the night.

Strategies *for* Change

How to Sleep Like a Baby

✔ Keep regular hours for going to bed and getting up in the morning. Stay as close as possible to this schedule on weekends as well as weekdays.

✔ Develop a sleep ritual—such as stretching, meditation, yoga, prayer, or reading a not-too-thrilling novel—to ease the transition from wakefulness to sleep.

✔ Don't drink coffee late in the day. The effects of caffeine can linger for up to eight hours. And don't smoke. Nicotine is an even more powerful stimulant—and sleep saboteur—than caffeine.

✔ Don't rely on alcohol to get to sleep. Alcohol disrupts normal sleep stages; so you won't sleep as deeply or as restfully as you normally would.

✔ Don't nap during the day if you're having problems sleeping through the night.

Connecting with Others

At every age, people who feel connected to others tend to be healthier physically and psychologically. College students are no exception: Those who have a supportive, readily available network of relationships are less psychologically distressed and more satisfied with life. (See Chapter 8 for a comprehensive discussion of communication, friendship, and intimacy.)

The opposite of *connectedness* is **social isolation,** a major risk factor for illness and early death. Individuals with few social contacts face two to four times the mortality rate of others. The reason may be that their social isolation weakens the body's ability to ward off disease. Medical students with higher-than-average scores on a loneliness scale had lower levels of protective immune cells.[50] The end of a long-term relationship—through separation, divorce, or death—also dampens immunity.[51]

It is part of our nature as mammals and as human beings to crave relationships. But invariably we end up alone at times. Solitude is not without its own quiet joys—time for introspection, self-assessment, learning from the past, and looking toward the future. Each of us can cultivate the joy of our company, of being alone without crossing the line and becoming lonely.[52]

Overcoming Loneliness

More so than many other countries, we are a nation of loners. Recent trends—longer work hours, busy family schedules, frequent moves, high divorce rates—have created even more lonely people. Only 23 percent of Americans say they're never lonely. Loneliest of all are those who are divorced, separated, or widowed and those who live alone or solely with children. Among sin-

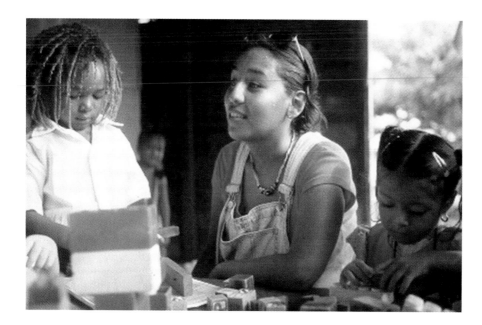

Volunteering is a rewarding way of connecting with others, giving of yourself, and feeling connected to your community.

gle adults who have never been married, 42 percent feel lonely at least sometimes. However, loneliness is most likely to cause emotional distress when it is a chronic rather than an episodic condition.[53]

To combat loneliness, people may join groups, fling themselves into projects and activities, or surround themselves with superficial acquaintances.[54] Others avoid the effort of trying to connect, sometimes limiting most of their personal interactions to chat groups on the Internet.

The Internet may actually make people feel lonelier. In the first study of the social and psychological effects of Internet use at home, researchers at Carnegie Mellon University found that people who spend even a few hours a week online have higher levels of depression and loneliness than those who use the Internet less frequently. "Virtual" communication, it seems, does not provide the same benefits as old-fashioned, face-to-face relationships.[55]

The true keys to overcoming loneliness are developing resources to fulfill our own potential and learning to reach out to others. In this way, loneliness can become a means to personal growth and discovery.[56]

Race and gender also affect the experience of loneliness. In a study of 100 African American undergraduates, having a best friend was the most important factor in low levels of emotional loneliness in men and high levels of feeling in control in women.[57] Some studies have found that men are lonelier than women. Others find no gender differences in loneliness, but researchers note that men, particularly those who score high on measures of masculinity, are more hesitant than women to admit that they're lonely.[58]

In cross-cultural studies, married people of all ages generally report less loneliness than single individuals and than unmarried individuals living together. In most nations, having children has little or no effect on how lonely people feel.[59] Even in middle and old age, the childless are not more vulnerable to loneliness or depression. Widowed and divorced men and women report higher levels of loneliness and depression than married people, regardless of whether they have children.[60]

Loneliness also affects positive health practices among college students. Those who do not have a network of supportive relationships report feeling a sense of utter aloneness, of living in a barren environment, of feeling empty and hollow, and of frequently experiencing

Strategies *for* Prevention

How to Avoid Feeling Lonely

✔ Learn to be by yourself. Enjoying your own company helps make you the sort of person others enjoy.

✔ Pursue some interests on your own—hiking in the woods, perhaps, or joining a singing group.

✔ Keep in touch with old friends, even when miles or years may separate you.

✔ Give of yourself as a volunteer. Nothing warms the spirit more than reaching out to those who need you.

boredom and aimlessness. These are also the students who feel least motivated to take the best possible care of their minds and bodies.

Facing Social Anxieties

Many people are uncomfortable meeting strangers or speaking or performing in public. In some surveys, as many as 40 percent of people describe themselves as shy, or *socially anxious*.[61] Some shy people—an estimated 10 to 15 percent of children—are born with a predisposition to social anxieties.[62] Others become shy because they don't learn proper social responses or because they experience rejection or shame. As a result, normal apprehension intensifies in situations in which they might be watched or criticized by others. They feel extremely self-conscious, embarrassed, and nervous. When attention is on them alone, they may tremble, breathe very rapidly (hyperventilate), sweat, or develop a dry mouth or nausea.

Social anxieties often become a problem in late adolescence. Students may develop symptoms when they go to a party at a fraternity or sorority or are called on in class. Some experience symptoms when they try to perform any sort of action in the presence of others, even such everyday activities as eating in public, using a public restroom, or writing a check. In a severe form of social anxiety, called **social phobia,** individuals typically fear and avoid various social situations. In performance anxiety—a subtype of social phobia—the main fear is of performing in front of others. The key difference between these problems and normal shyness and self-consciousness is the degree of distress and impairment that individuals experience.

If you're shy, you can overcome much of your social apprehensiveness on your own, in much the same way as you might set out to stop smoking or lose weight. For example, you can improve your social skills by pushing yourself to introduce yourself to a stranger at a party or to chat about the weather or the food selections with the person next to you in a cafeteria line. Gradually you'll acquire a sense of social timing and a verbal ease that will take the worry out of close encounters with others.

Those with more disabling social anxiety may do best with professional guidance, which has proven highly effective. One common technique used by experts is role playing, in which individuals act out situations that normally produce butterflies in the stomach, such as returning a defective product to a store or calling for a date. With practice and time, most individuals are able to emerge from the walls that shyness has built around them and take pleasure in interacting with others.

Strategies *for* Change

Developing Social Skills

✔ If you want to get to know someone you see on campus or at work, write down what you want to say, and rehearse on your own or with a friend.

✔ Use a mirror to practice making eye contact and smiling. Talk into a tape-recorder to improve your speaking voice and volume.

✔ Observe and copy the behavior of people who handle social situations well, perhaps those who make clear what they want without being obnoxious.

✔ Every two weeks, invite someone to accompany you on an inexpensive outing, such as a visit to a museum.

✔ When you're with others, focus on them and what they're saying. Try not to think about how you look or what you're saying.

 ## How Should I Deal with Difficult People?

Sooner or later we all have to deal with relatives, friends, roommates, colleagues, or bosses who annoy, attack, blame, manipulate, or infuriate us. Some simply have habits or behaviors that "push our buttons," grating on our nerves and clashing with our way of doing things. Others consistently irritate almost everyone they encounter. What makes them so difficult to deal with?

"Chances are that the most frustrating people in your life have personality disorders," says psychiatrist John Oldham, coauthor of *The Personality Self-Portrait,* who notes that the difference between ordinary orneriness or eccentricity and **personality disorders** is a matter of degree.[63] These common conditions are not difficulties that people *have*—like depression or anxiety—but fundamental problems with who they *are*: how they feel, how they see themselves, how they relate to others.

These extremely difficult people don't just make themselves miserable; they exasperate everyone around them. Since you can't avoid them, you have to know how to cope with them—and the first step is understanding that they aren't being difficult on purpose. They really can't help themselves. This realization may help friends and family members, who are often confused and hurt by the difficult people in their lives, find ways to work around them.

It can help to keep some emotional distance and not take annoying behavior personally. Most obnoxious behavior has more to do with the other person's insecurities than with you. When difficult people behave badly, they typically blame others for "making" them do so. A personality disorder may be an explanation for obnoxious, inconsiderate, annoying behavior, but it's not an excuse. Respect your own rights as a person, and expect others to do the same.

If you need to confront a difficult person for any reason, simply state how you feel or what you observe without judging. Exquisitely sensitive to rejection or disapproval, many such individuals overreact to any comment that could be construed as a criticism or challenge. You also can try to give them some of what they need. You don't have to cave in, but be pragmatic. If a friend or coworker is always suspicious, keep plans out in the open so it's clear that you're not hiding anything. If all else fails, you may have to write off a difficult person. Some individuals are so incorrigibly deceitful, manipulative, or destructive that a healthy relationship with them is impossible. Even if they feign remorse and swear to behave better, they actually feel little, if any, guilt.

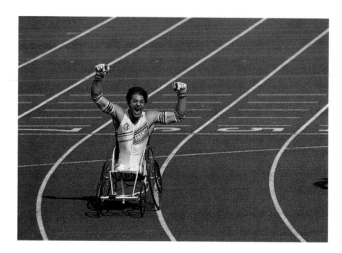

The characteristics of psychological health include a feeling of self-worth, an acceptance of life's possibilities, and a sense of fulfillment. We may not be in touch with these feelings all the time, but when we are, we also feel joy that we're alive.

Across the Lifespan: Psychological Well-Being in Middle and Old Age

Optimal aging demands a redefinition of who a person is and what makes his or her life worthwhile. Some sources of satisfaction, such as physical challenges or professional achievements, diminish later in life. Yet older people in general feel psychologically better than young people, with fewer worries about themselves and how they look to other people, higher self-esteem, and less loneliness.

The secret of emotional well-being in old age doesn't seem to be professional success or a happy marriage but the ability to cope with life's setbacks without blame or bitterness. In general, psychiatric disorders do not occur more frequently in the elderly. Even depression—which is not uncommon among the elderly—strikes less often in old age than at earlier stages of the life cycle. Those most likely to become depressed often have lost a spouse and have few social supports. The social ties of the elderly are most likely to fray as they retire, move, or lose spouses and close friends.

Making This Chapter Work for You

A Guide to Psychological Wellness

- Emotional health and mental health are both components of psychological health, our ability to be in touch with our feelings, to perceive reality as it is, and to work toward personal fulfillment.

- The psychologically healthy person is reasonable, self-aware, productive, realistic, and has an appreciation of self and life and the capacity to love others and maintain relationships.

- According to humanist theorist Abraham Maslow, we must first satisfy basic physiological needs—such as those for food, shelter, and sleep—before striving to fulfill higher needs for security, love and affection, and *self-actualization*, the state of functioning at the highest possible level and deriving the greatest possible satisfaction from life.

- Our attitudes and behavior are based on two types of values. Instrumental values represent ways of thinking and acting that we hold important, such as being loving or loyal. Terminal values represent goals, achievements, or ideal states toward which we strive.

- Self-esteem is belief or pride in ourselves, based on a sense of self-respect and acceptance that develops over time. Positive thinking and self-talk, through which we send complimentary or encouraging messages to ourselves, are the most useful techniques for bolstering self-esteem.

- While we all tend to experience bad moods, it is possible to manage, or *regulate*, mood through a variety of strategies. The most effective focus on the problem that caused the bad mood; others aim at dispelling negative feelings.

- Happiness is a sense of subjective well-being that tends to be highest when people combine frequent good experiences with occasional very intense pleasures. It is not based on wealth, beauty, or fame, but on characteristics such as high self-esteem, optimism, and the ability to form close relationships.

■ Optimism involves the conscious decision to seek out and expect positive experiences from life. Along with savoring life's pleasures, large and small, and looking for the humor in daily living, it is a key to finding happiness and achieving good psychological health.

■ We find meaning and fulfillment in life in various ways, including the experiences of loving and being loved, of developing our own spirituality, and of reaching out to help others.

■ Autonomy (a sense of independence) and assertiveness (making your needs and desires clear to others) are keys to a feeling of mastery and being in control of one's life.

■ The essential requirements for feeling energetic are regular exercise, good nutrition, and adequate sleep.

A good night's sleep consists of cycles of both REM (rapid-eye-movement) sleep and quiet, deep (non-REM) sleep. Many Americans do not get adequate sleep and consequently are not functioning at their best.

■ Social isolation is a major risk factor for illness and early death. While loneliness and social anxieties—fears of interacting with others or being observed by others—are common, they can be overcome.

■ Many people who are difficult to get along with suffer from personality disorders, long-standing conditions that reflect their lack of flexibility in adapting to new situations. Since these people are not likely to change, it is best to find ways to work around their often irritating personality characteristics.

Like physical health, psychological well-being is not a fixed state of being, but a process. The way you live

health / ONLINE

What's Your Emotional I.Q.?
http://www.utne.com/azEQ.tmpl
This ten-question online assessment lets you test your "emotional I.Q." and compare it with the national average.

Volunteering Opportunities
http://libraryspot.com/volunteerfeature.htm
Volunteering is a great way to do good for both yourself and for your community. This site includes links to volunteering opportunities with nonprofit organizations such as the Salvation Army, Habitat for Humanity, the Peace Corps, and much more. It also lets you search for volunteering opportunities by zip code, category, or date.

Strategies for Building Self-Esteem
http://www.utexas.edu/student/lsc/handouts/1914.html
The University of Texas at Austin offers students these suggestions for building self-esteem.

Please note that links are subject to change. If you find a broken link, use a search engine like http://www.yahoo.com *and search for the web site by typing in key words.*

 Campus Chat: What does spirituality mean to you? Share your thoughts on our online discussion forum at **http://health.wadsworth.com**

Find It On InfoTrac: You can find additional readings related to stress via InfoTrac College Edition, an online library of more than 900 journals and publications. Follow the instructions for accessing InfoTrac that came packaged with your textbook; then search for articles using a key word search.

• **Suggested article:** "Body Image and Self-Esteem: A Comparison of African-American and Caucasian Women," by Beth L. Molloy and Sharon D. Herzberger. *Sex Roles: A Journal of Research*, April 1998, Vol. 38, No. 7–8, p. 631.

(1) Compared to Caucasian women, why do African-American women have higher self-esteem when it comes to body image?

(2) How does one's socioeconomic status influence the incidence of low self-esteem?

For additional links, resources, and suggested readings on InfoTrac, visit our Health & Wellness Resource Center at **http://health.wadsworth.com**

every day affects how you feel about yourself and your world. Here are some basic guidelines that you can rely on to make the most of the process of living:

■ **Accept yourself.** As a human being, you are, by definition, imperfect. Come to terms with the fact that you are a worthwhile person despite your mistakes.

■ **Respect yourself.** Recognize your abilities and talents. Acknowledge your competence and achievements, and take pride in them.

■ **Trust yourself.** Learn to listen to the voice within you, and let your intuition be your guide.

■ **Love yourself.** Be happy to spend time by yourself. Learn to appreciate your company and to be glad you're you.

■ **Stretch yourself.** Be willing to change and grow, to try something new and dare to be vulnerable.

■ **Look at challenges as opportunities for personal growth.** "Every problem brings the possibility of a widening of consciousness," psychologist Carl Jung once noted. Put his words to the test.

■ **Think of not only where but also who you want to be a decade from now.** The goals you set, the decisions you make, the values you adopt now will determine how you feel about yourself and your life as you enter the twenty-first century.

 Mindful Living. What are the characteristics of "mindful" living?

Key Terms

The terms listed here are used within the chapter. Page numbers are included for each term. A definition of each term is given in the Glossary pages at the end of this book.

altruism   82
assertive   83
autonomy   83
culture   68
emotional health   68
emotional intelligence   69
locus of control   83
mental health   68

mood   77
moral   74
optimism   78
personality disorder   88
rapid-eye-movement (REM) sleep   85
self-actualization   73
self-esteem   75

social isolation   86
social phobia   88
spiritual health   68
spiritual intelligence   70
values   73
victimology   69

Critical Thinking Questions

1. Read over the Campus Focus box in this chapter. Why do you think students' volunteer activity drops between high school and college?

2. Are you aware of your ability to view life positively or negatively? Which way do you most often describe your life? What could you do to become more psychologically healthy?

3. What are some things you can do to achieve happiness? Of these, which have you done before? Have you been successful? Can you think of other ways to achieve happiness not mentioned in the text?

References

1. Diener, Ed, et al. "Subjective Well-being: Three Decades of Progress." *Psychological Bulletin*, Vol. 125, No. 2, March 1999.
2. Shapiro, Deane, and Walsh, Roger. *Beyond Health and Normalcy.* New York: Van Nostrand Reinhold, 1983.
3. Moore, Thomas. *Care of the Soul.* New York: Harper Perennial, 1994.
4. Proffitt, Steve. "Pursuing Happiness with a Positive Outlook, Not a Pill." *Los Angeles Times,* January 24, 1999.
5. Seligman, Martin. Presidential Address. American Psychological Association Annual Meeting, San Francisco, August 1998.
6. Seligman, Martin. "What Is the 'Good Life'?" *APA Monitor,* Vol. 29, No. 10, October 1998.
7. Seligman, Martin. "Building Human Strength: Psychology's Forgotten Mission." *APA Monitor,* Vol. 29, No. 1, January 1998.

8. Seligman, Martin. "Positive Social Science." *APA Monitor,* Vol. 29, No. 4, April 1998.

9. Goleman, Daniel. *Emotional Intelligence.* New York: Bantam Books, 1997.

10. Goleman, Daniel. *Working with Emotional Intelligence.* New York: Bantam Books, 1999.

11. Segal, Jeanne. *Raising Your Emotional Intelligence: A Practical Guide.* New York: Henry Holt, 1997.

12. Goleman, *Working with Emotional Intelligence.*

13. Sloan, R. P., et al. "Religion, Spirituality, and Medicine." *Lancet,* Vol. 353, No. 9153, February 20, 1999.

14. Harris, T. George. "Spiritual Intelligence." Symposium at American Psychological Association Annual Meeting, San Francisco, August 1998.

15. Ornish, Dean. Personal interview.

16. Rokeach, M. *Understanding Human Values: Individual and Society.* New York: Free Press, 1979.

17. Kohlberg, L. *The Psychology of Moral Development.* San Francisco: Harper & Row, 1983.

18. Burley, Rosalynn, et al. "The Relationship Between Goal Orientation and Age Among Adolescents and Adults." *Journal of Genetic Psychology,* Vol. 160, No. 1, March 1999.

19. Stephanie Marston. Personal interview.

20. McGuire, Patrick. "The Link Between Pessimism and Depression Begins in the Way We Talk to Our Inner Selves." *APA Monitor,* Vol. 29, No. 10, October 1998.

21. Randy Larsen. Personal interview.

22. Ibid.

23. Catanzo, Salvatore, and Gregory Greenwood. "Expectancies for Negative Mood Regulation, Coping and Dysphoria Among College Students." *Journal of Counseling Psychology,* Vol. 41, No. 1, 1994.

24. Lyubomirsky, Sonja, and Susan Nolen-Hoeksema. "Self-Perceptuating Properties of Dysphoric Rumination." *Journal of Personality and Social Psychology,* Vol. 63, No. 2, 1993.

25. Cervone, Daniel, et al. "Mood, Self-Efficacy, and Performance Standards: Lower Moods Induce Higher Standards for Performance." *Journal of Personality and Social Psychology,* Vol. 67, No. 3, September 1994.

26. Myers, David. *The Pursuit of Happiness: Who Is Happy—and Why.* New York: William Morrow, 1992.

27. Freeman, Leslie, et al. "The Relationship Between Adult Happiness and Self-Appraised Childhood Happiness and Events." *Journal of Genetic Psychology,* Vol. 160, No. 1, March 1999.

28. Ibid.

29. Chamberlin, Jamie. "People Need Help Finding What Makes Them Happy." *APA Monitor,* Vol. 29, No. 10, October 1998.

30. Freeman, "The Relationship Between Adult Happiness and Self-Appraised Childhood Happiness and Events."

31. Lane, Richard, et al. "Neuroanatomical Correlates of Happiness, Sadness, and Disgust." *American Journal of Psychiatry,* Vol. 154, No. 7, July 1997.

32. Niedenthal, Paula, et al. "Being Happy and Seeing 'Happy': Emotional State Mediates Visual Word Recognition." *Cognition & Emotion,* Vol. 11, No. 4, July 1997.

33. McIntosh, William, et al. "Goal Beliefs, Life Events, and the Malleability of People's Judgments of Their Happiness." *Journal of Social Behavior & Personality,* Vol. 12, No. 2, June 1997.

34. Ornstein, Robert, and David Sobel. *Healthy Pleasures.* Reading, MA: Addison-Wesley, 1990.

35. Seligman, Martin. April, 1988.

36. Brami, Elisabeth, and Philippe Bertran. *Little Moments of Happiness.* New York: Stewart Tabori & Chang, 1997.

37. McGuire, Patrick. "More Psychologists Are Finding That Discrete Uses of Humor Promote Healing in Their Patients." *APA Monitor,* Vol. 30, No. 3, March 1999.

38. Grensing-Pophal, Lin. "Getting Your Dose of Laughter." *Nursing,* Vol. 29, No. 2, February 1999.

39. Ornish, Dean. *Love & Survival: The Scientific Basis for the Healing Power of Intimacy.* New York: HarperCollins, 1999.

40. Moore, *Care of the Soul.*

41. George, Jennifer, and Arthur Brief. "Feeling Good-Doing Good: A Conceptual Analysis of the Mood at Work—Organizational Spontaneity Relationship." *Psychological Bulletin,* Vol. 112, No. 2, 1992.

42. Giles, Dwight, and Janet Eyler. "The Impact of a College Community Service Laboratory on Students' Personal, Social and Cognitive Outcomes." *Journal of Adolescence,* Vol. 17, No. 4, August 1994.

43. Larsen, Randy. Interview.

44. Kowalski, Kathiann. "How to Assert Yourself." *Current Health,* Vol. 25, No. 4, December 1998.

45. Trankina, Michele. "Linking Food to Moods." *World and I,* Vol. 13, No. 3, March 1998.

46. Hales, Dianne, and Robert E. Hales. "Sleep Disorders." In *Caring for the Mind: The Comprehensive Guide to Mental Health.* New York: Bantam Books, 1995.

47. Zepf, Bill. "Problem Sleepiness: An Often Unrecognized Condition." *American Family Physician,* February 15, 1999.

48. Voelker, Rebecca. "Sleep and Hypertension. *Journal of the American Medical Association,* Vol. 281, No. 10, March 10, 1999.

49. Teran-Santo, J., et al. "The Association Between Sleep Apnea and the Risk of Traffic Accidents." *New England Journal of Medicine,* Vol. 340, No. 11, March 18, 1999.

50. Schwartz, Richard. "Loneliness." *Harvard Review of Psychiatry,* Vol. 5, No. 2, July–August 1997.

51. "Health: That's What Friend & Family Are For." *Facts of Life: An Issue Briefing for Health Reporters from the Center for Advancement of Health,* Vol. 2, No. 6, November–December 1997.

52. Bucholz, Ester. *The Call of Solitude: Alonetime in a World of Attachment.* New York: Simon & Schuster, 1997.

53. Rokach, Ami, and Heather Brock. "Loneliness and the Effects of Life Changes." *Journal of Psychology,* Vol. 131, No. 3, May 1997.

54. Nurmi, Jari-Erik, and Katarina Salmela-Aro. "Social Strategies and Loneliness." *Personality & Individual Differences,* Vol. 23, No. 2, August 1997.

55. Preboth, Monica, and Shyla Wright. "Does the Internet Make People Unhappy?" *American Family Physician,* Vol. 59, No. 6, March 15, 1999.

56. Rokach, Ami. "Relations of Perceived Causes and the Experience of Loneliness." *Psychological Reports,* Vol. 80, No. 3, June 1997.

57. Clinton, Monique, and Lynn Anderson. "Social and Emotional Loneliness: Gender Differences and Relationships with Self-Monitoring and Perceived Control." *Journal of Black Psychology,* Vol. 25, No. 1, February 1999.

58. Cramer, Kenneth, and Kimberley Neyedley. "Sex Differences in Loneliness: The Role of Masculinity and Feminity." *Sex Roles: A Journal of Research,* Vol. 38, No. 7–8, April 1998.

59. Stack, Stephen. "Marriage, Family, and Loneliness: A Cross-National Study." *Sociological Perspectives,* Vol. 41, No. 2, Summer 1998.

60. Koropeckyj-Cox, Tanya. "Loneliness and Depression in Middle and Old Age: Are the Childless More Vulnerable?" *Journals of Gerontology,* Vol. 53, No. 6, November 1998.

61. Mannuzza, Salvatore, et al. "Generalized Social Phobia." *Archives of General Psychiatry,* Vol. 52, No. 3, March 1995.

62. Potts, Nicholas, and Jonathan Davidson. "Epidemiology and Pharmacotherapy of Social Phobia." *Psychiatric Times,* February 1995. Morris, Lois. "Social Anxiety." *American Health,* January–February 1995.

63. John Oldham. Personal interview.

64. Kass, J. (1998) *The Inventory of Positive Psychological Attitudes: Measuring attitudes which buffer stress and facilitate primary prevention.* In C. Zalaquett, R. Wood (Ed.) *Evaluating stress: A book of resources,* Vol. 2. Lanham, MD: Scarecrow Press/University Press of America.
Kass, J. Friedman, R., Leserman, J., Caudill, M., Zuttermeister, P., Benson, H. (1991). An inventory of positive psychological attitudes with potential relevance to health outcomes: Validation and preliminary testing. *Behavioral Medicine,* Fall, 17(3), 121–129.

4

Caring for the Mind

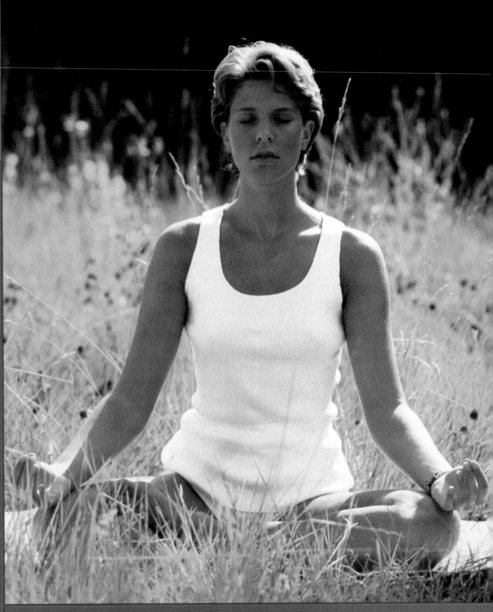

After studying the material in this chapter, you should be able to:

- **Identify** the major psychological problems experienced by members of our society.
- **Describe** the symptoms and risk factors associated with depression, anxiety disorders, attention disorders, and schizophrenia.
- **List** strategies to help prevent suicide.
- **Discuss** behaviors indicating the need for professional help and how to find such help.
- **Explain** why the brain is considered the last frontier.
- **Explain** some of the approaches used by professional therapists.

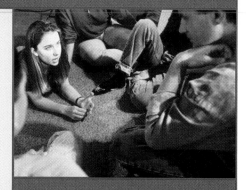

W e all live through bad days, sad times, crushing setbacks, heartbreaking losses. We may eat too much, sleep too little, reach too often for a drink or drug. At some point in life, one of every three people develops an emotional disorder. Young adulthood—the years from the late teens to the mid-twenties—is a time when many serious disorders, including bipolar illness (manic depression) and schizophrenia, often develop. The saddest fact is not that so many feel so bad, but that so few realize they can feel better. Only one out of every five men and women who could use treatment ever seeks help. Yet 80 to 90 percent of those treated for psychological problems recover, most within a few months.[1]

The problems of the mind can be far more perplexing than the ailments of the body. If the problem were an aching knee or a queasy stomach, we might know—or could easily find out—its cause, what we can do about it, whether to see a doctor. But because psychological pain can't be seen, touched, X-rayed, or biopsied, we can't always be sure how serious distress is. Yet, if ignored, emotional aches and pains can become more severe and more difficult to overcome—and can increase the risk and cost of physical illness.

By learning about psychological disorders, you may be able to recognize early warning signals in yourself or your loved ones so you can deal with potential difficulties or seek professional help for more serious problems.

 FREQUENTLY ASKED QUESTIONS

FAQ: **What is a mental disorder? p. 97**

FAQ: **How common are mental disorders? p. 97**

FAQ: **Does mental health affect physical health? p. 97**

FAQ: **What leads to suicide? p. 107**

FAQ: **Where can I turn for help? p. 111**

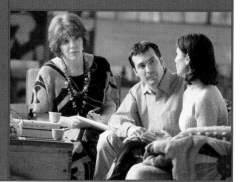

What Is Mental Health?

Mental health is not an absence of distress, but rather the capacity to think rationally and logically and to cope with life's transitions, stresses, traumas, and losses in a way that allows for emotional stability and growth. As described in Chapter 3, mentally healthy individuals value themselves, perceive reality as it is, accept their limitations and possibilities, carry out their responsibilities, establish and maintain close relationships, pursue work that suits their talent and training, and feel a sense of fulfillment that makes the efforts of daily living worthwhile (see Figure 4-1).

The Mental State of College Students

Many people assume that bright, young college students, at the peak of physical health, are immune from serious mental illness. This is not the case. Many mental disorders first develop in adolescence and young adulthood (See Campus Focus: "When Mental Disorders Begin"). Some students already suffer from problems like attention disorders or panic attacks (both discussed later in this chapter) when they arrive as freshmen. Others, as noted in Chapter 2, become overwhelmed by the stresses of being on their own and facing intense academic pressures. Those who experiment with drugs or alcohol may become addicted to these substances. Some develop other

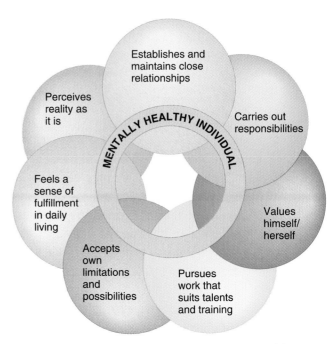

■ Figure 4-1 Mental well-being is a combination of factors.

addictive behaviors, such as compulsive buying (which affects an estimated 6 percent of undergraduates).[2]

Only recently, however, have researchers begun to study the mental state of undergraduates in depth. In the past, even faculty and administrators shared the common misconception that mental disorders strike only the old, the poor, the sick, and the disadvantaged.

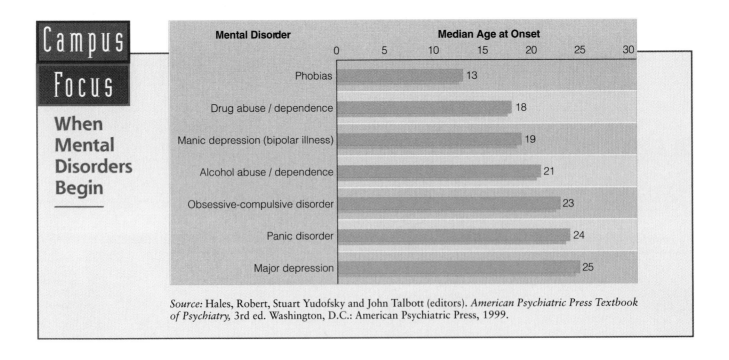

Campus Focus

When Mental Disorders Begin

Mental Disorder	Median Age at Onset
Phobias	13
Drug abuse / dependence	18
Manic depression (bipolar illness)	19
Alcohol abuse / dependence	21
Obsessive-compulsive disorder	23
Panic disorder	24
Major depression	25

Source: Hales, Robert, Stuart Yudofsky and John Talbott (editors). *American Psychiatric Press Textbook of Psychiatry,* 3rd ed. Washington, D.C.: American Psychiatric Press, 1999.

But no one—not even one who is young, bright, and fit—is immune to mental illness, and its consequences can be devastating. Each year 6 of every 100,000 college students in the United States kill themselves. A small but growing number assault and sometimes even kill other students.[3]

Awareness of mental health issues on campus is increasing, and many schools are expanding their psychological services and offering screenings for stress, **anxiety,** and depression. Students too must learn to recognize early symptoms and take steps to get help quickly for themselves or for a troubled friend. The good news, as you'll learn in this chapter, is that most mental disorders can be treated successfully. (See Table 4-1.)

 ## What Is a Mental Disorder?

While lay people may speak of "nervous breakdowns" or "insanity," these are not scientific terms. The U.S. government's official definition states that a serious mental illness is "a diagnosable mental, behavioral, or emotional disorder that interferes with one or more major activities in life, like dressing, eating, or working."[4]

The mental health profession's standard for diagnosing a mental disorder is the pattern of symptoms, or diagnostic criteria, spelled out for the almost 300 disorders in the American Psychiatric Association's *Diagnostic and Statistical Manual,* 4th edition (DSM-IV). It defines a **mental disorder** as "a clinically significant behavioral or psychological syndrome or pattern that occurs in an individual and that is associated with present distress (a painful symptom) or disability (impairment in one or more important areas of functioning) or with a significantly increased risk of suffering death, pain, disability, or an important loss of freedom."[5] (See Self-Survey: "Is Something Wrong?")

 ## How Common Are Mental Disorders?

Individuals with mental and emotional problems often feel terribly alone, as if no one else experiences or understands the misery they feel. Yet, as careful epidemiologic studies conducted in recent years have shown, mental disorders are much more common than had long been assumed. Approximately 52 million Americans aged 15 to 54 suffer from some form of mental illness.[6] During any given year, 30% of Americans suffer from at least one mental disorder.[7] The most common single mental disorder is major **depression,** while the anxiety disorders are the most prevalent group

of mental illnesses. Other common problems are alcohol dependence and abuse, drug dependence and abuse, and dysthymia (chronic mild depression).

Many individuals suffer from several mental disorders: 14 percent reported three or more disorders during their lifetime while an additional 13 percent had at least two mental disorders. Yet only 42 percent of those with a lifetime history of one or more mental disorders ever received any professional care. Just one in every four (26 percent) obtained treatment from a mental health professional.[8]

 ## Does Mental Health Affect Physical Health?

Mental disorders affect not just the mind, but also the body. Depression can have an impact on treatment and recovery from many physical conditions, including asthma, stroke, and cancer. It is a major risk factor for heart disease in healthy adults and exacerbates existing heart problems. In women, it accelerates the changes in bone mass that lead to osteoporosis.[9] In individuals who have a serious physical illness, depression doubles the length of time that they require hospitalization.[10] Anxiety can lead to intensified asthmatic reactions, skin conditions, and digestive disorders. As discussed in Chapter 2, stress can play a role in hypertension, heart attacks, sudden cardiac death and immune disorders.

By some estimates, as many as 60 percent of those who seek help from physicians suffer primarily from a psychological problem. Treating mental health problems leads not only to improved health but also to lower health-care costs. According to various studies, mental health care has reduced annual medical costs by 9.5 to 21 percent. Psychiatric treatment reduces hospitalizations, cuts medical expenses, and reduces work disability. The American Psychiatric Association's Commission on Psychotherapy by Psychiatrists estimates that every dollar spent on psychotherapy may save four dollars in medical costs.[11]

The Brain: The Last Frontier

The brain has intrigued scientists for centuries, but only recently have its explorers made dramatic progress in unraveling its mysteries. Leaders in **neuropsychiatry**—the field that brings together the study of the brain and the mind—remind us that 95 percent of what is known about brain anatomy, chemistry, and physiology has been learned in the last decade. These discoveries have reshaped our understanding of the organ that is central

■ **Table 4-1** The Top Four Mental Disorders of Young Adulthood

	Depression	**Bipolar Disorder**	**Anxiety Disorders**	**Schizophrenia**
Who Is Affected	One in 8 adolescents and young adults; women are twice as likely to become depressed.	One-third of young people diagnosed with major depression will also be diagnosed with bipolar disorder.	One in 10 adolescents have one or more anxiety disorders, including generalized anxiety disorder, panic disorder, or obsessive-compulsive disorder.	Three in 1,000 adolescents and young adults.
Symptoms	These symptoms must be consistent and last for two weeks or longer: pervasive sadness, anxiety and hopelessness; oversleeping or insomnia; sudden lack of interest in school; falling grades; social isolation; dropping once-loved activities; overeating or loss of appetite; drug or alcohol abuse; questions or comments about suicide; extreme irritability.	Bipolar disorder can send individuals plunging from a "high" state, where they believe they have superhuman energy and abilities, into a pit of despair. Symptoms of the manic/high state include grandiosity; pressured or rapid speech; racing thoughts; decreased need for sleep; distractibility; hyperactivity; impulsive behavior.	Symptoms include exaggerated and chronic worry; frequent fatigue, headache or nausea (generalized anxiety disorder); unrealistic worry or fear of dying accompanied by chest pain, shortness of breath, heart palpitations and abdominal discomfort (panic disorder); repetitive, intrusive thoughts and/or rituals such as washing, touching, counting, organizing, checking, hoarding (OCD).	The following symptoms must be present for at least six months for the disease to be diagnosed: delusions; hallucinations; disorganized thinking; paranoia; sudden lack of drive or initiative; social withdrawal; apathy; and emotional unresponsiveness.
Family Risk	Those with a depressed parent are twice as likely to become depressed. If both parents had the illness, the risk quadruples.	A family history of bipolar disorder increases risk, though it's not clear how much.	There are indications that an imbalance of the brain chemical serotonin seems to run in families; it may contribute to anxiety-related illnesses.	Risk increases if relatives have the disorder. Recent brain-imagery research shows an imbalance in dopamine and serotonin in those with schizophrenia.
Treatments	Psychotherapy is usually recommended for milder forms and may be used in combination with antidepressants. Occasionally, hospitalization in a psychiatric unit may be required for teens with severe depression or those at risk for suicide.	Psychotherapy is usually used in combination with mood-stabilizing medications such as Lithium or Depakote.	Cognitive behavioral therapy, which offers specific techniques to reduce anxiety and minimize compulsions, is recommended along with family therapy. Medications such as Prozac, Paxil, and Anafranil are frequently prescribed.	Atypicals, a new class of drugs including Clozaril, Risperdal, and Zyprexa, treats symptoms with fewer side effects and is especially helpful for young adults. Psychotherapy is also recommended to help teens remain medication compliant.
Resources	**National Institute of Mental Health** Depression Awareness, Recognition and Treatment Program; 800-421-4211; www.nimh.nih.gov **American Foundation for Suicide Prevention;** 888-333-AFSP; www.afsp.org	**National Depressive and Manic Depressive Association;** 800-826-3632; www.ndmda.org **Depression and Related Affective Disorders Association** in Baltimore; 410-955-4647; www.med.jhu.edu/drada/; E-mail: drada@welchlink.welch.jhu.edu	**National OCD Information Hotline:** 800-NEWS-4-OCD **Anxiety Disorders Association of America** in Rockville, MD; 301-231-9350; www.adaa.org **National Anxiety Foundation** in Lexington, KY; 606-272-7166; www.lexington-on-line.com/naf.html	**National Alliance for Research on Schizophrenia and Depression;** 800-829-8289; www.mhsource.com/narsad.html

Source: American Health for Women, November/December 1998.

Self-*Survey* Is Something Wrong?

Which of the following apply to you? Think about how you've been feeling over the past month, and check all that apply. Be honest with yourself.

- feel depressed or sad for several weeks ❑
- lack energy or feel tired all the time ❑
- take no joy or pleasure in normally enjoyable activities ❑
- think or talk about suicide ❑
- experience extreme mood swings ❑
- feel helpless or hopeless ❑
- feel excessively anxious ❑
- abuse alcohol or drugs ❑
- show a marked change in personality ❑

- feel unable to cope with problems and daily activities ❑
- show marked changes in eating or sleeping patterns ❑
- feel extremely angry, hostile, or violent ❑
- express bizarre or grandiose ideas ❑
- be unable to control or stop destructive behavior, like gambling or drinking ❑
- develop troubling physical symptoms that have no known medical cause ❑
- see things, experience sensations, or hear voices that don't exist ❑

The more of these boxes that describe what you (or someone close to you) have been experiencing in recent weeks, the more reason you have to be concerned that something may be wrong. This chapter provides information on common mental disorders, as well as guidance on finding and evaluating a therapist and advice on coping with everyday problems.

Psychological symptoms don't mean that you're "crazy," but they do indicate you need help in sorting out your life. Just as your body sometimes breaks down under the normal strain of day-to-day living, your mind also is vulnerable to dysfunction. Seeking help is the first step to feeling better and finding solutions to your problems. If you are struggling with a problem, you may want to schedule an appointment with a mental health professional at your school's counseling or student health-services facility.

Making Changes

Deciding If You Need Help

If you are still unsure about whether to seek help, the following questions may help in making the decision:

- Are emotional problems getting in the way of your work, relationships, or other aspects of your personal life?

- Have you been feeling less happy, less confident, and less in control than usual for a period of several weeks or longer?
- Have you reached the point of being so unhappy that you want to do something about it?
- Have close, trusted friends or family members commented on changes in your behavior and personality?
- Have your own efforts to deal with a problem failed to resolve the situation?
- Is dealing with everyday problems more of a struggle than it used to be?
- Do you feel emotionally "stuck" and helpless to change your own behavior or the circumstances you are in?

The key question to ask yourself is not, "Am I mentally ill?" or "Do I have serious problems?" but "Could I use some help right now?" If the answer is yes, do it. Therapy may turn out to be a catalyst and tool for change or a source of support when you need it most. At the very least, the psychological equivalent of a checkup can make sure that a problem isn't more serious than you may have realized.

to our identity and well-being and have fostered great hope for more effective therapies for the more than 1,000 disorders—psychiatric and neurologic—that affect the brain and nervous system.

Inside the Brain

Each human brain contains hundreds of billions of nerve cells, or **neurons,** and support cells called **glia.**

Most are present at birth, when the brain weighs less than a pound. In the first six years of life—the period when we acquire more knowledge more rapidly than ever again—the brain reaches its full weight of about 3 pounds (see Figure 4-2). From birth, male and female brains differ in a variety of ways. (See The X & Y Files: "Do Men's Brains Differ from Women's?")

The neurons are the basic working units of the brain. Like snowflakes, no two are exactly the same. Each consists of a cell body containing the **nucleus;** a long fiber, called the **axon,** which can range from less than an inch to several feet in length; an **axon terminal,** or ending; and multiple branching fibers called **dendrites.** The glia serve as the scaffolding for the brain, separate the brain from the bloodstream, assist in the growth of neurons, speed up the transmission of nerve impulses, and engulf and digest damaged neurons.

As the master control center for the body, the brain is constantly receiving information from the senses and relaying messages to various parts of the body. Some of these messages travel through the spinal cord, which extends from the neck about two-thirds of the way down the backbone. Other signals are carried by nerves that connect the brain directly with certain parts of the body.

Historically, scientists have focused on the anatomy or structures of the brain in their attempts to understand how it functions and why it sometimes malfunctions. Modern neuropsychiatrists have shifted much of their attention to biochemical processes within the brain, particularly those involved in communication between neurons.

Communication Within the Brain

Neurons "talk" with each other by means of electrical and chemical processes (see Figure 4-3). An electric charge, or impulse, travels along an axon to the terminal, where packets of chemicals called **neurotransmitters** are stored. When released, these messengers flow out of the axon terminal and cross a **synapse,** a specialized site at which the axon terminal of one neuron comes extremely close to a dendrite from another neuron. On the surface of the dendrite are **receptors,** protein molecules designed to bind with neurotransmitters. It takes only about a ten-thousandth of a second for a neurotransmitter and a receptor to come together—a union that neuropsychiatrist Richard Restak, author of *Receptors,* has lyrically compared to an embrace between two lovers. Neurotransmitters that do not connect with receptors may remain in the synapse until they are reabsorbed by the cell that produced them—a process called **reuptake**—or broken down by enzymes.

A malfunction in the release of a neurotransmitter, in its reuptake or elimination, or in the receptors or secondary messengers may result in abnormalities in think-

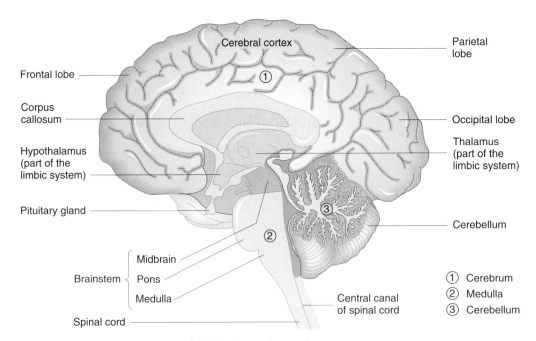

■ Figure 4-2 The brain. The three major parts of the brain are the cerebrum, cerebellum, and brainstem. The cerebrum is divided into two hemispheres—the left which regulates the right side of the body and the right, the left side. The cerebellum plays the major role in coordinating movement, balance, and posture. The brainstem contains centers that control breathing, blood pressure, heart rate, and other "autonomic" physiological functions.

The X&Y Files — Do Men's Brains Differ from Women's?

he brain is not an organ of sex," the pioneering feminist and economist Charlotte Perkins Gilman declared in 1898. "[We might] as well speak of the female liver." These days, gender scientists do indeed speak of the female liver, describing it as one of the most sexually distinctive of organs. What then of the brain? Consider these recent findings:

- **Men's brains are bigger; women use more neurons.** Overall, a woman's brain, like her body, is 10 to 15 percent smaller than a man's, yet the regions dedicated to higher cognitive functions such as language are more densely packed with neurons—and women use more of them. When a male puts his mind to work, neurons turn on in highly specific areas. When females set their minds on similar tasks, cells light up all over the brain.

- **Male and female brains perceive light and sound differently.** A man's eyes are more sensitive to bright light and retain their ability to see well at long distances longer in life. A woman hears a much broader range of sounds, and her hearing remains sharper longer.

- **The female brain responds more more intensely to emotion.** According to neuroimaging studies, the sexes clearly respond differently to emotions, especially sad-ness, which activates, or turns on, neurons in an area eight times larger in women than men.

- **Male and female brains age in different ways.** The male brain loses tissue at almost three times the rate of the female brain. Because of this gender difference, men's all-important frontal lobes, which are larger in youth and early adulthood, reach approximately the same size by the time both sexes reach their forties. Other parts of men's brains—including the corpus callosum and the left hemisphere—also atrophy more rapidly.

- **Neither sex's brain is "better."** Intelligence per se appears equal in both. The greatest gender differences appear both at the top and bottom of the intelligence scales. Men outnumber women both as geniuses and as morons. Nevertheless, more than half the time, regardless of the type of test, most women and men perform more or less equally—even though they may well take different routes to arrive at the same answers. And there is greater variability in cognitive skills both among women and among men than there is between the sexes. The best evaluation of all may have come from the essayist Samuel Johnson. When asked whether women or men are more intelligent, he responded, "Which man? Which woman?"

---

ing, feeling, or behavior. Some of the most promising and exciting research in neuropsychiatry is focusing on correcting such malfunctions. Serotonin and its receptors have been shown to affect mood, sleep, behavior, appetite, memory, learning, sexuality, and aggression and to play a role in several mental disorders.

The discovery of a possible link between low levels of serotonin and some cases of major depression has already led to the development of more precisely targeted **antidepressant** medications that boost serotonin to normal levels. In the next decade, neuropsychiatric research may yield a new generation of breakthrough medications for an ever-growing number of mental disorders.[12]

Anxiety Disorders

The most common type of mental illness, anxiety disorders may involve inordinate fears of certain objects or situations (**phobias**), episodes of sudden, inexplicable terror (**panic attacks**), chronic distress (**generalized anxiety disorder, or GAD**), or persistent, disturbing thoughts and behaviors (**obsessive compulsive disorder**). Over a lifetime, according to the National Comorbidity Survey, as many as one in four Americans may experience an **anxiety disorder**. Only one of every four of these individuals is ever correctly diagnosed and treated. Yet most who do get treatment, even for severe and disabling problems, improve dramatically.[13]

Phobias

Phobias—the most prevalent type of anxiety disorder—are out-of-the-ordinary, irrational, intense, persistent fears of certain objects or situations. About two million Americans develop such acute terror that they go to extremes to avoid whatever it is that they fear, even though they realize that these feelings are excessive or unreasonable.[14] The most common phobias involve animals, particularly dogs, snakes, insects, and mice; the sight of blood; closed spaces (*claustrophobia*); heights (*acrophobia*); air travel and being in places or situations from which they perceive it would be difficult or embarrassing to escape (*agoraphobia*).

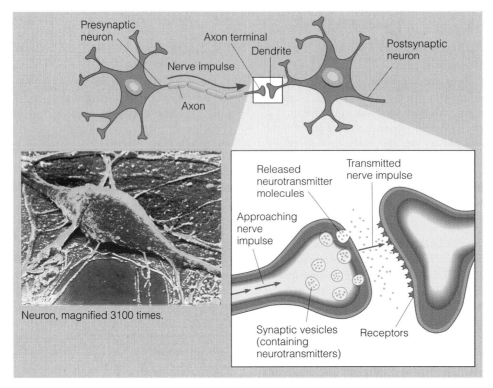

■ **Figure 4-3** The neuron is the basic working unit of the brain. Neurotransmitters released across the synapse transmit the chemical nerve impulse from one neuron to another.

Although various medications have been tried, none is effective by itself in relieving phobias. The best approach is behavior therapy, which consists of gradual, systematic exposure to the feared object (a process called *systematic desensitization*). Numerous studies have proven that exposure—especially in-vivo exposure, in which individuals are exposed to the actual source of their fear rather than simply imagining it—is highly effective; medical hypnosis—the use of induction of an altered state of consciousness—also can help.[15]

The characteristic symptoms of a phobia include:

- Excessive or unreasonable fear of a specific object or situation.
- Immediate, invariable anxiety when exposed to the object or situation.
- Recognition that the fear is excessive or unreasonable.
- Avoidance of the feared object or situation or enduring it only with intense anxiety or distress.
- Inability to function as usual at school or work or in social relationships because of the phobia.

Panic Attacks and Panic Disorder

Individuals who have had panic attacks describe them as the most frightening experiences of their lives.

Without reason or warning, their hearts race wildly. They may become light-headed or dizzy. Because they can't catch their breath, they may start breathing rapidly and hyperventilate. Parts of their bodies, such as their fingers or toes, may tingle or feel numb. Worst of all is the terrible sense that something horrible is about to happen: that they will die, lose their minds, or have a heart attack. Most attacks reach peak intensity within

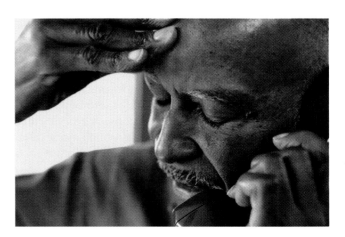

Most panic attacks occur during normal everyday activities. Observing someone having a panic attack, you may get no indication that the person is experiencing a high degree of distress.

ten minutes. Afterward, individuals live in dread of another one. **Panic disorder** develops when attacks recur or apprehension about them becomes so intense that individuals cannot function normally.

About one-third of all young adults experience at least one panic attack between the ages of 15 and 35. Full-blown panic disorder occurs in about 1.6 percent of all adults in the course of a lifetime and usually develops before age 30. Women are more than twice as likely as men to experience panic attacks, although no one knows precisely why. Parents, siblings, and children of individuals with panic disorders also are more likely to develop them than are others.

The two primary treatments for panic disorder are cognitive-behavioral therapy, which teaches specific strategies for coping with symptoms like rapid breathing, and medication. Treatment helps as many as 90 percent of those with panic disorder either improve significantly or recover completely, usually within six to eight weeks. Individuals who receive cognitive-behavioral therapy as well as medication are less likely to suffer relapses than those taking medication alone.[16]

The characteristic symptoms of panic attacks are:

- Palpitations, pounding heart, or accelerated heart rate.
- Sweating.
- Trembling or shaking.
- Sensations of shortness of breath or smothering.
- Feeling of choking.
- Chest pain or discomfort.
- Nausea or abdominal distress.
- Feeling dizzy, unsteady, lightheaded, or faint.
- Feelings of unreality or being detached from oneself.
- Fear of losing control or going crazy.
- Fear of dying.
- Numbness or tingling sensations.
- Chills or hot flushes.

Generalized Anxiety Disorder

The hallmark of a generalized anxiety disorder (GAD) is excessive or unrealistic apprehension that causes physical symptoms and lasts for six months or longer. Unlike fear, which helps us recognize and avoid real danger, GAD is an irrational or unwarranted response to harmless objects or situations of exaggerated danger. The most common symptoms are faster heart rate, sweating, increased blood pressure, muscle aches, intestinal pains, irritability, sleep problems, and difficulty concentrating.

Chronically anxious individuals worry—not just some of the time, and not just about the stresses and strains of ordinary life—but constantly, about almost everything: their health, families, finances, marriages, potential dangers. Treatment for GAD may consist of a combination of psychotherapy, behavioral therapy, and antianxiety drugs.

Obsessive-Compulsive Disorder

As many as 1 in 40 Americans has a type of anxiety called obsessive-compulsive disorder (OCD). Some of these individuals suffer only from an *obsession*, a recurring idea, thought, or image that they realize, at least initially, is senseless. The most common obsessions are repetitive thoughts of violence (e.g., killing a child), contamination (becoming infected by shaking hands), and doubt (wondering whether one has performed some act, such as having hurt someone in a traffic accident). Most people with OCD also suffer from a *compulsion*, repetitive behavior performed according to certain rules or in a stereotyped fashion. The most common compulsions involve handwashing, cleaning, hoarding useless items, counting, or checking (for example, making sure dozens of times that a door is locked).

Individuals with OCD realize that their thoughts or behaviors are bizarre, but they cannot resist or control them. Eventually, the obsessions or compulsions consume a great deal of time and significantly interfere with normal routine, job functioning, or usual social activities or relationships with others. A young woman who must follow a very rigid dressing routine may always be late for class, for example; a student who must count each letter of the alphabet as he types may not be able to complete a term paper.

OCD is believed to have biological roots. It may be a result of gene abnormalities, head injury, or even an autoimmune reaction after childhood infection with strep bacteria. Treatment may consist of cognitive therapy to correct irrational assumptions, behavioral techniques such as progressively limiting the amount of time someone obsessed with cleanliness can spend washing and scrubbing, and medication. About 70 to 80% of those with OCD improve with treatment.

Depressive Disorders

Depression, the world's most common mental ailment, affects the brain, the mind, and the body in complex ways. Stress-related events may trigger half of all depressive episodes; great trauma in childhood can increase vulnerability to depression later in life.[17] Individuals who develop major depression in adolescence are at especially high risk of suffering recurrences in young adulthood. (See Table 4-2.)[18]

Comparing everyday "blues" to a **depressive disorder** is like comparing a cold to pneumonia. Major depression can destroy a person's joy for living. Food, friends, sex, or any form of pleasure no longer appeals. It is impossible to concentrate on work and responsibilities. Unable to escape a sense of utter hopelessness, depressed individuals may fight back tears throughout the day and toss and turn through long, empty nights. Thoughts of death or suicide may push into their minds.

But there is good news: Depression is a treatable disease; psychotherapy is remarkably effective for mild depression. In more serious cases, antidepressant medication can lead to dramatic improvement in 40 to 80 percent of depressed patients.[19]

Major Depression

The simplest definition of **major depression** is sadness that does not end. The incidence of major depression has soared over the last two decades, especially among young adults. The National Comorbidity Survey found that major depression is the most widespread mental disorder, affecting 10.3 percent of Americans in any given year.

The characteristic symptoms of major depression include:

- Feeling depressed, sad, empty, discouraged, tearful.
- Loss of interest or pleasure in once-enjoyable activities.
- Eating more or less than usual and either gaining or losing weight.
- Having trouble sleeping or sleeping much more than usual.
- Feeling slowed down or restless and unable to sit still.
- Lack of energy.
- Feeling helpless, hopeless, worthless, inadequate.
- Difficulty concentrating, forgetfulness.
- Difficulty thinking clearly or making decisions.
- Persistent thoughts of death or suicide.
- Withdrawal from others, lack of interest in sex.
- Physical symptoms (headaches, digestive problems, aches and pains).

Most cases of major depression can be treated successfully, usually with psychotherapy, medication, or both. Psychotherapy alone works in more than half of mild-to-moderate episodes of major depression. Psychotherapy helps individuals pinpoint the life problems that contribute to their depression, identify negative or distorted thinking patterns, explore behaviors that contribute to depression, and regain a sense of control and pleasure in life.[20] Two specific psychotherapies—cognitive-behavioral therapy and interpersonal therapy (described later in this chapter)—have proved as helpful as antidepressant drugs in treating mild cases of depression, although they take longer than medication to achieve results.

Antidepressant medications work for more than half of those with moderate-to-severe depression and may be useful in treating mild depression in individuals who do not improve with psychotherapy alone (see the section on psychiatric drug therapy, later in this chapter). These prescription drugs generally take three or four weeks to produce significant benefits and may not have their full impact for up to eight weeks.

Newer antidepressants that boost levels of the neurotransmitter serotonin—the selective serotonin recep-

---

■ Table 4-2 The Natural History of Depression

Likelihood that a person will develop major depression or dysthymia in his/her lifetime: **6.1%**
Likelihood that a person will suffer some depressive symptoms in his/her lifetime: **23.1%**
Average age of first onset of major depression: **25–29**
Average duration of all depressive episodes: **20 weeks**
Percent of patients who recover within a year after onset of symptoms: **74%**
Likelihood of a second or more episodes of major depression: **80%**
Likelihood of a second or more episodes of minor depression: **100%**
Median number of major depressive episodes during a patient's lifetime: **4**
Percent of patients whose depression takes a chronic unremitting course: **12%**
Incidence of depression in women vs men: **3.62 vs 1.98** per 1,000 per year
Female:male ratio of depression incidence in cultures with low rates of alcoholism: **1:1**
Rank of unipolar major depression in the world league of disabling diseases in 1990: **4**
Rank of unipolar major depression among disabling diseases in westernized countries: **2**
Rank of depression among disabling diseases the world over, projected, in 2020: **2**

Source: Psychology Today, March/April 1999.

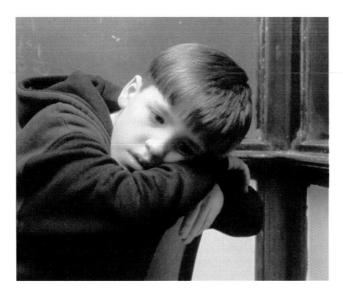

An increasing number of children suffer from bouts of depression, experiencing feelings of overwhelming hopelessness, helplessness, and sadness.

tor inhibitors (SSRIs)—have proven equally effective as older medications, but their side effects are different. The older drugs are more likely to adversely affect the heart and blood pressure and to cause dry mouth, constipation, dizziness, blurred vision, and tremors. Patients taking SSRIs report higher rates of diarrhea, nausea, insomnia, and headache.[21]

Eighty percent of people who have one episode of depression are likely to have another. Because of this high risk of recurrence, many psychiatrists now view depression as a chronic disease and advise ongoing treatment with antidepressants. However, little is known about the long-term effects of these medications.[22]

In individuals who cannot take antidepressant medications because of medical problems, or who do not improve with psychotherapy or drugs, *electroconvulsive therapy (ECT)*—the administration of a controlled electrical current through electrodes attached to the scalp—remains the safest and most effective treatment. About 50 percent of depressed individuals who do not get better with antidepressant medication and psychotherapy improve after ECT.

Manic Depression (Bipolar Disorder)

Manic depression, or **bipolar disorder,** consists of mood swings that may take individuals from *manic* states of feeling euphoric and energetic to depressive states of utter despair. In episodes of full mania, they may become so impulsive and out of touch with reality that they endanger their careers, relationships, health, or even survival. One percent of the population—about 2 million American adults—suffer from this serious but treatable disorder, which affects both genders and all races equally.

The characteristic symptoms of manic depression include mood swings (from happy to miserable, optimistic to despairing, and so on); changes in thinking (thoughts speeding through one's mind; unrealistic self-confidence; difficulty concentrating; delusions; hallucinations); changes in behavior (sudden immersion in plans and projects; talking very rapidly and much more than usual; excessive spending; impaired judgment; impulsive sexual involvement); and changes in physical condition (less need for sleep; increased energy; fewer health complaints than usual). During "manic" periods, individuals may make grandiose plans or take dangerous risks. But they often plunge from this highest of highs to a horrible low depressive episode, in which they may feel sad, hopeless, and helpless, and develop other symptoms of major depression. The risk of suicide is very real.

Professional therapy is essential in treating bipolar disorders. Mood-stabilizing medications are the keystone of treatment, although psychotherapy plays a critical role in helping individuals understand their illness and rebuild their lives. Most individuals continue taking medication indefinitely after remission of their symptoms because the risk of recurrence is high.[23]

Other Forms of Depression

In **seasonal affective disorder (SAD),** annual episodes of depression usually begin at the same time each year, most often from the beginning of October through November, and end in March or April, with the coming of spring. January and February, often cloudy and dark, are usually the worst months. According to National Institute of Mental Health (NIMH) estimates, some 10 million Americans have SAD. Although the gloomy gray days of winter can dampen anyone's spirits, these individuals feel helpless, guilt-ridden, and hopeless and have difficulty thinking and making decisions. Typically, they eat more and gain weight. In particular, many crave rich carbohydrates. They spend many more hours asleep, yet feel chronically exhausted.

SAD often improves with a specialized treatment: exposure to bright light, known as *phototherapy,* in which individuals sit in front of a specially designed light box every day during winter months. For severe forms of seasonal depression, therapists may combine phototherapy with antidepressant medications.

Dysthymia is the clinical term for chronic mild depression. Dysthymia, which usually develops in childhood, adolescence, or early adult life, occurs equally in boys and girls, but in adults it is more common among women. Individuals with this disorder experience symptoms of depression most of the day, and more days than not, for a period of at least two years. They also may have low self-esteem, eat and sleep more or less than usual, lack energy, have problems concentrating or making decisions, and feel a sense of hopelessness. Their symptoms, however, are less intense than those of major depression. A combination of drug and talk therapy has proven more effective than either treatment alone in treating dysthymia.[24] Aerobic exercise seems to be an especially helpful form of adjunctive, or additional, therapy.

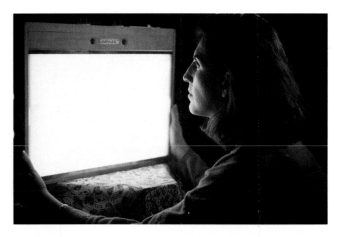

People with seasonal affective disorder (SAD), a form of depression, can be treated with bright-light therapy.

Suicide

Suicide is not in itself a psychiatric disorder, but it can be the tragic consequence of emotional and psychological problems. Every year 30,000 Americans—among them many young people who seem to have "everything to live for"—commit suicide. Ten times this many individuals attempt to take their own lives.

In the last thirty years, there have been significant increases in reported suicides among young adults between the ages of 15 and 24, children between the ages of 10 and 14, and young African-American men.[25] The suicide rate among males of all ages and races has increased fivefold since 1950.[26] College students commit suicide at about half the rate of young people their age who are not in school. Suicide rates at highly competitive schools are not significantly different from those at less rigorous ones. However, college students do think about suicide and, in lesser numbers, make specific plans for taking their own lives.

Among all young people under age 25, firearms-related deaths account for 65 percent of suicides. Among those aged 15 through 19, firearm-related suicides account for 81 percent of the increase in the overall suicide rate since 1980. Other stresses that may contribute to the soaring suicide rates among the young are psychological problems, mental disorders, drug abuse, school pressures, social difficulties, concern and confusion about sexual orientation, and family problems.

At all ages, men commit suicide three times more frequently than women, but women attempt suicide much more often than men. Elderly men are ten times more likely to take their own lives than older women; teenage boys kill themselves more than twice as often as girls. The suicide rate is generally higher for whites than other races, although it is rising among young African Americans in inner-city neighborhoods, who commit suicide twice as often as white men of their age. Native Americans have a suicide rate five times higher than that of the general population.

But suicide is not inevitable. Appropriate treatment can help as many as 70 to 80 percent of those at risk for suicide. Among young people, early recognition and treatment for depressive disorders and alcohol and drug use could save thousands of lives each year.

Strategies *for* Prevention

Helping to Prevent Suicide

If someone you know has talked about suicide, behaved unpredictably, or suddenly emerged from a severe depression into a calm, settled state of mind, don't rule out the possibility that he or she may attempt suicide.

✔ Encourage your friend to talk. Ask concerned questions. Listen attentively. Show that you take the person's feelings seriously and truly care.

✔ Don't offer trite reassurances. List reasons to go on living, try to analyze the person's motives, or try to shock or challenge him or her.

✔ Suggest solutions or alternatives to problems. Make plans. Encourage positive action, such as getting away for a while to gain a better perspective on a problem.

✔ Don't be afraid to ask whether your friend has considered suicide. The opportunity to talk about thoughts of suicide may be an enormous relief, and—contrary to a long-standing myth—will not fix the idea of suicide more firmly in a person's mind.

✔ Don't think that people who talk about killing themselves never carry out their threat. Most individuals who commit suicide give definite indications of their intent to die.

✔ If you feel that you aren't making any headway, suggest that both you and your friend talk to an expert.

✔ Stay close until you can get help. If you must leave your friend alone, negotiate with him or her. Have your friend promise that he or she won't do anything to harm himself or herself without first calling you. If your friend does call, get to him or her as soon as possible. Call for help immediately.

Why Do People Want to Kill Themselves?

Why? This question haunts partners, parents, children, relatives, friends, coworkers. There may never be a good enough explanation for what happened. Usually a suicide attempt is a desperate cry for help, a last attempt at communication. To people who take their own lives, death seems the best, if not the only, solution—not only for themselves, but also for their families and friends.

Many of those who kill themselves suffer from mental disorders. Some cannot cope any more; cannot think rationally; or feel ashamed, lonely, or helpless. Those with debilitating or terminal diseases may think of suicide as a welcome end to their struggle with infirmity and pain. Older individuals, who are faced with the loss of their own good health, of the people they love most, or of the activities that gave them decades of satisfaction, may see suicide as an alternative to a future without hope. (Physician-assisted suicide is discussed in Chapter 19.)

The reasons adolescents give most often for attempting suicide are to die, to escape, and to find relief. Less frequently they say that they wanted to make others feel sorry.[27] Suicidal teenagers tend to view death as a more pleasant state than do other teens, although they realize it is final. Younger suicidal children view death as both pleasant and temporary and believe that killing themselves would resolve all their worries.[28]

Understanding suicide in the young is especially hard. Substance abuse may play a major role. Naturally impulsive, young people who drink or take drugs may be especially likely to act without thinking and take their lives in a burst of rage or frustration. Those who first turned to drugs or alcohol as a way of easing their anxiety or escaping pressures may feel increasingly desperate as they realize that their problems haven't gone away or that they are losing control over their drinking or drug use.

More than half of all young people who attempt suicide may be clinically depressed. Often they feel that no one needs them or cares. Many have suffered a loss: the end of a romance or friendship, the death of a loved

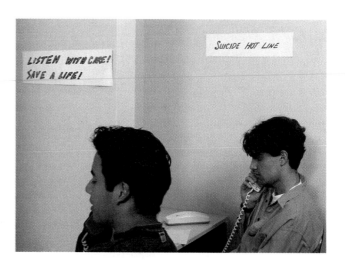

Suicide rates for young adults have risen dramatically in the last three decades. Talking with a mental health professional or calling a suicide hotline can help deal with feelings of despondency.

one, their parents' separation or divorce. According to studies comparing adolescents who attempt suicide, and those considered at risk, with normal teens, youths who try to kill themselves feel more hopeless and are more likely to say that life just isn't worth living.

Parents tend to underestimate the seriousness of their teenagers' psychological problems. In one study, 57 percent of adolescents who had attempted suicide suffered from major depression, but only 13 percent of the parents thought their child might be depressed.[29]

In some circumstances, the thought of suicide seems to capture the imagination of young people. When one suicide occurs in a community, it can spark a cluster of similar teen deaths. Studies of the impact of television movies on teen suicides have produced conflicting results, but some therapists feel that teens, who are especially prone to the effects of peer influence, may feel inspired to kill themselves after watching televised movies that portray suicide victims sympathetically.

What Leads to Suicide?

Researchers have looked for explanations for suicide by studying everything from phases of the moon to seasons (suicides peak in the spring in most young people and adults) to birth order in the family. They have found no conclusive answers. A constellation of influences—mental disorders, personality traits, biologic and genetic vulnerability, medical illness, and psychosocial stressors—may combine in ways that lower an individual's threshold of vulnerability. No one factor in itself may ever explain fully why a person chooses death.

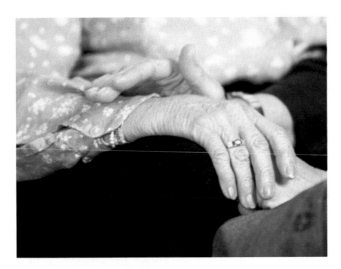

Depression and suicidal thoughts are closely linked. Educating close friends and relatives about depression prepares them to offer help and comfort during difficult times.

Mental Disorders

More than 95 percent of those who commit suicide have a mental disorder. Two in particular—depression and alcoholism—account for two-thirds of all suicides. Suicide also is a risk for those with other disorders, including schizophrenia and personality disorders.

Substance Abuse

Many of those who commit suicide drink beforehand, and their use of alcohol may lower their inhibitions. Since alcohol itself is a depressant, it can intensify the despondency suicidal individuals are already feeling. Alcoholics who attempt suicide often have other risk factors, including major depression, poor social support, serious medical illness, and unemployment. Drugs of abuse also can alter thinking and lower inhibitions against suicide.

Hopelessness

The sense of utter hopelessness and helplessness may be the most common contributing factors in suicide. When hope dies, individuals view every experience in negative terms and come to expect the worst possible outcomes for their problems. Given this way of thinking, suicide often seems a reasonable response to a life seen as not worth living.

Family History

One out of every four people who attempt suicide has a family member who also tried to commit suicide. While a family history of suicide is not in itself considered a predictor of suicide, two mental disorders that can lead to suicide—depression and bipolar disorder (manic depression)—do run in families.

Physical Illness

People who commit suicide are likely to be ill or to believe that they are. About 5 percent actually have a serious physical disorder, such as AIDS or cancer. While suicide may seem to be a decision rationally arrived at in persons with serious or fatal illness, this may not in fact be the case. Depression, not uncommon in such instances, can warp judgment. When the depression is treated, the person may no longer have suicidal intentions.

More than 80 percent of those who commit suicide have seen a physician about a medical complaint within the six months preceding suicide. To help general physicians identify people at risk of suicide, researchers at Johns Hopkins University developed a set of four crucial questions:

- Have you ever had a period of two weeks or more when you had trouble falling asleep, staying asleep, waking up too early, or sleeping too much?
- Have you ever had two weeks or more during which you felt sad, blue, depressed or when you lost interest and pleasure in things you usually cared about or enjoyed?
- Has there been a period of two weeks or more when you felt worthless, sinful, or guilty?
- Has there ever been a period of time when you felt that life was hopeless?

Anyone who answers yes to these questions should be referred immediately to a mental health professional.

Brain Chemistry

Investigators have found abnormalities in the brain chemistry of individuals who complete suicide, especially low levels of a metabolite of the neurotransmitter serotonin. There are indications that individuals with a deficiency in this substance may have as much as a ten times greater risk of committing suicide than those with higher levels.

Access to Guns

For individuals already facing a combination of predisposing factors, access to a means of committing suicide, particularly to guns, can add to the risk. Unlike other methods of suicide, guns almost always hit their mark. States with stricter gun-control laws have much lower rates of suicides than states with more lenient laws. Health professionals are urging parents whose children undergo psychological treatment or assessment to remove all weapons from their homes and to make sure their youngsters do not have access to potentially lethal medications and to alcohol.[30]

Other Factors

Individuals who kill themselves often have gone through more major life crises—job changes, births, financial reversals, divorce, retirement—in the previous six months, compared with others. Long-standing, intense conflict with family members or other important people may add to the danger. In some cases, suicide may be an act of revenge that offers the person a sense of control—however temporary or illusory. For example, a husband whose wife has had an affair may rationalize that he can get back at her, and have the final word, by killing himself. Others may feel that, by rejecting life, they are rejecting a partner or parent who abandoned or betrayed them.

Strategies *for* Prevention

If You Start Thinking About Suicide

At some point, the thought of ending it all—the disappointments, problems, bad feelings—may cross your mind. This experience isn't unusual. But if the idea of taking your life persists or intensifies, you should respond as you would to other warnings of potential threats to your health—by getting the help you need:

✔ Talk to a mental health professional. If you have a therapist, call immediately. If not, call a suicide hot line.

✔ Find someone you can trust and talk with honestly about what you're feeling. If you suffer from depression or another mental disorder, educate trusted friends or relatives about your condition so they are prepared if called upon to help.

✔ Write down your more uplifting thoughts. Even if you are despondent, you can help yourself by taking the time to retrieve some more positive thoughts or memories. A simple record of your hopes for the future and the people you value in your life can remind you of why your own life is worth continuing.

✔ Avoid drugs and alcohol. Most suicides are the results of sudden, uncontrolled impulses, and drugs and alcohol can make it harder to resist these destructive urges.

✔ Go to the hospital. Hospitalization can sometimes be the best way to protect your health and safety.

Attention Disorders

Approximately 10 percent of boys and 2 percent of girls in the United States have attention **deficit/hyperactivity disorder (ADHD)**, the most common psychiatric diagnosis of childhood.[31] Its causes are complex and include genetic and biological factors, including differences within the brain. New research has shown that children with ADHD often have smaller overall brain volumes than others, particularly in the right frontal region, an area of the brain associated with the processes of paying attention and focusing concentration.[32]

The diagnosis of ADHD in childhood remains controversial. Some critics charge that children with a variety of temperaments, neurological delays, and behavioral difficulties are being lumped together and labeled as being hyperactive or attention-disordered.[33] Others feel that attention disorders are still underdiagnosed, especially in girls, who tend to develop a type of ADHD primarily characterized by inability to concentrate.[34]

One-half to two-thirds of youngsters with ADHD do not outgrow their restless, reckless ways at puberty. In all, 1 to 2 percent of adult men and women—at least 5 million Americans—have problems sustaining attention or controlling their movements and impulses.

Adults with ADHD have one or more of three primary symptoms: hyperactivity, impulsivity, and distractibility. Rather than scooting around a room, they may tap their fingers or jiggle their feet. Some appear calm and organized but cannot concentrate long enough to finish reading a paragraph or follow a list of directions. Others, on a whim, go on buying sprees or take wild dares.

An estimated 1 percent of college students have an attention disorder that can have a significant impact on their academic performance. At one large midwestern university, for instance, the counseling service estimates that students with attention disorders have an average GPA of 2.4, compared to a university average mean of 3.1.

There is no specific test for detecting attention disorders, and diagnosis, based on the patient's history and a therapist's interview, can be difficult. Adults with ADHD may take the same medications that children do—stimulant drugs that, paradoxically, can aid concentration and reduce restlessness. Some antidepressants are effective in treating adult ADHD and may be an alternative to stimulants.[35] Medication often makes it possible for adults with ADHD to benefit from other treatments, such as psychotherapy, general counseling, vocational rehabilitation, and academic tutoring.

Schizophrenia

Schizophrenia, one of the most debilitating mental disorders, profoundly impairs an individual's sense of reality. As the National Institute of Mental Health (NIMH) puts it, schizophrenia, which is characterized by abnormalities in brain structure and chemistry, destroys "the inner unity of the mind" and weakens "the will and drive that constitute our essential character." It affects every aspect of psychological functioning, including the ways in which people think, feel, view themselves, and relate to others.

The characteristic symptoms of schizophrenia include:

- Hallucinations.
- Delusions.
- Inability to think in a logical manner.
- Talking in rambling or incoherent ways.
- Making odd or purposeless movements or not moving at all.
- Repeating others' words or mimicking their gestures.
- Showing few, if any, feelings; responding with inappropriate emotions.
- Lacking will or motivation to complete a task or accomplish something.
- Functioning at a much lower level than in the past at work, in interpersonal relations, or in taking care of themselves.

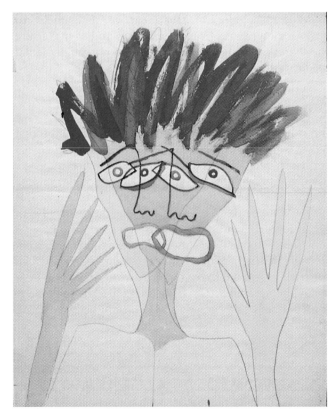

"My Head Is Going Round and Round." This drawing by a patient suffering from schizophrenia expresses the anxiety and agitation that may occur with this brain abnormality.

Individuals with schizophrenia may hear, see, or feel things that do not exist—a voice telling them to jump from a bridge, a statue crying tears of blood, a spaceship beaming a light upon them. Frightened and vulnerable, they may devote all their energy to warding off the demons within. Unable to take care of themselves, they may look messy and disheveled. They often move in unusual ways, such as rocking or pacing, or repeat certain gestures again and again. They may believe that someone or something, such as the devil, is putting thoughts into their heads or controlling their actions. Some think they are reincarnations of Christ or Napoleon. About a third attempt to take their own lives, often in response to a command they hear inside their heads.

Schizophrenia is most likely to occur between the ages of 17 and 24. One-half to 1 percent of the population—about 1 in every 150 people—suffers from this disorder. Danish researchers have found that children born during late winter or in urban areas appear to be at greater risk of schizophrenia, possibly because their mothers were more likely to contract a viral infection during pregnancy that could have affected the developing fetal brain.[36] According to NIMH's epidemiological data, the total lifetime prevalence for schizophrenia in the United States ranges from 1 to 1.9 percent. This means that between 2.5 million and 4.75 million Americans may have schizophrenia at any one time.

Schizophrenia typically consists of several stages. During the *prodromal phase,* a period ranging from months to years, individuals withdraw from social interactions, pay less attention to keeping clean or dressing appropriately, or act in peculiar ways. In the acute, or *active phase,* individuals develop "positive symptoms." They may experience delusions and become convinced that space aliens have taken control of their bodies or hallucinate and hear voices mocking them. Some talk nonstop, rambling on without making any clear point; others repeatedly shake their heads, tap their feet, or assume odd postures or positions. After positive symptoms subside, individuals enter the *residual phase,* which is characterized by "negative" symptoms, such as general apathy, flattened emotions, or inappropriate emotional reactions (for example, laughing when someone is hurt).

For centuries, the quest for a cure for this frightening and often tragic disease led to desperate methods, including spraying a strong stream of water at a patient's spine, injecting the patient with horse serum, and administering huge doses of vitamins. Today, for the vast majority of individuals with schizophrenia, antipsychotic drugs are the foundation of treatment. They make most people with schizophrenia feel more comfortable and in control of themselves, help organize chaotic thinking, and reduce or eliminate delusions or hallucinations, allowing fuller participation in normal activities. Those who do not improve significantly on medication almost invariably do even worse without it.[37]

Most of the antipsychotic drugs have a similar mode of action. While some may act more quickly than others, almost all are equally effective. But they can have problematic side effects, including uncontrollable facial tics, tongue tremors, and jaw movements known as tardive dyskinesia. Nearly one-third of individuals given conventional antipsychotics continue to have residual symptoms, such as apathy. In the past, little, if anything, could be done to relieve these negative symptoms. However, new antipsychotics, such as Clozaril (clozapine) and Zyprexa (olanzapine), can relieve such symptoms and help individuals who do not improve with standard medications or who develop intolerable side-effects.[38]

Some individuals with schizophrenia recover completely. However, many thousands—perhaps as many as 200,000—live on the street or in homeless shelters.

Overcoming Problems of the Mind

Mental illness costs our society an estimated $150 billion a year in lost work time and productivity, employee turnover, disability payments, and death. Yet many Americans do not have access to mental health services, nor do they have insurance for such services. Despite the fact that treatments for mental disorders have a higher success rate than those for many other diseases, employers often restrict mental health benefits. HMOs and health insurance plans (discussed in Chapter 11) are much more likely to limit psychotherapy visits and psychiatric hospitalizations than treatments for medical illnesses.[39]

Even when cost is not a barrier, many people do not seek treatment because they see psychological problems as a sign of weakness rather than illness. They also may not realize that scientifically proven therapies can bring relief, often in a matter of weeks or months.

Because an individual's perception of a problem is "culture-specific"—that is, influenced by his or her cultural, social, and religious beliefs—those who've immigrated to the United States from other countries may treat symptoms of psychological distress in different ways. For instance, Asian-American college students tend to seek medical care for physical symptoms, such as aches, pains, or sleep problems, but forego counseling for a mental disorder, because it is more appropriate in their native cultures to do so.

Where Can I Turn for Help?

As a student, your best contact for identifying local services may be your health education instructor or department. The health instructors can tell you about general and mental health counseling available on campus, school-based support groups, community-based programs, and special emergency services. On campus, you can also turn to the student health services or the office of the dean of student services or student affairs.

Within the community, you may be able to get help through the city or county health department and neighborhood health centers. Local hospitals often have special clinics and services; and there are usually local branches of national service organizations, such as United Way or Alcoholics Anonymous, other 12-step programs, and various support groups. You can call the psychiatric or psychological association in your city or state for the names of licensed professionals. (Check the telephone directory for listings.) Your primary physician may also be able to help.

The telephone book is another good resource. Special programs are often listed either by the nature of the service, by the name of the neighborhood or city, or by the name of the sponsoring group. In some places, the city's name may precede a listing: the New York City Suicide Hot Line, for instance. In addition to suicide-prevention programs, other listings usually include crisis intervention, violence prevention, and child-abuse prevention programs; drug-treatment information; shelters for battered women; senior citizen centers; and self-help and counseling services. Many services have special hot lines for coping with emergencies. Others provide information as well as counseling over the phone. (See Pulsepoints: "Ten Ways to Help a Troubled Friend or Relative.")

Types of Therapists

Many people refer to anyone in the mental health field as a "psychotherapist," but this is not an official designation, and anyone can advertise as one. Only professionally trained individuals who have met state licensing requirements are certified as psychiatrists, psychologists, or social workers. Before selecting any of these mental health professionals, be sure to check the person's background and credentials.

The most common types of mental health professionals are psychiatrists, psychologists, social workers, psychiatric nurses, and marriage and family therapists. **Psychiatrists** are licensed medical doctors (M.D.s) who complete medical school; a year-long internship (including at least four months of internal medicine and usually two months of neurology); and a three-year

PULSE points

Ten Ways to Help a Troubled Friend or Relative

1. **Take your loved one seriously.** Troubled individuals need to know you are willing to listen without lecturing or criticizing them.

2. **Don't try to treat the problem yourself.** Well-intentioned comments like "You'll feel better after a good rest" may make matters worse.

3. **Encourage openness and honesty.** Discussing troubling issues frankly can help a person realize that he or she is facing very real difficulties and may require some assistance to work through them.

4. **Seek out information.** The more you know, the more insight you'll have. Educate yourself about mental disorders and their treatments.

5. **Maintain as normal a relationship as possible.** Acknowledge the person's pain, but try to preserve your usual ways of relating to each other.

6. **Give and expect respect.** Psychological distress may explain hurtful behavior, but it does not excuse it.

7. **Resist the temptation to "overfunction."** If you take on his or her responsibilities, the person

will feel even more helpless and inadequate.

8. **Foster the will to be well.** Talk in positive terms about the future, though not at the expense of honesty about current feelings and fears.

9. **Live your own life.** Though it may be difficult, you must pursue your own interests for the sake of your own psychological well-being.

10. **Be patient. Recovery can take time.** Don't be discouraged by temporary setbacks. The mind, like the body, heals slowly and cannot be rushed.

---

residency that provides training in various forms of psychotherapy (including couples, family, and group therapy), psychopharmacology (the study of drugs that affect the mind), and both outpatient and inpatient treatment of mental disorders. They can prescribe medications and make medical decisions. *Board-certified* psychiatrists have passed oral and written examinations following completion of residency training. Child psychiatrists undergo additional academic and clinical training to work with children and adolescents; geriatric psychiatrists have special expertise in the problems of older men and women.

Psychologists complete a graduate program (including clinical training and internships) in human psychology but do not study medicine and cannot prescribe medication. They must be licensed in most states in order to practice independently. An increasing number have a doctorate (either a Ph.D. or Psy.D.) plus post-doctoral training, and are trained in a variety of psychotherapeutic techniques rather than in one particular school or theory. Some have additional training in working with children and families.

Certified social workers or licensed clinical social workers (LCSWs) usually complete a two-year graduate program and have specialized training in helping people with mental problems in addition to conventional social work. Some have doctoral degrees. Most states certify or license social workers as an independent profession and require two years of supervised postgraduate clinical work and a qualifying examination.

Psychiatric nurses have nursing degrees and have passed a state examination. They usually have special training and experience in mental health care, although no specialty licensing or certification is required.

Marriage and family therapists, licensed in some but not all states, usually have a graduate degree, often in psychology, and at least two years of supervised clinical training in dealing with relationship problems. Psychiatrists, psychologists, and clinical social workers may specialize in marriage and family counseling or devote much of their practices to helping couples and families.

Other therapists include pastoral counselors, members of the clergy who offer psychological counseling; hypnotherapists, who use hypnosis for problems such as smoking and obesity; stress-management counselors, who teach relaxation methods; and alcohol and drug counselors, who help individuals with substance abuse problems. Anyone can use these terms to describe themselves professionally, and there are no licensing requirements.

Options for Treatment

The term **psychotherapy** refers to any type of counseling based on the exchange of words in the context of the unique relationship that develops between a mental health professional and a person seeking help. The process of talking and listening can lead to new insight, relief from distressing psychological symptoms, changes

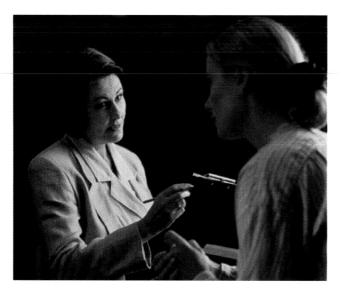

A therapist's education, title, and qualifications may vary. The qualities of compassion and caring are also important in choosing the right therapist.

in unhealthy or maladaptive behaviors, and more effective ways of dealing with the world.

Most mental health professionals today are trained in a variety of psychotherapeutic techniques and tailor their approach to the problem, personality, and needs of each person seeking their help. Because skilled therapists may combine different techniques in the course of therapy, the lines between the various approaches often blur.

Because insurance companies and health-care plans often limit the duration of psychotherapy, many mental health professionals are adopting a *time-limited* format in order to make the most of every session, regardless of the length of treatment. Brief or short-term psychotherapy typically focuses on a central theme, problem, or topic and may continue for several weeks to several months. The individuals most likely to benefit are those who are interested in solving immediate problems rather than changing their characters, can think in psychological terms, and are motivated to change.

Psychodynamic Psychotherapy

For the most part, today's mental health professionals base their assessment of individuals on a **psychodynamic** understanding that takes into account the role of early experiences and unconscious influences in *actively* shaping behavior. (This is the *dynamic* in psychodynamic.) Psychodynamic treatments work toward the goal of providing greater insight into problems and bringing about behavioral change. Therapy may be brief, consisting of 12 to 25 sessions, or may continue

for several years. According to current thinking, psychotherapy can actually rewire the network of neurons within the brain in ways that ease distress and improve functioning in many areas of daily life. Classical psychoanalysis, developed by Sigmund Freud, is a complex, lengthy process that deals with long-repressed feelings and issues. Less widely used than briefer forms of psychotherapy, it remains an option best suited for mentally healthy, high-functioning individuals who want to explore distressing patterns in their lives, such as a series of failed relationships.

Interpersonal Therapy (IPT)

Interpersonal therapy (IPT), originally developed for research into the treatment of major depression, focuses on relationships in order to help individuals deal with unrecognized feelings and needs and improve their communication skills. IPT does not deal with the psychological origins of symptoms but rather concentrates on current problems of getting along with others. The supportive, empathic relationship that is developed with the therapist, who takes an even more active role than in psychodynamic psychotherapy, is the most crucial component of this therapy. The emphasis is on the here and now and on interpersonal—rather than intrapsychic—issues. Individuals with major depression, chronic difficulties developing relationships, dysthymia, or bulimia (see Chapter 7 on eating disorders) are most likely to benefit. IPT usually consists of 12 to 16 sessions.

Cognitive-Behavioral Therapy

This approach, which focuses on inappropriate or inaccurate thoughts or beliefs, aims to help individuals break out of a distorted way of thinking. The techniques of **cognitive therapy** include identification of an individual's beliefs and attitudes, recognition of negative thought patterns, and education in alternative ways of thinking. Individuals with major depression or anxiety disorders are most likely to benefit, usually in 15 to 25 sessions.

Behavior therapy strives to substitute healthier ways of behaving for maladaptive patterns used in the past. Its premise is that distressing psychological symptoms, like all behaviors, are learned responses that can be modified or unlearned. Some therapists believe that changing behavior also changes how people think and feel. As they put it, "Change the behavior, and the feelings will follow." Behavior therapies work best for disorders characterized by specific, abnormal patterns of acting—such as alcohol and drug abuse, anxiety disorders, and phobias—and for individuals who want to change bad habits.

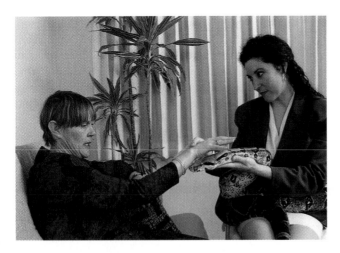

Systematic desensitization is one of the behavior therapies used to treat phobias.

Psychiatric Drug Therapy

Medications that alter brain chemistry and relieve psychiatric symptoms have brought great hope and help to millions of people. Thanks to the recent development of a new generation of more precise and effective **psychiatric drugs,** success rates for treating many common and disabling disorders—depression, panic disorder, schizophrenia, and others—have soared. Often used in conjunction with psychotherapy, sometimes used as the primary treatment, these medications have revolutionized mental health care.

At some point in their lives, about half of all Americans will take a psychiatric drug. The reason may be depression, anxiety, a sleep difficulty, an eating dis-

order, alcohol or drug dependence, impaired memory, or another disorder that disrupts the intricate chemistry of the brain. (See Consumer Health Watch: "What You Need to Know about Mind-Mood Medications.")

In the last decade alone, the number of available psychiatric drugs has doubled. These medications are now among the most widely prescribed drugs in the United States. Three of the top ten prescription drugs sold in this country are serotonin-boosting antidepressants—best known by their trade names Prozac, Paxil, and Zoloft—that are used to treat a variety of problems, including obsessive-compulsive disorder, premenstrual syndrome and attention deficits, as well as depression.

Psychiatric medications affect every aspect of a person's physical, mental, and emotional functioning. Some take effect immediately; others take several weeks to relieve symptoms; a few continue to exert their effects even after an individual discontinues their use. When taken appropriately, psychiatric agents can alleviate tremendous suffering and reduce the financial and personal costs of mental illness by lessening the need for hospitalization and by restoring an individual's ability to function normally, to work, and to contribute to society. But they do have side effects and must be used with care. This is especially true for their use in children. More than 500,000 serotonin-boosting drugs are written for children and adolescents each year, even though the FDA approved these medications only for patients over age 18. Although researchers note that these drugs are potentially helpful, their safety and effectiveness have not been assessed in young people, and there are no clear age and dosage guidelines.[40]

Consumer Health Watch

What You Need to Know About Mind-Mood Medications

Before taking any "psychoactive" drug (one that affects the brain), talk to a qualified health professional. Here are some points to raise:

• What can this medication do for me? What specific symptoms will it relieve? Are there other possible benefits?

• Are there any risks? What about side effects? Do I have to take it before or after eating? Will it affect my ability to study, work, drive, or operate machinery?

• When will I notice a difference? How long does it take for the medicine to have an effect?

• How will I be able to tell if the medication is working? What are the odds that it will help me?

• How long will I have to take medication? Is there any danger that I'll become addicted?

• What if it doesn't help?

• Is there an herbal or natural alternative? If so, has it been studied? What do you know about its possible risks and side effects?

Alternative Mind-Mood Products

Increasingly consumers are trying "natural" products, such as herbs and enzymes, that claim to have psychological effects. However, because they are not classified as drugs, they have not undergone the rigorous scientific testing required of psychiatric medications, and little is known about their safety or efficacy. "Natural" doesn't mean risk-free. Heroin and cocaine are "natural" substances that have dramatic and potentially deadly effects on the mind.[41]

The most popular herbal mood booster is St. John's Wort, named after St. John the Baptist because the yellow flowers of the *Hypericum perforatum* plant bloom in June, the anniversary month of his execution. Used to treat anxiety and depression in Europe for many years, St. John's Wort is believed to enhance the activity of several neurotransmitters, including serotonin. A *British Medical Journal* review of studies based on data from 1,008 patients concluded that it is effective in treating mild to moderate depression. In Germany, St. John's Wort is prescribed for depression four times as often as Prozac. A major clinical trial in the United States is underway. Side effects include dizziness, abdominal pain and bloating, constipation, nausea, fatigue, and dry mouth. St. John's Wort should not be taken in combination with other prescription antidepressants.[42]

Other substances are widely used despite little or no scientific evaluation of their risks and benefits. Valerian, derived from the root of *Valeriana officinalis,* is taken primarily for insomnia and may help induce sleepiness. Kava, from a pepper tree native to the South Pacific, is thought to have a naturally soothing effect that can relieve anxiety and tension. Gingko biloba, long used in Chinese medicine, is considered a natural brain booster that can improve memory and concentration. In several small studies, researchers have documented cognitive improvements in healthy seniors and those with mild to moderate forms of dementia who tried gingko.[43]

 ## Does Treatment Work?

According to the National Mental Health Advisory Council and the American Psychiatric Association, treatments for severe mental disorders—such as major depression, bipolar (manic-depressive) illness, panic disorder, and schizophrenia—are as or more effective than those available in other branches of medicine, including surgery. Treatments tailored to each individual's condition and needs can help 80 to 90 percent of those suffering from depression and bipolar disorder and 70 to 80 percent of those with panic disorder. In certain cases, such as panic disorder, specific types of psychotherapy,

such as cognitive behavioral techniques, have proven more effective as a long-term treatment than medications. In other disorders, such as depression, the combination of medication and psychotherapy may be most beneficial.[44] In schizophrenia, new antipsychotic drugs have had the greatest impact.

Across the Lifespan: Changes and Challenges

The way you are today, as an undergraduate, may determine your emotional well-being later in life. In a long-term study of 173 Harvard College graduates begun in the 1940s, childhood problems, such as being poor or orphaned, had almost no effect on psychological health at age 65. Many things that had seemed so important at college age, such as making friends easily, became unimportant later in life. However, students who had been good at practical organization were among the mentally healthiest at 65, as were those whom psychiatrists described as "steady, stable, dependable, thorough, sincere, and trustworthy." Although these individuals changed through the years, their psychological core remained the same.[45]

While the fullness of the years can bring great richness to our psychological lives, time also brings new challenges, physical as well as mental. Our bodies change; our brains change; our view of who we are and what matters most changes too.

The Aging Brain

Not long ago, scientists thought that the aging brain, once worn out, could never be fixed. They've since learned that the brain can and does repair itself. When neurons (brain cells) die, the surrounding cells develop "fingers" to fill the gaps and establish new connections, or synapses, between surviving neurons. Although self-repair occurs more quickly in young brains, the process continues in older brains. Even victims of Alzheimer's disease, the most devastating form of senility, have enough healthy cells in the diseased brain to regrow synapses. Scientists hope to develop drugs that someday may help the brain repair itself. (See the section on Alzheimer's disease later in this chapter.)

Mental ability does not decline along with physical vigor. Researchers have been able to reverse the supposedly normal intellectual declines of 60- to 80-year-olds by tutoring them in problem solving. Reaction time, intellectual speed and efficiency, nonverbal intelligence, and maximum work rate for short periods may diminish by age 75. However, understanding, vocabulary, ability to remember key information, and verbal intelligence remain about the same.

Memory

Some memory skills, particularly the ability to retrieve names and process information quickly, inevitably diminish over time. What normal changes should you expect? Here is a preview:

- *Recalling information takes longer.* As individuals reach their mid- to late sixties, the brain slows down, but usually just by a matter of milliseconds. As long as they're not rushed, older adults eventually adapt and perform just as well as younger ones.

- *Distractions become more disruptive.* Teenagers can study and listen to the stereo at the same time. Thirty-something moms can soothe the baby, field her baby's big brother's questions on homework, and put together a dinner all at once. But as individuals pass age 50, they find it much more difficult to divide their attention or to remember details of a story after having switched their attention to something else.

- *"Accessing" names gets harder.* "The ability to remember names—especially those that you don't use frequently—diminishes by as much as 50 percent between ages 25 and 65. Preventive strategies, such as repeating a person's name when introduced, writing down the name as soon as possible and making obvious associations (the Golden Gate for a man named Bridges) can help.

- *Learning new information is harder.* The quality of memory doesn't change, just the speed at which we receive, absorb, and react to information. That's why strategies like taking notes or outlining material become critical for older students, especially when learning brand-new skills. However, adding to existing knowledge remains as easy as ever.

- *Wisdom matters.* In any memory test involving knowledge of the world, vocabulary or judgment, older people outperform younger ones.

At any age, occasional forgetfulness, memory lapses, and misplacing everyday objects are common. What's *not* normal are any of the following:

- Frequent difficulty completing a sentence because of forgetting what you want to say or the words with which to say it.

- Misplacing important items, such as money or bank records.

- Frequent confusion.

- Forgetting how to use common items or perform simple tasks.

- Getting lost or disoriented in familiar places, especially at home.

- Difficulty identifying the month or season.

- Dizzy spells or severe headaches accompanying memory loss.

A number of illnesses, including depression, kidney disease, alcoholism, and Alzheimer's disease, can cause these symptoms. Only thorough medical and neurological examinations can pinpoint the specific problem.

Alzheimer's Disease

About 15 percent of older Americans lose previous mental capabilities, a brain disorder called **dementia.** Sixty percent of these—a total of 4 million men and women over age 65—suffer from the type of dementia called **Alzheimer's disease,** a progressive deterioration of brain cells and mental capacity.

Women are more likely to develop Alzheimer's than men. (Look again at The X & Y Files: "Do Men's Brains Differ from Women's?") By age 85, as many as 28 to 30 percent of women suffer from Alzheimer's, and women with this form of dementia perform significantly worse than men in various visual, spatial, and memory tests.

Hormone replacement therapy (HRT) has shown promise in keeping women's brains healthy as they age. In several small studies, the risk of Alzheimer's disease declined by 40 percent among women on HRT. Other reports have noted some cognitive improvement in women with Alzheimer's when they begin estrogen replacement therapy. However, a recent analysis of 27 studies of estrogen and its effect on intellectual function and Alzheimer's disease concluded that many of these investigations had not been well done in terms of scientific rigor. Before estrogen can be recommended as a means of protecting the postmenopausal brain, large-scale clinical trials will have to provide more convincing proof of its benefits.[46]

Often Alzheimer's progresses slowly, stealing bits of a person's mind and memory a little at a time. Its victims may withdraw into a world of their own, become quarrelsome or irritable, and say or do inappropriate things. The personalities of individuals with Alzheimer's often change. Some become more stubborn or impulsive; others may become increasingly apathetic, withdrawn, irritable, or suspicious, accusing others of thefts, betrayal, or plotting against them. As cognitive impairment worsens, inhibitions often loosen; they may masturbate or take off their clothes in public. Some become aggressive or violent. Eventually, individuals may forget the names of their close relatives, their own occupations, occasionally even their own names.

The early signs of dementia—insomnia, irritability, increased sensitivity to alcohol and other drugs, and decreased energy and tolerance of frustration—are usually subtle and insidious. Diagnosis requires a comprehensive assessment of an individual's medical history, physical health, and mental status, often involving brain scans and a variety of other tests. Using brain-imaging techniques, researchers have found what may be the first clearly recognizable early warning sign of Alzheimer's: damage in the hippocampus, a region of the brain that plays a key role in memory. This finding could help doctors begin treatments earlier and distinguish Alzheimer's from other forms of mental deterioration.[47]

Even though no one can restore a brain that is in the process of being destroyed by an organic brain disease like Alzheimer's, medications can control difficult behavioral symptoms and enhance or partially restore cognitive ability. Often physicians find other medical or psychiatric problems, such as depression, in these patients; recognizing and treating these conditions can have a dramatic impact.

Depression and the Elderly

According to a report by the National Institutes of Health Consensus Development Panel on Depression in Later Life, about 15 percent of men and women over 65 living in the community experience depression. In nursing homes, the rate is higher: 15 to 25 percent. Moreover, recurrences are common, with 40 percent of older persons suffering repeat bouts with depression.[48]

Late-life depression can be particularly hard to spot because older men and women often do not display the typical symptoms, or their symptoms are mistaken for normal signs of aging. Elderly people with physical problems are most prone to depression. Some classic signs of depression—appetite changes, a gain or loss of 5 percent of body weight in a month, insomnia or excessive sleep, fidgeting or extremely slow movements or speech, fatigue, or loss of energy—may be attributed to medical problems, medications, or old age itself. Depression that develops following an illness or injury, if not identified and treated, can hinder recovery.

The consequences of not recognizing and treating depression late in life can be tragic. Older Americans have the highest suicide rates in our society, with some 8,500 elderly persons killing themselves every year. The suicide rate is five times higher for those aged 65 than for younger individuals. And depressed older men and women are also more likely to die of other causes. However, late-life depression can be overcome. With treatment, more than 70 percent of the depressed elderly improve dramatically. Since loneliness and loss are often important contributing factors, psychiatrists often combine counseling, such as brief psychotherapy, with medication. Because of various physiological differences in the elderly, they usually respond more slowly to antidepressants than younger persons, and the benefits thus may not be apparent for 6 to 12 weeks.

Making This Chapter Work for You

Preventing and Solving Psychological Problems

- Mental health is not an absence of distress, but rather the capacity to think rationally and logically and to cope with life's transitions, stresses, traumas, and losses in a way that allows for emotional stability and growth.

- As defined by the American Psychiatric Association's *Diagnostic and Statistical Manual*, 4th edition (*DSM-IV*), a mental disorder is "a clinically significant behavioral or psychological syndrome or pattern that occurs in an individual and that is associated with present distress (a painful symptom) or disability (impairment in one or more important areas of functioning) or with a significantly increased risk of suffering death, pain, disability, or an important loss of freedom."

- During any given year, 30 percent of Americans suffer from at least one mental disorder. According to the National Comorbidity Survey, the most common single mental disorder is major depression, while the anxiety disorders are the most prevalent group of mental disorders. Only 42 percent of those with a lifetime history of one or more mental disorders ever receive any professional care.

- Psychological distress can contribute to major health problems, including high blood pressure, heart disease, cancer, and immune-related disorders. Treating mental disorders often reduces medical care costs.

- The brain contains hundreds of billions of nerve cells, or neurons, which are the basic working units of the brain.

- Communication with the brain involves a process called neurotransmission, in which an electric charge or impulse travels along a neuron's axon to the terminal, where packets of chemicals, called neurotransmitters, are released.

- The most common type of mental disorders, anxiety disorders may involve episodes of sudden, inexplicable terror (panic attacks), inordinate fears of certain objects or situations (phobias), chronic distress (generalized anxiety disorder, or GAD), or persistent, disturbing thoughts and behaviors (obsessive-compulsive disorder).

- Major depression, the most widespread mental disorder, has increased among young adults. Symptoms include a sense of helplessness or hopelessness, lack of energy, sleep disturbances, and loss of interest in food, sex, and work. Depression can be successfully treated with psychotherapy, drug therapy, or a combination.

- Other forms of depression include manic depression (or bipolar disorder), characterized by extreme mood swings; seasonal affective disorder, which develops only at certain times of the year; and dysthymia, chronic mild depression. All can be effectively treated by different therapies.

- The number of suicides is growing, especially among young people. The degree of hopelessness is a key variable in determining which students actually attempt to take their own lives.

- Many factors may contribute to suicide: depression, other mental disorders, substance abuse, feelings of loss or failure, physical illness, family history, altered brain chemistry, and access to guns. If the danger of suicide is recognized and individuals receive professional help, suicide can be prevented.

- Attention disorders are common among adults, affecting 1 to 2 percent of men and women. Their three primary symptoms are hyperactivity, impulsivity, and distractibility, and they often interfere with school and work performance. Medication is highly effective for adults, as it is for children with attention disorders.

- Schizophrenia profoundly impairs an individual's sense of reality. Individuals in the active phase of schizophrenia develop positive symptoms, such as hallucinations and delusions. In the residual phase, individuals suffer symptoms, such as general apathy or inappropriate emotional reactions. Although there is no cure for schizophrenia, powerful antipsychotic drugs can reduce confusion, anxiety, delusions, and hallucinations.

- There are many types of mental health professionals—psychiatrists, psychologists, licensed social workers, psychiatric nurses, and marriage and family therapists—and many options for treatment of mental disorders. Options for treatment include psychodynamic psychotherapy, interpersonal therapy, cognitive-behavioral therapy, and psychiatric drugs.

health **/ ONLINE**

National Institute of Mental Health
http://www.nimh.nih.gov/
This site includes information on anxiety disorders, depression, advances in mental illness treatment, and more.

American Psychological Association Help Center
http://helping.apa.org/index.html
The APA Help Center contains advice on when and how to access psychological services, several online readings on how to handle problems in one's professional and personal lives, and information about how the mind and body can work together to improve one's health.

National Mental Health Association
http://www.nmha.org
This site includes current news releases on mental health-related topics as well as an "information center" with online facts sheets and pamphlets about anxiety disorders, depression, childrens' disorders, Alzheimer's, and more.

Please note that links are subject to change. If you find a broken link, use a search engine like http://www.yahoo.com *and search for the web site by typing in key words.*

 Campus Chat: Is there still a stigma attached to mental illness? Share your thoughts on our online discussion forum at **http://health.wadsworth.com**

Find It On InfoTrac: You can find additional readings related to stress via InfoTrac College Edition, an online library of more than 900 journals and publications. Follow the instructions for accessing InfoTrac that came packaged with your textbook; then search for articles using a key word search.

- **Suggested article:** "Melancholy Nation." *U.S. News & World Report*, March 8, 1999, Vol. 126, issue 9, p. 56.

  (1) To what extent have pharmacological treatments for depression succeeded? How have they fallen short?
  (2) List at least three different types of depression.

For additional links, resources, and suggested readings on InfoTrac, visit our Health & Wellness Resource Center at **http://health.wadsworth.com**

Many consumers also try alternative mind-mood medications, such as the herb St. John's Wort. Little is known about the safety or efficacy of such "natural" agents.

■ Although the brain changes over time, many cognitive functions remain intact. Memory skills, such as recalling names and new information, can be improved by practical strategies, such as making associations and taking notes while learning new material. Alzheimer's disease, a progressive deterioration of brain cells and mental capacity, affects millions of older men and women. There is no cure, but various treatments can enhance a person's ability to function.

There is one primary rule for evaluating your own emotional mental health: If your problems are interfering with the way you function, it's time to seek help. If you feel less happy, less confident, and less in control for a prolonged period, or if others comment on changes in your behavior and personality, ask for help. "Seeing a therapist is giving yourself the opportunity to create options," says one psychotherapist, "and that may be the greatest gift we can give to ourselves or the people who love us."

 St. John's Wort. What is known about the effectiveness of St. John's Wort?

Key Terms

The terms listed here are used within the chapter. Page numbers are included for each term. A definition of each term is given in the Glossary pages at the end of this book.

Alzheimer's disease   116
antidepressant   101
anxiety   97
anxiety disorders   101
attention deficit/hyperactivity disorder (ADHD)   109
axon   100
axon terminal   100
behavior therapy   113
bipolar disorder   105
certified social worker   110
cognitive therapy   113
dementia   116
dendrites   100
depression   97
depressive disorders   104
dysthymia   105

generalized anxiety disorder (GAD)   101
glia   99
hormone replacement therapy (HRT)   116
interpersonal therapy (IPT)   113
licensed clinical social worker (LCSW)   112
major depression   104
marriage and family therapist   112
mental disorder   97
neurons   99
neuropsychiatry   97
neurotransmitters   100
nucleus   100
obsessive-compulsive disorder (OCD)   101

panic attack   101
panic disorder   103
phobia   101
psychiatric drugs   114
psychiatric nurse   112
psychiatrists   111
psychodynamic   113
psychologists   112
psychotherapy   112
receptors   100
reuptake   100
schizophrenia   110
seasonal affective disorder (SAD)   105
synapse   100

Critical Thinking Questions

1. Paula went to a therapist when she was feeling depressed and was given a prescription for an antidepressant called fluoxetine (trade name Prozac). Her therapist recommended the drug because it causes fewer side effects than other medications. However, Paula later read in a news magazine that some patients, claiming that Prozac had made them violent or suicidal, had sued the drug's manufacturers. Their suits didn't win in court, but Paula was less certain about taking the prescribed medication. What do you think she should do? How would you weigh the risks and benefits of taking a psychiatric drug?

2. Research has indicated that many homeless men and women are in need of outpatient psychiatric care, often because they suffer from chronic mental illnesses or alcoholism. Yet government funding for the mentally ill is inadequate, and homelessness itself can make it difficult, if not impossible, for people to gain access to the care they need. How do you feel when you pass homeless individuals who seem disoriented or out of touch with reality? Who should take responsibility for their welfare? Should they be forced to undergo treatment at psychiatric institutions?

References

1. Hales, Robert, and Stuart Yudofsky. *The American Psychiatric Press Textbook of Psychiatry.* 3rd ed. Washington, DC: American Psychiatric Press, 1999.

2. Roberts, James. "Compulsive Buying Among College Students." *Journal of Consumer Affairs*, Vol. 32, No. 2, Winter 1998.

3. Chisholm, Margaret. "Colleges Need to Provide Early Treatment of Students' Mental Illnesses." *Chronicle of Higher Education,* May 15, 1998.

4. Hales, Dianne, and Robert Hales. *Caring for the Mind: The Comprehensive Guide to Mental Health.* New York: Bantam Books, 1995.

5. American Psychiatric Association. *Diagnostic and Statistical Manual of Mental Disorders.* 4th ed. Washington, DC: American Psychiatric Association, 1994. Andreasen, Nancy. "The Validation of Psychiatric Diagnosis: New Models and Approaches." *American Journal of Psychiatry,* Vol. 152, No. 2, February 1995.

6. Shaw, Elizabeth. "Minding our Mental Health." *American Health,* March 1999.

7. Gliatto, Michael, et al (editors). *Psychiatry for Family Care Practitioners.* Washington, DC: American Psychiatric Press, 1999.

8. Hales, Robert, and Stuart Yudofsky (editors). *Essentials of Clinical Psychiatry.* Washington, DC: American Psychiatric Press, 1999.

9. Marano, Hara Estroff. "Depression: Beyond Serotonin." *Psychology Today,* March–April 1999.

10. Sloan, Denise. "Depression with Physical Illness Doubles Psychiatric Hospital Stays." *Psychomatic Medicine,* news release, January 29, 1999.

11. Carlat, Daniel. "The Psychiatric Review of Symptoms: A Screening Tool for Family Physicians." *American Family Physician,* November 1, 1998.

12. Hales, Robert, and Dianne Hales. *The Mind-Mood Pill Book.* New York: Bantam Books, 2000.

13. National Institute of Mental Health. "Anxiety Disorders Research at NIMH." November 1998.

14. Gard, Carolyn. "Coping with the Fear of Fear." *Current Health,* Vol. 25, No. 5, January 1999.

15. Kulkarni, Nitin, and Richard Ross. "Anxiety Disorders." *Psychiatry for Family Care Practitioners.* Washington, DC: American Psychiatric Press, 1999.

16. Hollander, Eric, et al. "Anxiety Disorders." In *The American Psychiatric Press Textbook of Psychiatry.* 3rd ed. Washington, DC: American Psychiatric Press, 1999.

17. Marano, "Depression: Beyond Serotonin."

18. Lewinsohn, Peter, et al. "Continuity into Adulthood (Natural Course of Adolescent Major Depressive Disorder, Part I). *Journal of the American Academy of Child and Adolescent Psychiatry,* Vol. 38, No. 1, January 1999.

19. Ilivicky, Howard. "Mood Disorders." *Psychiatry for Family Care Practitioners.* Washington, DC: American Psychiatric Press, 1999.

20. American Psychological Association Practice Directorate. "How Psychotherapy Helps People Recover from Depression." October 1998.

21. Mulrow, Cynthia, et al. " Agency for Health Policy and Research Evidence Report on Treatment of Depression—New Pharmacotherapies." *Psychopharmacology Bulletin,* Vol. 34, No. 4, March 1999.

22. Frank, Christina. "Skirmish or Siege?" *Psychology Today,* March–April 1999.

23. Hales, Robert, and Dianne Hales. *Caring for the Mind.* New York: Bantam Books, 1995.

24. "Dysthymia." *Harvard Health Letter,* Vol. 24, No. 6, March 1999.

25. Campbell, E. Cabrina, et al. "Suicide and Violence." *Psychiatry for Family Care Practitioners.* Washington, DC: American Psychiatric Press, 1999.

26. Simpson, Michael. "Suicide Prevention: What You Can Do." *NEA Today,* Vol. 17, No. 5, February 1999.

27. Boergers, Julie, et al. "Reasons for Adolescent Suicide Attempts: Associations with Psychological Functioning." *Journal of the American Academy of Child and Adolescent Psychiatry,* Vol. 37, No. 12, December 1998.

28. Gothelf, Doron, et al. "Death Concepts in Suicidal Adolescents." *Journal of the American Academy of Child and Adolescent Psychiatry,* Vol. 37, No. 12, December 1998.

29. "Keep Your Eye On." *Brown University Child and Adolescent Behavior Letter,* Vol. 15, No. 4, April 1999.

30. Kruesi, Markus, et al. "Suicide and Violence Prevention: Parent Education in the Emergency Department." *Journal of the American Academy of Child and Adolescent Psychiatry,* Vol. 38, No. 3, March 1999.

31. Popper, Charles, and Scott West. "Disorders Usually Diagnosed in Infancy, Childhood or Adolescence." *American Psychiatric Press Textbook of Psychiatry.* 3rd ed. Washington, DC: American Psychiatric Press, 1999.

32. Mostofsky, Stewart. "Brain Abnormalities in Children with ADHD." American Academy of Neurology, annual meeting, Toronto, April 1999.

33. Carey, William. "Problems in Diagnosing Attention and Activity." *Pediatrics,* Vol. 103, No. 3, March 1999.

34. Neuman, R.J., et al. "Evaluation of ADHD Typology in Three Contrasting Samples: A Latent Class Approach." *Journal of the American Academy of Child and Adolescent Psychiatry,* Vol. 38, No. 1, January 1999.

35. Huffman, Grace Brooke. "Antidepressants Are Effective in Treatment of Adult ADHD." *American Family Physician,* Vol. 59, No. 6, March 15, 1999.

36. Mortensen, Preben Bo. "Effects of Family History and Place and Season of Birth on the Risk of Schizophrenia." *Journal of the American Medical Association,* Vol. 281, No. 14, April 14, 1999.

37. Black, Donald, and Nancy Andreasen. "Schizophrenia, Schizophreniform Disorders and Delusional (Paranoid) Disorders." *Essentials of Clinical Psychiatry,* Washington, DC: American Psychiatric Press, 1999.

38. Wickelgren, Ingrid. "A New Route to Treating Schizophrenia." *Science,* Vol. 281, No. 5381, August 28, 1998.

39. Shaw, "Minding our Mental Health."

40. Hales and Hales, *The Mind-Mood Pill Book.*

41. Ibid.

42. Dickstein, Leah. "Nature's Pharmacy Is Full of Surprises." *Psychology Today,* March–April 1999.

43. Kinoshita, June. "Beyond Gingko Mania: The New Memory Cures." *American Health,* September 1998.

44. Kopta, S. Mark, et al."Individual Psychotherapy Outcome and Process Research." *Annual Review of Psychology,* 1999.

45. Hales and Hales, *Caring for the Mind.*

46. Hoff, Kristine, et al. "Estrogen Therapy in Postmenopausal Women: Effects on Cognitive Function and Dementia." *Journal of the American Medical Association,* Vol. 179, No. 9, March 4, 1998.

47. Small, Scott. "Early Warning Signs of Alzheimer's." American Academy of Neurology, annual meeting, Toronto, April 1999.

48. Blazer, Daniel. "Geriatric Psychiatry." *American Psychiatric Press Textbook of Psychiatry.* 3rd ed. Washington, DC: American Psychiatric Press, 1999.

SECTION

II

Healthy Lifestyles

You have enormous influence over your health and vitality. This section provides information about the tools you have at hand to become healthier and feel stronger and more energetic throughout your lifetime. By learning how to eat a balanced and varied diet, how to manage your weight, and how to become physically fit, you can get started on a lifelong journey of becoming all you can be. And as you take better care of your body today, you'll build the foundation for feeling your best for many tomorrows to come.

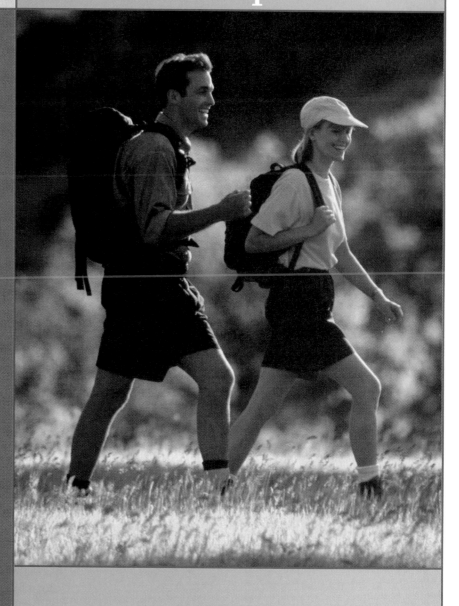

5

The Joy of Fitness

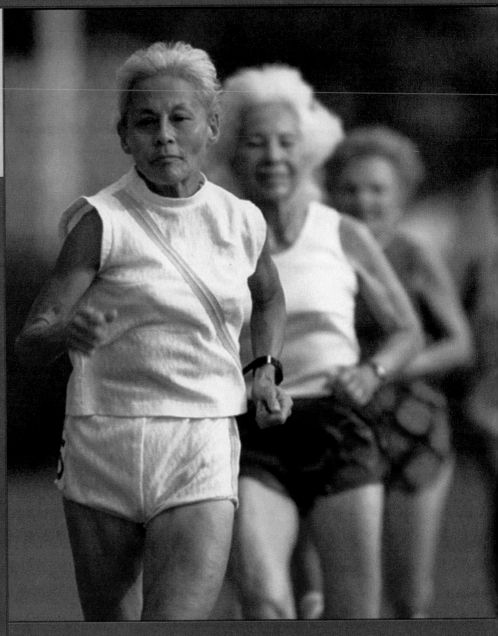

After studying the material in this chapter, you should be able to:

- **List** and **explain** the components of physical fitness.
- **Explain** the benefits of exercise as a strategy for health prevention.
- **Compare** and **contrast** aerobic exercises and strength or muscular exercises.
- **Design** a personal total fitness program.
- **List** the potential health effects of using anabolic steroids.
- **Plan** a personal exercise program, and **list** nutritional and safety strategies that you should also pursue.

Y ou are designed to move. In ways far more complex than the fastest airplane or sleekest car, your body runs, stretches, bends, swims, climbs, glides, and strides—day after day, year after year, decade after decade. While mere machines break down from constant wear and tear, your body thrives on physical activity. The more you use your body, the stronger and fitter you can become.

Unfortunately, most people never reach their physical potential. Consider these findings from the U.S. Surgeon General and *Healthy People 2000:*

- More than 60 percent of adults do not exercise regularly. An estimated 150 million Americans are sedentary and do not exercise at all.[1]

- Only 14 percent of Americans engage in high-intensity physical activity on a regular basis; 20 percent engage in moderate-intensity exercise.

- Education and economics affect activity levels. The higher their income and the more years of schooling they've had, the more likely Americans are to exercise regularly.[2]

- Americans have met or exceeded only 1 of the 13 physical activity and fitness goals of *Healthy People 2000:* They've instituted more employer-sponsored fitness programs.[3] Although overall physical activity in adults has increased, there has been no change in the percentage of sedentary persons, and fewer adults are combining regular physical activity with sound dietary practices to maintain a healthy body weight.

- America's young people are less fit than children were two decades ago. School-age children have more body fat and weigh more than their counterparts did 20 years ago. Fewer youngsters participate in daily physical education at school. An alarming 60 percent of U.S. children exhibit at least one risk factor for coronary heart disease by age 12; one of the most prevalent is physical inactivity.[4]

Often the college years represent a turning point in personal fitness. The most rapid declines in physical activity occur during late adolescence and early adulthood. According to the Surgeon General's report, from ages 18 through 21, the frequency of exercising vigorously three or more times a year declines 6.2 percentage points in men and 7.3 percentage points in women. This trend continues after graduation. In one survey of recent graduates, 47 percent reported a drop in physical activity.[5]

The choices you make and the habits you develop *now* can affect how long and how well you'll live. As you'll see in this chapter, exercise can help you reduce stress, boost your spirits, feel better, live longer, and lower your risk of serious disease. To get these benefits, you don't have to turn into a jock or fitness fanatic. All you have to do is get moving. This chapter can help. It presents the latest activity recommendations, documents the benefits of exercise, describes types of exercise, and provides guidelines for getting into shape and exercising safely. ❖

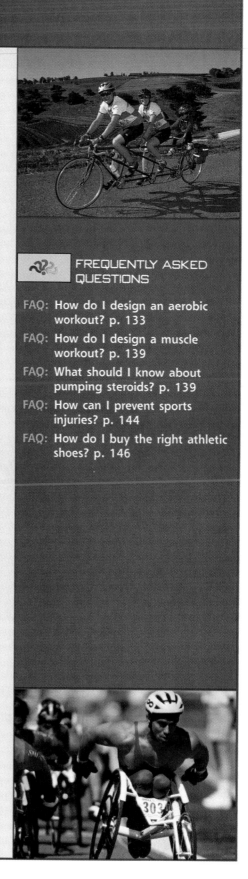

FREQUENTLY ASKED QUESTIONS

FAQ: **How do I design an aerobic workout? p. 133**

FAQ: **How do I design a muscle workout? p. 139**

FAQ: **What should I know about pumping steroids? p. 139**

FAQ: **How can I prevent sports injuries? p. 144**

FAQ: **How do I buy the right athletic shoes? p. 146**

Four components of physical fitness. (a) Cardiovascular fitness. (b) Muscular strength and endurance. (c) Body composition. (d) Flexibility.

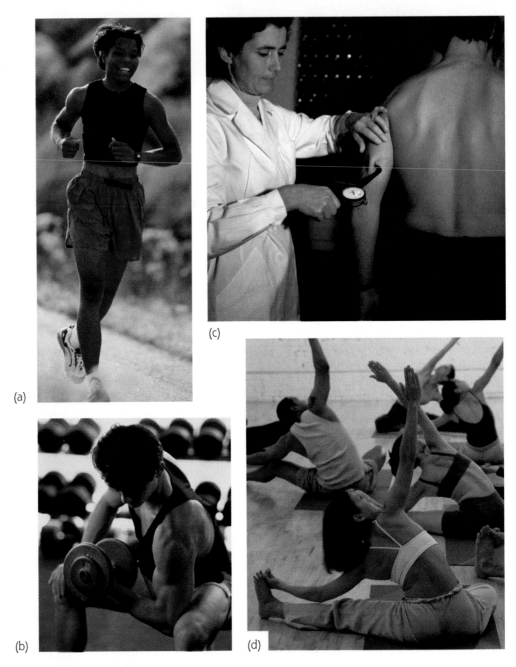

(a)

(b)

(c)

(d)

What Is Physical Fitness?

The simplest, most practical definition of **physical fitness** is the ability to respond to routine physical demands, with enough reserve energy to cope with a sudden challenge. You can consider yourself fit if you meet your daily energy needs; can handle unexpected extra demands; have a realistic but positive self-image; and are protecting yourself against potential health problems, such as heart disease.

Fitness is important both for health and for athletic performance. The health-related components of physi-

cal fitness, which this chapter emphasizes, include aerobic or cardiovascular endurance, muscular strength and endurance, flexibility, and body composition (the ratio of fat and lean body tissue). Athletic performance depends on additional skills, such as agility, coordination, balance, and speed, which vary with specific sports. While many amateur and professional athletes are in superb overall condition, you do not need athletic skills in order to keep your body operating at maximum capacity throughout life.

Cardiovascular fitness refers to the ability of the heart to pump blood through the body efficiently. It is achieved through **aerobic exercise**—any activity, such as brisk walking or swimming, in which the amount of oxygen taken into the body is slightly more than, or equal to, the amount of oxygen used by the body. In other words, aerobic exercise involves working out strenuously without pushing to the point of breathlessness. **Anaerobic exercise** is any activity in which the amount of oxygen taken in by the body cannot meet the demands of the activity; there is thus an oxygen deficit that must be made up later. An example of an anaerobic exercise is sprinting the quarter-mile, which leaves even the best-trained athletes gasping for air. In *nonaerobic exercise,* there is frequent rest between activities, as happens in bowling, softball, and doubles tennis. The body easily takes in all the oxygen needed for these activities, so your heart and lungs don't really get a workout.

Muscular fitness has two components: strength and endurance. **Strength** refers to the force within muscles; it is measured by the absolute maximum weight that we can lift, push, or press in one effort. **Endurance** is the ability to perform repeated muscular effort; it is measured by counting how many times you lift, push, or press a given weight. Both are equally important. It's not enough to be able to hoist a shovelful of snow; you've got to be able to keep shoveling until the entire driveway is clear.

Body composition refers to the relative amounts of fat and of lean tissue (bone, muscle, organs, water) in the body. As discussed in detail in Chapter 7, a high proportion of body fat has serious health implications, including increased incidence of heart disease, high blood pressure, diabetes, stroke, gall bladder problems, back and joint problems, and some forms of cancer. College-age men average 15 percent body fat; college-age women, 23 percent. Men with a body fat level higher than 25 percent and women with 32 percent or higher body fat are considered obese.

A combination of regular exercise and good nutrition is the best way to maintain a healthy body composition. Aerobic exercise helps by burning calories and increasing metabolic rate (the rate at which the body uses calories) for several hours after a workout. Strength training increases the proportion of lean body tissue by building muscle mass, which also increases the metabolic rate.

Flexibility is the range of motion around specific joints—for example, the stretching you do to touch your toes or twist your torso. Flexibility depends on many factors: your age, gender, and posture; bone spurs; and how fat or muscular you are. As children develop, their flexibility increases until adolescence. Then a gradual loss of joint mobility begins and continues throughout adult life. Both muscles and connective tissue, such as tendons and ligaments, shorten and become tighter if not used at all or not used through their full range of motion.

Physical **conditioning** (or training) refers to the gradual building up of the body to enhance cardiovascular or aerobic fitness, muscular strength and endurance, or flexibility.

Why Should I Exercise?

If exercise could be packed into a pill, it would be the single most widely prescribed and beneficial medicine in the nation. Why? Because nothing can do more to help your body function at its best (Figure 5-1). With regular activity, your heart muscles become stronger and pump blood more efficiently. Your heart rate and resting pulse slow down. Your blood pressure may drop slightly from its normal level.

Regular physical activity thickens the bones and can slow the loss of calcium that normally occurs with age. Exercise increases flexibility in the joints and improves digestion and elimination. It speeds up metabolism, so the body burns up more calories and body fat decreases. It heightens sensitivity to insulin (a great benefit for diabetics) and may lower the risk of developing diabetes.[6] In addition, exercise enhances clot-dissolving substances in the blood, helping to prevent strokes, heart attacks, and pulmonary embolisms (clots in the lungs). Regular, vigorous exercise can actually extend the lifespan. (See Pulsepoints: "Ten Reasons to Get Moving.")

Here is a summary of the benefits of getting in shape:

Longer Life

Longevity has more to do with one's level of physical activity than with genetics. In a 19-year study tracking the health and lifestyles of twins, the risk of death was 56 percent lower for those who exercised at least 30 minutes, six or more times per month, and 34 percent lower for occasional exercisers.[7]

A Hardier Heart and Stronger Lungs

Officials at the Centers for Disease Control and Prevention (CDC) have identified insufficient exercise as one of the leading preventable causes of coronary death in this country. Sedentary people are about twice as likely to die of a heart attack as people who are physically active. (See Chapter 13 for a detailed discussion of exercise and the prevention of heart disease.) In addition to its effects on the heart, exercise makes the lungs more efficient. They take in more oxygen, and their vital capacity (ability to take in and expel air) is increased, providing more energy for you to use.

■ **Figure 5-1 The Benefits of Exercise**
Exercise improves your body and mind
more than you might expect.

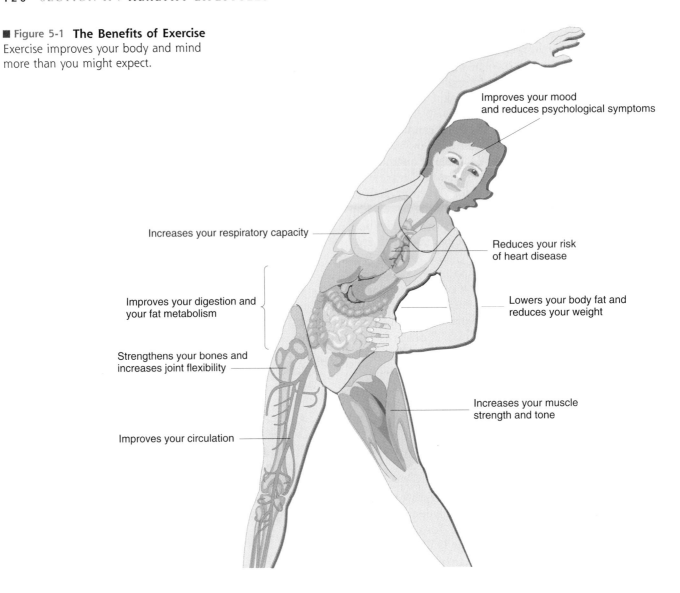

Improves your mood
and reduces psychological symptoms

Increases your respiratory capacity

Reduces your risk
of heart disease

Improves your digestion and
your fat metabolism

Lowers your body fat and
reduces your weight

Strengthens your bones and
increases joint flexibility

Increases your muscle
strength and tone

Improves your circulation

Better Bones

Weak and brittle bones are common among people who
don't exercise. **Osteoporosis,** a condition in which
bones lose their mineral density and become increasingly soft and susceptible to injury, affects a great many
older people. Women, in particular, are more vulnerable
because their bones are less dense to begin with.

Brighter Mood

Exercise makes people feel good from the inside out. As
discussed in Chapters 2 and 3, exercise boosts mood,
increases energy, reduces anxiety, improves concentration and alertness, and enables people to handle stress
better. During long workouts, some people experience
what is called "runner's high," which may be the result
of increased levels of mood-elevating brain chemicals
called **endorphins.**

Better Mental Health

Exercise has also proven an effective—but under-
used—treatment for mild to moderate depression and
may help in treating other mental disorders. A recent
review of more than 20 years of studies found that
aerobic exercise and strength training are equally
effective in relieving depression. They also reduce
anxiety in patients with panic disorder and can be
an important part of treatment for people with
schizophrenia.[8]

Protection Against Certain Cancers

Exercise reduces the risk of colon and rectal cancers,
possibly by enhancing digestion and elimination. In women, exercise also may help reduce
the risk of cancer of the breast and reproductive
organs.

PULSE *points*

Ten Reasons to Get Moving

1. **Improve cardiovascular fitness.** Regular activity strengthens the heart so it pumps blood more efficiently.
2. **Tone muscles.** With exercise, muscles become firmer, function more smoothly, and are capable of withstanding much more strain.
3. **Reduce stress.** Working out releases tensions and enhances your ability to deal with daily challenges.
4. **Improve mood.** Exercise may be the single most effective strategy for changing a bad mood. It also works wonders for reducing anxiety and depression.
5. **Burn calories.** Exercise speeds up metabolism, so the body uses more calories during and after a workout.
6. **Increase flexibility.** Exercise stretches and lengthens muscles and increases flexibility in the joints.
7. **Enhance strength and stamina.** Muscle workouts improve the circulation of blood in the tissues and increase the body's ability to do sustained work.
8. **Keep bones strong.** Regular physical activity (especially weight-bearing activities) thickens the bones, possibly preventing the slow loss of calcium that normally occurs with age.
9. **Lower the risk of disease.** Exercise helps prevent many serious health problems, including high blood pressure, strokes, heart attacks, and certain cancers.
10. **Put more life in your years—and possibly more years in your life.** Physical activity slows the aging process, so you remain healthier and more active for a longer time. And if you work out often and vigorously enough, you can actually extend your lifespan.

Lower Weight

Aerobic exercise burns off calories during your workout, because as your body responds to the increased demand from your muscles for nutrients, your metabolic rate rises. Moreover, this surge persists for as long as 12 hours after exercise, so you continue to use up more calories than usual even after you've stopped sweating. In addition, aerobic exercise suppresses appetite, so you aren't as tempted to eat. It also helps dieters lose fat rather than lean muscle tissue when they cut back on calories.[9] (See Chapter 7 for information on exercise and weight control.)

A More Active Old Age

Exercise slows the changes that are associated with advancing age: loss of lean muscle tissue, increase in body fat, and decrease in work capacity. In addition to lowering the risk of heart disease and stroke, exercise also helps older men and women retain the strength and mobility needed to live independently. Male and female runners over age 50 have much lower rates of disability and much lower health care costs than less active seniors.

How Much Exercise Do I Need?

When it comes to exercise, less is not more—but it's definitely better than none. Physical inactivity accounts for as many as 23 percent of all deaths from major chronic diseases, yet almost one of every three Americans is sedentary. (See Self-Survey: "Test Your Physical Activity IQ.") According to the CDC, 29.4 percent of those surveyed report no leisure-time physical activity at all. City dwellers tend to be more active than country folks, with 27.4 percent saying they are sedentary, compared with 36.6 percent of those in rural areas. Westerners also are more active than Americans in other regions.[10]

Even light exercise—activity that increases oxygen consumption less than three times the level burned by the body at rest—can improve physical and mental well-being. While light activity is good, moderate is even better, and health experts encourage everyone to accumulate at least 30 minutes a day of moderate physical activity. But you don't have to head to a gym or hit the bike path to do so. As recent studies have confirmed, "lifestyle" activities, such as walking, housecleaning, and gardening, are as effective as a structured exercise program in improving heart function, lowering blood pressure, and maintaining or losing weight.[11] (See Figure 5-2.)

In one study, overweight, sedentary middle-aged men and women who learned behavioral skills to make them more physically active (such as walking around airports or train stations while waiting for a departure) reduced their body fat percentage and improved their blood pressure and heart function as much as individuals participating in structured programs at a fitness center.[12] In another study, obese women ranging in age from 21 to

Self-*Survey* Test Your Physical Activity IQ

1. In general, what percentage of the calories you eat should come from carbohydrates if you are physically active?
   a. 60–65 percent
   b. 40 percent
   c. 50 percent
2. The most effective physical activity plan is:
   a. strength (resistance) training
   b. aerobic workouts at moderate intensity three or more times a week.
   c. combination of strength training and aerobic activity
3. *True or False?* Certain activities can help you to selectively remove fat from your waist, thighs, or other specific areas of your body.
   a. True
   b. False
4. *True or False?* Women tend to have a lower metabolic rate than men.
   a. True
   b. False
5. How long does it take to see improvements in fitness level if you are doing moderate intensity (somewhat hard) aerobic activity for 30 minutes three times a week?
   a. a day or two
   b. a week or two
   c. a month or two

6. What type of workout maximizes fat burning?
   a. low intensity
   b. moderate intensity
   c. high intensity
7. *True or False?* A person who weighs more burns more calories doing the same exercise as someone who weighs less.
   a. True
   b. False
8. *True or False?* Because we start losing muscle mass every year after about 30 years of age, physical activity has only a small benefit for older individuals.
   a. True
   b. False
9. What are the key components of physical activity that are important for improving your fitness?
   a. frequency, intensity, duration
   b. calorie intake, altitude, humidity
   c. temperature, time, type of activity
10. *True or False?* People who want bigger muscles should take protein supplements.
    a. True
    b. False

Answers: 1) a; 2) c; 3) False; 4) True; 5) b; 6) b; 7) True; 8) False; 9) a; 10) False

Source: U.S. Government, Shape Up America! (www.shapeup.org.)

---

60 who adapted a more active lifestyle lost as much weight as women in a low-impact aerobics program—and regained fewer pounds in the following year.[13]

Recognizing the value of different levels and types of activity, the American College of Sports Medicine has changed its recommendations on quantity and quality of exercise to include flexibility as well as aerobic and muscle workouts and to acknowledge that multiple short bouts of exercise during the day are nearly as beneficial as one long session.[14] Here are the current recommendations:

Cardiorespiratory Fitness

- Individuals who have not been active and are not fit should perform lower-intensity exercise (such as walking) for 30 minutes or more three to five days a week.

- To maintain fitness, individuals should engage in more intense aerobic exercise three to five days a week for 20 to 60 minutes or substitute two to six 10-minute periods of aerobic activity throughout the day. (The section on aerobic fitness discusses recommended intensity of aerobic workouts.)

Muscular Fitness

- One set of 8 to 10 exercises that work the major muscle groups should be performed two or three days a week. For most adults, the guidelines suggest 8 to 12 repetitions (or to a near-fatigue level) of each exercise. Persons who are older or frail may benefit from 10 to 15 repetitions.

Flexibility Training

- Flexibility exercises should be performed two or three days a week, with at least four repetitions per muscle group.[15]

■ Figure 5-2 **Getting Physical**

The benefits you can get from longer sessions of moderately intense activities are similar to the ones you would get from shorter sessions of more strenuous activities. Here are some examples of different activities that can boost your fitness level:

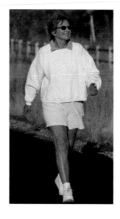
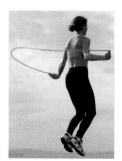
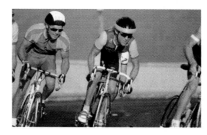

Less vigorous activities (done for longer periods of time)
    Washing and waxing a car for 45–60 minutes
    Washing windows or floors for 45–60 minutes
    Playing volleyball for 45 minutes
    Playing touch football for 30–45 minutes
    Gardening for 30–45 minutes
    Wheeling yourself in a wheelchair for 30–40 minutes
    Walking 1¾ miles in 35 minutes (20 minutes per mile)
    Basketball (shooting baskets) for 30 minutes
    Bicycling 5 miles in 30 minutes
    Dancing fast (social dancing) for 30 minutes
    Pushing a stroller 1½ miles in 30 minutes
    Raking leaves for 30 minutes
    Walking 2 miles in 30 minutes (15 minutes per mile)
    Doing water aerobics for 30 minutes

More vigorous activities (done for shorter periods of time)
    Swimming laps for 20 minutes
    Playing wheelchair basketball for 20 minutes
    Basketball (playing a game) for 15–20 minutes
    Bicycling 4 miles in 15 minutes
    Jumping rope for 15 minutes
    Running 1½ miles in 15 minutes (10 minutes per mile)
    Shoveling snow for 15 minutes
    Stairwalking for 15 minutes

Source: U.S. Department of Health and Human Services. *Physical Activity and Health: A Report of the Surgeon General.* Atlanta: U.S. Department of Health and Human Services, 1996.

Motivation

You know exercise is good for you—but do you work out regularly? As "Campus Focus: How Active Are College Students?" indicates, most students don't. Men are more likely than women to exercise on college campuses, and more white and Hispanic students work out than do African-American undergraduates. According to the Surgeon General's report on fitness, nearly half of Americans between the ages of 12 and 21 are not vigorously active on a regular basis.

What keeps you from working out? When that question was posted on a national chat board students listed a variety of excuses: "Gym membership is too expensive." "I'm not going to run in the snow!" "I don't have enough time." "I don't like the school gym—it stinks, people are trying too hard, and it takes too long to get a machine." "The workout room in my dorm is always crowded." Others revealed ways they had managed to overcome these barriers and motivate themselves, including:

- Sign up for a fitness "class," such as spinning or step-aerobics, so that exercise is built into your weekly schedule.

- Go to the gym with friends. "Even if it's rainy and cold, I know they're waiting for me so I go," one woman explained.

- Find a fun workout. "I love working out when it's something different—like water aerobics, ice skating, or swing dance," said one student.

- Use humor. One student put this sign on the wall: "You think flu season is scary? Wait till bathing suit season hits!"

- Build activity into your day. Many students walk to classes or always take the stairs rather than the elevator in their dorms.

- Do double-duty. Some students read class notes while on a Stairmaster or stationary bicycle. Others listen to audiocassettes of required reading books as they work out.

The course in which you're using this text may help you get motivated and moving. In a study that compared college alumni who had taken a health and physical education course with others who had not, those who'd taken the course were more likely to engage in aerobic exercise. Not coincidentally, they also were less likely to smoke and had lower intakes of dietary fat, cholesterol,

Campus Focus

How Active Are College Students?

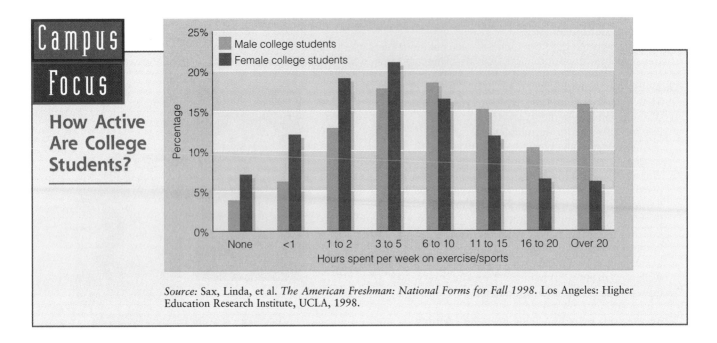

Source: Sax, Linda, et al. *The American Freshman: National Forms for Fall 1998.* Los Angeles: Higher Education Research Institute, UCLA, 1998.

and sodium.[16] In a recent study called "Project Grad," researchers at an urban university in Southern California developed a special course, "Fitness as a Lifestyle," designed to teach seniors to adopt and maintain physical activity. Did this "intervention" change the students' activity levels? For men, the answer was no. For women, it was yes. The women significantly increased their total energy expenditure and physical activity in their leisure hours and specifically increased strengthening and flexibility exercises. The men showed no significant changes, perhaps because they were already far more active than the women when they began the course.[17]

This gender difference is important because, at all ages, women are less physically active than men. According to the Surgeon General, 25 percent of women are sedentary, and more than 60 percent do not exercise regularly. Yet women have every reason to be more active. In addition to exercise's unisex benefits—such as lowering the risk of dying from coronary heart disease and of developing high blood pressure, colon cancer, and diabetes—physical activity helps women keep their bones healthy and strong, controls weight, builds lean muscle, reduces body fat, helps control joint swelling and pain associated with arthritis, eases symptoms of anxiety and depression, fosters improvements in mood and feelings of well-being, and can help reduce blood pressure in some women with hypertension.[18]

Getting Started

Most people don't need to see a doctor before beginning a gradual, sensible exercise program. However, you

should seek medical advice if you match any of the following descriptions:

- You've had a heart attack; your doctor has told you that you have heart trouble or a heart murmur; or your father, mother, brother, or sister had a heart attack before age 50.
- You often have pains or pressure in your left or midchest area or in your left neck, shoulder, or arm during or right after exercise, or you feel faint or have spells of dizziness, or you experience extreme breathlessness after mild exertion (such as a short walk at a moderate pace).
- Your doctor has told you that you have high blood pressure that is not under control or bone or joint problems, such as arthritis.
- You have a medical condition, such as diabetes, that might need special attention in an exercise program.
- You should also check with your doctor if you are over 40 and haven't been exercising two or three times a week.

Sticking with It: What Works

By some estimates, as many as half of all people who start an exercise program drop out within a year. According to the Surgeon General, you are more likely to keep up a healthy level of physical activity if you:

- think that, overall, you will benefit from exercise
- include activities that you enjoy
- feel you can do the activities safely and correctly
- have access to the activities on a regular basis
- can fit the activities into your daily schedule

The X&Y Files

Does One Sex Have an Athletic Advantage?

The classic advantage that men bring to athletics remains size. Their bigger hearts pump more blood with each beat. Their larger lungs take in 10 to 20 percent more oxygen. Their longer legs cover more distance with each stride. Their greater proportion of muscle generates more energy. The average adult male has roughly twice the percentage of muscle mass and half the percentage of body fat as a woman. If a man jogs along at 50 percent of capacity, a woman has to push to 73 percent of hers to keep up.

Overall, men are about 30 percent stronger, particularly above the waist. A woman's upper body power is usually only one half to two-thirds that of an equally well-conditioned man, while her legs have about 70 percent of his strength. With training, a woman's leg strength, compared pound for pound, can equal or surpass a man's. However, the best female sprinters aren't likely to outrun the best males, for anatomic reasons. The angle of the upper leg bone (femur) to the pelvis is greater in a woman, so her legs are less efficient at running. But this doesn't mean she can't run very, very fast.

Differences in body fat and muscle also affect performance. Adult women have 10 to 15 more pounds of fat and 45 pounds less muscle than men. Even with conditioning, women's bodies remain fatter. Female cadets at the United States Military Academy at West Point—who are stronger, fitter, and leaner than most women—have roughly twice the percentage of body fat (18 to 19 percent) of their male classmates (9 to 10 percent).

Women's smaller muscle mass also affects their potential strength. With muscular training, women will increase their strength and then plateau after 4 to 6 months, when they approach the limits of their genetic potential for improvement. Men continue to make progress for 8 to 12 months. There is a similar limitation in aerobic conditioning. Although training improves oxygen capacity for both sexes, a woman's maximum oxygen intake remains about 27 percent lower than that of an equally well-conditioned man.

But there are advantages as well as disadvantages to female anatomy and physiology. Because they are shorter and smaller, women have a lower sense of gravity and better balance—pluses in sports like gymnastics and diving. Because their tissues and joints are more elastic (another of estrogen's gifts), women are more flexible. And, in ways exercise physiologists are just beginning to appreciate, the body of a woman may be superbly designed—physiologically, biochemically, anatomically—to go the distance.

The longer the race—on land, water, or ice—the better that women perform. In an analysis of world-record times in running, swimming, and speed skating, researchers at Northeastern University observed that in all three sports the superiority of men's performances diminished with increasing distance. A study of female and male runners, conducted at South Africa's University of the Witwatersrand, found that women were able to maintain a higher rate of exertion for longer periods than men at distances of 90 kilometers or greater. Another South African study showed that women ultra-marathon runners—who run cross-country races of 30 miles or more—have greater resistance to fatigue than equally trained men.

What accounts for women's surprising stamina? The answer may lie in that most maligned form of body tissue: fat. According to studies at Ball State University, women are more efficient than men at using fat as an energy source—and they have a higher percentage of fat available for such use. It may be that by burning fat first, women can put off the depletion of their stores of carbohydrate energy that can cause overwhelming muscle fatigue. In the water, female fat has even more advantages. A woman's larger amount of hip fat makes her more buoyant so her body stays higher in the water. It also insulates her from the cold so her body temperature doesn't fall as much as a man's. This may explain why no man has managed to break the world record for swimming the English channel, which was set in 1978 by Penny Dean.

Source: Hales, Dianne. *Just Like a Woman.* New York: Bantam Books, 2000.

• feel that the activities don't impose financial or social costs you aren't willing to take on

• think that the activities have few negative consequences, such as injury or lost time

Strategies for Change: "Psyching Yourself Up to Work Out" on page 132 offers additional suggestions that can help you stick with a shape-up program.

Cardiovascular or Aerobic Fitness

Your heart and lungs need regular work to reach peak efficiency. If you haven't been exercising regularly, even mild forms of exertion, such as climbing stairs, can

Strategies *for* Change

Psyching Yourself Up to Work Out

Here are some additional suggestions that can help you stick with a shape-up program.

✔ Set goals. People who keep their eyes on a prize—whether it's lowering blood pressure or improving their time on a 10K run—are more likely to stick with an exercise plan.

✔ Go for 12. The most noticeable fitness gains come in the first 6 to 12 weeks of an exercise program. If you stick with it that long, you're more likely to keep working out.

✔ Alternate athletic activities. If you mainly jog, try step aerobics as a change of pace. Switching activities breaks the monotony and also gives muscles you've been using time to recover.

✔ Keep a log. If you chart your mood and energy levels on days with or without exercise, you'll probably see the emotional payoff of being physical.

✔ If you don't feel like exercising, tell yourself you'll just work out for ten minutes. Chances are that when you reach that point you'll want to continue.

✔ Reward yourself. An occasional new running shirt or jacket can feel well earned after you've reached a certain milestone in your shape-up regimen.

seem rigorous. As you get in shape, however, your body will be able to handle greater challenges with ease.

Your Target Heart Rate

The best way you can be sure you're working hard enough to condition your heart and lungs but not overdoing it is to use your pulse, or heart rate, as a guide. One of the easiest places to feel your pulse is in the carotid artery in your neck. Tilt your head back slightly and to one side. Use your middle finger or forefinger, or both, to feel for your pulse. (Do not use your thumb; it has a beat of its own.) To determine your heart rate, count the number of pulses you feel for 10 seconds and multiply that number by six, or count for 30 seconds and multiply that number by two. Learn to recognize the pulsing of your heart when you're lying or sitting down. On your fitness record, make note of your **resting heart rate.**

Start taking your pulse during, or immediately after, exercise, when it's much more pronounced than when you're at rest. Three minutes after heavy exercise, take your pulse again. The closer that reading is to your resting heart rate, the better your condition. If it takes a long time for your pulse to recover and return to its resting level, your body's ability to handle physical stress is poor. As you continue working out, however, your pulse will return to normal much more quickly.

You don't want to push yourself to your maximum heart rate; yet you must exercise at about 60 to 85 percent of that maximum to get cardiovascular benefits from your training. This range is called your **target heart rate.** If you don't exercise intensely enough to raise your heart rate at least this high, your heart and lungs won't benefit from the workout. If you push too hard, on the other hand, and exercise at or near your absolute maximum heart rate, you run the risk of placing too great a burden on your heart.

Table 5-1 lists target heart rates for various ages. The following formulas can also be used to calculate your maximum and target heart rates (in beats per minute).

For men, the formula is as follows:

$$220 - \text{Age} = \text{Maximum Heart Rate} \times .60 \, (\text{Target Zone for Beginners}) = \text{Target Heart Rate}$$

Example for a 20-year-old man:

$$220 - 20 = 200 \; \text{Maximum Heart Rate} \times .60 = 120 \; \text{Target Heart Rate}$$

For women, the formula is as follows:

$$225 - \text{Age} = \text{Maximum Heart Rate} \times .60 \, (\text{Target Zone for Beginners}) = \text{Target Heart Rate}$$

Example for a 20-year-old woman:

$$225 - 20 = 205 \; \text{Maximum Heart Rate} \times .60 = 123 \; \text{Target Heart Rate}$$

In the initial stages of training, aim for the lower end of your target zone (the 60 percent calculated above), and gradually build up to 75 percent of your maximum heart rate. After six months or more of regular exercise, you can push up to 85 percent of your maximum heart rate if you wish, though you don't have to work that hard just to stay in shape. As long as you use your target heart rate as your guide, your exercise intensity should be just right.

■ **Table 5-1** Target Heart Rate

	Men			Women		
Age	Average Maximum Heart Rate (100%)	Target Heart Rate (60–85%)		Average Maximum Heart Rate (100%)	Target Heart Rate (60–85%)	
20	200	120	170	205	123	174
25	195	117	166	200	120	170
30	190	114	162	195	117	166
35	185	111	157	190	114	162
40	180	108	153	185	111	157
45	175	105	149	180	108	153
50	170	102	145	175	105	149
55	165	99	140	170	102	145
60	160	96	136	165	99	140
65	155	93	132	160	96	136
70	150	90	128	155	93	132

 ## How Do I Design an Aerobic Workout?

Whatever activity you choose, your aerobic workout should consist of several stages:

Warm-Up

Just as you don't get in your car and gun your engine to 60 miles per hour, you shouldn't do the same with your body. You need to prepare your cardiovascular system for a workout, speed up the blood flow to your lungs, and increase the temperature and elasticity of your muscles and connective tissue to avoid injury.

Start by walking briskly for about five minutes. This helps your body make the transition from inactivity to exertion. Follow this general warm-up with about five minutes of simple stretches of the muscles you'll be exercising most. Before a jog, for instance, you can stretch the muscles in your ankle and the back of your leg by leaning against a wall, with one leg bent and tilted forward and the other straight. Lean forward until you feel the stretch and hold.

Aerobic Activity

The two key components of this part of your workout are intensity and duration. As described above, you can use your target heart rate to make sure you are working at the proper intensity. The American College of Sports Medicine recommends an intensity that achieves 55 to 90 percent of the maximum heart rate and a duration of 20 to 60 minutes in one session or two to six briefer sessions (each lasting at least 10 minutes) during the course of the day.

Cool-Down

After you've pushed your heart rate up to its target level and kept it there for a while, the worst thing you can do is slam on the brakes. If you come to a sudden stop, you put your heart at risk. When you stand or sit immediately after vigorous exercise, blood can pool in your legs. You need to keep moving—though at a slower pace—to ensure an adequate supply of blood to your heart. Ideally, you should walk for five to ten minutes at a comfortable pace before you end your workout session.

Your Long-Term Plan

One of the most common mistakes people make is to push too hard too fast. Often they end up injured or discouraged and quit entirely. If you are just starting an aerobic program, think of it as a series of phases: beginning, progression, and maintenance:

- *Beginning (4–6 weeks):* Start slow and low (in intensity). If you're walking, monitor your heart rate and aim for 55 percent of your maximal heart rate. Another good way to make sure you're moving at the right pace is this rule of thumb: If you can sing as you walk, you're going too slow; if you can't talk, you're going too fast.

- *Progression (16–20 weeks):* Gradually increase the duration and/or intensity of your workouts. For instance, you might add five minutes every two weeks to your walking time. You also gradually can pick up your pace, using your target heart rate as your guide. Keep a log of your workouts so you can chart your progress until you reach your goal.

- *Maintenance (lifelong):* Once you've reached the stage of exercising at your target heart rate for 20 to

60 minutes three to five days a week, there's little added benefit—and increased risk of injury—if you push harder or farther. You may want to develop a repertoire of aerobic activities you enjoy and combine or alternate to avoid monotony and keep up your enthusiasm. This is called cross-training.

Walking

More men and women—an estimated 65 million in all, according to the National Sporting Goods Association—are taking to their feet. Some, casualties of high-intensity sports, can no longer withstand the wear-and-tear of rigorous workouts. Others want to shape up, slim down, or ward off heart disease and other health problems. The good news for all is that walking may well be the perfect exercise.

According to recent studies, walking at an easy to moderate pace for 40 to 60 minutes is actually better than exercising hard for just 20 minutes. While both approaches enhance fitness, walking is less likely to lead to injuries. Walking develops cardiovascular fitness, builds up endurance, burns fat, and strengthens muscles in the lower body. Recent research at the University of Pittsburgh Graduate School of Public Health found that women who began a walking program 10 to 15 years ago were more likely to remain active and reported fewer cases of heart disease than their sedentary counterparts.[19] Another bonus is stress reduction. Since you can do it during a break or at lunch time, walking builds relaxation into your day.

Treadmills are a good alternative to outdoor walks—and not just in bad weather. They keep you moving at a certain pace, they're easier on the knees, and they allow you to exercise in a climate-controlled, pollution-free environment—a definite plus for many city dwellers.

Waterwalking in a pool or at a lake or beach is another alternative—and an excellent exercise. Because of the water's resistance, you don't have to walk as fast in water as you would on land to burn the same number of calories. Walking two miles per hour in thigh-high water is equivalent to three miles per hour on land.

In race-walking, or striding (as its noncompetitive form is called), you must keep your lead foot on the ground as your trailing leg pushes off, and your knee remains straight as your body passes over that leg. As a result, one foot is always supporting the body, so the maximum impact per step is much lower than when you run and the injury rate is low.

Because their stride is shorter, race-walkers have to stretch their hips forward and backward, which is good for flexibility. Because of the extra effort, they can get an added bonus: they burn up more calories than they would running at the same speed over the same distance.

Here are some guidelines for putting your best foot forward:

- Walk very slowly for five minutes, and then do some simple stretches.
- Maintain good posture. Focus your eyes ahead of you, stand erect, and pull in your stomach.
- Use the heel-to-toe method of walking. The heel of your leading foot should touch the ground before the ball or toes of that foot do. When you push off with your trailing foot, bend your knee as you raise your heel. You should be able to feel the action in your calf muscles.
- Pump your arms back and forth to burn 5 to 10% more calories and get an upper-body workout as well.
- End your walk the way you started it—let your pace become more leisurely for the last five minutes.

Jogging and Running

The difference between jogging and running is speed. You should be able to carry on a conversation with someone on a long jog or run; if you're too breathless to talk, you're pushing too hard.

If your goal is to enhance aerobic fitness, long, slow, distance running is best. If you want to improve your speed, try *interval training*, which consists of repeated hard runs over a certain distance, with intervals of relaxed jogging in between. Depending on what suits you and what your training goals are, you can vary the distance, duration, and number of fast runs, as well as the time and activity between them. Interval training is usually done on a track and should not be attempted unless you're in top shape.

If you have been sedentary, it's best to launch a walking program before attempting to jog or run. Start by walking for 15 to 20 minutes three times a week at a comfortable pace. Continue at this same level until you no longer feel sore or unduly fatigued the day after exercising. Then increase your walking time to 20 to 25 minutes, speeding up your pace as well.

When you can handle a brisk 25-minute walk, alternate fast walking with slow jogging. Begin each session walking, and gradually increase the amount of time you spend jogging. If you feel breathless while jogging, slow down and walk. Continue to alternate in this manner until you can jog for 10 minutes without stopping. If you gradually increase your jogging time by 1 or 2 minutes with each workout, you'll slowly build up from 10 to 20 or 25 minutes per session. For optimal fitness, you should jog at least three times a week.

Here's how to be sure you're running right:

- As you run, keep your back straight and your head up. Run tall, with your buttocks tucked in. Look straight ahead. Hold your arms slightly away from your body. Your elbows should be bent slightly so that your forearms are almost parallel to the ground. Move your arms rhythmically to propel yourself along.

- Have your heels hit the ground first. Land on your heel, rock forward, and push off the ball of your foot. If this is difficult, try a more flat-footed style.

- Avoid running on the balls of your feet; this produces soreness in the calves because the muscles must contract for a longer time. To avoid shin splints (a dull ache in the lower shins), stretch regularly to strengthen the shin muscles and to develop greater flexibility in your ankles.

- Avoid running on hard surfaces and making sudden stops or turns.

- Breathe through your nose and mouth to get more volume. Learn to "belly breathe": When you breathe in, your belly should expand; when you breathe out, it should flatten. If your breathing becomes labored, try exhaling with resistance through pursed lips so that your body utilizes more oxygen per breath.

- When you approach a hill, shorten your stride. Lift your knees higher; pump your arms more. If the hill is really steep, lean forward. When you start downhill, lean forward, and run as if you were on a flat surface. Don't lean back, because doing so could strain your knees and the muscles in your legs.

Swimming

More than 100 million Americans dive into the water every year. What matters for our heart's health, however, is getting a good workout, not just getting wet. Swimming is an excellent exercise for cardiovascular fitness and also rates fairly high for weight control, muscular function, and flexibility. However, it's not as effective as activities such as walking and running for building strong bones and preventing osteoporosis.

For aerobic conditioning, you have to swim laps, using a freestyle, butterfly, breast-, or backstroke. (The sidestroke is too easy.) You've also got to be a good enough swimmer to keep churning through the water for at least 20 minutes. Your heart will beat more slowly in water than on land, so your heart rate while swimming is not an accurate guide to exercise intensity. You should try to keep up a steady pace that's fast enough to make you feel pleasantly tired, but not completely exhausted, by the time you get out of the pool.

Swimming is good for people of all ages, particularly those over 50 or with physical handicaps. Swimming facilities are available in nearly all communities. Check your college gym; your local YWCA, YMCA, or JCC; your city recreation department; and other schools in your area.

Here are some guidelines for smart swimming:

- Start by swimming 50 yards and rest when you feel breathless.

- Try to swim 100 yards, rest for a minute, and then swim another 100 yards.

- Increase your distance slowly. See if you can work up to 700 yards in 18 minutes.

- Stick to the crawl, the butterfly, the breaststroke, or the backstroke.

Cycling

Bicycling, indoors and out, can be an excellent cardiovascular conditioner, as well as an effective way to control weight—provided you aren't just along for the ride. If you coast down too many hills, you'll have to ride longer up hills or on level ground in order to get a good workout. Half of all bikes now sold in the United States are mountain bikes, sturdy cycles with knobby tires that allow bikers to climb up and zoom down dirt trails and explore places traditional racing bikes couldn't go. However, an 18-speed bike can make pedaling too easy, unless you choose gears carefully. To gain aerobic benefits, mountain bikers have to work hard enough to raise their heart rates to their target zone and keep up that intensity for at least 20 minutes.

Using a one-wheel stationary cycle with a tension-control knob, you can adjust the amount of effort

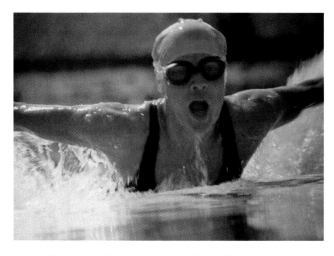

Swimming is good exercise for people of all ages—particularly for cardiovascular fitness and flexibility.

required; start with low resistance, then increase the tension until you're working at your target heart rate. You can put the cycle in front of a television set or look out the window if you feel the need for some scenery— or you can read or simply meditate while pedaling.

Here's a guide to smart cycling:

- If you're not used to cycling, start slowly. Work up from 5 minutes of steady pedaling (interrupted by rest periods if necessary) to 10, 15, 20, and 25 minutes. Limit your rides to 5–10 minutes the first week. Increase your time and speed gradually to avoid sore thigh muscles. Rest when you feel breathless.

- Keep your elbows slightly bent to allow for a more relaxed upper body. Change your hand positions periodically to avoid numbness.

- Monitor your heart rate to make sure you're working within your target range.

- When riding outdoors, be sure to wear a helmet. Look for proof that it conforms to either the Snell or ANSI standard for head protection.

- Make yourself visible. Wear reflective clothing if you can. If you cannot, remember that drivers see bright pink, yellow, and orange most easily.

- Always follow the rules of the road—stick to the right, stop at stop signs, heed one-way signs, and so on.

Cross-country Skiing

One of the most effective forms of aerobic exercise, cross-country or Nordic skiing, has become an increasingly popular winter sport. Thanks to machines that simulate the moves of Nordic skiing, it's now possible to "ski" in any season. Because almost every muscle in the body gets a workout, cross-country skiing is excellent for all-around conditioning. Using the poles works the arms, shoulders, back, and abdomen, while the kick-and-glide action of skiing involves virtually all the muscles of the legs, thighs, and abdomen. Also, as exercisers breathe faster and more deeply, their rib, abdominal, and shoulder muscles get a workout. Another plus: The risk of joint and ligament injury while cross-country skiing is lower than for many other impact-aerobic activities (and much lower than for downhill skiing).

Other Aerobic Activities

Because variety is the spice of an active life, many people prefer different forms of aerobic exercise. All can provide many health benefits. Among the popular options:

- *Spinning.*™ Spinning is a cardiovascular workout for the whole body that utilizes a special stationary bicy-

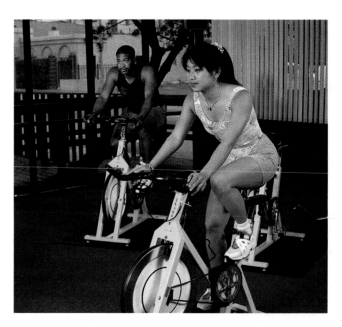

"Spinning" is an increasingly popular way to get a cardiovascular workout.

cle. Led by an instructor, a group of bikers listen to music and modify their bikes' resistance and their own pace according to the rhythm. An average spinning class lasts 45 minutes and has between 20 and 40 participants.

   Unlike an ordinary stationary bike, a spinning bike has a larger saddle area and a heavier fly wheel to create greater resistance; the rider, rather than a built-in computer, monitors performance. Introduced in 1987, this indoor cycling program has become enormously popular. More than 150,000 people in 60 countries worldwide participate in "spinning" classes every day, burning an average of 500 calories in each workout. Spinning has grown in appeal because it is time efficient and nonimpact and because people of all ages, skills, and fitness levels can participate in the same class.[20]

- *Skipping rope.* This is essentially a form of stationary jogging with some extra arm action thrown in. It is excellent both as a heart conditioner and as a way of losing weight. Always warm up before starting and cool down afterward. To alleviate boredom, try skipping to music, and vary the steps: both feet together, alternating left and right feet, or jumping up and down on one leg.

- *Aerobic dancing.* This activity combines music with kicking, bending, and jumping. A typical class (you can also dance at home to a video or TV program) consists of stretching exercises and sit-ups, followed by aerobic dances and cool-down exercises. A particular benefit of aerobic dance is that people get enjoyment and stimulation from the music; they're also able to move their bodies without worrying about skill and technique. "Soft," or low-impact, aerobic dancing doesn't put as much strain on the joints as "hard," or high-impact, routines.

- *Step training or bench aerobics.* This low-impact workout combines step, or bench, climbing with music and choreographed movements. Basic equipment consists of a bench 4 to 12 inches high. The fitter you are, the higher the bench—but the higher the bench, the greater the risk of knee injury. A 40-minute step workout is equivalent to running at seven miles an hour in terms of oxygen uptake and calories burned.

- *Stair-climbing.* An estimated 4 million Americans are stepping up to fitness, according to the American Sports Data Institute. You could run up the stairs in an office building or dormitory, but most people use stair-climbing machines available in home models and at gyms and health clubs. On most versions of these machines, exercisers push a pair of pedals up and down—much easier on the feet and legs than many other activities.

- *Rollerblading.* In-line skating can increase aerobic endurance and muscular strength and is less stressful on joints and bones than running or high-impact aerobics. Rollerbladers can adjust the intensity of their workout by varying the terrains. (Obviously, they'll have to work harder while going up hills, and less so on the slide down.) They can also buy special training wheels and weights to increase resistance and make muscles work harder. One caution: Protective gear, including a helmet, knee and elbow pads, and wrist guards, is essential.

Muscular Strength and Endurance

Although aerobic workouts condition your insides (heart, blood vessels, and lungs), they don't exercise many of the muscles that shape your outsides and provide power when you need it. Strength workouts are important because they enable muscles to work efficiently and reliably. Conditioned muscles function more smoothly and contract somewhat more vigorously and with less effort. With exercise, muscle tissue becomes firmer and can withstand much more strain—the result of toughening the sheath protecting the muscle and developing more connective tissue within it (see Figure 5-3).

Muscular strength and endurance are critical for handling everyday burdens, such as cramming a 20-pound suitcase into an overhead luggage bin or hauling a trunk down from the attic. Prolonged exercise prepares the muscles for sustained work by improving the circulation of blood in the tissue. The number of tiny blood vessels, called capillaries, increases by as much as 50 percent in regularly exercised muscles; and existing capillaries open wider so that the total circulation increases by as much as 400 percent, thus providing the muscles with a much greater supply of nutrients. This increase occurs after about 8 to 12 weeks in young persons, but takes longer in older individuals. Inactivity reverses the process, gradually shutting down the extra capillaries that have developed.

The latest research on fat-burning shows that the best way to reduce your body fat is to add muscle-strengthening exercise to your workouts. Muscle tissue is your very best calorie-burning tissue, and the more you have, the more calories you burn, even when you are resting. You don't have to become a serious body builder. Using handheld weights (also called free weights) two or three times a week is enough. Just be sure you learn how to use them properly because you can tear or strain muscles if you don't practice the proper weight-lifting techniques.

A balanced workout regimen of muscle-building and aerobic exercise does more for you than just burn fat. It gives you more endurance by promoting better distribution of oxygen to your tissues and increasing the blood flow to your heart.

Exercise and Muscles

Your muscles never stay the same. If you don't use them, they atrophy, weaken, or break down. If you use them rigorously and regularly, they grow stronger. The only way to develop muscles is by demanding more of them than you usually do. This is called **overloading.** As you train, you have to increase the number of repetitions or the amount of resistance gradually and work the muscle to temporary fatigue. That's why it's important not to quit when your muscles start to tire. Some exercise enthusiasts believe that the experience of pain—the "burn"—signals that exercise is paying off; however, others contend that it means you're pushing too hard and risking injury.

You need to exercise differently for strength than for endurance. To develop strength, you do a few repetitions with heavy loads. As you increase the load, object, or weight your muscles must move, you increase your strength. To increase endurance, you do many more repetitions with lighter loads. If your muscles are weak and you need to gain strength in your upper body, you may have to work for weeks to do a half-dozen regular pushups. Then you can start building endurance

Strength workouts increase circulation

The heart's right half pumps oxygen-poor blood to capillary beds in lungs. There, O_2 diffuses into blood and CO_2 diffuses out. The oxygenated blood flows into the heart's left half where it is then pumped to capillary beds throughout the body

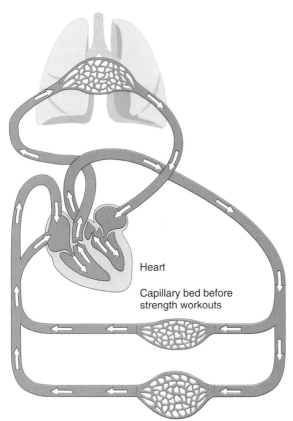

Heart

Capillary bed before strength workouts

Capillary bed after 8–12 weeks of strength workouts (extra capillaries develop, circulation increases)

Strength workouts build muscles

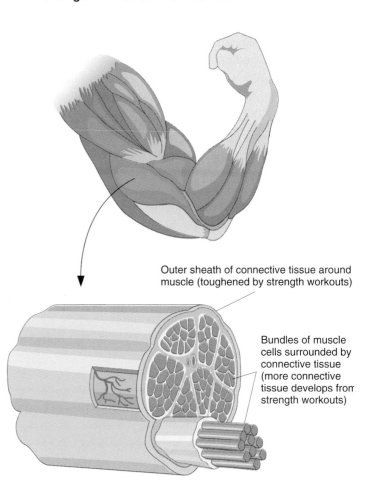

Outer sheath of connective tissue around muscle (toughened by strength workouts)

Bundles of muscle cells surrounded by connective tissue (more connective tissue develops from strength workouts)

■ **Figure 5-3** Strength training in combination with aerobic exercise develops muscles, burns fat, and increases blood circulation and oxygen supply to body tissues.

by doing as many pushups as you can before collapsing in exhaustion.

Isometric exercises are those in which you push or pull against an immovable object, with each muscle contraction being held for five to eight seconds and being repeated five to ten times daily. Isometric exercises seem to raise blood pressure in some people, which can be dangerous; they're not generally used to develop muscle strength.

Isotonic exercises are those in which the muscle moves a moderate load several times, as in weight-lifting or calisthenics. The kind of isotonic exercise best for producing muscular strength involves high resistance and a low number of repetitions. On the other hand, you can develop the greatest flexibility, coordination, and endurance with isotonic exercises that incorporate lower resistance and frequent repetitions.

For isotonic exercise, you can use free weights (such as barbells and dumbbells) or Nautilus or Universal equipment, found in most gyms and health clubs. Nautilus and Universal weight-training machines use the principle of progressive resistance. The Universal equipment is a system of cables, pulleys, and weights. Nautilus machines have a special cam (a pulley with an off-center axis) that adjusts the resistance for exercise in all positions.

Isokinetic exercises that use special machines provide resistance to overload muscles throughout the entire range of motion. These exercises are highly effective in strengthening specific muscle groups; but the sophisticated mechanical devices are expensive, elaborate, and generally available only at commercial fitness clubs.

Muscular training is highly specific, which means that you have to exercise certain muscles for certain results. If you want to build up your leg muscles to run a marathon, pushups won't help—just as running a marathon won't develop your upper body. If you're training with specific goals in mind, you have to tailor your exercise program to make sure you meet them.

How Do I Design a Muscle Workout?

A workout with weights should exercise your body's primary muscle groups: the *deltoids* (shoulders), *pectorals* (chest), *triceps* and *biceps* (back and front of upper arms), *quadriceps* and *hamstrings* (front and back of thighs), *gluteus maximus* (buttocks), and *abdomen* (see Figure 5-4). Various machines and free-weight routines focus on each muscle group, but the principle is always the same: Muscles contract as you raise and lower a weight, and you repeat the lift-and-lower routine until the muscle group is tired.

A weight-training program is made up of both **sets** (set numbers of repetitions of the same movement) and **reps** (the single performance of exercises, such as lifting 75 pounds once). You should allow your breath to return to normal before moving on to each new set. Pushing yourself to the limit builds strength.

Maintaining proper breathing techniques during weight training is crucial. To breathe correctly, inhale when muscles are relaxed, and exhale when you push or lift. Don't ever hold your breath because oxygen flow helps prevent muscle fatigue and injury.

Remember that your muscles need sufficient time to recover from a weight-training session. Allow no less than 48 hours, but no more than 96 hours, between training sessions, so that your body can recover from the workout and so that you'll avoid overtraining. Workouts on consecutive days do more harm than good, because the body can't recover that quickly. Two or three 30-minute training sessions a week should be sufficient for building strength and endurance. Indeed, you can obtain 70 to 80 percent as much improvement by strength training twice a week as three times a week. However, your muscles will begin to

atrophy if you let more than three or four days pass without exercising them. For total fitness, you may want to schedule aerobic workouts for your days off from weight training.

What Should I Know About Pumping Steroids?

Steroids

Anabolic steroids, synthetic derivatives of the male hormone testosterone, are approved for medical use in treating severe burns and injuries. However, some competitive athletes seeking an extra edge, those trying to transform their bodies and look strong, and the "fighting elite"—gang members, police, and bouncers who want to increase their size and strength—use steroids, usually in dangerous forms and doses, to gain weight and strength. (See Chapter 15 for a further discussion of steroid abuse.)

■ Figure 5-4 **The Body's Primary Muscle Groups**
Different exercises can strengthen and stretch different muscle groups.

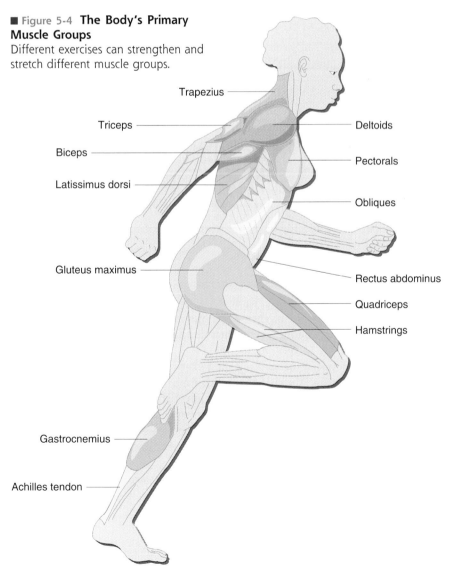

Strategies *for* Prevention

Working with Weights

If you plan to work with free weights, here are some guidelines for using them safely and effectively:

✔ Don't train alone—for safety's sake. Work with a partner so you can serve as spotters for each other and help motivate each other as well.

✔ Always warm up and stretch before weight training; also be sure to stretch after training.

✔ Begin with relatively light weights (50 percent of the maximum you can lift), and increase the load slowly until you find the weight that will cause muscle failure at anywhere from eight to twelve repetitions. (Muscle failure is the point during a workout at which you can no longer perform or complete a repetition through the entire range of motion.)

✔ In the beginning, don't work at maximum intensity. Increase your level of exertion gradually over two to six weeks to allow your body to adapt to new stress without soreness.

✔ Always train your entire body, starting with the larger muscle groups. Don't focus only on specific areas, although you may want to concentrate on your weakest muscles.

✔ Always use proper form. Unnecessary twisting, lurching, lunging, or arching can cause serious injury. Remember, quality matters more than quantity. One properly performed set of lifts can produce a greater increase in strength and muscle mass than many sets of improperly performed lifts.

Some users inject high doses of steroids intended only for horses. Others, in a practice called "stacking," take several different steroids at the same time. Steroids do increase weight and muscle strength; but they have dangerous side effects on the liver, reproductive organs, and the mind (see Chapter 15 on substance abuse). Long-term use also reduces levels of beneficial high-density lipoproteins, thereby increasing the risk of heart disease.[21]

In addition, the sharing of needles to inject steroids could result in transmission of HIV from an infected person to others. Anabolic steroids also have profound psychological effects. Long-term, high-dose use may lead to a preoccupation with steroid use, difficulty stopping despite side effects, drug craving, and withdrawal symptoms (including depression).

Some athletes and bodybuilders are experimenting with alternatives to steroids, including human growth hormone (HGH) and gamma hydroxybutyrate (GHB).

Neither substance is safe, and they should never be taken in the mistaken belief that they can add bulk to muscles. The use of HGH, an injectable form of the hormone that produces normal growth, carries the risk of hepatitis or HIV infection from tainted needles, as well as other medical complications. GHB, a substance naturally found in the central nervous system, can cause sudden sleepiness, short-term coma, vomiting, dizziness, headache, nausea, vomiting, and seizures.

Ergogenic Aids

They sound too good to be true: dietary supplements that boost strength and enhance athletic performance. Teenage boys and men in their twenties are the heaviest users. Do they work? Or are users endangering their health for an unproven benefit? Here's what we know—and don't know—about some popular energy-boosting, or ergogenic, aids:

* *Androstenedione* (a testosterone precursor normally produced by the adrenal glands and gonads). After home-run record holder Mark McGwire admitted that he used this supplement, androstenedione use increased fivefold among young people.[22] Seen as a natural alternative to anabolic steroids, androstenedione has not been proven safe or effective. In a study of its effects on men between the ages of 19 and 29, androestenedione did not show any effect on muscle strength but did increase concentrations of estrogen, which is associated with breast enlargement and increased risk of cardiovascular and pancreatic cancer in men.[23]

* *Creatine* (an amino acid that provides energy for muscular activity). While tests show creatine may increase strength and endurance, other effects on the body remain unknown. In a study of college football players randomly assigned to placebo or creatine treatment groups, the participants who took creatine gained significantly in their fat-free/bone-free mass, isotonic lifting volume, and sprint performance. They weighed more, found themselves able to move greater weight volume, and cycled faster for short periods of time. However, little is known about the medical safety of short-term or long-term creatine supplementation.[24]

* *GBL* (gamma butyrolactone). This unapproved drug, being studied as a treatment for narcolepsy, a disabling sleep disorder, is also marketed on the Internet and in some professional gyms as a muscle-builder and performance-enhancer. In 1999 the FDA warned consumers to avoid any products containing GBL, noting that they have been associated with at least 55 reports of adverse health effects, including 1 death and 19 incidents in which users became comatose or unconscious.[25]

• *Glycerol* (a natural element derived from fats). Some sports-drink manufacturers are testing formulations that include glycerol, which they claim can lower heart rate and stave off exhaustion in marathon events. However, glycerol-induced hyperhydration (holding too much water in the blood) can have a negative impact on performance and may be hazardous to health.[26]

• *Sodium bicarbonate* (baking soda). This everyday substance is believed to delay fatigue by neutralizing lactic acid in the muscles. However, while it can enhance performance in brief, high-intensity exercise, you have to use so much that you're likely to experience a most unpleasant side effect: explosive diarrhea.

• *Energy bars.* Sold in supermarkets, energy bars come in tantalizing flavors like java chip and chocolate-banana, and promise performance-boosting proteins, amino acids, and antioxidants. Some do indeed provide high protein and carbohydrates in munchable form, but they tend to be the least tasty. Sweeter and chewier energy bars often contain as many as 300 calories and 6 grams of fat—more than a candy bar. (See Figure 5-5.)

Flexibility

By simplest definition, *flexibility* refers to your ability to go through the complete range of motion that your joints allow in a comfortable, fluid fashion. Some people seem to be born more flexible than others. Other factors that affect flexibility include age, gender, posture, and how fat or muscular you are.

Of all the components of fitness, flexibility is the one most likely to be overlooked—until problems start. Unused muscles hold more tension, which can lead to muscle strain. And muscles shorten and tighten if they aren't used. If you spend a lot of time sitting in front of a computer, for instance, the hamstring muscles in your legs get shorter, and that can lead to lower back pain.

Everyone needs to work on overall flexibility, regardless of general fitness or activity level. But if you exercise, flexibility can be critical. Stiffness in one area (the shoulders, for instance) can increase the risk of injury in others (such as the knees and ankles during a run). Different sports require flexibility in different parts of the body. For swimming, flexible shoulders are crucial; for tennis and golf, the lower back has to be limber. Cyclists should be sure to stretch their quadriceps (front thigh muscles) and calves, while runners should concentrate on their hamstrings and feet.

Keep in mind that warming up and stretching are not the same thing. A warm-up involves getting the heart beating, breaking a sweat, and readying the body for more vigorous activity. Stretching, on the other hand, is

Snack	Energy bar	Candy bar	Orange (1 medium)
Calories	220	280	65
Fat (grams)	5	14	.1
Vitamin A*	100%	0%	0%
Vitamin C*	100%	0%	More than 100%
Vitamin E*	100%	0%	0%

* Percentage of the Daily Values for women aged 25 to 50.

■ **Figure 5-5 Which Snack Boosts Energy Most?**
Fresh fruit provides a no-fat pick-me-up. Energy bars and candy bars can be high in calories and fat, but at least the energy bars provide nutrients.

a specific activity intended to elongate muscles and keep joints limber, not simply a prelude to some other activity, such as a game of tennis or a three-mile run.

Stretching and warming up can prevent the soreness that occurs in surrounding connective tissue when muscle fibers are injured. Stretching actually may be more important after your workout. It helps move lactic acid out of your muscles, increases your range of motion, decreases soreness, and helps get blood, oxygen, and other nutrients to the muscle tissues.

An extra benefit of stretching is that, like a body yawn, it loosens you up and relieves tension. Even a brief stretch break during the day can be relaxing. However, although stretching is one of the safest activities, it's important that you do it properly so you don't end up hurting instead of helping yourself. Always practice *static*, or passive, stretching—moving gradually into a stretch that you hold for a short time (6 to 60 seconds). An example of such a stretch is letting your hands slowly slide down the front of your legs (keeping your knees in a soft, unlocked position) until you reach your toes and holding this final position for several seconds before slowly straightening up.

Ballistic stretching, by comparison, is characterized by rapid bouncing or jerking movements, such as a series of up-and-down bobs as you try again and again to touch your toes with your hands. These bounces can stretch muscle fibers too far, causing the muscle to contract rather than stretch; they can also tear ligaments and weaken or rupture tendons, the strong fibrous cords connecting muscles to bones.

To avoid problems, think of the muscle as a rubber band. If you abruptly stretch it out and release it, a

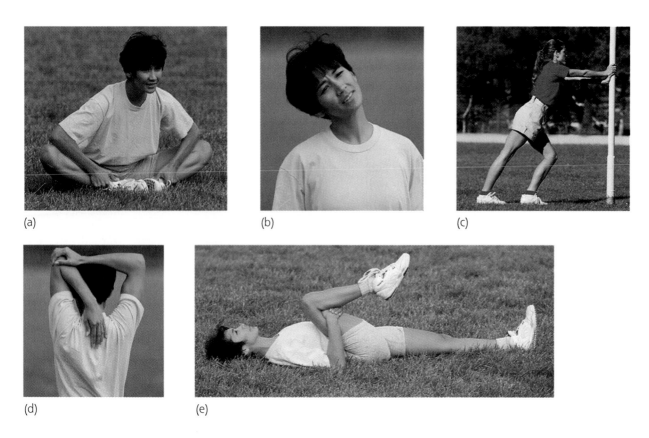

Some simple stretching exercises. (a) *Foot pull for the groin and thigh muscles.* Sit on the ground and bend your legs so that the sole of your feet touch. Pull your feet closer as you press on your knees with your elbows. Hold for 10 seconds; repeat. (b) *Lateral head tilt.* Gently tilt your head to each side. Repeat several times. (c) *Wall stretch for the Achilles tendon.* Stand 3 feet from a wall or post with your feet slightly apart. Keeping your heels on the ground, lean into the wall. Hold for 10 seconds; repeat. (d) *Triceps stretch for the upper arm and shoulder.* Place your right hand behind your neck and grasp it above the elbow with your left hand. Gently pull the elbow back. Repeat with the left elbow. (e) *Knee-chest pull for lower back muscles.* Lying on your back, clasp one knee and pull it toward your chest. Hold for 15–30 seconds; repeat with the other knee.

rubber band snaps back. If you stretch it too hard or too far, it can break. But if you pull it gently, hold it, and gently release it, the rubber band stretches with far less strain. That's how you want to stretch your muscles.

Always move slowly into a stretch position. You should never feel pain, although you will feel a slight tugging as you extend your stretch. Reach to this point of discomfort and then back off slightly, relaxing and allowing your muscles to adjust. You should hold this stretch until the feeling of tension diminishes. Concentrate on the feeling of the stretch itself, not on the flexibility you want to attain. Perform stretching exercises regularly. "Use it or lose it" is the motto to keep in mind when it comes to flexibility.

Total Fitness

No one single exercise can stretch and strengthen your muscles and also enhance your cardiovascular fitness.

That's why **cross-training** (alternating two or more different types of fitness activities) and **aerobic circuit training** (combining aerobic and strength exercises to build both cardiovascular fitness and muscular strength and endurance) have become increasingly popular:

• *Cross-training.* The pioneers of contemporary cross-training were triathletes, who run, swim, and cycle. Depending on the specific sports, cross-training can yield various benefits. Alternating aerobic workouts with weight-lifting, for example, can increase speed and performance. Alternating running with a low-impact aerobic exercise, such as swimming, lessens the risk of knee, ankle, or shin injuries. Cross-training also helps exercisers avoid boredom and offers the pleasures of variety.

There's no one cross-training combination that's right for everyone. To plan a program, first identify your fitness goals: Do you want to control your weight, get stronger, feel better about yourself, improve your

Strategies *for* Change

Safe Stretching

Before you begin, increase your body temperature by slowly marching or running in place. Sweat signals that you're ready to start stretching.

✔ Don't force body parts beyond their normal range of motion. Stretch to the point of tension, back off, and hold for ten seconds to a minute.

✔ Do a minimum of five repetitions of each stretch, with equal repetitions on each side.

✔ Don't hold your breath. Continue breathing slowly and rhythmically throughout your stretching routine. To strengthen muscles, tighten the muscles opposite the ones you're stretching. For example, when you're stretching your hamstrings, the major muscles in the backs of your thighs, you should tighten your quadriceps, the major muscles in the front of your thighs.

✔ Don't do any stretches that require deep knee bends or full squats. These positions can harm your knees and lower back.

general health, and improve your performance in a particular competitive sport? Your unique fitness goals will dictate the cross-training program that's right for you.

• *Aerobic circuit training.* Done individually or in a group at a gym or health club, aerobic circuit training generally involves weight-training equipment (such as free weights or Nautilus or Universal machines) and aerobic stations (treadmills, stationary bikes, stair-climbing machines, or cross-country skiing machines). By alternating weight and aerobic stations and moving quickly from one station to the next, exercisers can get a total-body workout. Some aerobic circuit trainers have reported significant improvements in aerobic capacity as well as enhanced toning and shaping of muscles.

Nutrition for Exercise

A balanced diet that follows the Food Guide Pyramid described in Chapter 6 can supply everything most exercisers need to perform well. However, endurance athletes whose workouts last an hour or more do best with a diet high in complex carbohydrates, which help keep the level of sugar in the blood steady and increase the amount of available glycogen, the body's fuel reserve, which is stored in the liver. This prevents sudden drops in blood glucose, weakness, and lightheadedness.

The American Dietetic Association recommends that physically active adults get 60–65 percent of their total calories from carbohydrate. Athletes who train to exhaustion or who compete in endurance events (like a marathon) should consume a diet that provides 65–70 percent of calories from carbohydrate.

Because muscles are made of protein, many exercisers think that more protein will make their muscles stronger. Yet heavy workouts don't significantly increase your body's need for protein, and high-protein diets don't lead to high performance. In fact, the American Dietetic Association has warned that too much protein can actually impair athletic performance by placing an excessive burden on the kidneys and liver.

If you're interested in high-octane nutrition to enhance your athletic performance, you may be tempted to try "body building" or "high-energy" foods, drugs, or dietary supplements, such as amino acids. Don't. You'll be wasting a lot of money, and you might end up feeling worse, rather than better, because of a nutritional imbalance.

What you do need before and during a workout is water. On a hot day, some athletes lose 2 pounds during a training session; that amounts to a quart of sweat. And as their bodies become dehydrated, their hearts find it more difficult to satisfy the demands of their muscles for oxygen and nutrients.

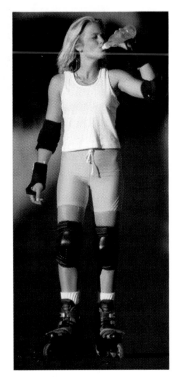

Water works best to prevent dehydration, because it's absorbed more quickly than any athletic drink or beverage containing sugar, sodium, potassium, or other ingredients. The American Dietetic Association dictates "plain cool water" as the fluid of choice for "most persons undertaking moderate exercise in moderate temperature conditions."

Although you may have heard a great deal about salt tablets, stay away from them. They're unnecessary and potentially dangerous. You do lose some salt in sweat, but the

Plain water before and during a workout is the best way to prevent dehydration.

loss is minimal—and more than made up for by the huge amounts of sodium most Americans get in their daily diet.

Sports Safety

Whenever you work out, you don't want to risk becoming sore or injured. Starting slowly when you begin any new fitness activity is the smartest strategy. Keep a simple diary to record the time and duration of each workout. Get accustomed to an activity first and then begin to work harder or longer. In this way, you strengthen your musculoskeletal system so you're less likely to be injured, you lower the cardiovascular risk, and you build the exercise habit into your schedule.

Even seasoned athletes should "listen to their bodies." If you develop aches and pains beyond what you might expect from an activity, stop. Never push to the point of fatigue. If you do, you could end up with sprained or torn muscles.

 ## How Can I Prevent Sports Injuries?

According to the American Physical Therapy Association, the most common exercise-related injury sites are the knees, feet, back, and shoulders, followed by the ankles and hips. **Acute injuries**—sprains, bruises, and pulled muscles—are the result of sudden trauma, such as a fall or collision. **Overuse injuries,** on the other hand, are the result of overdoing a repetitive activity, such as running. When one particular joint is overstressed—such as a tennis player's elbow or a swimmer's shoulder—tendinitis, an inflammation at the point where the tendon meets the bone, can develop. Other overuse injuries include muscle strains and aches and stress fractures, which are hairline breaks in a bone, usually in the leg or foot.

To prevent injuries and other exercise-related problems before they happen, use common sense and take appropriate precautions, including the following:

- Get proper instruction and, if necessary, advanced training from knowledgeable instructors.
- Make sure you have good equipment and keep it in good condition. Know how to check and do at least basic maintenance on the equipment yourself. Always check your equipment prior to each use (especially if you're renting it).
- Always make sure that stretching and exercises are preventing, not causing, injuries.
- Use reasonable protective measures, including wearing a helmet when cycling.
- For some sports, such as boating, always go with a buddy.

- Take each outing seriously—even if you've dived into this river a hundred times before, even if you know this mountain like you know your own backyard. Avoid the unknown under adverse conditions (for example, hiking unfamiliar terrain during poor weather or kayaking a new river when water levels are unusually high or low) or when accompanied by a beginner whose skills may not be as strong as yours.
- Never combine alcohol or drugs with any sport.

Extreme Sports

Many people are trying exciting, exhilarating sports that, by their very nature, entail some risk. If you choose these activities, you're responsible for learning how to stay safe as you push to the limit. Here are some sport-specific guidelines:

- *Inline skating.* This may seem the easiest and safest of "adventure" sports, but inline skating requires good aerobic fitness and strong leg and back muscles. The most common injuries are to the wrists. Skaters should always wear protective gear, including a helmet, wrist guards, and knee pads, and should warm up before strapping on their skates. Learn how to fall: Relax, go down to your knees, and roll to one side.
- *Mountain biking.* Off-road biking requires skills that go beyond biking, including knowing how to shift your weight to keep a bike stable on rough trails. Know the limits of your endurance and of your equipment. Wear a helmet, bicycle gloves, and glasses or goggles to protect your eyes from dirt and overhanging branches. Be sure to carry a bike repair kit and a first aid kit if you head for a remote area.
- *Rock climbing.* In addition to overall fitness, rock climbing takes strength, balance, and hand-eye coordination. Training with a qualified instructor is essential to learn proper technique. The best place to learn is indoors, with supervised instruction and controlled conditions.
- *Snowboarding.* This winter sport requires aerobic fitness, muscular strength, and excellent flexibility. Well-fitted snowboarding boots are essential, as is training in how to fall. The most common injuries are to the wrist or thumb, which can fracture if snowboarders put out their palms to break a fall. Sunburn and frostbite are both risks, and snowboarders should wear sunscreen and monitor weather conditions closely.

Thinking of Temperature

Prevention is the wisest approach to heat problems. Always dress appropriately for the weather and be aware of the health risks associated with temperature extremes.

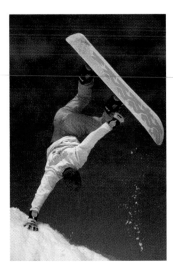
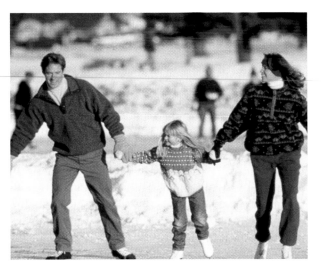

All sports carry a risk of injury. Participants should take responsibility for their own safety by having the proper equipment and training for their sport.

a noontime workout. Exposure to ground-level ozone, produced as sunlight reacts with exhaust fumes, can irritate the lungs and constrict bronchial tubes. An ozone level of 0.12 part per million causes, on the average, a 13 percent decline in lung capacity. This level is the maximum considered safe under the Clean Air Act, but it is often surpassed in New York, Los Angeles, and other urban areas.

Heeding Heat

Always wear as little as possible when exercising in hot weather. Choose loose-fitting, lightweight, white or light-colored clothes. Cotton is good because it absorbs perspiration. Never wear rubberized or plastic pants and jackets to sweat off pounds. These sauna suits will cause you to lose water only—not fat—and, because they don't allow your body heat to dissipate, they can be dangerous. On humid days, carry a damp washcloth to wipe off perspiration and cool yourself down. Be sure to drink plenty of fluids while exercising (especially water), and watch for the earliest signs of heat problems, including cramps, stress, exhaustion, and heatstroke. (See Chapter 18 for a further discussion of safety precautions.)

Coping with Cold

Protect yourself in cold weather (or cold indoor gyms) by covering as much of your body as possible, but don't overdress. Wear one layer less than you would if you were outside but not exercising. Don't use warm-up clothes of waterproof material because they tend to trap heat and keep perspiration from evaporating. Make sure your clothes are loose enough to allow movement and exercise of the hands, feet, and other body parts, thereby maintaining proper circulation. Choose dark colors that absorb heat. And because 40 percent or more of your body heat is lost through your head and neck, wear a hat, turtleneck, or scarf. Make sure you cover your hands and feet as well; mittens provide more warmth and protection than gloves.

Toxic Workouts

If you live in a large city, you may have to consider the risks of exercising in polluted air. On smoggy days, avoid

Overtraining

About half of all people who start an exercise program drop out within six months. One common reason is that they **overtrain,** pushing themselves to work too intensely too frequently. Signs of overdoing it include persistent muscle soreness, frequent injuries, unintended weight loss, nervousness, and an inability to relax. If you're pushing too hard, you may find yourself unable to complete a normal workout, or have difficulty recovering afterward.

If you develop any of the symptoms of overtraining, reduce or stop your workout sessions temporarily. Make gradual increases in the intensity of your workouts. Allow 24 to 48 hours for recovery between workouts. Make sure you get adequate rest. Check with a physical education instructor, coach, or trainer to make sure your exercise program fits your individual needs.

Evaluating Fitness Products and Programs

In the last decade fitness has become part of the American lifestyle. In a recent report, the Fitness Products Council identified eight major fitness trends in the 1990s:

- An increase in the use of exercise machines, especially cardiovascular machines such as treadmills, elliptical trainers, and stair climbers.

- A boom in the use of free weights, especially by women. Working out with free weights has become the number one fitness activity in the nation.

- An increase in treadmill popularity. In 1987, 4.4 million Americans reported exercising on a treadmill. By 1997, the number had grown by 720 percent to 31.7 million.

- An increase in health club popularity. Health-club memberships rose more than 63 percent in the last decade.

- Increased use of home equipment. The Fitness Products Council reports that exercise equipment is owned and used in nearly one-third of American households.

- Enduring commitment. Baby boomers, the creators of the fitness movement, have not surrendered to middle age but remain committed to working out.

- An evolution in exercise forms. New devices include spinning bikes, stair climbers, abdominal trainers, and elliptical motion machines.

- More personal trainers. Personal trainers, once employed only by movie stars and sports heroes, are now accessible to almost anyone.[27]

Just as you have to be a savvy health-care consumer (see Chapter 11), you should be a smart fitness consumer as well. Whatever activity you choose—even one as simple as walking—you'll find plenty of products to choose from. Make sure you judge them according to function, not fanciness or form.

 ## How Do I Buy the Right Athletic Shoes?

For many aerobic activities, good shoes are the most important purchase you'll make. Take the time to choose well. Here are some basic guidelines:

- Shop for shoes in the late afternoon, when your feet are most likely to be somewhat swollen—just as they will be after a workout.

- For walking shoes, look for a shoe that's lightweight, flexible, and roomy enough for your toes to wiggle, with a well-cushioned, curved sole; one that has good support at the heel; and one with an upper that is made of a material that breathes (allows air in and out).

- For running shoes (see Figure 5-6), look for good cushioning, support, and stability. You should be able to wiggle your toes easily, but the front of your foot shouldn't slide from side to side, which could cause blisters. Your toes should not touch the end of the shoe because your feet will swell with activity. Allow about half an inch from the longest toe to the tip of the shoe.

- For racquetball shoes, look for reinforcement at the toe for protection during foot drag. The sole should allow minimal slippage. There should be some heel elevation to lessen strain on the back of the leg and Achilles tendon. The shoe should have a long "throat" to ensure greater control by the laces.

- For tennis shoes, look for reinforcement at the toe. The sole at the ball of the foot should be well padded, because that's where most pressure is exerted. The sides of the shoe should be sturdy, for stability during continuous lateral movements. The toe box should allow ample room and some cushioning at the tips. A long throat ensures greater control by the laces.

Don't wear wet shoes for training. Let wet shoes air-dry, because a heater will cause them to stiffen or shrink. Use powder in your shoes to absorb moisture, lessen friction, and prevent fungal infections. Break in new shoes for several days before wearing them for a long-distance run or during competition.

Exercise Equipment

Always try out equipment before buying it. If you decide to purchase a stationary bicycle, for instance, read all the product information. Ask someone in your physical education department or at a local gym for recommendations. Try out a bicycle at the gym. Make sure any equipment you purchase is safe and durable.

Think about your fitness goals. If you're primarily interested in aerobic fitness, try out stationary bicycles, stair-climbing machines, rowing machines, treadmills, and cross-country skiing machines. Spend five to ten minutes working at moderate intensity. How do your movements on this particular piece of equipment feel to you—awkward or fluid, extremely difficult or surprisingly easy?

If you're considering strength-training equipment, remember that free weights are your least expensive option. The best resistance machines are also the most expensive, with prices soaring over $1,000. Would you use one often enough to justify that cost? Or would an annual health-club membership be more cost-effective?

Your exercise style is also an important consideration. Are you going to find sitting at a stationary bicycle for 30 minutes too boring? Are you motivated enough to hoist free weights on your own several times a week? The best home exercise equipment will do you no good unless you use it.

Fitness Centers and Trainers

If you decide to join a gym or health club, find out exactly what facilities and programs it offers. The club should be located close to home, campus, or work and should be open at convenient hours. Think about your schedule and when you'll have time to work out. Visit the club at the times you're most likely to use it: during peak hours, you might have to wait half an hour for a turn on the Nautilus machines.

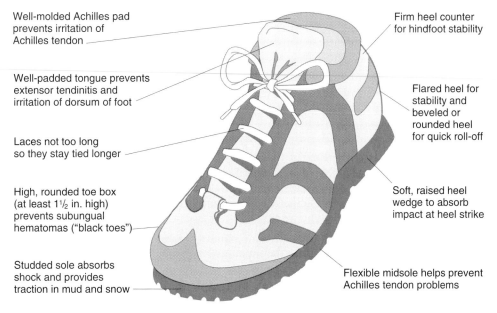

Well-molded Achilles pad prevents irritation of Achilles tendon

Well-padded tongue prevents extensor tendinitis and irritation of dorsum of foot

Laces not too long so they stay tied longer

High, rounded toe box (at least 1½ in. high) prevents subungual hematomas ("black toes")

Studded sole absorbs shock and provides traction in mud and snow

Firm heel counter for hindfoot stability

Flared heel for stability and beveled or rounded heel for quick roll-off

Soft, raised heel wedge to absorb impact at heel strike

Flexible midsole helps prevent Achilles tendon problems

■ Figure 5-6 **What to Look for When You Buy Running Shoes**

Source: Canadian Podiatric Sports Medicine Academy.

A club should have facilities for a complete workout, including both aerobic and muscle workouts: exercycles, rowing machines, treadmills, stair-climbing machines, stationary bicycles, a running track, aerobics classes, a swimming pool, strength-training equipment, and, if that's what you're looking for, racquetball and squash courts and a large gym for basketball and volleyball.

Find out whether all facilities are available to all members at all times. Some clubs reserve the pool for families only or kids' lessons at certain times. Ask if you can try out the club before joining. Find out what the membership includes. Will you end up paying extra for lockers, towels, classes, and the like? Are student discounts offered? Beware of long-term memberships; many clubs go out of business or change ownership often. Pay attention to cleanliness and to the atmosphere and people. Do the members seem to be significantly older or younger, or in much better or worse shape, than you are? You're more likely to work out regularly in a place, and with people, you like.

Across the Lifespan:
Turning Back the Clock

Once everyone, even the medical experts, thought of aging in terms of weakness, frailty, and declining strength. Now we know better: No one is ever too old to get in shape. Rather than encouraging seniors to take it easy, the American College of Sports Medicine now encourages them to engage in the full range of physical activities, including flexibility exercises, aerobic conditioning, and strength training.[28] (See Table 5-2 on page 149.)

Throughout life exercise is so effective in preserving well-being that gerontologists describe it as "the closest thing to an anti-aging pill." It slows many changes associated with advancing age, such as loss of lean muscle tissue, increase in body fat, and decreased work capacity. Aerobic activities lower the risk of heart disease and stroke in the elderly—and greatly improve general health. Male and female runners over age 50 have much lower rates of disability and much lower health-care costs than less active seniors. Strength training also yields significant benefits, including increased bone mass, stronger muscles, improved balance, better sleep, greater mobility, and brighter mood. Flexibility exercises lessen the risks of strains, sprains, and injuries.

Despite these potential benefits, many seniors are not active. By age 75, about one in three men and one in two women engage in no physical activity. However, even sedentary individuals in their eighties and nineties can participate in an exercise program—and gain significant benefits.

For aerobic fitness, federal health officials recommend a moderate amount of physical activity, either in longer sessions of moderately intense activities (such as walking) or in shorter sessions of more vigorous activities (such as fast walking or stairwalking). Seniors can gain additional health benefits by increasing the duration, intensity, or frequency of their workouts, but should avoid overdoing their training because of the risk of injury. Older adults should always consult with a physician before beginning a new physical activity program.

According to the Surgeon General, the additional benefits of physical activity for older Americans include:

● greater ability to live independently

● reduced risk of falling and fracturing bones

● lower risk of dying from coronary heart disease and of developing high blood pressure, colon cancer, and diabetes

● reduced blood pressure in some people with hypertension

● greater stamina and muscle strength in people with chronic, disabling conditions

● fewer symptoms of anxiety and depression

● improvements in mood and feelings of well-being

● relief of joint swelling and pain associated with arthritis[29]

Consumer Health Watch

Selecting a Personal Trainer

A personal trainer can help you design a workout that will meet your needs or work with you regularly, motivating you through each workout. Here are some factors to consider in choosing a trainer:

- Does the trainer have a solid background in exercise physiology, anatomy, injury prevention, and monitoring of exercise intensity? Ideally, a trainer should have a degree in a related medical or physical science field or certification through a nationally recognized organization.

- Does the trainer have experience in fitness training?

- Does he or she keep current with research through associations and educational programs and publications?

- Is the trainer certified in CPR and first aid?

- Does the trainer require a health screening or release from your doctor?

- Can the trainer provide you with references from other clients?

- Does the trainer keep a record of your workouts and update your medical history periodically?

- Does the trainer have liability insurance in case you get injured through negligence on the trainer's part?

- Does the trainer provide clear-cut policies on cancellation and billing in writing?

- Is the trainer within your budget? Trainers charge a broad range of fees depending on length of workout, location, and the trainer's experience.

- Does the trainer listen to what you want and communicate well with you?

- Is the trainer willing to put his or her workout methods in writing and explain the reasoning behind your exercise program?

- Do you feel you will get along well with the trainer? Are your personalities compatible?

- Is the trainer interested in helping you maintain a balanced, healthy lifestyle in addition to exercise?

Making This Chapter Work for You

Shaping Up

- A physically fit person has enough energy to meet routine physical demands, with enough reserve energy to cope with unexpected challenges. Fitness itself has four basic components: cardiovascular fitness, body composition, muscular strength and endurance, and flexibility.

- The preventive benefits of physical activity include a healthier heart, greater lung capacity, increased metabolism, stronger bones, better mood and mental health, protection against certain forms of cancer, lower weight, and a more active old age.

- Habitual inactivity increases death rates from all causes, especially heart disease. But increasing activity level, even in middle age, can reduce the risk of an early death. Even light exercise can improve physical and emotional well-being, but moderate to rigorous activity produces greater benefits.

- The CDC and the American College of Sports Medicine currently recommend a minimum of 30 minutes a day of moderate physical activity at least five days a week. This can take almost any form—gardening, walking, dancing, housework, playing

actively with children—and can help lower the risk of many chronic health problems, including heart disease, high blood pressure, diabetes, osteoporosis, colon cancer, anxiety, and depression.

- To achieve optimal fitness and function at your physiological best, the American College of Sports Medicine recommends a regular program of aerobic activities for the cardiovascular system, strength-training exercises for the muscles, and flexibility exercises.

- Although they may be aware of exercise's potential benefits, many Americans remain inactive. Among the most common obstacles to exercise are: a lack of time; a lack of affordable, accessible, or safe places to exercise; scheduling difficulties; injury or other physical limitations; bad weather; a dislike of rigorous exertion; and a lack of confidence in individual physical abilities.

- Different types of exercise produce different benefits. Stretching can improve flexibility. Aerobic exercises, which cause the heart and lungs to work harder and more efficiently, improve cardiovascular fitness. Building up strength and endurance through strength workouts ensures muscular fitness. A complete fitness program should include exercises for flexibility, aerobic fitness, and muscular strength.

- Among the many options for aerobic exercise are brisk walking; race-walking; jogging or running; swimming; indoor and outdoor cycling; cross-

■ Table 5-2 Exercise: Special Benefits for Specific Groups

Teenagers and Young Adults
Regular physical activity improves strength, builds lean muscle, and decreases body fat. It can build stronger bones to last a lifetime.

Dieters
Regular physical activity burns calories and preserves lean muscle mass. It is a key component of any weight loss effort and is important for controlling weight.

People with High Blood Pressure
Regular physical activity helps lower blood pressure.

People Who Feel Anxious, Depressed, or Moody
Regular physical activity improves mood, helps relieve depression, and increases feelings of well-being.

People with Arthritis
Regular physical activity can help control joint swelling and pain. Physical activity of the type and amount recommended for health has not been shown to cause arthritis.

People with Disabilities
Regular physical activity can help people with chronic, disabling conditions improve their stamina and muscle strength. It can also improve their psychological well-being and quality of life by increasing their ability to perform the activities of daily life.

Older Adults
No one is too old to enjoy the benefits of regular physical activity. Of special significance to older adults is evidence that muscle-strengthening exercises can reduce the risk of falling and fracturing bones and can improve the ability to live independently.

Children
Parents can help their children maintain a physically active lifestyle by providing encouragement and opportunities for physical activity. Family events can be designed to allow everyone in the family to be active.

country skiing, skipping rope; aerobic dancing; low-impact aerobics; and various new activities, such as stair climbing, rollerblading, and step training.

■ A weight-training program for muscular fitness should exercise the body's primary muscle groups. One particularly dangerous shortcut to building up muscles is the use of anabolic steroids, which can damage the cardiovascular system, liver, reproductive organs, and mental abilities.

■ To get the most of physical activity, you need to eat a balanced diet, use common sense to prevent injuries, protect yourself from heat and cold, and avoid potential risks—such as pollution and overtraining.

Even though fitness products and facilities can make exercise more appealing, getting physical doesn't mean joining a health club, buying designer sportswear, or working out on expensive bodybuilding equipment. All you need, other than some good shoes for your feet, is a genuine desire to make the most of your body and a strategy for getting started.

Becoming more active is, above all else, a matter of making a commitment to make more of your body.

Here are some guidelines to get you going:

■ Add a new sport or physical activity you genuinely enjoy to your schedule.

■ Carve out time for this activity. Write "Running" or "Tennis" (or whatever) on your calendar.

■ Always try to exercise at the same time of day. For instance, you could jog in the morning before breakfast or in the evening before dinner.

■ Get someone to go out with you, if that helps.

■ As you aim for optimal fitness, start out slowly and proceed gradually, and be aware that there will be plateaus in your progress. Some days you'll exercise more slowly than others; that's okay. Some days you may not be able to exercise at all because of illness or bad weather; that, too, is okay. Just keep in mind that when you start exercising regularly again, you should build up slowly to reach your prior fitness level.

■ Be sure you don't overwork your body so that it becomes fatigued or injured. If your muscles persistently feel sore and stiff, if you have headaches, continuing fatigue, loss of appetite or weight, or cessation of menstruation; or if you develop emotional symptoms, such as depression or a lack of interest in your sport, you may be exercising too hard.

After a few months of leading a more active life, stop and take stock. Think of how much more energy you have at the end of the day. Ask if you're feeling any less stressed, despite the push and pull of daily pressures. Focus on the unanticipated rewards of exercise. Savor the exhilaration of an autumn morning's walks; the thrill of feeling newly toughened muscles bend to your will; or the satisfaction of a long, smooth stretch after a stressful day. Enjoy the pure pleasure of living in the body you deserve.

 The Fittest City in the U.S. How fitness-conscious are people in your city?

health / ONLINE

The Internet's Fitness Resource
http://www.netsweat.com/
Includes fitness advice, news, and links to fitness-related sites such as research centers, specific sports pages, general fitness sites, nutrition and weight loss sites, and more.

Shape Up America!
http://www.shapeup.org/
This web site provides information about safe weight management, healthy eating, and physical fitness. It includes an online library, a weight management support center, and more.

Spinning on the Internet
http://www.spinning.com
This web site provides answers to frequently asked questions about the growing sport of spinning.

Please note that links are subject to change. If you find a broken link, use a search engine like http://www.yahoo.com *and search for the web site by typing in key words.*

 Campus Chat: Should schools focus solely on educating students' brains, or should physical fitness be a significant part of students' education as well? What arguments can you give for your position? Share your thoughts on our online discussion forum at **http://health.wadsworth.com**

Find It On InfoTrac: You can find additional readings related to fitness via InfoTrac College Edition, an online library of more than 900 journals and publications. Follow the instructions for accessing InfoTrac that came packaged with your textbook; then search for articles using a key word search.

- **Suggested article:** "Take It Off, Keep It Off," by Cris Beam, *Vegetarian Times*, August 1999, p. 52.
  (1) What are the three basic kinds of metabolism?
  (2) What steps can you take toward raising your metabolic rate?

For additional links, resources, and suggested readings on InfoTrac, visit our Health & Wellness Resource Center at **http://health.wadsworth.com**

Key Terms

The terms listed here are used within the chapter. Page numbers are included for each term. A definition of each term is given in the Glossary pages at the end of this book.

Critical Thinking Questions

1. Shelley knows that exercise is good for her health, but she figures she can keep her weight down by dieting, and worry about her heart and health when she gets older. "I look good. I feel okay. Why should I bother exercising?" she asks. What would you say in reply?

2. When he started working out, Jeff simply wanted to stay in shape. But he felt so pleased with the way his body looked and responded that he kept doing more. Now he runs ten miles a day (longer on weekends), lifts weights, works out on Nautilus equipment almost every day, and plays racquetball or squash whenever he gets a chance. Is Jeff getting too much of a good thing? Is there any danger in his fitness program? What would be a more reasonable approach?

References

1. Carter, Marcia Jean. "Moving Beyond the Surgeon General's Report: An HPERD Challenge?" *Journal of Physical Education, Recreation & Dance*, Vol. 70, Issue 2, February 1999.
2. U.S. Department of Health and Human Services. *Physical Activity and Health: A Report of the Surgeon General*. Atlanta: U.S. Department of Health and Human Services, 1996.
3. Francis, Kennon. "Status of the Year 2000 Health Goals for Physical Activity and Fitness." *Physical Therapy*, Vol. 79, Issue 4, April 1999.
4. Ibid.
5. Sallis, James, et al. "Evaluation of a University Course to Promote Physical Activity: Project GRAD (Graduate Ready for Activity Daily)." *Research Quarterly for Exercise and Sport*, Vol. 70, No. 1, March 1999.
6. Liu, Jian. "Physical Activity and Insulin Resistance." Presentation, Society for Epidemiologic Research, Baltimore, June 1999.
7. Ljungquist, Birgit, et al. "The Effect of Genetic Factors for Longevity: A Comparison of Identical and Fraternal Twins in the Swedish Twin Registry." *Journal of Gerontology*, Vol. 53A, No. 6, November, 1998.
8. Tkachuk, Gregg, and Garry Martin. "Exercise Therapy for Patients with Psychiatric Disorders: Research and Clinical Implications." *Professional Psychology: Research and Practice*, Vol. 30, No. 3, June 1999.
9. Pinkowish, Mary. "Exercising to Keep Weight Off." *Patient Care*, Vol. 31, No. 19, November 30, 1997.
10. Rose, Verna. "CDC Report on Physical Inactivity." *American Family Physician*, Vol. 59, Issue 6, March 15, 1999.
11. "Moderate Activity Keeps Heart, Waistline in Shape." *Harvard Health Letter*, Vol. 24, No. 7, April 1999.
12. Dunn, Andrea, et al. "Comparison of Lifestyle and Structured Interventions to Increase Physical Activity and Cardiorespiratory Fitness." *Journal of the American Medical Association*, Vol. 281, No. 4, January 27, 1999.
13. Anderson, Ross, et al. "Effects of Lifestyle Activity vs. Structured Aerobic Exercise in Obese Women." *Journal of the American Medical Association*, Vol. 281, No. 4, January 27, 1999.
14. "How much exercise do you need?" *University of California, Berkeley Wellness Letter*, Vol. 15, No. 7, April 1999.

15. Scott, Sharon Morey. "ACSM Revises Guidelines for Exercise to Maintain Fitness." *American Family Physician*, Vol. 59 Issue 2, January 15, 1999.
16. Pearman, Silas, et al. "The Impact of a Required College Health and Physical Education Course on the Health Status of Alumni." *American Journal of College Health*, Vol. 46, September 1997.
17. Sallis, James, et al. "Evaluation of a University Course to Promote Physical Activity: Project GRAD (Graduate Ready for Activity Daily)."
18. U.S. Department of Health and Human Services. *Physical Activity and Health: A Report of the Surgeon General*.
19. "Walk Your Way to Total Health." *Amercian Health*, March 1999.
20. "Spinning on the Internet." http://www.spinning.com
21. Sachtleben, Thomas, et al. "Serum Lipoprotein Patterns in Long-Term Anabolic Steroid Users." *Research Quarterly for Exercise and Sport*, Vol. 68, No. 1, March 1997.
22. King, Douglas, et al. "Effect of Oral Androstenedione on Serum Testosterone and Adaptations to Resistance Training in Young Men." *JAMA*, Vol. 281, No. 21, June 2, 1999.
23. Birchard, Karen. "Body-Building Supplement Fails to Strengthen Muscle and May Harm Health." *Lancet*, Vol. 353, No. 9168, June 5, 1999.
24. Feldman, Elaine. "Creatine: A Dietary Supplement and Ergogenic Aid." *Nutrition Reviews*, Vol. 57, No. 2, February 1999.
25. Bradbury, Jane. "US FDA Issues Warning on Dietary Supplement." *Lancet*, Vol. 353, No. 9150, January 30, 1999.
26. Wagner, Dale. "Hyperhydrating with Glycerol: Implications for Athletic Performance." *Journal of the American Dietetics Association*, Vol. 99, No. 2, February 1999.
27. Howe, D. K. "Fitness & Exercise." *American Fitness*, Vol. 17, Issue 2, March 1999.
28. "Medicine's Fitness Guidelines for People over 50." *Harvard Health Letter*, Vol. 23, No. 12, October 1998.
29. National Institute on Aging. *Exercise: A Guide from the National Institute on Aging*. Gaithersburg, Md.: NIA Information Center, 1998.

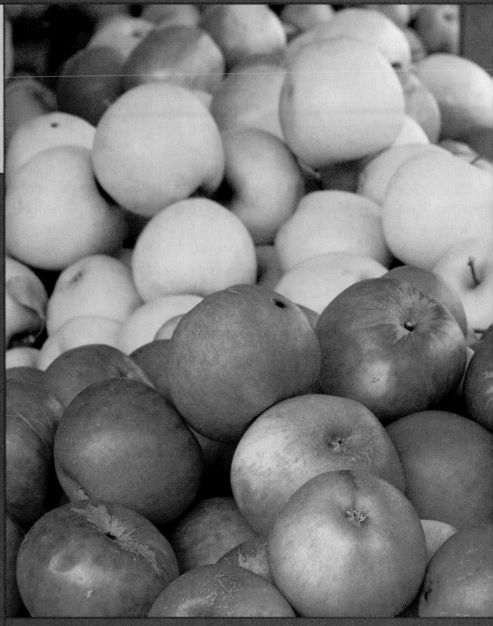

Nutrition for Life

After studying the material in this chapter, you should be able to:

- **List** and **define** the basic nutrients necessary for a healthy body.
- **Describe** the Food Guide Pyramid and **explain** its significance.
- **Explain** current recommendations for healthy eating, and **use** the nutritional information provided on the new food labels to make healthy choices.
- **Compare** the advantages and disadvantages of various alternative diets and ethnic foods.
- **Explain** the importance of food safety to personal health.
- **Develop** a personal plan for healthy nutritional choices.

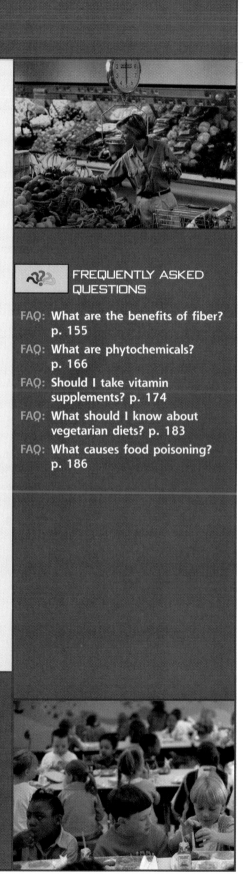

We are indeed what we eat—and it shows in everything from our stamina and strength to the sheen of our hair and the glow in our cheeks. Eating well helps us live well and feel well. As shown by recent advances in **nutrition**—the science that explores the connections between our bodies and the food we eat—our daily diet affects both how long and how healthfully we live. Diet-related diseases cost more than $250 billion annually in medical expenses and lost productivity.[1]

Americans are changing the way we eat. In a national survey conducted in 1999, three of four respondents said they've made an effort to trim fat from their diets, often by switching to low-fat versions of favorite foods. Nearly half say they are consuming fewer calories than in the past, while four in ten have reduced their intake of sugar and about a third have increased their fiber. Two-thirds say that when they shop, finding healthy, nutritious foods is very or extremely important.[2]

Yet making good food choices isn't always easy. Advertising claims are often confusing, and it can be hard to sort out which to believe. Research, too, keeps changing the way we view certain foods. Some nutrients that once were touted for their health benefits, such as beta carotene, have not lived up to their promise. Others that have long been considered nutritional outcasts, such as dietary fats, are being reevaluated.

But deciding what to eat involves more than selecting nutrients and weighing their advantages and disadvantages. Food can, and should, be a source of pleasure and satisfaction. This chapter translates the latest information on good nutrition into specific advice that you can use to make smart food choices for the twenty-first century—choices that will enable you both to eat well and feel well throughout your life. ❖

What You Need to Know About Nutrients

We all need the same essential **nutrients** to form muscles, bones, and other tissues and to provide energy for work and play. These nutrients include water, protein, carbohydrates, fiber, fats, vitamins, and minerals, each of which will be covered in this chapter.

Nutrients reach our body's structures through the process of digestion (see Figure 6-1). Each of the organs of the digestive system contributes to the process by either mechanically or chemically breaking down foods into small molecules capable of being absorbed into body cells.

Nutritionists have conducted thousands of studies to determine the types and amounts of nutrients that individuals of different ages, genders, sizes, and levels of activity need in order to feel and perform at their best. Epidemiological studies assess the dietary habits and health status of a particular population, while metabolic studies examine the effects of different nutrients in animal or human metabolism.

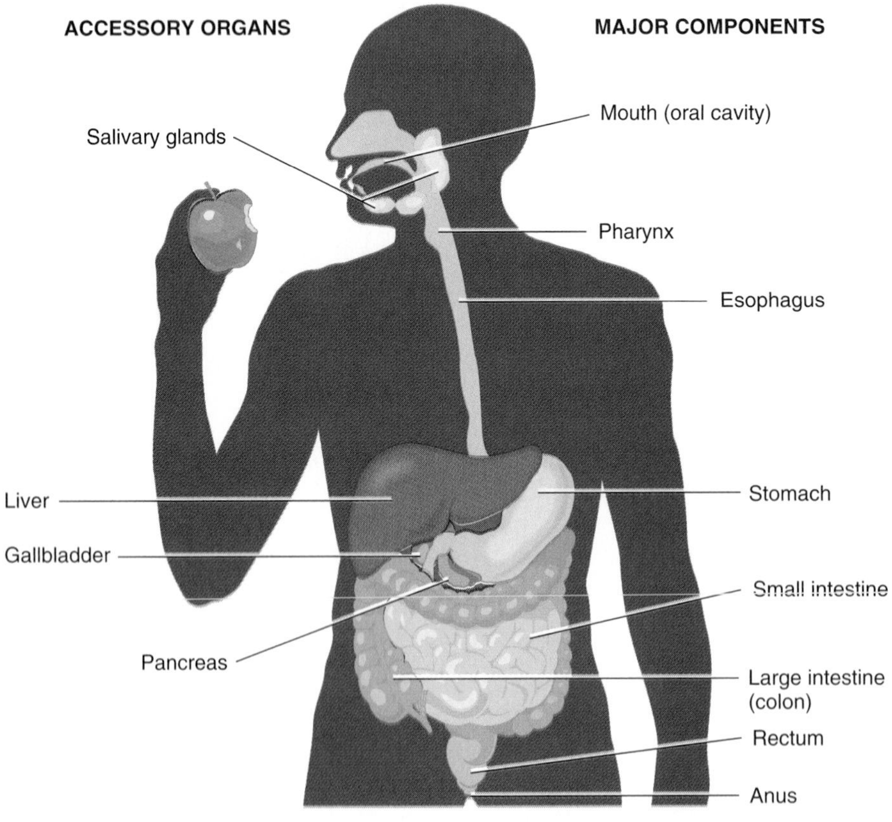

Water

Water makes up 85 percent of the blood, 70 percent of the muscles, and about 75 percent of the brain.[3] It carries nutrients, maintains temperature, lubricates joints, helps with digestion of food, and helps rid your body of waste through urine. Although we can live for several weeks without food, we would die after a few days without water. A loss of 5 percent of the body's water causes dizziness, fatigue, headache, and weakness; a 15 to 20 percent loss can be fatal. Water is an important element in the production of sweat, which evaporates from the skin to cool the body.

You lose about 64 to 80 ounces of water a day—the equivalent of eight to ten 8-ounce glasses—through urine, perspiration, bowel movements, and normal exhalation.[4] You lose water more rapidly if you're ill, live in a dry climate, are at a high altitude, drink a lot of coffee or alcohol (which increase urination), skip a meal, exercise, or travel on an airplane. It's important to drink water before and during exercise to prevent dehydration. A general guideline is to drink one or two 8-ounce glasses of water 30 minutes to an hour before exercising and half to three-quarters of a glass of water every 10 to 20 minutes during a workout.

To keep up your water supply, try these tips:

- Don't substitute soft drinks, coffee, tea, or alcoholic beverages for water.

- Take regular water breaks to prevent mild dehydration. Keep a water bottle or pitcher nearby whenever possible.

- Respond quickly to thirst, which is a good but not foolproof indicator of dehydration. If you're ill, exercising, or at a high altitude, you need more fluid than usual, even if you don't feel thirsty.

- Check your urine. Dark yellow urine means your kidneys had to concentrate waste material into a smaller volume of water, while pale urine is a sign of good hydration.

Protein

Protein forms the basic framework for our muscles, bones, blood, hair, and fingernails and is essential for growth and repair.

ACCESSORY ORGANS   MAJOR COMPONENTS

Salivary glands

Mouth (oral cavity)

Pharynx

Esophagus

Liver

Gallbladder

Stomach

Pancreas

Small intestine

Large intestine (colon)

Rectum

Anus

■ Figure 6-1 **Digestive System**
The organs of the digestive system break down food into nutrients the body can use.

The main source of protein in the American diet is animal protein. Meat, fish, and poultry make up 42 percent of the protein in our diets, while dairy products constitute 20 percent. Grains contribute the most (18 percent) to plant protein consumption.[5]

Various racial and ethnic groups and both genders get a similar percentage of their calories from protein, but their sources are different (see The X & Y Files: "His Plate, Her Plate" on page 183). African Americans eat a higher percentage of poultry and pork protein and a lower percent of dairy protein than do whites and Mexican Americans. Mexican Americans consume a higher percentage of legume and egg protein than do whites and blacks. Whites consume a higher percentage of grain protein than do blacks and Mexican Americans.[6]

Carbohydrates

Carbohydrates are organic compounds that provide our brains and bodies with glucose, their basic fuel. The major sources are plants, including grains, vegetables, fruits, and beans, and milk. The three types of carbohydrates are complex carbohydrates (starches), simple carbohydrates (sugars), and fiber.

Both **simple** and **complex carbohydrates** have 4 calories per gram. Sugars, which provide little more than a quick spurt of energy, comprise 16 percent of the average American's calories and 20 percent of the average teenager's calories. According to nutritional analysis, adults age 25 to 50 who consume the most added sugars are less likely to get recommended amounts of key vitamins and minerals. Foods rich in added sugars, which are "calorie-dense" rather than "nutrient-dense," also may contribute to obesity and heart disease. Some nutritionists are calling for a dietary guideline to limit added sugars to 6 teaspoons a day if you eat about 1,600 calories, 12 teaspoons at 2,200 calories, or 18 teaspoons at 2,800 calories.[7]

Complex Carbohydrates: Going for the Grain

Americans get most of their complex carbohydrates from refined grains, which have been stripped of fiber and many nutrients. Far more nutritious are whole grains, which are made up of all components of the grain—the bran (or fiber-rich outer layer), the endosperm (middle layer), and the germ (the nutrient-packed inner layer). However, only 1 percent of what the average American eats comes from whole grain. To encourage more consumption of whole grains, the U.S. Food and Drug Administration (FDA) has authorized a new health claim allowing food companies to promote the health benefits of whole grains, such as those in Cheerios, Wheaties, and Total breakfast cereals, which

can protect against cardiovascular disease and are associated with a reduced risk for colon, rectal, gastric, endometrial, oral, pharyngeal, tongue, and esophageal cancer.[8]

Increasing whole grain consumption has become a public health priority. Four national health organizations—the American Heart Association, the American Cancer Society, the National Institutes of Health, and the American Society for Clinical Nutrition—have joined in recommending that Americans increase their consumption of whole grain foods to at least three servings every day. Numerous studies show that those who habitually eat whole grain products each day have about a 15 to 25 percent reduction in death from all causes, including heart disease and cancer. To identify whole-grain products, check the ingredient list; the first ingredient on the list should be a whole grain, such as "whole grain oats," "whole grain wheat," or "whole wheat."

 ## What Are the Benefits of Fiber?

The indigestible leaves, stems, skins, seeds, and hulls of grains and plants contain dietary **fiber**. *Insoluble fibers*—cellulose, lignin, and some hemicellulose—increase bulk in feces, prevent constipation and diverticulosis (a painful inflammation of the bowel), and may lower the risk of heart disease and stroke. Good sources of insoluble fiber are wheat and corn bran (the outer layer), leafy greens, and the skins of fruits and root vegetables. *Soluble fibers*—pectin, gums, and some hemicellulose—lower blood cholesterol and may help control blood sugar levels. Good sources of soluble fiber are oats, beans, barley, and the pulp of many fruits and vegetables, such as apples and citrus fruits.

Contrary to a long-held assumption, dietary fiber does not appear to protect against the development of colorectal cancer. A 1999 report on almost 90,000 women found that those who ate the most dietary fiber had the same risk of developing colorectal cancer as women who ate the least dietary fiber.[9] However, the link between fiber and colon cancer is complex, and researchers have yet to sort it out. In the meantime, nutritionists continue to urge people to add fiber to their diets, because fiber-rich foods are an important source of other nutrients and can lower heart-attack risk and prevent digestive problems.[10]

Despite the benefits of fiber, few Americans eat enough. The National Cancer Institute recommends that a person consume 20 to 35 grams a day, but the average intake is about 11 to 13 grams. More servings of fruit and vegetables could make a big difference in fiber intake. One apple or half a grapefruit can add 2 grams of fiber to your diet. (See Table 6-1 for good fiber sources.)

■ **Table 6-1** Putting the Fiber into Meals and Snacks

High-Fiber Options for Breakfast

Whole-grain toast		2 g per slice
Bran cereal:		
Bran flakes	1 cup	7 g
All Bran	⅓ cup	10 g
Raisin bran	¾ cup	5 g
Oat bran	⅓ cup	5 g
Bran muffin, with fruit	1 small	3 g
Strawberries	10	2 g
Raspberries	½ cup	3 g
Bananas	1 medium	2 g

Lunches that Include Fiber

Whole-grain bread		2 g per slice
Baked beans	½ cup	10 g
Carrot	1 medium	2 g
Raisins	¼ cup	2 g
Peas	½ cup	6 g
Peanut butter	2 tablespoons	2 g

Fiber on the Menu for Supper

Brown rice	½ cup	2 g
Potato	1 medium	3 g
Dried cooked beans	½ cup	8 g
Broccoli	½ cup	3 g
Corn	½ cup	5 g
Tomato	1 medium	2 g
Green beans	½ cup	3 g

Fiber-Filled Snacks

Peanuts	¼ cup	3 g
Apple	1 medium	2 g
Pear	1 medium	4 g
Orange	1 medium	3 g
Prunes*	3	2 g
Sunflower seeds	¼ cup	2 g
Popcorn	2 cups	2 g

*Prunes contain fiber, but their laxative effect is primarily due to a naturally occurring chemical substance that causes an uptake of fluid into the intestines and the contraction of muscles that line the intestines.

Source: From Brown, *Nutrition Now* (Wadsworth, 1999).

If you have not been eating a high-fiber diet, increase grains, fruits, and vegetables gradually. A sudden increase in fiber intake can result in intestinal gas, bloating, cramps, and diarrhea—the consequences of fermentation of fiber and sugars in the colon. Try to spread out your fiber intake throughout the day and increase total consumption gradually to avoid these effects. An extremely high-fiber diet may block absorption of some minerals, such as zinc, iron, and calcium, but most nutritionists feel that high-fiber foods are rich enough in nutrients to compensate for any such losses. Individuals taking fiber pills or powders, which contain no nutrients, are more likely to suffer mineral deficiencies.

Fats

Fats, which provide energy and serve as carriers for certain vitamins, are made up of a mixture of saturated and unsaturated fatty acids. The predominant type of fatty acid determines whether a fat is solid or liquid and whether it is characterized as saturated or unsaturated. (See Table 6-2 for the different forms of dietary fats.) **Saturated fats** such as lard and butter, which are harder at room temperature, contain higher levels of saturated fatty acids. Oils such as soybean, canola, cottonseed, corn, and other vegetable oils, which are liquid at room temperature, contain higher levels of unsaturated fatty acids and are considered **unsaturated fats.** Unsaturated fats can be monounsaturated or polyunsaturated.

Trans fats are unsaturated fatty acids formed when vegetable oils are processed and made more solid or into a more stable liquid. This processing is called hydrogenation. Most trans fats come from processed foods; about one-fifth come from animal sources such as meats and dairy products. Trans fats are found in most foods made with partially hydrogenated oils, such as baked goods and fried foods, and some margarine products. Fats and oils containing trans fat, such as palm and coconut oil, are used in place of baking and frying fats, such as butter and lard, that have higher levels of saturated fats.

Initially, manufacturers switched to partially hydrogenated oils in response to consumer and health professionals' demand for less saturated fat in the food supply. However, even though trans fats are unsaturated, they appear similar to saturated fats in terms of raising total and LDL (low-density lipoprotein) cholesterol levels. Epidemiological studies have suggested a possible link between cardiovascular disease risk and high intakes of trans fats, and researchers have concluded that they are, gram for gram, twice as damaging as saturated fat.[11]

When you do use them, which fats should you choose? Olive oil, which is high in monounsaturated fats, is one of the best vegetable oil for salads and cooking. It has been used for thousands of years in countries around the Mediterranean, which have relatively low levels of heart disease.[12] Canola oil is lowest in saturated fat and can be used for baking, stir-frying, and salad dressings. Table 6-3 shows the percentage of fat calories in different foods.

■ Table 6-2 Forms of Dietary Fats

Fat	Sources	What It Does
Saturated fat	Red meat, dairy products, egg yolks, coconut and palm oils	Provides energy; triggers production of cholesterol and LDL
Unsaturated fats		
Monounsaturated fats	Some fish, avocados, olive, canola and peanut oils	Also provides energy, but triggers more HDL production and less cholesterol and LDL production
Polyunsaturated fats	Some fish, corn, sesame, soybean, and safflower oils	Similar to monounsaturated fats
Omega-3 fatty acids	Fish (tuna, salmon, sardines, bluefish, trout)	Reduce the risk of clotting by thinning the blood; may protect against hardening of arteries
Trans-fatty acids	Shortening, stick margarine, baked goods	Promote production of LDL and cholesterol
Triglycerides	Any food that contains fat	Not fully broken down by the liver, they have effects similar to those of saturated fats

Strategies *for* Change

Cutting Down on Trans Fats

✔ Choose soybean, canola, corn, olive, safflower, and sunflower oils, which are naturally lower in saturated fats and are trans fat-free.

✔ Try reduced-fat, low-fat, fat-free, and trans fat-free versions of frequently consumed foods that otherwise would be made with saturated fats or trans fats.

✔ Choose soft margarines. In a study that compared the effects of soybean oil, shortening, semiliquid, soft, and stick margarine on cholesterol, ratios of total cholesterol to HDL cholesterol were lowest after the consumption of the soybean-oil diet and semiliquid-margarine diet and highest after the stick-margarine diet.

The Cholesterol Connection

Blood **cholesterol,** or lipid, or fat, reflects the amount of three major classes of lipoproteins in the blood: very-low-density lipoprotein (VLDL); low-density lipoprotein (LDL), which contains most of the cholesterol found in the blood; and high-density lipoprotein (HDL). LDL seems to be the culprit in heart disease and is associated with cholesterol deposits on artery walls.

In the body, cholesterol is essential for the production of many hormones, the formation of the outer membranes protecting our body cells, and the functioning of the liver. However, when blood cholesterol levels become too high, the excess cholesterol can build up within the arteries (a condition called *atherosclerosis,* discussed in Chapter 10). Foods high in saturated fats and trans fats raise blood cholesterol levels more than any other foods, even those high in cholesterol.

Cholesterol-lowering margarines contain compounds that may help lower LDL cholesterol for some individuals. The American Heart Association describes the margarines as "another tool to help lower elevated levels of LDL cholesterol, especially when consumed as part of a health plan that includes physical activity and a balanced diet."[13] However, they can lower LDL cholesterol levels only 7 to 10 percent and should be combined with a diet that is low in saturated fat. For many people, cholesterol-lowering drugs may still provide the best means of lowering LDL cholesterol levels. Children and adults who have not been diagnosed as having elevated levels of LDL cholesterol should not consume the product as a "preventive" measure. While cholesterol-lowering margarines may be used as part of a treatment plan, they do not prevent the underlying cause of elevated LDL cholesterol levels.

How Much Fat Is Okay?

The 1990 and 1995 Dietary Guidelines advised Americans to limit total fat consumption to 30 percent or less of total caloric intake and saturated fat intake to less than 10 percent of total caloric intake. Americans haven't quite reached that goal, but they've gotten

■ **Table 6-3** Percentage of Fat Calories in Foods

Type of Food	Less Than 15% of Calories from Fat	15%–30% of Calories from Fat	30%–50% of Calories from Fat	More Than 50% of Calories from Fat
Fruits and Vegetables	Fruits, plain vegetables, juices, pickles, sauerkraut		French fries, hash browns	Avocados, coconuts, olives
Bread and Cereals	Grains and flours, most breads, most cereals, corn tortillas, pita, matzoh, bagels, noodles and pasta	Corn bread, flour tortillas, oatmeal, soft rolls and buns, wheat germ	Breakfast bars, biscuits and muffins, granola, pancakes and waffles, donuts, taco shells, pastries, croissants	
Dairy Products	Nonfat milk, dry curd cottage cheese, nonfat cottage cheese, nonfat yogurt	Buttermilk, low-fat yogurt, 1% milk, low-fat cottage cheese	Whole milk, 2% milk, creamed cottage cheese	Butter, cream, sour cream, half & half, most cheeses (including part-skim and lite cheeses)
Meats		Beef round; veal loin, round, and shoulder; pork tenderloin	Beef and veal, lamb, fresh and picnic hams	All ground beef, spareribs, cold cuts, beef, hot dogs, pastrami
Poultry	Egg whites	Chicken and turkey (light meat without skin)	Chicken and turkey (light meat with skin, dark meat without skin), duck and goose (without skin)	Chicken/turkey (dark meat with skin), chicken-turkey hot dogs and bologna, egg yolks, whole eggs
Seafood	Clams, cod, crab, crawfish, flounder, haddock, lobster, perch, sole, scallops, shrimp, tuna (in water)	Bass and sea bass, halibut, mussels, oyster, tuna (fresh)	Anchovies, catfish, salmon, sturgeon, trout, tuna (in oil, drained)	Herring, mackerel, sardines
Beans and Nuts	Dried beans and peas, chestnuts, water chestnuts		Soybeans	Tofu, most nuts and seeds, peanut butter
Fats and Oils	Oil-free and some lite salad dressings			Butter, margarine, all mayonnaise (including reduced-calorie), most salad dressings, all oils
Soups	Bouillons, broths, consomme	Most soups	Cream soups, bean soups, "just add water" noodle soups	Cheddar cheese soup, New England clam chowder
Desserts	Angel food cake, gelatin, some new fat-free cakes	Pudding, tapioca	Most cakes, most pies	
Frozen Desserts	Sherbet, low-fat frozen yogurt, sorbet, fruit ices	Ice milk	Frozen yogurt	All ice cream
Snack Foods	Popcorn (air popped), pretzels, rye crackers, rice cakes, fig bars, raisin biscuit cookies, marshmallows, most hard candy, fruit rolls	Lite microwave popcorn, Scandinavian "crisps," plain crackers, caramels, fudge, gingersnaps, graham crackers	Snack crackers, popcorn (popped in oil), cookies, candy bars, granola bars	Most microwave popcorn, corn and potato chips, chocolate, buttery crackers

Source: American Heart Association/USDA.

closer. In the last three decades they've reduced the percent of calories from total fat from about 45 percent to about 34 percent. Many Americans are not necessarily eating less fat, however, but rather consuming more calories, largely in the form of carbohydrates and to a lesser extent, soft drinks and alcoholic beverages.[14] As a result, the percentage of calories from fat is lower, but less than 20 percent of the population is actually meeting the government's recommendations for total and saturated fat intake.[15]

Some health experts, such as Dean Ornish, M.D., who first demonstrated that a combination of a very low-fat diet, exercise, and psychological change could actually reverse atherosclerotic plaque, advocate cutting dietary fat down to 10 percent of daily calories. However, their success with reversing atherosclerosis may have depended on an entire program of dietary and behavioral change, rather than on simply eating more low-fat foods.

Others have questioned the benefits of a drastic reduction in dietary fats. Although high-fat diets have long been linked with various cancers, this association does not seem valid for breast cancer. A 1999 analysis of the diets of almost 90,000 women participating in the Nurses' Health Study over a 14-year period found that those eating diets with 20 percent fat or less were just as likely to get breast cancer as those eating diets with 30 percent to 35 percent fat. It made no difference whether the dietary fat was saturated, polyunsaturated, or monounsaturated or animal or vegetable in origin.[16]

High-fat diets also are associated with a higher risk of heart disease, but it is not clear whether an extreme reduction in dietary fat invariably lowers this risk. At least in some individuals, a low-fat diet can lead to an increase in a particularly dangerous form of low-density lipoprotein (LDL), the heart-harming form of cholesterol.[17] A one-year study of men with high cholesterol examined the cholesterol-lowering effects of diets that ranged from 30 percent to 18 percent fat. The men who aggressively restricted their dietary fat intake incurred two worrisome changes: higher triglycerides, fats that circulate in the bloodstream and provide energy, and a reduction of "good" HDL cholesterol. People who eat a high-carbohydrate diet—including excessive hard candies, fat-free cookies, and fat-free frozen yogurt—often have high triglyceride levels even if their fat intake is low.

Even athletes need some fat in their diet. In recent research, trained runners who severely limited their fat intake suppressed their immune system and increased their susceptibility to infections and inflammation.[18] Other research has shown that incorporating the right types of fat in daily diet can actually improve athletic performance—not just by providing calories, but by replenishing intramuscular fat stores (fat stored within the muscle and used to fuel extended exercise).[19]

Depending on how they reduce the fat in their diet, some Americans who cut way back on fat may end up shortchanging themselves of essential nutrients. In a study that analyzed the diets of individuals who cut back on fat by choosing skim rather than whole-fat milk, ate lean rather than fatty meat, or used fat-modified products, the diets of all improved when compared with those of individuals who did not try to reduce fat at all. However, the skim milk users had the highest ratings of

PULSE *points*

Top Ten Ways to Cut Fat

1. **Eat less meat.** Rather than making meat the heart of a meal, think of it as a flavoring ingredient.

2. **Forget frying.** Instead, steam, boil, bake, or microwave vegetables or meats.

3. **Switch to reduced-fat and non-fat dairy products.** Rather than buying whole-fat dairy products, choose skim milk, fat-free sour cream, and low- or nonfat yogurts.

4. **Season with herbs and spices.** Avoid using fatty sauce, butter, or margarine over your vegetables, pastas, or other dishes.

5. **Avoid high-fat fast foods.** Hot dogs, fried foods, packaged snack foods, and pastries are most likely to be high in fat.

6. **Say no to ice cream.** As a tasty treat, try frozen ices and nonfat frozen yogurt instead.

7. **Read labels carefully.** Remember that "cholesterol-free" doesn't necessarily mean fat-free. Avoid products that contain highly saturated coconut oil, palm oil, or lard.

8. **Check the numbers.** When buying prepared foods, choose items

that contain no more than 3 grams of fat per 100 calories.

9. **Remove all visible fat.** When you do serve meat, make sure to choose lean cuts and trim fat before and/or after cooking.

10. **Think small.** Remember that a dinner-size serving of meat should be about the size of a deck of cards or the palm of your hand. As you cut back on meat portions, serve larger amounts of fresh fruits and vegetables, grains, and beans.

micronutrients in their daily diets, while switching to lean meat led to inadequate zinc levels in men and eating lean meat or using fat-modified products resulted in low levels of zinc and of vitamin E in women.[20]

Fat Substitutes

The craze for low- and no-fat food peaked in the mid-1990s, but products made with fat substitutes remain popular. One of the most controversial is olestra, a non-absorbable fat substitute that passes through the human body without being digested, so it adds no fat or calories to foods cooked with it. Olestra causes gastrointestinal upset in some people and interferes with the absorption of vitamins and nutrients from foods eaten about the same time.

The Food and Drug Administration requires a warning label on snacks that contain olestra, and consumer activists continue to campaign against it. However, studies have not found a significantly higher rate of digestive problems among olestra consumers. In one, 38.2 percent of those eating olestra chips reported at least one gastrointestinal symptom—as did 36.9 percent of those who ate regular chips.[21]

Vitamins and Minerals

Vitamins and **minerals** are nutrients that are essential to regulating growth, maintaining tissue, and releasing energy from foods. Vitamins help put proteins, fats, and carbohydrates to use. Together with the enzymes in the body, they help produce the right chemical reactions at the right times. They're also involved in the manufacture of blood cells, as well as hormones and other compounds.

Some vitamins are produced within the body. Vitamin D, for example, is manufactured in the skin after exposure to sunlight, and then changed to an active form through processes in the liver and then kidney. However, most vitamins must be ingested. Vitamins such as A, D, E, and K are *fat-soluble*—absorbed through the intestinal membranes and stored in the body. The B vitamins and vitamin C are *water-soluble*—absorbed directly into the blood and then used up or washed out of the body in urine and sweat. They must be replaced daily. (See Table 6-4.)

The elements carbon, oxygen, hydrogen, and nitrogen make up 96 percent of our body weight. The other 4 percent consists of minerals, which help build bones and teeth, aid in muscle function, and help our nervous systems transmit messages. We need daily about a tenth of a gram (100 milligrams) or more of each of the *major minerals*: sodium, potassium, chloride, calcium, phosphorus, and magnesium. We also need daily about a hundredth of a gram (10 milligrams) or less of each of

the *trace minerals*: iron (more than that for premenopausal women), zinc, selenium, molybdenum, iodine, copper, manganese, fluoride, and chromium (see Table 6-5).

What Are Antioxidants?

Antioxidants are substances that prevent the harmful effects caused by oxidation within the body. There has been great general and scientific interest in the antioxidant vitamins, particularly vitamin C, vitamin E, and beta-carotene (a form of Vitamin A). The proven health benefits of these vitamins are many. Vitamin C speeds healing, helps prevent infection, and prevents scurvy. Vitamin E helps prevent heart disease by stopping the oxidation of low-density lipoprotein (the harmful form of cholesterol), strengthens the immune system, and may help prevent Alzheimer's disease, cataracts, and some forms of cancer. Beta-carotene aids eyesight and resistance to infection and keeps skin, hair, teeth, gums, and bones healthy.

Antioxidants also may prevent damage to our cells caused by *free radicals* (oxygen molecules formed by normal metabolic processes) as well as by smog, smoke, radiation, and cancer-promoting chemicals. For example, free radicals may alter a cell's DNA (deoxyribonucleic acid), the basic genetic blueprint, in ways that could lead to uncontrolled cell growth—that is, to cancer. They also may play a role in the buildup of cholesterol in the arteries.[22]

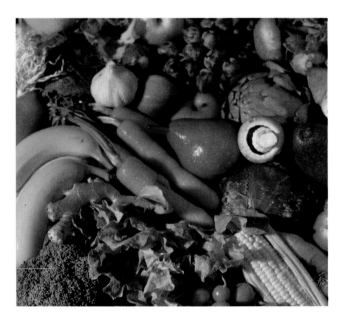

Antioxidant salad. Believe it or not, it's easy to get your daily antioxidant fix directly from food. Just eat an orange for breakfast and half a carrot for lunch and you'll have all the vitamin A (1,000 retinal equivalents) and vitamin C (60 milligrams) you need for the day.

"Don't underestimate the threat free radicals pose to our health," says Lester Packer of Lawrence Berkeley National Laboratory, a pioneer in antioxidant research. "They are major culprits in the aging process and in nearly every known disease, from cardiovascular disease to cancer to cataracts to arthritis.[23]

Like tiny thugs, free radicals constantly roam through the body and attack cells in the brain, heart, blood stream and immune system. Antioxidants rush to the rescue, limit damage, and help repair any harm that's been done. Like bouncers in a nightclub, antioxidants wrap up the troublemakers and carry them away.

Do antioxidants, as their ardent advocates claim, also protect the heart, prevent cancer, and forestall aging? "There is a great deal of sound scientific evidence that antioxidants play a critical role in promoting health," says Jeffrey Blumberg, chief of the USDA's antioxidants research lab at Tufts University. "But antioxidants are not a single compound. There are lots of different antioxidants that work together as a network. They're important preventive factors as part of a total dietary plan, but they are not the be-all and end-all of good health."[24]

Keeping Hearts Healthy. In the cardiovascular system, free radicals combine with cholesterol and dangerous low-density lipoprotein (LDL) to damage the inner lining of blood vessels. Vitamin E, a fat-soluble vitamin found in wheat germ, vegetable oils and nuts, short-circuits this process. In various clinical studies, it has generally lowered the risk of heart attacks and strokes by 40 to 60 percent.[25] Because it is difficult to get adequate levels of vitamin E in a daily diet, many experts recommend supplements of 100 to 400 IU (international units) a day.[26]

"Of all the antioxidants, the strongest scientific case can be made for vitamin E as a means of preventing heart disease," says William Pryor, director of Louisiana State University's Biodynamics Institute. "We're as close now to having enough data to support vitamin E supplements as we'll ever be, even though the benefit is statistical. Not everyone taking vitamin E will benefit, but most people will." Higher doses are considered safe for most individuals, although those taking anti-coagulation medications should check with their doctors because of the risk of internal bleeding.[27]

Other antioxidants, particularly vitamin C and beta-carotene, have not proved as helpful in protecting the heart.[28] In one study of 22,000 male physicians, 20 milligrams of beta-carotene, either alone or combined with vitamin E, did not reduce the risk of heart attacks. However, in epidemiological studies, individuals eating lots of dark green, yellow, and orange fruits and vegetables (good sources of vitamin C and beta-carotene) consistently have lower rates of coronary disease.

Preventing Cancer. At least in theory, antioxidants can block genetic damage induced by free radicals that could lead to some cancers. Diets high in antioxidant-rich fruits and vegetables have been linked with lower rates of esophageal, lung, colon, and stomach cancer. "We have reams of data on the benefits of foods, but not on supplements," says nutritionist Linda Nebeling of the National Cancer Institute. "Fruits and vegetables contain a cornucopia of antioxidant vitamins and phytochemicals," she says. "A supplement pill provides just one piece of this very large puzzle."[29]

Scientific studies have not proven conclusively that any specific antioxidant, particularly in supplement form, can prevent cancer. In studies of beta-carotene, this carotenoid did not reduce overall cancer rates or mortality. In two studies of smokers, beta-carotene actually was associated with increased mortality from lung cancer. "It may be that taking too high a dose of any one antioxidant is like trying to fit a piece 50 times the usual size into a puzzle," says Nebeling. "It throws off the balance. If you take huge doses, antioxidants become pro-oxidant and may actually induce damage."

Slowing Down the Aging Process. Over time, the cumulative effect of free radicals may be responsible for many diseases associated with age, including memory impairment, cataracts, macular degeneration (deterioration of the central part of the eye), and arthritis.[30] Can antioxidants stop or slow their progress? "They may not be able to turn back the clock, but they certainly can affect it," says Packer. "Even after a chronic, degenerative disorder is recognized, we've shown that antioxidants can slow its progression. In the future, we're going to see them used more and more to improve the quality of everyday life for older people."

In laboratory and animal studies, vitamin E has shown particular promise in slowing neurological aging and improving cognitive function. While there is no evidence that E can prevent Alzheimer's disease, high doses have modestly slowed progression of this form of dementia. Earlier this year, in the first large-scale American study of vitamin E's impact on human memory, biostatistician Siu Hui and her colleagues at Indiana University found that higher blood concentrations of vitamin E—but not of beta-carotene, vitamins A or C, or the mineral selenium—correlated with better performance on simple recall tests. "Our study doesn't prove that vitamin E preserves or improves memory, but it adds to the supporting evidence," she says.[31]

Certain antioxidants have proven be a boon for aging eyes. In the Baltimore Longitudinal Study of Aging, vitamin E, vitamin C, and beta-carotene all provided protection against age-related macular degeneration.[32] Other studies indicate that individuals with

■ **Table 6-4** Key Information about Vitamins

Vitamin	Significant Sources	Chief Functions	Signs of Severe, Prolonged Deficiency	Signs of Extreme Excess
Fat Soluble Vitamin A	Fortified milk, cheese, cream, butter, fortified margarine, eggs, liver; spinach and other dark, leafy greens, broccoli, deep orange fruits (apricots, cantaloupes) and vegetables (squash, carrots, sweet potatoes, pumpkins)	Antioxidant, needed for vision, health of cornea, epithelial cells, mucous membranes, skin health, bone and tooth growth, hormone synthesis and regulation, immunity	Anemia, painful joints, cracks in teeth, tendency toward tooth decay, diarrhea, depression, frequent infections, night blindness, keratinization, corneal degeneration, rashes, kidney stones	Nosebleeds, bone pain, growth retardation, headaches, abdominal cramps and pain, nausea, vomiting, diarrhea, weight loss, overreactive immune system, blurred vision, pain in calves, fatigue, irritability, loss of appetite, dry skin, rashes, loss of hair, cessation of menstruation
Vitamin D	Fortified milk or margarine, eggs, liver, sardines; exposure to sunlight	Promotes calcium and phosphorus absorption	Abnormal growth, misshapen bones (bowing of legs), soft bones, joint pain, malformed teeth	Raised blood calcium, excessive thirst, headaches, irritability, loss of appetite, weakness, nausea, kidney stones, stones in arteries, mental and physical retardation
Vitamin E	Margarine, salad dressings, shortenings, green and leafy vegetables, wheat germ, whole-grain products, nuts, seeds	Antioxidant, needed for stabilization of cell membranes, regulation of oxidation reactions	Red blood cell breakage, anemia, muscle degeneration, weakness, difficulty walking, leg cramps, fibrocystic breast disease	Augments the effects of anticlotting medication; general discomfort
Vitamin K	Liver, green leafy vegetables, cabbage-type vegetables, milk	Needed for synthesis of blood-clotting proteins and a blood protein that regulates blood calcium	Hemorrhage	Interference with anticlotting medication; jaundice
Water-Soluble Vitamin B-6	Green and leafy vegetables, meats, fish, poultry, shellfish, legumes, fruits, whole grains	Part of a coenzyme needed for amino acid and fatty acid metabolism, helps make red blood cells	Anemia, smooth tongue, abnormal brain wave pattern, irritability, muscle twitching, convulsions	Depression, fatigue, impaired memory, irritability, headaches, numbness, damage to nerves, difficulty walking, loss of reflexes, weakness, restlessness
Vitamin B-12	Animal products (meat, fish, poultry, milk, cheese, eggs)	Part of a coenzyme used in new cell synthesis, helps maintain nerve cells	Anemia, smooth tongue, fatigue, nervous system degeneration progressing to paralysis, hypersensitivity	None reported

■ Table 6-4 Key Information about Vitamins (continued)

Vitamin	Significant Sources	Chief Functions	Signs of Severe, Prolonged Deficiency	Signs of Extreme Excess
Vitamin C	Citrus fruits, cabbage-type vegetables, dark green vegetables, cantaloupe, strawberries, peppers, lettuce, tomatoes, potatoes, papayas, mangoes	Antioxidant, collagen synthesis (strengthens blood vessel walls, forms scar tissue, matrix for bone growth), amino acid metabolism, strengthens resistance to infection, aids iron absorption	Anemia, pinpoint hemorrhages, frequent infections, bleeding gums, loosened teeth, muscle degeneration and pain, hysteria, depression, bone fragility, joint pain, rough skin, blotchy bruises, failure of wounds to heal	Nausea, abdominal cramps, diarrhea, excessive urination, headache, fatigue, insomnia, rashes, aggravation of gout symptoms; deficiency symptoms may appear at first on withdrawal of high doses
Thiamin	Pork, ham, bacon, liver, whole grains, legumes, nuts; occurs in all nutritious foods in moderate amounts	Part of a coenzyme needed for energy metabolism, normal appetite function, and nervous system	Edema, enlarged heart, abnormal heart rhythms, heart failure, nervous/muscular system degeneration, wasting, weakness, pain, low morale, difficulty walking, loss of reflexes, mental confusion, paralysis	None reported
Riboflavin	Milk, yogurt, cottage cheese, meat, leafy green vegetables, whole-grain or enriched breads and cereals	Part of a coenzyme needed for energy metabolism, supports normal vision and skin health	Cracks at corner of mouth, magenta tongue, hypersensitivity to light, reddening of cornea, skin rash	None reported
Niacin	Milk, eggs, meat, poultry, fish, whole-grain and enriched breads and cereals, nuts, and all protein-containing foods	Part of a coenzyme needed for energy metabolism, supports skin health, nervous system, and digestive system	Diarrhea, black smooth tongue, irritability, loss of appetite, weakness, dizziness, mental confusion, flaky skin rash on areas exposed to sun	Diarrhea, heartburn, nausea, ulcer irritation, vomiting, fainting, dizziness, painful flush and rash, sweating, abnormal liver function, low blood pressure
Folate	Leafy green vegetables, legumes, seeds, liver, enriched bread, cereal, pasta, and grains	Part of a coenzyme needed for new cell synthesis	Anemia, heartburn, diarrhea, constipation, frequent infections, smooth red tongue, depression, mental confusion, fainting	Masks Vitamin B-12 deficiency
Panothenic Acid	Widespread in foods	Part of a coenzyme used in energy metabolism	Vomiting, intestinal distress, insomnia, fatigue	Water retention (rare)
Biotin	Widespread in foods	Used in energy metabolism, fat synthesis, amino acid metabolism, and glycogen synthesis	Abnormal heart action, loss of appetite, nausea, depression, muscle pain, weakness, fatigue, drying, rash, loss of hair	None reported

Source: Adapted from Sizer/Whitney, *Nutrition: Concepts and Controversies,* 8th ed. Belmont, Calif.: Wadsworth, 2000.

■ **Table 6-5** Key Information about Essential Minerals

Mineral	Significant Sources	Chief Functions	Signs of Severe, Prolonged Deficiency	Signs of Extreme Excess
Major Minerals				
Sodium	Foods processed with salt, cured foods (corned beef, ham, bacon, pickles, sauerkraut), table and sea salt, bread, milk, cheese, salad dressing	Needed to maintain acid-base balance in body fluids, helps regulate water in blood and body tissues, needed for muscle and nerve activity	Weakness, apathy, poor appetite, muscle cramps, headache, swelling	High blood pressure, kidney disease, heart problems
Potassium	Plant foods (potatoes, squash, lima beans, tomatoes, bananas, oranges, avocados), meats, milk and milk products, coffee	Needed to maintain acid-base balance in body fluids, helps regulate water in blood and body tissues, needed for muscle and nerve activity	Weakness, irritability, mental confusion, irregular heartbeat, paralysis	Irregular heartbeat, heart attack
Chloride	Foods processed with salt, cured foods (corned beef, ham, bacon, pickles, sauerkraut), table and sea salt, bread, milk, cheese, salad dressing	Aids in digestion, needed to maintain acid-base balance in body fluids, helps regulate water in the body	Muscle cramps, apathy, poor appetite, long-term mental retardation in infants	Vomiting
Calcium	Milk and milk products, broccoli, dried beans	Component of bones and teeth, needed for muscle and nerve activity, blood clotting	Weak bones, rickets, stunted growth in children, convulsions, muscle spasms, osteoporosis	Drowsiness, calcium deposits in kidneys, liver, and other tissues, suppression of bone remodeling, decreased zinc absorption
Phosphorus	Milk and milk products, meats, seeds, nuts	Component of bones and teeth, energy formation, needed to maintain the right acid-base balance of body fluids	Loss of appetite, nausea, vomiting, weakness, confusion, loss of calcium from bones	Loss of calcium from bones, muscle spasms
Magnesium	Plant foods (dried beans, tofu, peanuts, potatoes, green vegetables)	Component of bones and teeth, nerve activity, energy and protein formation	Stunted growth in children, weakness, muscle spasms, personality changes	Diarrhea, dehydration, impaired nerve activity
Trace Minerals				
Iron	Liver, beef, pork, dried beans, iron-fortified cereals, prunes, apricots, raisins, spinach, bread, pasta	Aids in transport of oxygen, component of myoglobin, energy formation	Anemia, weakness, fatigue, pale appearance, reduced attention span, resistance to infection, developmental delays in children	"Iron poisoning," vomiting, abdominal pain, blue coloration of skin, shock, heart failure, diabetes, decreased zinc absorption
Zinc	Meats, grains, nuts, milk and milk products, cereals, bread	Protein reproduction, component of insulin	Growth failure, delayed sexual maturation, slow wound healing, loss of	Nausea, vomiting, weakness, fatigue, susceptibility to infection, copper

■ **Table 6-5** Key Information about Essential Minerals (continued)

Mineral	Significant Sources	Chief Functions	Signs of Severe, Prolonged Deficiency	Signs of Extreme Excess
			taste and appetite; in pregnant women, low-birth-weight infants and preterm delivery	deficiency, metallic taste in mouth
Selenium	Meats and seafood, eggs, grains	Acts as an antioxidant in conjunction with vitamin E	Anemia, muscle pain and tenderness, Keshar disease, heart failure	Hair and fingernail loss, weakness, liver damage, irritability, "garlic" or "metallic" breath
Molybdenum	Dried beans, grains, dark green vegetables, liver, milk and milk products	Aids in oxygen transfer from one molecule to another	Rapid heartbeat and breathing, nausea, vomiting, coma	Loss of copper from the body, joint pain, growth failure, anemia, gout
Iodine	Iodized salt, milk and milk products, seaweed, seafood, bread	Component of thyroid hormones that help regulate energy production and growth	Goiter, cretinism in newborns (mental retardation, hearing loss, growth failure)	Pimples, goiter, decreased thyroid function
Copper	Bread, potatoes, grains, dried beans, nuts and seeds, seafood, cereals	Component of enzymes involved in the body's utilization of iron and oxygen; functions in growth, immunity, cholesterol, and glucose utilization; brain development	Anemia, seizures, nerve and bone abnormalities in children, growth retardation	Wilson's disease (excessive accumulation of copper in the liver and kidneys); vomiting, diarrhea, tremors, liver disease
Manganese	Whole grains, coffee, tea, dried beans, nuts	Formation of body fat and bone	Weight loss, rash, nausea and vomiting	Infertility in men, disruptions in the nervous system, muscle spasms
Fluoride	Fluoridated water, foods, and beverages; tea; shrimp; crab	Component of bones and teeth (enamel)	Tooth decay and other dental diseases	Fluorosis, brittle bones, mottled teeth, nerve abnormalities
Chromium	Whole grains, liver, meat, beer, wine	Glucose utilization	Poor blood glucose control, weight loss	Kidney and skin damage

Source: Adapted from Brown, *Nutrition Now.* Belmont, Calif.: Wadsworth, 1999.

low antioxidant levels are more likely to develop cataracts, while those with higher levels have a lower risk. "There is compelling evidence that vitamin C may reduce the risk of cataracts by as much as 80 percent," reports Blumberg.

Folic Acid

Beginning in 1998, food manufacturers began adding folic acid, or folate, a B vitamin, to America's food. The primary reason is that insufficient levels of folic acid increase the risk of neural tube defects (abnormalities of the brain and spinal cord), such as spina bifida, in which a piece of the spinal cord protrudes from the spinal column.

Neural tube defects occur in about 4,000 pregnancies every year; 50 to 70 percent could be prevented with a daily intake of 4,000 micrograms of folic acid. In a national Gallup poll, 68 percent of women of childbearing age said they had heard or read about folic acid. However, only 13 percent knew that folic acid helps prevent birth defects. About a third of women (32 percent) take a vitamin supplement containing folic acid every day.[33]

Folate, when obtained both from a diet high in vegetables and citrus fruit and from supplements, also reduces blood levels of homocysteine, a chemical associated with increased risk of cardiovascular disease.[34] Folic acid also reduces the excess risk of breast cancer associated with alcohol consumption.[35]

Calcium

Calcium, the most abundant mineral in the body, builds strong bone tissue throughout our lives and plays a vital role in heart and brain functioning. Adequate calcium is especially critical for pregnant or nursing women, who need it to meet the additional needs of their babies' bodies. (See Chapter 10 for a complete discussion of diet and pregnancy.) Calcium may also help control high blood pressure and prevent colon cancer in adults.

Experts do not agree on how much calcium is enough. The NIH (National Institutes of Health) guidelines call for higher intakes for pregnant and nursing women and women over age 50 who are not using hormone replacement therapy. The Food and Nutrition Board of the National Academy of Sciences does not take age or gender differences into account. (See Table 6-6.) The new USDA Food Pyramid for Older Americans recommends dietary supplements of calcium and vitamins B-12 and D for all men and women over age 70.

Adequate calcium intake during the teens and twenties may be crucial to prevent osteoporosis, the bone-weakening disease that strikes one out of every four women over the age of 60. Dietary calcium can significantly increase the bone density of children, safeguarding against osteoporosis in later life. Research has shown that elderly men and women who consume adequate calcium can keep their bones strong and prevent fractures.

Iron

Iron is an essential ingredient of **hemoglobin**, the protein that makes the blood red and carries oxygen to all our tissues. Because oxygen is needed to convert food into energy, too little iron—and thus too little hemoglobin—can trigger an internal energy crisis. Getting enough iron can be a big problem for women, whose iron stores are drained by menstruation, pregnancy, and nursing. Half of all women of childbearing age get less than the RDA of 15 milligrams, and 5 percent suffer from iron-deficiency anemia.

The symptoms of iron deficiency are sensitivity to cold, chronic fatigue, edginess, depression, sleeplessness, and susceptibility to colds and infections. To boost

■ **Table 6-6** How Much Calcium?

National Academy of Sciences Recommendations

Age Group	Milligrams per Day
0–6 months	210 (solely from human milk)
7–12 months	270 (human milk and solid foods)
1–3 years	500
4–8 years	800
9–18 years	1,300
19–50 years	1,000
51 and older	1,200

NIH Recommendations

Age Group	Milligrams per Day
Infants	
Birth–6 months	400
6 months–1 year	600
Children	
1–5 years	800
6–10 years	800–1,200
Adolescents/Young Adults	
11–24 years	1,200–1,500
Men	
25–65 years	1,000
65 and older	1,500
Women	
25–50 years	1,000
Postmenopausal	
Taking/not taking H.R.T.	1,000/1,500
65 years and older	1,500
Pregnant/nursing	1,200–1,500

Source: Food and Nutrition Board, Institute of Medicine of the National Academy of Sciences; NIH Consensus Development Panel on Optimal Calcium Intake.

your iron, use the strategies on page 167. Don't take supplements unless you've had a blood test that indicates you should. Excess iron can cause severe constipation and other complications.

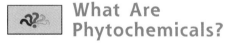 ## What Are Phytochemicals?

Phytochemicals are substances that exist naturally in plants. The thousands of phytochemicals serve many functions, including helping a plant protect itself from bacteria and disease. Phytochemicals have a range of effects on human health. Some, such as solanine, an insect-repelling chemical found in the leaves and stalks of potato plants, are natural toxins. However, many are beneficial. Although research has yet to show a cause-and-effect relationship between consumption of phyto-

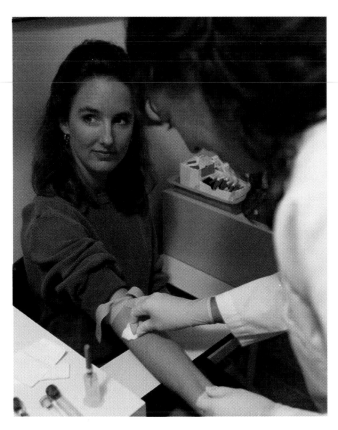

A blood test is necessary to diagnose iron-deficiency anemia. A healthy diet that includes whole-grain cereals, broccoli, and foods rich in vitamin C is a good way to boost iron stores.

Strategies *for* Prevention

Getting More Iron in Your Diet

✔ Eat vegetables and starches high in iron: whole-grain cereals (such as bran flakes), broccoli, soybeans, and red kidney beans.

✔ To increase the amount of iron your body absorbs from these plant foods, eat foods high in vitamin C at the same meal.

✔ Eat iron-rich lean red meats two or three times a week. Oysters are also a good iron source.

✔ Don't drink tea with your meal, because the tannin in it may interfere with iron absorption.

chemicals and prevention of a specific disease,[36] phytochemicals are associated with a reduced risk of heart disease, certain cancers, age-related macular degeneration, adult-onset diabetes, stroke, and other diseases.

Some phytochemicals act as antioxidants and limit and repair damage caused by free radicals. Others act as hormone-like substances to prevent cancer or block the enzymes that promote the development of cancer and other diseases. Flavonoids, found in apples, strawberries, grapes, onions, green and black tea, and red wine, may decrease atherosclerotic plaque and DNA damage related to cancer developments. Carotenoids (beta-carotene, lutein, zeaxanthin, cryptoxanthin, and lycopene) protect the eye from harmful oxidation reactions. Lignans, found in flaxseed, seaweed, soybeans, bran, and dried beans, are "phytoestrogens" that interfere with the action of the sex hormone estrogen and may help prevent hormone-related cancers, slow the growth of cancer cells, and lower the risk for heart disease.

Phytochemicals appear to work together to enhance health and prevent disease. Studies of supplements of individual phytochemicals, such as beta-carotene, have proven disappointing. There is no solid evidence that specific phytochemicals extracted from foods can benefit health. Nevertheless, some researchers are recommending that phytochemicals, such as carotenoids, and antioxidant vitamins be added to foods and beverages to transform them into "nutraceuticals" or foods that serve a therapeutic function.[37] A better option, nutritionists say, is eating more fruits and vegetables. (See Table 6-7.) Among the foods recognized as rich in beneficial phytochemicals are:

Tomatoes: They, along with tomato products, are a rich source of the carotenoid lycopene, which may lower the risk of prostate cancer.

Garlic: Rich in a variety of phytochemicals, garlic has shown strong antibacterial and antioxidant activity.

Oranges: Along with other citrus fruits, oranges contain a wealth of flavonoids, vitamin C, and other antioxidant compounds.

Broccoli: This cruciferous vegetable contains many phytochemicals, including flavonoids, carotenoids (highest concentration in the florets), vitamin C, dietary fiber, selenium, and vitamin E.

Green Tea: Green tea is a good source of flavonoids and antioxidants.

Soybeans (and soy foods): These are a prime source of isoflavonoids, flavonoids, lignans, phytoesterols, phytic acid, and dietary fiber. Soy oil is a nonfish source of essential fatty acids and one of the richest sources in the American diet of vitamin E because so many margarines, salad dressings, and packaged baked goods rely on soybean oil. Soy foods include soy milk, miso, tofu, and tempeh.

Brussels Sprouts: This cruciferous vegetable has phytochemicals, including flavonoids, and vitamin C.

■ **Table 6-7** Some Foods Rich in Antioxidants and Phytochemicals

Antioxidant	Food	Phytochemical	Food
Beta-carotene	Apricots, Asparagus, Brussels sprouts, Cantaloupe, Carrot, Peach, Romaine lettuce, Spinach, Sweet potato	Capsaicin	Hot peppers
		Coumarins	Citrus fruit, Tomatoes
Selenium	Lean meat, 100% whole wheat bread, Nonfat milk, Skinless chicken, 100% whole-grain cereal, Seafood	Flavonoids	Berries, Carrots, Citrus fruit, Peppers, Tomatoes
		Genistein	Beans, Peas, Lentils
Vitamin C	Asparagus, Broccoli, Brussels sprouts, Cabbage, Collard greens, Grapefruit, Green pepper, Orange juice, Strawberries, Tomato juice	Indoles	Broccoli, Cabbage family
		Isothiocyanates	Broccoli, Cabbage, Mustard, Horseradish
		Ligands	Barley, Flaxseed, Wheat
Vitamin E	Almonds, 100% whole wheat bread, Wheat germ, 100% whole-grain cereal, Safflower oil	Lycopene	Pink grapefruit, Tomatoes
		S-allycysteine	Chives, Garlic, Onions
		Triterpenoids	Citrus fruit, Licorice root

Eating for Good Health

Recognizing the importance of diet, the U.S. government formulates dietary guidance and maintains a nutrition monitoring system to assess the healthfulness of Americans' diet. Since 1980, the U.S. Departments of Agriculture and Health and Human Services have produced Dietary Guidelines for Americans. Here are their recommendations:

- *Eat a variety of foods.* Choosing among different types of foods every day helps ensure that you get the protein, vitamins, and minerals you need.

- *Maintain a healthy weight.* Excess pounds can increase your risk of high blood pressure, heart disease, stroke, certain cancers, and the most common kind of diabetes. (See Chapter 7 for more on weight management.)

- *Choose a diet low in fat, saturated fat, and cholesterol.* Fat contains more than twice the calories of an equal amount of protein or carbohydrates, and increases your risk of certain diseases.

- *Choose a diet with plenty of vegetables, fruits, and grain products.* These foods provide vitamins, minerals, fiber, and complex carbohydrates.

- *Use sugars only in moderation.* Sugars, or simple carbohydrates, provide few nutrients for their calories and can contribute to tooth decay.

- *Use salt and sodium only in moderation.* Excessive sodium intake, as discussed in Chapter 13 on cardiovascular illness, may increase your risk of high blood pressure. The Food and Drug Administration recommends that all adults restrict sodium to no more than 2,400 milligrams a day.

- *If you drink alcoholic beverages, do so only in moderation.* Alcohol, which has a very low nutrient density (nutritional value compared to calories), can lead to dependence and other health problems. (See Chapter 16 for a thorough discussion of alcohol consumption.)

The Food Guide Pyramid

The USDA's Food Guide Pyramid (see Figure 6-2), adopted in 1992, replaced the traditional basic four food groups—meats, milk products, fruits and vegetables, breads and cereals—with five categories. These categories are not considered nutritional equals. For the sake of good health, you need some food from all the groups every day, but in different amounts.

"The idea of the pyramid is to get people to eat more of the foods at its base (grains, fruits, and vegetables) and fewer of those toward the top (meat, milk products, sugars, and fats)," says Ann Shaw, a nutritionist with the federal Agriculture Research Service.[38] Foods in one group cannot substitute for those in another. Although the new guide doesn't ban any foods from plates or palates, the pyramid clearly advises less of some favorites, including meat. "Your maximum daily protein intake should be 5 to 7 ounces, with no more than half of that coming from red meat," says Shaw. "We're trying to get people to eat fewer servings of meat and to eat smaller ones—the size of a deck of cards, not half the dinner plate."

College students generally do not eat well-balanced diets. According to the National College Health Risk Behavior Survey, only 25 percent of undergraduate women and 28 percent of undergraduate men eat five or

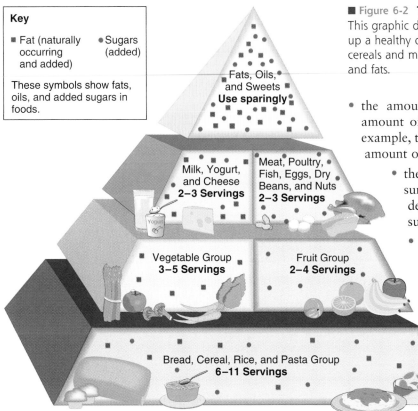

Key

■ Fat (naturally occurring and added)   ● Sugars (added)

These symbols show fats, oils, and added sugars in foods.

Fats, Oils, and Sweets
Use sparingly

Milk, Yogurt, and Cheese
2–3 Servings

Meat, Poultry, Fish, Eggs, Dry Beans, and Nuts
2–3 Servings

Vegetable Group
3–5 Servings

Fruit Group
2–4 Servings

Bread, Cereal, Rice, and Pasta Group
6–11 Servings

■ Figure 6-2 **The USDA's Food Guide Pyramid**
This graphic demonstrates the daily food choices that make up a healthy diet, with a broad foundation of grains and cereals and more modest amounts of meat, dairy products, and fats.

- the amount of food that provides a comparable amount of key nutrients from that food group; for example, the amount of cheese that provides the same amount of calcium as a cup of milk

  - the amount of food recognized by most consumers or easily multiplied or divided to describe how much food is actually consumed

    - the amount traditionally used in previous food guides to describe servings

A food label "serving" is a specific amount of food that contains the quantity of nutrients described on the Nutrition Facts label.

For many foods, the serving size in the Food Guide Pyramid and on the food label are the same (for example, half a cup of canned fruit or one slice of bread), but in other cases they differ. The pyramid describes serving units for each food group in ways that consumers find easy to remember (for example, a cup of leafy raw vegetables), while the food label is meant to help consumers compare nutrient information on a number of food products within a category (for example, frozen dinner entrees containing foods from several food groups).

A "portion" is the amount of a specific food that an individual eats at one time. Portions can be bigger or smaller than the servings on food labels or in the Food Guide Pyramid. According to research by the USDA, portion sizes tend to be bigger for men than women, but to decrease for both sexes with age.[39] Particularly if you are trying to balance your diet or control your weight, it's important to keep track of the size of your portions so that you do not exceed the recommended serving. For instance, a three-ounce "serving" of meat is about the size of a pack of cards or a computer "mouse." If you eat a larger amount, count it as more than one serving.

more servings of fruit or vegetables every day. Yet 84.9 percent of the women and 69.6 percent of the men have two or more servings of high-fat foods.

Although following the pyramid may seem complicated at first, it doesn't have to be. Simple changes in what you eat can transform a lopsided eating plan into a well-balanced one. (See Self-Survey: "Rate Your Diet.")

Food Portions and Servings

Consumers often are confused by what a "serving" actually is, especially since many American restaurants have "supersized" the amount of food they put on their customers' plates. Very often a "serving" at a restaurant, in a cafeteria, or at home is much larger than those referred to in the Food Guide Pyramid and on the Nutrition Facts Label—and higher in calories.

A Food Guide Pyramid "serving" describes the total amount of foods recommended *daily* from each of the food groups. It does not describe the size of an individual portion. The size of the daily serving is determined by four criteria:

- the amount of foods from a food group typically reported in surveys as consumed on one eating occasion

Breads, Cereals, Rice, and Pasta (6–11 servings a day)

These foods are the foundation of a healthy diet because they are a good source of complex carbohydrates. Both simple and complex carbohydrates (starches) have 4 calories per gram. Sugars provide little more than a

Self-*Survey*   Rate Your Diet

Step 1

For a week, write down everything you eat and drink for meals and snacks. Include the approximate amount eaten (for example, ½ cup, 1 large, 12 oz. can, and so on).

	Mon	Tues	Wed	Thurs	Fri	Sat	Sun
Grains							
Vegetables							
Fruits							
Milk, yogurt, cheese							
Meat, poultry, dry beans, eggs, nuts							
Fats, oil, sweets, cheese							

Step 2: Are You Getting Enough Vegetables, Fruits, and Grains?

How often do you eat:	Seldom/never	1–2 times a week	3–5 times a week	Almost daily
At least three servings of vegetables a day?				
Starchy vegetables like potatoes, corn, or peas?				
Foods made with dry beans, lentils, or peas?				
Dark green or deep yellow vegetables (broccoli, spinach, collards, carrots, sweet potatoes, squash)?				
At least two servings of fruit a day?				
Citrus fruits and 100% fruit juices (oranges, grapefruit, tangerines)?				
Whole fruit with skin or seeds (berries, apples, pears)?				
At least six servings of breads, cereals, pasta, or rice a day?				

The best answer for each of the above is "almost daily." Use your food diary to see which foods you should be eating more often.

Step 3: Are You Getting Too Much Fat?

How often do you eat:	Seldom/never	1–2 times a week	3–5 times a week	Almost daily
Fried, deep-fat fried, or breaded food?				
Fatty meats, such as sausages, luncheon meat, fatty steaks or roasts?				
Whole milk, high-fat cheeses, ice cream?				
Pies, pastries, rich cakes?				
Rich cream sauces and gravies?				
Oily salad dressings or mayonnaise?				
Butter or margarine on vegetables, rolls, bread, or toast?				

Ideally, you should be eating these foods no more than one or two times a week. If your food diary indicates that you're eating them more frequently, your fat intake may well be too high.

Step 4: Are You Getting Too Much Sodium?

How often do you eat:	Seldom/never	1–2 times a week	3–5 times a week	Almost daily
Cured or processed meats, such as ham, sausage, frankfurters, or luncheon meats?				
Canned vegetables or frozen vegetables with sauce?				
Frozen TV dinners, entrees, or canned or dehydrated soups?				
Salted nuts, popcorn, pretzels, corn chips, or potato chips?				
Seasoning mixes or sauces containing salt?				
Processed cheese?				
Salt added to table foods before you taste them?				

Ideally, you should be eating these high-sodium items no more than one or two times a week. If your food diary indicates that you're eating them more frequently, your sodium intake may well be too high.

Making Changes

How to Improve Your Diet
- Follow the Food Guide Pyramid in planning your daily meals.
- Read food nutritional labels carefully. Always check fat and sodium content.
- Rethink your meal choices. Have cereal or whole-grain toast instead of eggs for breakfast, salad in place of a burger for lunch, rice or pasta dishes rather than meats as a main course for dinner.
- Include a green or orange food at both lunch and dinner. Add extra vegetables to every recipe that calls for them.
- Serve fresh fruit or vegetable salsas instead of sauces for meat, poultry or fish.
- Peel and slice fruit at home and take it along to work in a plastic bag for a snack.
- Rather than sipping a soda at your desk or drinking gatorade after working out, choose water or 100% fruit juice instead.
- Use herbs and spices as seasonings for vegetables and meats instead of salt.

Source: Adapted from materials prepared by the USDA Human Nutrition Information Service.

quick spurt of energy, whereas complex carbohydrates are rich in vitamins, minerals, and other nutrients. Less than 25 percent of the daily calories in a typical American diet comes from complex carbohydrates; ideally, they should account for 50 to 60 percent.

A typical serving in this category might be one slice of bread, and one ounce of ready-to-eat cereal (or one-half cup of cooked cereal, rice, or pasta). Although many people think of these foods as fattening, it's actually what you put on them, such as butter on a roll or cream sauce on pasta, that adds extra calories.

Here are suggestions for getting more grains in your diet:

- Add brown rice or barley to soups.
- Check labels of rolls and bread, and choose those with at least 2 to 3 grams of fiber per slice. Grain products made with white or refined wheat flour have

had most of their fiber-rich bran mechanically removed. However, if fiber has been added, some white breads may actually have more fiber than multigrain breads.

- Go for pasta power. Pasta has 210 calories per cooked cup and only 9 calories from fat. Like whole-grain breads, whole-grain pastas may provide more nutrients than those made with refined flour.

Vegetables (3–5 servings a day)

Naturally low in fat and high in fiber, vegetables provide crucial vitamins (such as A and C) and minerals (such as iron and magnesium). A serving in this category consists of one cup of raw leafy vegetables, one-half cup of other vegetables (either cooked or raw), three-quarters cup of vegetable juice, or one potato or

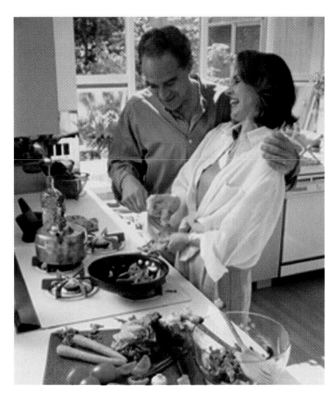

Including more vegetables in your diet has many health benefits and can help lower your risk of developing cancer.

ear of corn. Since different types of vegetables provide different nutrients, it's best to eat a variety. Dark green vegetables are especially good sources of vitamins and minerals; certain greens (such as collards, kale, turnip, and mustard) provide calcium and iron. Winter squash, carrots, and the plant family that includes broccoli, cabbage, kohlrabi, and cauliflower (the **crucifers**) are high in fiber, rich in vitamins, and excellent sources of **indoles**, chemicals that help lower cancer risk.

Here are ways to increase your vegetable intake:

- Make or order sandwiches with extra tomatoes or other vegetable toppings.
- Add extra vegetables whenever you're preparing soups, sauces, and so on.
- If you can't find fresh vegetables, use frozen. They contain less salt than canned veggies.
- Use raw vegetables for dipping, instead of chips.

Fruit (2–4 servings a day)

Like whole grains and vegetables, fruits are excellent sources of vitamins, minerals, and fiber. Along with vegetables, fruits may protect against cancer; those who eat little produce have a cancer rate twice that of people who eat the most fruits and vegetables. A serving consists of a medium apple, banana, or orange; a half-cup of chopped, cooked, or canned fruit; or three-quarters of a cup of fruit juice.

Try the following suggestions to get more fruit into your daily diet:

- Carry a banana, apple, or package of dried fruit with you as a healthy snack.
- Eat fruit for dessert or a snack. Try poached pears, baked apples, or fresh berries.
- Start the day with a daily double: a glass of juice and a banana or other fruit on cereal.
- Add citrus fruits (such as slices of grapefruit, oranges, or apples) to green salads, rice, grains, and chicken, pork, or fish dishes.
- Squeeze fresh lemon or lime juice over seafood, fruit salads, or vegetable dishes.

Meat, Poultry, Fish, Dry Beans, Eggs, and Nuts (2–3 servings a day)

A serving in this category consists of 2 or 3 ounces of lean, cooked meat, fish, or poultry (roughly the size of an average hamburger or the amount of meat on half a medium chicken breast). An egg or one-half cup of cooked dry beans can substitute for 1 ounce of lean meat. Thus, one day's total protein intake might include an egg at breakfast, a serving of beans or 2 ounces of sliced chicken in a sandwich at lunch, and 3 ounces of fish for dinner.

Recent research indicates that eating as much as an egg a day doesn't appear to increase your risk of developing heart disease or suffering a stroke. Eggs, it turns out, do not significantly raise cholesterol levels in blood, except for individuals whom physicians call "responders," who churn out cholesterol when they eat eggs. However, medical experts still caution against eating eggs in ways that contain lots of saturated fats, such as fried or served with bacon.[40]

To pick the best protein, follow these recommendations:

- Choose the leanest meats, such as beef round or sirloin, pork tenderloin, or veal. Broil or roast instead of fry. Trim fat before cooking, which can lower the fat content of the meat you eat by more than 10 percent. Marinate low-fat cuts to increase tenderness.
- Cook stews, boiled meat, or soup stock ahead of time; refrigerate; and remove the hardened fat before using. Drain fat from ground beef after cooking.

- Watch out for processed chicken and turkey products; for example, bolognas and salamis made from turkey can contain 45 to 90 percent fat.
- Select small chickens when you shop: They're leaner than large ones. Broiler-fryers are lowest in fat, followed by roasters. Remove skin before eating poultry.
- Choose fish as a leaner alternative to meat. It's high in protein, and packed with vitamins and minerals.
- Substitute bean-based dishes, such as chili or lentil stew, for meat entrees.

Milk, Yogurt, and Cheese (2–3 servings a day)

Most milk products are high in calcium, riboflavin, protein, and vitamins A and B-12. The Food Guide Pyramid recommends two servings of milk, yogurt, or cheese for most adults and three for women who are pregnant or breast-feeding. In addition, teenagers and young adults up to age 24 should also get three servings of milk products a day. Dairy products, such as milk and yogurt, are the best calcium sources, but be sure you choose products that are lowfat, or preferably nonfat. A serving in this category consists of an 8-ounce cup of milk, one cup of plain yogurt, 1½ ounces of hard cheese, or one tablespoon of cheese spread. An 8-ounce glass of nonfat milk is a more nutritious choice than a tablespoon of a high-fat cheese spread.

A growing concern is the problem of lactose intolerance, or inability to digest milk products, which is particularly common in nonwhite minority groups (see Figure 6-3). In individuals who do not produce adequate amounts of the intestinal enzyme lactase, milk products travel through the stomach undigested and ferment in the small bowel, causing gas, cramps, and diarrhea. Overall, 25 percent of Americans have trouble digesting dairy products. Over-the-counter medicines can help, and many dairy products are available in special forms for the lactose-intolerant.[41]

To make sure you get more milk with less fat, try the following:

- Gradually switch from whole milk to 2%-fat (reduced fat) milk, then to 1%-fat (low-fat) milk, then to nonfat (skim) milk.
- Substitute fat-free sour cream or nonfat plain yogurt for sour cream.
- Use part-skim or low-fat cheeses whenever possible.
- Note that cottage cheese is lower in calcium than most cheeses. Thus, one cup of cottage cheese counts as only one-half serving of milk.

Fats, Oils, and Sweets (small amounts each day)

The Food Guide Pyramid places fats, oils, and sweets at the very top so that Americans will realize they should use them only in very small amounts. These foods supply calories but little or no vitamins or minerals.

Added sugars include sweeteners used in processing or at the table (such as jams, jellies, syrups, corn sweetener, molasses, fruit-juice concentrate, and the sugar in candy, cake, and cookies). These foods often are hidden in favorites—such as soft drinks (9 teaspoons of sugar per can), low-fat fruit yogurt (7 teaspoons per cup), fruit pie (6 teaspoons per serving), and catsup (a teaspoon in every tablespoon).

Try the following:

- Avoid temptation by not keeping a stash of cookies or candies.
- Put a small, child-sized spoon in the sugar bowl.
- When you crave a sweet, reach for nature's candy: fruit.
- If you want a daily sweet, have it as dessert, when you'll eat less of it, rather than as a snack.
- Drink fruit juices and water instead of sugar-laden soft drinks.

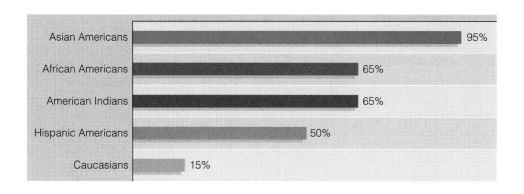

■ Figure 6-3 Percentage of Population Who Are Lactose Intolerant

Source: Dr. Richard Grand, Tufts University Medical School. In *The New York Times*, June 29, 1999. Reprinted by permission.

Asian Americans	95%
African Americans	65%
American Indians	65%
Hispanic Americans	50%
Caucasians	15%

DRIs, RDAs, and Daily Values

Set by the Food and Nutrition Board of the National Academy of Sciences, the **Recommended Dietary Allowances (RDAs)** were developed fifty years ago to establish suggested levels of intake of essential nutrients. Last updated in 1989, the RDAs are being folded into (and eventually replaced by) **Dietary Reference Intakes (DRIs)**. Informed by the most current scientific knowledge, DRIs reflect a new approach to establishing suggested nutrient intake levels. DRIs include:

- *Estimated Average Requirements (EAR)*—These are population-wide average nutrient requirements for nutrition research and policymaking. They are the basis upon which RDA values are set.
- *Recommended Daily Allowances (RDA)*—These are the nutrient intake goals for individuals, derived from EARs.
- *Adequate Intakes (AI)*—These are nutrient intake goals for individuals, set when there is not enough scientific data to establish EAR or RDA values.
- *Tolerable Upper Intake Levels (UL)*—ULs suggest the upper limits of safe intake for nutrients that have the potential to be toxic if taken in too large dosages.

See Table 6-8 for the most recent DRIs available. Additionally, Table 6-9 shows the RDAs of nutrients for which DRIs are not yet available.

A third set of nutrient guidelines are **Daily Values (DV)**. These are the values you will find on food labels at grocery stores. Daily Values differ from DRIs in that they provide one set of general recommendations for everyone, whereas DRIs provide more individualized recommendations based on factors like age and gender. For more on Daily Values, see "What Should I Look for on Nutrition Labels?" later in this chapter.

Dietary Supplements

Would you take a pill that promises to make you stronger, smarter, younger, healthier? More than half of Americans regularly use nutritional and dietary supplements—vitamins, minerals, and botanical and biological substances that have not been approved for sale as drugs.[42] There are serious questions about the safety and efficacy of these products.[43] (See Chapter 5 for a discussion of strength-building and performance-enhancing supplements, such as androstenedione.)

Marketed as foods, supplements do not have to undergo the same rigorous testing required of drugs. They can carry "structure/function" claims—claims that a product may affect the structure or functioning of the body—but not claims that they can treat, diagnose, cure, or prevent a disease. For example, statements such as "helps maintain a healthy cholesterol level" are acceptable, while statements such as "lowers cholesterol levels" are not.

The FDA has issued new rules for dietary supplement labeling. Labels must now include an information panel titled "Supplement Facts" (similar to the "Nutrition Facts" panel that appears on processed foods), a clear identity statement, and a complete list of ingredients. Specifically, the "Supplement Facts" panel must show the manufacturer's suggested dose/serving size; information on nutrients that are present in significant levels (such as vitamins A and C, calcium, iron and sodium) and the percent Daily Value where a reference has been established; and all other dietary ingredients present in the product, including botanicals and amino acids. Herbal products are identified by the common or usual name and the part of the plant used (such as root, stem, or leaf).

Should I Take Vitamin Supplements?

Many health experts feel that the best way to make sure your body gets the vitamins and minerals it needs is to eat a wide variety of foods. If you rely on vitamin/mineral pills and fortified foods to make up for poor nutrition, you may shortchange yourself.

Even though there's little proof that multivitamin supplements can help them, many people figure that taking them certainly can't hurt. As they see it, supplements serve as a nutritional insurance policy, something to fall back on in case they don't get everything they need from whole foods. For the most part, this is true. "If you have a good diet and you take a multivitamin supplement, there's probably no danger," says nutritionist Ann Shaw. "But if you take megadoses of a single vitamin or several different vitamins, you could run into problems."[44] See Table 6-10 for a summary of what we know about different supplements.

As scientists note, most health benefits and dangers stem from more than one source, so it's unlikely that changing any one nutrient will in itself produce great benefits—and may, by interfering with the complex balance of nutrients, do harm. This is particularly true for the fat-soluble vitamins, primarily A and D, which can build up in our bodies and cause serious complications, such as damage to the kidneys, liver, or bones. Large doses of water-soluble vitamins, including the B vitamins, also may be harmful. Excessive intake of vitamin B-6 (pyridoxine), often used to relieve premenstrual bloating, can cause neurological damage, such as numbness in the mouth and tingling in the hands. (An

■ Table 6-8 1997–2000 Dietary Reference Intakes (DRI)

Age (yr)	Thiamin (mg)	Riboflavin (mg)	Niacin (mg NE)	Vitamin B₆ (mg)	Folate (µg DFE)	Vitamin B₁₂ (µg)	Vitamin E (mg)	Vitamin C (mg)	Phosphorus (mg)	Magnesium (mg)	Selenium (µg)	Vitamin D (µg)	Pantothenic acid (mg)	Biotin (µg)	Choline (mg)	Calcium (mg)	Fluoride (mg)
Infants[a]																	
0.0–0.5[b]	0.2	0.3	2	0.1	65	0.4	4	40	100	30	15	5	1.7	5	125	210	0.01
0.5–1.0	0.3	0.4	4	0.3	80	0.5	6	50	275	75	20	5	1.8	6	150	270	0.5
Children																	
1–3	0.5	0.5	6	0.5	150	0.9	6	15	460	80	20	5	2.0	8	200	500	0.7
4–8	0.6	0.6	8	0.6	200	1.2	7	25	500	130	30	5	3.0	12	250	800	1.1
Males																	
9–13	0.9	0.9	12	1.0	300	1.8	11	45	1250	240	40	5	4.0	20	375	1300	2.0
14–18	1.2	1.3	16	1.3	400	2.4	15	75	1250	410	55	5	5.0	25	550	1300	3.2
19–30	1.2	1.3	16	1.3	400	2.4	15	90	700	400	55	5	5.0	30	550	1000	3.8
31–50	1.2	1.3	16	1.3	400	2.4	15	90	700	420	55	5	5.0	30	550	1000	3.8
51–70	1.2	1.3	16	1.7	400	2.4	15	90	700	420	55	10	5.0	30	550	1200	3.8
>70	1.2	1.3	16	1.7	400	2.4	15	90	700	420	55	15	5.0	30	550	1200	3.8
Females																	
9–13	0.9	0.9	12	1.0	300	1.8	11	45	1250	240	40	5	4.0	20	375	1300	2.0
14–18	1.0	1.0	14	1.2	400	2.4	15	65	1250	360	55	5	5.0	25	400	1300	2.9
19–30	1.1	1.1	14	1.3	400	2.4	15	75	700	310	55	5	5.0	30	425	1000	3.1
31–50	1.1	1.1	14	1.3	400	2.4	15	75	700	320	55	5	5.0	30	425	1000	3.1
51–70	1.1	1.1	14	1.5	400	2.4	15	75	700	320	55	10	5.0	30	425	1200	3.1
>70	1.1	1.1	14	1.5	400	2.4	15	75	700	320	55	15	5.0	30	425	1200	3.1
Pregnancy	1.4	1.4	18	1.9	600	2.6	15	85	*	+40	60	*	6.0	30	450	*	*
Lactation	1.5	1.6	17	2.0	500	2.8	19	120	*	*	70	*	7.0	35	550	*	*

The first eleven nutrient columns (Thiamin through Selenium) are **Recommended Dietary Allowances (RDA)**; the last six columns (Vitamin D through Fluoride) are **Adequate Intakes (AI)**.

*Values for these nutrients do not change with pregnancy or lactation. Use the value listed for women of comparable age.

[a]For all nutrients, values for infants are AI; for the B vitamins and choline, the age groupings are 0 through 5 months and 6 through 11 months.

[b]The AI for niacin for this age group is stated as milligrams of preformed niacin instead of niacin equivalents.

Source: Adapted with permission from *Recommended Dietary Allowances*, 10th Edition, and the first two of the *Dietary Reference Intakes* series, National Academy Press. Copyright 1989, 1997, and 1998, respectively, by the National Academy of Sciences. Courtesy of the National Academy Press, Washington, D.C.

Tolerable Upper Intake Levels (UL) for Selected Nutrients (per day)

Age (yr)	Vitamin D (µg)[a]	Niacin (mg)	Vitamin B₆ (mg)	Folate (µg)	Choline (mg)	Vitamin C (mg)	Vitamin E (mg)	Calcium (mg)	Phosphorus (mg)	Magnesium (mg)	Fluoride (mg)	Selenium (mg)
Infants												
0.0–0.5	25	—[b]	—[b]	—[b]	—[b]	—[b]	—[b]	—[b]	—[b]	—[b]	0.7	45
0.5–1.0	25	—[b]	—[b]	—[b]	—[b]	—[b]	—[b]	—[b]	—[b]	—[b]	0.9	60
Children												
1–3	50	10	30	300	1000	400	200	2500	3000	65	1.3	90
4–8	50	15	40	400	1000	650	300	2500	3000	110	2.2	150
9–13	50	20	60	600	2000	1200	600	2500	4000	350	10.0	280
14–18	50	30	80	800	3000	1800	800	2500	4000	350	10.0	400
Adults												
19–70	50	35	100	1000	3500	2000	1000	2500	4000	350	10.0	400
>70	50	35	100	1000	3500	2000	1000	2500	3000	350	10.0	400
Pregnancy	50	35	100	1000	3500	2000	1000	2500	3500	350	10.0	400
Lactation	50	35	100	1000	3500	2000	1000	2500	4000	350	10.0	400

[a]To convert µg to IU, multiply by 40. For example, 50 µg × 40 = 2000 IU.

[b]Upper Levels were not established for many nutrients in the infant category because of a lack of data.

Source: Adapted from the first two of the *Dietary Reference Intakes* series, National Academy Press. Copyright 1997 and 1998, by the National Academy of Sciences. Courtesy of the National Academy Press, Washington, D.C. Search for *Dietary Reference Intakes* online at: http//www.nap.edu/readingroom.

■ **Table 6-9** 1989 Recommended Dietary Allowances (RDA)

Age (yr)	Energy (kcal)	Protein (g)	Vitamin A (µg RE)	Vitamin K (µg)	Iron (mg)	Zinc (mg)	Iodine (µg)
Infants							
0.0–0.5	650	13	375	5	6	5	40
0.5–1.0	850	14	375	10	10	5	50
Children							
1–3	1300	16	400	15	10	10	70
4–6	1800	24	500	20	10	10	90
7–10	2000	28	700	30	10	10	120
Males							
11–14	2500	45	1000	45	12	15	150
15–18	3000	59	1000	65	12	15	150
19–24	2900	58	1000	70	10	15	150
25–50	2900	63	1000	80	10	15	150
51+	2300	63	1000	80	10	15	150
Females							
11–14	2200	46	800	45	15	12	150
15–18	2200	44	800	55	15	12	150
19–24	2200	46	800	60	15	12	150
25–50	2200	50	800	65	15	12	150
51+	1900	50	800	65	10	12	150
Pregnancy	+300	60	800	65	30	15	175
Lactation							
1st 6 mo.	+500	65	1300	65	15	19	200
2nd 6 mo.	+500	62	1200	65	15	16	200

excessive amount in this case is 250 to 300 times the recommended dose.) High doses of vitamin C can produce stomachaches and diarrhea. Niacin, often taken in high doses to lower cholesterol, can cause jaundice, liver damage, and irregular heartbeats as well as severe, uncomfortable flushing of the skin. Table 6-4 provides more information about the effects of vitamin excess.

Large doses of vitamins can be especially dangerous for individuals with certain health conditions. Excessive intake of vitamin C or D may precipitate the formation of kidney stones in the urinary tract. Too much vitamin B-6 may inhibit milk production in breast-feeding mothers. In individuals suffering from epilepsy, folate may interfere with their drug therapy. However, if you belong to any of the following groups, check with your doctor about the potential pluses of adding vitamins or vitamin-rich foods to your daily diet:

- Pregnant, breast-feeding, and menopausal women.
- People at risk for heart attack, especially smokers.
- Strict vegetarians.
- People with chronic illnesses that may interfere with appetite or the body's use of nutrients.

- Individuals taking medications that affect appetite or digestion.
- The elderly.

Knowing What You Eat

For years, many manufacturers advertised products as "nutritious," "healthy," or otherwise good for you, but offered little or no proof to back up such claims. Today, thanks to the Nutrition Labeling and Education Act, enacted in 1994, food manufacturers must provide information about fat, calories, and ingredients in large type on packaged food labels that must show how a food item fits into a daily diet of 2,000 calories. The law also restricts nutritional claims for terms such as *healthy, low-fat,* or *high-fiber.*

In evaluating food labels and claims, keep in mind that, while individual foods vary in their nutritional value, what matters is your total diet. If you eat too much of any one food—regardless of what its label states—you may not be getting the variety and balance of nutrients that you need.

■ Table 6-10 Do Dietary Supplements Work?

Supplement	Claims	What We Know
Amino acids	Increase muscle mass.	No solid evidence that amino acid supplements promote muscle building. Little known about the side effects of high doses of single or combination amino acid supplements.
Beta-carotene (converted into vitamin A in the body)	Reduces your risk of cancer.	No evidence that beta-carotene supplements reduce cancer risk.
B complex vitamins	Provide energy; help relieve stress and may help reduce heart disease risk.	No evidence that B vitamins relieve stress. Long thought to be nontoxic, some B vitamins such as B6 and niacin may have serious side effects when taken in very high doses.
Vitamin C	Prevents colds, certain cancers, and heart disease.	Vitamin C supplements can lessen the severity of colds but not prevent them. Observational studies have shown that vitamin C may help prevent cancer and heart disease, but too few clinical trials have been conducted to substantiate those results.
Calcium	Prevents osteoporosis and colon cancer and reduces high blood pressure.	Calcium plays a critical role in preventing osteoporosis if taken with vitamin D. Results of research on calcium's role in preventing colon cancer are still preliminary. It may help regulate blood pressure in some people, but there is no way of knowing who might benefit.
Chromium picolinate	Reduces body fat, builds muscle, and improves overall fitness.	Scientists have found that this popular nutritional and dietary supplement causes DNA breakage and may be a cancer risk.
Vitamin E	Reduces the risk of heart disease and cancer.	Supplements of 400–800 IU may protect against heart disease. Very few side effects have been reported, but high doses of vitamin E supplements should not be used by anyone taking anticoagulation medication.
Niacin	Helps lower cholesterol.	Niacin, in the form of nicotinic acid, is an inexpensive alternative to cholesterol-lowering drugs but should be prescribed by a doctor. Side effects include flushing and itching and gastrointestinal distress. Time-released niacin can be toxic to the liver.
Zinc	Boosts immunity, wards off colds, and improves sex drive.	Zinc taken at the onset of a cold can lessen its severity. High doses of zinc, however, may *suppress* immune function. No evidence that zinc supplements affect sexual performance.

What Should I Look for on Nutrition Labels?

As Figure 6-4 shows, the "Nutrition Facts" on food labels present a wealth of information—if you know what to look for. The label focuses on those nutrients most clearly associated with disease risk and health: total fat, saturated fat, cholesterol, sodium, total carbohydrate, dietary fiber, sugar, and protein.

- *Calories.* Calories are the measure of the amount of energy that can be derived from food. Science defines a **calorie** as the amount of energy required to raise the temperature of one gram of water by one degree Celsius. In the laboratory, the caloric content of food is measured in 1,000-calorie units called *kilocalories*. The "calorie" referred to in everyday usage is actually the equivalent of the laboratory kilocalorie.

  The label lists two numbers for calories: calories per serving and calories from fat per serving. This allows consumers to calculate how many calories they'll consume and to determine the percentage of fat in an item.

- *Serving size.* Rather than the tiny portions manufacturers sometimes used in the past to keep down the number of calories per serving, the new labels reflect more realistic portions. Serving sizes, which have been defined for approximately 150 food categories,

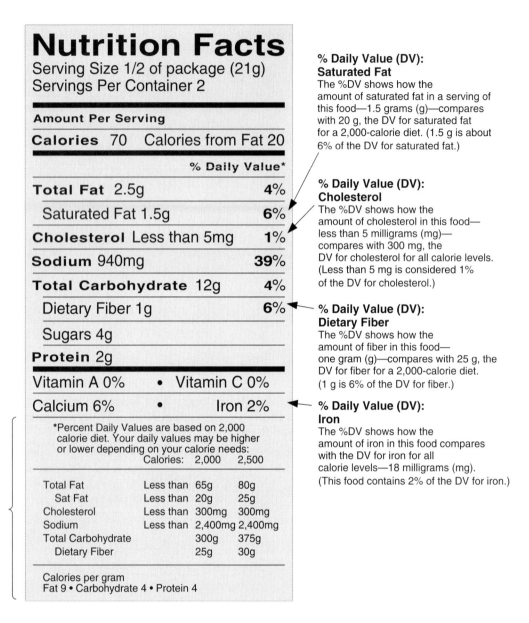

Facts
Detailed food labels allow you to compare foods and remind you of serving size and health concerns, such as fat and cholesterol content.

Larger packages may carry this expanded version of the new label, which includes Daily Values (DVs) for these six nutrients based on both 2,000-calorie and 2,500-calorie diets. The DVs for other nutrients are not shown on the label.

must be the same for similar products (for example, different brands of potato chips) and for similar products within a category (for example, snack foods such as pretzels, potato chips, and popcorn). This makes it easier to compare the nutritional content of foods.

- *Daily Values (DVs).* DVs refer to the total amount of a nutrient that the average adult should aim to get or not exceed on a daily basis. The DVs for cholesterol, sodium, vitamins, and minerals are the same for all adults. The DVs for total fat, saturated fat, carbohydrate, fiber, and protein are based on a 2,000-calorie daily diet—the amount of food ingested by many American men and active women.

- *Percent Daily Values (%DV).* The goal for a full day's diet is to select foods that together add up to 100 percent of the DVs. The %DVs show how a particular food's nutrient content fits into a 2,000-calorie diet.

Individuals who consume (or should consume) fewer than 2,000 total calories a day have to lower their DVs for total fat, saturated fat, and carbohydrates—for example, if their caloric intake is 10 percent less than 2,000 calories, they would lower the DV by 10 percent. Similarly, those who consume more than 2,000 calories should adjust the DVs upward.

- *Calories per gram.* The bottom of the food label lists the number of calories per gram for fat, carbohydrates, and protein.

What Should You Look For?

According to national surveys, consumers most often look at nutrition labels for information on fat. Only one-third of them read the other information on the

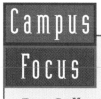

Campus Focus

Do College Students Read Nutrition Labels?

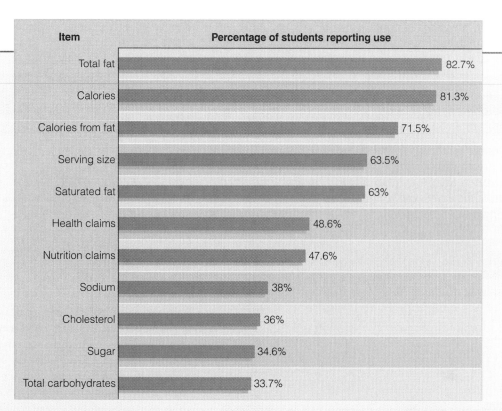

In a survey of 208 undergraduates at a midwestern university, 70.2 percent said they look at the Nutrition Facts label, at least sometimes, when considering a new food product. The information they use most is depicted above.

Source: Marietta, Anne et al. "Knowledge, Attitudes and Behaviors of College Students Regarding the 1990 Nutrition Labeling Education Act Food Labels," *Journal of the American Dietetic Association,* Vol. 99, No. 4, April 1999.

label. More than 72 percent said they would purchase a product with a health claim on the label rather than a product with no such claim. (See Campus Focus: "Do College Students Read Nutrition Labels?") Yet even though 95 percent of students say that nutrition labels are useful, the information they get from them plays only a minor role in their daily diet planning.[45]

Different people may zero in on different figures on the food label—for example, calories if they're watching their weight, specific ingredients if they have **food allergies.** Among the useful items to check are the following:

- *Calories from fat.* Get into the habit of calculating the percentage of fat calories in a food before buying or eating it.
- *Total fat.* Since the average person munches on 15 to 20 food items a day, it's easy to overload on fat. Saturated fat is a figure worthy of special attention because of its reported link to several diseases.
- *Cholesterol.* Cholesterol is made by and contained in products of animal origin only. Many high-fat products, such as potato chips, contain 0 percent choles-

terol because they're made from plants and are cooked in vegetable fats. However, the vegetable fats they contain can be processed and made into saturated fats that are more harmful to the heart than cholesterol itself.

- *Sugars.* There is no DV for sugars because health experts have yet to agree on a daily limit. The figure on the label includes naturally present sugars, such as lactose in milk and fructose in fruit, as well as those added to the food, such as table sugar, corn syrup, or dextrose.
- *Fiber.* A "high-fiber" food has 5 or more grams of fiber per serving. A "good" source of fiber provides at least 2.5 grams. "More or added" fiber means at least 2.5 grams more per serving than similar foods— 10 percent more of the DV for fiber.
- *Calcium.* "High" equals 200 milligrams (mg) or more per serving. "Good" means at least 100 mg, while "more" indicates that the food contains at least 100 mg more calcium—10 percent more of the DV—than the item usually would have.

- *Sodium.* Since many foods contain sodium, most of us routinely get more than we need. It's important to read labels carefully to avoid excess sodium, which can be a health threat.
- *Vitamins.* A DV of 10 percent of any vitamin makes a food a "good" source; 20 percent qualifies it as "high" in a certain vitamin.

Nutrition labeling for fresh produce, fish, meat, and poultry remains voluntary. Packages too small for a full-sized label must provide an address or phone number so that consumers can obtain information from the manufacturer.

What You Should Watch Out For

Almost everything in the supermarket has something good to say about itself: fiber-rich, fat-free, light or "lite," 98 percent fat-free, enriched, high-fiber. You can't believe everything you read on the packages of the food you buy. Table 6-11 provides a guide to the required meaning of "front of the package" nutrition terms.

The Way We Eat

For centuries, Native Americans ate a diet of corn, beans, fish, game, wild greens, wild fruits, squash, and tomatoes. Over time the United States—a nation of immigrants—has imported a wide variety of ethnic cuisines. Although many people think of foods such as hamburgers, steak, potatoes, and cheesecake or ice cream as "all-American" favorites, in most cities across the country, it is possible to taste dozens of different cultural cuisines.

Dietary Diversity

Whatever your cultural heritage, you have probably sampled Chinese, Mexican, Indian, Italian, and Japanese foods. If you belong to any of these ethnic groups, you may eat these cuisines regularly. Each type of ethnic cooking has its own nutritional benefits and potential drawbacks.

The African-American Diet

African-American cuisine traces some of its roots to food preferences from West Africa (for example, peanuts, okra, and black-eyed peas), as well as to traditional American foods, such as fish, game, greens, and sweet potatoes. Cajun cuisine, most closely associated with New Orleans, blends both African and French tra-

ditions in dishes such as gumbos (thick spicy soups), sausage, red beans, and seafood. African-American cooking uses many nutritious vegetables, such as collard greens and sweet potatoes, as well as legumes. However, some dishes include high-fat food products such as peanuts and pecans or involve frying, sometimes in saturated fat.

The Chinese Diet

The mainland Chinese diet, which is plant-based, high in carbohydrates, and low in fats and animal protein, is considered one of the healthiest in the world. However, Chinese food is prepared differently in America. Chinese restaurants here serve more meat and sauces than are generally eaten in China. According to laboratory tests of typical take-out dishes from Chinese restaurants, many have more fats and cholesterol than hamburger or egg dishes from fast-food outlets.

To eat healthfully when you choose Chinese cuisine, select boiled, steamed, or stir-fried dishes, mix entrees with steamed rice, and lift food out of a container with chopsticks or a fork and transfer it to serving bowls to leave excess sauce behind. Order wonton soup rather than egg rolls or pork spareribs. To avoid the cholesterol in egg yolks, steer away from items made with lobster or egg foo yung sauces. If you are prone to high blood pressure, watch out for the high sodium content of soy and other sauces, and of a seasoner called MSG (monosodium glutamate). Some people are sensitive to MSG, and most restaurants offer some MSG-free dishes or will leave out MSG on request.

The Japanese Diet

The traditional Japanese diet is very low in fat, which may be why the incidence of heart disease is low in Japan. Dietary staples include soybean products, fish, vegetables, noodles, and rice. A variety of fruits and vegetables are also included in many dishes. However, Japanese cuisine is high in salted, smoked, and pickled foods. Watch out for deep-fried dishes such as tempura, and salty soups and sauces (which you can ask for on the side). Ask for broiled entrees in a restaurant or non-fried dishes made with tofu, a soybean curd protein, which has no cholesterol.

The Mediterranean Diet

Several years ago epidemiologists noticed something unexpected in the residents of regions along the Mediterranean: a lower incidence of deaths from heart disease. They speculated that the plant-based "Mediterranean diet," which is rich in fruits, vegetables, legumes, cereal, wine, and olive oil, may be the reason.

■ Table 6-11 What Food Labels Really Mean

Term	Examples	Means That a Serving of the Product Contains:
Extra-lean	Extra-lean pork, extra-lean hamburger	Fewer than 5 g of fat, fewer than 2 g of saturated fat *and* fewer than 95 mg of cholesterol per serving (applies to meats only).
Extra, More	Bread with added fiber, fortified foods	At least 10% more of the Daily Value of a nutrient per serving than in a similar food.
Fat-free	Skim milk, no-fat salad dressing	Less than 0.5 g of fat per serving.
Free	Sugar-free, sodium-free	No or negligible amounts of sugars, sodium, or fat.
Good source	Good source of fiber, good source of calcium	10 to 19% of the Daily Value for a particular nutrient.
Healthy	Healthy burritos, canned vegetables	No more than 60 mg of cholesterol, 3 grams of fat, and 1 gram of saturated fat per serving; and more than 10% of the Daily Value of vitamin A, vitamin C, iron, calcium, protein, or fiber per serving. "Healthy" foods must also contain 360 mg or less sodium per serving.
High	High in iron, high in vitamin C	20% or more of the Daily Value for a particular nutrient.
Lean	Lean beef, lean turkey	Fewer than 10 g of fat, fewer than 4 g of saturated fat, *and* fewer than 95 mg of cholesterol per serving (applies to meats only).
Less	Less saturated fat, less cholesterol	25% less of a nutrient than a comparable food.
Light or lite	Light in sodium, lite in fat, light brown sugar, light and fluffy	33% fewer calories or half the fat as the regular product, or 50% or less sodium than usual in a low-calorie, low-fat food. "Light" can also be used on labels to describe the texture or color of a food.
Low-calorie	Low-calorie cookies, low-calorie fruit drink	40 calories or fewer per serving.
Low-fat	Low-fat cheese, low-fat ice cream	3 g or less fat per serving.
Low-saturated fat	Low-saturated fat pancake mix, low-saturated fat eggnog	1 g or less saturated fat per serving.
Low-sodium	Low-sodium soup, low-sodium hot dogs	140 mg or less sodium per serving.
Percent fat-free	95% fat-free; 98% fat-free	The specified percentage of fat on a weight basis (only low-fat foods can use this label).
Reduced	Reduced calories, reduced cholesterol	25% less of a nutrient or calories than the regular product.

Subsequent research has confirmed that heart disease is much less common in countries along the Mediterranean than in other Western nations. In one four-year study of more than 400 men and women in France who had already suffered one heart attack, about half switched to a Mediterranean diet while the others ate a more traditional Western diet relatively low in fat, saturated fat, and cholesterol. Those following the Mediterranean diet were 50 to 70 percent less likely to experience a recurrence of heart disease, including strokes and fatal and nonfatal heart attacks.

No one knows exactly what makes the Mediterranean diet so heart-healthy. As illustrated by the Mediterranean Food Pyramid (see Figure 6-5), the diet features lots of fruits and vegetables, legumes, nuts, and grains. Meat is used mainly as a condiment rather than as

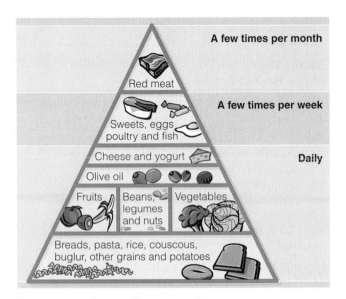

A few times per month
Red meat

A few times per week
Sweets, eggs poultry and fish

Daily
Cheese and yogurt

Olive oil

Fruits | Beans, legumes and nuts | Vegetables

Breads, pasta, rice, couscous, buglur, other grains and potatoes

■ Figure 6-5 **The Mediterranean Diet**
The Mediterranean diet relies heavily on fruits, vegetables, grains, and potatoes. It also includes considerable olive oil, and regular exercise is suggested.

Source: Oldways Preservation & Exchange Trust. Reprinted by permission of *The New York Times.*

ease differs according to whether they are eating a Mediterranean or a Western diet.[47]

The French Diet

Traditional French cuisine, which includes rich, high-fat sauces and dishes, has never been considered healthful. Yet nutritionists have been stumped to explain the so-called French paradox. Despite a diet high in saturated fats, the French have had one of the lowest rates of coronary artery disease in the world.

Recent reports indicate that the French diet is changing. Until 1990 the French ate much less animal fat and had significantly lower blood cholesterol levels than Americans and Britons.[48] Fat consumption in France has since risen as the French have begun eating more meat and fast foods, snacking more, eating fewer relaxed meals, exercising less, and drinking less wine.[49] They've also been getting fatter, and some researchers contend that their rates of heart disease will inevitably rise in the coming decades. The French diet increasingly resembles the American diet, but French portions tend to be one-third to one-half the size of American portions.

The Mexican Diet

The cuisine served in Mexico features rice, corn, and beans, which are low in fat and high in nutrients. However, the dishes Americans think of as Mexican are far less healthful. Burritos, especially when topped with cheese and sour cream, are very high in fat. Although guacamole has a high fat content, it contains mostly monounsaturated fatty acids, a better form of fat.

a main course, and fish, yogurt, and low-fat feta cheese are the predominant animal foods. The diet is relatively high in fat, but the main source is olive oil, an unsaturated fat.[46] Wine, an essential component of the Mediterranean diet, may be one of the factors responsible for the lower incidence of heart disease. Some researchers have found that wine's effect on blood platelets in men with heart dis-

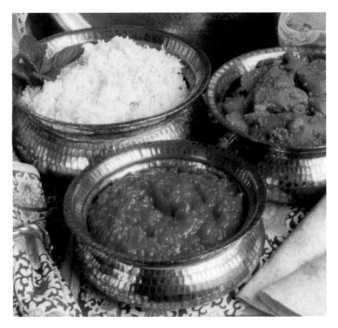

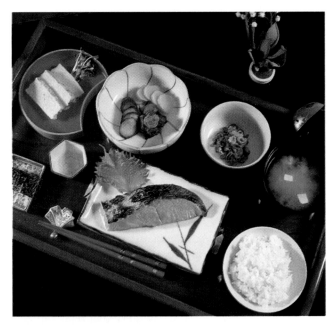

All-American diversity. The rice and beans of Mexico are healthy and high in protein, but too much cheese can cancel some of the benefits. The Japanese diet is high in seafood and rice and low in fats, cheese, and meat.

His Plate, Her Plate

J ake and Clarissa go out to dinner. He orders a burger and a beer. She has a salad and mineral water with lime. Back at her apartment, she takes out a pint of mocha mint chip and eats the entire thing. An anthropology professor describes this eating pattern as "classic dating behavior." In public and in private, men and women tend to put different things on their plates. Here is what research has found about men and women's eating habits:

- Men tend to be more comfortable about the kinds of foods they eat. Women tend to think of certain foods as "good" and others as "bad." While to a man, chocolate may simply be a sweet, to a woman, it's likely to be viewed as a sinful indulgence.
- Both male and female college students eat high-fat diets, but in different forms. Men tend to prefer their fat with protein in foods such as steaks, burgers, and pizza. Women tend to like their fats fixed with sugar and crave candy, ice cream, cookies, and cake.
- Women consume a lower percentage of beef (14 percent) and pork (7 percent) protein than men (18 percent and 9 percent, respectively) and a higher percentage of poultry (13 percent), dairy (22 percent), and fruit and

vegetable (11 percent) protein than men (11, 19, and 9 percent, respectively).
- Women are more likely to eat the recommended five servings of fruit and vegetables every day. According to the National Cancer Institute, 21 percent of women are getting their "five a day," compared with only 14 percent of men.
- In reading nutrition labels, women are more likely than men to look for information on total calories, calories from fat, total grams of fat and saturated fat on nutrition labels. Men are more likely than women to look for information about protein and vitamin A.
- College-age men are most likely to take dietary supplements to perform better in sports; women take them to make up for inadequacies in their diet.

Sources: Bailey, Stephen. *Body Maps.* Nicklas, Theresa, et al. "Impact of Breakfast Consumption on Nutritional Adequacy of the Diets of Young Adults in Bogalusa, La.: Ethnic and Gender Contrasts," *Journal of the American Dietetic Association,* Vol. 98, No. 12, December 1998. Schulman, Evelyn. "'Get Fit with 5' During National 5 a Day Week," NCI Office of Cancer Communications, May 5, 1999. Pierce, Colleen. "Conquer Your Cravings." *American Health,* April 1999. Driskell, Judy. "Vitamin and Mineral Supplementation Habits and Beliefs of Male and Female Graduate Students." *Journal of Family and Consumer Sciences,* Vol. 99, January 1999.

When eating at Mexican restaurants, ask that cheese and sour cream be served on the side. Avoid refried beans, which are usually cooked in lard. Hold back on guacamole, quesadillas, and enchiladas. Nutritious choices include rice, beans, and shrimp or chicken tostadas on unfried corn meal tortillas.

The Indian Diet

Many Indian dishes highlight healthful ingredients such as vegetables and legumes (beans and peas). However, many also use "ghee" (a form of butter) or coconut oil, which is rich in harmful saturated fats. The best advice in an Indian restaurant is to ask how each dish is prepared. Good choices include daal or dal (lentils), karbi or karni (chickpea soup), and chapati (tortilla-like bread). Hold back on bhatura (fried bread), coconut milk, and samosas (fried meat or vegetables in dough).

The Southeast Asian Diet

A rich variety of fruits and vegetables—bamboo shoots, bok choy, cabbage, mangoes, papayas, cucumbers—provides a sound nutritional basis for this diet. In addi-

tion, most foods are broiled or stir-fried, which keeps fat low. However, coconut oil and milk, used in many sauces, are high in fat. The use of MSG and pickled foods means the sodium content is high. At Thai or Vietnamese restaurants, choose salads (larb is a chicken salad with mint) or seafood soup (po tak).

What Should I Know About Vegetarian Diets?

Not all vegetarians avoid all meats. Some, who call themselves "lact-ovo-pesco-vegetarians," eat dairy products, eggs, chicken, and fish, but not red meat. **Lacto-vegetarians** eat dairy products as well as grains, fruits, and vegetables; **ovo-lacto-vegetarians** also eat eggs. Pure vegetarians, called **vegans,** eat only plant foods; often they take vitamin B-12 supplements, because that vitamin is normally found only in animal products. If they select their food with care, vegetarians can get sufficient amounts of protein, vitamin B-12, iron, and calcium without supplements (see Figure 6-6).

The key to getting sufficient protein from a vegetarian diet is understanding the concept of **complementary**

New York Medical College Vegetarian Pyramid

Vegans Must Consume Daily
Blackstrap Molasses, Vegetable Oil, Brewer's Yeast

Milk and Milk Substitutes Group
Milk, Yogurt, Cheese and Fortified Soy Milk
2–4 Servings

Meat/Fish Substitutes Group
Dry beans, Nuts, Seeds, Peanut butter, Tofu, and Eggs
2–3 Servings

Vegetable Group
3+ Servings

Fruit Group
2–4 Servings

Grains and Starchy Vegetables Group
Bread, Cereal, Rice, Pasta, Potatoes, Corn, and Green Peas
6–11 Servings

proteins. Meat, poultry, fish, eggs, and dairy products are **complete proteins** that provide the nine essential **amino acids**—substances containing carbon, hydrogen, oxygen, and nitrogen that the human body cannot produce itself. **Incomplete proteins,** such as legumes or nuts, may have relatively low levels of one or two essential amino acids, but fairly high levels of others. By combining complementary protein sources, you can make sure that your body makes the most of the nonanimal proteins you eat. (See Figure 6-7.) Many cultures rely heavily on complementary foods for protein. In Middle Eastern cooking, sesame seeds and chickpeas are a popular combination; in Latin American dishes, beans and rice, or beans and tortillas; in Chinese cuisine, soy and rice.

Vegetarian diets have proven health benefits. Studies show that vegetarians' cholesterol levels are low, and vegetarians are seldom overweight. As a result, they're less apt to be candidates for heart disease than those who consume large quantities of meat. Vegetarians also have lower incidences of breast, colon, and prostate cancer; high blood pressure; and osteoporosis. When combined with exercise and stress reduction, vegetarian diets have led to reductions in the buildup of harmful plaque within the blood vessels of the heart. (See Chapter 13 for

a further discussion of the connections between diet and heart disease.)

Fast Food: Nutrition on the Run

Not all fast foods are junk foods—that is, high in calories, sugar, salt, and fat, and low in nutrients. But while it's not all bad, fast food has definite disadvantages. A meal in a fast-food restaurant may cost twice as much as the same meal prepared at home and may provide half your daily calorie needs. The fat content of many items is extremely high. A Burger King Whopper with cheese contains 723 calories and 48 grams of fat, 18 grams from saturated fat. A McDonald's Sausage McMuffin with egg has 517 calories and 33 grams of fat, 13 grams from saturated fat. Many fast-food chains have switched from beef tallow or lard to unsaturated vegetable oils for frying, but the total fat content of the foods remains the same (see "Counting Your Calories and Fat" in the Hales Health Almanac at the back of this book).

In response to criticism by health professionals and consumers in general, many fast-food outlets have also added lighter menu items, such as salads, grilled chicken sandwiches on whole-grain buns, and nonfat yogurt. Some have reduced sodium in their products, removed additives from fish breading, and taken MSG out of sausages.

At regular restaurants or cafeterias, with a little extra attention, you can usually get a better nutritional value for the calories you consume. For example, you can request that your entree be baked or broiled without fat. You can also ask that fresh vegetables be steamed without salt or butter. When possible, ask for luncheon rather than dinner-sized portions. Or order appetizers and side dishes instead of an entree, for instance, tomato soup, a salad, and vegetables. Ask for your salad dressing on the side, request low-calorie dressing if available, or make your own dressing with lemon juice or vinegar.

Food Safety

Increasingly, Americans are concerned not just with whether the food they eat is nutritious, but whether it's safe. Many unsuspected safety hazards have been identified by **food toxicologists,** specialists who detect toxins (potentially harmful substances) and treat the conditions they produce.

Food combinations that supply complete protein are shown below:

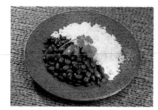
Rice and black beans.

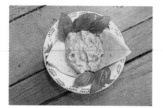
Hummus and bread.

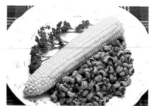
Corn and black-eyed peas.

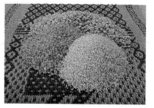
Bulgur (whole wheat) and lentils.

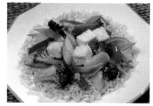
Tofu and rice.

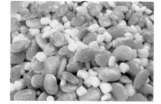
Corn and lima beans (succotash).

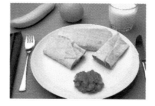
Tortilla with refried beans (e.g., a bean burrito).

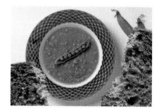
Pea soup and bread.

■ Figure 6-7 **Vegetarian Food Combinations That Supply Complete Protein**
Source: From Brown, *Nutrition Now,* Wadsworth, 1999.

Strategies *for* Prevention

A Guide to Fast Foods

✓ For breakfast, avoid croissants or muffins stuffed with eggs or meat; they pack as many as 700 calories. Better options include plain scrambled eggs (150–180 calories), pancakes without butter or syrup (400 calories), and English muffins (185 calories each).

✓ For lunch or dinner, if you want meat, go for plain hamburgers (no cheese), which average 275 to 350 calories. An even better choice is roast beef, which is lower in fat and calories.

✓ Be wary of fast-food fish. With frying oil trapped in the breading and creamy tartar sauce on top, fried-fish sandwiches supply more calories (425–500) and fat than regular hamburgers.

✓ Avoid fried chicken; the coatings tend to retain grease. If you want bite-sized chicken, select bites made of chicken breast, not processed chicken (which contains fatty, ground-up skin).

✓ Ask for unsalted items; they are available. (Many chains have also reduced the amount of sodium used in cooking.)

✓ If you sample the salad bar, steer clear of mayonnaise, bacon bits, oily vegetable salads, and rich dressings.

Pesticides, Processing, and Irradiation

Plants and animals naturally produce compounds that act as pesticides to aid in their survival. The vast majority of the pesticides we consume are therefore natural, not added by farmers or food processors. As discussed in depth in Chapter 20, *commercial* pesticides save billions of dollars of valuable crops from pests, but they also may endanger human health and life.

Fearful of potential risks in pesticides, many consumers are purchasing **organic** foods. The term *organic* refers to foods produced without the use of commercial chemicals at any stage. Some independent certifying groups certify foods as organic if they have no detected residues of pesticides, even though pesticides may have been used in their cultivation. Foods that are truly organic are cleaner and have much lower levels of residues than standard commercial produce. There's no guarantee that the organic produce you buy at a grocery or health-food store is more nutritious than other produce. However, buying organic foods is one way in which you can work toward a healthier environment.

Irradiation is the use of radiation, either from radioactive substances or from devices that produce X rays, on food. It doesn't make the food radioactive. Its primary benefit is to prolong the shelf life of food. Like the heat in canning, irradiation can kill all the microorganisms that might grow in a food, and the sterilized food can then be stored for years in sealed containers at room temperature without spoiling. Are irradiated foods safe to eat? The best available answer is a qualified yes, because we don't have complete data yet. Most of the research conducted so far has focused on low-dose irradiation to delay ripening and destroy insects. In 1997 the FDA approved the irradiation of red meat as a means of eliminating dangerous bacteria that could cause food poisoning. Irradiation had previously been approved for poultry, where it was used to kill disease-causing bacteria like Salmonella and fruits and vegetables, where it is used in low doses to kill funguses and molds.[50]

Genetically engineered foods—custom built to improve quality or remove unwanted traits—may become an important part of our diets in the future. By modifying the genetic makeup of plants, engineers will be able to produce apples that resist insects, raspberries that last longer, and potatoes that absorb less fat in cooking. Will these items be as tasty and healthful as foods grown the old-fashioned way? And will they have unforeseen health hazards? That's yet to be seen.

Additives: Risks Versus Benefits

Additives are substances added to foods to lengthen storage time, change taste in a way the manufacturer thinks is better, alter color, or otherwise modify them to make them more appealing. The average American takes in approximately 160 pounds of food additives per year: more than 140 pounds of sweeteners, 15 pounds of table salt, and 5 to 10 pounds of all others.

Additives provide numerous benefits. Sodium and calcium propionate, sodium benzoate, potassium sorbate, and sulfur dioxide prevent the growth of bacteria, yeast, and mold in baked goods. BHA (butylated hydroxyanisole), BHT (butylated hydroxytoluene), propyl gallate, and vitamin E protect against the oxidation of fats (rancidity). Other additives include leavening agents, emulsifiers, stabilizers, thickeners, dough conditioners, and bleaching agents.

Some additives can pose a risk to eaters. For example, nitrites—used in bacon, sausages, and lunch meats to inhibit spoilage, prevent botulism, and add color—can react with other substances in your body or in food to form potentially cancer-causing agents called *nitrosamines*. In the last decade, the food industry has reduced the amount of nitrite used to cure foods, so there should be less danger than in the past. Sulfites, used to prevent browning, can produce severe, even fatal, allergic reactions in sensitive individuals. The FDA has required the labeling of sulfites in packaged foods and has banned the use of sulfites on fresh fruits and vegetables, including those in salad bars.

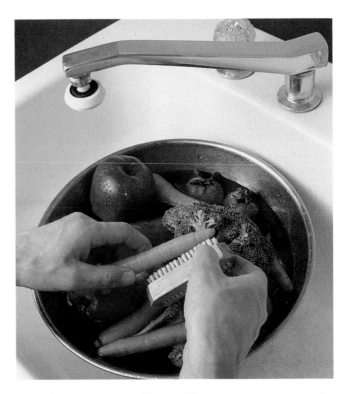

Clean food from a clean kitchen. Wash produce thoroughly in fresh water to remove dirt and any pesticide residue, scrubbing when necessary to clean off soil.

 ## What Causes Food Poisoning?

Someone in the United States is stricken with food poisoning approximately every second of every day, says the Council for Agricultural Sciences and Technology. Every year as many as 35 million Americans suffer from food poisoning; some 9,000 die as a result. In a study of food-borne illnesses, the General Accounting Office estimated that such illnesses cost the economy some $22 billion annually. The World Health Organization describes food as "the major source of exposure to disease-causing agents—biological and chemical—from which no one in either the developing or developed countries is spared."[51] (See Chapter 12 for an in-depth discussion of infectious illnesses.)

Food-borne infections generally produce nausea, vomiting, and diarrhea from twelve hours to five days after infection. The symptoms and severity depend on the specific microorganism and the victim's overall health. Although the illnesses tend to be short-term and not usually severe, they can be fatal to those whose immune systems are impaired or whose general health is poor. (See Table 6-12.)

Salmonella is a bacterium that contaminates many foods, particularly undercooked chicken, eggs, and sometimes processed meat. Eating contaminated food can result in Salmonella poisoning, which causes diarrhea and vomiting. The Centers for Disease Control and Prevention (CDC) estimates that there are approximately 40,000 reported cases of Salmonella poisoning a year; the actual number of cases could be anywhere from 400,000 to 4 million. Another bacterium, *Campylobacter jijuni,* may cause even more stomach infections than Salmonella. Found in water, milk, and some foods, *Campylobacter* poisoning causes severe diarrhea and has been implicated in causing stomach ulcers.

Bacteria can also cause illness by producing toxins in food. *Staphlycoccus aureus,* the most common cause of food-borne intoxication, occurs when cooked foods are cross-contaminated with the bacteria from raw foods and not stored properly. Staph infections cause nausea and abdominal pain anywhere from thirty minutes to eight hours after ingestion.

Bacteria account for two-thirds of food–borne infections, and thousands of suspected cases of infection

■ **Table 6-12** Food Poisoning: Common Culprits

	Source	Symptoms	Onset	Prevention
Bacterial				
Campylobacter Jejuni	Bacteria on poultry, cattle, and sheep that can contaminate the meat or milk of these animals.	Diarrhea, abdominal cramping, fever and/or bloody stools.	2 to 5 days	Cook foods thoroughly; drink pasteurized milk.
Escherichia coli (E.coli)	Water, raw or under-cooked meat and cross-contaminated foods.	Watery or bloody diarrhea, abdominal cramps, or vomiting.	10 to 72 hours	Cook foods thoroughly; wash hands well.
Listeria	Deli meats, hot dogs, soft cheese, raw meat, unpasteurized milk.	Headache, fever, and nausea.	24 hours to 12 days	Cook meats thoroughly; buy pasteurized milk; wash hands well.
Salmonella	Raw or undercooked meat, poultry or eggs, and unpasteurized milk.	Fever, muscle aches, nausea, abdominal cramps, diarrhea, fever, and/or headache.	5 hours to 4 days	Cook meats and leftovers thoroughly; wash hands well.
Staphylococcus aureus	Food left too long at room temperature, including meat, poultry, or egg products, tuna, potato salad, and cream-filled pastries. Unlike other bacteria, staphylo-cocci grow well in foods that are high in sugar or salt; any food can be contaminated by infected food handlers.	Vomiting, nausea, diarrhea, abdominal pain, and/or cramps.	30 minutes to 8 hours	Cook foods thoroughly; refrigerate leftovers immediately; wash your hands before and after handling food.
Nonbacterial				
Hepatitis A virus	Oysters, clams, mussels, or scallops that come from waters polluted with untreated sewage, and improper food handling with unwashed hands.	Weakness, appetite loss, nausea, vomiting, and fever; jaundice may develop.	15 to 50 days	Buy seafood from reputable markets; wash hands well.
Trichinella spiralis	(causes trichinosis) A parasite found in raw or undercooked pork or carnivorous animals.	Muscle pain, swollen eyelids, and/or fever; can be fatal.	8 to 15 days	Cook meat thoroughly.

Source: USDA.

with *Escherichia coli,* or **E. coli** bacteria in undercooked or inadequately washed food have been reported. (See Chapter 12 on infectious diseases.) In one outbreak in Washington State the failure of fast-food restaurants to cook hamburger meat to a temperature high enough to kill *Escherichia coli* bacteria led to the hospitalization of 151 people and three deaths.[52]

Even many "healthy" foods can pose dangers. In 1999 the FDA urged consumers to avoid eating raw sprouts because of the risk of getting sick. Sprouts, particularly alfalfa and clover, can be contaminated by the salmonella or *E.coli* bacteria, which can cause nausea, diarrhea and cramping in healthy adults. Children and senior citizens can experience effects that can lead to kidney failure and compromised immune systems. The FDA advises people to either cook sprouts before eating them or request that they be left off sandwiches and other food ordered in restaurants. Homegrown sprouts can also present a risk if they come from contaminated seeds. The FDA also has warned consumers about the dangers of unpasteurized orange juice because of the risk of salmonella contamination.

Strategies *for* Prevention

Protecting Yourself from Food Poisoning

✓ Clean food thoroughly. Wash produce thoroughly. Wash utensils, plates, cutting boards, knives, blenders, and other cooking equipment with very hot water and soap after preparing raw meat, poultry, or fish to avoid contaminating other foods or the cooked meat.

✓ Drink only pasteurized milk. Raw or unpasteurized milk increases the danger of microbial infections.

✓ Don't eat raw eggs. Since raw eggs can be contaminated with Salmonella, don't use them in salad dressings, eggnog, or other dishes.

✓ Cook chicken thoroughly. About a third of all poultry sold contains harmful organisms. Thorough cooking eliminates any danger.

✓ Cook pork to an internal temperature of 170°F to kill parasites called Trichina occasionally found in the muscles of pigs.

✓ Keep foods hotter than 140°F or colder than 40°F. The temperatures in between are a danger zone. If you must leave foods out—perhaps at a buffet or picnic—don't let them stay in the temperature danger zone for more than two hours. After that time, throw the food away.

✓ Refrigerate leftovers as soon as possible and use them within three days. If frozen, use leftovers within two to three months.

An uncommon but sometimes fatal form of food poisoning is **botulism,** caused by the *Clostridium botulinum* organism. Improper home-canning procedures are the most common cause of this potentially fatal problem.

There have been several outbreaks of listeriosis, caused by the bacteria **listeria,** commonly found in deli meats, hot dogs, soft cheeses, raw meat, and unpasteurized milk. At greatest risk are pregnant women, infants, and those with weakened immune systems. You can reduce your risk by cooking meats and leftovers thoroughly and by washing everything that may come into contact with raw meat.

Food Allergies

A woman nibbles on a strawberry and collapses. A boy develops hives immediately after eating a peanut butter sandwich. A baby vomits after swallowing some regular milk. In each case, the body has responded as if the food being consumed were a threatening invader and has mobilized its internal forces to fight against it.

Physicians disagree as to which foods are the most common triggers of food allergies. Cow's milk, eggs, seafood, wheat, soybeans, nuts, seeds, and chocolate have all been identified as culprits. The symptoms they provoke vary. One person might sneeze if exposed to an irritating food; another might vomit or develop diarrhea; others might suffer headaches, dizziness, hives, or a rapid heartbeat. Symptoms may not develop for up to 72 hours, making it hard to pinpoint which food was responsible. (See Chapter 12 for a further discussion of allergies.)

If you suspect that you have a food allergy, see a physician with specialized training in allergy diagnosis. Medical opinion about the merits of many treatments for food allergies is divided. Once you've identified the culprit, the wisest and sometimes simplest course is to avoid it.

Nutritional Quackery

The American Dietetic Association describes nutritional quackery as a growing problem for unsuspecting consumers. Yet, because so much nutritional nonsense is garbed in scientific-sounding terms, it can be hard to recognize bad advice when you get it. One basic rule: If the promises of a nutritional claim sound too good to be true—they probably are. (See Consumer Health Watch: "Becoming a Smart Nutrition Consumer.")

If you seek the advice of a nutrition consultant, check his or her credentials and professional associations carefully. Because licensing isn't required in all states, almost anyone can call him- or herself a nutritionist, regardless of qualifications. Be wary of diplomas from obscure schools and organizations that allow anyone who pays dues to join. (One physician obtained a membership for his dog!) Registered dietitians (R.D.s), who have bachelor's degrees

Consumer Health Watch

Becoming a Smart Nutrition Consumer

- Don't believe everything you read. A quick way to spot a bad diet book is to look in the index for a diet to prevent or treat rheumatoid arthritis (none exists). If you find one, don't buy the book.
- Before you try any new nutritional approach, check with your doctor or a registered dietitian or call the ADA consumer hot line.
- Don't believe ads or advisers basing their nutritional recommendations on hair analysis, which is not accurate in detecting nutritional deficiencies.
- Be wary of anyone who recommends megadoses of vitamins or nutritional supplements, which can be

dangerous. High doses of vitamin A, which some people take to clear up acne, can be toxic.
- Question personal testimonies about the powers of some magical-seeming pill or powder, and be wary of "scientific articles" in journals that aren't reviewed by health professionals.
- Be wary of any nutritional supplements sold in health stores or through health and bodybuilding magazines that contain ingredients that have not been tested and proven safe.

---

from approved programs and specialized training (including an internship), and who pass a certification examination, are usually members of the American Dietetic Association (ADA), which sets the standard for quality in diets. Nutrition experts with M.D.s or Ph.D.s generally belong to the ADA, the American Institute of Nutrition, or the American Society of Clinical Nutrition; all have stringent membership requirements.

Across the Lifespan: Changing Nutritional Needs

Good nutrition is important at every age, but nutritional needs change as bodies grow—and grow older. The USDA has tailored its nutritional guidelines specifically for children and older adults. Figures 6-8 and 6-9 present the USDA food pyramids for those two groups.

Children's nutrition and eating patterns are important because they can have a lifelong effect on children's health. According to one recent study, children who gain a lot of weight as youngsters develop more risk factors for heart disease as adults. Other research has shown that, as a group, Hispanic and African-American children eat significantly more fat than white youngsters, which may contribute to the higher percentage of heart disease in adults in these minority groups.

Like adults, children should base their diet on whole grains, fruits, and vegetables and should limit fats and sweets, including soda. According to the USDA, 37 percent of children ages 3 to 5 drink carbonated beverages, which account for about 40 percent of their fluid intake. Because soda contains few if any nutrients, this may mean they drink fewer healthier drinks.[53] Incidentally, the USDA guidelines include a wholehearted endorsement of physical activity. Kids who play hard not only get strong but also develop an appetite for a wider variety of foods.

Older people, who need fewer daily calories, often do not get adequate nutrients from their daily diets. The food pyramid for older americans was designed specifically for adults over age 70, but the USDA urges anyone age 50 or older to heed its recommendations.[54] The new guidelines advise eight or more eight-ounce glasses of water daily to reduce the risk of dehydration and constipation, which become increasing risks because of decreased thirst sensation in the elderly. The pyramid also calls for dietary supplements of calcium and vitamins B-12 and D.[55]

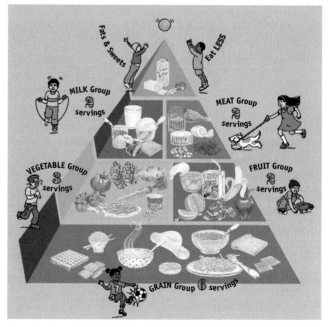

■ Figure 6-8 **Food Pyramid for Kids**
(USDA-recommended daily servings for 2- to 6-year-olds)

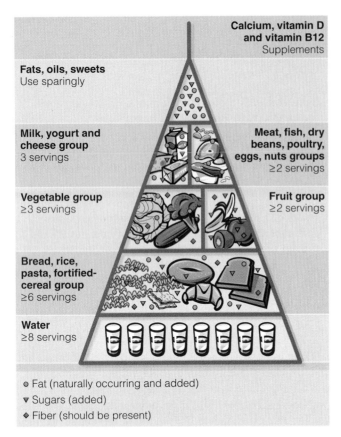

Figure 6-9 Food Pyramid for Older Adults
(USDA-recommended daily servings for adults 70 or older)

Making This Chapter Work for You

A Food Guide for the Twenty-First Century

- Nutrition—the science that explores the connections between our bodies and the food we eat—has shown that our daily diet affects our long-term health prospects more than any other factor within our control.

- Health officials recommend that Americans reduce fat intake, eat more grains, fruits, and vegetables, and consume only moderate amounts of salt, sugar, and alcohol.

- Saturated fats, found in meat and animal products, can increase the risk of heart disease and certain cancers, including those of the colon and breast. When converted to liquid form in vegetable oils, polyunsaturated fats form potentially harmful substances known as trans fatty acids. Monounsaturates, the most beneficial form of fat, are found in olive and canola oils. Dietary fats, especially saturated and trans fatty ones, can increase blood levels of cholesterol.

- Fiber (found in whole grains, vegetables, and fruit) helps keep the intestines healthy and aids elimination; prevents diverticulosis; is low in calories; and may lessen the risks of certain illnesses, such as heart disease, colon cancer, and diabetes.

- The Nutrition Labeling and Education Act requires food manufacturers to provide substantial information about fat, calories, and ingredients. Food labels must state serving size, calories per serving, fat per serving, daily values (the total amount of a nutrient that the average adult should not exceed on a daily basis), and percent daily values (an indication of how a particular food's nutrition content fits into a 2,000-calorie diet).

- Vitamins and minerals may play an important role in preventing disease. Certain antioxidant vitamins (particularly vitamin C, vitamin E, and beta-carotene, a form of Vitamin A) may prevent damage to our cells by free radical oxygen molecules.

- Most people eating a balanced diet don't need vitamin supplements. However, certain people may benefit from a supplement of folic acid, calcium, iron, or a multivitamin.

- The USDA's Food Guide Pyramid reflects scientific recognition of the health benefits of complex carbohydrates (plant-based foods such as whole grains, vegetables, and fruits), which should form the core of our daily diet. Americans should eat fewer servings of animal products, such as dairy products, meats, poultry, and eggs. Added fats and sugars should be used sparingly.

- Because of its rich cultural diversity, American diets include foods from many different countries, including China, Mexico, India, Italy, France, and Japan. Each type of cuisine has its own nutritional benefits and potential drawbacks. The plant-based Mediterranean diet is associated with a much lower rate of heart disease.

- An increasing number of people are cutting down on meats or adopting a vegetarian diet, which may or may not include dairy products, fish, or poultry.

- Because of their concern about pesticides, some Americans prefer organic foods, even though there's no guarantee that these foods haven't been exposed to existing contaminants in the air, water, or soil.

- Food safety has become an increasingly important issue because of the possible dangers of food-borne illnesses, additives, antibiotics and hormones in meat, pesticides, and irradiation.

- Food allergies and nutritional gimmicks can also endanger health. In each case, you have to seek out available information, weigh the risks versus the benefits, and make the choices that seem best for your health.

Nutritional needs change as bodies grow—and grow older. The USDA has tailored its nutritional guidelines specifically for children and older adults and developed food pyramids for young people and for older Americans.

After reading this chapter, you may well conclude that eating isn't simple anymore. You're right. Every time you grill bacon for breakfast, grab a quick cheeseburger for lunch, or heat up a burrito for dinner, you're making a choice that could have a long-term negative impact on your health. But responsibility for wise food choices extends beyond the individual. In studies of interventions designed to promote better nutrition, simple changes—such as adding more salads in a cafeteria or giving out informational literature in a supermarket—have led to healthful changes in individuals' food choices and eating habits. The more you learn about what you eat, the more likely you are to choose wisely and eat well.

While we must eat to live, eating can also bring a special joy and satisfaction to living. Here are some guidelines for eating for physical and psychological well-being:

- Eat with people whom you like.
- Talk only of pleasant things while eating.
- Eat slowly. Focus on the taste of each food you're eating.
- When you eat, eat—don't write, work, or talk on the phone.
- Eat because you're hungry, not to change how you feel.
- After eating, take time to be quiet and rest.

 Can Veggies Keep You Young? What has research shown about foods high in antioxidants?

health / ONLINE

Nutrition Navigator: A Rating Guide to Nutrition Web Sites
http://navigator.tufts.edu/
This site ranks nutrition web sites based on accuracy, depth of information, currency, and user-friendliness. A great resource for finding and evaluating nutrition information on the web.

The American Dietetic Association
http://www.eatright.org/
The official web site of the American Dietetic Association provides nutrition news, consumer resources, information for nutrition professionals, and a dietician referral service.

What Does It Take to Be Healthy?
http://www.5aday.gov
Take this online assessment to find out how your eating and exercise habits stack up to experts' recommendations. Sponsored by the National Cancer Institute and the Centers for Disease Control and Prevention.

Please note that links are subject to change. If you find a broken link, use a search engine like **http://www.yahoo.com** *and search for the web site by typing in key words.*

 Campus Chat: What do you eat during a typical day? How nutritious is your diet? Share your thoughts on our online discussion forum at **http://health.wadsworth.com**

Find It On InfoTrac: You can find additional readings related to fitness via InfoTrac College Edition, an online library of more than 900 journals and publications. Follow the instructions for accessing InfoTrac that came packaged with your textbook; then search for articles using a key word search.

- **Suggested article:** "8 Cellular Bodyguards for your Health," by Victoria Dolby Toews. *Better Nutrition*, May 1999, Vol. 61, Issue 5, p. 36(1).

  (1) What are eight nutrients that can help protect your cells from damage?

For additional links, resources, and suggested readings on InfoTrac, visit our Health & Wellness Resource Center at **http://health.wadsworth.com**

Key Terms

The terms listed here are used within the chapter. Page numbers are included for each term. A definition of each term is given in the Glossary pages at the end of this book.

additives   186
amino acids   184
antitoxidants   160
botulism   188
calorie   177
carbohydrates   169
cholesterol   157
complementary proteins   183
complete proteins   184
complex carbohydrates   155
crucifers   172
Daily Values (DV)   174
Dietary Reference Intakes
   (DRIs)   174

E. coli   188
fiber   155
food allergies   188
food toxicologists   184
hemoglobin   166
incomplete proteins   184
indoles   172
irradiation   185
lacto-vegetarians   183
listeria   188
minerals   160
nutrients   154
nutrition   153
organic   185

ovo-lacto-vegetarians   183
phytochemicals   166
protein   154
Recommended Dietary Allowances
   (RDAs)   174
saturated fat   156
simple carbohydrates   155
trans fats   156
unsaturated fat   156
vegans   183
vitamins   160

Critical Thinking Questions

1. Scientists are using genetic engineering to develop foods, such as tomatoes that won't bruise easily, cows that will produce more milk, or corn that will grow larger ears. Some consumer advocates argue that these items shouldn't be put on the market because they haven't been studied carefully enough. What do you think of these foods? Would you eat them?

2. Which alternative or ethnic diet do you think has the best-tasting food? Which is the most healthy? Why?

3. Is it possible to meet nutritional requirements on a limited budget? Have you ever been in this situation? What would you recommend to someone who wanted to eat healthfully on $30 a week?

4. Consider the number of times a week you eat fast food. How much money would you have saved if you had eaten home-prepared meals? What different foods from the bottom levels of the Food Guide Pyramid might you have eaten instead?

References

1. Anand, Rajen, and Peter P. Basiotis. "Is Total Fat Consumption Really Decreasing?" *Family Economics and Nutrition Review,* Vol. 11, No. 3, Summer, 1999.

2. Clements, Mark. "What America Eats." New York: NFO Research, 1999.

3. Conkling, Winifred. "Water: How Much Do We Need?" *American Health,* May 1995.

4. Ibid.

5. Smit, Ellen, et al. "Estimates of Animal and Plant Protein Intake in U.S. Adults." *Journal of the American Dietetic Association,* Vol. 99, July 1999.

6. Ibid.

7. Liebman, Bonnie. Center for Science in the Public Interest. Testimony, Hearings for the RDA, March 1999.

8. Johnson, Tim. "U.S. Food and Drug Administration Includes Whole Grains in Fight Against Heart Disease and Cancer." U.S. FDA Press release, July 8, 1999.

9. Fuchs, Charles, et al. "Dietary Fiber and the Risk of Colorectal Cancer and Adenoma in Women." *New England Journal of Medicine,* Vol. 340, No. 3 , January 21, 1999.

10. "Fiber: Still the Right Choice." *University of California, Berkeley Wellness Letter,* Vol. 15, No. 7, April 1999.

11. Lichtenstein, Alice, et al. "Effects of Different Forms of Dietary Hydrogenated Fats on Serum Lipoprotein Cholesterol Levels." *New England Journal of Medicine,* Vol. 340, No. 25, June 24, 1999.

12. "Olive Oil: Beyond the Hype." *University of California, Berkeley Wellness Letter,* Vol. 15, No. 5, February 1999.

13. American Heart Association Media Advisory. "Cholesterol Lowering Margarines." Statement. May 25, 1999.

14. Anand Basiotis. "Is Total Fat Consumption Really Decreasing?"

15. Peterson, Sharon, et al. "Impact of Adopting Lower-Fat Food Choices on Energy and Nutrient Intakes of American Adults." *Journal of the American Dietetic Association,* Vol. 99, No. 2 , February 1999.

16. Holmes, Michelle, et al. "Association of Dietary Intake of Fat and Fatty Acids With Risk of Breast Cancer." *JAMA,* Vol. 281, No. 10, March 10, 1999.

17. Raloff, J. "Why Cutting Fats May Harm the Heart." *Science News,* Vol. 155, No. 12, March 20, 1999.

18. Venkatraman, Jaya. "Very-Low-Fat Diet May Compromise Immunity." International Society for Exercise and Immunology Symposium, Rome, May 20, 1999.

19. Clark, Nancy. "Fat Facts and Fads." *American Fitness*, Vol. 17, Issue 3, May 1999.

20. Peterson et al. "Impact of Adopting Lower-Fat Food Choices on Energy and Nutrient Intakes of American Adults."

21. Sandler, Robert. "Gastrointestinal Symptoms in 3181 Volunteers Ingesting Snack Foods Containing Olestra or Triglycerides: A 6-Week Randomized, Placebo-Controlled Trial." *JAMA*, Vol. 281, No. 20, May 26, 1999.

22. "Antioxidants: Separating Hope from Hype." *Harvard Health Letter*, Vol. 24, Issue 5, February 1999.

23. Packer, Lester. Personal interview.

24. Blumberg, Jeffrey. Personal interview.

25. Nuovo, James. "AHA Statement on Antioxidants and Coronary Disease." *American Family Physician*, Vol. 59, Issue 10, May 15, 1999.

26. Tribble, D. L. "Antioxidant Consumption and the Risk of Coronary Heart Disease: Emphasis on Vitamin C, Vitamin E and Beta-Carotene. A Statement for Health Care Professionals from the American Heart Association." *Circulation*, Vol. 99, February 2, 1999.

27. Pryor, William. Personal interview.

28. Omenn, Gilbert. "An Assessment of the Scientific Basis for Attempting to Define the Dietary Reference Intake for Beta Carotene." *Journal of the American Dietetic Association*, Vol. 98, Issue 12, December 1998.

29. Nebeling, Linda. Personal interview.

30. McBride, Judy. "Can Foods Forestall Aging?" *Agricultural Research*, Vol. 47, Issue 2, February 1999.

31. Hui, Siu. Personal interview.

32. Pelton, Ross. "Keeping a Watch on Vision." *American Druggist*, Vol. 216, No. 5, May 1999. Lyle, Barbara, et al. "Antioxidant Intake and Risk of Incident Age-Related Nuclear Cataracts in the Beaver Dam Eye Study." *American Journal of Epidemiology*, Vol. 149, No. 9, May 1, 1999.

33. Petrini, J. R., et al. "Knowledge and Use of Folic Acid by Women of Childbearing Age." *JAMA*, Vol. 281, No. 20, May 26, 1999.

34. Brouwer, Ingeborg, et al. "Dietary Folate from Vegetables and Citrus Fruit Decreases Plasma Homocysteine Concentrations in Humans in a Dietary Controlled Trial." *Journal of Nutrition*, Vol. 129, No. 6, June 1999.

35. Zhang, S. M., et al. "A Prospective Study of Folate Intake and the Risk of Breast Cancer." *JAMA*, Vol. 281, No. 17 , May 5, 1999.

36. McBride, Judy. "Can Foods Forestall Aging?" *Agricultural Research*, Vol. 47, No. 2, February 1999.

37. Elliott, James. "Application of Antioxidant Vitamins in Food and Beverages." *Food Technology*, Vol. 53, No. 2, February 1999.

38. Ann Shaw. Personal interview.

39. "Food Portions and Servings: How Do They Differ?" *Nutrition Insights*, Vol. 11, March 1999.

40. "Are Eggs Really Okay?" *Tufts University Health and Nutrition Newsletter*, 1999.

41. France, David. "Groups Debate Role of Milk in Building a Better Pyramid." *New York Times*, June 19, 1999.

42. Schwartz, Ronald. "Henney Defends FDA on Dietary Supplements." *American Druggist*, Vol. 216, No. 5, May, 1999.

43. American Chemical Society. "Popular Diet Supplement May be a Cancer Risk." April 1, 1999.

44. Ann Shaw. Personal interview.

45. Marietta, Anne, et al. "Knowledge, Attitudes and Behaviors of College Students Regarding the 1990 Nutrition Labeling Education Act Food Labels." *Journal of the American Dietetic Association*, Vol. 99, No. 4, April 1999.

46. Pinkowish, Mart. "Effects of the Mediterranean Diet in MI Prevention." *Patient Care* , Vol. 33, No. 7, April 15, 1999.

47. Seppa, N. "Mediterranean Diet Proves Value Again." *Science News*, Vol. 155, No. 8, February 20, 1999.

48. Brody, Jane. "Paradox or Not, Cholesterol in France Is on the Rise." *The New York Times*, June 22, 1999.

49. de Lorgeril, Michel and Salen, Patricia. "Wine, Ethanol, Platelets, and Mediterranean Diet." *Lancet*, Vol. 353, No. 9158, March 27, 1999.

50. Kolata, Gina. "F.D.A., Saying Process Is Safe, Approves Irradiating Red Meat." *New York Times*, December 3, 1997.

51. Gavzer, Bernard. "We Can Make Our Food Safer." *Parade*, October 19, 1997.

52. Stoeckle, Mark, and Douglas R. Gordon. "Infectious Diseases." *Journal of the American Medical Association*, Vol. 273, No. 13, June 7, 1995.

53. www.usda.gov/cnpp

54. Russell, Robert, et al. "Modified Food Guide Pyramid for People over Seventy Years of Age." *Journal of Nutrition*, Vol. 29, No. 3, March 1999.

55. "New Food Guide Pyramid Specifically for People 70 and Older." *Tufts University Health & Nutrition Letter*, Vol. 17, No. 2, April 1999.

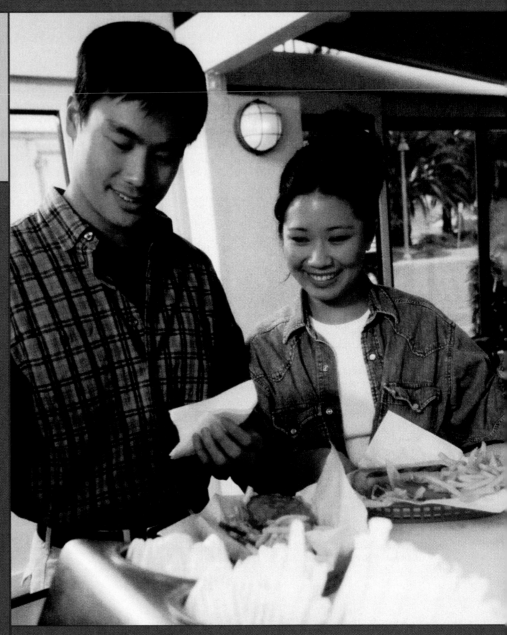

CHAPTER

7

Eating Patterns and Problems

After studying the material in this chapter, you should be able to:

- **Define** body mass and know your BMI (body mass index).
- **Identify** several factors that influence food consumption.
- **Identify** and **describe** the symptoms and dangers associated with abnormal eating behaviors and eating disorders.
- **Define** obesity and **describe** its relationship to genetics, lifestyle, and major health problems.
- **Assess** various approaches to weight loss.
- **Design** a personal plan for sensible weight management.

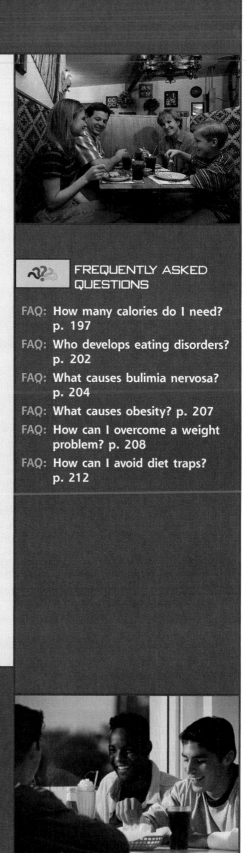

W ith more food choices than ever before in history, Americans are eating more—and gaining more weight. According to revised federal guidelines, 55 percent of all Americans aged 20 and older are overweight. In the last 30 years, the prevalence of obesity in adults increased from nearly 13 percent to 22.5 percent of the population.[1]

Ironically, as average weights have increased, the quest for thinness has become a national obsession. In a society in which slimmer is seen as better, anyone who is less than lean may feel like a failure. Individuals—especially young women—who are overweight or embarrassed by their appearance often assume that they would be happier, sexier, or more successful in thinner bodies. And so they diet. Each year, 15 to 35 percent of Americans go on diets, but no matter how much they lose, 90 to 95 percent regain extra pounds within five years.[2]

This chapter explores our national preoccupation with slimness; explains body mass index (BMI); examines unhealthy eating patterns and eating disorders; tells what obesity is and why excess pounds are dangerous; shows why fad diets don't work; and offers guidelines for how to control weight safely, sensibly, and permanently. ❖

FREQUENTLY ASKED QUESTIONS

FAQ: **How many calories do I need?** p. 197

FAQ: **Who develops eating disorders?** p. 202

FAQ: **What causes bulimia nervosa?** p. 204

FAQ: **What causes obesity?** p. 207

FAQ: **How can I overcome a weight problem?** p. 208

FAQ: **How can I avoid diet traps?** p. 212

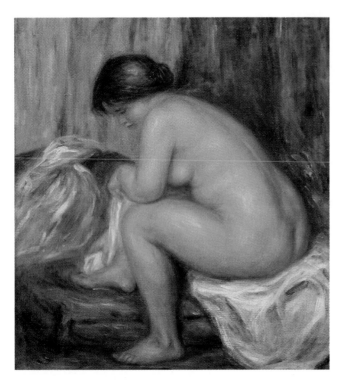

The body beautiful. "Thinner is better" is not the worldwide standard, and in past centuries more flesh rather than less was considered healthy and beautiful. This painting by Renoir, from the late 1880s, shows a rounded feminine ideal.

Body Image

Throughout most of history, bigger was better. The great beauties of centuries past, as painted by such artistic masters as Rubens and Renoir, were soft and fleshy, with rounded bellies and dimpled thighs. Many developing countries still regard a full figure, rather than a thin one, as the ideal standard for health and beauty. "Fattening huts," in which brides-to-be eat extra food to plump up before marriage, still exist in some African cultures. Among certain Native Americans of the Southwest, if a girl is thin at puberty, a fat woman places her foot on the girl's back so she will magically gain weight and become more attractive.

At the beginning of the twenty-first century in the United States, men and women are paying more attention to their body image than ever before. (See The X & Y Files: "Real Versus Ideal Body Images in Men and Women.") Even though studies show that men don't necessarily consider the slimmest women the most attractive, young women—especially white women—grow up thinking that thin is better. African-American women often have more positive attitudes toward their bodies, feeling more satisfied with their weight and seeing themselves as more attractive. However, there are no significant differences between African-American and white women *dieters* in terms of self-esteem and body dissatisfaction.

As men and women age, their attitudes about their bodies change. The elderly feel less positively about their facial appearance, but older women express greater satisfaction than young ones with their weight. Throughout life men generally have more positive body attitudes than women, but this gender difference becomes less pronounced with age.[3]

What Should I Weigh?

Many factors determine what you weigh: heredity, eating behavior, food selection, amount of daily exercise. For any individual of a given height, there is no single best weight, but a range of healthy weights. The federal government and medical experts have replaced "ideal weight tables" with a better measure—body mass index (BMI).

Body Mass Index (BMI)

Body mass index (BMI), a ratio between weight and height, is a mathematical formula that correlates with body fat. The BMI numbers apply to both men and women. (See Table 7-1.) In general, BMI is a better predictor of disease risk than body weight alone. However, certain people should not rely on BMI to estimate their body fat. These include competitive athletes and body builders, whose BMI is high because of a relatively larger amount of muscle, and women who are pregnant or nursing. BMI also is not intended for use in growing children or in frail and sedentary elderly individuals.

If your BMI is high, you may be at increased risk of developing certain diseases, including hypertension, cardiovascular disease, adult-onset diabetes (Type II), sleep apnea, osteoarthritis, and other conditions. (The section on Being Overweight or Obese discusses the health risks associated with a high BMI.)

You can also calculate your body mass index by following these three simple steps:

1. Multiply your weight in pounds by 703.
2. Multiply your height in inches by itself.
3. Divide the first number by the second and then round up to the nearest whole number. This is your body mass index.

Other Ways of Weighing In

Another way of assessing weight is by measuring body fat. The lowest health risks are associated with a body fat percentage of weight below 20 for men and 25 for women. Body fat may be assessed in different ways. **Skin calipers,** which pinch skin folds at the arms, waist,

The X&Y Files

Real Versus Ideal Body Images in Men and Women

W omen have long been bombarded by the media with idealized images of female bodies that bear little resemblance to the way most women look. Increasingly, more advertisements and men's magazines are featuring idealized male bodies. Sleek, strong, and sculpted, they too do not resemble the bodies most men inhabit. In fact, the gap between reality and ideal is getting bigger for both sexes.

In the last decade, numerous studies have shown that women in *Playboy* centerfolds and Miss America pageants weigh less than they did in the 1970s. In one analysis, 29 percent of *Playboy* centerfolds and 17 percent of Miss America Pageant winners had BMIs below 17.5, one of the criteria for anorexia nervosa and a definite indication of being severely underweight.

By comparison, reality may be healthier. In a sampling of Canadian and American women between ages 18 and 24, all had BMIs in the low-risk zone between 18 and 24—although the average American woman was at the higher end of that zone. Yet most women do not feel satisfied with their weight until they drop to 90 percent of the ideal for their height. (Men don't feel dissatisfied with their weight until it climbs to 105 percent of their ideal.)

As beauty pageant queens and female models have been shrinking, the men featured in *Playgirl* centerfolds have been bulking up. Their BMIs are higher than in the past—as are the BMIs of a sample of Canadian and American men between the ages of 18 and 24. Researchers do not know if the higher BMIs are the result of an increase in lean body mass or body fat. Their theory: The models have gotten more muscular over time, accounting for their high BMIs, while real guys may simply have gotten fatter.

Bigger does seem better to many young males. About half of high school boys say they would like to have larger biceps, wrists, shoulders, and chests, while male college undergraduates want bigger chests and arms. The greatest body dissatisfaction occurs in thin males. Underweight college age men are as dissatisfied with themselves as overweight college women. The desire for a larger, more muscular body has been associated with use of anabolic steroids and other body-building aids (discussed in Chapter 5). The incidence of high school senior boys using anabolic steroids is estimated to be 7 percent—higher than the incidence of anorexia nervosa among high school girls.

In youth and young adulthood, men—except for the very thin and the very fat—generally report higher levels of body satisfaction than women. As men age, their body satisfaction declines, and by the time they are in their forties and fifties they are as dissatisfied with their body shape as women. This change seems to result from older men holding onto body image ideals identical to those of younger males.

The "ideals" for female and male bodies are clearly different, but researchers consider both dangerous. The gap between the average woman's body size and the thin female ideal in the media may fuel the greater body dissatisfaction reported by women. "Today's female body ideal is harmful psychologically and physically," concluded one research team, noting that the new muscular male ideal may be just as dangerous as a risk factor for steroid use in young men. "It may prove to be as difficult to attain, restrictive, and potentially harmful as women's ideals."

Sources: Malkin, Amy, et al. "Women and Weight: Gendered Messages on Magazine Covers." *Sex Roles: A Journal of Research,* Vol. 40, No. 7–8, April 1999. Spitzer, Brenda, et al. "Gender Differences in Population Versus Media Body Sizes: A Comparison over Four Decades." *Sex Roles: A Journal of Research,* Vol. 40, No. 7–8, April 1999.

---

and back, are the most widely used, although they may be less accurate than other techniques. Proper use of these instruments by trained personnel is critical in getting a precise reading. **Hydrostatic weighing**—weighing a person in water to distinguish buoyant fat from denser muscle—is far more precise. Other methods include whole-body counting, which measures the total amount of K-40, a naturally occurring form of potassium found primarily in lean tissue; imaging methods, such as computerized tomography (CT) and magnetic resonance imaging (MRI); ultrasonography, which uses high-frequency sound waves; and bioelectrical imped-

ance assessment (BIA), which measures the resistance of the body to a flow of alternating electric current.

 ## How Many Calories Do I Need?

Calories are the measure of the amount of energy that can be derived from food. Science defines a **calorie** as the amount of energy required to raise the temperature of 1 gram of water by one degree Celsius. In the laboratory, the caloric content of food is measured in 1,000-calorie

■ **Table 7-1** Body Mass Index (BMI)

	18	19	20	21	22	23	24	25	26	27	28	29	30	31	32	33	34	35	36	37	38	39	40
Height												**Body Weight (pounds)**											
4'10"	86	91	96	100	105	110	115	119	124	129	134	138	143	148	153	158	162	167	172	177	181	186	191
4'11"	89	94	99	104	109	114	119	124	128	133	138	143	148	153	158	163	168	173	178	183	188	193	198
5'0"	92	97	102	107	112	118	123	128	133	138	143	148	153	158	163	168	174	179	184	189	194	199	204
5'1"	95	100	106	111	116	122	127	132	137	143	148	153	158	164	169	174	180	185	190	195	201	206	211
5'2"	98	104	109	115	120	126	131	136	142	147	153	158	164	169	175	180	186	191	196	202	207	213	218
5'3"	102	107	113	118	124	130	135	141	146	152	158	163	169	175	180	186	191	197	203	208	214	220	225
5'4"	105	110	116	122	128	134	140	145	151	157	163	169	174	180	186	192	197	204	209	215	221	227	232
5'5"	108	114	120	126	132	138	144	150	156	162	168	174	180	186	192	198	204	210	216	222	228	234	240
5'6"	112	118	124	130	136	142	148	155	161	167	173	179	186	192	198	204	210	216	223	229	235	241	247
5'7"	115	121	127	134	140	146	153	159	166	172	178	185	191	198	204	211	217	223	230	236	242	249	255
5'8"	118	125	131	138	144	151	158	164	171	177	184	190	197	203	210	216	223	230	236	243	249	256	262
5'9"	122	128	135	142	149	155	162	169	176	182	189	196	203	209	216	223	230	236	243	250	257	263	270
5'10"	126	132	139	146	153	160	167	174	181	188	195	202	209	216	222	229	236	243	250	257	264	271	278
5'11"	129	136	143	150	157	165	172	179	186	193	200	208	215	222	229	236	243	250	257	265	272	279	286
6'0"	132	140	147	154	162	169	177	184	191	199	206	213	221	228	235	242	250	258	265	272	279	287	294
6'1"	136	144	151	159	166	174	182	189	197	204	212	219	227	235	242	250	257	265	272	280	288	295	302
6'2"	141	148	155	163	171	179	186	194	202	210	218	225	233	241	249	256	264	272	280	287	295	303	311
6'3"	144	152	160	168	176	184	192	200	208	216	224	232	240	248	256	264	272	279	287	295	303	311	319
6'4"	148	156	164	172	180	189	197	205	213	221	230	238	246	254	263	271	279	287	295	304	312	320	328
6'5"	151	160	168	176	185	193	202	210	218	227	235	244	252	261	269	277	286	294	303	311	319	328	336
6'6"	155	164	172	181	190	198	207	216	224	233	241	250	259	267	276	284	293	302	310	319	328	336	345

Under-weight	Healthy Weight	Overweight	Obese
BMI (<18.5)	BMI (18.5–24.9)	BMI (25–29.9)	BMI (≥30)

Find your height along the lefthand column and look across the row until you find the number that is closest to your weight. The number at the top of that column identifies your BMI.

Source: From Brown, *Nutrition Now,* 2nd ed. Belmont, Calif.: Wadsworth, © 2000.

units called *kilocalories*. The calorie referred to in everyday usage is actually the equivalent of the laboratory kilocalorie. (The Hales Health Almanac at the back of this book contains calorie counts for many foods.)

The number of calories you need every day depends on your gender, age, size, and activity level. An "average" adult woman—with a median height of 5 feet 4 inches and a weight of 138 pounds—generally needs 1,900 to 2,200 calories. An average man—with a median height of 5 feet 10 inches and a weight of 174 pounds—generally consumes 2,300 to 2,900 calories. How many calories you need depends on your gender, age, body-frame size, weight, percentage of body fat, and your **basal metabolic rate (BMR)**—the number of calories needed to sustain your body at rest.

Your activity level also affects your calorie requirements. Regardless of whether you consume fat, protein, or carbohydrates, if you take in more calories than required to maintain your size and don't work them off in some sort of physical activity, your body will convert the excess to fat (Table 7-2).

Hunger, Satiety, and Set Point

Why do you wake up starving or feel your stomach rumbling during a late afternoon lecture? The simple answer is **hunger**: the physiological drive to consume food. More than a dozen different signals may influence and control our desire for food. Researchers at the National Institutes of Health have discovered appetite receptors within the hypothalamus region of the brain that specifically respond to hunger messages carried by chemicals. Hormones, including insulin and stress-related epinephrine (adrenaline), may also stimulate or suppress hunger. Hunger, recent studies show, activates parts of the brain involved with emotions, thinking, and feeling.[4] Even the size of our fat cells may affect how hungry we feel. (Many overweight people have fat cells two to two-and-a-half times larger than normal.)

Appetite—the psychological desire to eat—usually begins with the fear of the unpleasant sensation of hunger. We learn to avoid hunger by eating a certain amount of food at certain times of the day, just as dogs

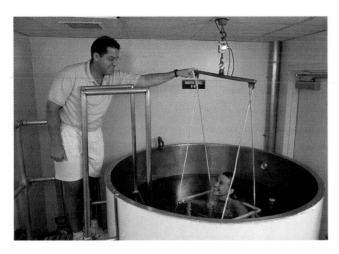

Measuring body fat. The most accurate way of measuring body fat is hydrostatic weighing in an immersion tank.

■ **Table 7-2**	How Many Calories Do You Need Daily?		
Desirable Weight (lb)	**High Activity**	**Medium Activity**	**Low Activity**
Women			
99	1700	1500	1300
110	1850	1650	1400
121	2000	1750	1550
128	2100	1900	1600
132	2150	1950	1650
143	2300	2050	1800
154	2400	2150	1850
165	2550	2300	1950
Men			
121	2400	2150	1850
132	2550	2300	1950
143	2700	2400	2050
154	2900	2600	2200
165	3100	2800	2400
176	3250	2950	2500
187	3300	3100	2600

in the laboratory learn to avoid electric shocks by jumping at the sound of a warning bell. But appetite is easily led into temptation. In one famous experiment, psychologists bought bags of high-calorie goodies—peanut butter, marshmallows, chocolate-chip cookies, and salami—for their test rats. The animals ate so much on this "supermarket diet" that they gained more weight than any laboratory rats ever had before. The snack-food diet that fattened up these rats was particularly high in fats. Biologists speculate that creamy, buttery, or greasy foods may cause internal changes that increase appetite and, consequently, weight.

We stop eating when we feel satisfied; this is called **satiety,** a feeling of fullness and relief from hunger. According to the **set-point theory,** each individual has an unconscious control system for regulating appetite and satiety to keep body fat at a predetermined level, or *set point.* If our fat stores fall too low, our appetite gnaws at us, so we eat more. Conversely, appetite subsides if we overeat.

From this perspective, diets are doomed to fail because they pit the dieter against tireless internal enemies: the set point and its enforcer, appetite. The only effective alternative is lowering, or resetting, the set point. And the safest, most effective way to do so is through physical activity, which dampens appetite in the short run and lowers the set point for the long term. As discussed later in this chapter, moderate activity not only works up an appetite but also helps work it off.

Unhealthy Eating Behavior

Sooner or later many people *don't* eat the way they should. They may skip meals, thereby increasing the likelihood that they'll end up with more body fat, a higher weight, and a higher blood cholesterol level. Others live on "diet" foods, but consume so much of them that they gain weight anyway. Yet others engage in more extreme forms of what health professionals call "disordered eating." They continuously go on and off diets, eat compulsively, or binge on high-fat treats. Such behaviors can be warning signs of potentially serious eating disorders that should not be ignored.

Disordered Eating in Children and Adolescents

Unhealthy eating behavior is developing at earlier ages, often stemming from a fear of getting fat. Among 10-year-old girls, 31 percent say they're afraid of being fat. More than 50 percent of adolescent girls diet to lose weight, while 13 percent engage in bulimic or anorexic behaviors.[5]

According to the National Longitudinal Study of Adolescent Health, many teens are concerned about their weight, try to change it, and often use inappropriate means either to lose or to gain weight. In the national sample of more than 6,500 adolescents in grades seven to twelve, almost two-thirds of girls and one-sixth of boys were attempting to lose weight, while almost one-tenth of girls and more than one-fourth of boys were trying to gain weight.[6]

The reasons teens try to change their weight have little to do with health. Some want to gain weight to

Campus Focus

Eating Disorders and College Students

Have you ever had an eating disorder?
Yes: 11%
No: 89%

Do you know one or more students with an eating disorder?
Know one student: 55%
Know two students: 52%
Know three or more students: 33%

If you had an eating disorder, to whom would you go for help?
Friends: 85%
Family: 75%
Private physician: 12%
College health service: 8%

If you had an eating disorder and did not seek help, whom would you want to intervene?
Friend or relative: 92%
College counselor: 54%

What is the best source of information about eating disorders?
College health service: 35%
Classes at school: 22%
Student counselors: 15%
Magazine articles: 15%
School lectures and seminars: 12%
Friends: 11%
TV news: 10%

Source: These answers come from a national poll of 500 college women conducted by *People* magazine and published in "Thin Is In, No Matter the Toll," *People,* April 12, 1999. Respondents were allowed to select one or more answers.

look older and stronger and improve athletic prowess and performance. Others diet for complex psychological and social reasons. A key factor that distinguishes teen dieters from nondieters is poor self-esteem.[7] While most adolescent boys have higher self-esteem than girls, overweight teens of both sexes rank lower in self-esteem and consider themselves less socially acceptable.[8] Among both white girls and African-American girls with college-educated mothers, body fat correlates with dieting, dissatisfaction with their weight, and probability of dating (which declines as body fat rises, even in nonobese girls).[9]

For adolescents, dieting is the most important predictor of eating disorders. In a study that followed 14- and 15-year-old teens for three years, girls who went on extreme weight loss diets were 18 times more likely to develop an eating disorder than those who did not diet. Those who followed moderate diets were 5 times as likely. Boys were a little less than a third as likely as girls to develop an eating disorder.[10]

Disordered Eating in College Students

College students—particularly women—are at risk for unhealthy eating behaviors. (See Campus Focus: "Eating Disorders and College Students.") The prevalence of disordered eating symptoms and eating disorders has increased dramatically in the last 20 years. One reason may be the pressure some young women feel to attain what some have called the "Super Woman" ideal. As they try to excel in multiple roles, they diet, induce vomiting, or restrict food intake for the sake of meeting their idealized standards for appearance.

Extreme Dieting

"Extreme" dieters go beyond cutting back on calories or increasing physical activity and become preoccupied with what they eat and weigh. Although their weight never falls below 85 percent of normal, their weight loss is severe enough to cause uncomfortable physical consequences, such as weakness and sensitivity to cold. Technically, these dieters do not have *anorexia nervosa* (discussed later in the chapter), but they are at increased risk for it.

Extreme dieters may think they know a great deal about nutrition, yet many of their beliefs about food and weight are misconceptions or myths. For instance, they may eat only protein because they believe complex carbohydrates, including fruits and breads, are fattening. When they're anxious, angry, or bored, they focus on food and their fear of fatness. Dieting and exercise become ways of coping with any stress in their lives.

Sometimes nutritional education alone can help change this eating pattern. However, many avid dieters who deny that they have a problem with food may need counseling (which they usually agree to only at their family's insistence) to correct dangerous eating behavior and prevent further complications.

Compulsive Overeating

Individuals who eat compulsively cannot stop putting food in their mouths. They eat fast; they eat a lot; they eat even when they're full; and they may eat round the clock rather than at set meal times—often in private because of embarrassment over how much they consume.

Some mental health professionals describe compulsive eating as a food addiction that is much more likely to develop in women. According to Overeaters Anonymous (OA), an international support agency, many women who eat compulsively view food as a source of comfort against feelings of inner emptiness, low self-esteem, and fear of abandonment.

The following behaviors may signal a potential problem:

- Turning to food when depressed or lonely, when feeling rejected, or as a reward.
- A history of failed diets and anxiety when dieting.
- Thinking about food throughout the day.
- Eating quickly and without pleasure.
- Frequent talking about food, or refusing to talk about food.
- Fear of not being able to stop eating once you start. Continuing to eat even when you're no longer hungry.

Recovery from compulsive eating can be challenging because people with this problem cannot give up entirely the "substance" they abuse. Like everyone else, they must eat. However, they can learn new eating habits and ways of dealing with underlying emotional problems. An OA survey found that most of its members joined to lose weight but later felt the most important effect was their improved emotional, mental, and physical health. As one woman put it, "I came for vanity but stayed for sanity."

Binge Eating

Binge eating—the rapid consumption of an abnormally large amount of food in a relatively short time—often occurs in compulsive eaters. Individuals with a binge-eating disorder typically eat a larger-than-ordinary amount of food during a relatively brief period, feel a lack of control over eating, and binge at least twice a week for at least a six-month period. During most of these episodes, individuals experience at least three of the following:

- Eating much more rapidly than usual.
- Eating until they feel uncomfortably full.
- Eating large amounts of food when not feeling physically hungry.
- Eating large amounts of food throughout the day with no planned mealtimes.
- Eating alone because they are embarrassed by how much they eat and by their eating habits.

It is not clear whether dieting leads to binge eating—or vice versa. Binge-eaters may spend up to several hours eating, and consume 2,000 or more calories-worth of food in a single binge—more than many people eat in a day. After such binges, they usually do not induce vomiting, use laxatives, or rely on other means (such as exercise) to control weight. They simply get fatter. As their weight climbs, they become depressed, anxious, or troubled by other psychological symptoms to a much greater extent than others of comparable weight.

About 2 percent of Americans—some 5 million in all—may have binge-eating disorder.[11] It is most common among young women in college and, increasingly, in high school. Persons who binge-eat may require professional help to change their behavior. Treatment includes education, behavioral approaches, cognitive therapy, and psychotherapy. As they recognize the reasons for their behavior and begin to confront the underlying issues, individuals usually are able to resume normal eating patterns.

Eating Disorders

Just a few decades ago there was no official psychiatric diagnosis for behaviors that are now collectively called **eating disorders.** They are much more common in women. The best known are anorexia nervosa, which affects fewer than 1 percent of adolescent women, and bulimia nervosa, which strikes 2 to 3 percent. Many more young women do not have the characteristic symptoms of these disorders, but are preoccupied with their weight or experiment with unhealthy forms of dieting. According to the Harvard Eating Disorders Center, 5 to 10 percent of young people have some form of disordered eating. These problems usually develop between ages 12 and 15; the average age is 17.[12]

 ## Who Develops Eating Disorders?

Eating disorders affect an estimated 5 to 10 million women and 1 million men. Most people with these problems are young (from ages 14 to 25), white, and affluent, with perfectionistic personalities. According to the Eating Disorders Awareness and Prevention Group of Seattle, 5 to 7 percent of American undergraduates suffer from eating disorders.[13] In one recent poll, one in ten undergraduates said they suffered from an eating disorder. (See Campus Focus: "Eating Disorders and College Students.") Although white women are considered at higher risk, recent studies indicate that more African-American women are developing eating disorders.[14]

In a survey of health care professionals at the country's largest colleges and universities, 70 percent said that eating disorders are common among their undergraduates; 11 percent said they were widespread; 19 percent described them as rare. Almost half (45 percent) felt that the incidence of eating disorders on their campuses had increased over the last five years; just 2 percent felt that the incidence had decreased. While 99 percent of the schools surveyed provide general mental health services, 69 percent have professionals on staff who specialize in diagnosing and treating eating disorders. Of all the hurdles to helping students with eating disorders, 39 percent said denial is the biggest , while 24 percent felt it was unwillingness to seek treatment, and 20 percent blamed pressure from peers and the media to stay thin.[15]

Eating disorders affect every aspect of college students' lives, including dating. Both men and women tend to avoid dating individuals with eating disorders, but men are far less accepting of obesity than women. In one study, 74 percent of men and 60 percent of women reported being uncomfortable dating someone who is obese. A smaller percentage—53 percent of the men and 59 percent of the women—said they wouldn't want to date a person with an eating disorder.[16]

More men are seeking treatment for eating disorders. According to a recent study, there are more similarities than differences between men and women with eating disorders—in age of onset of the problem, current age, and other factors. However, diet pill and laxative abuse is much less common in men than in women with bulimia.[17]

Athletes, both male and female, also are vulnerable to eating disorders, either because of the pressure to maintain ideal body weight or to achieve a weight that might enhance their performance. Many female athletes, particularly those participating in sports or activities that emphasize leanness (such as gymnastics, distance running, diving, figure skating, and classical ballet) have "subclinical" eating disorders that could undermine their nutritional status and energy levels.[18] However, there is often little awareness or recognition of their disordered eating. A recent survey found that collegiate coaches generally lack knowledge about recognizing and responding to eating disorders in young athletes.[19]

If someone you know has an eating disorder, let your friend know you're concerned and that you care. Don't criticize or make fun of his or her eating habits. Encourage your friend to talk about other problems and feelings, and suggest that he or she talk to the school counselor or someone at the mental health center, the family doctor, or another trusted adult. Offer to go along if you think that will make a difference.

Anorexia Nervosa

Although *anorexia* means loss of appetite, most individuals with **anorexia nervosa** are, in fact, hungry all the time. For them, food is an enemy—a threat to their sense of self, identity, and autonomy. In the distorted mirror of their mind's eye, they see themselves as fat or flabby even at a normal or below-normal body weight. Some simply feel fat; others think that they are thin in some places and too fat in others, such as the abdomen, buttocks, or thighs.

The incidence of anorexia nervosa has increased in the last three decades in most developed countries. An estimated 0.5 to 1 percent of young women in their late teens and early twenties develop anorexia. According to the American Psychiatric Association (APA)'s Work Group on Eating Disorders, cases are increasing among males, minorities, women of all ages, and possibly preteens.

In the *restricting* type of anorexia, individuals lose weight by avoiding any fatty foods, and by dieting, fasting, and exercising. Some start smoking as a way of controlling their weight. In the *binge eating/purging* type, they engage in binge eating, purging (through self-induced vomiting, laxatives, diuretics, or enemas), or both. Obsessed with an intense fear of fatness, they may weigh

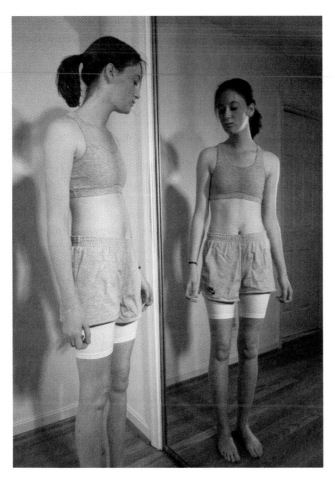

Anorexia nervosa is complex in its causes, and successful treatment usually involves medical, nutritional, and behavioral therapy.

themselves several times a day, measure various parts of their body, check mirrors to see if they look fat, and try on different items of clothing to see if they feel tight.

What Causes Anorexia Nervosa?

Many complex factors interact and contribute to this disorder, including biological, psychological, and social ones. Anorexia is more common among close relatives, particularly sisters, than it is in the general population. The relatives of anorexics also have a higher than expected frequency of depressive disorders.

Anorexia is associated with changes within the brain, including abnormalities in the stress-hormone cortisol, the neurotransmitters dopamine, serotonin, and norepinehprine—all of which influence appetite and satiety—and the peptide cholecystokinin, which affects feelings of fullness. It is not clear whether these changes are a cause or a consequence of this disorder.

Anorexia also may be a response to a personal loss or a sign of a driven, perfectionist personality. Often

young anorexics have above-average grades and an unwarranted fear of failure. Some theorists speculate that young teenage girls may starve themselves because of fear of their budding sexuality. By drastically reducing their weight, they can prevent or stop menstruation and breast development.

Girls who develop anorexia often have little insight or awareness of their feelings, needs, and wants. After years of reacting to the expectations of others, they may feel inadequate as they approach the age of independence. In some ways, starvation may serve as a way of creating an identity and asserting independence. In one study that followed 21 college women with eating disorders for six years, 11 got better during their postcollege years, while 10 continued to struggle with disordered eating. The major difference between the two groups revolved around issues of autonomy and relation. These who could better negotiate the tension between being independent and relating to others had higher self-esteem, a more positive self-concept, and a healthier relationship with food.[20]

About one-third of those with anorexia initially were mildly overweight and cut back on food just to lose a few pounds. Others had normal weights but began to diet to look more attractive or, in the case of male and female athletes and dancers, to gain a performance advantage. Sometimes, illness, stress, or surgery triggers weight loss. Often the initial response to their weight loss—from parents, coaches, or friends—is positive. However, starvation seems to take on a life of its own, and anorexics cannot return to a healthy eating pattern. In time, they may place so much value on thinness that they cannot recognize the dangers to their health.

Recognizing and Treating Anorexia Nervosa

The characteristics of anorexia nervosa include:

- A refusal to maintain normal body weight.
- An intense fear of gaining weight or becoming fat, even though underweight.
- A distorted body image, so that the person feels fat even when emaciated.
- In women, the absence of at least three menstrual cycles.

The medical consequences of anorexia nervosa are serious: Menstrual periods stop in women; testosterone levels decline in men. Adolescents with this disorder do not undergo normal sexual maturation, such as breast development, and may not reach their anticipated height. Even individuals who look and feel reasonably healthy may have subtle or hidden abnormalities, including heart irregularities and arrhythmias that can increase their risk of sudden death. Women who do not menstruate for six months or more may develop osteoporosis and suffer irreversible weakening and thinning of their bones as a result. (See Table 7-3.)

Even when they realize that they are jeopardizing their health, people with anorexia tend to fear that treatment will make them worse—that is, fatter. They need repeated reassurance that they will not become overweight and that they can and will find healthier ways of coping with life.

According to current practice guidelines, treatment of anorexia nervosa includes medical therapy (such as "refeeding" to overcome malnutrition) and behavioral, cognitive, psychodynamic, and family therapy (described in Chapter 4). Antidepressant medication sometimes can help, particularly when there is a personal or family history of depression. Most people who get help do return to normal weight, but it can take a long time for their eating behaviors to become normal and for them to deal with troubling body image issues.

Bulimia Nervosa

Individuals with **bulimia nervosa** go on repeated eating binges and rapidly consume large amounts of food, usu-

---

■ **Table 7-3** Medical Complications of Eating Disorders

Related to Weight Loss
Loss of fat and muscle mass, including heart muscle
Increased sensitivity to cold
Irregular heartbeats
Bloating, constipation, abdominal pain
Amenorrhea (absence of menstruation)
Growth of fine babylike hair over body
Abnormal taste sensations
Osteoporosis
Depression
Sudden death

Related to Purging
Abnormal levels of crucial chemicals
Inflammation of the salivary glands and pancreas
Erosion of the esophagus and stomach
Severe abdominal pain
Erosion and decay of dental enamel, particularly of front teeth
Fatigue and weakness
Seizures

Sources: Hales, Robert, et al. *American Psychiatric Press Textbook of Psychiatry,* 3rd ed. Washington, DC: American Psychiatric Press, 1998.

---

ally sweets, stopping only because of severe abdominal pain or sleep, or because they are interrupted. Those with *purging* bulimia induce vomiting or take large doses of laxatives to relieve guilt and control their weight. In *non-purging* bulimia, individuals use other means, such as fasting or excessive exercise, to compensate for binges.

According to the DSM-IV, 1 to 3 percent of adolescent and young American women develop bulimia. Some experiment with bingeing and purging for a few months and then stop when they change their social or living situation. Others—an estimated 1 to 3 percent of adolescent and young adult females—develop longer-term bulimia. Among males, this disorder is about one-tenth as common. The average age for developing bulimia is 18.

What Causes Bulimia Nervosa?

Bulimia usually begins after a rigid diet that lasted from several weeks to a year or more. Strict dieting may affect brain chemistry in such a way as to disrupt the normal mechanisms for appetite and satiety. Semi-starvation eventually sets off a binge; bingeing leads to purging. Once dieters realize that vomiting reduces the anxiety triggered by gorging, they no longer fear overeating. When this happens, bingeing may become more frequent and severe until, in time, it becomes an all-purpose way of coping with stress. However, the driving force in this disorder may not be the overeating but the vomiting or laxative use. If individuals felt they couldn't get rid of food, they might not overeat.

Obesity in adolescence may increase the likelihood of bulimia in adulthood. Extremely obese individuals may lose weight by vomiting and not want to stop because they fear regaining it. Sometimes bulimia develops after recovery from anorexia. Purging becomes an alternative way of staying thin.

As with anorexia, bulimia is associated with changes in brain chemistry, particularly low levels of the peptide cholescystokinin, which produces feelings of satiety. The cycle of bingeing and purging seems to wreak havoc on the biological controls that keep weight at a certain level.

Family conflicts, life stresses such as going away to school, and struggles with the transition to independent adulthood also may play a role. Bulimia also may be a symptom of depression. About 20 to 30 percent of those with this problem are chronically depressed; others have a history of depressive episodes. Bulimic individuals also are more likely to experience other problems, including anxiety disorders, substance abuse, and impulse disorders, such as shoplifting (kleptomania) and cutting themselves. A significant percentage of bulimics—from to a quarter to a half, by some estimates—may have been victims of incest, sexual molestation, or rape, but this correlation is controversial.[21]

Recognizing and Treating Bulimia Nervosa

The characteristics of bulimia nervosa include:

- Repeated binge eating.
- A feeling of lack of control over eating behavior.
- Regular reliance on self-induced vomiting, laxatives, or diuretics.
- Strict dieting or fasting, or vigorous exercise, to prevent weight gain.
- A minimum average of two bingeing episodes a week for at least three months.
- A preoccupation with body shape and weight.

Bulimia may continue for many years, with binges alternating with periods of normal eating. Often dentists are the first to detect bulimia because they notice damage to teeth and gums, including erosion of the enamel from the stomach acids in vomit. Repeated vomiting can lead to other complications as it robs the body of essential nutrients and fluids, causes dehydration and electrolyte imbalances, and impairs the ability of the heart and other muscles to function. Bulimia can trigger cardiac arrhythmias and, occasionally, sudden death.

Most mental health professionals treat bulimia with a combination of nutritional counseling, psychodynamic, cognitive-behavioral therapy, individual or group psychotherapy, and medication. The drug most often prescribed is an antidepressant medication such as Prozac or fluoxetine, which increases levels of the neurotransmitter serotonin. About 70 percent of those who complete treatment programs reduce their bingeing and purging, although flareups are common in times of stress.

Being Overweight or Obese

The federal government has developed clinical guidelines, first released in 1998, that have changed the meaning of what it means to be overweight or obese. Based on the most extensive review ever of the scientific evidence, the guidelines shift focus away from body weight—the numbers on the scale—to body mass index (BMI), waist circumference, and individual risk factors for diseases and conditions associated with obesity.[22]

The guidelines define "overweight" as a BMI of 25 to 29.9 and "obese" as a BMI of 30 and above (see Figure 7-1). According to these definitions, a person with a BMI of 30 is about 30 pounds overweight—the equivalent of 221 pounds in a 6-foot person or 186 pounds in someone who is 5 foot 6 inches. As noted earlier, very muscular individuals may have a high BMI yet not be overweight or obese.

The risk for cardiovascular and other disease rises significantly in individuals with BMIs above 25; the risk of premature death increases when BMI reaches 30 or above. As BMI levels rise, average blood pressure and total cholesterol levels increase, and average "good" or HDL cholesterol decline. Men in the highest obesity category have more than twice the risk of hypertension, high blood cholesterol, or both compared with men whose BMI's are

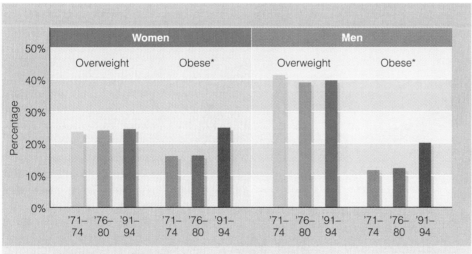

Overweight is defined as 25 to just under 30 pounds over the recommended weight for a person's height. **Obese** is defined as 30 pounds or more over the recommended weight for a person's height.

*Figures for obesity do not include figures for people who are overweight.

■ Figure 7-1 **Overweight Americans**
According to the most recent government survey, 55 percent of the adult population (97 million people) is overweight or obese, with the figures for obesity having grown sharply since the previous survey. Above are the breakdowns for men and women.

Source: National Heart, Lung and Blood Institute. Reprinted by permission of *The New York Times.*

in the healthy range. Women in the highest obesity category have four times the risk.[23]

In addition to BMI, individuals also should be aware of any other risk factors, such as a family history of obesity-related disease, and discuss them with a physician. These additional risks may require more vigilance about weight and more intensive efforts to keep BMI in a healthy range.

Although more people in certain regions of the country are likely to be heavy, obesity affects all racial and ethnic groups. A third of white American women are obese—as are nearly 50 percent of African-American and Mexican-American women. In some Native American communities, up to 70 percent of all adults are dangerously overweight. Differences in metabolic rates may be one factor.[24]

Weight Problems in Children and Adolescents

Youngsters of both sexes are getting heavier. According to estimates from the Centers for Disease Control and Prevention, 10 to 15 percent of American children are overweight. In one study of more than 18,000 children ages 10 to 14, boys and girls of all ethnic backgrounds had higher weights and body mass indexes than their counterparts did a decade before. They also had higher blood pressures, a troubling trend because elevated pressure often continues into adulthood, increasing the risk of hypertension and heart disease.[25] Another major investigation, the Bogalusa Heart Study, found that over half of overweight children and adolescents had at least one additional risk factor for heart disease, such as elevated total cholesterol or high blood pressure readings.[26] Researchers also have found that accumulation of excess abdominal fat in childhood and adolescence increases the risk of this dangerous pattern of fat storage later in life.[27]

Preventing childhood obesity has become a national health priority. Starting early may be the key. According to recent research, babies who are breast-fed have a lower risk of becoming obese. In one study, the overall rate of obesity among children breast-fed during infancy was half that of children who were bottle-fed. In those breast-fed for at least six months, the risks of being overweight or obese were reduced by more than 30 to 40 percent.[28] Another common risk factor for childhood obesity is physical inactivity. However, its effects are reversible—with moderate exercise. In one study, eight weeks of exercise led to beneficial changes in teenagers' body composition.[29]

Waist-Hip Ratio: Apples Versus Pears

The distribution of weight and the location of excess fat also are important. Excess weight around the abdominal area, creating an "apple shaped" silhouette, is associated with increased cardiovascular risk for both men and women.[30] A waist circumference of over 40 inches in men and over 35 inches in women signifies an increased risk in those with BMIs over 25.

Many women accumulate excess pounds in their hips and thighs, giving them a "pear" shape. This fat, stored primarily for special purposes such as pregnancy and nursing, is

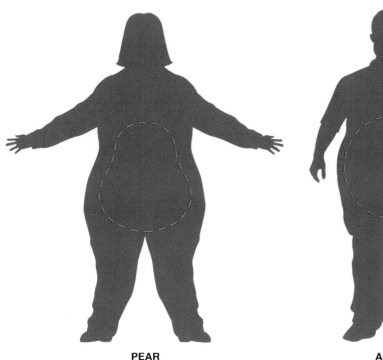
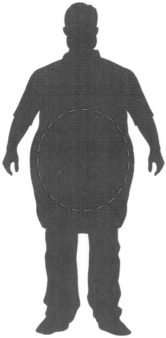

PEAR
Fat stores around hips
predominate

APPLE
Fat stores around waist
predominate

■ Figure 7-2 **Pear versus Apple Shaped Bodies**

more difficult to lose. When men and women diet, men lose more visceral fat located around the abdominal area. This produces more cardiovascular benefits for men, including a decrease in triglycerides (fats circulating in the blood) and an increase in the "good" form of cholesterol, high-density lipoprotein (HDL).[31]

What Causes Obesity?

Are some people fated to be fat? Scientists have identified a gene for a protein that signals the brain to halt food intake or to step up metabolic rate to make use of extra calories. If this gene is defective or malfunctions, it could contribute to weight problems. The discovery of a genetic predisposition to excess weight could explain, at least in part, why children with obese parents tend to be obese themselves, especially if both parents are obese.[32] A protein named leptin also may play a role. When laboratory mice are injected with high doses of leptin, they initially decrease their food intake, increase their metabolic rate, and become much thinner. Eventually, the body adapts to the high levels of leptin and becomes resistant to its effects. However, human studies have had contradictory results.[33] Some suggest that increased leptin does not cause, but is caused by, obesity.[34]

Yet genes are not the sole culprits. As scientists now realize, obesity is a complex and serious disorder with multiple causes. These include

- *Developmental factors.* Some obese people have a high number of fat cells, others have large fat cells, and the most severely obese have both more *and* larger fat cells. Whereas the size of fat cells can increase at any time in life, the number is set during childhood, possibly as the result of genetics or overfeeding at a young age.

- *Social determinants.* In affluent countries, people in lower socioeconomic classes tend to be more obese. For reasons unknown, those in the upper classes, who can afford as much food as they want, tend to be leaner. Education may be one factor; another is that a healthy, nonfattening diet with plenty of fresh fruits and vegetables is more expensive.

- *Physical activity.* Obesity tends to go with a sedentary lifestyle. In those countries where many people tend to work at physically demanding jobs, obesity is rare. Physical activity prevents obesity by increasing caloric expenditure, decreasing food intake, and increasing metabolic rate.

- *Emotional influences.* Obese people are neither more nor less psychologically troubled than others. Psychological problems, such as irritability, depres-

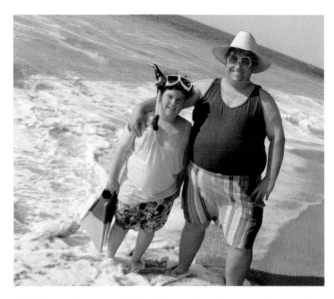

Obesity tends to run in families, so heredity may play a role in your weight. But environment and behavior also play roles: If you choose to eat high-calorie, high-fat foods, you're likely to become overweight.

sion, and anxiety, are more likely to be the result of obesity than the cause. However, emotions do play some role in weight problems. Just as some people reach for a drink or a drug when they're upset, others cope by overeating, bingeing, or purging.

- *Lifestyle.* People who watch more than three hours of TV a day are twice as likely to be obese as those who watch less than an hour. Even those who log between one and two hours are fatter than those who watch just one. Researchers don't know if TV watching causes obesity or if obese people watch more TV, but they have found that the more TV that viewers watch, the less physically active and fit they are.

The Dangers of Obesity

Obesity has long been singled out as a major health threat that increases the risk of many chronic diseases. Obese people have three times the normal incidence of high blood pressure and diabetes. Very heavy women have a threefold higher risk of heart attack and chronic chest pain than very lean women. Excess weight in women has been linked with an increased incidence of high blood pressure, ovarian cancer, and breast cancer. Obese men have an increased chance of heart disease and cancer of the colon, rectum, and prostate. If overweight individuals have surgery, they're more likely to develop complications. Even relatively small amounts of excess fat—as little as 5 pounds—can add to the dangers in those already at risk for hypertension and diabetes. Obesity also causes alterations in various measures of immune function.[35]

In our calorie-conscious and thinness-obsessed society, obesity can be a heavy psychological burden and is often seen as a sign of failure, laziness, or inadequate willpower. As a result, overweight men and women often blame themselves for becoming heavy, and feel guilty and depressed as a result. In fact, the psychological problems once considered the cause of obesity may be its consequence.

Does obesity lead to a shorter life? The answer is far from clear—and intensely controversial. Studies have shown that overweight middle-aged men and women have a higher risk of dying from all causes, especially from heart disease and certain cancers, than those who are normal weight or underweight. Among men who have smoked, the risk of dying is almost two times higher for those with the highest body weight than for those with the lowest body weight. Researchers have found an association between greater Body Mass Index and higher death rates. However, the relative risk of being heavy declines with age.[36]

In responding to such findings, some experts have argued that the data linking overweight and death are "limited, fragmentary, and inconclusive" and that doctors may campaign against obesity because of a tendency to "medicalize behavior" they do not approve of. In some cases, they note, the means to which individuals turn in their attempts to lose weight may be riskier than any dangers posed by the excess pounds they

carry.[37] However, other experts counter that obesity indirectly contributes to as many as 318,000 deaths a year.[38] What is even less clear is the actual danger of being mildly to moderately overweight.

 ## How Can I Overcome a Weight Problem?

Each year an estimated 15 to 35 percent of Americans go on a diet, but no matter how much weight they lose, 95 percent gain it back within five years.[39] Most dieters cut back on food, not because they want to *feel* better, but because they want to *look* better. Individuals who drastically reduce their food intake and make weight loss a major part of their lives may be jeopardizing their physical and psychological well-being.

The best approach to a weight problem depends on how overweight a person is. For extreme obesity, medical treatments, including surgery, may be necessary to overcome the danger to a person's health and life. People who are moderately or mildly obese can lose weight through different approaches, including behavioral modification (monitoring food intake, altering eating style, avoiding eating "triggers," and similar strategies); cognitive therapy (changing thoughts or beliefs that lead to overeating); and social support (participating in groups such as Overeaters Anonymous).[40] The keys to overcoming obesity are acknowledging biological limits, addressing individual differences, altering unrealistic expectations, and individualizing treatment. (See Pulsepoints: "Top Ten Ways to Lose Weight.")

Severe Obesity

A BMI higher than 40 (or higher than 35 for those with other conditions) indicates a life-threatening condition. Because of the medical dangers they face, some severely obese men and women, as a last resort, may undergo surgery to reduce the volume of their stomachs and to tighten the passageway from the stomach to the intestine. Others opt for a "gastric bubble," a soft, polyurethane sac placed in the stomach to make the person feel full while following a low-calorie diet. It is not yet clear whether people who lose weight with this bubble will be able to keep it off. Diet pills, discussed later in this chapter, are another treatment approach.

Mild to Moderate Obesity

For individuals with a BMI of 30 to 39, doctors recommend a six-month trial of "lifestyle therapy," including a supervised diet and exercise. The initial goal should be a 10 percent reduction in weight, an amount that

---

Strategies *for* Change

Building Better Body Image

Here are some ways of improving your body esteem if you're overweight:

✔ Don't put off special plans until you reach a certain magical weight: do what you want to do now.

✔ Start being the person you want to be—your body will catch up with you.

✔ Focus on the parts of your body you like. Maybe you have beautiful brown eyes or powerful shoulders.

✔ Don't put yourself down or joke about your weight.

✔ Treat yourself with the respect you'd like to receive from others.

✔ Try new activities. Don't let weight loss be the center of your life. Take up folk dancing, sailing, gardening, or some other hobby. And the more active your new interest, the better.

PULSE *points*

Top Ten Ways to Lose Weight

1. **Take charge of your weight.** Successful dieters often simply decide that they no longer are going to be fat.

2. **Make a commitment.** Join a group, such as an on-campus support group.

3. **Bite and write.** As an exercise, for a week, record every morsel that goes into your mouth. Reread your diary to find out what, how much, when, and where you eat—and why.

4. **Don't skip meals.** People who eat three meals a day burn off 10% more calories than meal skippers.

5. **Snack sensibly.** Avoid high-fat snack foods. Reach for plain popcorn, rice cakes, vegetables, and fruit instead.

6. **Eat at a moderate pace.** Slow down and savor each bite. And avoid that second helping—the "little bit more" you don't really need.

7. **Narrow your options.** While you should eat an assortment of food, be wary of too many tempting tastes at one meal. We eat more when offered many different foods at once.

8. **Graze, don't gorge.** Spread calorie intake over the day rather than stuffing yourself at any one meal. Potential payoffs include better performance, greater stamina, and less likelihood of a weight gain.

9. **Get a buddy.** If you want to lose weight, don't go it alone. Dieters who double up with a friend or spouse lose more weight and are more likely to keep it off.

10. **Move it and lose it.** Don't lie down when you can sit; don't sit when you can stand; don't stand when you can walk; don't walk when you can run. The more active you are, the more calories you use up.

---

reduces obesity-related risks. With success and if warranted, individuals can attempt to lose more weight.

Weight loss drugs approved by the FDA also may be part of a comprehensive weight management program for the moderately obese. However, drug safety and effectiveness beyond one year of total treatment have not been established.

Overweight

Rather than going on low-calorie diets, people with BMIs of 25 to 29 should cut back moderately on their food intake and concentrate on developing healthy eating and exercise habits. Many moderately to mildly overweight people turn to national organizations such as Weight Watchers, or to other commercial weight-loss groups. Most of these programs offer behavior-modification techniques, inspirational lectures, and carefully designed nutritional programs, but dropout rates are high. As many as half the members drop out in six weeks.

A Practical Guide to Weight Management

Even experienced dieters who've tried dozens of ways of losing weight often know little about the most effective ways to shed pounds and keep them off. (See Self-Survey: "Do You Know How to Lose Weight?") In studies of successful dieters, those who were highly motivated, who monitored their food intake, increased their activity, set realistic goals, and received social support from others were most likely to lose weight. Another key to long-term success is tailoring any weight-loss program to an individual's gender, lifestyle, and cultural, racial, and ethnic values.[41]

A Customized Weight-Loss Plan

"If there's one thing we've learned in decades of research into weight management, it's that the one-diet-fits-all approach doesn't work," says clinical psychologist David Schlundt of Vanderbilt University.[42] The key is recognizing the ways you tend to put on weight and developing strategies to overcome them. Here are some examples:

- Do you simply like food and consume lots of it? If so, keep a diary of everything you put in your mouth and tally up your daily total in calories and fat grams. The numbers may stun you. Look for where most of the calories come from—probably high-fat foods such as whole milk, chocolate, cookies, fried foods, potato chips, steaks—and cut down on how much and how often you eat them.

- Do you eat when you're bored, sad, frustrated, or worried? If so, you may be especially susceptible to "cues" that trigger eating. "People get in the habit of using food to soothe bad feelings or cope with boredom,"

Self-*Survey* Do You Know How to Lose Weight?

When it comes to weight control, willpower isn't enough: A sound knowledge of exercise, nutrition, and healthy eating behavior is essential. To test your weight-loss know-how, try this quiz, which was developed by Dr. Kelly Brownell, director of the Yale University Center for Eating and Weight Disorders.

Instructions:

In each section, mark the statements True or False.

Section I: Nutrition

1. The calorie is a measure of the amount of fat in a food. _____
2. If you eat an equal number of servings from each of the five food groups in the Food Guide Pyramid, you'll get a balanced diet. _____
3. The recommended daily intake of dietary fat is 30 percent or less of total calories. _____
4. Carbohydrates aren't as important as other nutrients are, and they should make up only about 30 percent of your daily diet. _____
5. One gram of fat contains more than twice the calories of one gram of carbohydrate or protein. _____

Section II: Behavior

1. Keeping a daily record of what you eat is essential for weight loss. _____
2. Ordering à la carte at restaurants is a better idea than ordering package meals. _____
3. It's best to take all of what you'll eat in one serving so that you won't need additional helpings. _____
4. When you're trying to lose weight, it's a good idea to go food shopping when you're hungry so you can test your willpower. _____
5. Controlling how much you eat at a special event is easier if you eat a low-calorie snack before you go. _____

Section III: Exercise

1. Walking one mile burns almost as many calories as running one mile. _____
2. Exercise can help keep you from losing muscle tissue when you're trying to lose weight. _____
3. Climbing stairs requires more energy per minute— and therefore burns more calories per minute—than many more popular forms of exercise, such as swimming or jogging. _____
4. No exercise can help you lose fat in specific parts of the body. _____
5. Exercise must be done in specific amounts—say, at least 30 minutes at a stretch—to help you lose weight. _____

Section IV: Myths

1. The most important factor in weight reduction is discovering the psychological roots of your weight problem. _____

2. There's no such thing as a slow or underactive metabolism. _____
3. Since excess dietary fat has been linked to heart disease and other health problems, it's best to eliminate all fat from your diet. _____
4. Eating quickly helps you enjoy food more because your taste buds get more stimulation. _____
5. The calorie level necessary to lose weight is the same for all people. _____

Answers

Section I: Nutrition

1. **False.** The calorie is a measure of the energy your body gets from a food. Fat supplies some of the calories in some foods, but so do carbohydrates and protein.
2. **False.** You should eat the following every day: 2 to 3 servings of dairy products; 2 to 3 servings of meat, poultry or other high-protein foods (fish, beans, eggs, and nuts); 2 to 4 servings of fruit; 3 to 5 servings of vegetables; and 6 to 11 servings of breads and cereals (including rice and pasta).
3. **True.** If you follow the Food Guide Pyramid, you should be able to keep your fat calories under 30 percent.
4. **False.** Carbohydrates should make up the largest portion of your daily diet (between 55 and 60 percent of total calories).
5. **True.** One gram of fat contains nine calories, while one gram of carbohydrate or protein contains only four calories.

Section II: Behavior

1. **True.** People who have lost weight and kept it off generally report that record keeping was one key to their success.
2. **True.** If you order a package meal—say, a hamburger with french fries and coleslaw—you'll probably end up with more calories than you want or need.
3. **False.** It's best to take one portion at a time, because it interrupts the tendency to eat without thinking and gives you time to consider whether you really need more food.
4. **False.** Shopping on an empty stomach is asking for trouble. You'll do less impulse buying if you shop *after* eating.
5. **True.** Eating a low-calorie food before you go will take the edge off your hunger and help you resist

the high-calorie snacks, such as chips and nuts, typically served at parties.

Section III: Exercise

1. **True.** How far you go is more important than how fast you go, so walking helps with weight control.
2. **True.** Exercise can prevent muscle loss while maximizing fat loss. For weight loss, exercise combined with dieting is preferable to dieting alone.
3. **True.** Climbing stairs is an excellent way to burn calories.
4. **True.** You can reduce fat in general, but you cannot dictate where it will come off.
5. **False.** Any amount of exercise helps, so do what you can.

Section IV: Myths

1. **False.** Psychological problems are at the root of some, but not all, cases of overweight. And there's no evidence that uncovering these causes helps with weight loss.
2. **False.** There are wide variations in metabolic rate—how fast calories are used by the body for energy—among different people.
3. **False.** Fat plays an important role in the body, including protecting vital organs and preventing excessive heat loss, so it shouldn't be totally eliminated from your diet.
4. **False.** Your taste buds catch nothing but a blur if the food shoots past. If you slow down, the food will taste better, and you may feel more satisfied and therefore eat less.
5. **False.** There are large differences in how much weight people lose when they have the same caloric intake. Some women, for example, lose weight on 2,000 calories a day while others don't lose any on 1,000.

Scoring

Give yourself one point for each correct answer and total the points for each section.

Section I: Nutrition

5 You're a nutrition nabob! With so many food facts at your fingertips, controlling your weight should be no heavy task.

3 or 4 Your food choices could use a dash more nutrition know-how if you want to keep your weight at a palatable level.

1 or 2 You need to be enlightened on food if you want to scale down.

Section II: Behavior

5 You ain't misbehavin': Your eating and food shopping habits are right on target.

3 or 4 You may want to brush up on your p's and q's: Some of your habits may be hindering your efforts.

1 or 2 If you don't break your bad habits, you'll always be fighting the battle of the bulge.

Section III: Exercise

5 You've got a leg up on controlling your weight.

3 or 4 You should work out the kinks in your workout to help keep your weight in check.

1 or 2 Shape up, or you'll never like the shape of things to come!

Section IV: Myths

5 It's no myth that you know what you're talking about.

3 or 4 Watch out: If you don't separate food fact from food fiction, you may be led astray.

1 or 2 When it comes to weight control, don't believe everything you read.

Making Changes

Long-Term Weight Management

If you decide to change your eating habits in order to lower your weight, try following these steps:

- *Establish your goals.* Subtract your target weight from your actual weight and calculate how long it will take you to lose the difference, based on a weekly loss of 1½ pounds.
- *Never say diet.* Going on a diet implies going off a diet sooner or later.
- *Be realistic.* Trying to shrink to an impossibly low weight dooms you to defeat. Start off slowly and make steady progress. If your weight creeps up 5 pounds, go back to the basics of your program. Take into account normal fluctuations, but watch out for an upward trend. If you let your weight continue to creep up, it may not stop until you have a serious weight problem—again.
- *Recognize that there are no quick fixes.* Ultimately, quick-loss diets are very damaging physically and psychologically because when you stop dieting and put the pounds back on you feel like a failure.
- *Note your progress.* Make a graph, with your initial weight as the base, to indicate your progress. View plateaus or occasional gains as temporary setbacks rather than disasters.
- *Adopt the 90 percent rule.* If you practice good eating habits 90 percent of the time, a few indiscretions won't make a difference. In effect, you should allow for occasional cheating, so that you don't have to feel guilty about it.
- *Try, try again.* Remember, dieters don't usually keep weight off on their first attempt. The people who eventually succeed try various methods until they find the plan that works for them.

Source: American Health, November 1994:29–31.

says Schlundt. "Sometimes the real issue is a self-esteem or body-image problem." Dealing with these concerns is generally more helpful in the long run than dieting.

- Do you "graze," nibbling on snacks rather than eating regular meals? If so, limit yourself to low-calorie, low-fat foods, like carrots, celery, grapes, or air-popped popcorn. Take sips of water regularly to freshen your mouth. Even if you're only having a few crackers or carrots, put them on a plate, and try to eat in the same place, preferably while seated. This helps you break the habit of putting food in your mouth without thinking.

How Can I Avoid Diet Traps?

Whatever your eating style, there are only two effective strategies for losing weight: eating less and exercising more. Unfortunately, most people search for easier alternatives that almost invariably turn into dietary dead ends. The following are among the most common traps to avoid.

Diet Foods

According to the Calorie Control Council, 90 percent of Americans choose some foods labeled "light." But even though these foods keep growing in popularity, Americans' weight keeps rising. There are several rea-

sons: Many people think choosing a food that's lower in calories, fat-free, or "light" gives them a license to eat as much as they want. What they don't realize is that many foods that are low in fat are still high in sugar and calories. Refined carbohydrates, rapidly absorbed into the bloodstream, raise blood glucose levels. As they fall, appetite increases.[43]

What about the artificial sweeteners and fake fats that appear in many diet products? Nutritionists caution to use them in moderation, and not to substitute them for basic foods, such as grains, fruits, and vegetables (see Chapter 6). Foods made with fat substitutes may have fewer grams of fat, but they don't necessarily have significantly fewer calories. Many people who add reduced-fat, fat-free or sugar-free sodas, cookies, chips, and other snacks to their diet often cut back on more nutritious foods, such as fruits and vegetables. They also tend to eat more of low- or no-fat foods so that their daily calorie intake either stays the same or actually increases.[44]

The Yo-Yo Syndrome

On-and-off-again dieting, especially by means of very-low-calorie diets (under 800 calories a day), can be self-defeating and dangerous. Some studies have shown that "weight cycling" may make it more difficult to lose weight or keep it off. Repeated cycles of rapid weight loss followed by weight gain may even change food preferences. Chronic crash dieters often come to

Consumer Health Watch

Consumer Health Watch: Evaluating a Diet

If you hear about a new diet that promises to melt away fat, don't try it until you get answers to the following questions:

- Does it include a wide variety of nutritious foods?
- Does it provide at least 1,200 calories a day?
- Is it designed to reduce your weight by one-half to two pounds per week?
- Does it emphasize moderate portions?
- Does it use foods that are easy to find and prepare?
- Can you follow it wherever you eat—at home, work, restaurants, or parties?
- Is its cost reasonable?

If the answer to any of these questions is no, don't try the diet; then ask yourself one more question: Is losing weight worth losing your well-being?

The National Council Against Health Fraud cautions dieters to watch for warnings of dangerous or fraudulent programs, including:

- Promises of very rapid weight loss.
- Claims that the diet can eliminate "cellulite" (a term used to refer to dimply fatty tissue on the arms and legs).
- "Counselors" who are really salespersons pushing a product or program.
- No mention of any risks associated with the diet.
- Unproven gimmicks, such as body wraps, starch blockers, hormones, diuretics, or "unique" pills or potions.
- No maintenance program.

prefer foods that combine sugar and fat, such as cake frosting.

There is a way to avoid weight cycling and overcome its negative effects: exercise. Researchers at the University of Pennsylvania found that when overweight women who also exercised went off a very-low-calorie diet, their metabolisms did not stay slow but bounced back to the appropriate level for their new, lower body weights.[45] The reason may be exercise's ability to preserve muscle tissue. The more muscle tissue you have, the higher your metabolic rate.

Very-Low-Calorie Diets

Any diet that promises to take pounds off fast can be dangerous. For reasons that scientists don't fully understand, rapid weight loss is linked with increased mortality. Most risky are very-low-calorie diets that provide fewer than 800 calories a day. Whenever people cut back drastically on calories, they immediately lose several pounds because of a loss of fluid. As soon as they return to a more normal way of eating, they regain this weight.

On a very-low-calorie diet, as much as 50 percent of the weight you lose may be muscle (so you'll actually look flabbier). Because your heart is a muscle, it may become so weak that it no longer can pump blood through your body. In addition, your blood pressure may plummet, causing dizziness, lightheadedness, and fatigue. You may develop nausea and abdominal pain. You may lose hair. If you're a woman, your menstrual cycle may become irregular, or you may stop menstruating altogether. As you lose more water, you also lose essential vitamins, and your metabolism slows down. Even reaction time slows, and crash dieters may not be able to respond as quickly as usual.[46]

Once you go off an extreme diet—as you inevitably must—your metabolism remains slow, even though you're no longer restricting your food intake. The human body appears to alter its energy use to compensate for weight loss. These metabolic changes may make it harder for people to maintain a reduced body weight after dieting.

Diet Pills and Products

In their search for a quick fix to weight problems, millions of people have tried often-risky remedies. In the 1920s, some women swallowed patented weight-loss capsules that turned out to be tapeworm eggs. In the 1960s and 1970s, addictive amphetamines were common diet aids. In the 1990s, appetite suppressants known as fen-phen ("fen" referring to fenfluramine [Pondimin] or dexfenfluramine [Redux], appetite depressants, and "phen" referring to phentermine, a

type of amphetamine) became popular. They were taken off the market after being linked to heart valve problems.

Many people rely on meal replacements, usually shakes or snack bars, to lose or keep off weight. If used appropriately—as actual replacements rather than supplements to regular meals and snacks—they can be a useful strategy for weight loss.[47]

More weight-loss drugs have won FDA approval, including Meridia (sibutramine) and Xenical (orlistat). Both are intended only for people with a BMI of at least 30 or a BMI of 27 and additional risk factors.

Unlike fenfluramine and Redux, which fooled patients into feeling full by boosting production of the brain chemical serotonin, Meridia slows the body's dissipation of the serotonin it naturally produces. The FDA describes Meridia as "moderately effective" at helping obese people shed pounds—in studies, they lost about 7 to 11 more pounds than mere dieters—but it can cause increases in blood pressure and pulse rate that may endanger certain patients. No one who has poorly controlled hypertension, heart disease, or an irregular heartbeat or who has survived a stroke should use the drug. Meridia users should not only see a doctor for regular blood pressure but should also check themselves regularly with an at-home blood pressure monitor.

Xenical is the first drug in a new class known as lipase inhibitors, which work by preventing gastrointestinal and pancreatic enzymes from breaking down fat for absorption by the body. Combined with a supervised diet, it has proven effective in promoting weight loss, lessening weight re-gain, and improving some obesity-related risk factors.[48] Its long-term effects are unknown.[49] Wellbutrin (bupropion), an antidepressant and anti-smoking drug, also has shown potential for weight loss. In one study women who took the drug and followed a moderate-calorie diet lost four times more weight than women taking a placebo and following the same diet.[50]

Although available only by prescription, Xenical and Meridia are being marketed over the Internet to anyone who fills out a computerized form reviewed by a company doctor. As a result, many people are taking this medication without medical supervision. Such misuse could cause health risks. Xenical causes side effects, including bloating, flatulence, diarrhea, and fecal incontinence. Because it blocks absorption of the fat-soluble vitamins A, D, E and K, a daily vitamin supplement is necessary. And there may be additional risks for individuals with eating disorders.[51]

The search for the perfect diet drug continues—with plenty of economic incentives for drug makers. By some estimates, the potential market for weight-loss pills totals at least $5 billion. Other diet products, including diet sodas and low-fat foods, also are a very big business. Yet people who use these products aren't necessarily sure to slim down. In fact, people who consume such products often gain weight because they think that they can afford to add high-calorie treats to their diet.

Liquid Diets

Liquid diets, such as Optifast, Medifast, and other programs, supply 420 to 800 calories a day and include sufficient protein to preserve muscle tissue. For several months, dieters on these plans eat no solid food, consuming only the special liquid formula and water. These extreme diets, generally reserved for those at least 40 percent or more overweight, do result in rapid loss, but they can be hazardous.

Today's liquid diets contain more protein, carbohydrates, vitamins, and minerals than the formulas that led to at least 58 deaths in the late 1970s. However, programs that rely solely on liquid formulas should be supervised by a doctor or hospital that provides weekly screening of blood pressure, heart function, electrolyte levels, urine content, and potassium—all indicators of how the body is coping without real food. The side effects of liquid diets include dry skin, hair loss, constipation, gum disease, sensitivity to cold, and mood swings. Only 10 to 20 percent of those who enroll in liquid-diet programs manage to stay within ten pounds of their target weight a year and a half after entering the program.

Exercise: The Best Solution

You may think that exercise will make you want to eat more. Actually, it has the opposite effect. The combination of exercise and cutting back on calories may be the most effective way of taking weight off and keeping it off. As research has shown, exercise keeps your metabolic rate up while you're dieting—and afterward. Exercise, along with a healthy diet, can lead to weight losses of up to 10 pounds.

Exercise has other benefits: it increases energy expenditure, builds up muscle tissue, burns off fat stores, and stimulates the immune system.[52] Exercise also may reprogram metabolism so that individuals burn up more calories during and after a workout. (See Chapter 5 for a complete discussion of exercise.)

Moderate physical activity also can help control weight. Recent studies have found that everyday activities, such as walking, gardening, and heavy household chores, are as effective as a structured exercise program in maintaining or losing weight.[53] Scientists use the acronym **NEAT**—for **non-exercise activity thermogenesis**—to

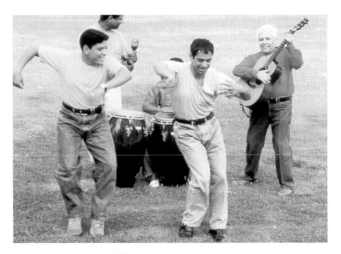

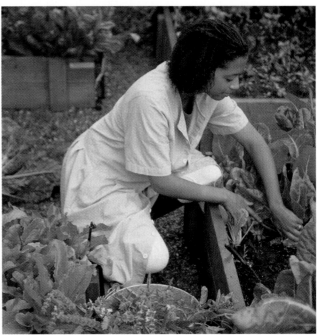

Exercise isn't just tennis or jogging. You can increase your daily exercise by such simple changes as taking the stairs instead of the escalator. Walking, gardening, hiking, and other not-so-strenuous activities can provide enjoyment as well as exercise.

describe such "non-volitional" movements and have verified that it can be an effective way of burning calories. In a study of 16 nonobese adults, "intentional" exercise and metabolic rate had little effect on variations in weight gain, whereas NEAT did.[54] One form of NEAT, fidgeting, turns out to play a more important role in daily energy expenditure—and may be particularly useful in preventing weight gain after overeating.[55]

Once you start an exercise program, keep it up. Individuals who've started an exercise program during or after a weight-loss program are consistently more successful in keeping off most of the pounds they've shed.

Strategies *for* Change

Working Off Weight

✓ *Get moving.* Take the stairs instead of the elevator. Get off the bus a few blocks from your home and walk the rest of the way.

✓ *Walk.* Most people find it hard to make excuses for not walking 15 minutes every day. Once you start, increase gradually so that you go farther and faster.

✓ *Exercise daily.* You're more likely to lose and keep weight off if you exercise regularly. Try to burn 1,800 to 2,000 calories a week through exercise—the equivalent of 18 to 20 miles of walking or jogging.

✓ *Get physical.* There are more ways to burn calories than traditional exercise activities: Dancing, hiking, gardening can all help you get in shape. Check your campus bulletin boards and newspapers for information on rock-climbing, kayaking, skiing, and other fun forms of working out.

Making This Chapter Work for You

Weighing In for a Healthy Future

■ According to recent government statistics, 97 million Americans are overweight or obese.

■ Weight has become a central preoccupation in many people's lives. However, an obsession with appearance can be dangerous to physical and psychological well-being. People who want to look or be thinner may develop unhealthy eating behaviors, such as extreme dieting and bingeing, that can undermine their health and diminish their self-esteem.

■ Many factors determine what a person should weigh: heredity, eating behavior, food selection, amount of daily exercise. The federal government defines healthy weights in terms of body mass index (BMI), a standard method for assessing the ratio of a person's weight to height. A BMI of 19 to 25 is considered a "healthy weight target" and poses a minimal risk to your health, but a BMI higher than 26 begins to increase your risk for a variety of serious health problems. A BMI of 25 to 29.9 is considered overweight while 30 or above is considered obese.

■ The number of calories you need every day depends on your gender, age, size, and activity level. An "average" adult woman—with a median height of 5 feet 4 inches and a weight of 138 pounds—generally needs 1,900 to 2,200 calories. An average man—with a median height of 5 feet 10 inches and a weight of 174 pounds—generally needs 2,300 to 2,900 calories.

■ Hunger, the physiological drive to consume food, stimulates our appetite or desire for food. We stop eating when we achieve a state of satisfaction called satiety. According to the set-point theory, each individual has an unconscious control system for regulating appetite and satiety to keep body fat at a predetermined level, or set point.

■ Unhealthy eating behaviors, such as extreme or chronic dieting, compulsive overeating, and binge eating (the rapid consumption of an abnormally large amount of food in a relatively short time) can be early warning signals of more serious eating disorders.

■ The eating disorders anorexia nervosa and bulimia nervosa are most common among young women.

■ The causes of anorexia nervosa are complex; genetic, biochemical, and developmental factors may play a role. Its consequences include extreme weight loss, cessation of menstrual periods in women, decline in testosterone levels in men, heart irregularities, and arrhythmias that can increase the risk of sudden death. Because of their fear of fatness, many people with this disorder resist seeking help. A combination of medical therapy and psychotherapy can lead to recovery.

■ Individuals with bulimia nervosa go on repeated eating binges and rapidly consume large amounts of food, usually sweets. Those with purging-type bulimia induce vomiting or take large doses of laxatives to control their weight. Individuals with non-purging bulimia use other means, such as fasting or excessive exercise, to compensate for binges. Complications include damaged tooth enamel, dehydration, electrolyte imbalance, cardiac arrhythmias, and even sudden death. Most mental health professionals treat bulimia with a combination of nutritional counseling, psychotherapy, and medication.

■ People gain weight whenever they take in more calories than they burn off. Many different factors contribute to obesity, including heredity, environment, culture, and development.

■ A person's waist-hip ratio can indicate health risks. Abdominal fat seems more dangerous than fat stored on the hips, thighs, and buttocks. The bigger the waist and belly, the higher the risk of various diseases, such as diabetes, heart disease, and stroke.

■ Obese people are at risk for developing high blood pressure, diabetes, heart disease, certain kinds of cancer, and other life-threatening conditions. Severely obese people can be treated by stomach reduction surgery and medications; moderately and mildly obese individuals do best with diet, exercise, and behavior modification.

■ In studies of successful dieters, those who were highly motivated, who monitored their food intake, set realistic goals, and received social support from others were most likely to lose weight.

■ Many people fall into diet traps, such as an overreliance on low or reduced fat and other "light" foods, a pattern of off-and-on or yo-yo dieting, very-low-calorie diets, appetite suppressants, diet aids (such as gum, powders, or potions, and low- or no-calorie soft drinks and snacks), and liquid diets.

■ Exercise in combination with diet is the most effective means of losing excess pounds and keeping them off. Exercise increases energy expenditure, builds up muscle tissue and burns off fat stores. Exercise and other forms of activity also may reprogram your metabolism so that you burn up more calories during and after a workout.

 New Weight Loss Drugs. How do drugs like Xenical and phentermine work?

health **/ ONLINE**

Body Mass Index Calculator
http://www.shapeup.org/bmi/index.html
This site instantly calculates your body mass index and explains the health implications associated with your BMI.

Weight-Control Information Network
http://www.niddk.nih.gov/health/nutrit/win.htm
The Weight-Control Information Network provides online publications on several weight-related topics, including binge eating, dieting, and obesity treatment. It also includes information about university-based eating disorder programs and services by state.

American Anorexia Bulimia Association
http://www.aabainc.org/
This site contains general information about eating disorders and information on support services for eating disorder sufferers, family/friends, and professionals.

Please note that links are subject to change. If you find a broken link, use a search engine like **http://www.yahoo.com** *and search for the web site by typing in key words.*

 Campus Chat: What factors do you think lead to eating disorders? How would you help a friend who was suffering from an eating disorder? Share your thoughts on our online discussion forum at **http://health.wadsworth.com**

Find It On InfoTrac: You can find additional readings related to health via InfoTrac College Edition, an online library of more than 900 journals and publications. Follow the instructions for accessing InfoTrac that came packaged with your textbook; then search for articles using a key word search.

• **Suggested article:** "Gender Differences in Weight Reduction," *Nutrition Research Newsletter,* Vol. 18, Issue 2, p. 2(1), February 1999.
  (1) According to the research, in what parts of the body do men lose body fat to a greater extent when compared to women?
  (2) Why do men lose more weight and body fat when dieting than do women, after adjusting for all other variables?

For additional links, resources, and suggested readings on InfoTrac, visit our Health & Wellness Resource Center at **http://health.wadsworth.com**

Key Terms

The terms listed here are used within the chapter. Page numbers are included for each term. A definition of each term is given in the Glossary pages at the end of this book.

anorexia nervosa   202
appetite   198
basal metabolic rate (BMR)   198
binge eating   201
body mass index (BMI)   196
bulimia nervosa   204

calorie   197
eating disorders   201
hunger   198
hydrostatic weighing   197
non-exercise activity thermogenesis
   (NEAT)   214

obese   205
obesity   207
satiety   199
set-point theory   199
skin calipers   197
waist-hip ratio   206

Critical Thinking Questions

1. Ask your friends—particularly your women friends—how they feel about their bodies. Chances are they'll mention something they hate: their hair, their hips, their height, and, most often of all, their weight. What do you think leads to such dissatisfaction? What can individuals do to feel better about the way they look?

2. Different cultures have different standards for body weight and attractiveness. Within our society, even men and women often seem to follow different standards. What influences have shaped your personal feelings about desired weight?

3 If you could choose skin calipers or hydrostatic immersion testing, which would you select to determine your body fat? Explain the reasons for your choice.

References

1. NHLBI Communications Office. "First Federal Obesity Clinical Guidelines Released." Bethesda, Md.: National Heart, Lung, and Blood Institute, June 17, 1998.

2. Hales, Dianne. "A Way that Really Works." *Parade Magazine,* October 11, 1998.

3. Franzoi, Stephen, and Virginia Koehler. "Age and Gender Differences in Body Attitudes: A Comparison of Young and Elderly Adults." *International Journal of Aging & Human Development,* Vol. 47, No. 1, July–August 1998.

4. Bovsun, Mara. "Brain Scans Shed Light on Hunger." News release, National Institute of Diabetes and Digestive and Kidney Disease, April 12, 1999.

5. Ellin, Abby. "Their Bodies, Their Selves." *New York Times,* April 4, 1999.

6. Kilpatrick, Marcus, et al. "Adolescent Weight Management and Perceptions: An Analysis of the National Longitudinal Study of Adolescent Health." *Journal of School Health,* Vol. 69, Issue 4, April 1999.

7. Pesa, Jacqueline. "Psychosocial Factors Associated with Dieting Behaviors Among Female Adolescents." *Journal of School Health,* Vol. 69, No. 5, May 1999.

8. O'Dea, Jennifer, and Abraham, Suzanne. "Association Between Self-Concept and Body Weight, Gender and Pubertal Development Among Male and Female Adolescents." *Adolescence,* Vol. 34, No. 133, Spring 1999. Paxton, Susan, et al. "Friendship Clique and Peer Influences on Body Image Concerns, Dietary Restraint, Extreme Weight-Loss Behaviors, and Binge Eating in Adolescent Girls." *Journal of Abnormal Psychology,* Vol. 108, No. 2, May 1999.

9. Halpern, Carolyn Tucker, et al. "Effects of Body Fat on Weight Concerns, Dating, and Sexual Activity: A Longitudinal Analysis of Black and White Adolescent Girls." *Developmental Psychology,* Vol. 35, No. 3, May 1999.

10. Patton, G. C., et al. "Onset of Adolescent Eating Disorders: Population-based Cohort Study over Three Years." *British Medical Journal,* Vol. 318, Issue 7186, March 20, 1999.

11. Hales, Dianne, and Robert E. Hales. *Caring for the Mind.* New York: Bantam Books, 1997.

12. "The Weight of Eating Disorders and Women's Health." *National Women's Health Report,* Vol. 21, No. 2, April 1999.

13. Hubbard, Kim, et al. "Out of Control." *People,* April 12, 1999.

14. Lester, Regan, and Trent Petrie. "Physical, Psychological and Societal Correlates of Bulimic Symptomatology Among African-American College Women." *Journal of Counseling Psychology,* Vol. 45, No. 3, July 1998.

15. Hubbard, Kim, et al. "Out of Control."

16. Lang, Susan. "Obesity, Eating Disorders Discourage College Dates." *Human Ecology Forum,* Vol. 26, No. 4, Fall 1998.

17. Braun, Devra, et al. "More Males Seek Treatment for Eating Disorders." *International Journal of Eating Disorders,* May 1999.

18. Beals, Katharine, and Melinda Manore. "Nutritional Status of Female Athletes with Subclinical Eating Disorders." *Journal of the American Dietetic Association,* Vol. 98, No. 4, April 1998.

19. Turk, Joanne, et al. "Collegiate Coaches' Knowledge of Eating Disorders." *Journal of Athletic Training,* Vol. 34, No. 1, January–March 1999. Vinci, Debra. "Effective Nutrition Support Programs for College Athletes." *International Journal of Sport Nutrition,* Vol. 8, No. 3, September 1998.

20. Hesse-Biber, Sharlene, et al. "A Longitudinal Study of Eating Disorders Among College Women: Factors that Influence Recovery." *Gender & Society,* Vol. 13, No. 3, June 1999.

21. Hales, Dianne, and Robert E. Hales. *Caring for the Mind.*

22. NHLBI Communications Office. "First Federal Obesity Clinical Guidelines Released."

23. Ibid.

24. Weyer, Christian. "Basal Metabolic Rate in African-American Women." *Journal of Clinical Nutrition,* July 1999.

25. Luepker, Russell. "Adolescent Weights, Blood Pressure Rising." *Journal of Pediatrics,* Vol. 134, June 1999.

26. Hensley, Tim. "New Study Finds Overweight Children and Adolescents Are at Risk for Cardiovascular Problems." New release, CDC Division of Nutrition and Physical Activity, June 4, 1999.

27. Goran, Michael, and Robert Maline. "Fat Distribution During Childhood and Adolescence." *American Journal of Human Biology,* Vol. 11, No. 2, March–April 1999.

28. von Kries, Rudiger, et al. "Breastfeeding Prevents Obesity." *British Medical Journal,* Vol. 319, July 17, 1999.

29. Sadowsky, H. S., et al. "The Effect of Moderate Intensity Exercise on Adolescent Body Composition." *Physical Therapy,* Vol. 79, Issue 5, May 1999.

30. Seidell, Jacob, et al. "Abdominal Adiposity and Risk of Heart Disease." *JAMA,* Vol. 281, No. 24, June 23, 1999. Rexrode, K. M., et al. "Abdominal Adiposity and Coronary Heart Disease in Women." *JAMA,* Vol. 280, 1998.

31. "Gender Differences in Weight Reduction." *Nutrition Research Newsletter,* Vol. 18, Issue 2, February 1999.

32. Magid, Barry. "Is Biology Destiny After All?" *Journal of Psychotherapy Practice & Research,* Vol. 4, No. 1, Winter 1995.

33. Heymsfield, Steven, et al. "Recombinant Leptin for Weight Loss in Obese and Lean Adults." *JAMA,* Vol. 282, No. 16, October 27, 1999.

34. Gaven, Safak. "Plasma Leptin and Insulin Levels in Weight-Reduced Obese Women." *JAMA,* Vol. 282, No. 16, October 27, 1999.

35. Nieman, David, et al. "Influence of Obesity on Immune Function." *Journal of the American Dietetic Association,* Vol. 99, No. 3, March 1999.

36. Bender, Ralf, et al. "Effect of Age on Excess Mortality in Obesity." *JAMA,* Vol. 281, April 28, 1999.

37. Kassirer, Jerome, and Marcia Angell. "Losing Weight: An Ill-fated New Year's Resolution?" *New England Journal of Medicine,* Vol. 338, No. 1, January 1, 1998.

38. Kolata, Gina. "The Fat's in the Fire, Again." *New York Times,* January 11, 1998.

39. Hales, Dianne. "A Way that Really Works."

40. "Weight Management: Maintaining a Healthy Weight." *JAMA,* Vol. 281, January 20, 1999.

41. Mattfeldt-Bernan, Mildred, et al. "Participants' Evaluation of a Weight-Loss Program." *Journal of the American Dietetic Association,* Vol. 99, Issue 1, January 1999.

42 David Schlundt. Personal interview.

43. "Eating Less Fat, More of Some Carbs May Make Us Hungrier, Heavier." *Focus: News from Harvard Medical, Dental and Public Health Schools,* March 19, 1999.

44. Lang, Susan. "Fat and Sugar Substitutes Don't Take Off Weight." Cornell University Press Release, July 8, 1999. Keenan, Debra Palmer, et al. "Factors Perceived to Influence Dietary Fat Reduction Behaviors." *Journal of Nutrition Education,* Vol. 31, No. 3, May–June, 1999.

45. Brownell, K. D., and Judy Rodin. "Medical, Metabolic, and Psychological Effects of Weight Cycling." *Archives of Internal Medicine,* June 27, 1994.

46. "Cutting Calories Too Much Can Slow Reaction Time." *Tufts University Health & Nutrition Letter,* Vol. 14, No. 6, August 1997.

47. Ditschuneit, Herwig, et al. "Are Meal Replacements Effective for Weight Loss Maintenance?" *Nutrition Research Newsletter,* Vol. 18, Issue 4, April 1999.

48. "Another Weight-Loss Drug Approved." *Harvard Women's Health Watch,* Vol. 6, No. 11, July, 1999.

49. "Orlistat Promotes Weight Loss and Keeps It Off for Years." *JAMA,* Vol. 281, January 20, 1999.

50. Voelker, Rebecca. "New Weight Loss Tool." *JAMA,* Vol. 281, No. 24, June 23, 1999.

51. Canedy, Dana. "Almost Anyone Can Easily Get Pill Meant for the Truly Obese." *New York Times,* May 11, 1999.

52. "Dieters, Get Up and Get Moving or Risk Immune Decline." *Environmental Nutrition,* Vol. 22, Issue 3, March 1999.

53. "Moderate Activity Keeps Heart, Waistline in Shape." *Harvard Health Letter,* Vol. 24, No. 7, April 1999.

54. Ravussin, Eric, and Danforth, Eliot. "Beyond Sloth—Physical Activity and Weight Gain." *Science,* Vol. 283, Issue 5399, January 8, 1999.

55. Levine, James, et al. "Role of Nonexercise Activity Thermogenesis in Resistance to Fat Gain in Humans." *Science,* Vol. 283, Issue 5399, January 8, 1999.

III

Responsible Sexuality

Our most special relationships are those that bring us closer to others—our friends, partners, spouses, parents, and children. Such intimacy is the most rewarding and often the most demanding of human involvements. The giving of ourselves to another—sharing thoughts, feelings, experiences, and sexual pleasure—touches the essence of what it means to be human. This section provides a comprehensive philosophical and practical view of relating to others. Each of the chapters focuses on the unique form of personal responsibility involved in every close relationship: a responsibility that looks beyond the self to those we care for and love.

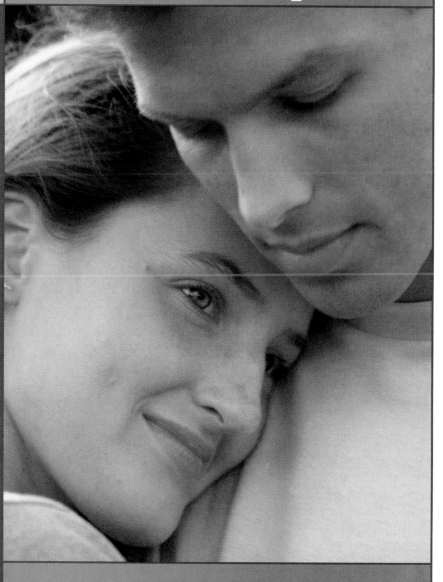

8

Communication and Relationships

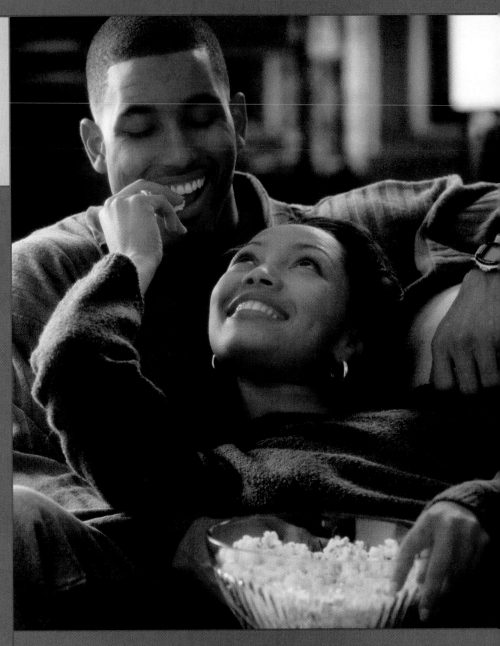

After studying the material in this chapter, you should be able to:

- **Define** friendship and **explain** how friendship grows.
- **Compare** and **contrast** the behavioral expectations for friendship, dating, and mature love.
- **Describe** the typical progress of a relationship from dating to mature love.
- **List** and **explain** three living arrangements today's adults might choose.
- **Explain** how some of the problems likely to affect long-term relationships can be prevented.
- **Name** some of the major issues facing parents in the world today.

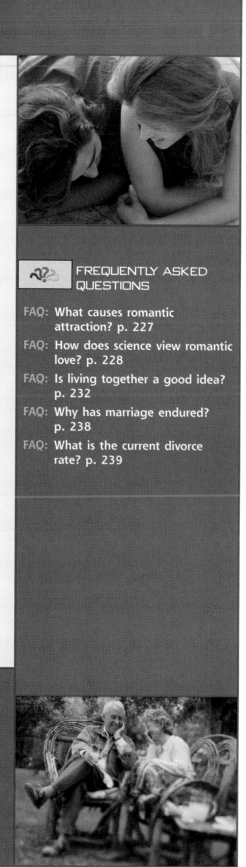

e are born social. From our first days of life, we reach out to others, struggle to express ourselves, strive to forge connections. People make us smile, laugh, cry, hope, dream, pray. The fabric of our personalities and lives becomes richer as others weave through it the threads of their experiences.

How we feel about ourselves affects how others feel about us. But we also must be able to communicate our feelings and needs. Relationships begin with signals: yes, no, and maybe. From the first, we should try to make our signals clear. As we progress to messages, we should try to respond honestly and naturally and to express our feelings as precisely as we can. As individuals and as part of society, we need to care about others and to know that others care about us, to feel for others and have others feel for us, to share what we know and to learn from what others know.

Sending clear messages through words, gestures, expressions, and behaviors is the essence of good communication. The more effectively we communicate, the more likely we are to create good relationships built on honesty, understanding, and mutual trust. Such relationships can infuse our lives with a richness no solitary pleasure can match.

This chapter discusses the social needs we all share, the ways some of us respond to those needs, and the possibilities that exist for coming together from our solitude to warm ourselves in each other's glow of life. ❖

FREQUENTLY ASKED QUESTIONS

FAQ: **What causes romantic attraction? p. 227**

FAQ: **How does science view romantic love? p. 228**

FAQ: **Is living together a good idea? p. 232**

FAQ: **Why has marriage endured? p. 238**

FAQ: **What is the current divorce rate? p. 239**

Personal Communication

Getting to know someone is one of life's greatest challenges and pleasures. When you find another person intriguing—as a friend, as a teacher, as a colleague, as a possible partner—you want to find out as much as you can about him or her and to share more and more information about yourself. Roommates may talk for endless hours. Friends may spend years getting to know each other. Partners in committed relationships may delight in learning new things about each other.

Communication stems from a desire to know and a decision to tell. Each of us chooses what information about ourselves we want to disclose and what we want to conceal or keep private. But in opening up to others, we increase our own self-knowledge and understanding.

Communicating Feelings

A great deal of daily communication focuses on facts: on the who, what, where, when, and how. Information is easy to convey and comprehend. Emotions are not. Some people have great difficulty saying "I appreciate you" or "I care about you," even though they are genuinely appreciative and caring. Others find it hard to know what to say in response and how to accept such expressions of affection.

Some people feel that relationships shouldn't require any effort, that there's no need to talk of responsibility between people who care about each other. Yet responsibility is implicit in our dealings with anyone or anything we value—and what can be more valuable than those with whom we share our lives? Friendships and other intimate relationships always demand an emotional investment, but the rewards they yield are great.

Sometimes people convey strong emotions with a kiss or a hug, a pat or a punch, but such actions aren't precise enough to communicate exact thoughts. Stalking out of a room and slamming the door may be clear signs of anger, but they don't explain what caused the anger or suggest what to do about it. You must learn how to communicate all feelings clearly and appropriately if you hope to become truly close to another person.

As two people build a relationship, they must sharpen their communication skills so that they can discuss all the issues they may confront. They must learn how to communicate anger as well as affection, hurt as well as joy—and they must listen as carefully as they speak. If and when love grows, they will find themselves as concerned with the other as with the self.

Every man and every woman is unique, but researchers who've carefully observed each gender have

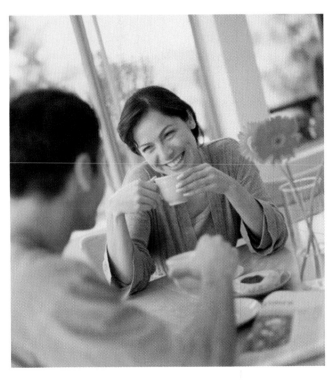

Good communication is essential to a healthy and successful relationship.

observed differences in the way many—but not necessarily all—men and women use language. (See The X & Y Files: "Gender Differences in Communication.")

Strategies *for* Change

How to Enhance Communication

✔ *Use "I" statements.* Describe what's going on with you. Say, "I worry about being liked" or "I get frustrated when I can't put my feelings into words." Avoid generalities such as "You never think about my feelings," or "Nobody understands me."

✔ *Gently ask how the other person feels.* If your friend or partner describes thoughts rather than feelings, ask for more adjectives. Was he or she sad, excited, angry, hurt?

✔ *Become a very good listener.* When another person talks, don't interrupt, ask why, judge, or challenge. Nod your head. Use your body language and facial expression to show you're eager to hear more.

✔ *Respect confidences.* Treat a friend's or partner's secrets with the discretion they deserve. Consider them a special gift entrusted to your care.

The X&Y Files

Gender Differences in Communication

Only recently have scientists begun to explore gender differences in the way women and men use language. In ongoing research, psychologist James Pennebaker of the University of Texas developed a computer program to analyze four 450-word essays by more than 900 university students. The preliminary findings suggest that sex differences in written language are huge—larger, in fact, than many other psychological and personality characteristics.

In writing, women use more words overall, more words related to emotion (positive and negative), more idea words, more hearing, feeling, and sensing words, more causal words, such as *because,* and more modal words (*would, should, could*). Men use more numbers, more prepositions, and more articles, such as *an* and *the, that,* Pennebaker notes, "make language more concrete." Women use more question marks, more pronouns (especially *I*), and more references to other people. Men use more body words and, even in an academic assignment, twice as many swear words. Women write more about the past and present; males mention the future more often. Women use more motion words and more occupational words related to either school or work and write more about home. Men write more about sports, TV, and money.

When men and women speak, other gender differences emerge. In her insightful studies of language, linguist Deborah Tannen has noted that men speak more often and for longer periods in public, often as a way of putting themselves in a "one-up" situation; women speak more in private, usually to build better connections to others. In a male's hierarchical social order, she explains, conversations "are negotiations in which people try to achieve and maintain the upper hand if they can and protect themselves from others' attempts to put them down and push them around." To women, who see the world as a network of connectedness, conversations are something else entirely: "negotiations for closeness in which people try to seek and give confirmation and support, and to reach consensus." While men use words to preserve independence, women talk to draw others closer.

Perhaps this is why, in public and private, women generally are better listeners, "facilitating" conversation by nodding, asking questions, and signaling interest by saying "uh-huh," or "yes." Men interrupt more, breaking in on another's monologue if they aren't getting the information they need. Women are more likely to wait for the speaker to finish. "There's more than one interpretation for why a woman is less likely to interrupt," says psychologist Judith Hall. "It could show that she's being submissive and not playing the aggressive role. But it also could mean that she is less of a social blunderer and is more adept at reading the other person's signals."

Beginning in their preteen and teen years, women consistently outsmile men in all sorts of situations—with children, other women, or men—when they're in positions of authority or power. They even manage to grin under stress. "If you put a man and a woman in an equally nerve-wracking situation, the woman will laugh and smile," notes Hall. In hospitals, women physicians smile considerably more than their male colleagues.

Women also look more at others' faces. In experimental studies that measure "gaze," females of all ages consistently look at others more than males do. When engaged in conversation, a woman's gaze shifts in a remarkably predictable way: She glances at her companion as she starts to speak and looks away when nearing the end of her comment; then she glances back to check the effect of her words.

In social interactions, two white women talking together look into each other's eyes far more often than two men; African-American women are less likely to do so. When a man and a woman are together, the man gazes into the woman's eyes more often than he would a man's, while a woman makes eye contact less often than she would if she were with another woman—a nice exercise in reciprocity. "A man talking with a woman will act more like a woman, and a woman will act more like a man," observes Hall. "It's as if they're adjusting to accommodate each other's cultural norm."

Source: Personal interviews with James Pennebaker and Judith Hall. Hales, Dianne. *Just Like a Woman.* New York: Bantam Books, 2000.

Nonverbal Communication

More than 90 percent of communication may be nonverbal. While we speak with our vocal cords, we communicate with our facial expressions, tone of voice, hands, shoulders, legs, torsos, posture. "Body language is a very elementary level of communication that people react to without realizing why," observes Albert Mehrabian, a professor of psychology at the University of California, Los Angeles (UCLA) and author of *Silent Messages.* "It's the building block upon which more advanced verbal forms of communication rest."[1]

In fact, learning to interpret what people *don't* say can reveal more than what they *do* say. "Understanding nonverbal communication is probably the best tool there is for a good life of communicating, be it personally or

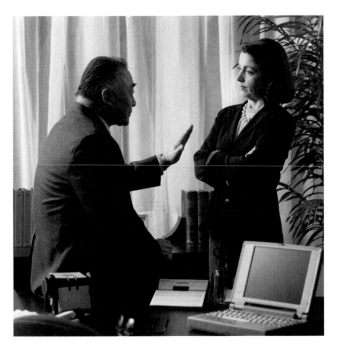

Learning to interpret nonverbal messages and being aware of your own body language are key to successful communication.

professionally," says Marilyn Maple, an educator at the University of Florida. "It's one of the most practical skills you can develop. When you can consciously read what others are saying unconsciously, you can deal with issues before they become problems."[2]

Culture has a great deal of influence over body language. In some cultures, for example, establishing eye contact is considered hostile or challenging; in others, it conveys friendliness. A person's sense of personal space—the distance he or she feels most comfortable in keeping from others—also varies in different societies. Nonverbal messages also reveal something important about the individual. "Nonverbal messages come from deep inside of you, from your own sense of self-esteem," says Maple. "To improve your body language, you have to start from the inside and work out. If you're comfortable with yourself, it shows. People who have good self-esteem, who give themselves status and respect, who know who they are, have a relaxed way of talking and moving and always come across best."

Forming Relationships

We first learn how to relate in our families, as children. Our relationships with parents and siblings change dramatically as we grow toward independence. In college,

students can choose to spend their leisure time socializing or engaging in solitary activities, like watching TV. (See Campus Focus: "The Social Life of College Students.") Relationships between friends also change as they move or develop different interests; between lovers, as they come to know more about each other; between spouses, as they pass through life together; and between parents and children, as youngsters develop and mature. But throughout life, close relationships, tested and strengthened by time, allow us to explore the depths of our souls and the heights of our emotions.

I, Myself, and Me

The way each of us perceives himself or herself affects all the ways we reach out and relate to others. If we feel unworthy of love, others may share that opinion. Self-esteem and self-love (discussed in Chapter 3) provide a positive foundation for our relationships with others. Self-love doesn't mean vanity or preoccupation with our own needs; rather, it is a genuine concern and respect for ourselves so that we remain true to our own feelings and beliefs. We can't know or love or accept others until we know and love and accept ourselves, however imperfect we may be.

If we're lacking in self-esteem, our relationships may suffer. According to research on college students by psychologists at the University of Texas, individuals with negative views of themselves seek out partners (friends, roommates, dates) who are critical and rejecting—and who confirm their low opinions of their own worth.[3]

Friendship

Friendship has been described as "the most holy bond of society." Every culture has prized the ties of respect, tolerance, and loyalty that friendship builds and nurtures. An anonymous writer put it well:

A friend is one who knows you as you are,
Understands where you've been,
Accepts who you've become,
And still gently invites you to grow.

Friends can be a basic source of happiness, a connection to a larger world, a source of solace in times of trouble. Although we have different friends throughout life, often the friendships of adolescence and young adulthood are the closest we ever form. They ease the normal break from parents and the transition from childhood to independence.

Campus Focus

The Social Life of College Students

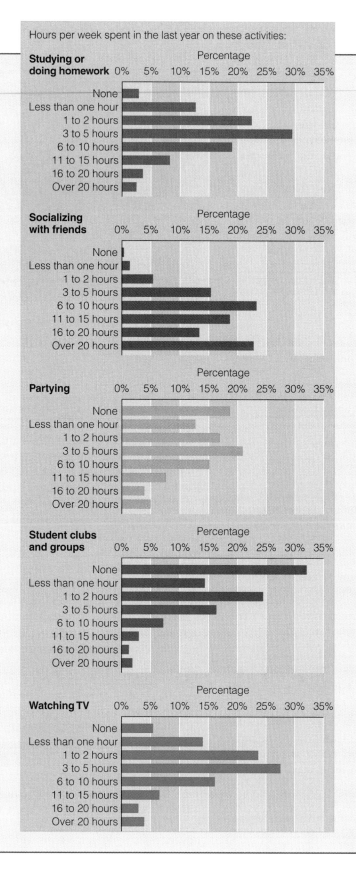

Hours per week spent in the last year on these activities:

Studying or doing homework

Socializing with friends

Partying

Student clubs and groups

Watching TV

Responses are from two-year colleges, four-year colleges, and universities. Statistics are weighted national norms for the Class of 2002.

Source: Sax, Linda, et al. *The American Freshman: National Norms for Fall 1998.* Los Angeles: Higher Education Research Institute, UCLA, 1998.

Friendship transcends all boundaries of distance and differences and enhances feelings of warmth, trust, love, and affection between two people. It is a common denominator of human existence that cuts across major social categories: In every country, culture, and language, human beings make friends. Friendship is both a universal and a deeply satisfying experience.

"Wishing to be friends," Aristotle wrote, "is quick work, but friendship is a slowly opening fruit." The qualities that make a good friend include honesty, acceptance, dependability, empathy, and loyalty. More than anything else, good friends are there when we need them. They see us at our worst but never lose sight of our best. They share our laughter and tears, our triumphs and tragedies.

Strategies *for* Change

Being a Good Friend

✓ *Be willing to open up.* The more you share, the deeper the bond between you and your friend will become.

✓ *Be sensitive to your friend's feelings.* Keep in mind that, like you, your friend has unique needs, desires, and dreams.

✓ *Express appreciation.* Be generous with your compliments. Let your friends know you recognize their kindnesses.

✓ *Know that friends will disappoint you from time to time.* They, too, are only human. Accept them as they are. Admitting their faults need not reduce your respect for them.

✓ *Talk about your friendship.* Evaluate the relationship periodically. If you have any gripes or frustrations, air them.

Dating

A date is any occasion during which two people share their time. It can be a Friday night dance, a bicycle ride, a dinner for two, or a walk in the park. Friends and lovers go on dates; so do complete strangers. Some men date other men; some women date other women. We don't expect to love, or even like, everyone we date. Yet the people you date reveal something about the sort of person you are.

While in school, you may go out with people you meet in class or on campus. However, with more people remaining single longer, the search for a good date has become more complex. Singles bars have become less popular because of the dangers of excessive drinking

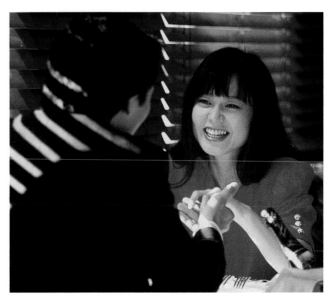

Dating refers to any occasion during which two people share their time. Your dating experiences can help you explore your social and sexual identity.

and casual sex. Cafes, laundromats, health clubs, and bookstores have become more acceptable as places to meet new people. Personal ads and "cyberspace"—the electronic web linking people through computers—are alternative ways to meet potential dates. (See Consumer Health Watch: "Do's and Don'ts of Online Dating.")

Dating can do more than help you meet people. By dating, you can learn how to make conversation, get to know more about others as well as yourself, and share feelings, opinions, and interests. In adolescence and young adulthood, dating also provides an opportunity for exploring your sexual identity. Some people date for months and never share more than a good-night kiss. Others may fall into bed together before they fall in love or even "like."

It's often difficult to sort out your emotional feelings about someone you're dating from your sexual desires. The first step to making responsible sexual decisions is respecting your sexual values and those of your partner. If you care about the other person—not just his or her body—and the relationship you're creating, sex will be an important, but not the all-important, factor while you're dating. (Chapter 9 discusses sexual decision making and etiquette.)

Most longitudinal studies on dating relationships have shown little change in love over time, although love has been found to increase for individuals who advance to a deeper, more long-lasting commitment. Romantic partners in enduring relationships generally perceive their love, commitment, and satisfaction as increasing over time. A four-year study of romantic cou-

Consumer Health Watch

Do's and Don'ts of Online Dating

Forget personal ads or single bars. If you're looking for love in the new millennium, the place more people are turning is cyberspace. Since America Online launched a relationship/matchmaking site called LOVEAOL in 1996, more than 130,000 singles have logged on, searching for friendship, romance, maybe more. Some estimate that thousands, perhaps millions of people, are using the Internet to find a companion.

Email flirtations can be fun, but they also entail some risks, particularly if you decide to go off-line and meet in person. Here are some guidelines:

- Be careful of what you type. Anything you put on the Internet can end up almost anywhere. To avoid embarrassment, don't say anything you wouldn't want to see in newspaper print.

- Don't give out your address, telephone number, or any other identifying information. The people you meet online are strangers, and you should keep your guard up.

- Don't "date" on an office or university computer. You could end up supplying your professors, classmates, or coworkers with unintentional entertainment. Also, many organizations and institutions consider email messages company property.

- Remember that you have no way of verifying if a correspondent is telling the truth about anything—sex, age, occupation, marital status. If your online partner seems insincere or strange in any way, stop corresponding.

- If you do decide to meet, make your first face-to-face encounter a double or group date, and make it somewhere public, like a cafe or museum. Don't plan a full-day outing. Coffee or a drink in a crowded place makes the best transition from emails.

- Make sure you tell a friend or family member your plans and have your own way of getting home. It's also a good idea to schedule the first meeting in the afternoon or early in the evening rather than later at night.

- Don't let your expectations run wild. Finding Mr. or Ms. Right is no easier in cyberspace than anywhere else, so be realistic about where your relationship might lead.

- Don't rely on the Internet as your only method of meeting people. Continue to get out in the real world and meet potential dates the old-fashioned ways.

ples, all dating as the study began, found that those who remained together perceived that their love, satisfaction, and commitment had grown.[4]

 ## What Causes Romantic Attraction?

What draws two people to each other and keeps them together: chemistry or kismet, survival instincts or sexual longings? "Probably it's a host of different things," reports sociologist Edward Laumann, coauthor of *Sex in America*, a landmark survey of 3,432 men and women conducted by the National Opinion Research Center at the University of Chicago.[5] "But what's remarkable is that most of us end up with partners much like ourselves—in age, race, ethnicity, socioeconomic class, education."

Why? "You've got to get close for sexual chemistry to occur," says Laumann. "Sparks may fly when you see someone across a crowded room, but you only see a preselected group of people—people enough like you to

be in the same room in the first place. This makes sense because initiating a sexual relationship is very uncertain. We all have such trepidations about being too fat, too ugly, too undesirable. We try to lower the risk of rejection by looking for people more or less like us."

Scientists have tried to analyze the combination of factors that attract two people to each other. In several studies of college students, four predictors ranked as the most important reasons for attraction: warmth and kindness, desirable personality, something specific about the person, and reciprocal liking.[6]

In the University of Chicago survey, most men and women chose sexual and marital partners of the same race, the same or similar religion and socioeconomic class, and within five years of their own age. More than 75 percent selected partners of similar education levels.[7]

Evolutionary Factors

In his cross-cultural research, psychologist David Buss, author of *The Evolution of Desire*, found that men in

37 sample groups drawn from Africa, Asia, Europe, North and South America, Australia, and New Zealand rated youth and attractiveness as more important in a possible mate than did women. Women placed greater value on potential mates who were somewhat older, had good financial prospects, and were dependable and hardworking. Many said physical appearance did matter—not as much as financial responsibility and dependability.[8]

The reason for this gender difference could be evolutionary. Throughout time, men have sought fertile females of "high reproductive value." Two outward signs of female fertility are youth and a more subtle factor: waist-to-hip ratio. When researchers analyzed the physical dimensions of the women considered most attractive by men in various studies, those with the slimmest waists and roundest hips were consistently rated as most desirable.

From an evolutionary perspective, women have had to look for mates who could provide greater security for their offspring. For them, a man's power, wealth, and status—which require more time to assess—mattered more than appearance. But today's women may have different criteria: In a survey of over 1,500 *Psychology Today* readers, women said a man's ability to empathize or talk about feelings, his intelligence, and his sense of humor mattered most—far more than his facial appearance and body build. Women also indicated that they usually accept the way their men look, even if they fail to match up to their ideal.[9]

Intimate Relationships

The term **intimacy**—the open, trusting sharing of close, confidential thoughts and feelings—comes from the Latin word for *within*. Intimacy doesn't happen at first sight, or in a day or a week or a number of weeks. Intimacy requires time and nurturing; it is a process of revealing rather than hiding, of wanting to know another and to be known by that other. (See Figure 8-1 for the elements of love.) Although intimacy doesn't require sex, an intimate relationship often includes a sexual relationship, heterosexual or homosexual.

All of our close relationships, whether they're with parents or friends, have a great deal in common. We feel we can count on these people in times of need. We feel that they understand us and we understand them. We give and receive loving emotional support. We care about their happiness and welfare. However, when we choose one person above all others to share a life with, there is something even deeper and richer—something we call romantic love.

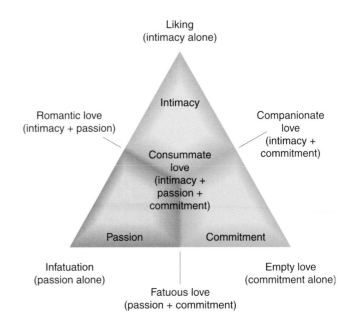

■ **Figure 8-1** Sternberg's love triangle: (a) the three components of love and (b) the various kinds of love as reflected in different combinations of the three components. *Note:* Non-love is the absence of all three components.

How Does Science View Romantic Love?

Falling in love is an intense, dizzying experience. A person not only enters our life but takes possession of it as well. We are intrigued, flattered, delighted—but is this love, or a love of loving? At the time you're experiencing it, you may not care. You're in such a state of giddy elation that it doesn't matter, at least for the moment, whether it stems from a strong sexual attraction, a fear of loneliness, loneliness itself, or a hunger for approval.

"We use the word love in such a sloppy way that it can mean almost nothing or absolutely everything," observes Diane Ackerman, author of *A Natural History of Love*, who notes that "love" is such a small word to convey "an idea so immense and powerful that it has altered the flow of history, calmed monsters, kindled works of art, cheered the forlorn, turned tough guys to mush, consoled the enslaved, driven strong women mad, glorified the humble, fueled national scandals, bankrupted robber barons, and made mincemeat of kings."[10]

We like to think of this powerful force, this source of both danger and delight, as something that defies analysis. However, in recent years, as scientists have attempted to study love objectively, they have provided new perspectives on its nature.

An Anthropological View

When you first fall in love, you may be sure that no one else has ever known the same dizzying, wonderful feelings. Yet, while every romance may be unique, romantic love is anything but. In a comprehensive study of societies around the world, anthropologists William Jankowiak of the University of Nevada-Las Vegas and Edward Fischer of Tulane University found evidence of romantic love in at least 147 of the 166 cultures they studied. The experience of an "intense attraction that involves the idealization of the other, within an erotic context, with the expectation of enduring for some time in the future," they concluded, "constitutes a human universal, or at the least, a near-universal."

Another anthropologist, Helen Fisher, author of *Anatomy of Love: The Natural History of Monogamy, Adultery and Divorce,* describes romantic love "as a very primitive, basic human emotion, as basic as fear, anger or joy." As she explains, it pulled men and women of prehistoric times into the sort of partnerships that were essential to child rearing. But after about four years—just "long enough to rear one child through infancy," says Fisher—romantic love seemed to wane, and primitive couples tended to break up and find new partners. This "four-year itch" may well have endured through the centuries, contends Fisher, who notes that divorce statistics from most of the 62 cultures she has studied still show a pattern of restlessness four years into a marriage.[11]

A Biochemical View

The heart is the organ we associate with love, but the brain may be where the action really is. According to research on **neurotransmitters** (messenger chemicals within the brain), love sets off a chemical chain reaction that causes our skin to flush, our palms to sweat, and our lungs to breathe more deeply and rapidly. The "love chemicals" within the brain—dopamine, norepinephrine, and phenylethylamine (PEA)—have effects similar to those of amphetamines, stimulant drugs that intensify physiological reactions (see Chapter 15).[12]

Infatuation may indeed be a natural high, but like other highs, this rush doesn't last—possibly because the body develops tolerance for love-induced chemicals, just as it does with amphetamines. However, as the initial lovers' high fades, other brain chemicals may come into play: the endorphins, morphinelike chemicals that can help produce feelings of well-being, security, and tranquility. These feel-good molecules may increase in partners who develop a deep attachment.

The hormone **oxytocin,** best known for its role in inducing labor during childbirth (see Chapter 10), seems particularly important in our ability to bond with others.

By measuring blood levels of women as they recalled positive and negative relationships, researchers have found that women whose oxytocin levels rose when remembering a positive relationship reported having little difficulty setting appropriate boundaries, being alone, or trying too hard to please others. Women whose oxytocin levels fell in response to remembering a negative emotional relationship reported greater anxiety in close relationships. "It seems that having this hormone 'available' during positive experiences, and not being depleted of it during negative experiences, is associated with well-being in relationships," the researchers concluded.[13]

Mature Love

Social scientists have distinguished between passionate love—characterized by intense feelings of elation, sexual desire, and ecstasy—and companionate love, which is characterized by friendly affection and deep attachment. (See Self-Survey: "How Strong is the Communication and Affection in Your Relationship?") Often relationships begin with passionate love and evolve into a more companionate love. Sometimes the opposite happens and two people who know each other well discover that their friendship has "caught fire" and the sparks have flamed an unexpected passion.

A romantic relationship shows definite promise if:

- You feel at ease with your new partner.
- You feel good about your new partner both when you're together and when you're not.
- Your partner is open with you about his or her life—past, present, and future.
- You can say no to each other without feeling guilty.
- You feel cared for, appreciated, and accepted as you are.
- Your partner really listens to what you have to say.

Mature love is a complex combination of sexual excitement, tenderness, commitment, and—most of all—an overriding passion that sets it apart from all other love relationships in one's life. This passion isn't simply a matter of orgasm, but also entails a crossing of the psychological boundaries between oneself and one's lover. You feel as if you're becoming one with your partner while simultaneously retaining a sense of yourself. (For other characteristics of mature, healthy love, see Pulsepoints: "Ten Characteristics of a Good Relationship.")

When Love Ends

Breaking up is indeed hard to do. Sometimes two people grow apart gradually, and both of them realize that

Self-*Survey* — How Strong Is the Communication and Affection in Your Relationship?

Effective, caring communication and loving affection markedly enhance a couple's relationship. The following self-test may help you to assess the degree of good communication, love, and respect in your intimate relationship. If you agree or mostly agree with a statement, answer yes. If you disagree or mostly disagree, answer no. You may wish to have your partner respond to this assessment as well. If so, mark your answers on a separate sheet.

1. My partner seeks out my opinion.	Yes	No
2. My partner cares about my feelings.	Yes	No
3. I don't feel ignored very often.	Yes	No
4. We touch each other a lot.	Yes	No
5. We listen to each other.	Yes	No
6. We respect each other's ideas.	Yes	No
7. We are affectionate toward one another.	Yes	No
8. I feel my partner takes good care of me.	Yes	No
9. What I say counts.	Yes	No
10. I am important in our decisions.	Yes	No
11. There's lots of love in our relationship.	Yes	No
12. We are genuinely interested in one another.	Yes	No
13. I love spending time with my partner.	Yes	No
14. We are very good friends.	Yes	No
15. Even during rough times, we can be empathetic.	Yes	No
16. My partner is considerate of my viewpoint.	Yes	No
17. My partner finds me physically attractive.	Yes	No
18. My partner expresses warmth toward me.	Yes	No
19. I feel included in my partner's life.	Yes	No
20. My partner admires me.	Yes	No

Scoring: A preponderance of yes answers indicates that you enjoy a strong relationship characterized by good communication and loving affection. If you answered yes to fewer than seven items, it is likely that you are not feeling loved and respected and that the communication in your relationship is decidedly lacking.

Source: Gottman, John. *Why Marriages Succeed or Fail.* New York: Simon & Schuster, 1994. See Hyde and DeLameter, 1997, 6th ed., p. 272.

Getting Your Signals Straight

- *Tune into your body talk.* Notice details about the way you speak, gesture, and move. If possible, watch yourself on videotape. Analyze the emotions you're feeling at the time and think of how they may be influencing your body language.

- *Learn to establish good eye contact, but don't glare or stare.* If you sense that someone feels uncomfortable with an intense eye grip, shift your focus so that your gaze hits somewhere between the eyes and the chin, rather than pupil-to-pupil.

- *Avoid putting up barriers.* If you fold your arms across your chest, you'll look defensive or uninterested in contact. Crossing your legs or ankles also can seem like a way of keeping your distance.

- *Identify the little things you characteristically do when you're tense.* Some people pat their hair or pick at their ears; others rub their necks, twist a ring or watch, twirl a lock of hair, or play with a pen. Train yourself to become aware of what you're doing (have a friend give you a signal, if necessary) and to control your mannerisms.

---

they must go their separate ways. More often, one person falls out of love first. It hurts to be rejected; it also hurts to inflict pain on someone who once meant a great deal to you. In surveys, college students say it's more difficult to initiate a breakup than to be rejected. Those who decided to end a relationship reported greater feelings of guilt, uncertainty, discomfort, and awkwardness than those with whom they broke up.

Research suggests that people do not end their relationships because of the disappearance of love. Rather a sense of dissatisfaction or unhappiness develops, which may then cause love to stop growing. The fact that love does not dissipate completely may be one of the reasons why breakups are so painful.[14] While the pain does ease over time, it can help both parties if they end their relationship in a way that shows kindness and respect. Your basic guideline should be to think of how you would like to be treated if someone were breaking up with you. Would it hurt more to find out from someone else? Would it be more painful if the person you cared for lied to you or deceived you, rather than admitted the truth? Saying, "I don't feel the way I once did about you; I don't want to continue our relationship," is hard, but it's also honest and direct.

PULSE *points*

Ten Characteristics of a Good Relationship

1. **Trust.** Partners are able to confide in each other openly, knowing their confidences will be respected.
2. **Togetherness.** In a healthy relationship, two people create a sense of both intimacy and autonomy. They enjoy each other's company but also pursue solitary interests.
3. **Expressiveness.** Partners in healthy relationships say what they feel, need, and desire.
4. **Staying power.** Couples in committed relationships keep their bond strong through tough times by proving that they will be there for each other.
5. **Security.** Because a good relationship is strong enough to absorb conflict and anger, partners know they can express their feelings honestly. They also are willing to risk vulnerability for the sake of becoming closer.
6. **Laughter.** Humor keeps things in perspective—always crucial in any sort of ongoing relationship or enterprise.
7. **Support.** Partners in good relationships continually offer each other encouragement, comfort, and acceptance.
8. **Physical affection.** Sexual desire may fluctuate or diminish over the years, but partners in loving, long-term relationships usually retain some physical connection.
9. **Personal growth.** In the best relationships, partners are committed to bringing out the best in each other and have the other's best interests at heart.
10. **Respect.** Caring partners are aware of each other's boundaries, need for personal space, and vulnerabilities. They do not take each other or their relationship for granted.

Strategies *for* Change

Dealing with Rejection

✔ Remind yourself of your own worth. You are no less attractive, intelligent, interesting, or lovable because someone ends his or her relationship with you.

✔ Accept the rejection as a statement of the other person's preference rather than trying to debate or defend yourself.

✔ Think of other people who value or have valued you, who accept and even see as appealing the same characteristics the rejecting person viewed as undesirable.

✔ Don't withdraw from others. Although you may not want to risk further rejection, it's worth the gamble to get involved again. The only individuals who've never been rejected are those who've never reached out to connect with another.

Living Arrangements

Today's adults have many choices to explore regarding how and with whom they might live: returning to one's primary family, staying single, living with one or more friends, living in a long-term relationship with a lover of the same or opposite sex, or getting married. Increasingly, men and women in their twenties are spending more time considering all their options before committing themselves to an exclusive relationship.

Living with Parents

According to the Census Bureau, young adults between the ages of 18 and 24 are more likely to be living in their parents' homes in the 1990s than young people were in the 1970s. (See Figure 8-2.) One in eight adults between the ages of 25 and 34 is still living with parents—compared with one in eleven in 1980. Their reasons include the high cost of housing and the low incomes most men and women earn in their early twenties. People also are getting married later in life. In 1999, the median age for a first-time groom was 26.7 years; for a first-time bride, 25 years—significantly older than in decades past.[15] (See Figure 8-3.)

Single Life

In young adulthood, single men outnumber single women; after age 40, however, there are more single women than single men. Perhaps because there are so many singles, more and more Americans are living alone. Approximately one-quarter of the households in the nation are one-person homes, and approximately 10 percent of today's young men and women will never marry. Among Americans between 25 and 34 years old,

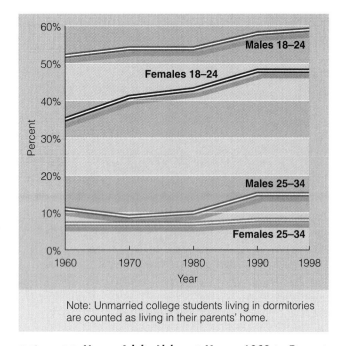

Note: Unmarried college students living in dormitories are counted as living in their parents' home.

■ Figure 8-2 **Young Adults Living at Home: 1960 to Present**

Source: U.S. Bureau of the Census. Internet release date: January 7, 1999. Data based on Current Population Survey (CPS).

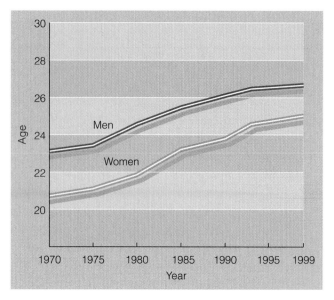

■ Figure 8-3 **Median Age at First Marriage**
Age at first marriage has continued to rise for both women and men

Source: Bureau of the Census. "Estimated Mean Age at First Marriage by Sex." January 7, 1999.

about 35 percent (14 million) have never been married. Of African Americans in this age group, 53 percent have never been married.[16] Being single no longer marks a transition phase between living with parents and living with a spouse, but is an accepted, appealing lifestyle for millions of men and women.

The number-one reason people remain single is not being able to find the right person, according to psychologist Florence Kaslow, director of the Florida Couples and Family Institute. For women, the next two reasons for staying single are their careers and independence. For men, independence and resolving personal issues are the second and third reasons for not marrying. Most of the women and all of the men in her study said that they would like to get married—someday.

Only 5 percent of bachelors over age 40 ever marry. Never-married men in this age group tend to avoid emotional intimacy, fear conflict, and shy away from challenges in life, according to a study of 30 lifelong bachelors. In general, the men didn't hate women, but they seemed reluctant to get involved, make demands, or assert their needs in relationships.

Increasing numbers of single people, including those living alone or with heterosexual or homosexual partners, claim that they are discriminated against in housing, credit, insurance, membership groups, and medical services. Those who oppose the concept of singles' rights say that extending spousal benefits to singles or "domestic partners" would erode the institution of marriage and cause a bureaucratic mess. Despite such opposition, the campaign for singles' rights is winning increasing support.

Strategies *for* **Change**

How to Stay Single and Satisfied

✓ Fill your life with meaningful work, experiences, and people.

✓ Build a network of supportive friends who care for and about you.

✓ Be open to new experiences that can expand your feelings about yourself and your world.

✓ Don't miss out on a special event because you don't have someone to accompany you: Go alone.

✓ Volunteer to help others less fortunate, or become involved in church and social organizations.

 ## Is Living Together a Good Idea?

Although couples have always shared homes in informal relationships without any official ties, "living together," or **cohabitation,** has become more common, increasing by 80 percent in the last two decades. There are about 7 unmarried couples for every 100 married ones. Often young people live together in a trial marriage, getting to know each other better to see whether they're compatible—although this does not necessarily lead to a more successful marriage. People who have been married and divorced may be content just sharing their lives with one another.

More than 4 million unmarried heterosexual couples live together, in contrast to only half a million 30 years ago.[17] (See Figure 8–3.) For many young adults, particularly children of divorced parents, living together seems like a good way to achieve some of the benefits of marriage as they get to know each other and find out if they're suited to each other. According to surveys, most young people say it is a good idea to live with a person before marrying.

That's not the case, argues a controversial recent report. Researchers for the National Marriage Project of Rutgers University in New Jersey reviewed all available research and concluded that living together is not a good way to prepare for marriage or to avoid divorce. Though living together has become common, they found that these unions, in comparison to marriages, tend to have more episodes of domestic violence of women, and more physical and sexual abuse of children. Unmarried couples also report lower levels of happiness and well-being than married couples. Annual rates of depression among unmarried couples are more than three times those of married couples. The divorce rate among couples who eventually marry is also higher.[18]

According to the report, cohabitation is probably least harmful (though not necessarily helpful) when it is prenuptial—when both partners are definitely planning to marry, have formally announced their engagement, and have picked a wedding date. The longer that two people live together, the more likely they are to have problems. The reason, the researchers suggest, is that individuals develop a "low-commitment ethic" that is the opposite of what is required for a successful marriage.

Multiple living-together experiences also have a negative impact, both for an individual's own sense of well-being and for the likelihood of establishing a strong lifelong partnership. Rather than teaching people to have better relationships, repeated cohabiting is a strong predictor of the failure of future relationships.

Cohabitation poses particular risks to children. Since cohabiting parents break up at a much higher rate than married parents, children face a greater likelihood of a potentially devastating breakup. Moreover, youngsters living in cohabiting unions are at higher risk of sexual abuse and physical violence, including lethal violence, than are children living with married parents.[19]

Unmarried couples are gaining legal recognition. Some U.S. cities have "domestic partnership" laws that grant a variety of spousal rights—such as insurance benefits and bereavement leave—to partners, heterosexual or homosexual, who live together.

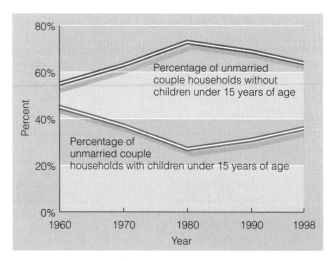

■ **Figure 8-4** **Unmarried Couple Households, by Presence of Children: 1960 to Present**

Source: U.S. Bureau of the Census. Figures have been rounded to nearest percentages.

Committed Relationships

Even though men and women today may have more sexual partners than in the past, most still yearn for an intense, supportive, exclusive relationship, based on mutual commitment and enduring over time. In our society, most such relationships take the form of heterosexual marriages, but partners of the same sex or heterosexual partners who never marry also may sustain long-lasting, deeply committed relationships. These couples are much like married people: They make a home, handle daily chores, cope with problems, celebrate special occasions, plan for the future—all the while knowing that they are not alone, that they are part of a pair that adds up to far more than just the sum of two individual souls.

Marriage

Like everything which is not the involuntary result of fleeting emotion but the creation of time and will, any marriage, happy or unhappy, is infinitely more interesting and significant than any romance, however passionate.

W. H. Auden

Contemporary marriage has been described as an institution that everyone on the outside wants to enter and everyone on the inside wants to leave. About 56 percent of all American adults (111 million people) are married and living with their spouses. The marriage rate has dropped dramatically: a lower percentage of couples tied the knot in the 1990s than in previous decades. In fact, the national marriage rate has dropped over the last four decades to its lowest point ever. In 1960, the number of marriages per 1,000 women age 14 and older was 66 percent; by the late 1990s, it had fallen to 55 percent.[20] (See Figure 8–5.)

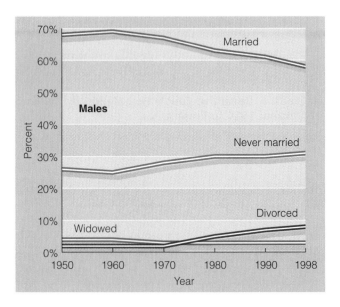

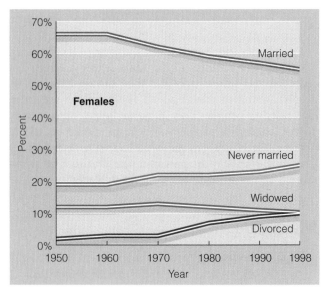

■ Figure 8-5 **Marital Status of the Population 15 Years and Over, by Sex: 1950 to Present**

Source: U.S. Bureau of the Census. Internet release date: January 7, 1999. Note: 1950 and 1960 data are for the population 15 years and older. Figures have been rounded to the nearest whole number percentages. Source of CPS data: U.S. Bureau of the Census, Current Population Reports, Series P20-514, "Marital Status and Living Arrangements: March 1998 (Update)" and earlier reports.

Not only are fewer people getting married, but fewer marital partners describe themselves as "very happy" in their relationships. In a recent report on "the social health of marriage in America," researchers at Rutgers University found that more couples are choosing to live together outside of marriage or are putting off vows until later in life. Young people also have grown disenchanted with the prospect of marriage. The percentage of teenagers who thought they would be happier married than not married has fallen over the last two decades.[21]

Not too long ago, marriage was often a business deal, a contract made by parents for economic or political reasons when the spouses-to-be were still very young. Today, in some countries, it is still culturally acceptable to arrange marriages in this manner. Even in America, certain ethnic groups, such as Asians who have recently immigrated to the United States, plan marriages for their children. In such arrangements, the marriage partners are likely to have similar values and expectations. However, the newlyweds also start out as strangers who may not even know whether they like— let alone love—each other. Sometimes arranged marriages do lead to loving unions; sometimes they trap both partners in loneliness and longing.

Most of today's marriages aren't arranged, but even in this day and age, partners often marry because they have to: One out of every six brides is pregnant on her wedding day. Other young couples marry as a way to escape from their parents' homes and authority. But most people say they marry for one far-from-simple reason: love.

Preparing for Marriage

With more than half of all marriages ending in divorce, there's little doubt that modern marriages aren't made in heaven. Are some couples doomed to divorce even before they swap "I do's"? Could counseling before a marriage increase its odds of success? According to recent research findings, the answer to both questions is yes.

Finding Mr. or Ms. Right

Generally, men and women marry people from the geographical area they grew up in and from the same social background. Differences in religion and race can add to the pressures of marriage, but they also can enrich the relationship if they aren't viewed as obstacles. In our culturally diverse society, interracial and crosscultural marriages are becoming more common and widely accepted. (See Figure 8-6.) According to the Census Bureau, there are six times as many interracial couples today than there were in 1960.

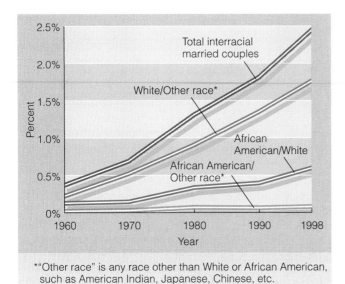

■ Figure 8-6   Interracial Married Couples: 1960 to Present

Source: U.S. Bureau of the Census. Internet release date: January 7, 1999. 1980–1998 data taken from the Current Population Survey (CPS): 1960 and 1970 data taken from the Decennial Census. Source of CPS data: U.S. Bureau of the Census, Current Population Reports, Series P20-514, "Marital Status and Living Arrangements: March 1998 (Update)" and earlier reports. Source of Decennial Census data: U.S. Bureau of the Census, 1990 Census of the Population.

ality issues, communication, conflict resolution, financial management, leisure activities, sex, children, family and friends, egalitarian roles, and religious orientation. In longitudinal studies in which couples took the assessment prior to marriage and then were interviewed three years after they married, the PREPARE inventory was about 80 percent accurate in predicting which couples would divorce and which would have happy marriages.[23] Couples who become aware of potential conflicts by means of the inventory may be able to resolve them through professional counseling. In some cases, they may want to reconsider or postpone their wedding.

Other common predictors of marital discord, unhappiness, and separation are:

• A high level of arousal during a discussion.
• Defensive behaviors such as making excuses and denying responsibility for disagreements.
• A wife's expressions of contempt.
• A husband's stonewalling (showing no response when a wife expresses her concerns).

By looking for such behaviors, researchers have been able to predict with better than 90 percent accuracy whether a couple will separate within the first few years of marriage.

Some of the things that appeal to us in a date become less important when we select a mate; others become key ingredients in the emotional cement holding two people together. According to psychologist Robert Sternberg of Yale University, the crucial ingredients for commitment are the following:

• Shared values.
• A willingness to change in response to each other.
• A willingness to tolerate flaws.
• A match in religious beliefs.
• The ability to communicate effectively.

The single best predictor of how satisfied one will be in a relationship, according to Sternberg, is not how one feels toward a lover, but the difference between how one would like the lover to feel and how the lover actually feels. Feeling that the partner you've chosen loves too little or too much is, as he puts it, "the best predictor of failure."[22]

Premarital Assessments

There are scientific ways of predicting marital happiness. One is a premarital assessment inventory called PREPARE that uses 125 items to identify strengths and weaknesses in 11 aspects of a relationship: realistic expectations, person-

---

Strategies *for* Prevention

When to Think Twice About Getting Married

Don't get married if:

✔ You or your partner is constantly asking the other such questions as "Are you sure you love me?"

✔ You spend most of your time together disagreeing and quarreling.

✔ You're both still very young (under the age of 20).

✔ Your boyfriend or girlfriend has behaviors (such as nonstop talking), traits (such as bossiness), or problems (such as drinking too much) that really bother you and that you're hoping will change after you're married.

✔ Your partner wants you to stop seeing your friends, quit a job you enjoy, or change your life in some other way that diminishes your overall satisfaction.

Types of Marriage

Sociologists have categorized marriages as traditional or companion-oriented. In **traditional marriages,** the

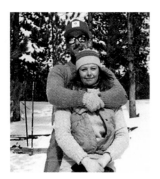 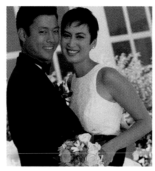 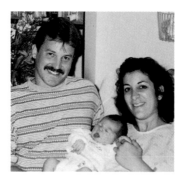 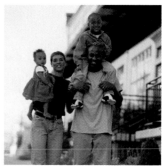

A relationship is just as alive as the individuals who create it. It grows if there is caring; it can blossom if there is emotional nourishment, and it endures if there is commitment.

couples assume prescribed societal roles. In **companion-oriented marriages,** the partnership and its rewards—rather than the roles of fathering, mothering, and breadwinning—are primary. In addition, there are **romantic marriages,** in which sexual passion never seems to die, and **rescue marriages,** in which one partner suffered a traumatic childhood and sees marriage as a way of healing. Regardless of type, a marriage can succeed if it fulfills basic tasks, such as providing a sense of intimacy and autonomy and providing a safe haven that is strong enough to absorb inevitable conflicts.

Issues in Marriage and Other Committed Relationships

No two people can live together in perfect harmony all the time. Some of the issues that crop up in any long-term relationship include the following:

Unrealistic Expectations

Partners may think that their significant others should always be as attractive, charming, and tolerant as they were when they were dating. They may assume that their partners will always agree with them or will automatically see their point of view; or they may believe that their one true love will always be able to meet all their needs. Because no one could ever live up to such expectations, the partners are doomed to disappointment.

Settling Differences

Contrary to what you may assume, arguments can be good for the health of a relationship. According to the National Institute of Mental Health, couples who learn how to fight fairly and effectively have a 50 percent lower divorce rate than those who haven't mastered the art of disagreeing. Results of a study of 150 couples from premarriage through the first ten years of marriage

(the highest risk period for divorce) led researchers to conclude that "nondestructive" arguing lowers the likelihood for physical violence, helps couples stay together longer, and benefits children by preparing them to build good intimate relationships as adults.

Money

Money may make the business world go around, but it has the opposite effect on relationships: It knocks them off their tracks, brings them to a halt, twists them upside down. However, even though almost all couples quarrel about money, they rarely fight over how much they have. What matters more—whether they make $10,000 or $100,000 a year—is what money means to both partners. How does each person use money to meet emotional needs? Who decides how the money is spent? Who keeps track? Until they resolve these issues, couples may quarrel over money as long as they're together.

To avoid fighting over money, understand that having different money values or expectations doesn't make

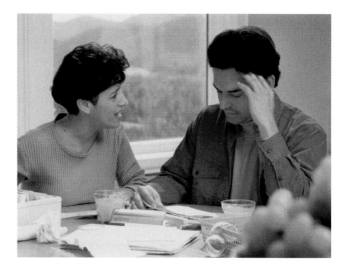

Fight fairly. You can learn to argue effectively, without attacking others or damaging relationships.

Strategies *for* Change

How to Fight Fairly

The art of arguing is a skill, like bicycle riding, that anyone can master with time, patience, and plenty of practice. Here are some basic ground rules:

✔ Learn to listen. Rather than thinking about what you're going to say next, tune in to your partner. Think before you open your mouth. Taking a few deep breaths gives you time to weigh your words.

✔ Use the speaker/listener technique. When one person has the floor, the other listens. Start sentences with "I," not "You." Instead of attacking with a statement such as "You're jealous and immature," say, "I feel hurt when you quiz me about my old relationships."

✔ Make sure you're arguing about the right issue. Are you angry simply because your partner is never on time? Or because you don't seem to be the top priority?

✔ Don't embarrass each other by fighting in front of others. Don't attack each other so viciously that one of you is backed into a corner. Be fair. Whenever there's a cheap shot, one of you should stop the fight by crying "Foul!"

✔ If you can't come to terms on a particular issue, agree to disagree, or to keep talking in the future.

one of you right and the other wrong. Recognize the value of unpaid work. A partner who's finishing school or taking care of the children is making an important contribution to the family and its future. It also helps to go over your finances together, so you have a firm basis in reality for what you can and can't afford. Talk about the financial goals you hope to attain five years from now. Set priorities to meet them. Also, set aside money for each of you to spend without asking or answering to the other. Even a small amount can make each partner feel more independent.

Sex

Like every other aspect of a relationship, sex evolves and changes over the course of marriage. The redhot sexual chemistry of the early stages of intimacy invariably cools down. Even so, the happiest couples have sex more often than unhappily married pairs do.[24]

What matters most isn't quantity alone, but the quality of sexual activity and intimacy (discussed in Chapter 9). Are both partners satisfied with their sexual relationship? Does one partner always initiate sex? Do the partners talk about their preferences and pleasures? Sexuality, like personality, is dynamic and changes throughout life. Do the partners acknowledge and adapt to these changes? Do they feel sufficiently at ease with each other to discuss anxieties about sex? The answers to these questions can determine how sexually gratifying a marriage is for both spouses.

Extramarital Affairs

How faithful are American mates? The answer depends on the questions researchers ask and whom they ask. In face-to-face interviews with 3,432 Americans, aged 18 to 59, University of Chicago researchers found that 25 percent of men and 15 percent of women had had affairs, and that 94 percent of the married subjects had been monogamous in the last year.[25] Another survey of 1,049 Americans, aged 18 to 65, found that one out of six had had an extramarital relationship—19 percent of the men and 15 percent of the women.[26]

High or low, numbers are little comfort when affairs do occur. A husband or wife who learns about a spouse's affair typically feels a devastating sense of betrayal as well as deep feelings of shame, fear of abandonment, depression, and anger. Two crucial questions determine whether a marriage can survive: Do the spouses still feel a serious commitment to each other? And do they love each other and want to grow old together?

Two-Career Couples

More than 75 percent of women with children work— a dramatic increase from the 1960s, when only 30 percent of mothers worked outside the home. (See Figure 8-7.) Two careers can bring pressure to a relationship: Both individuals may come home tired and irritable; both may have to spend a great deal of time on their jobs; both may have to travel or work on weekends. It becomes even more important for partners to discuss their problems openly.

Couples pursuing individual careers sometimes face difficult choices. What happens, for example, if the husband is offered a promising job in another city? Does the wife quit her job, pack up, and move? What if she's offered a promising job elsewhere? Does her husband automatically pack up and go? Some couples resolve such dilemmas by working in different cities and spending weekends together. Others try to alternate career and home priorities. However imperfect these arrangements may be, they work for some couples.

The working couples most likely to stay together are those who are not tightly tied to traditional gender roles. Because neither spouse has very narrow expectations of

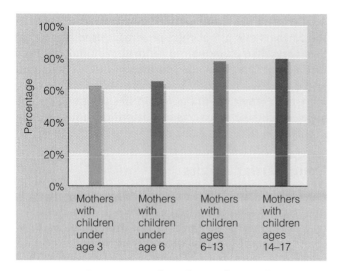

■ Figure 8-7 Percentage of Mothers Who Work

Source: Women's Bureau, Department of Labor Statistics, 1999.

what the other should or shouldn't be doing, both are free to pursue individual interests outside the home.

 ## Why Has Marriage Endured?

Despite its problems, marriage endures because it is a fulfilling way for two people to live. As researchers have proven, good marriages make people happy and healthy. For years researchers thought that marriage was especially beneficial to men. Married men have lower rates of alcohol and drug abuse, depression, and risk-taking behavior than divorced men. They also earn more money—possibly because they have more incentive to do so.

However, recent research has shown that marriage also is good for women. Both married men and women live longer than single or divorced individuals. In one national survey, about 90 percent of husbands and wives survived until at least age 65, compared with only about 60 to 70 percent of divorced and never-married men and women. Married people also have healthier behaviors: They drink less alcohol and use fewer illicit drugs. Happily married men and women rate themselves as happier than the divorced or never-married. However, women in unhappy unions—but not their husbands—have higher rates of depression and unhappiness than single women.[27]

Married people, who have sex about twice as often, consistently report greater satisfaction than unmarried partners. Cohabiting couples also have active sex lives, but they get less emotional satisfaction from it than married lovers—especially women. For married men, researchers report, satisfaction stems from sexual frequency, fidelity, and emotional commitment. These factors are equally important to women, but just being married adds an extra kick to their sexual satisfaction.

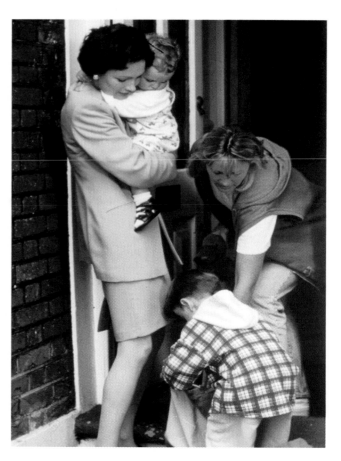

Two-career couples cope with balancing family and work in various and sometimes imperfect ways.

Although there has been much research on same-sex committed relationships, most experts believe that gay couples are likely to enjoy similar benefits, as long as they remain together and receive social support for doing so.

Couples Therapy

According to the Association of Family and Marital Therapists, at least one of every five couples in this country needs professional counseling—and increasing numbers are seeking help. An estimated five million couples—married or not—now turn to the 50,000 licensed family therapists in the United States, a dramatic increase since 1980. The relationships of about two-thirds of those who get counseling do improve, according to both the couples' own judgments and objective measures of satisfaction.

A well-trained counselor can spot destructive behavior patterns and help couples see their situations in a new light. Therapy often helps stop spouses from hurting each other so badly that they can't stay together. If nothing else, it can help both partners decide whether to continue or end the relationship.

Strategies *for* Prevention

Making the Most of a Committed Relationship

✓ Focus on what's right with your partner. Be kinder to your partner. Don't take for granted the nice things your spouse does.

✓ Learn to negotiate for what you want. One effective approach is offering your mate what he or she wants in return.

✓ Look for the problem behind the problem. Often an affair or a lack of sexual interest is merely a symptom; the real question is why this problem has developed.

✓ Keep your perspective. Uncapped toothpaste tubes or food not prepared exactly to your taste may be annoying, but are they worth a fight?

✓ Rather than thinking of all the things your partner is or isn't doing, look for things you can do to make your marriage better.

What Is the Current Divorce Rate?

More than one in every five men and women who have ever been married have been divorced. About 10 percent of American adults (19.4 million) are currently divorced.[28] The divorce rate, once up to 55 percent in the United States, has dropped, and the Census Bureau now estimates that most new marriages will endure, with a mere (at least relatively) 40 percent predicted to fail. Increasingly, therapists and family counselors are urging couples to try to work out their differences—for their own and their children's sake. As many people have discovered, divorce hurts.

Even after their hopes for happiness with one spouse end, men and women still yearn to mesh two personalities, two life histories, and two persons' dreams into a marriage. Eighty percent of divorced men and women remarry, and the remarriage rate increases with the number of times an individual has been divorced. The remarriage rate after a second divorce is 90 percent; after a third divorce, it's even higher.

Family Ties

The structure of American families changed dramatically from 1970 to 1990, as the proportion of households made up of married couples with children fell. The rate of change continued but slowed considerably in the 1990s. Today about seven in ten of the 102.5 million households (defined as a person or group of persons living in a housing unit) in the United States are family households. About half (49 percent) of family households contain children under 18, down from 56 percent in 1970s. The average family household consists of 3.18 people, down from 3.58 in 1970, but unchanged from 1990. Hispanic families are larger, with an average of 3.92 members, than either white or African-American families.[29]

Diversity Within Families

The "all-American" **family**—as portrayed on television and in movies—is typically white and middle-class. But families of different cultures—Italian to Indian to Indonesian—reflect different traditions, beliefs, and values. Within African-American families, for instance, traditional gender roles are often reversed, with women serving as head of the household, a kinship bond uniting several households, and a strong religious commitment or orientation. In Chinese-American families, both spouses may work and see themselves as breadwinners, but the wife may not have an equal role in decision making. In Latino families, wives and mothers are acknowledged and respected as healers and dispensers of wisdom. At the same time, they are expected to defer to their husbands, who see themselves as the strong, protective, dominant head of the family. As time passes and families from different cultures become more integrated into American life, traditional gender roles and decision-making patterns often change, particularly among the youngest family members.

American families also are diverse in other ways. About 4 million children, nearly 6 percent of all children under 18, live with their grandparents. This 77-percent increase since 1970 is attributed to rising divorce rates, teen pregnancy, child abuse, and imprisonment of a parent or parents.[30] Three of every ten households consist of blended families, formed when one or both of the partners getting married bring children from a previous union. In the future, social scientists predict, American families will become even more diverse, or pluralistic. But even as norms or expectations about the configurations of families have changed, values or ideas about the intents and purposes of families have not. American families of every type still support each other and strive toward values such as commitment and caring.

Becoming Parents

Parenting is a 24-hour-a-day, 7-day-a-week, 52-week-a-year job, with no sabbaticals or sick leaves and no opportunity to renegotiate the contract. Having a child is an experience that deeply affects, involves, and changes a man and a woman.

When Baby Makes Three

New parents are likely to feel proud one moment and anxious the next. The infant may fascinate them both, but the adjustment to a baby-centered life can cause resentment. The husband who feels that his wife is more concerned with the baby than with him often feels jealous, which in turn makes him feel guilty. The mother, still recovering from childbirth, may feel overwhelmed by new responsibilities and the daunting physical demands of caring for a newborn.

Experts in family development, who have been studying the changes a baby brings to a marriage, note that marital satisfaction invariably declines, if only slightly, while the number of separations and divorces rises after a baby's arrival. However, couples who stick together as partners through the process of becoming parents can keep their marriages strong.

As Children Grow

A child's greatest need is for love—the feeling of being wanted and cared for, of being special, and of realizing that the parents like the child for him- or herself. According to a study that followed 379 kindergarten-aged children for 36 years, warm, loving parenting—the kind that supplies plenty of hugs, kisses, and cuddles—has more influence on adult social adjustment than any other parental or childhood factor. The individuals whose mothers and fathers were openly affectionate were able to sustain long and relatively happy marriages, raise children, develop close friendships, and enjoy varied activities outside their marriage.

Children have other needs, too. They need security—assurance that their parents will be there when needed most; protection; confidence; and a feeling of belonging. They need role models to learn behavior from and a sense of clear limits and controls. Parents are responsible for establishing values of what is right or wrong and for guiding by example as well as with words.

With each year that passes in a child's life, the conflict between independence and dependence becomes more intense. Children are drawn into the larger world outside the family and home, and their parents are torn between clinging to them and pushing them out of the nest. It's not enough to set rules; parents must also advise a child on how to make decisions within those rules.

The teen years—the transition from childhood to adulthood—are, for parents and children, the best and worst of times. Children becoming teenagers develop more responsibility, a greater sense of self, and more

independence. Simultaneously, they may rebel, challenging and testing their parents. Setting limits—such as curfews and dating guidelines—may set off a confrontation instead of being a simple matter of stating policy. A teen's emerging sexuality may be difficult for the parents to acknowledge and accept. (Chapter 9 discusses adolescent sexuality.)

Siblings

The ways in which siblings relate as children often affect their interactions with each other—and with others, including their mates—when they grow up. Sibling rivalry, for instance, though normal, can lead to unhealthy ways of relating to others. For example, siblings who had to compete fiercely for parental attention or affection may remain competitive throughout life, doing anything necessary in order to come out on top. And youngsters who feel that their parents clearly prefer another child in the family may come to think that they're inadequate or somehow unworthy of love.

Siblings typically grow more distant during adolescence, as they focus on developing their own identities. This separation continues during early adulthood. However, in middle age, most adults report positive relationships with siblings. Some are bound by loyalty, even if they don't feel friendly toward a brother or sister. Others socialize with siblings but are closer to friends. In old age, sisters and brother-sister pairs have more positive relationships than brothers; elderly African Americans tend to have more positive relationships with their siblings than do elderly whites.

Working Parents: The New Collaborators

Throughout the world, mothers have taken on increased economic responsibility for their families. As a result, they are working longer hours at home and on the job. In the United States, nearly half of employed married women contribute half or more of their family's income. Most women with children are working either full- or part-time, including those with very young children.

Marital roles continue to change with the times. The supermoms of the eighties tried to do it all—at home and at work. The "jugglers" of the nineties were always struggling to keep something up in the air. Now trend-watchers have a different term for millennium mates: the new collaborators.

From 1965 to 1985, demographers have calculated, married mothers reduced the time devoted to housework by ten hours a week (from 30 hours to 20); husbands doubled theirs (from 5 to 10). Couples who could afford them hired cleaning services. Those who couldn't lowered their standards from the spic-and-span perfection of the 1950s. But as recently as the 1980s, many women were stilling putting in a second shift of domestic toil, and "chore wars" were erupting in sticky-countered kitchens across the land.

In the last decade, things changed. One in four men now does most of the grocery shopping, up from 15 percent of men in 1986. The Family and Work Institute of New York calculates that American husbands put in 75 percent as much time as wives on workday chores—a dramatic rise from 30 percent in 1977. In actual clocktime, the gender difference in domestic "scut-work" amounts to just 45 minutes a day.

Plenty of sociologists—and lots of weary women still doing the lioness share of chores—doubt whether all men in all income groups are doing as much. However, the trend toward greater husbandly involvement is real—and likely to continue. Researchers have actually calculated the exact percentage of shared work that equals a "fair share": Among employed husbands and wives, those who each reported doing less than half—45.8 percent each, to be precise—also reported the highest levels of psychological well-being and lowest levels of distress.[31]

The basis of the new collaboration goes beyond shared chores to shared values. In a study of 300 dual-earner couples in the Boston area, women and men showed remarkable similarities in how they felt about their relationships with each other and with their children. Contrary to the old assumption that family problems were female concerns and work issues male concerns, both spouses showed equal sensitivity to stress at home, problems in the marital relationships, and work concerns. Another study found that gender has virtually no bearing on how parents respond, physically or psychologically, to situations in which work interferes with family life or family life interferes with work. Mothers *and* fathers care—and care deeply—about both.[32]

Fathers' Changing Roles

Traditionally, many fathers were spectators in their children's lives. As parents of both sexes have redefined their roles and responsibilities, more fathers have moved to center stage within their families.

Single Fathers

The number of single fathers has grown 25 percent since 1995, from 1.7 million to 2.1 million, while the number of single mothers has remained constant at about 9.8 million. Men now comprise 1 in 6 of the nation's 11.9 million single parents, up from 1 in 7 in 1995 and one in ten in 1980.

The typical single father is 38 years old. One in 9 is under age 25; and 1 in 70 is 60 or older. About 5 of every 6 (83 percent) of the nation's single fathers are white. African Americans and Hispanics each constitute about 13 percent. About half of single fathers reside in suburban areas, and most (85 percent) maintain their own households. Of single fathers raising their own children, 63 percent care for only one child under 18 and 11 percent care for 3 or more. In 1998, 44 percent of single fathers were divorced, 35 percent had ever married, 12 percent were separated, and about 5 percent each were widowed or separated due to reasons other than marital discord.

An estimated 3.1 million children in one-parent homes live with their fathers, triple the number in 1980. Their median family income is significantly lower than the median for two-parent families. Twenty percent are poor, compared with 9 percent of two-parent families. Half live in rental housing, compared with one-quarter of two-parent families.

Fathers as Child-Care Providers

In the 6.2 million married, two-career families with preschoolers, 27 percent of the fathers care for the children during the mother's work hours.[33] This number is expected to grow—and the trend toward more active, hands-on fathering may have a profound effect, both on children and their dads. In a study of 95 school-aged youngsters from mostly middle-class families in New England, fathers who were more involved with their children had sons and daughters who expressed fewer gender-stereotyped emotions.[34]

Child care also changes fathers. Men who take primary responsibility for raising their children are more nurturing and affectionate and disclose more feelings than others. "Their emotional expressiveness resembles what we stereotypically associate with women," says psychologist Leslie Brody of Boston University. In her studies, taking care of young children seems to elicit feelings that have less to do with being female or male than with the nature of nurturing.[35]

Children of Divorce

Each year divorce separates more than a million children from their parents. The breakup of a marriage has an enormous impact on many aspects of a child's life, including his or her standard of living. Very young children may become more babyish, irritable, and dependent. Preschool or young school-age children may blame themselves, feeling that "Daddy left because I was bad." School-age children may feel lonely, helpless, and depressed; they may develop illnesses or have problems in their friendships. Preteens may experiment with alcohol, drugs, and sex. For teenagers, divorce may make separating from the family and establishing an adult identity even harder.

Long-term studies show that the impact of divorce on children varies. According to one of the largest and most comprehensive studies of children of divorce, most youngsters fare well academically. In an analysis of data collected on 1,700 children, ages 5 to 8, from divorced households, the key factor in their academic achievement was not the absence of their father but the education of their mothers. The children of more highly educated moms consistently did better in school than those whose mothers had less formal education.[36] Psychologically, divorce can take a greater toll. According to various reports, 15 to 20 percent of all children whose parents divorce may require professional therapy. However, the odds that children of divorce will end their own marriages has declined by almost 50 percent since 1973.[37]

Strategies *for* Change

Helping Children of Divorce

✔ Don't give youngsters everything they want just to get them to like you more than the other parent.

✔ Be honest, but spare your children the gory details. Don't fight in front of them.

✔ Let children know it's okay for them to love both their parents. Give them a chance to talk about how they feel.

✔ Let them know that you love them and that they are not responsible for the breakup.

Single-Parent and Blended Families

While more households continue to be headed by single mothers and single fathers, their numbers are rising more slowly than in previous years. One-parent families comprise 27 percent of family households with children, up from 24 percent in 1990 and 11 percent in 1970. About 28 percent (20 million) of all children under 18 years of age in the United States live with just one parent. The majority of children who live with just one parent live with their mother (84 percent). No other adults are present in the household for 56 percent of children living with single parents.[38]

Each year about half a million children become part of new, **blended families** when their parents remarry. Over

the years many studies have found significant differences in family and relationship processes in these families. However, improved communication and problem solving can help blended families work through their problems.

Children can also be encouraged to spend time with members of the extended family or friends to experience other role models.

Dysfunctional Relationships

Relationships that don't promote healthy communication, honesty, and intimacy are sometimes called **dysfunctional**. Individuals with addictive behaviors or dependence on drugs or alcohol (see Chapters 14 and 15), and the children or partners of such people, are especially likely to find themselves in such relationships.

Often partners have magical, unrealistic expectations (e.g., they expect that a relationship with the right person will make their life okay), and one person uses the other almost as if he or she were a mood-altering drug. The partners may compulsively try to get the other to act the way they want. Both persons may not trust or may deceive each other. Often they isolate themselves from others, thus trapping themselves in a recurring cycle of pain.

Dysfunctional families exist in every economic, social, educational, religious, and racial group. They inflict emotional pain on children through destructive behaviors, such as physical, emotional, verbal, or sexual abuse; physical or emotional neglect; and alcoholism or drug use. Although alcohol or drugs do not in themselves create dysfunctional families, they can push parents over a psychological brink. The results can be emotionally devastating. The children of alcoholics, drug users, and parents with other addictive behaviors are prone to learning disabilities, eating disorders, compulsive achievement, and addiction.

Codependence

As used by contemporary therapists, the term **codependence** (or coaddiction) refers to the tendency of the spouses, partners, parents, and friends of individuals with addictive behaviors to allow or *enable* their loved ones to continue their self-destructive habits. Codependent individuals focus on their loved ones, even to the extent of giving up their own lives. They change who they are and what they feel in order to please others, feel responsible for meeting others' needs, have low self-esteem, and frequently have compulsions of their own. However, codependent behaviors need to be evaluated in the context of an individual's culture. For example, the emphasis on family values and support that is part of the value system of many Latinos would not be considered codependent behavior.

Codependents Anonymous, founded in 1986 for men and women whose common problem is an inability to maintain functional relationships, is one of the fastest-growing support programs in the country. Other self-help groups for codependents include Al-Anon (for adult family members of alcoholics), Alateen (for the teenaged children of addicts), Nar-Anon (for people in relationships with individuals who abuse drugs), O-Anon (for those whose family members have eating disorders), and Gam-Anon (for those living with people who have gambling problems). Local chapters of these groups can be found in the white pages of the telephone book. Through such groups, codependent individuals can learn how to leave behind guilt feelings, how to become less judgmental and moralistic, how to understand their powerlessness over their loved one's problem, and how to do what needs to be done for themselves as well as the addict.

If you wonder if you may be codependent, read through the following list of characteristics of codependence and check any that apply to you:

- I find myself covering for another person's alcohol or drug use, eating or work habits, gambling, sexual escapades, or general behavior.

- I spend a great deal of time talking about and worrying about other people's behavior/problems/future instead of living my own life.

- I have marked or counted bottles, searched for a hidden stash, or in other ways monitored someone else's behavior.

- I find myself taking on more responsibility at home or in a relationship, even though I resent it.

- I ignore my own needs in favor of meeting someone else's.

- I'm afraid that if I get angry, the other person will leave or not love me.

- I worry that if I leave a relationship or stop controlling the other person, that person will fall apart.

- I spend less time with friends and more with my partner/parent/child in activities that I wouldn't normally choose.

- My self-esteem depends on what others say and think of me, or on my possessions or job.

- I grew up in a family in which there was little communication, in which expressing feelings wasn't acceptable, and in which there were either rigid rules or none at all.

If you identify with more than three of these statements, you may be codependent. There are many useful books on codependence at libraries and bookstores. You may also wish to visit a support group on campus or in your area or talk with a counselor.

Enabling

Experts on the subject of addiction first identified traits of codependence in spouses of alcoholics, who followed a predictable pattern of behavior: While intensely trying to control the drinkers, the codependent mates would act in ways that allowed the drinkers to keep drinking. For example, if an alcoholic found it hard to get up in the morning, his wife would wake him up, pull him out of bed and into the shower, and drop him off at work. If he was late, she made excuses to his boss. The husband was the one with the substance-abuse problem, but without realizing it, his wife was enabling him to continue drinking. In fact, he might not have been able to keep up his habit without her unintentional cooperation.

The different styles or components of **enabling** include the following:

- *Shielding.* Codependents may cover up for abusers, preventing them from experiencing the full impact of the harmful consequences of their behavior—for example, by dropping off a paper or report so that the addicted person can avoid a missed deadline.

- *Controlling.* A codependent may try to control the significant other—for instance, by withholding sex or using sex as a reward for cutting down on an addictive behavior.

- *Taking over responsibilities.* The codependent may take over such household chores as shopping or running errands.

- *Rationalizing.* Codependents try to rationalize their partners' addiction by telling themselves that a compulsive behavior pattern, like workaholism, is making the person more successful, or that drinking helps him or her relax.

- *Cooperating.* Sometimes codependents become involved in the person's compulsion, perhaps placing bets for a gambler or buying alcohol for a drinker.

- *Rescuing.* The codependent may become overprotective—for example, by allowing the user to use drugs at home to avoid the risk of an accident or arrest.

Codependence progresses just as an addiction does, and codependents excuse their own behavior with many of the same defense mechanisms used by addicts, such as rationalization ("I cut class so I could catch up on my reading, not to keep an eye on my partner") and denial ("He likes to gamble, but he never loses more than he can afford"). In time, just as an addict's world becomes smaller and smaller, codependents lose sight of everything but their loved one. They feel that if they can only "fix" this person, everything will be fine.

Making This Chapter Work for You

Building Better Relationships

- Sending clear messages through words, gestures, expressions, and behaviors is the essence of good communication. Effective communication helps cre-

ate good relationships built on honesty, understanding, and mutual trust.

- Nonverbal communication refers to the unspoken messages people send with their gestures, expressions, and body movements.

- A genuine concern and respect for ourselves helps us remain true to our own feelings and beliefs and enhances the likelihood that we will seek out healthy, positive relationships.

- Friendships are among the most cherished bonds among people. In today's society, friends often become our extended family, providing acceptance, warmth, and loyalty.

health / ONLINE

Family & Relationships - APA
http://helping.apa.org/family/index.html
This site from the American Psychological Association provides advice for dealing with family conflicts and maintaining healthy relationships.

Marriage Support/Couples Place
http://marriagesupport.com/
Provides articles, polls, quizzes, advice, and skills training to help people succeed at marriage and other couple relationships.

Relationship Web
http://relationshipweb.com/index.shtml
First aid for relationships, links to thousands of related sites, discussion forums, and more.

Please note that links are subject to change. If you find a broken link, use a search engine like http://www.yahoo.com *and search for the web site by typing in key words.*

 Campus Chat: How do you feel about cohabiting with a boyfriend/girlfriend? Would you ever live with someone without being married to him/her? Why or why not? Share your thoughts on our online discussion forum at **http://health.wadsworth.com**

Find It On InfoTrac: You can find additional readings related to communication and relationships via InfoTrac College Edition, an online library of more than 900 journals and publications. Follow the instructions for accessing InfoTrac that came packaged with your textbook; then search for articles using a key word search.

- **Suggested reading:** "The Social Origins and Maintenance of Gender: Communication Styles, Personality Types and Grid-Group Theory," by Gregg Franzwa and Charles Lockhart. From *Sociological Perspectives*, Spring 1998, Vol. 41, No. 1, p. 185 (24) [hint: use "communication styles" as your key words to search for this article]

  (1) According to Deborah Tannen's work, how do the communication styles of men differ from those of women?

  (2) How can the results of the Myers-Briggs Personality Type Indicator help improve our communications with family members? With coworkers?

For additional links, resources, and suggested readings on InfoTrac, visit our Health & Wellness Resource Center at **http://health.wadsworth.com**

- Dating provides opportunities to get to know other people, to practice social skills, and to explore one's sexuality.

- Sexual attraction usually involves many different factors, including similarity in age, race, ethnicity, and socioeconomic class.

- Romantic love is characterized by intense passion. This type of bond, which anthropologists have found in almost all societies, may help pull men and women into the sort of partnerships needed to care for children. From a biochemical view, infatuation may trigger a rise in certain neurotransmitters that create a natural high that is very pleasurable—but not long-lasting.

- Mature love combines sexual excitement, tenderness, a sincere commitment to bringing out the best in each other, the encouragement of mutual growth, a willingness to risk vulnerability, and the ability to enjoy solitude or separateness from one's partner.

- Increasingly, young adults are spending longer periods of time living on their own, with their parents, or with a partner, before deciding about marriage.

- If they do marry, most couples do so for love. The older and more similar two people are, the more likely they are to have a successful marriage. Premarital assessments can identify behavior patterns that can predict the likelihood of divorce.

- Even happily married couples must contend with many complex issues and pressures, including dual careers, money, sex, and day-to-day disagreements.

- For all its challenges, marriage provides many rewards. Married people are more likely to be healthier, to live longer, and to be better able to cope with stress than are single people.

- Divorce rates have remained fairly stable, and more people are seeking help to make their marriages work. However, more marriages around the world are ending in divorce.

- Parenthood is among the most demanding, difficult, and gratifying responsibilities a person will ever have. Today more fathers are actively involved with their children, and more mothers have careers. Both parents must work together to meet the physical and psychological needs of growing children.

- The number and percentage of traditional two-parent families has fallen, while the number of single-parent homes has skyrocketed.

- The response of children to the divorce of their parents depends on their age and on the amount of fighting before and after the divorce.

- Dysfunctional relationships do not promote healthy communication, honesty, and intimacy and can be emotionally destructive, especially for children.

 Working Relationships. Do you value your work and your relationships equally? If not, why?

Key Terms

The terms listed here are used within the chapter. Page numbers are included for each term. A definition of each term is given in the Glossary pages at the end of this book.

blended family   242
codependence   242
cohabitation   232
companion-oriented marriage   236
dysfunctional   242

enabling   243
family   239
intimacy   228
neurotransmitters   229
oxytocin   229

rescue marriage   236
romantic marriage   236
traditional marriage   235

Critical Thinking Questions

1. Flip back to The X&Y Files in this chapter, and think about your own communication style. How does the way you communicate compare to the patterns Pennebaker and Tannen have revealed for your gender? Do your personal experiences support or contest the research results?

2. While our society has become more tolerant, marriages between people of different religious and racial groups still face special pressures. What issues might arise if a Christian marries a Jewish or Muslim man or woman? What about the issues facing partners of different races? How could these issues be resolved? What are your own feelings about mixed marriages? Would you date someone of a different religion or race? Why or why not?

3. What are your personal criteria for a successful relationship? Develop a brief list of factors you consider important, and support your choices with examples or experiences from your own life.

References

1. Mehrabian, Albert. Personal interview.
2. Maple, Marilyn. Personal interview.
3. Swann, William, et al. "Socialization Patterns of Depressed and Non-Depressed College Students." *Journal of Abnormal Psychology,* Vol. 104, 1992.
4. Sprecher, Susan. "Insiders' Perspectives on Reasons for Attraction to a Close Other." *Social Psychology Quarterly*, Vol. 61, No. 4, December 1998.
5. Laumann, Edward. Personal interview.
6. Sprecher, Susan. "Insiders' Perspectives on Reasons for Attraction to a Close Other."
7. Laumann, Edward, et al. *The Social Organization of Sexuality.* Chicago: University of Chicago Press, 1994.
8. Buss, David. *The Evolution of Desire.* New York: Basic Books, 1994.
9. "The Beefcaking of America." *Psychology Today,* November/ December 1994.
10. Ackerman, Diane. *A Natural History of Love.* New York: Vintage Books, 1995.
11. Fisher, Helen. Personal interview.
12. Ackerman, *A Natural History of Love.*
13. Nowlis, Rebecca Sladek. "Hormone Involved in Reproduction May Have Role in Maintenance of Relationships." News release, UCSF News Service, July 14, 1999.
14. Sprecher, Susan. "'I Love You More Today than Yesterday': Romantic Partners' Perceptions of Changes in Love and Related Affect Over Time." *Journal of Personality and Social Psychology,* Vol. 76, No. 1, January 1999. Simon, Robin. "Strength of Beliefs Intensify Sense of Loss." News release, Center for the Advancement of Health, June 20, 1999.
15. Bureau of the Census.
16. Ibid.
17. Labi, Nadya. "A Bad Start? Living Together, a Report Claims, May Be the Road to Divorce." *Time,* Vol. 153, No. 6, February 15, 1999. Popenoe, David, and Barbara Dafoe Whitehead. *Should We Live Together? What Young Adults Need to Know About Cohabitation Before Marriage.* Rutgers, N.J.: National Marriage Project, 1999. "U.S. Marriage Is Weakening, Study Reports." *New York Times,* July 4, 1999.
18. Popenoe, David. *The State of Our Unions: The Social Health of Marriage in America.* Rutgers, N.J.: National Marriage Project, 1999.
19. Ibid.
20. Bureau of the Census.
21. Popenoe, David. *The State of Our Unions: The Social Health of Marriage in America.*
22. Sternberg, Robert. Personal interview.
23. Larsen, A., and Olson, D. "Predicting Marital Satisfaction Using PREPARE: A Replication Study." *Journal of Marital and Family Therapy,* Vol. 15, 1989.
24. Robinson, John, and Geoffrey Godbey. "No Sex, Please … We're College Graduates." *American Demographics,* February 1998.
25. Laumann et al., *The Social Organization of Sexuality.*
26. Clemens, Mark. "Sex in America." *Parade,* August 7, 1993.
27. Marano, Hara. "Debunking the Marriage Myth: It Works for Women Too." *New York Times,* August 4, 1998.
28. Bureau of the Census.
29. Ibid.
30. Ibid.
31. Bird, Chloe. "Doing Housework: The 'Ideal' Fair Share." *Journal of Health and Social Behavior,* March 1999.
32. Barnett, Rosalind. Personal interview.
33. Bureau of the Census.
34. Hales, Dianne. *Just Like a Woman.* New York: Bantam Books, 1999. O'Neil, John. "For Women, Ideal Man Has Two Faces, Study Finds." *New York Times,* June 24, 1999.
35. Brody, Leslie. Personal interview.
36. Mott, Frank. Director of the Center for Human Resources Research, Ohio State University. Personal interview.
37. Wolfinger, Nicholas. "Coupling and Uncoupling: Changing Marriage Patterns and the Intergenerational Transmission of Divorce." American Sociological Association annual meeting, August 1999.
38. Bureau of the Census.

9

Personal Sexuality

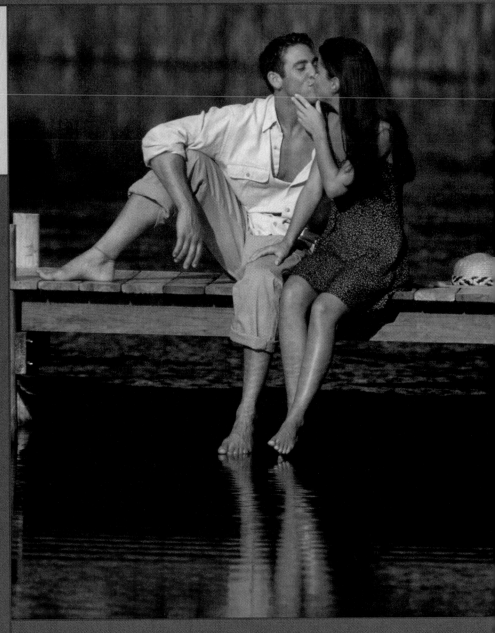

After studying the material in this chapter, you should be able to:

- **Describe** the male and female reproductive systems and the functions of the individual components of each system.

- **Define** sexual health and sexually healthy relationships.

- **Describe** some conditions or issues unique to women's sexual health and men's sexual health.

- **Describe** some methods for preventing infection from HIV and other sexually transmitted diseases.

- **List** the common concerns of men and women about sexual performance difficulties.

Human **sexuality**—the quality of being sexual—is as rich, varied, and complex as life itself. Along with our **sex,** or biological maleness or femaleness, it is an integral part of who we are, how we see ourselves, and how we relate to others. Of all of our involvements with others, sexual **intimacy,** or physical closeness, can be the most rewarding. But while sexual expression and experience can provide intense joy, they also can involve great emotional turmoil.

You are ultimately responsible for your sexual health and behavior. You make decisions that affect how you express your sexuality, how you respond sexually, and how you give and get sexual pleasure. Yet most sexual activity involves another person. Therefore, your decisions about sex—more so than those you make about nutrition, drugs, or exercise—have important effects on other people. Recognizing this fact is the key to responsible sexuality.

Sexual responsibility means learning about your body, your partner's body, your sexual development and preferences, and the health risks associated with sexual activity. This chapter is an introduction to your sexual self and an exploration of sexual issues in today's world. It provides the information and insight you can use in making decisions and choosing behaviors that are responsible for all concerned. ❖

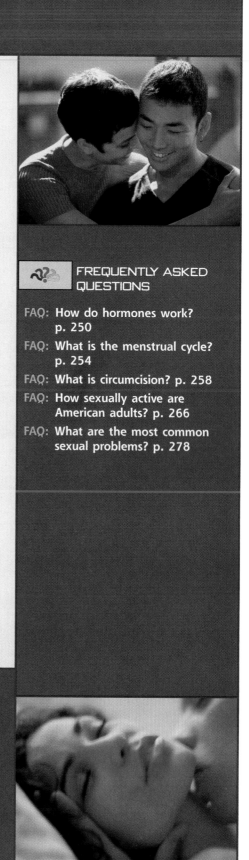

FREQUENTLY ASKED QUESTIONS

FAQ: **How do hormones work? p. 250**

FAQ: **What is the menstrual cycle? p. 254**

FAQ: **What is circumcision? p. 258**

FAQ: **How sexually active are American adults? p. 266**

FAQ: **What are the most common sexual problems? p. 278**

Becoming Male or Female

Physiological maleness or femaleness, or biological sex, is indicated by the sex chromosomes, hormonal balance, and genital anatomy. **Gender** refers to the psychological and sociological, as well as the physical, aspects of being male or female. You are born with a certain *sexual identity* based on your sexual anatomy and appearance; you, your parents, and society mold your *gender identity*.

Are You an X or a Y?

Biologically, few absolute differences separate the sexes: Males alone can make sperm and contribute the chromosome that causes embryos to develop as males; females alone are born with sex cells (eggs or ova), menstruate, give birth, and breast-feed babies. But the process of becoming male or female is a long and complex one.

In the beginning, all human embryos have undifferentiated sex organs. Only after several weeks do the sex organs differentiate, becoming either male or female **gonads** (testes or ovaries), the structures that produce the future reproductive cells of an individual. This initial differentiation process depends on genetic instructions in the form of the sex chromosomes, referred to as X and Y. If a Y (or male) chromosome is present in the embryo, about seven weeks after conception, it signals the sex organs to develop into testes. If a Y chromosome isn't present, an embryo begins developing ovaries in the eighth week. From this point on, the sex hormones produced by the gonads, not the chromosomes, play the crucial role in making a male or female.

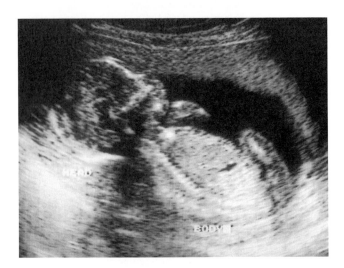

Sex hormones begin their work early in an embryo's development.

 ## How Do Hormones Work?

In Greek, *hormone* means "set into motion"—and that's exactly what our **hormones** do. These chemical messengers, produced by various organs in the body, including the sex organs, and carried to target structures by the bloodstream, arouse cells and organs to specific activities and influence the way we look, feel, develop, and behave.

The group of organs that produce hormones is referred to as the **endocrine system.** Except for the sex organs, males and females have identical endocrine systems. Directing the endocrine system is the *hypothalamus,* a pea-sized section of the brain. The pituitary gland, directly beneath the hypothalamus, turns the various glands on and off in response to messages from it.

The ovaries produce the sex hormones most crucial to women, **estrogen** and **progesterone.** The primary sex hormone in men is **testosterone,** which is produced by the testes and the adrenal glands. However, both men and women have small amounts of the hormones of the opposite sex. Estrogen, in fact, is crucial to male fertility and gives sperm what researchers describe as their "reproductive punch."

The sex hormones begin their work early in an embryo's development. As soon as the testes are formed, they start releasing testosterone, which stimulates the development of other structures, such as the penis. The absence of testosterone in an embryo causes female genitals to form. (If the testes of a genetic male don't produce testosterone, the fetus will develop female genitals. Similarly, if a genetic female is exposed to excessive testosterone, the fetus will have ovaries but will also develop male genitals.)

As puberty begins, the pituitary gland initiates the changes that transform boys into men and girls into women. When a boy is about 14 years old and a girl about 12, their brains stimulate the hypothalamus to secrete a hormone called *gonadotropin releasing hormone (GnRH).* This substance causes the pituitary gland to release hormones called **gonadotropins.** These, in turn, stimulate the gonads to make sex hormones. (See Figure 9-1.)

The gonadotropins are *follicle-stimulating hormone (FSH)* and *luteinizing hormone (LH).* In girls, these hormones travel to the ovary and stimulate the production of estrogen. As estrogen increases, a girl's **secondary sex characteristics** develop. Her breasts become fuller, her external genitals enlarge, and fat is deposited on her hips and buttocks. Estrogen keeps her hair thick and skin smooth. She begins menstruating because she has begun ovulating, the process that prepares her body to conceive and carry a baby.

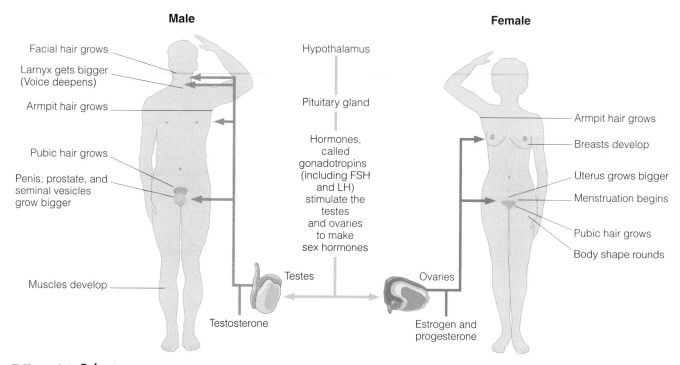

Figure 9-1 Puberty
The body's endocrine system produces hormones that trigger body changes in males and females. Additional body changes include growth spurts and changes to the skeleton.

According to biologist Martha McClintock of the University of Chicago, the maturing of the adrenal glands also brings about the first flicker of sexual desire. After years of being oblivious to physical charms, boys and girls suddenly look around a crowded classroom and, as McClintock puts it, start to "notice—with a capital N" that someone, whether of the same or the other sex, looks particularly good to them. They feel a zing that may not be sexual in the adult sense but definitely carries a charge. A year and a half to two years later, as the reproductive glands churn out much greater amounts of sex hormones, desire kicks in. In the University of Chicago analysis, this happened at a mean age of 11.9 for girls and 11.2 for boys, with first sexual activity beginning more than three years later for girls (at age 15.2) and two years later for boys (at 13.1).[1]

In addition to the adrenals, a girl's ovaries also begin to mature—again, at an earlier age than many had assumed. In an analysis of growth charts from 17,077 girls from ages 3 to 12, researchers at the University of North Carolina at Chapel Hill found that, by age 8, 15 percent of white girls and 48 percent of African-American girls show signs of sexual development. (The reasons for this racial discrepancy are not known.) The mean ages for breast development are 8.87 years for African-American girls and 9.96 years for white girls; for pubic hair, they are 8.78 years and 10.51 years, respectively. African-American girls begin

menstruating at 12.16 years; white girls, at 12.88 years.[2] **Menarche** is the term for a girl's first menstrual cycle.

Cultural influences affect a girl's response to menarche. In a cross-cultural study of college students, the most common emotions expressed by American women at menarche were embarrassment, pride, and anxiety. Malaysian women cited fear, embarrassment, and worry. Lithuanian women described themselves as happy or scared, while Sudanese women cited fear, anxiety, embarrassment, and anger. The Lithuanian women reported feeling more valuable and believing they had entered the world of women. American girls worried about whether they could still play sports, felt superior to friends who had not reached menarche, and became eager to learn about sex. Malaysians described feeling wise, respected, and mature. Sudanese women felt more beautiful and aware that they could now have children.[3]

In boys, the gonadotropins stimulate the testes to produce testosterone, which triggers the development of male secondary sex characteristics. Their voices deepen, hair grows on their faces and bodies, their penises become thicker and longer, and their muscles become stronger.

The sex hormones released during puberty change the growth pattern of childhood, so that a boy or girl may now spurt up 4 to 6 inches in a single year. The skeleton matures very rapidly until, at the end of puberty (usually around age 18), the growth centers at the ends of the bones close off. Estrogen causes girls' bones to stop growing at an earlier age than boys' bones.

Sexual Stereotypes

Being male is not the same as being masculine, and being female is not the same as being feminine. Today more men and women are breaking out of traditional stereotypes. Men are acknowledging their feelings and fears and taking on what were formerly women's jobs—becoming nurses and secretaries at work, and doing the grocery shopping and laundry at home. Although there still aren't any female linebackers in the National Football League (and no one expects that there will be), women have taken their places among astronauts, truck drivers, engineers, pilots, coal miners, physicians, and executives.

An alternative to both male and female sexual type-casting is the concept of **androgyny,** a word that literally translates (from the Greek) as "man woman." Androgynous individuals combine aspects of both masculinity and femininity into their personalities and lifestyles. They act in ways that seem appropriate to a given relationship or situation—instead of in ways that seem appropriately masculine or feminine. Such behaviors can enhance compatibility and satisfaction in a relationship.

Women's Sexual Health

Only recently has medical research devoted major scientific investigations to issues in women's health. In fact, until 1993, the National Institutes of Health routinely excluded women from experimental studies because of concerns about menstrual cycles and pregnancy. In clinical settings, women are more likely to have their symptoms dismissed as psychological and not to be referred to a specialist than are men with identical complaints. Some physicians are suggesting the creation of a new medical specialty (distinct from obstetrics and gynecology) that would be devoted to women's health to provide more comprehensive care and overcome the current gender gap in health services.

Female Sexual Anatomy

As illustrated in Figure 9-2A, the **mons pubis** is the rounded, fleshy area over the junction of the pubic bones. The folds of skin that form the outer lips of a woman's genital area are called the **labia majora.** They cover soft flaps of skin (inner lips) called the **labia minora.** The inner lips join at the top to form a hood over the **clitoris,** a small elongated erectile organ, and the most sensitive spot in the entire female genital area. Below the clitoris is the **urethral opening,** the outer opening of the thin tube that carries urine from the bladder. Below that is a larger opening, the mouth of the

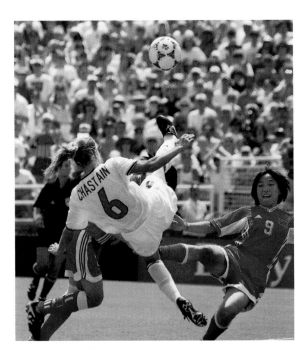

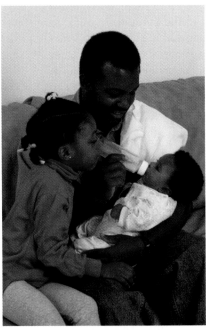

In today's world, women and men are increasingly succeeding in jobs and roles that break the old sexual stereotypes.

A. External structure

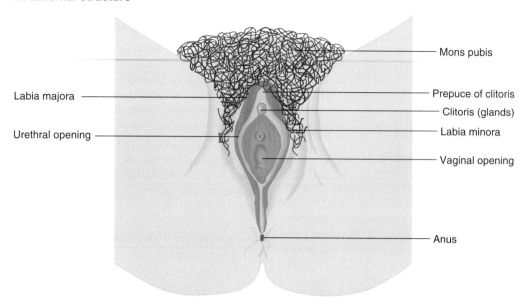

Mons pubis

Prepuce of clitoris

Clitoris (glands)

Labia minora

Vaginal opening

Labia majora

Urethral opening

Anus

B. Internal structure

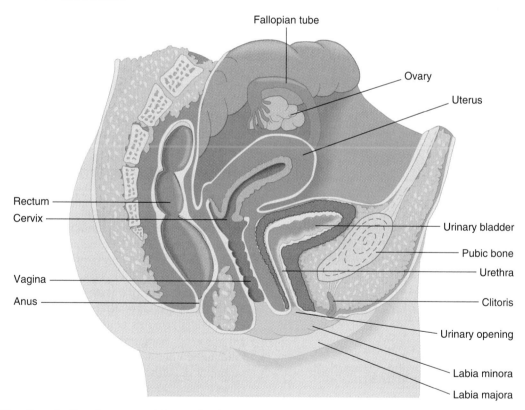

Fallopian tube

Ovary

Uterus

Urinary bladder

Pubic bone

Urethra

Clitoris

Urinary opening

Labia minora

Labia majora

Rectum

Cervix

Vagina

Anus

■ Figure 9-2 **The Female Sex Organs and Reproductive Structure**

vagina, the canal that leads to the primary internal organs of reproduction. The **perineum** is the area between the vagina and the anus (the opening to the rectum and large intestine).

At the back of the vagina is the **cervix,** the opening to the womb, or **uterus** (see Figure 9-2B). The uterine walls are lined by a layer of tissue called the **endometrium.** The **ovaries,** about the size and shape of almonds, are located on either side of the uterus, and contain egg cells called **ova** (singular, **ovum**). Extending outward and back from the upper uterus are the **fallopian tubes,** the canals that transport ova from the ovaries to the uterus. When an egg is released from an ovary, the fingerlike ends of the adjacent fallopian tube "catch" the egg and direct it into the tube.

 ## What Is The Menstrual Cycle?

As shown in Figure 9-3, the hypothalamus monitors hormone levels in the blood and sends messages to the pituitary gland to release follicle stimulating hormone (FSH) and luteinizing hormone (LH). In the ovary, these hormones stimulate the growth of a few of the immature eggs, or ova, stored in every woman's body. Usually, only one ovum matures completely during each monthly cycle. As it does, it increases its production of the female sex hormone estrogen, which in turn triggers the release of a larger surge of LH.

At midcycle, the increased LH hormone levels trigger **ovulation,** the release of the egg cell, or ovum. Estrogen levels drop, and the remaining cells of the follicle then enlarge, change character, and form the **corpus luteum,** or yellow body. In the second half of the menstrual cycle, the corpus luteum secretes estrogen and larger amounts of progesterone. The endometrium (uterine lining) is stimulated by progesterone to thicken and become more engorged with blood in preparation for nourishing an implanted, fertilized ovum.

If the ovum is not fertilized, the corpus luteum disintegrates. As the level of progesterone drops, **menstruation** occurs; the uterine lining is shed during the course of a menstrual period. If the egg is fertilized and pregnancy occurs, the cells that eventually develop into the placenta secrete *human chorionic gonadotropin (HCG),* a messenger hormone that signals the pituitary not to start a new cycle. The corpus luteum then steps up its production of progesterone. Many women experience physical or psychological changes, or both, during their monthly cycles. Usually the changes are minor, but more serious problems can occur.

Premenstrual Syndrome (PMS)

Women with **premenstrual syndrome (PMS)** experience bodily discomfort and emotional distress for up to two weeks, from ovulation until the onset of menstruation. Three to 15 percent of these women develop very severe symptoms. In some studies, as many as 40 to 45 percent of women have reported at least one premenstrual symptom.

Once dismissed as a psychological problem, PMS has been recognized as a very real physiological disorder that may be caused by a hormonal deficiency; abnormal levels of thyroid hormone; an imbalance of estrogen and progesterone; changes in brain chemicals; or social and environmental factors, particularly stress. Because there are no consistent or objective ways of diagnosing premenstrual complaints, it's hard to know precisely how many women are affected.

The most common symptoms of PMS are mood changes, anxiety, irritability, difficulty concentrating, forgetfulness, impaired judgment, tearfulness, digestive symptoms (diarrhea, bloating, constipation), hot flashes, palpitations, dizziness, headache, fatigue, changes in appetite, cravings (usually for sweets or salt), water retention, breast tenderness, and insomnia. For a diagnosis to be made, women—using a self-rating symptom scale or calendar—must report troubling premenstrual symptoms in the period before menstruation in at least two successive menstrual cycles.

Treatments for PMS depend on specific symptoms. Diuretics (drugs that speed up fluid elimination) can relieve water retention and bloating. Relaxation techniques have led to a 60 percent reduction in anxiety symptoms. Sleep deprivation, or the use of bright light to adjust a woman's circadian or daily rhythm, also has proven beneficial. Behavioral approaches, such as exercise or charting cycles, help by letting women know when they're vulnerable. Calcium supplements and psychiatric drugs that boost the neurotransmitter serotonin, such as the antidepressants Prozac and Zoloft, also have provided significant relief for symptoms such as tension, depression, irritability, and mood swings.[4]

Premenstrual Dysphoric Disorder (PMDD)

Premenstrual dysphoric disorder, which is not related to PMS, occurs in an estimated 1 to 3 percent of all menstruating women. It is characterized by regular symptoms of depression (depressed mood, anxiety, mood swings, diminished interest or pleasure) during the last week of the menstrual cycles. Women with PMDD cannot function as usual at work, school, or home. They feel better a few days after menstruation begins.

PMDD remains controversial, primarily for political reasons. Some women's advocacy groups oppose labeling women with menstruation-linked symptoms as mentally ill. Others contend that a diagnosis of PMDD simply recognizes the distress some women experience and may make it easier for them to obtain needed help.

Menstrual Cramps

Dysmenorrhea is the medical name for the discomforts—abdominal cramps and pain, back and leg pain, diarrhea, tension, water retention, fatigue, and depression—that can occur during menstruation. About half of all men-

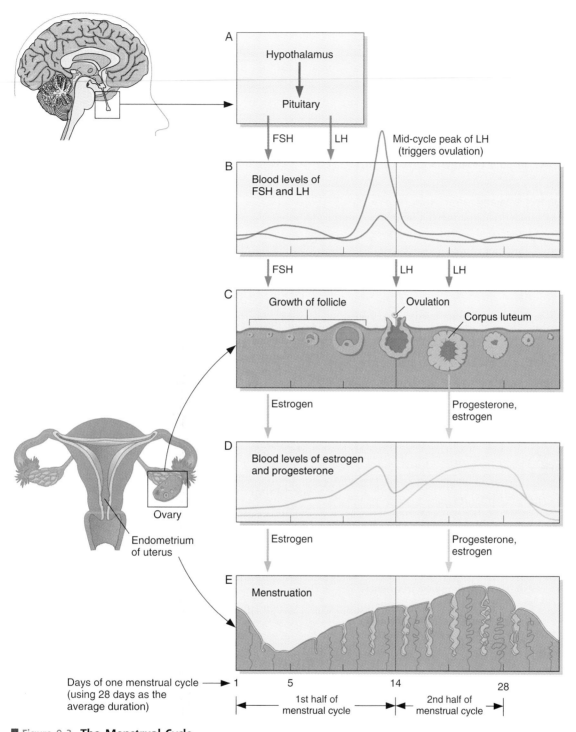

A Hypothalamus → Pituitary

FSH   LH

B Blood levels of FSH and LH

Mid-cycle peak of LH (triggers ovulation)

FSH   LH   LH

C Growth of follicle   Ovulation   Corpus luteum

Estrogen   Progesterone, estrogen

D Blood levels of estrogen and progesterone

Estrogen   Progesterone, estrogen

E Menstruation

Ovary

Endometrium of uterus

Days of one menstrual cycle (using 28 days as the average duration) → 1   5   14   28

1st half of menstrual cycle   2nd half of menstrual cycle

■ Figure 9-3 **The Menstrual Cycle**

Levels of the gonadotropins (FSH and LH) rise and then fall to stimulate the cycle. These changes affect the levels of the hormones estrogen and progesterone, which in turn react with LH and FSH. As a result, the lining of the uterus prepares to receive a fertilized egg while the ovarian follicle matures and then ruptures, releasing the ova (eggs) into the fallopian tube. If a fertilized egg is deposited, pregnancy begins. But if the egg is not fertilized, progesterone production decreases and the uterine lining is shed (menstruation). At this point both estrogen and progesterone levels have dropped, so the pituitary responds by producing FSH, and the cycle beings again.

Strategies *for* Prevention

Preventing Premenstrual Problems

✓ *Get plenty of exercise.* Physically fit women usually have fewer problems both before and during their periods.

✓ *Eat frequently and nutritiously.* In the week before your period, your body doesn't regulate the levels of sugar, or glucose, in your blood as well as it usually does.

✓ *Swear off salt.* If you stop using salt at the table and while cooking, you may gain less weight premenstrually, feel less bloated, and suffer less from headaches and irritability.

✓ *Cut back on caffeine.* Coffee, colas, diet colas, chocolate, and tea can increase breast tenderness and other symptoms.

✓ *Don't drink or smoke.* Some women become so sensitive to alcohol's effects before their periods that a glass of wine hits with the impact of several stiff drinks. Nicotine worsens low blood sugar problems.

✓ *Watch out for sweets.* Premenstrual cravings for sweets are common, but try to resist. Sugar may pick you up, but later you'll feel worse than before.

struating women suffer from dysmenorrhea. The cause seems to be an overproduction of bodily substances called *prostaglandins,* which typically rise during menstruation.

Women who produce excessive prostaglandins have more severe menstrual cramps. During a cramp, the uterine muscles may contract too strongly or frequently, and temporarily deprive the uterus of oxygen, causing pain. Medications that inhibit prostaglandins can reduce menstrual pain, and exercise can also relieve cramps.

Amenorrhea

Women may stop menstruating—a condition called **amenorrhea**—for a variety of reasons, including a hormonal disorder, drastic weight loss, strenuous exercise, or change in environment. "Boarding-school amenorrhea" is common among young women who leave home for school. Distance running and strenuous exercise also can lead to amenorrhea. The reason may be a drop in body fat from the normal 18 to 22 percent to 9 to 12 percent. To be considered amenorrhea, a woman's menstrual cycle is typically absent for three or more consecutive months. Prolonged amenorrhea can have serious health consequences, including a loss of bone density that may lead to stress fractures or osteoporosis.

In recent years scientists have discovered that the menstrual cycle actually begins in the brain with the production of gonadotropin-releasing hormone (GnRH). Each month a surge of GNRH sets into motion the sequence of steps that lead to ovulation, the potential for conception, and, if conception doesn't occur, menstruation. This understanding has led to the development of chemical mimics, or analogues, of GnRH—usually administered by nasal spray—that trigger ovulation in women who don't ovulate or menstruate normally.

Toxic Shock Syndrome (TSS)

This rare, potentially deadly bacterial infection primarily strikes menstruating women under the age of 30 who use tampons. Both *Staphylococcus aureus* and group A *Streptococcus pyogenes* can produce toxic shock syndrome (TSS). Symptoms include a high fever; a rash that leads to peeling of the skin on the fingers, toes, palms, and soles; dizziness; dangerously low blood pressure; and abnormalities in several organ systems (the digestive tract and the kidneys) and in the muscles and blood. Treatment usually consists of antibiotics and intense supportive care; intravenous administration of immunoglobulins that attack the toxins produced by these bacteria also may be beneficial. (See Chapter 12 for more on TSS.)

Menstruating women should follow these guidelines to reduce their risk of TSS:

- Use sanitary napkins instead of tampons.
- If you do use tampons, check the labels for information on absorbency (which the FDA has required manufacturers to provide), and avoid superabsorbent brands.
- Change tampons three or four times during the day.
- Use napkins during the night or for some time during each day of menstrual flow.

Midlife Changes

As the baby-boom generation ages, more people are focusing their attention on the major changes that occur in a woman's middle years. In the next decade, the number of women between the ages of 45 and 54 will increase by half, from 13 million to 19 million. Thus, a large segment of the population will be entering **perimenopause,** the period from a woman's first irregular cycles to her last menstruation.

Perimenopause

During this time, the egg cells, or oocytes, in a woman's ovaries start to "senesce" or die off at a faster rate.

Eventually, the number of egg cells drops to a tiny fraction of the estimated 2 million packed into her ovaries at birth. Trying to coax some of the remaining oocytes to ripen, the pituitary gland churns out extra follicle-stimulating hormone (FSH). This surge is the earliest harbinger of menopause, occurring six to ten years before a woman's final periods. Eventually the other menstrual messenger, luteinizing hormone (LH), also increases, but at a slower rate.

These hormonal shifts can trigger an array of symptoms. The most common are nighttime awakenings, caused by a spike in temperature (a subdromal hot flash, in medical terms) that is just intense enough to disrupt sleep. About 10 to 20 percent of perimenopausal women also experience daytime hot flashes—a symptom that becomes more prevalent with the more drastic and enduring hormonal changes of menopause itself.

Even in women who have never suffered from premenstrual syndrome (PMS), perimenopause can trigger its classic symptoms: irritability, tearfulness, fatigue, migraines, mood swings, anxiety. The suspected culprits are changes both in reproductive hormones and in neurochemistry. Some women report headaches, heart palpitations, dizziness, insomnia, tingling sensations in the skin, chills, restlessness, listlessness, headaches, or stress incontinence (release of urine when running, laughing, or sneezing).

While many women feel no need to seek help with such perimenopausal problems, an array of options can ease the way through this physiological prelude to menopause. More and more women are trying herbal and nutritional remedies, such as plant-based estrogens (phytoestrogens), including those found in soy products, and lifestyle changes, like exercise and relaxation, to promote better health. Physicians often suggest low-dose oral contraceptives, which relieve symptoms like night sweats and offer protection from pregnancy—a not insignificant benefit. Among women in their forties, the rate of unplanned pregnancies is almost as high as among teenagers.

Menopause

Menopause, defined as the complete cessation of menstrual periods for 12 consecutive months, officially arrives generally at age 51 or 52. About 10 to 15 percent of women breeze through this transition with only trivial symptoms. Another 10 to 15 percent are virtually disabled. The majority fall somewhere in between these extremes.

Dwindling levels of estrogen subtly affect many aspects of a woman's health, from her mouth (where dryness, unusual tastes, burning, and gum problems can develop) to her skin (which may become drier, itchier,

and overly sensitive to touch). The drop in estrogen levels also may cause hot flashes (bursts of perspiration that last from a few seconds to 15 minutes), which often happen at night, disturbing sleep and causing fatigue. With less estrogen to block them, a woman's androgens, or male hormones, may have a greater impact, causing acne, hair loss, and, according to some anecdotal reports, surges in sexual appetite. (Other women, however, report a drop in sexual desire.)

At the same time, a woman's clitoris, vulva, and vaginal lining begin to shrivel, sometimes resulting in pain or bleeding during intercourse. Since the thinner genital tissues are less effective in keeping out bacteria and other pathogens, urinary tract infections may become more common. Some women develop breast or ovarian cysts, which usually go away on their own. Eventually, a woman's ovaries don't respond at all to her pituitary hormones. After the last ovulatory cycle, progesterone is no longer secreted, and estrogen levels decrease rapidly.

Hormone Replacement Therapy

Hormone replacement therapy, or HRT, comes in different combinations, forms, and doses. Many regimens use much lower doses of estrogen than in the past; some use plant-based phytoestrogens or substitute natural progesterone for synthetic progestins; special formulations add testosterone to estrogen and progesterone.

HRT entails side effects and risks: Some women who try HRT become depressed (particularly if they had a similar reaction to birth control pills), develop gallstones, or experience a worsening of breast tenderness, migraines, fibroids, or endometriosis.

The biggest concern for women—and the primary reason they refuse or discontinue HRT—is the threat of breast cancer. Research studies, using different forms and doses of estrogen in different groups of women over varying periods of time, have produced contradictory findings. In general, breast cancer rates generally increase among women who have taken replacement hormones for prolonged periods (five, seven, or ten or more years in various studies). However, it is not certain if mortality rates from breast cancer also increase, or if every formulation presents an equal risk.

Countering HRT's risk of breast cancer are some major health benefits, including a greater than 50 percent reduction in heart disease, the number-one killer of women. Because of this potentially life-saving advantage, in statistical analyses, the presence of a single risk factor for heart disease, such as a family history of cardiovascular problems or hypertension, even among women at high risk of breast cancer, tips the risk-benefit balance in favor of HRT. (See Chapter 13.)

HRT also prevents the dramatic loss of bone density that begins after menopause and that can lead to osteoporosis. Women who start HRT within five years of menopause decrease their risk of hip, wrist, and non-spinal fractures when compared with women who have never used estrogen.

In addition to its benefits for heart and skeleton, HRT may also benefit the brain. Some studies suggest that HRT users score higher on tests of verbal and spatial memory, language, and attention (although the insomnia caused by hot flashes in women not on HRT may in itself lower their scores). Estrogen may increase production of acetylcholine, a neurotransmitter that regulates memory, learning, and other cognitive functions.

HRT also provides many short-term "QOL" or quality of life benefits that make living in a menopausal body more comfortable, although many women report that plant-based estrogens and herbal and nutritional remedies, though scientifically untested and unproven, can do the same. HRT relieves hot flashes, improves sleep, alleviates sexual symptoms, makes intercourse more enjoyable, and lessens urinary tract problems. Women on HRT report that they think better, remember more, and feel more energetic. They're also less prone to many age-related problems, such as tooth loss and driving accidents (possibly a consequence of improved concentration).

For these varied reasons, an increasing number of women are trying HRT. According to current estimates, 25 percent of all postmenopausal American women use HRT (up from 16 percent a decade ago); among those aged 50 to 54, the rate approaches 50 percent. The future should bring more and better choices. A new generation of selective estrogen receptor modulators (SERMS), including the anticancer drug tamoxifen and the osteoporosis drug raloxifene, which target only certain parts of the body, may greatly reduce the cancer risks associated with standard hormone replacement with long-term use. Other SERMS, currently being tested in the United States and Europe, may offer the benefits of estrogen, progesterone, and testosterone with few of their drawbacks. However, SERMS, like all medications, have side effects of their own, and it will take a number of years to sort out which ones may be most helpful to which women.

Men's Sexual Health

Because the male reproductive system is simpler in many ways than the female, it's often ignored—especially by healthy young men. However, just like women, men should make regular self-exams (including checking their penises, testes, and breasts, as described in Chapter 14) part of their routine.

Male Sexual Anatomy

The visible parts of the male sexual anatomy are the **penis** and **scrotum,** the pouch that contains the **testes** (see Figure 9-4). The testes manufacture testosterone and **sperm,** the male reproductive cells. Immature sperm are stored in the **epididymis,** a collection of coiled tubes adjacent to each testis.

The penis contains three hollow cylinders loosely covered with skin. The two major cylinders, the *corpora cavernosa,* extend side by side through the length of the penis. The third cylinder, the *corpus spongiosum,* surrounds the **urethra,** the channel for both seminal fluid and urine (see Figure 9-4).

When hanging down loosely, the average penis is about 3¾ inches long. During erection, its internal cylinders fill with so much blood that they become rigid, and the penis stretches to an average length of 6¼ inches. About 90 percent of all men have erect penises measuring between 5 and 7 inches in length. There is no relation, however, between penis size and female sexual satisfaction: A woman's vagina naturally adjusts during intercourse to the size of her partner's penis.

Inside the body are several structures involved in the production of seminal fluid, or **semen,** the liquid in which sperm cells are carried out of the body during ejaculation. The **vas deferens** are two tubes that carry sperm from the epididymis into the urethra. The **seminal vesicles,** which make some of the seminal fluid, join with the vas deferens to form the **ejaculatory ducts.** The **prostate gland** produces some of the seminal fluid, which it secretes into the urethra during ejaculation. The **Cowper's glands** are two pea-sized structures on either side of the urethra (just below where it emerges from the prostate gland) and connected to it via tiny ducts. When a man is sexually aroused, the Cowper's glands often secrete a fluid that appears as a droplet at the tip of the penis. This fluid is not semen, although it occasionally contains sperm.

 ## What Is Circumcision?

In its natural state, the tip of the penis is covered by a fold of skin called the foreskin. About 60 percent of baby boys in the United States undergo **circumcision,** the surgical removal of the foreskin. However, increasingly more parents are opting for the natural look.

An estimated 1.2 million newborn males are circumcised in the United States annually for reasons that vary from religious traditions to preventive health measures. Until the last half century, there was limited scientific evidence to support or repudiate routine circumcision.

A. External structure

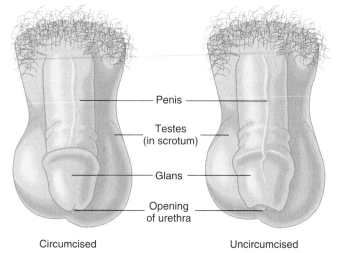

Penis

Testes
(in scrotum)

Glans

Opening
of urethra

Circumcised   Uncircumcised

B. Internal structure

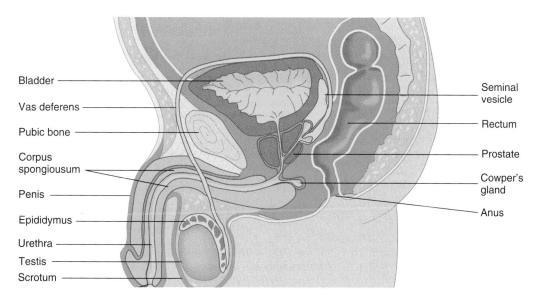

Bladder

Vas deferens

Pubic bone

Corpus
spongiousum

Penis

Epididymus

Urethra

Testis

Scrotum

Seminal
vesicle

Rectum

Prostate

Cowper's
gland

Anus

■ Figure 9-4 **The Male Sex Organs and Reproductive Structure**

cumcision include the risk of complications (which tend to be uncommon and minor) and pain. The AAP recommends that, when circumcision is performed, analgesic creams or anesthetic shots be used to minimize discomfort.

Parents who choose not to have their sons circumcised should not attempt to retract the foreskin. This could lead to infection, bleeding, or scarring. As a boy gets older, gradual retraction of the foreskin during bath time helps it dilate, with full retraction possible by age two to four. There is little consensus on what impact the presence or absence of a foreskin has on sexual functioning or satisfaction.

Prostate Problems

The chestnut-sized prostate gland, which surrounds the urethra at the base of the bladder, is a common source of concern. The most common problem in younger men is infection, or **prostatitis,** which can cause fever, pain during bowel movements, pain during a rectal exam, and pus in the urine. Infrequent sexual activity is one cause of prostatitis, and occasional bursts of sexual activity between long periods of abstinence are also likely to produce this problem. Prostatitis is usually treated with antibiotics, such as sulfa medications.

After age 40, the prostate enlarges; this condition, called **benign prostatic hypertrophy,** occurs in every man. By age 50, half of all men have some enlargement of the gland; after 70, three-quarters do. As it expands, the prostate tends to pinch the urethra, decreasing urinary flow and creating a sense of urinary urgency, particularly at night. Other warning signs of prostate problems include difficult urination, blood in the urine, painful ejaculation, or constant lower-back pain.

The drug Proscar (generic name, finasteride), which shrinks an enlarged prostate, has provided an alternative

In 1999, the American Academy of Pediatrics reviewed 40 years of data and concluded that, while there are potential medical benefits, the data are not strong enough to recommend routine neonatal circumcision. Since the procedure is not essential to the child's current well-being, the academy concluded that parents should determine what is in the best interest of the child.[5]

Circumcision does provide some benefits: Boys who are not circumcised are four times as likely to develop urinary tract infections in their first year; however, such infections develop in only 1 percent of uncircumcised boys. Uncircumcised men are three times as likely to develop penile cancer, but the absolute risk is low. (Only about nine in every million American men ever gets cancer of the penis.) Circumcised men also are at lower risk of becoming infected after exposure to HIV or other sexually transmitted diseases. The drawbacks of cirto corrective surgery for many men. Other drugs and treatments are being tried experimentally.

The older a man gets, the more likely he is to develop prostate cancer, which now affects one in every eleven American men and claims 30,000 lives each year (see Chapter 14). Second only to lung cancer in terms of mortality, prostate cancer is more common in African Americans than in white Americans. Scientists have developed a screening test that measures levels of a protein called *prostate-specific antigen (PSA)* in the blood. The test, designed to detect prostate cancer at its earliest, most curable stage, is not precise and often indicates cancer where none exists. Men over age 50 should also receive annual rectal examinations, in which a doctor inserts a (gloved) finger into the rectum and feels the prostate for abnormal growths that may indicate cancer.

Midlife Changes

Although men don't experience the dramatic hormonal upheaval that women do at midlife, they do experience a decline by as much as 30 to 40 percent in their primary sex hormone, testosterone, between the ages of 48 and 70. This drop may cause a range of symptoms, including decreased muscle mass, greater body fat, loss of bone density, flagging energy, lowered fertility, and impaired virility. Some researchers are experimenting with testosterone supplements, which, in tests with young men, have been shown to increase lean body mass and decrease body fat—at least temporarily. However, other researchers warn that, particularly in older men, excess testosterone might raise the risk of prostate cancer and heart disease.

While the production of testosterone diminishes with age, sexual ability and enjoyment do not. However, men should expect some differences in their sexual response as they grow older, including the following:

- A need for more time and arousal to achieve erection.
- A longer time before ejaculation.
- A briefer orgasm.
- A decrease in the force of expulsion of the semen at orgasm.
- A smaller volume of ejaculate.
- A more rapid loss of erection after orgasm.
- A lengthening of the time after ejaculation until a man is again capable of intercourse and orgasm.

Responsible Sexuality

The World Health Organization defines **sexual health** as "the integration of the physical, emotional, intellectual, and social aspects of sexual being in ways that are positively enriching, and that enhance personality, communication, and love . . . every person has a right to receive sexual information and to consider sexual relationships for pleasure as well as for procreation."

Characteristics of a Sexually Healthy Adult

SIECUS has worked with nongovernmental organizations around the world to develop a consensus about the life behaviors of a sexually healthy adult. These include:

- Appreciating one's own body.
- Seeking information about reproduction as needed.
- Affirming that sexual development may or may not include reproduction or genital sexual experience.
- Interacting with both genders in respectful and appropriate ways.
- Affirming one's own sexual orientation and respecting the sexual orientation of others.
- Expressing love and intimacy in appropriate ways.
- Developing and maintaining meaningful relationships.
- Avoiding exploitative or manipulative relationships.
- Making informed choices about family options and lifestyles.
- Enjoying and expressing one's sexuality throughout life.
- Expressing one's sexuality in ways congruent with one's values.
- Discriminating between life-enhancing sexual behaviors and those that are harmful to self and/or others.
- Expressing one's sexuality while respecting the rights of others.
- Seeking new information to enhance one's sexuality.
- Using contraception effectively to avoid unintended pregnancy.
- Preventing sexual abuse.
- Seeking early prenatal care.
- Avoiding contracting or transmitting a sexually transmitted disease, including HIV.

- Practicing health-promoting behaviors, such as regular check-ups, breast and testicular self-exam, and early identification of potential problems.
- Demonstrating tolerance for people with different sexual values and lifestyles.
- Exercising democratic responsibility to influence legislation dealing with sexual issues.
- Assessing the impact of family, cultural, religious, media, and societal messages on one's thoughts, feelings, values, and behaviors related to sexuality.
- Promoting the rights of all people to accurate sexuality information.
- Avoiding behaviors that exhibit prejudice and bigotry.
- Rejecting stereotypes about the sexuality of diverse populations.[6]

Sexually Healthy Relationships

A sexually healthy relationship, as defined by SIECUS, is based on shared values and has five characteristics: It is consensual, nonexploitative, honest, mutually pleasurable, and protected against unintended pregnancy and sexuality transmitted diseases (STDs), including HIV/AIDS. All individuals also have sexual rights, which include the right to the information, education, skills, support, and services they need to make responsible decisions about their sexuality consistent with their own values, as well as the right to express one's sexual orientations without violence or discrimination.

Sexual decision making always takes place within the context of an individual's values (discussed in Chapter 3) and perceptions of right and wrong behavior. Making sexually responsible decisions means considering all the possible consequences of sexual behavior for both yourself and your partner. It must always take into account, not just personal preferences and desires, but the very real risks of unwanted pregnancy, sexually transmitted diseases (STDs) and long-term medical consequences (such as impaired fertility). You also must consider the emotional consequences of a sexual relationship—not just for yourself but also for your partner.

The following sections may help ensure that the sexual decisions you make are responsible ones.

Sexuality Education

Public support for sexuality education has grown. In a national SIECUS poll, 93 percent of Americans said they support teaching about sexuality in high school, while 84 percent support sexuality instruction in middle or junior high schools. More than eight in ten believe young people should be given information to protect themselves from unplanned pregnancies and STDs as well as learning about abstinence.[7]

The CDC estimates that 91.5 percent of American students have been taught about AIDS or HIV infection in school.[8] By the end of 2002, the federal government will have allocated nearly half a billion dollars in funds for programs that teach abstinence only until marriage.[9] According to studies of the impact of sexuality programs, learning about sex and protection from STDs does not increase sexual activity and can delay the age of first intercourse, reduce the frequency of intercourse, and decrease the number of sexual partners.[10]

The most effective educational programs provide accurate information about the risks of unprotected intercourse and methods of avoiding them; focus on one or more sexual behaviors that lead to unintended pregnancy or HIV/STD infection; give a clear and consistent message; address social pressures on sexual behaviors; and provide modeling and practice of communication, negotiation, and refusal skills.[11] Studies comparing programs that emphasize abstinence with those emphasizing either abstinence or safer sex found that both reduce HIV sexual risk behaviors, but that safer sex programs may be especially effective with sexually experienced adolescents and may have longer-lasting effects for all teens.[12] In one study that interviewed participants a year after completing "sex ed," African-American adolescents who completed a safer-sex educational program reported more frequent condom use than peers who received abstinence-only or general health education. Those who began having sex prior to entering the program had intercourse and unprotected intercourse less often. Those in the abstinence-only program reported more frequent condom use than those in the general health programs.[13]

Sexuality education is a lifelong process. Your own knowledge about sex may not be as extensive as you might assume. Most people grow up with a lot of myths and misconceptions about sex. (See Self-Survey: "How Much Do You Know About Sex?") Rather than relying on what peers say or what you've always thought was true, find out the facts. This textbook is a good place to start. The student health center and the library can provide additional materials on sexual identity, orientation, behavior, and health, as well as on options for reducing your risk of acquiring sexually transmitted diseases (discussed in Chapter 12) or becoming pregnant.

Self-*Survey* — How Much Do You Know About Sex?

Mark each of the following statements True or False:

1. Men and women have completely different sex hormones. _____
2. Premenstrual syndrome (PMS) is primarily a psychological problem. _____
3. Circumcision diminishes a man's sexual pleasure. _____
4. Sexual orientation may have a biological basis. _____
5. Masturbation is a sign of emotional immaturity. _____
6. Only homosexual men engage in anal intercourse. _____
7. Despite their awareness of AIDS, many college students do not practice safe sex. _____
8. After age 60, lovemaking is mainly a fond memory, not a regular pleasure of daily living. _____
9. Doctors advise against having intercourse during a woman's menstrual period. _____
10. Only men ejaculate. _____
11. It is possible to be infected with HIV during a single sexual encounter. _____
12. Impotence is always a sign of emotional or sexual problems in a relationship. _____

Answers:

1. False. Men and women have the same hormones, but in different amounts.
2. False. PMS has been recognized as a very real physiological disorder that may be caused by a hormonal deficiency, abnormal levels of thyroid hormone, changes in brain chemicals, or social and environmental factors, such as stress.
3. False. Sex therapists have not been able to document differences in sensitivity to stimulation between circumcised and uncircumcised men.
4. True. Researchers documented structural differences in the brains of homosexual men and women.
5. False. Throughout a person's life, masturbation can be a form of sexual release and pleasure.
6. False. As many as one in every four married couples under age 35 have reported that they occasionally engage in anal intercourse.
7. True. In one recent study, more than a third of college students had engaged in vaginal or anal intercourse at least once in the previous year without using effective protection from conception or sexually transmitted diseases (STDs).
8. False. More than a third of American married men and women older than 60 make love at least once a week as do 10% of those older than 70.
9. False. There's no medical reason to avoid intercourse during a woman's menstrual period.
10. False. Stimulation of the Grafenberg spot in a woman's vagina may lead to a release of fluid from her urethra during orgasm.
11. True. Although the risk increases with repeated sexual contact with an infected partner, an individual can contract HIV during a single sexual encounter.
12. False. Many erection difficulties have physical causes.

Making Changes

Informing Yourself About Sex

Your score on this self-survey may indicate that you know a lot more—or less—about sex than you thought you did. Part of sexual responsibility is being informed about sexuality, including reproductive anatomy, sexual orientation, the range of sexual behaviors, and ways of protecting yourself from sexually transmitted diseases.

How can you get good information about sex? If you have questions about sexual biology or behavior, you can usually get accurate and understandable answers from college-level human sexuality textbooks. If you're concerned about birth control or protection from sexually transmitted diseases, your college health clinic and your local Planned Parenthood clinic are excellent resources. For questions regarding your own sexual and reproductive health and organs, visit a health care professional for a thorough examination.

Knowledge about sex can help free you from misconceptions that could be dangerous to your health. There's an added psychological benefit as well: The more you know, the less confused you'll feel about your own sexuality.

Talking About Sex

Prior to any sexual activity that involves a risk of sexually transmitted infection or pregnancy, both partners should talk about their prior sexual histories (including number of partners and exposure to STDs) and other high-risk behavior, such as the use of injection drugs. They should also discuss the issue of birth control and which methods might be best for them to use. If you know someone well enough to consider having sex with that person, you should be able to talk about such sensitive subjects. If a potential partner is unwilling to talk or hedges on crucial questions, you shouldn't be engaging in sex. (See Pulsepoints: "Top Ten Rules of Sexual Etiquette.")

Styles of communicating vary among white Americans, African Americans, Hispanic Americans, and Asian Americans. While white and African Americans may openly discuss sex with partners, Hispanic-American couples generally do not discuss their sexual relationship. Asian Americans also are less inclined to discuss sex and to value nonverbal, indirect, and intuitive communication over explicit verbal interaction.[14]

Here are some questions to consider as you think and talk about the significance of becoming sexually intimate with a partner:

- What role do we want relationships and sex to have in our life at this time?

- What are my values and my potential partner's values as they pertain to sexual relationships? Does each of us believe that intercourse should be reserved for a permanent partnership or committed relationship?

- Will a decision to engage in sex enhance my positive feelings about myself or my partner? Does either of us have questions about sexual orientation or the kinds of people we are attracted to?

- Do I and my partner both want to have sex? Is my partner pressuring me in any way? Am I pressuring my partner? Am I making this decision for myself or my partner?

- Have my partner and I discussed our sexual histories and risk factors? Have I spoken honestly about any STDs I've had in the past? Am I sure that neither my partner nor I have a sexually transmitted infection?

- Have we taken precautions against unwanted pregnancy and STDs?

Whether couples are on a first date or have been married for years, each partner always has the right *not* to have sex. Unfortunately, "no" sometimes seems to mean different things to men and women. At some campuses, such as Antioch College in Ohio, freshmen must attend workshops on sexual consent and adhere to a campus policy that requires "willing and verbal consent" for each sexual act. (Chapter 18 also discusses sexual coercion.)

PULSE *points*

Top Ten Rules of Sexual Etiquette

1. **Be sure sexual activity is consensual.** Coercion can take many forms: physical, emotional and verbal. All cause psychological damage and undermine trust and respect.

2. **No means no.** At any point in a relationship, whether the couple is dating or married, either individual has the right to say "no."

3. **In sexual situations, always think ahead.** For the sake of safety, think about potential dangers—parking in an isolated area, going into a bedroom with someone you hardly know, and the like—and options to protect yourself.

4. **Be aware of your own and your partner's alcohol and drug intake.** The use of such sub-

stances impairs judgment and reduces the ability to say no. While under their influence, you may engage in sexual behavior you'll later regret.

5. **Be prepared.** If there's any possibility that you may be engaging in sex, be sure you have the means to protect yourself against unwanted pregnancy and sexually transmitted diseases.

6. **Communicate openly.** If you or your partner cannot talk openly and honestly about your sexual histories and contraception, you avoid having sex. For the sake of protecting your sexual health, you have to be willing to ask—and answer—questions that may seem embarrassing.

7. **Share responsibility in a sexual relationship.** Both partners should be involved in protecting

themselves and each other from STDs and, if heterosexual, unwanted pregnancy.

8. **Respect sexual privacy.** Revealing sexual activities violates the trust between two partners. Bragging about a sexual conquest demeans everyone involved.

9. **Do not sexually harass others.** Pinches, pats, sexual comments or jokes, and suggestive gestures are offensive and disrespectful. (See Chapter 18 for more on harassment.)

10. **Be considerate.** A public display of sexual affection can be extremely embarrassing to others. Roommates, in particular, should be sensitive and discrete in their sexual behavior.

Source: Adapted from: Hatcher, Robert, et al. *Sexual Etiquette 101.* Atlanta, GA: Emory University School of Medicine.

The X&Y Files

An Evolutionary View of Sex Differences in Attraction

hat triggers sexual attraction? For heterosexuals, the answer is likely to depend on whether they are male or female. These differences may have evolved millions of years ago—and may have helped guarantee the survival of our species.

What attracts a man to a woman? In various surveys in the past decades, men consistently rate one factor as most important: appearance. However, even though men usually report that they notice a woman's bosom or legs, psychologists who carefully measured the proportions of pin-ups of yesteryear, as well as of contemporary *Playboy* centerfolds, homecoming queens, and beauty contestants, found one anatomical feature that most attracted men: the ratio of a woman's waist to her hips. Regardless of the actual measurements, women whose hips were about a third larger than their waists ranked as most desirable.

According to evolutionary theorists, men may have unconsciously learned to assess a woman's waist-hip ratio—or WHR—eons ago. Why? Waist-hip ratio may be a good guarantee of a woman's ability to deliver a healthy infant safely. A slim-hipped woman may be unable to do so; a large-waisted woman may, in fact, already be pregnant with another man's child. As it turns out, WHR also testifies to a woman's health. According to contemporary analyses of apple and pear shapes, women whose hips measure about a third larger than their waists are less likely to develop high blood pres-

sure, diabetes, gall bladder problems, and other diseases. Other features that attract men—shiny hair, white teeth, glowing skin, full lips—also testify to youth, health, and fertility, essentials for guaranteeing their genetic future.

Appearance has never ranked highly in determining which men women find attractive. After studying female preferences in various cultures around the world, evolutionary biologist David Buss of the University of Texas concluded that women primarily want good providers of resources for their children. From the perspective of a woman's evolutionary mandate, nothing may have mattered more than finding a mate who would help ensure the survival of her child.

The human baby is born more helpless than any other, explains anthropologist Nina Jablonsky of the California Academy of Sciences. Women must have realized very early on that they would not be able to protect it all by themselves. They needed partners who would provide them and their children with shelter, adequate food, and protection from predators and other dangers.

Do these evolutionary drives still make sense in the modern world? No, say many experts, who note that, nonetheless, knowing about the evolutionary roots of behavior may help contemporary men and women understand each other better.

Sources: Hales, Dianne. *Just Like a Woman.* New York: Bantam Books, 2000. Buss, David. *The Evolution of Desire.* New York: HarperCollins, 1994. Allman, William. *The Stone Age Present.* New York: Simon & Schuster, 1994.

Across the Lifespan: Sexual Behavior

From birth to death, we are sexual beings. Our sexual identities, needs, likes, and dislikes emerge in adolescence and become clearer as we enter adulthood, but we continue to change and evolve throughout our lives. In men, sexual interest is most intense at age 18; in women, it reaches a peak in the 30s. Although age brings changes in sexual responsiveness, we never outgrow our sexuality.

Sexuality in Childhood

For infants, the mouth is the principal source of sensual pleasure, but they are also sensitive to genital and general body contact. By the age of 3 or 4, children recognize the genital differences between males and females, and may develop childhood romances. Curiosity about

adults' and other children's genitals, about where babies come from, and about breasts on women and beards on men continues until age 8 or 9. At that time, interest in sex play becomes less common; but curiosity about sex and where babies come from remains high.

"Unless they don't watch TV, don't go to movies and don't talk with friends, children will be curious about sex," says Nancy Adler, professor of medical psychology at the University of California, San Francisco. "Even if they didn't, they'd probably still want to know about sex." It is crucially important for today's parents to answer children's questions about sex as honestly as they can. The primary message to convey, Adler suggests, is simple: Sex is a normal part of life that's done responsibly by two people in a loving relationship.[15] While some awkwardness may be inevitable, parents can master the art of honest, open, and comfortable conversation.

Strategies *for* Change

How to Say No to Sex

✓ First of all, recognize your own values and feelings. If you believe that sex is something to be shared only by people who've already become close in other ways, be true to that belief.

✓ If you're at a loss for words, try these responses: "I like you a lot, but I'm not ready to have sex." "You're a great person, but sex isn't something I do to prove I like someone." "I'd like to wait until I'm married to have sex."

✓ If you're feeling pressured, let your date know that you're uncomfortable. Be simple and direct. Watch out for emotional blackmail. If your date says, "If you really liked me, you'd want to make love," point out that if he or she really liked you, he or she wouldn't try to force you to do something you don't want to do.

✓ If you're a woman, monitor your sexual signals. Men impute more sexual meaning to gestures (such as casual touching) that women perceive as friendly and innocent.

✓ Communicate your feelings to your date sooner rather than later. It's far easier to say, "I don't want to go to your apartment," than to fight off unwelcome advances once you're there.

✓ Remember that if saying no to sex puts an end to a relationship, it wasn't much of a relationship in the first place.

Adolescent Sexuality

Early in adolescence, sexual curiosity explodes, and sexual exploration—both alone and with a partner—takes on new meaning and intensity. Sexual education programs can make a difference by helping young people become sexually responsible, enable them to form satisfying relationships, help them assess their own attitudes toward sex, and give them information on sexuality. Good programs can clarify values and enhance communication.[16]

It's not unusual for teenage boys to experience frequent erections during the day and night, including **nocturnal emissions,** or wet dreams, during which ejaculation occurs. **Masturbation** (discussed later in this chapter) is the primary form of sexual expression for many teenagers, especially boys. Self-stimulation helps teens learn about their bodies and their sexual potential and serves as an outlet for sexual tension. By the end of

adolescence, the majority of teens have masturbated to orgasm.

Other common sexual activities during adolescence include kissing and petting—erotic physical contact that may include holding, touching, manual stimulation of the genitals, and oral sex. As many as 25 percent of teens experience some same-sex attractions. Although many experiment with heterosexual and homosexual sexual experiences, adolescent sexual behavior does not always foretell sexual orientation. Young people, who often feel confused about their sexual identity, may engage in sexual activity with members of the same or the other sex as a way of testing how they really feel.[17]

According to the CDC, today's teens are less sexually active than in the past.[18] (See Figure 9-5.) More than half remain virgins until they are at least 17 years of age. By age 20, 20 percent of males and 24 percent of females have not had sexual intercourse. In the 1990s, the percentage of male sexually active high school students dropped significantly, as did the prevalence of multiple sexual partners among males. Condom use increased among sexually active students.[19]

Nonetheless, the United States continues to have the highest rate of teen pregnancy in the Western world. Of the 11 million unmarried adolescent females who are sexually active, about 1 million become pregnant each year. An estimated 40 percent of these pregnancies end in abortion; 50 percent, in live births; the others, in miscarriage.[20] (See the discussion of teen pregnancy in Chapter 10.)

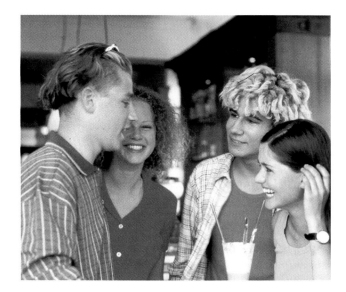

Sexuality has biological and psychological components. During adolescence sexuality develops rapidly: teens explore different social and intimate relationships as they begin to develop a sexual identity.

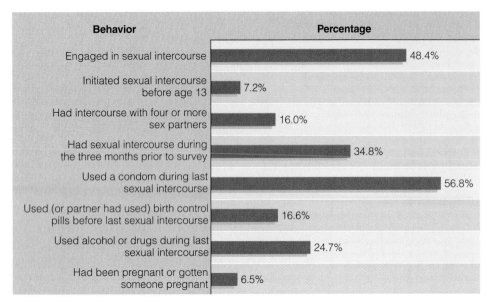

■ Figure 9-5 **The Sex Life of High School Students**

Sex on Campus

As Campus Focus: "The Sex Life of College Students" indicates, many college students engage in a variety of sexual behaviors. This sort of activity begins prior to first intercourse. In a recent study of 311 students at several northeastern colleges and universities, the men reported somewhat more frequent sexual behavior before first intercourse than the women (by about 5 to 8 percent). However, the majority of both men (70 percent) and women (57 percent) reported at least one experience with oral genital contact; more than 25 percent reported more frequent experiences.[21]

A substantial proportion of college students—male and female—report that they engage in unwanted sexual activity. Sometimes this is the result of sexual coercion (a problem discussed in Chapter 18) or alcohol use.[22] However, some students admit to feigning desire and consenting to an unwanted sexual activity for various reasons, including satisfying a partner's needs, promoting intimacy, and avoiding relationship tension.[23]

Even when well informed about safer sex and the risk of HIV infection and other STDs, many college students engage in risky behaviors. According to some researchers, the "typical" high-risk student is a non-Asian young male who became sexually active at a younger age than his peers, has more permissive attitudes toward sexuality, and is not religious. Interestingly, he also has greater knowledge about HIV, is more likely to have been tested for HIV, is more self-confident, and is somewhat more comfortable talking to sexual partners about past sexual history and AIDS testing.[24]

There are many reasons why college students, even when well informed, do not always take precautions to reduce the risk of STDs. Often they believe that HIV and other infections simply couldn't happen to them, or they use misleading criteria in assessing risk. In one experiment, college students, especially men, overrelied on a potential partner's physical attractiveness and gave less consideration to sexual history.[25] Women tend to insist on safe-sex practices with a new partner but, as they become more seriously involved, use protection less often—a potentially dangerous practice since knowing someone better doesn't make sex safer.

A study of 61 homosexual college men at a large mid-Atlantic state university found considerable concern about HIV infection. More than a quarter of the men had not engaged in homosexual activity. Of the 72 percent who had had sex with a man, some had made dramatic changes in their sexual behavior because of their fear of HIV: 7 percent had become celibate, and 14 percent no longer engaged in anal intercourse. About half had limited the number of people with whom they had sex and reported being more selective in choosing partners; 36 percent refused to have sex without a condom.

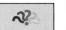 ## How Sexually Active Are American Adults?

The scientific study of Americans' sexual behavior began in 1938, when Alfred Kinsey, Ph.D., a professor of biology at the University of Indiana, and his colleagues asked some 5,300 white men and 5,940 white women about their sexual practices. In his landmark studies—*Sexual Behavior in the Human Male*, published in 1948, and *Sexual Behavior in the Human Female*, published in 1953—Kinsey reported that 73 percent of men and 20 percent of women had premarital intercourse by age 20, and 37 percent of men and 17 percent of women had some homosexual experience in their lifetime.

Even though Kinsey's research sample was not representative of the population as a whole, for decades his

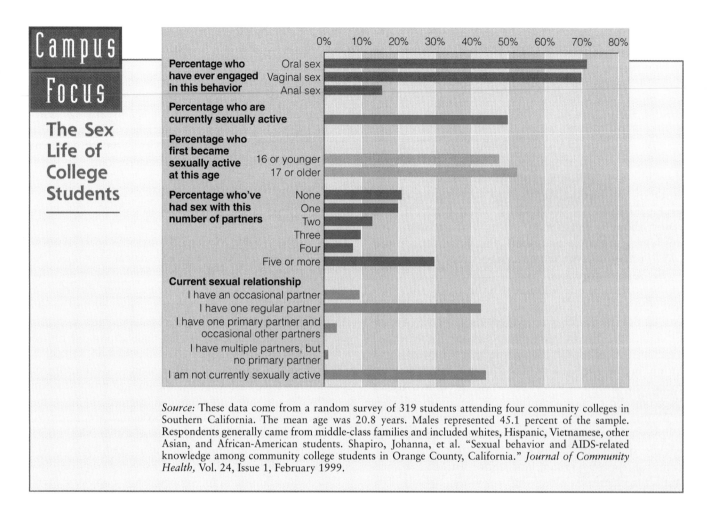

Campus Focus

The Sex Life of College Students

Percentage who have ever engaged in this behavior
- Oral sex
- Vaginal sex
- Anal sex

Percentage who are currently sexually active

Percentage who first became sexually active at this age
- 16 or younger
- 17 or older

Percentage who've had sex with this number of partners
- None
- One
- Two
- Three
- Four
- Five or more

Current sexual relationship
- I have an occasional partner
- I have one regular partner
- I have one primary partner and occasional other partners
- I have multiple partners, but no primary partner
- I am not currently sexually active

Source: These data come from a random survey of 319 students attending four community colleges in Southern California. The mean age was 20.8 years. Males represented 45.1 percent of the sample. Respondents generally came from middle-class families and included whites, Hispanic, Vietnamese, other Asian, and African-American students. Shapiro, Johanna, et al. "Sexual behavior and AIDS-related knowledge among community college students in Orange County, California." *Journal of Community Health,* Vol. 24, Issue 1, February 1999.

work remained the most definitive and revealing account of the sex lives of ordinary people. In the 1980s, after the emergence and recognition of the HIV epidemic, researchers and public health officials felt an urgent need for contemporary population-based studies that might help develop strategies to prevent HIV transmission. The last decade has seen several national surveys of sexual behavior.

The Janus Report on Sexual Behavior, published in 1993, was based on a survey of 2,765 individuals across the United States. A larger survey, conducted by researchers at the University of Chicago, was based on face-to-face interviews with 3,432 Americans, aged 18 to 59. It became the basis for two books published in 1994: *Sex in America,* aimed at a lay audience, and *The Social Organization of Sexuality,* a more scholarly work. Since then, the researcher's General Social Survey (GSS) database on sexual activity has grown to nearly 10,000 respondents, about three times larger than the 1992 study.

The GSS data indicate that overall sexual activity in America is relatively infrequent, with an average of 58 episodes per year, or slightly more than one a week. Yet there has been an increase in sexual activity in the 1990s, compared with earlier decades—even though the population is aging, works longer hours, and can choose among a growing number of distractions. About 15 percent of adults engage in half of all sexual activity; 42 percent of adults engage in 85 percent of all sex.[26]

The average adult reports having sex about once a week. However, 1 in 5 Americans has been celibate for at least a year, and 1 in 20 engages in sex at least every other day. Men report more sexual frequency than women—not because men are more boastful about their prowess, the researchers contend, but because the sample of women includes many widows and older women without partners. Among married people, the frequency reports of husbands and wives (not in the same couples) are within one episode per year—58.6 for married men and 57.9 for married women. And if other differences between men and women are statistically controlled (such as sexual preference, age, and educational attainment), married women actually report a slightly higher frequency than men.

People who are married, have children at home, and work long hours report having more sex. Those who work more than 60 hours a week are about 10 percent more sexually active than other workers, and even those who have preschool-aged children report having more sex than average. Even after their answers are controlled for differences in age, gender, and other factors, Americans with the longest work hours report higher sexual frequency.

The main reason why married people have sex more often is that they have easy access to a partner. Affluent, well-educated people, those in the top one-tenth of the income distribution, also report above-average sexual frequency. Even then, the rich only report about 5 percent more sex. In fact, adjustment for age and marital status reveals that Americans at the lower rungs of the income ladder may have slightly higher sexual frequency.

Sexual frequency peaks among those with some college education, then decreases among four-year college graduates, and declines even further among those with professional degrees. Americans who have attended graduate school are the least sexually active educational group in the population. These respondents may be more honest than others in reporting sexual activity, or they may be more precise in their definition of what counts as sex.

Sexual frequency increases among those who engage in other pleasurable pursuits, such as attending concerts, sporting events, and active forms of leisure. Yet it also increases along with television viewing. The more TV individuals watch, the more often they have sex. "It is not clear," the researchers observe, "whether the sexual response is stimulated by what is on the screen, or by boredom. And for some reason, watching PBS seems more positively related with increased sexual behavior than watching regular prime-time drama."

Sexual activity is higher among self-defined political liberals than among moderates or conservatives, and it is highest among those who describe themselves as "extreme liberals" and among "extreme conservatives." Catholics are slightly more sexually active than Protestants. But both Christian groups are about 20 percent less active than are Jews or agnostics. Among Protestant groups, Baptists are slightly above average and Presbyterians and Lutherans are slightly below average. Those who attend religious services of any sort at least once a week are less sexually active.

The most sexually active Americans are far more likely than average to approve of premarital or extramarital sex, to see positive benefits in pornography, to watch X-rated movies, and to favor giving birth control pills to teenagers. But those with liberal attitudes aren't the only sexually active individuals. People who own guns also have higher-than-average sexual frequency.

Does sex make people happier or healthier? Based on their analysis, the researchers concluded that the more sex a person has, the more likely he or she is to report having a happy life and a happy marriage. This connection is stronger among women than men. A second and more important predictor of sexual frequency is the feeling that one's life is exciting rather than routine or dull. "Being excited by life is most strongly associated with being happier," the researchers noted. "It seems that increased sexual activity is one of the many benefits of having a positive attitude."

Sex and Aging

In 1999 the AARP Modern Maturity Sexual Survey of 1,384 adults, one of the largest national studies ever done of middle-aged and older Americans, found that the number of people who view their partners as romantic and/or physically attractive does not decline with age but may actually increase. Six in ten men aged 45 to 59 gave their partners the highest possible ratings for being "physically attractive," as did 64 percent of 75-year-olds. About half of the women in their forties and fifties gave their partners the highest possible rating as "physically attractive," and 57 percent of those age 75 and over gave the same response.[27]

In terms of frequency, among those with sexual partners, more than 6 in 10 of men aged 45 to 59 (62 percent) and women 45 to 54 (64 percent) reported that they engage in sexual intercourse once a week or more, as do about one-quarter of those 75 and older (26 percent for men and 24 percent for women). Overall, 7 in 10 of those with partners (72 percent for men and 75 percent for women) reported engaging in intercourse at least once a month. However, only 21 percent of women 75 and older have partners, compared to 58 percent for men in the same age group.

Despite media hype over Viagra, few of those with self-reported problems took impotence drugs, and those who did said sexual frequency didn't increase, but the sex was better. Among men, 33 percent reported having sex once a week or more after using Viagra or another treatment, compared to 25 percent reporting weekly intercourse before treatment. However, 62 percent of men and 9 percent of women who used some drug or treatment said it enhanced their satisfaction with their sex life, and 54 percent of men and 57 percent of women said it had a "positive effect."

Health and sexuality interact in various ways as we age. In a review of sexual function in 1,202 aging men, both the men's health status and their partners' perceived responsiveness were key factors in sexual frequency. When they were in good health and had a willing partner, a substantial number of older men continued to be sexually active.[28] A recent study of a group of physically active men and women over age 50 found that the fittest men and women reported more frequent sexual activity; the fittest men (but not women) also showed the greatest sexual satisfaction.

Other research has found a relationship between sex and longevity. A Swedish study found that men, but not women, who had discontinued intercourse had higher death rates. A study of the entire male population of a small Welsh town found that the sexually active men had half the mortality of the inactive group. In a Duke University study, longevity in women correlated with enjoyment of sexual intercourse, rather than with its frequency.[29]

Aging does cause some changes in sexual response: Women produce less vaginal lubrication, and it takes longer for an older man to achieve an erection or orgasm and longer to attain another erection after ejaculating. Both men and women experience fewer contractions during orgasm. However, none of these changes reduces sexual pleasure or desire.

Sexual Diversity

Human beings are diverse in all ways—including sexual preferences and practices. Physiological, psychological, and social factors attract us to members of a certain sex; this attraction is our **sexual orientation**. Sigmund Freud argued that we all start off **bisexual**, or attracted to both sexes. But by the time they reach adulthood, most males prefer female sexual partners, and most females prefer male partners. **Heterosexual** is the term used for individuals whose primary orientation is toward members of the other sex. In virtually all cultures, some men and women are **homosexuals**, preferring partners of their own sex.

In our society, we tend to view heterosexuality and homosexuality as very different. In reality, these orientations are opposite ends of a spectrum of sexual preferences. Sex researcher Alfred Kinsey devised a seven-point continuum representing sexual orientation in American society. At one end of the continuum are those exclusively attracted to members of the opposite sex; at the other end are people exclusively attracted to members of the same sex. In between are varying degrees of homosexual and heterosexual orientation.

According to Kinsey's original data, 4 percent of men and 2 percent of women are exclusively homosexual. More recent studies have found lower numbers. For instance, in the University of Chicago's national survey, 2.8 percent of the men and 1.4 percent of the women defined themselves as homosexual. However, when asked if they'd had sex with a person of the same gender since age 18, about 5 percent of men and 4 percent of women said yes. If asked if they found members of the same sex sexually attractive, 6 percent of men and 5.5 percent of women said yes.

Bisexuality

Bisexuality—sexual attraction to both males and females—can develop at any point in one's life. In some cultures, bisexual activity is considered part of normal sexual experimentation. Among the Sambia Highlanders in Papua New Guinea, for instance, boys perform oral sex on one another as part of the rites of passage into manhood.[30]

Some people identify themselves as bisexual even if they don't behave bisexually. Some are "serial" bisexuals—that is, they are sexually involved with same-sex partners for a while and then with partners of the other sex, or vice versa. An estimated 7 to 9 million men, about twice the number thought to be exclusively homosexual, could be described as bisexual during some extended period of their lives. The largest group are married, rarely have sexual relations with women other than their wives, and have secret sexual involvements with men.

Fear of HIV infection has sparked great concern about bisexuality, particularly among heterosexual women who worry about becoming involved with a bisexual man. About 20 to 30 percent of women with AIDS were infected by bisexual partners, and health officials fear that bisexual men who hide their homosexual affairs could transmit HIV to many more women. (See Chapter 11.)

Homosexuality

Homosexuality—social, emotional, and sexual attraction to members of the same sex—exists in almost all cultures. Men and women homosexuals are commonly referred to as *gay;* women homosexuals are also called *lesbians.*

Homosexuality threatens and upsets many people, perhaps because homosexuals are viewed as different, or perhaps because no one understands why some people are heterosexual and others homosexual. Homophobia has led to an increase in "gay bashing" (attacking homosexuals) in many communities, including college campuses. Some blame the emergence of AIDS as a societal danger. However, researchers have found that fear of AIDS has not created new hostility but has simply given bigots an excuse to act out their hatred.

Violations of basic human rights for gays and lesbians remain common around the globe. Amnesty International has documented abuses, ranging from

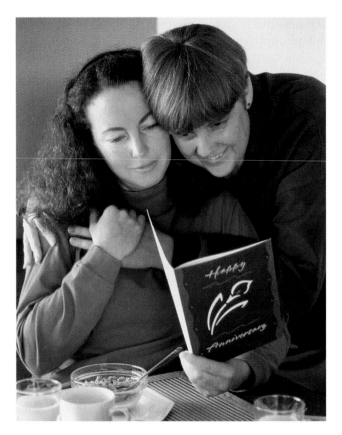

Happy together. Close-couple homosexual relationships are similar to stable heterosexual relationships.

exile to labor camps in China to "social cleansing" death squads in Colombia to the death penalty for homosexual acts in Iran.

The Roots of Homosexuality

For decades, behavioral and medical specialists have debated whether homosexuality is biologically or socially determined. Some say that sexual orientation is genetically determined. However, new research has cast doubt on the existence of a "homosexuality gene." Earlier studies had suggested that male homosexuality might be linked to a set of five DNA sequences located on a specific region of the X chromosome, which is passed down by mothers to their offspring. Gay brothers in earlier studies had tended to share these sequences, suggesting a genetic origin for homosexuality passed through the female line. But a study of 52 gay brothers drawn from 48 families found "no excess sharing for any of the four markers tested" above that which would normally be expected of any two brothers, regardless of sexual orientation. Other studies in families and twins do suggest that sexual orientation may be at least partially linked to genetics.[31]

Others contend that prenatal hormones influence sexual preference. Some psychotherapists have argued that mothers foster homosexuality by loving their sons too much and their daughters too little. Others have traced homosexuality to broken homes, seductive friends, and failure at "dating and mating." Today, questions and controversies persist about the roots and nature of sexual orientation.

Homosexual Lifestyles

Extensive studies of male and female homosexuals have shown that only a minority have problems coping with their homosexuality. The happiest and best adjusted tend to be those in close-couple relationships, the equivalent of stable heterosexual partnerships. An estimated 3 to 5 million gays and lesbians have conceived children in heterosexual relationships; others have become parents through adoption or artificial insemination. These men and women describe their families as much like any other; and studies of lesbian mothers have found that their children are essentially no different from average in self-esteem, gender-related issues and roles, sexual orientation, and general development.

Different ethnic groups respond to homosexuality in different ways. To a greater extent than white homosexuals, gays and lesbians from ethnic groups tend to stay in the closet longer rather than risk alienation from their families and communities. Often they feel forced to choose between their gay and ethnic identities.

In general, the African-American community has stronger negative views of homosexuals than whites, possibly because of the influence of strong fundamentalist Christian beliefs. Hispanic culture, with its emphasis on machismo, also has a very negative view of male homosexuality. Asian cultures, which tend to view an individual as a representative of his or her family, tend to view open declarations of sexual orientation as shaming the family and challenging their reputation and future.

Sexual Activity

Part of learning about your own sexuality is having a clear understanding of human sexual behaviors. Understanding frees us from fear and anxiety, so that we may accept ourselves and others as the natural sexual beings we all are.

Celibacy

A celibate person does not engage in sexual activity. Complete **celibacy** means that the person doesn't masturbate (stimulate himself or herself sexually) or engage in sexual activity with a partner. In partial celibacy, the person masturbates but doesn't have sexual contact with others. Many people decide to be celibate at certain times of their lives. Some don't have sex because of concerns about pregnancy or STDs; others haven't found a partner for a permanent, monogamous relationship. Many simply have other priorities, such as finishing school or starting a career and realize that sex outside of a committed relationship is a threat to their physical and psychological well-being.

Abstinence

Increasing numbers of adolescents and young adults are choosing to remain virgins and abstain from sexual intercourse until they enter a permanent, committed, monogamous relationship. Many people who were sexually active in the past also are choosing abstinence rather than getting involved with a new partner, because the risk of medical complications associated with STDs increases with the number of sexual partners a person has.

Abstinence is the safest, healthiest option for many. However, there is confusion about what it means to abstain, and individuals who think they are abstaining may still be engaging in behaviors that put them at risk for HIV and STDs.

What Does It Mean to Abstain?

The CDC defines **abstinence** as "refraining from sexual activities which involve vaginal, anal, and oral intercourse." This is not the same way that many college students think of abstinence. In a survey of more than 1,100 students at a large southeastern university, 10.2 percent of respondents classified engaging in vaginal

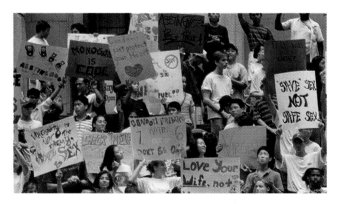

Abstinence is one sexual choice—the most risk-free in relation to sexually transmitted diseases (STDs). Deciding to abstain may also be a social choice, to wait until you are in a committed, permanent, monogamous relationship.

intercourse as being sexually abstinent. Even larger percentages defined it as engaging in anal intercourse (24.31 percent), having oral contact with another person's genitals (36.93 percent), and having oral-anal contact (47.14 percent).[32]

There also is confusion about virginity. In one study of urban high school students, 47 percent had never engaged in vaginal intercourse. However, more than a third of these "virgins" had engaged in some form of heterosexual genital activity in the preceding year, including masturbation of a partner. About 10 percent had engaged in oral sex.[33]

Sexuality and health educators have expressed concern about these findings, because behaviors such as anal intercourse and oral-anal contact put individuals at risk of HIV transmission.[34]

What Is Sex?

There also is confusion about what it means to "have sex." (See Table 9-1.) American college students, according to one survey at a large midwestern state university, almost universally agree that penile-vaginal intercourse qualifies as "having sex"; 81 percent considered penile-anal intercourse as sex, while 19 percent did not. Only 40 percent said they considered oral-genital contact "having sex," while 14 to 15 percent indicated that manual stimulation of the genitals constitutes sex. Men were more likely than women to consider various activities, including genital and breast contact, as sex. Those who had never engaged in penile-vaginal intercourse were less likely to say that oral-genital contact meant "having sex." One in five of the students surveyed did not count penile-anal intercourse as having sex.[35]

It's not just Americans whose sexual definitions vary. In a survey of Australian university students, more than 99 percent said that penis-vagina sex with ejaculation was sex; 97 percent thought it was sex even if no ejaculation occurred; 90 percent defined anal intercourse as sex. Far fewer considered other sexual activities as "sex": Only 58 percent regarded oral-sex with orgasm as having sex, while 54 percent thought of oral sex without orgasm as sex; 30 percent regarded touching or stroking as having sex, while 7 percent regarded tongue-kissing as sex.[36]

Fantasy

The mind is the most powerful sex organ in the body, and erotic mental images can be sexually stimulating. Sexual fantasies can accompany sexual activity or be pleasurable in themselves. Fantasies generally enhance sexual arousal, reduce anxiety, and boost sexual desire.

■ **Table 9-1** Is It "Sex"?

Would you say you "had sex" with someone if you engaged in one of the following intimate behaviors?

Behavior	Percentages Answering Yes		
	Total	Men	Women
Penile-vaginal intercourse	99.5	99.2	99.7
Penile-anal intercourse	81	79.1	82.3
Oral contact with your genitals	40.2	43.9	37.7
Oral contact with other's genitals	39.9	43.7	37.3
Person touches your genitals	15.1	19.2	12.2
You touch other's genitals	13.9	17.1	11.6
Oral contact on other's breasts/nipples	3.4	6.1	1.4
You touch other's breasts/nipples	3.4	5.7	1.7
Person touches your breasts/nipples	3	4.5	2.0
Oral contact on your breasts/nipples	3	4.1	2.3
Deep kissing	2	2.9	1.4

Source: Based on data presented in Sanders, Stephanie, and June Reinisch. "Would You Say You 'Had Sex' If . . . ?" *JAMA,* Vol. 281, No. 3, January 20, 1999.

They're also a way to anticipate and rehearse new sexual experiences, as well as to bolster a person's self-image and feelings of desirability. Part of what makes fantasies exciting is that they provide an opportunity for expressing forbidden desires, such as sex with a different partner or with a past lover.

In the University of Chicago survey, more than half the men (54 percent)—but only 19 percent of the women—said they thought about sex every day or several times a day. Men and women also have different types of sexy thoughts, with men's fantasies containing more explicit genital images and culminating in sexual acts more quickly than women's. In women's fantasies, emotional feelings play a greater role, and there is more kissing and caressing rather than genital contact. For many women, fantasy helps in reaching orgasm during intercourse; a loss of fantasy often is a sign of low sexual desire.

Sex in Cyberspace

The Internet, designed for communication of very different sorts, has become a new medium for relationships, including those that might be described as sexual. In certain chat rooms, individuals can share explicit sexual fantasies or engage in the cyberspace equivalent of mutual fantasizing. In some ways, the Internet is the perfect venue for a safe form of sexual risk-taking. Individuals can assume any name, gender, race, or personality and can pretend to lead lives entirely different from their actual existences.[37] (See Consumer Health Watch: "X-rated Online Sites.")

Many see cybersex as a harmless way of adding an extra erotic charge to their daily lives. In some cases, individuals who meet in cybersex chat rooms develop what they come to think of as a meaningful relationship and arrange to meet in person. Sometimes these meetings are awkward; sometimes they do lead to a real-life romance. However, they rarely survive the intrusive reality of everyday existence and sometimes they end disastrously in disappointment and danger.

For some individuals, particularly gays and lesbians, the Internet provides the opportunity to join a virtual community. In addition to sexual exchanges, they can find access to information and resources that may not be available elsewhere. For adolescents struggling with gender identity or for closeted homosexuals, going online can be their only opportunity to be open about their sexuality.

Masturbation

Not everybody masturbates, but most people do. Kinsey estimated that 7 out of 10 women and 19 out of 20 men masturbate (and admit they do). Their reason is simple: It feels good. Masturbation produces the same physical responses as sexual activity with a partner and can be an enjoyable form of sexual release.

Masturbation has been described as immature; unsocial; tiring; frustrating; and a cause of hairy palms, warts, blemishes, and blindness. None of these myths is true. Even Freud felt that masturbation was normal for children. Sex educators recommend masturbation to adolescents as a means of releasing tension and becom-

Consumer Health Watch

X-Rated Online Sites

Sex is the number-one word searched for online. About 15 percent of Americans logging onto the Internet visit sexually oriented sites. Men are the largest consumers of sexually explicit material and outnumber women by a ratio of six to one. However, while men look for visual erotica, women are more likely to visit chat rooms, which offer more interactions. Most people who check out sex sites on the Internet do not suffer any negative impact, but psychologists who surveyed Internet users warn of some potential risks, including the following:

- *Dependence.* Individuals who spend eleven hours or more a week online in sexual pursuits show signs of psychological distress and admit that their behavior interferes with some areas of their lives.

- *Interference with work.* While most individuals use their home computers when surfing the Internet for

sex-related sites, 5.8 percent of those surveyed use an office computer and 12.7 percent use computers at both home and work. Some corporations have strict policies barring such practices and may take punitive actions against employees who violate the rules.

- *Sexual compulsivity.* About 8 percent of those surveyed were found to be at risk of a serious problem as a result of their heavy Internet use.

- *Dishonesty.* Most respondents—61 percent—admitted that they occasionally "pretended" about their age on the net. Three of four said they kept secret how much time they spend on sexual pursuits in cyberspace.

Source: Cooper, Alvin, et al. "Sexuality on the Internet: From Sexual Exploration to the Pathological Expression." *Professional Psychology,* Vol. 30, No. 2, March 1999.

---

ing familiar with their sexual organs. Throughout adulthood, masturbation often is the primary sexual activity of individuals not involved in a sexual relationship and can be particularly useful when illness, absence, divorce, or death deprives a person of a partner. In the University of Chicago survey, about 25 percent of men and 9 percent of women said they masturbate at least once a week.

White men and women have a higher incidence of masturbation than African-American men and women. Latino women have the lowest rate of masturbation, compared with Latino men, white men and women, and black men and women. Individuals with a higher level of education are more likely to masturbate than those with less schooling, and people living with sexual partners masturbate more than those who live alone.[38]

Masturbation helps some people make better decisions about getting sexually involved with others. Self-stimulation also can aid women learning to experience orgasms or men experimenting with ways of delaying ejaculation. Some people find that masturbation enables them to relax and fall asleep more easily at night.

Kissing and Touching

A kiss is a universal sign of affection. A kiss can be just a kiss—a quick press of the lips—or it can lead to much more. Usually kissing is the first sexual activity that couples engage in, and even after years of sexual exper-

imentation and sharing, it remains an enduring pleasure for partners.

Touching is a silent form of communication between friends and lovers. Although a touch to any part of the body can be thrilling, some areas, such as the breasts and genitals, are especially sensitive. Stimulating these **erogenous** regions can lead to orgasm in both men and women. Though such forms of stimulation often

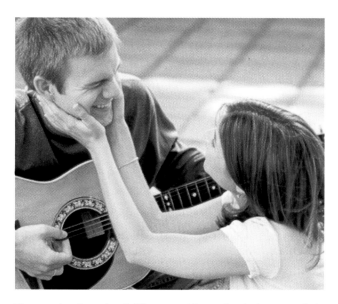

The magic of touch. Thrilling, soothing, stimulating—touch is a powerful nonverbal communication.

accompany intercourse, more couples are gaining an appreciation of these activities as primary sources of sexual fulfillment—and as safer alternatives to intercourse.

Intercourse

Vaginal **intercourse,** or coitus, refers to the penetration of the vagina by the penis (see Figure 9-6). This is the preferred form of sexual intimacy for most heterosexual couples, who may use a wide variety of positions. The most familiar position for intercourse in our society is the so-called missionary position, with the man on top, facing the woman. An alternative is the woman on top, either lying down or sitting upright. Other positions include lying side by side (either face to face or with the man behind the woman, his penis entering her vagina from the rear); lying with the man on top of the woman in a rear-entry position; and kneeling or standing (again, in either a face-to-face or rear-entry position). Many couples move into several different positions for intercourse during a single episode of lovemaking; others may have a personal favorite, or may choose different positions at different times.

Sexual activity, including intercourse, is possible throughout a woman's menstrual cycle. However, some women prefer to avoid sex while menstruating because of uncomfortable physical symptoms, such as cramps, or concern about bleeding or messiness. Others use a diaphragm or cervical cap (see Chapter 10) to hold back menstrual flow. Since different cultures have different views on intercourse during a woman's period, partners should discuss their own feelings and try to respect each other's views. If they choose not to have intercourse, there are other gratifying forms of sexual activity.

Vaginal intercourse, like other forms of sexual activity involving an exchange of bodily fluids, carries a risk of sexually transmitted diseases, including HIV infection. In many other parts of the world, in fact, heterosexual intercourse is the most common means of HIV transmission. (See Chapter 12.)

Oral-Genital Sex

Our mouths and genitals give us some of our most intense pleasures. Though it might seem logical to combine the two, some people are very uncomfortable with it. Some people consider oral-genital sex a perversion; it is against the law in many states, and a sin in some religions. However, others find it normal and acceptable. (The same comments apply to anal sex as well—see the next section.)

The formal terms for oral sex are **cunnilingus,** which refers to oral stimulation of the woman's genitals, and **fellatio,** oral stimulation of the man's genitals. For many couples, oral-genital sex is a regular part of their lovemaking. For others, it's an occasional experiment. Oral sex with a partner carrying a sexually transmitted disease, such as herpes or HIV infection, can lead to infection, so a condom should be used (with cunnilingus, a condom cut in half to lay flat can be used).

Different groups of the population have diverse views of oral sex. In one survey, more African-American than white men reported never having performed or received oral sex.[39] Among American women, career women are more likely than homemakers to consider oral sex a normal act.[40]

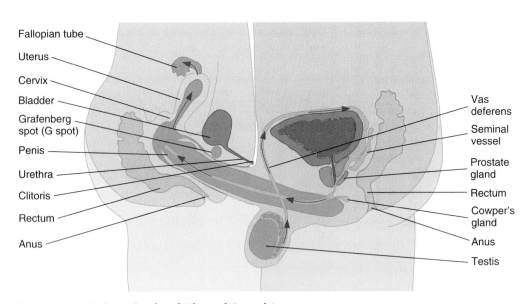

■ Figure 9-6 **A Cross-Sectional View of Sexual Intercourse**
Sperm are formed in each of the testes and stored in the epididymis. When a man ejaculates, sperm, in semen, travel up the vas deferens. (The prostate gland and seminal vesicles contribute components of the semen.) The semen is expelled from the penis through the urethra and deposited in the vagina, near the cervix. During sexual excitement and orgasm in a woman, the upper end of the vagina enlarges and the uterus elevates. After orgasm, these organs return to their normal states, and the cervix descends into the pool of semen.

Anal Stimulation and Intercourse

Because the anus has many nerve endings, it can produce intense erotic responses. Stimulation of the anus by the fingers or mouth can be a source of sexual arousal; anal intercourse involves penile penetration of the anus. An estimated 25 percent of adults have experienced anal intercourse at least once. However, anal sex involves important health risks, such as damage to sensitive rectal tissues, and the transmission of various intestinal infections, hepatitis, and STDs, including HIV.

Cultural Variations

While the biological mechanisms underlying human sexual arousal and response are essentially universal, the particular sexual stimuli or behaviors that people find arousing are greatly influenced by cultural conditioning. For example, in Western societies, where the emphasis during sexual activity tends to be heavily weighted toward achieving orgasm, genitally focused activities are frequently defined as optimally arousing. In contrast, devotees to Eastern Tantric traditions (where spirituality is interwoven with sexuality) often achieve optimal pleasure by emphasizing the sensual and spiritual aspects of shared intimacy rather than orgasmic release.

Kissing on the mouth, a universal source of sexual arousal in Western society, may be rare or absent in many other parts of the world. Certain North American Eskimo people and inhabitants of the Trobriand Islands would rather rub noses than lips, and among the Thonga of South Africa, kissing is viewed as odious behavior. The Hindu people of India are also disinclined to kiss because they believe such contact symbolically contaminates the act of sexual intercourse. One survey of 190 societies found that mouth kissing was acknowledged in only 21 societies and practiced as a prelude or accompaniment to coitus in only 13.

Oral sex (both cunnilingus and fellatio) is a common source of sexual arousal among island societies of the South Pacific, in industrialized nations of Asia, and in much of the Western world. In contrast, in Africa (with the exception of northern regions), such practices are likely to be viewed as unnatural or disgusting behavior.

Foreplay in general, whether it be oral sex, sensual touching, or passionate kissing, is subject to wide cultural variation. In some societies, most notably those with Eastern traditions, couples may strive to prolong intense states of sexual arousal for several hours. While varied patterns of foreplay are common in Western cultures, these activities often are of short duration as lovers move rapidly toward the "main event" of coitus. In still other societies, foreplay is either sharply curtailed or absent altogether. For example, the Lepcha farmers of the southeastern Himalayas limit foreplay to men briefly caressing their partners' breasts, and among the Irish inhabitants of Inis Beag, precoital sexual activity is reported to be limited to mouth kissing and rough fondling of the woman's lower body by her partner.[41]

Sexual Response

Sexuality involves every part of you: mind and body, muscles and skin, glands and genitals. The pioneers in finding out exactly how human beings respond to sex were William Masters and Virginia Johnson, who first studied more than 800 individuals in their laboratory in the 1950s. They discovered that sexual response is a well-ordered sequence of events, so predictable it could be divided into four phases: excitement, plateau, orgasm, and resolution (see Figure 9-7). In real life, individuals don't necessarily follow this well-ordered pattern. But the responses for both sexes are remarkably similar. And sexual response always follows the same sequence, whatever the means of stimulation.

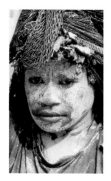 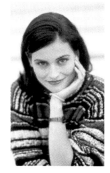 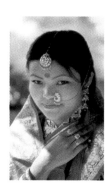 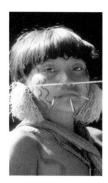 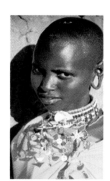 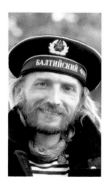

Our standards of physical attractiveness vary widely, as can be seen in these six photos of women and men from around the world who are considered in their cultures to be attractive.

Excitement

Stimulation is the first step: a touch, a look, a fantasy. In men, sexual stimuli set off a rush of blood to the genitals, filling the blood vessels in the penis. Because these vessels are wrapped in a thick sheath of tissue, the penis becomes erect. The testes lift.

Women respond to stimulation with vaginal lubrication within 10 to 20 seconds of exposure to sexual stimuli. The clitoris becomes larger, as do the vaginal lips (the labia), the nipples, and later the breasts. The vagina lengthens, and its inner two-thirds increase in size. The uterus lifts, further increasing the free space in the vagina.

Plateau

During this stage, the changes begun in the excitement stage continue and intensify. The penis further increases in both length and diameter. The outer one-third of the vagina swells. During intercourse, the vaginal muscles grasp the penis to increase stimulation for both partners. The upper two-thirds of the vagina become wider as the uterus moves up; eventually its diameter is 2½ to 3 inches.

Orgasm

Men and women have remarkably similar **orgasm** experiences. Both men and women typically have 3 to 12 pelvic muscle contractions approximately four-fifths of a second apart and lasting up to 60 seconds. Both undergo contractions and spasms of other muscles, as well as increases in breathing and pulse rates, and blood pressure. Both can sometimes have orgasms simply from kisses, stimulation of the breasts or other parts of the body, or fantasy alone.

The process of **ejaculation** (the discharge of semen by a male) requires two separate events. First, the vas deferens, the seminal vesicles, the prostate, and the upper portion of the urethra contract. The man perceives these subtle contractions deep in his pelvis just before the point of no return—which therapists refer to as the point of "ejaculatory inevitability." Then, seconds later, muscle contractions force semen out of the penis via the urethra.

Female orgasms follow several patterns. Some women experience a series of mini-orgasms—a response sometimes described as "skimming." Another pattern consists of rapid excitement and plateau stages, followed by a prolonged orgasm. This is the most frequent response to stimulation by a vibrator.

Female orgasms are primarily triggered by stimulating the clitoris. When stimulation reaches an adequate level, the vagina responds by contracting. Although it sometimes seems that vaginal stimulation alone can set off an orgasm, the clitoris is usually involved—at least indirectly during full penile penetration.

Some researchers have identified what they call the *Grafenberg (or G) spot* (or area) just behind the front wall of the vagina, between the cervix and the back of the pubic bone (see Figure 9-6). When this region is stimulated, women report various sensations, including slight discomfort, a brief feeling that they need to urinate, and increasing pleasure. Continued stimulation may result in an orgasm of great intensity, accompanied by ejaculation of fluid from the urethra. However, other researchers have failed to confirm the existence and importance of the G spot, and sex therapists disagree about its significance for a woman's sexual satisfaction.

Resolution

The sexual organs of men and women return to their normal, nonexcited state during this final phase of sexual response. Heightened skin color quickly fades after

---

Strategies *for* Change

Improving a Sexual Relationship

✓ Use "I" statements, such as "I really enjoy making love, but I'm so tired right now that I won't be a responsive partner. Why don't we get the kids to bed early tomorrow so we can enjoy ourselves a little earlier?"

✓ If your partner has temporarily lost interest in sex, express concern and ask what the two of you might do to make things better. Don't blame yourself.

✓ Speak up if something hurts during sex. Be specific.

✓ If you would like to try something different, say so. Practice saying the words first if they embarrass you. If your partner feels uncomfortable, don't force the issue, but do try talking it through.

✓ Set aside time for a regular sex talk. Take turns bringing up topics. Mention special pleasures or particular problems.

✓ If you want to request changes or tackle a touchy topic, start with positive statements. Let your partner know how much you enjoy having sex, and then express your desire to enjoy lovemaking more often or in different ways.

✓ Encourage small changes. If you want your partner to be less inhibited, start slowly, perhaps by suggesting sex in a different room or place.

Males

Excitement

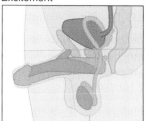

Testes enlarge and elevate, penis becomes partially erect

Plateau

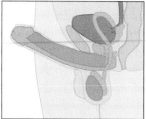

Testes are fully elevated; penis reaches full erection, glans swell, drops of fluid are released

Orgasm

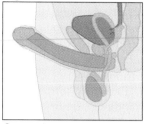

Contractions release semen into urethra; urethral sphincter relaxes, penile contractions occur, semen is ejaculated

Resolution

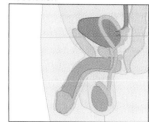

Erection disappears, testes descend

Females

Excitement

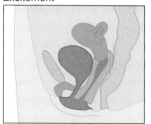

Inner vagina expands, clitoris swells, and labia swell

Plateau

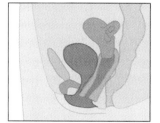

Inner vagina becomes fully expanded, outer vagina swells, and clitoris retracts under hood

Orgasm

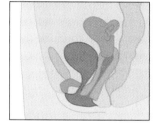

Anal sphincter contracts, uterus contracts, and outer vagina contracts

Resolution

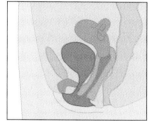

Uterus lowers, vagina returns to normal

■ Figure 9-7 **Human Sexual Response is a Well-Ordered Sequence: Excitement, Plateau, Orgasm, and Resolution**

orgasm, and the heart rate, blood pressure, and breathing rate soon return to normal. The clitoris also resumes its normal position and appearance very shortly thereafter, whereas the penis may remain somewhat erect for up to 30 minutes.

After orgasm, men typically enter a **refractory period,** during which they are incapable of another orgasm. The duration of this period varies from minutes to days, depending on age and the frequency of previous sexual activity. If either partner doesn't have an orgasm after becoming highly aroused, resolution may be much slower and may be accompanied by a sense of discomfort.

Sexual Concerns

Many sexual concerns stem from myths and misinformation. There is no truth, for instance, behind the misconception that men are always capable of erection, that sex always involves intercourse, that partners should experience simultaneous orgasms, or that people who truly love each other always have satisfying sex lives.

Cultural and childhood influences can affect our attitudes toward sex. Even though America's traditionally Puritanical values have eased, our society continues to convey mixed messages about sex. Some children, repeatedly warned of the evils of sex, never accept the sexual dimensions of their identity. Others—especially young boys—may be exposed to macho attitudes toward sex and feel a need to prove their virility. Young girls may feel confused by media messages that encourage them to look and act provocatively and a double standard that blames them for leading boys on. In addition, virtually everyone has individual worries. A woman may feel self-conscious about the shape of her breasts; a man may worry about the size of his penis; both partners may fear not pleasing the other.

The concept of sexual normalcy differs greatly in different times, cultures, or racial and ethnic groups. In certain times and places, only sex between a husband and wife has been deemed normal. In other circumstances, "normal" has been applied to any sexual behavior—alone or with others—that does not harm others or produce great anxiety and guilt. The following are some of the most common contemporary sexual concerns.

Safer Sex

Having sex is never completely safe; the only 100 percent risk-free sexual choice is abstinence. If you choose to be sexually active, you can greatly reduce your risk by restricting sexual activity to the context of a mutually exclusive, monogamous relationship in which both partners know, on the basis of laboratory testing, that neither has an STD or HIV antibodies.

For centuries, sexually transmitted diseases, such as gonorrhea and syphilis, caused great suffering and many deaths. Modern medicine has developed effective treatments for these health threats, but other STDs, such as herpes and chlamydia, have become serious health problems. No one is immune to STDs, including the young. A quarter of all STDs in the United States occur among adolescents, and a quarter of sexually active adolescents acquire an STD each year. The United States has the highest rate of STDs among all developed countries, yet there is no effective national system of STD prevention.[42] (Chapter 11 provides a complete discussion of the symptoms, diagnosis, and treatment of sexually transmitted diseases, including HIV infection and AIDS.)

Sex with a person who has never been exposed to HIV or to other STDs is safe (for you), regardless of what type of sexual activity you engage in. The only way of knowing for certain that a prospective partner doesn't have an STD or is not infected with HIV is through laboratory testing (see Chapter 11). Sex educators and health professionals strongly encourage couples to abstain from any sexual activity that puts them at risk for STDs until they both undergo medical examinations and testing for STDs. This process greatly reduces the danger of disease transmission and can also help foster a deep sense of mutual trust and commitment. Many campus and public health clinics provide exams or laboratory testing either free of charge or on a sliding scale determined by your income.

What Are the Most Common Sexual Problems?

A sexual difficulty may occur anywhere in the sexual response sequence. A man's penis may not become erect; a woman's vagina may not become moist. A man may lose his erection while attempting intercourse; the woman's vagina may become dry after penetration. Some men and women become excited, enjoy the plateau stage, but then don't achieve an orgasm; or their sexual cycle may be too long or too short for one of the partners. Sometimes the cause of the problem is alcohol or drugs (see Table 9-2), disease, injury, stress, or chronic pain. Often, however, it's fear or ignorance.

■ **Table 9-2** Sexual Effects of Some Drugs

Alcohol	Chronic alcohol abuse causes hormonal alterations (reduces size of testes and suppresses hormonal function) and permanent damage to the circulatory and nervous systems.
Marijuana	Reduces testosterone levels in men and decreases sexual desire.
Tobacco	Adversely affects small blood vessels in the penis and decreases the frequency and duration of erections (Mannino et al., 1994).
Cocaine	Causes erectile disorder and inhibited orgasm.
Amphetamines	In high doses and with chronic use, inhibits orgasm, decreases erection and lubrication.
Barbiturates	Causes decreased desire, erectile disorders, delayed orgasm.

Source: Finger et al., 1997.

One of the most common feelings associated with sex—along with curiosity, desire, and love—is anxiety. No one is born knowing about sex. Most of us learn from our experiences, and—as with most activities, from skiing to speaking French—our first attempts tend to be awkward. A caring, loving relationship can make all the difference.

Sexual Dysfunction

SIECUS defines **sexual dysfunction** as the inability to react emotionally and/or physically to sexual stimulation in a way expected of the average healthy person or according to one's own standards. Sexual dysfunctions, which have a wide range of psychological and physiological origins, can affect different stages in the sexual response cycle. They are not all-or-nothing problems but vary considerably in how severe they are and how frequently they occur. In as many as one-third of people with sexual problems, the partner also has a sexual dysfunction.[43]

Most men and women at one time or another experience some sort of sexual difficulty, but they tend to develop different types. Men are more likely to seek and receive treatment for sexual problems. Nevertheless, they find them very difficult to talk about and may delay or avoid seeking help.[44] In women, the most common sexual dysfunction is loss of desire for sexual activity.[45]

Problems with Arousal

Perfectly healthy couples with no physical impairment sometimes simply become bored with sex, even though they love each other and find each other attractive and enjoyable. Men and women may lose interest in sex, and often neither partner has had previous arousal or orgasm problems. Physical disorders, including neurological and endocrine diseases, can affect sexual desire, as can psychological conditions such as depression and fatigue. Many medications and drugs of abuse (see Table 9-2) also can inhibit desire.

Often stress—perhaps caused by a recent move, a new baby, or a high-pressure job—is the real culprit. Severe stress can short-circuit normal sexual response. Couples who try to unwind by drinking or using tranquilizers usually make the problem worse by further dampening their sexual responses.

Erectile Dysfunction

Erectile dysfunction (ED), or **impotence,** affect many men as they age. Virtually all men are occasionally unable to achieve or maintain an erection because of fatigue, stress, alcohol, or drug use. As clinically defined, impotence means that a man cannot get an erection more often than once in four attempts. Psychological factors, such as anxiety about performance, may cause impotence. But in as many as 80 percent of cases, the problem has physical origins. Diabetes and reactions to drugs—including an estimated 200 prescription medications—are the most frequent organic causes. Even cigarettes can create erection problems for men sensitive to nicotine. According to the Impotence Information Center, smoking ten or more cigarettes a day increases the likelihood of impotence.

A little blue pill called Viagra (sildenafil), which delays the breakdown of an enzyme involved in deflating the penis after ejaculation, has revolutionized therapy for ED. In its first two months on the market in the United States, approximately 2 million men tried Viagra, making it one of the the best-selling new drugs in history. For some men, particularly those with mild cases of impotence, Viagra has lived up to its promise. But Viagra works without side effects in only about one-third of the men who try it; another third benefit but also experience side effects (headache, nasal congestion, facial flushing); the final third do not respond at all.[46]

There are medical risks associated with Viagra use, and as many as 80 deaths have been associated with the drug. The U.S. Food and Drug Administration (FDA) requires health labels on bottles of Viagra that warn doctors and patients that men with heart problems and very high or very low blood pressure should be carefully examined before getting a prescription. Interactions with certain drugs, such as heart medications containing nitrate, have proven fatal. Other medications, including antifungal medications and the antibiotic erythromycin, also can affect Viagra's metabolism and excretion. Some users experience visual side effects, but these are temporary and are not considered serious.[47] However, despite the warnings and risks, many men have bought Viagra online after filling out an application reviewed by a medical doctor—a practice condemned by medical societies and by the drug's manufacturer.[48]

Women have tried Viagra to increase their sexual responsiveness, but there are no scientific data showing a benefit. However, female interest in Viagra has spurred new research into treatments that may enhance women's sexual satisfaction.[49]

Other treatments include vacuum devices that increase blood flow to the penis to induce erection; injectable drugs (such as Caverject) that produce an erection within 20 minutes of injection into the base of the penis; vascular reconstruction (grafts of arteries from the lower abdomen are placed around narrowed branches of the main artery leading to the penis to restore blood flow); and penile implants (some inflatable, some permanently rigid) that enable impotent men to have sexual intercourse.

Failure to Respond

Women probably fail to become aroused at least as often as men, but it doesn't seem to be as upsetting to them as the inability to become erect is to men, partly because it isn't as noticeable. Our culture is also more accepting of women who say they simply "don't feel like sex." The myth that a man should become aroused at every opportunity urges many men to have sex—or try to—regardless of how they feel.

Orgasm Problems in Men

About 20 percent of men complain of **premature ejaculation,** which is defined as ejaculating within 30 to 90 seconds of inserting the penis into the vagina, or after 10 to 15 thrusts.[50] Another definition is that a premature ejaculator cannot control or delay his ejaculation long enough to satisfy a responsive partner at least half the time. By this definition, a man may be premature with some women but not with others.

To delay orgasm, men may try to think of baseball or other sports, but this just makes sex boring. Others may masturbate before intercourse, hoping to take advantage of the refractory period, during which they cannot ejaculate again. Others may bite their lips or dig their nails into their palms—although usually this just results in premature ejaculators with bloody lips and scarred palms. Some physicians prescribe drugs, including antidepressants, and androgens (male sex hormones), to cure premature ejaculation. Topical anesthetics used to prevent climax dull pleasurable sensations for the woman as well as for the man.

Men can learn to control their ejaculation by concentrating on their sexual responses, rather than by trying to distract themselves or ignore their reactions. Some men find that they have greater control by lying on their backs with their partner on top, by relaxing during intercourse, and by communicating with their partner about when to stop or slow down movements.

Other techniques for delaying ejaculation include *stop-start*, in which a man learns to sense the feelings that precede ejaculation and stop his movements before the point of ejaculatory inevitability, allowing his arousal to subside slightly before restarting sexual activity. In the *squeeze technique*, a man's partner applies strong pressure with her thumb on the frenum and her second and third fingers on the top side of the penis, one above and one below the corona, until the man loses the urge to ejaculate.

Intercourse and Orgasm Problems in Women

Some women experience **dyspareunia**, or pain during intercourse. An extreme form of painful intercourse is **vaginismus**, in which involuntary contractions of the muscles of the outer third of the vagina are so intense that they totally or partially close the vaginal opening. This problem often derives from a fear of being penetrated. Relaxation techniques, such as *Kegel exercises* (alternately tightening and relaxing the muscles of the pelvic floor), or the use of fingers or dilators to gradually open the vagina, can make penetration easier.

The female orgasm has long been a controversial sexual topic. According to recent estimates, about 90 percent of sexually active women have experienced orgasm, but only a much smaller percentage achieve orgasm through intercourse alone. Even fewer reach orgasm if intercourse isn't accompanied by direct stimulation of the clitoris. Is intercourse without orgasm a sexual problem? The best answer is that it is a problem if a woman wants to experience orgasm during intercourse but doesn't.

Many counseling programs urge women who have never had orgasms to masturbate. They are then encouraged to share with their partners what they've learned, communicating with words or gestures what is most pleasing to them. Some women regularly want or need more than a single orgasm during intercourse. Partners can help by varying positions and experimenting with sexual techniques. However, in sexual response, more is not necessarily better, and the couple should keep in mind that no one else is counting.

Sex Therapy

Modern sex therapy, pioneered by Masters and Johnson in the 1960s, views sex as a natural, healthy behavior that enhances a couple's relationship. Their approach emphasizes education, communication, reduction of performance anxiety, and sexual exercises that enhance sexual intimacy.

Today most sex therapists, working either alone or with a partner, have modified Masters and Johnson's approach. Most see couples once a week for eight to ten weeks; the focus of therapy is on correcting dysfunctional behavior, not exploring underlying psychodynamics.

Contrary to common misconceptions, sex therapy does not involve conducting sexual activity in front of therapists. The therapist may review psychological and physiological aspects of sexual functioning and evaluate the couple's sexual attitudes and ability to communicate. The core of the program is the couple's "homework"—a series of exercises, carried out in private, that enhances their sensory awareness and improves nonverbal communication. These techniques have proven effective for couples regardless of their age or general health.

You and your partner should consider consulting a sex therapist if any of the following is true for you:

- Sex is painful or physically uncomfortable.
- You're having sex less and less frequently.
- You have a general fear of, or revulsion toward, sex.
- Your sexual pleasure is declining.
- Your sexual desire is diminishing.
- Your sexual problems are increasing in frequency or persisting for longer periods.

Drugs and Sex

Many recreational drugs, such as alcohol and marijuana, are believed to enhance sexual performance. However, none of the popular drugs touted as *aphrodisiac*—including amphetamines, barbiturates, cantharides ("Spanish fly"), cocaine, LSD and other psychedelics, marijuana, amyl nitrite ("poppers"), and L-dopa (a medication used to treat Parkinson's disease)—is truly a sexual stimulant. In fact, these drugs often interfere with normal sexual response. Researchers are studying one drug that may truly enhance sexual performance: yohimbine hydrochloride, which is derived from the sap of the tropical yohimbe tree that grows in West Africa.

Because many psychiatric problems can lower sexual desire and affect sexual functioning, medications appropriate to the specific disorders can help. In addition, psychiatric drugs may be used as part of therapy. Drugs such as certain antidepressants may be used to prolong sexual response in conditions such as premature ejaculation.

Medications can also cause sexual difficulty. In men, drugs that are used to treat high blood pressure, anxiety, allergies, depression, muscle spasms, obesity, ulcers, irritable colon, and prostate cancer can cause impotence, breast enlargement, testicular swelling, priapism (persistent erection), loss of sexual desire, inability to ejaculate, and reduced sperm count. In women, they can diminish sexual desire, inhibit or delay orgasm, and cause breast swelling or secretions.

Atypical Behavior

Although sexual desire and response are universal, some individuals develop sexual appetites or engage in activities that are not typical sexual behaviors.

Sexual Addiction

Some men and women can get relief from their feelings of restlessness and worthlessness only through sex (either masturbation or with a partner). Once the sexual high ends, however, they're overwhelmed by the same negative feelings and driven, once more, to have sex.

Some therapists describe this problem as **sexual addiction**; others, as **sexual compulsion**. Professionals continue to debate exactly what this controversial condition is, how to diagnose it, and how to overcome it. However, most agree that for some people, sex is more than a normal pleasure: It is an overwhelming need that must be met, even at the cost of their careers and marriages.

Sex addicts can be heterosexual or homosexual, male or female. Their behaviors include masturbation, phone sex, reading or viewing pornography, attending strip shows, having affairs, engaging in anonymous sex with strangers or prostitutes, exhibitionism, voyeurism, child molestation, incest, and rape. Many were physically and emotionally abused as children or have family members who abuse drugs or alcohol. They typically feel a loss of control and a compulsion for sexual activity, and they continue their unhealthy sexual behavior despite the dangers, including the risk of contracting STDs. Characteristics exhibited by sex addicts include:

- A preoccupation with sex so intense and chronic that it interferes with a normal sexual relationship with a spouse or lover.
- A compulsion to have sex again and again within a short period of time, and to engage in sexual behav-

ior that results in feelings of anxiety, depression, guilt, or shame.

- A great deal of time spent away from family or work, in order to look for sex partners or engage in sex.
- Use of sex to hide from troubles.

With help, sex addicts can deal with the shame that both triggers and follows sexual activity. Professional therapy may begin with a month of complete sexual abstinence, to break the cycle of compulsive sexual behavior. Several organizations, such as Sexaholics Anonymous and Sexual Addicts Anonymous, offer support from people who share the same problem.

Sexual Deviations

Sexual deviations listed by the American Psychiatric Association include the following:

- *Fetishism:* Obtaining sexual pleasure from an inanimate object or an asexual part of the body, such as the foot.
- *Pedophilia:* Sex between an adult and a child.
- *Transvestitism:* Becoming sexually aroused by wearing the clothing of the opposite sex.
- *Exhibitionism:* Exposing one's genitals to an unwilling observer.
- *Voyeurism:* Obtaining sexual gratification by observing people undressing or involved in sexual activity.
- *Sadism:* Becoming sexually aroused by inflicting physical or psychological pain.
- *Masochism:* Obtaining sexual gratification by suffering physical or psychological pain.

Another, increasingly common sexual variation, hypoxyphilia, involves attempts to enhance the pleasure of orgasm by reducing oxygen intake. Individuals who do so by tying a noose around the neck have accidentally killed themselves.[51]

Psychiatrists distinguish between passive sexual deviancy, which doesn't involve actual contact with another, and aggressive deviancy. Most voyeurs and obscene phone callers don't seek physical contact with the objects of their sexual desire. These behaviors are performed predominantly, but not exclusively, by males.

Transgenderism

Transgendered individuals, formerly called *transsexuals,* have gender identities opposite their biological sex. Most are males who feel deeply that they are more truly females. More than 3,000 Americans have undergone complex medical procedures to change their genital and secondary sex characteristics. Those who desire *sex-change operations* should be carefully screened and counseled to determine whether such extreme measures would be appropriate and beneficial.

The Business of Sex

Sex, without affection and individuality, becomes a product to be packaged, marketed, traded, bought, and sold. Two of the billion-dollar industries that treat sex as a commodity are prostitution and pornography.

Prostitution, described as the world's oldest profession, is a nationwide industry grossing more than $1 billion annually. In every state except Nevada (and in all but a few counties there), prostitution is illegal. Besides the threat of jail and fines, prostitutes and their clients face another danger: sexually transmitted diseases, including HIV infection and hepatitis B.

Pornography is a multimedia industry—books, magazines, movies, the Internet, phone lines, and computer games are available to those who find sexually explicit material entertaining or exciting. Most laws against pornography are based on the assumption that such materials can set off uncontrollable, dangerous sexual urges, ranging from promiscuity to sexual violence. Research indicates that exposure to scenes of rape or other forms of sexual violence against women, or to scenes of degradation of women, does lead to tolerance of these hostile and brutal acts.

Sex sells. Topless bars and strip clubs are among the businesses that cater to those who enjoy sexual stimulation outside a loving relationship.

Making This Chapter Work for You

Responsible Sexuality

- A person's gender is determined not only by his or her physiological sex, but also by psychological and sociological factors.

- Our sexual hormones—in the female, estrogen and progesterone; in the male, testosterone—play a key role in sexual development. At puberty, estrogen causes a girl to develop female secondary sex characteristics—including enlarged external genitals and full breasts and hips and prepares her body for conception and pregnancy. Testosterone stimulates the development of male secondary sex characteristics, which include a deeper voice, facial and body hair growth, and enlarged genitals.

- More women and men are shattering sexual stereotypes by choosing roles and occupations that have traditionally been closed to them. Individuals who allow themselves to express both their masculine and feminine traits are called androgynous.

- Women and men have different sexual organs, hormones, and different health problems. Awareness of these differences can help individuals take better care of their own sexual health and be more sensitive to the needs of their partners.

- A woman's menstrual cycle is a monthly process involving all her reproductive organs. Once a month, her ovary releases an egg cell, or ovum, that travels through the fallopian tube to the uterus. If the egg isn't fertilized, the uterine lining is shed during menstruation.

- Menstrual cycle problems include premenstrual syndrome, premenstrual dysphoric disorder, dysmenorrhea, and amenorrhea.

- In a woman's forties, she enters perimenopause. Her periods stop entirely at about age 51 to 52.

- Sexual health issues for males include circumcision, which has some health advantages as well as some potential complications, such as increased risk of urinary tract infection. As men grow older, they are at risk for prostatitis, prostate enlargement, and prostate cancer. At midlife, men often experience a period of change and possible crisis.

■ Making responsible sexual decisions—especially important in an age of sexual risks—requires accurate information, honest communication, consideration of all your options, determining whether you and your partner are ready for sex, and recognition of every individual's right to say no.

■ Sexual behavior, which begins with the sexual curiosity of childhood, changes over the life span. More adolescents are remaining virgins longer. Most college students are sexually active. Although concerned about HIV, many have not changed their sexual practices.

■ Several national surveys have shown that most Americans have had several sex partners, have inter-

course more often if they're married or under age 39, and engage in a range of sexual practices.

■ Sexual orientation may be predominantly heterosexual, bisexual, or homosexual. Regardless of sexual orientation, healthy sexuality involves an understanding of your own body, your partner's needs and desires, and responsible sexual behavior.

■ Sexual behaviors include celibacy, erotic fantasizing, cybersex, kissing and touching, masturbation, intercourse, and oral sex.

■ Whatever the type of sexual stimulation, the body's response always follows the same sequence: excitement, plateau, orgasm, and resolution.

■ The safest sex practices are abstinence or sexual relations with only one partner who has never been exposed to HIV or other STDs.

■ Sexual concerns include sexual anxiety, lack of sexual interest, sexual unresponsiveness, and sexual

health **/ ONLINE**

Go Ask Alice
http://www.goaskalice.columbia.edu/Cat6.html
You'll find answers to all of your most personal questions about sexuality at this Columbia University health site.

SIECUS: Sexuality Information and Education Council of the United States
http://www.siecus.org/
This site includes information for students, educators, and parents alike on sexuality-related topics. Includes fact sheets, information for educators of color, and issues related to sexuality and religion.

Online Sexual Disorders Screening
http://www.med.nyu.edu/Psych/public.html
This page from the NYU Department of Psychiatry includes online screening for sexual disorders for both men and women.

Please note that links are subject to change. If you find a broken link, use a search engine like http://www.yahoo.com *and search for the web site by typing in key words.*

 Campus Chat: Are schools doing enough, too little, or too much to educate students about sex? Share your thoughts on our online discussion forum at **http://health.wadsworth.com**

Find It On InfoTrac: You can find additional readings related to health via InfoTrac College Edition, an online library of more than 900 journals and publications. Follow the instructions for accessing InfoTrac that came packaged with your textbook; then search for articles using a key word search.

• **Suggested reading:** "Changing Attitudes to Sexual Morality: A Cross-national Comparison," by Jacqueline Scott. *Sociology,* Nov. 1998, Vol. 32, Issue 14, p. 815.

   (1) According to research, why are women generally more tolerant of homosexual relationships than are heterosexual men?

   (2) According to the author's research, what are the geographic trends regarding approval of premarital sex?

For additional links, resources, and suggested readings on InfoTrac, visit our Health & Wellness Resource Center at http://health.wadsworth.com

impairment due to the use of recreational drugs or medications. In men, common sexual problems include erectile disorders and premature ejaculation; women are more likely to have a lack of desire and orgasm difficulties.

■ Sexual addiction, transgenderism, and sexual deviations are considered atypical sexual behaviors. Prostitution and pornography strip sex of its emotional, deeply human meaning and transform it into a business.

By caring for your sexual health and treating your partner with respect, you prepare yourself to become a responsible, responsive sexual partner. By avoiding the dangers of sexually transmitted diseases, you assume responsibility for your safety and health. By dealing with any sexual problems that arise, you take charge of a key aspect of your health and behavior.

Key Terms

The terms listed here are used within the chapter. Page numbers are included for each term. A definition of each term is given in the Glossary pages at the end of this book.

abstinence   271
amenorrhea   256
androgyny   252
benign prostatic hypertrophy   259
bisexual   269
celibacy   270
cervix   253
circumcision   258
clitoris   252
corpus luteum   254
Cowper's glands   258
cunnilingus   274
dysmenorrhea   254
dyspareunia   280
ejaculation   276
ejaculatory duct   258
endocrine system   250
endometrium   253
epididymis   258
erogenous   273
estrogen   250
fallopian tubes   254
fellatio   274
gender   250
gonadotropins   250
gonads   250

heterosexual   269
homosexual   269
hormones   250
hormone replacement therapy   257
impotence   279
intercourse   274
intimacy   249
labia majora   252
labia minora   252
masturbation   265
menarche   251
menopause   257
menstruation   254
mons pubis   252
nocturnal emissions   265
orgasm   276
ova (ovum)   254
ovaries   253
ovulation   254
penis   258
perimenopause   256
perineum   253
premature ejaculation   279
premenstrual dysphoric disorder (PMDD)   254
premenstrual syndrome (PMS)   254

progesterone   250
prostate gland   258
prostatitis   259
refractory period   277
scrotum   258
secondary sex characteristics   250
semen   258
seminal vesicles   258
sex   249
sexual addiction   281
sexual compulsion   281
sexual dysfunction   278
sexual orientation   269
sexuality   249
sperm   258
testes   258
testosterone   250
transgendered   281
urethra   258
urethral opening   252
uterus   253
vagina   253
vaginismus   280
vas deferens   258

Critical Thinking Questions

1. Anita insists that her boyfriend, Bill, has never taken any sexual risks. But when she suggested that they get tested for STDs, he was furious and refused. Now Anita says she doesn't know what to believe. Is he telling the truth, or is he hiding something? She doesn't want to take any risks, but she doesn't want to lose him either. What would you advise her to say or do?

2. Do you think it's okay to read or look at pornographic books, magazines, web sites, and videos? Why or why not?

3. Some people support the legalization of homosexual marriages. Some gay people feel that they will never be fully accepted in society unless they can legally marry. Other gay people oppose the idea as too imitative of straight couples. Some heterosexuals think that gay marriages would violate the sanctity of marriage. Do you think homosexual marriages should be accepted? Why or why not?

References

1. McClintock, Martha, and Gilbert Herdt. "Rethinking Puberty: The Development of Sexual Attraction." *Current Directions in Psychological Science,* Vol. 9, No. 6, December 1996.

2. Herman-Giddens, Marcia, et al. "Second Sexual Characteristics and Menses in Young Girls Seen in Office Practice: A Study from the Pediatric Research in Office Settings Network." *Pediatrics,* Vol. 80, No. 4, April 1997.

3. Chrisler, J. C., and C. B. Zitell. "Menarche Stories: Reminiscences of College Students from Lithuania, Malaysia, Sudan and the United States." *Health Care for Women International,* Vol. 19, No. 4, July–August 1998.

4. Yonkers, Kimberly A.; Halbreich, Uriel; Freeman, Ellen; Brown, Candace; and others. " Symptomatic Improvement of Premenstrual Dysphoric Disorder with Sertraline Treatment: A Randomized Controlled Trial." *Journal of the American Medical Association,* Vol. 278, No. 12, September 24, 1997.

5. Task Force on Circumcision. "Circumcision Policy Statement." *Pediatrics,* Vol. 103, No. 3, March 1999.

6. SIECUS.

7. "Public Support for Sexuality Education Reaches Highest Level." SIECUS news release, 1999.

8. "Youth Risk Behavior Surveillance—United States, 1997." *Morbidity and Mortality Weekly Report,* Vol. 47, Issue 3, 1998.

9. "SIECUS Report Reads 'Between the Lines' of Federal Abstinence-only Education Program." SIECUS press release, April 5, 1999.

10. "Programs That Work for Reducing Risk Behaviors Among Adolescents." *School Health Opportunities and Progress (SHOP) Bulletin,* Vol. 4, Issue 4, April 30, 1999.

11. Kirby, D. "Reducing Adolescent Pregnancy: Approaches that Work." *Contemporary Pediatrics,* January 1, 1999.

12. Jemott, John, et al. "Abstinence and Safer Sex: HIV Risk-Reduction Interventions for African-American Adolescents." *JAMA,* Vol. 279, No. 19, 1998.

13. Schreck, L. "Safer-Sex Programs Increase Condom Use Among Black Adolescents." *Family Planning Perspectives,* Vol. 31, No. 1, January 1999.

14. Crooks and Baur, *Our Sexuality,* 7th ed. Pacific Grove, CA: Brooks/Cole, 1999.

15. Adler, Nancy. Personal interview.

16. Haffner, Debra W., and Goldfarb, Eva. "But Does It Work? Improving Evaluations of Sexuality Education." *SIECUS Report,* Vol. 25, No. 6, August–September 1997.

17. Campbell, Lisa. "Adolescent Sexual Behavior Does Not Always Foretell Sexual Orientation." *The Brown University Child and Adolescent Behavior Letter,* Vol. 10, No. 12, December 1994.

18. "National Survey of Teens on Dating, Intimacy and Sexual Experiences." *School Health Opportunities and Progress (SHOP) Bulletin,* Vol. 3, Issue 3, April 17, 1998.

19. "Decrease in Teen Intercourse Among Males." *School Health Opportunities and Progress (SHOP) Bulletin,* Vol. 3, Issue 16, October 16, 1998.

20. Alan Guttmacher Institute, 1994.

21. Schwartz, Israel. "Sexual Activity Prior to Coital Initiation: A Comparison Between Males and Females." *Archives of Sexual Behavior,* Vol. 28, No. 1, February 1999.

22. Ullman, Sarah, et al. "Alcohol and Sexual Assault in a National Sample of College Women." *Journal of Interpersonal Violence,* Vol. 14, No. 6, June 1999.

23. O'Sullivan, Lucia, and Elizabeth Rice Allgier. "Feigning Sexual Desire: Consenting to Unwanted Sexual Activity in Heterosexual Dating Relationships." *Journal of Sex Research,* Vol. 35, No. 3, August 1998.

24. Shapiro, Johanna, et al. "Sexual Behavior and AIDS-Related Knowledge Among Community College Students in Orange County, California." *Journal of Community Health,* Vol. 24, Issue 1, February 1999.

25. Agocha, Bede, and Cooper, Lynne. "Risk Perception and Safer-Sex Intentions: Does a Partner's Physical Attractiveness Undermine the Use of Risk-Relevant Information?" *Personality & Social Psychology Bulletin,* Vol. 25, No. 6, June 1999.

26. Robinson, John, and Geoffrey Godbey. "No Sex, Please ... We're College Graduates." *American Demographics,* February 1998.

27. "AARP's Modern Maturity Reveals Survey Results on Sexual Attitudes, Looks at the top issues affecting relationships," AARP Press Release, August 3, 1999.

28. Bortz, Walter, et al. "Sexual Function in 1,202 Aging Males." *Journal of Gerontology,* Vol. 54, No. 5, May 1999.

29. Bortz, Walter, et al. "Physical Fitness, Aging and Sexuality." *Western Journal of Medicine,* Vol. 170, Issue 3, March 1999.

30. Crooks and Baur, *Our Sexuality.*

31. Rice, George, et al. "Male Homosexuality: Absence of Linkage to Microsatellite Markers at Xq28." *Science,* Vol. 284, No. 5414, April 23, 1999.

32. Horan, P. F., et al. "The Meaning of Abstinence for College Students." *Journal of HIV/AIDS Prevention and Education for Adolescents and Children,* Vol. 2, No. 2, 1998.

33. "Fact Sheet: Adolescence and Abstinence." SIECUS.

34. "Concern About Meaning of 'Abstinence' for College Students." *School Health Opportunities and Progress (SHOP) Bulletin,* Vol. 4, Issue 7, June 11, 1999.

35. Sanders, Stephanie, and June Reinisch. "Would You Say You Had 'Had Sex' If . . . ? *JAMA,* Vol. 281, No. 3, January 20, 1999.

36. Richters, Juliet, and Angela Song. "Australian University Students Agree with Clinton's Definition of Sex." *British Medical Journal,* Vol. 318, Issue 7189, April 10, 1999.

37. Cooper, Alvin, et al. "Sexuality on the Internet: From Sexual Exploration to the Pathological Expression." *Professional Psychology,* Vol. 30, No. 2, March 1999.

38. Laumann, et al. *The Social Organization of Sexuality.*

39. Billy, J. O., et al. "The Sexual Behavior of Men in the United States." *Family Planning Perspectives,* Vol. 25, 1993.

40. Janus, Samuel, and Cynthia Janus. *The Janus Report on Sexual Behavior.* New York: Wiley, 1993.

41. Crooks Baur. *Our Sexuality.*

42. Horan, P. F., et al. "The Meaning of Abstinence for College Students."

43. Gregoire, Alain. "Assessing and Managing Male Sexual Problems." *British Medical Journal,* Vol. 318, Issue 7179, January 30, 1999.

44. Ibid.

45. Butcher, Josie. "Loss of Desire—What About the Fun?" *British Medical Journal,* Vol. 318, Issue 7175, January 2, 1999.

46. Parrish, Michael. "Viagra—Don't Expect Miracles." *American Health,* September 1998.

47. Newman, Nancy. "Retinal Side-Effects of Sildenafil." *American Journal of Ophthalmology,* Vol. 127, No. 6, June, 1999.

48. "Online Viagra Prescriptions Bring Disapproval." *Impotence & Male Health Weekly Plus,* May 17, 1999.

49. Eisenberg, Anne. "A Boost to Research on Women's Sexuality." *New York Times,* June 13, 1999.

50. Gregoire, Alain. "Assessing and Managing Male Sexual Problems."

51. de Silva, W. P. "Sexual Variations." *British Medical Journal,* Vol. 318, Issue 7184, March 6, 1999.

10

Reproductive Choices

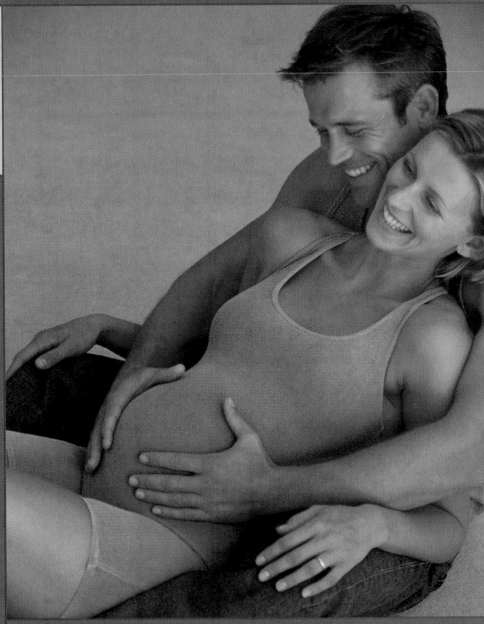

After studying the material in this chapter, you should be able to:

- **Explain** the process of conception in humans.
- **List** the major options available for contraception, and **explain** the advantages and risks of each.
- **Define** *abortion*, and **list** the commonly used abortion methods.
- **Define** and **give examples** of *preconception care.*
- **Describe** the physiological effects of pregnancy on a woman.
- Briefly **describe** the development of a fetus.
- **Describe** the three stages of labor and birth.
- **Explain** the options available to infertile couples wanting children.

As human beings, we have a unique power: the ability to choose to conceive or not to conceive. No other species on earth can separate sexual activity and pleasure from reproduction. However, simply not wanting to get pregnant is never enough to prevent conception, nor is wanting to have a child always enough to get pregnant. Both desires require individual decisions and actions.

Anyone who engages in vaginal intercourse must be willing to accept the consequences of that activity—the possibility of pregnancy and responsibility for the child who might be conceived—or take action to avoid those consequences. A heterosexual woman in Western countries spends 90 percent of her reproductive years trying to prevent pregnancy and 10 percent of these years trying to become or being pregnant.

Although many people are concerned about the risks associated with contraception, using birth control is safer and healthier than not using it. According to the Population Reference Bureau, the use of contraceptives, including oral contraceptives, saves millions of lives each year.[1] Some forms of contraception also reduce the risk of sexually transmitted diseases (STDs).

This chapter provides information on conception, birth control, abortion, infertility, and the processes by which a new human life develops and enters the world. ❖

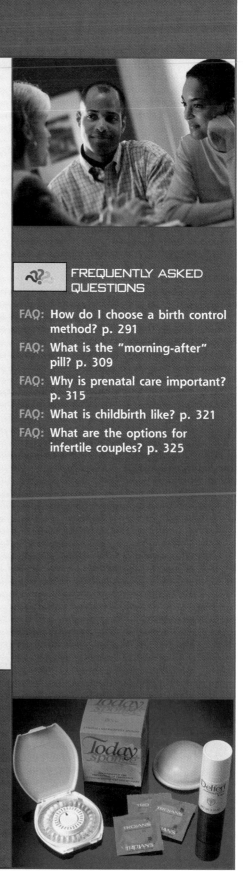

FREQUENTLY ASKED QUESTIONS

FAQ: **How do I choose a birth control method? p. 291**

FAQ: **What is the "morning-after" pill? p. 309**

FAQ: **Why is prenatal care important? p. 315**

FAQ: **What is childbirth like? p. 321**

FAQ: **What are the options for infertile couples? p. 325**

Conception

The equation for making a baby is quite simple: One sperm plus one egg equals one fertilized egg, which can develop into an infant. But the processes that affect or permit **conception** are quite complicated. The creation of sperm, or **spermatogenesis,** starts in the male at puberty. As discussed in Chapter 9, the production of sperm is regulated by hormones. Sperm cells form in the seminiferous tubules of the testes and are passed into the epididymis, where they are stored until ejaculation (see Figure 10-1); a single male ejaculation may contain 500 million sperm. Each of the sperm released into the vagina during intercourse moves on its own, propelling itself toward its target, an ovum.

To reach its goal, the sperm must move through the acidic secretions of the vagina, enter the uterus, travel up the fallopian tube containing the ovum, then fuse with the nucleus of the egg (**fertilization**). Just about every sperm produced by a man in his lifetime fails to accomplish its mission.

There are far fewer human egg cells than there are sperm cells. Each woman is born with her lifetime supply of ova, and between 300 and 500 eggs eventually mature and leave her ovaries during ovulation. As discussed in Chapter 9, every month, one or the other of the woman's ovaries releases an ovum to the nearby fallopian tube. It travels through the fallopian tube until it reaches the uterus, a journey that takes three to four days. An unfertilized egg lives for about 24 to 36 hours, disintegrates, and, during menstruation, is expelled along with the uterine lining.

Even if a sperm, which can survive in the female reproductive tract for two to five days, meets a ripe egg in a fallopian tube, its success is not assured. It must penetrate the layer of cells and a jellylike substance that surrounds each egg. Every sperm that touches the egg deposits an enzyme that dissolves part of this barrier. When a sperm bumps into a bare spot, it can penetrate the egg membrane and merge with the egg. (See Figure 10-2.) The fertilized egg travels down the fallopian tube, dividing to form a tiny clump of cells called a **zygote.** When it reaches the uterus, about a week after fertilization, it burrows into the endometrium, the lining of the uterus. This process is called **implantation.**

Conception can be prevented by **contraception.** Some contraceptive methods prevent ovulation or implantation, and others block the sperm from reaching the egg. Some methods are temporary; others permanently alter one's fertility.

The Quest for Contraception

Although many assume that birth control started with the pill, contraceptives date back to the earliest human

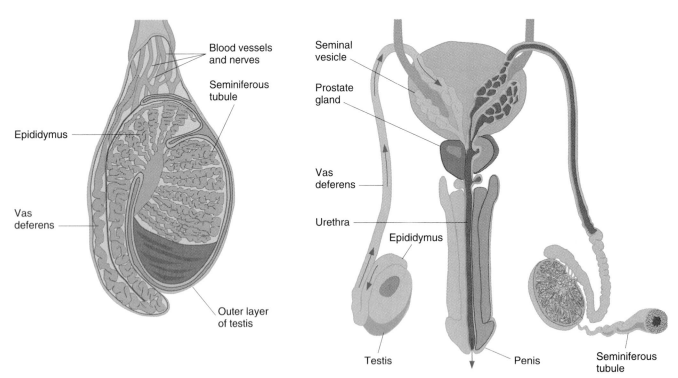

■ Figure 10-1 **The Testes**
Spermatogenesis takes place in the testes. Sperm cells form in the seminiferous tubules and are stored in the coils of the epididymis. Eventually, the sperm drain into the vasa deferentia ready for ejaculation.

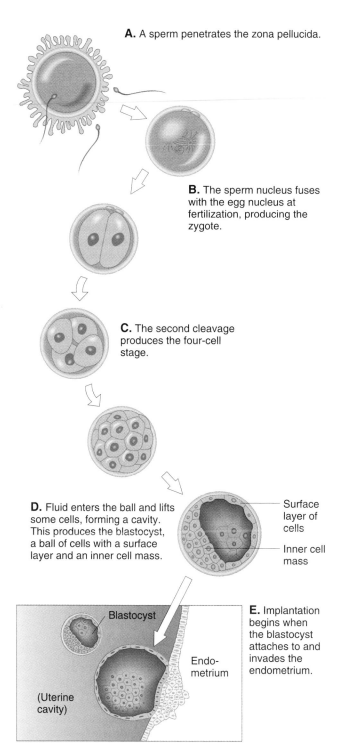

A. A sperm penetrates the zona pellucida.

B. The sperm nucleus fuses with the egg nucleus at fertilization, producing the zygote.

C. The second cleavage produces the four-cell stage.

D. Fluid enters the ball and lifts some cells, forming a cavity. This produces the blastocyst, a ball of cells with a surface layer and an inner cell mass.

Surface layer of cells

Inner cell mass

Blastocyst

Endo- metrium

(Uterine cavity)

E. Implantation begins when the blastocyst attaches to and invades the endometrium.

■ **Figure 10-2 Fertilization**
(A) The efforts of hundreds of sperm may allow one to penetrate the ovum's corona radiata, and outer layer of cells, and then the zona pellucida, a thick inner membrane. (B) The nuclei of the sperm and the egg cells approach. The nuclei merge, and the male and female chromosomes in the nuclei come together, forming a zygote. (C) The zygote divides into two cells, then four cells, and so on. (D) As fluid enters the ball, cells form a ball of cells called a blastocyst. (E) The blastocyst implants itself in the endometrium.

societies, when women tried all sorts of methods—the foam from a camel's mouth, alligator dung, gunpowder, opium, herbs, or alum (applied to the vagina before sex to make the cervix contract). They consulted healers, midwives, priests, practitioners of every form of the black arts and medical sciences. They held very still or stood during intercourse, jumped up and down or sneezed violently afterward, douched with poisons, endured horrible pain, and risked—and occasionally lost—their lives.

The Basics of Birth Control

Today birth control is safer, more effective, and more convenient than in the past—yet none of today's contraceptives is 100 percent safe, 100 percent effective, or 100 percent convenient. (See Pulsepoints: "Ten Ways to Avoid Getting Pregnant.") And even protection that is effective 95 percent of the time (which, some contend, is the best available in real-life use) isn't as good as it may sound. With just a 5 percent failure rate, statistically speaking, seven in ten women who want no more than two children would have to undergo one or more abortions in order to achieve their desired family size. (See Table 10-1, which shows the use of contraception around the world.)

Ideally, two partners should decide together which form of birth control to use. However, according to a national poll, more than 70 percent of men and women said men were "not responsible enough" to choose a birth control method. Both sexes believed that men were uninvolved because they "don't care" and because they consider birth control the "female's responsibility." Among those surveyed, 57 percent of the women using birth control said they were the ones who made sure contraception was used; 35 percent shared the decision with their male partners; the male took responsibility in the remaining instances.[2] The general lack of male involvement may account for 40 percent of each year's unwanted pregnancies.

Another barrier to birth control is cost. Many health insurers do not cover the cost of reversible methods of birth control—despite evidence that contraception, when used properly, is far more cost-effective than an unplanned pregnancy. Even when birth control is affordable and available, many college students do not use it consistently.

If you are engaging in sexual activity that could lead to conception, you have to be realistic about your situation. This may mean assuming full responsibility for your reproductive ability, whether you're a man or a woman. You also have to recognize the risks associated with various methods of contraception. If you're a woman, the risks are chiefly yours. Although most women never experience any serious complications, it's

PULSE points

Ten Ways to Avoid Getting Pregnant

1. **Abstain.** The only 100 percent safe and effective way to avoid unwanted pregnancy is not to engage in heterosexual intercourse.

2. **Limit sexual activity to "outercourse."** You can engage in many sexual activities—kissing, hugging, touching, massage, oral-genital sex—without risking pregnancy.

3. **Talk about birth control with any potential sex partner.** If you are considering sexual intimacy with a person, you should feel comfortable enough to talk about contraception.

4. **Know what doesn't work—and don't rely on it.** There are lots of misconceptions about ways to avoid getting pregnant, such as having sex in a standing position or during menstruation. Only the methods described in this chapter are reliable forms of birth control.

5. **Talk with a health care professional.** A great deal of information and advice is available—in writing, from family planning counselors, from physicians on the Internet. Check it out.

6. **Choose a contraceptive method that matches your personal habits and preferences.** If you can't remember to take a pill every day, oral contraceptives aren't for you. If you're constantly forgetting where you put things, a diaphragm might not be a good choice.

7. **Consider long-term implications.** Since you may well wish to have children in the future, find out about the reversibility of various methods and possible effects on future fertility.

8. **Resist having sex without contraceptive protection "just this once."** It only takes once—even the very first time—to get pregnant. Be wary of drugs and alcohol. They can impair your judgment and make you less conscientious about using birth control—or using it properly.

9. **Use backup methods.** If there's a possibility that a contraceptive method might not offer adequate protection (for instance, if it's been almost three months since your last injection of Depo-Provera), use an additional form of birth control.

10. **Inform yourself about emergency contraception.** Just in case a condom breaks or a diaphragm slips, find out about the availability of forms of after-intercourse contraception.

important to be aware of the potential for long-term risks. Risks that are acceptable to others may not be acceptable to you.

Unintended Pregnancy

The United States has the highest rate of unintended pregnancies in the world. Many of these, as seen in Campus Focus: "Unintended Pregnancy Among College Students," occur because couples do not have a method of contraception or do not use their usual form of birth control.[3] Yet 53 percent of the women who unintentionally become pregnant every year are using contraception.

Women between ages 20 and 24 have a higher rate of unintended pregnancy than women in any other age group, including teenagers. They are less likely to report uninterrupted use of an effective birth control method and more likely to use contraception sporadically than women aged 25 to 34. Such high-risk contraceptive behavior is more likely among women in less stable relationships, those having infrequent intercourse, and

■ **Table 10-1** Global Use of Contraception

Method of Contraception	Regularly Used By (approximate)	Most Popular in These Places
Sterilization	200 million	Asia, Latin America
Intrauterine device (IUD)	110 million	China, Arab states
The Pill	70 million	Latin America, USA, Europe
Injectable methods	10 million	Sub-Saharan Africa
Implants	1.5 million	Indonesia
Condom	> 25 million	Worldwide

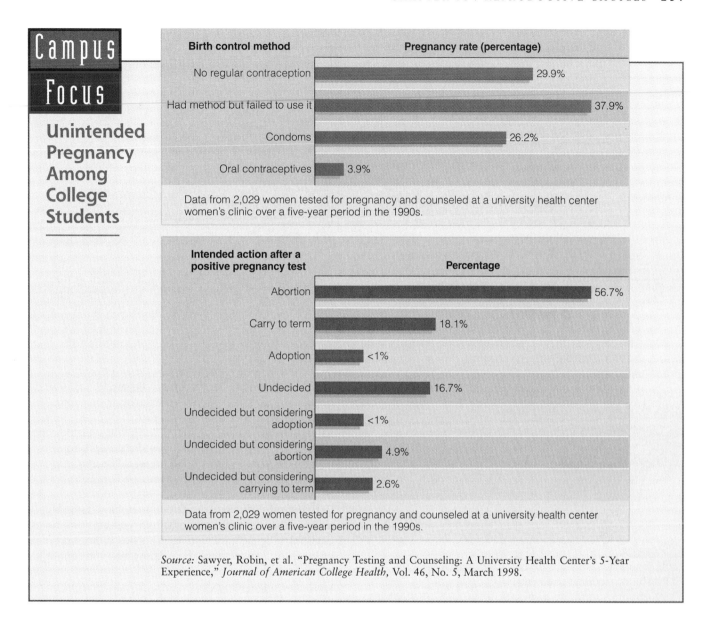

Campus
Focus

Unintended
Pregnancy
Among
College
Students

Birth control method	Pregnancy rate (percentage)
No regular contraception	29.9%
Had method but failed to use it	37.9%
Condoms	26.2%
Oral contraceptives	3.9%

Data from 2,029 women tested for pregnancy and counseled at a university health center women's clinic over a five-year period in the 1990s.

Intended action after a positive pregnancy test	Percentage
Abortion	56.7%
Carry to term	18.1%
Adoption	<1%
Undecided	16.7%
Undecided but considering adoption	<1%
Undecided but considering abortion	4.9%
Undecided but considering carrying to term	2.6%

Data from 2,029 women tested for pregnancy and counseled at a university health center women's clinic over a five-year period in the 1990s.

Source: Sawyer, Robin, et al. "Pregnancy Testing and Counseling: A University Health Center's 5-Year Experience," *Journal of American College Health*, Vol. 46, No. 5, March 1998.

those who recently experienced nonvoluntary intercourse for the first time.[4]

Most pregnancies among contraceptive users are the result of incorrect or inconsistent use. Among the factors that influence the way sexual partners use birth control are the degree of communication and cooperation between them, the predictability and frequency of intercourse, their attitudes about sexuality and fertility, experience or practice with a particular method, and the ease and affordability of contraception.[5] Many women temporarily discontinue birth control, primarily because they're dissatisfied with a particular method. In one recent study, 30 percent of women stopped using contraception after six months; approximately 45 percent stopped after a year. About 70 percent of women resumed birth control use within one to three months.[6]

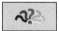 ### How Do I Choose a Birth Control Method?

When it comes to deciding which form of birth control to use, there's no one "right" decision. (See Self-Survey: "Which Contraceptive Method Is Best for You?") However, good decisions are based on sound information. You should consult a physician or family-planning counselor if you have questions or want to know how certain methods might affect existing or familial medical conditions, such as high blood pressure or diabetes.

As Table 10-3 indicates, contraception doesn't always work. As you evaluate any contraceptive, always consider its **effectiveness** (the likelihood that it will indeed prevent pregnancy). Inevitably, theoretical effectiveness, based on statistical estimates, is greater than actual

Self-*Survey* | Which Contraceptive Method Is Best for You?

Answer Yes or No to each statement as it applies to you and, if appropriate, your partner.

1. You have high blood pressure or cardiovascular disease. _____
2. You smoke cigarettes. _____
3. You have a new sexual partner. _____
4. An unwanted pregnancy would be devastating to you. _____
5. You have a good memory. _____
6. You or your partner have multiple sexual partners. _____
7. You prefer a method with little or no bother. _____
8. You have heavy, crampy periods. _____
9. You need protection against STDs. _____
10. You are concerned about endometrial and ovarian cancer. _____
11. You are forgetful. _____
12. You need a method right away. _____
13. You're comfortable touching your own and your partner's genitals. _____
14. You have a cooperative partner. _____
15. You like a little extra vaginal lubrication. _____
16. You have sex at unpredictable times and places. _____
17. You are in a monogamous relationship and have at least one child. _____

Scoring:
Recommendations are based on Yes answers to the following numbered statements:

The combination pill: 4, 5, 6, 8, 9, 16
The progestin-only pill: 1, 2, 5, 7, 16
Condoms: 1, 2, 3, 6, 9, 12, 13, 14
Norplant and Depo-Provera: 1, 2, 4, 7, 11, 16
Diaphragm or cervical cap: 1, 2, 13, 14
The IUD: 1, 2, 7, 11, 13, 16, 17
Spermicides: 1, 2, 12, 13, 14, 15
Sponge: 1, 2, 12, 13

Making Changes

Choosing a Contraceptive
Your responses may indicate that there's more than one appropriate method of birth control for you. Remember that you may choose different types of birth control at different stages of your life, or switch contraceptives for various reasons. Here are some factors you and your partner should always consider and discuss:

- **Effectiveness.** Keep in mind that your own conscientiousness will play an important role. If you forget to take your daily pill, or if you decide not to use a condom "just this once," you'll increase the odds of pregnancy by interfering with effective birth control.
- **Suitability.** If you don't have sex very often, a contraceptive with many risks and side effects, such as the pill, may be wrong for you. If you have many sexual partners and are at risk of contracting a sexually transmitted disease, a condom may provide protection against pregnancy and infection, especially if used with a diaphragm or cervical cap.
- **Side effects.** Some complications related to contraceptives are serious health threats. Be sure to ask questions and gather as much information as possible about what side effects to expect.
- **Safety.** The risks of certain contraceptives, such as the pill, may be too great to allow their use, if, for example, you have high blood pressure. Be honest in describing your medical history to your physician.
- **Future fertility.** Some women don't return to regular menstrual cycles for six months to a year after discontinuing oral contraceptives. This possibility may or may not be important to you now, but you should try to look ahead.
- **Cost.** The only free contraceptive methods are abstinence and rhythm methods. If you're on a tight budget, you might consider the relative costs of a year's prescription of oral contraceptives compared to a year's supply of condoms or spermicidal foam or jelly. However, you should also think about the long-term costs and consequences.
- **Reduced risk of sexually transmitted diseases.** Some forms of contraception, in particular barrier contraceptives and spermicides, help reduce the risk of transmission of some STDs. However, none provides complete protection.

■ Table 10-2 The Costs of Contraception

Method	Cost
Continuous abstinence	none
Outercourse (sex play without vaginal intercourse)	none
Sterilization	$1,000–$2,500 for tubal sterilization
Tubal: intended to permanently block women's tubes where sperm join egg	$240–$520 for vasectomy
Vasectomy: intended to permanently block man's tubes that carry sperm	(Vasectomy costs less because it is a simpler operation that can be done in the clinician's office)
Norplant	$500–$600 for exam, implants, and insertion $100–$200 for removal
Depo-Provera	$30–$75 per injection. May be less at clinics. $35–$125 for exam. Some family planning clinics charge according to income. $20–$40 for subsequent visits plus medication.
IUD (intrauterine device)	$150–$300: exam, insertion, and follow-up visit. Some family planning clinics charge according to income.
The Pill	$15–$25 per monthly pill-pack at drugstores. Often less at clinics $35–$125 for exam. Some family planning clinics charge according to income.
Male Condom	25 cents and up: dry 50 cents and up: lubricated $2.50 and up: plastic, animal tissue, or textured Some family planning centers give them away or charge very little.
Withdrawal	none
Diaphragm	$13–$25 $50–$125 for exam Often less at family planning clinics $4–$8 for supplies of spermicide jelly or cream
Cervical cap	$13–$25 $50–$125 for exam Often less at family planning clinics $4–$8 for supplies of spermicide jelly or cream
Female condom	$2.50
Spermicide	$8 for applicator kits of foam and gel $4–$8 for refills
Periodic Abstinence or FAMS (Fertility Awareness Methods)	$5–$8 and up for temperature kits (drugstores) Free classes often available in health and church centers

Source: Planned Parenthood web site © 1998 (**www.plannedparenthood.org**).

effectiveness. The **failure rate** for a contraceptive refers to the number of pregnancies that occur per year for every 100 women using a particular method of birth control.

The reliability of contraceptives in actual, real-life use is much lower than those reported in national surveys or clinical trials.[7] (See Table 10-3.) In general, failure rates are highest among cohabiting and other unmarried women, among very poor families, among black and Hispanic women, among adolescents, and among women in their twenties. Unmarried adolescent women

■ **Table 10-3** Failure Rates of Contraceptives in the First Year of Use

Spermicides	26%
Withdrawal	24%
Periodic abstinence	21%
Male condom	14%
Diaphragm, cervical cap	12%
Birth control pill	8%
Hormonal implant, injectables	2–3%

Source: Fu, Haishan, et al. "Contraceptive Failure Rates." *Family Planning Perspectives*, Vol. 31, No. 2, March 1999.

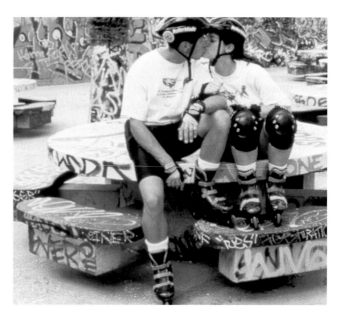

What does abstinence mean? Some couples refrain from intercourse but engage in "outercourse," or intimacy that includes kissing, hugging, and sensual touching.

who are living with a partner have an average failure rate of about 31 percent in the first year of contraceptive use, regardless of method of birth control, compared with a failure rate of 7 percent among married women aged 30 and older. The annual failure rate among black women is about 19 percent, regardless of family income. Among Hispanic women, the overall failure rate is 10 percent, but it is higher among poorer women than more affluent ones. Teenagers whose partners are three or more years older are less likely to use contraceptives regularly.

Some couples use withdrawal or **coitus interruptus,** removal of the penis from the vagina before ejaculation, to prevent pregnancy, even though it is not a reliable form of birth control. About half the men who have tried coitus interruptus find it unsatisfactory, either because they don't know when they're going to ejaculate or because they can't withdraw quickly enough. Also, the Cowper's glands, two pea-sized structures located on each side of the urethra, often produce a fluid that appears as drops at the tip of the penis any time from arousal and erection to orgasm. This fluid can contain active sperm and, in infected men, HIV.

As many as 3 million unintentional pregnancies each year in the United States are the result of contraceptive failure, either from problems with the drug or device itself or from improper use. Partners can lower the risk of unwanted pregnancy by using backup methods—that is, more than one form of contraception simultaneously. Emergency or post-intercourse contraception (discussed later in this chapter) could prevent as many as 2.3 million unwanted pregnancies each year.

Always discuss contraception with your partner. Men shouldn't automatically shift this responsibility to women simply because women are the ones who get pregnant. And women shouldn't assume that men don't want to be consulted or participate, nor should they hesitate to discuss sharing the costs with their partners. It takes two people to conceive a baby, and two people should be involved in deciding *not* to conceive a baby.

In the process, they can also enhance their skills in communication, critical thinking, and negotiating.

Abstinence and "Outercourse"

The contraceptive methods discussed in this chapter are designed to prevent pregnancy as a consequence of vaginal intercourse. Couples who choose abstinence make a very different decision—to abstain from vaginal intercourse and other forms of sexual activity (any in which ejaculation occurs near the vaginal opening) that could result in conception. Abstinence is the only form of birth control that is 100 percent effective and risk-free. It is also an important, increasingly valued lifestyle choice. A growing number of individuals, including some who have been sexually active in the past, are choosing abstinence until they establish a relationship with a long-term partner.

Individuals who choose abstinence from vaginal intercourse often engage in activities sometimes called "outercourse," such as kissing, hugging, sensual touching, and mutual masturbation. Outercourse can prevent pregnancy, but couples must be careful to avoid any penis-vagina contact. If the man ejaculates near the vaginal opening, sperm can swim up into the vagina and fallopian tubes to fertilize an egg. Except for oral-genital and anal sex, outercourse also may lower the risk of contracting sexually transmitted diseases. Some couples routinely restrict themselves to outercourse; others choose such sexual activities temporarily when it is inadvisable for them to have vaginal intercourse—for example, after childbirth.

Hormone-Based Contraceptives

These reversible forms of birth control for women use forms of estrogen and progesterone to inhibit ovulation, alter the mucus lining of the cervix so that it blocks the passage of sperm, or prevent successful implantation of the fertilized egg in the uterus.

The Birth Control Pill

"The pill"—the popular term for **oral contraceptives**—is the method of birth control preferred by unmarried women and by those under age 30, including college students. Women 18 to 24 years old are most likely to choose oral contraceptives. In use for 30 years, the pill is one of the most researched, tested, and carefully followed medications in medical history—and one of the most controversial. Although many women incorrectly think that the risks of the pill are greater than those of pregnancy and childbirth, long-term studies show that oral contraceptive use does not increase mortality rates. In a recent long-term British study, oral contraceptives significantly reduced the risk of ovarian and endometrial cancer and produced no increase in serious disease, including breast cancer, diabetes, multiple sclerosis, rheumatoid arthritis, and liver disease. There was an increased risk of cerebrovascular disease, pulmonary embolism, and blood clots for pill-users who were smokers and who took high-estrogen pills.[8]

Three types of oral contraceptives are currently widely used in the United States: the constant-dose combination pill, the multiphasic pill, and the progestin-only pill. The **constant-dose combination pill** releases two hormones, synthetic estrogen and progestin, which play important roles in controlling ovulation and the menstrual cycle, at constant levels throughout the menstrual cycle. The **multiphasic pill** mimics normal hormonal fluctuations of the natural menstrual cycle by providing different levels of estrogen and progesterone at different times of the month. Multiphasic pills reduce total hormonal dose and side effects. Both constant-dose combina-

tion and multiphasic pills block the release of hormones that would stimulate the process leading to ovulation. They also thicken and alter the cervical mucus, making it more hostile to sperm, and they make implantation of a fertilized egg in the uterine lining more difficult. Multiphasic pills may heighten a woman's sex drive.[9]

The **progestin-only,** or **minipill,** contains a small amount of progestin and no estrogen. Unlike women who take constant-dose combination pills, those using minipills probably ovulate at least occasionally. The minipills make the mucus in the cervix so thick and tacky, however, that sperm can't enter the uterus. Minipills also may interfere with implantation by altering the uterine lining.

Advantages. Birth control pills have several advantages: They are reversible, so a woman may easily stop using them. They do not interrupt sexual activity. Women on the pill have more regular periods, less cramping, and fewer tubal, or ectopic, pregnancies (discussed later in this chapter). After five years of use, the pill halves the risk of endometrial and ovarian cancer. It also reduces the risk of benign breast lumps, ovarian cysts, iron-deficiency anemia, and pelvic inflammatory disease (PID). In addition, the pill is one of the most effective forms of contraception. In actual use, the failure rate is 1 to 5 percent for estrogen/progesterone pills and 3 to 10 percent for minipills.

Disadvantages. The pill does not protect against HIV infection and other sexually transmitted diseases, so condoms and spermicide should also be used. In addition, the hormones in oral contraceptives may cause various side-effects, including spotting between periods, weight gain or loss, nausea and vomiting, breast tenderness, and decreased sex drive. Some women using the pill report emotional changes, such as mood swings and depression. Oral contraceptives can interact with other medications and diminish their effectiveness; women should inform any physician providing medical treatment that they are taking the pill.

Current birth control pills contain much lower levels of estrogen than early pills. As a result, the risk of heart disease and stroke among users is much lower than it once was; the danger may be lowest with the minipill. Yet there still is a risk of cardiovascular problems associated with use of the pill, primarily for women over 35 who smoke and those with other health problems, such as high blood pressure. Heart attacks strike an estimated 1 in 14,000 pill users between the ages of 30 and 39, and 1 in 1,500 between the ages of 40 and 44. Strokes occur five times more frequently among women taking oral contraceptives, and clots in the veins develop in 1 out of every 500 previously healthy women.

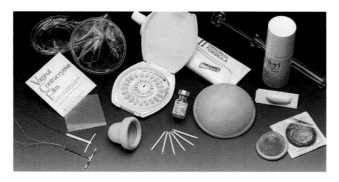

There is a wide variety of contraceptives available to couples.

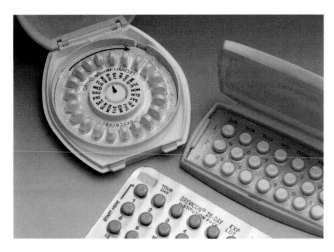

Oral contraceptives. The birth control pill.

Before starting on the pill, you should undergo a thorough physical examination that includes the following tests:

- Routine blood pressure test.
- Pelvic exam, including a Pap smear.
- Breast exam.
- Blood test.
- Urine sample.

You should also let your doctor know about any personal or family incidence of high blood pressure or heart disease, diabetes, liver dysfunction, hepatitis, unusual menstrual history, severe depression, sickle-cell anemia, cancer of the breast, ovaries, or uterus, high cholesterol levels, or migraine headaches.

How to Use Oral Contraceptives. The pill usually comes in 28-day packets: 21 of the pills contain the hormones, and 7 are "blanks," included so that the woman can take a pill every day, even during her menstrual period. If a woman forgets to take one pill, she should take it as soon as she remembers. However, if she forgets during the first week of her cycle or misses more than one pill, she should rely on another form of birth control until her next menstrual period.

Even if you experience no discomfort or side effects while on the pill, see a physician at least once a year for an examination, which should include a blood pressure test and a pelvic and breast exam. Notify your doctor at once if you develop severe abdominal pain, chest pain, coughing, shortness of breath, pain or tenderness in the calf or thigh, severe headaches, dizziness, faintness, muscle weakness or numbness, speech disturbance, blurred vision, a sensation of flashing lights, a breast lump, severe depression, or yellowing of your skin.

Generally, when a woman stops taking the pill, her menstrual cycle resumes the next month, but it may be irregular for the next couple of months. However, 2 to 4 percent of pill users experience prolonged delays. Women who become pregnant during the first or second cycle after discontinuing use of the pill may be at greater risk of miscarriage; they also are more likely to conceive twins. Most physicians advise women who want to conceive to change to another method of contraception for three months after they stop taking the pill.

Contraceptive Implants (Norplant)

About 1 percent of women use hormonal implants, such as Norplant, which prevent pregnancy for up to five years. Six thin silicone rubber capsules release a low, continuous dose of a synthetic form of progestin called levonorgestrel. Other implants are currently being developed.

Norplant works primarily by suppressing ovulation, but it also thickens the cervical mucus (which inhibits sperm migration), inhibits the development and growth of the uterine lining, and limits secretion of progesterone during the second or luteal half of the menstrual cycle. The best candidates for Norplant are women who desire reversible long-term contraception, those who don't want to have to insert or ingest a contraceptive regularly, those who cannot take estrogen-containing oral contraceptives, those who would face high medical risks if they did become pregnant, and those who are undecided about sterilization. Adolescents using Norplant are con-

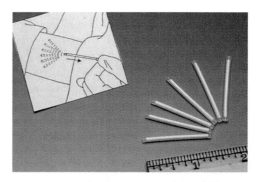

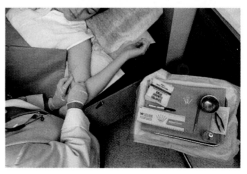

How Norplant works.

Consumer Health Watch

Health Risks of Birth Control Methods

For individuals with certain medical conditions, specific types of birth control can pose a health risk. To be safe, follow these guidelines:

- If you have high blood pressure (180/110 mmHg or higher), avoid birth control pills or injectables containing estrogen, which may increase your risk of a heart attack or stroke.

- If you've suffered episodes of depression, avoid products that contain progestin, such as Depo-Provera, Norplant, and the minipill. In some women with depression, progestin may worsen depressive symptoms. Also, check with your doctor if you are taking an antidepressant medication; it may affect or be affected by oral contraceptives and you may require a different dose.

- If you have a seizure disorder, avoid low-dose birth control pills. Some anti-seizure medications, such as

Dilantin, accelerate liver metabolism of all substances, including oral contraceptives, and make them less effective.

- If you've had an ectopic pregnancy, avoid IUDs. Although IUDs do not cause ectopic pregnancies, if your fallopian tubes have been scarred by a previous ectopic gestation, you're more likely to have another ectopic if you use an IUD.

- If you have any form of hepatitis (discussed in Chapter 12), avoid birth control pills or injectables containing estrogen, which is metabolized in the liver—an organ damaged by hepatitis.

Source: "Is Your Birth Control Safe for You?" *American Health,* September 1999.

---

siderably less likely than pill users to become pregnant unintentionally. An estimated 1.8 million women have used Norplant worldwide.

Advantages. Norplant has proven to be ten times more effective than the pill in preventing pregnancy, with a pregnancy rate of only four or five pregnancies per 1,000 users per year, compared with 20 to 50 pregnancies per 1,000 users of oral contraceptives. Norplant is most effective in women who weigh less than 110 pounds and somewhat less effective in those weighing more than 154 pounds. However, even in heavier women, Norplant is more effective than oral contraceptives. Like the pill, it may reduce the risk of endometrial and ovarian cancer.

For sexually active adolescents and young adults, who often do not use birth control pills and other forms of contraception consistently, Norplant's primary advantage is its long duration of action and the fact that they do not need to remember to use it. In clinical studies, teenagers reported more side effects with Norplant than with oral contraceptives.

Disadvantages. Common side effects of Norplant include menstrual irregularities, spotting, and amenorrhea; these are most likely to occur in the first year of use. Other possible complications include ovarian cysts, headaches, acne, weight changes, breast discharge, and hair growth. Because Norplant doesn't include estrogen (as birth control pills do), there is no risk of clotting or high blood pressure. However, the FDA advises women

with acute liver disease, unexplained vaginal bleeding, breast cancer, or blood clots in the lungs, legs, or eyes to avoid Norplant.

After Norplant became available in the United States in 1991, initial user satisfaction was high. However, satisfaction has declined, primarily because of side effects (cramps, headache, weight gain, and nausea are most common) and difficulties with removal of the implants. In one study, more than one in ten women had implants removed within one year because of side effects. Because of scarring and permanent nerve damage caused during implant removal, a class-action lawsuit was filed against Norplant's manufacturer. Physicians and nurse practitioners have subsequently

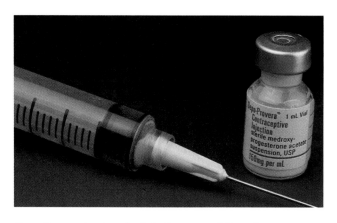

Depo-Provera is given by injection every 12 weeks.

developed removal techniques that they believe can lessen the risk of such complications.

Controversy also arose over the suggestion that women on welfare or convicted of child abuse be ordered or given incentives to use Norplant. The American Medical Association's board of trustees has stated its opposition to the involuntary use of long-acting contraceptives because such a policy inhibits a person's fundamental rights to refuse medical treatment, not to receive cruel and unusual punishment, and to procreate.

How to Use Norplant. A qualified health-care professional, using a local anesthetic, implants the Norplant capsules with a needle under the skin of a woman's upper arms. The simple surgical procedure generally takes about five to ten minutes. Once in place, the capsules can be felt and may be visible, particularly in slender women. Removal of the capsules again requires minor surgery, lasting 15 to 20 minutes, with a local anesthetic. Complications can occur during removal; the most common are bruising, slight bleeding, and pain at the removal site. After removal, fertility generally returns with the next menstrual cycle. According to various studies, most former users of Norplant began ovulating again within seven weeks of implant removal, and most of those who wished to conceive did so within one year.

Depo-Provera

One injection of Depo-Provera, a synthetic version of the natural hormone progesterone, provides three months of contraceptive protection. This long-acting hormonal contraceptive, approved for use in the United States in 1992, raises levels of progesterone, thereby simulating pregnancy. The pituitary gland doesn't produce FSH and LH, which normally cause egg ripening and release. The endometrial lining of the uterus thins, preventing implantation of a fertilized egg.

Advantages. Because Depo-Provera contains only progestin, it can be used by women who cannot take oral contraceptives containing estrogen (such as those who've had breast cancer). Its main advantage is that women do not need to take a daily pill or use a barrier method during sexual activity. It also may have some protective action against endometrial and ovarian cancer.

Disadvantages. Depo-Provera provides no protection against HIV and other STDs. It causes menstrual irregularities in most users; a delayed return of fertility; excessive endometrial bleeding; and other side effects, including decreased libido, depression, headaches, dizziness, weight gain, frequent urination, and allergic reactions in a small percentage of users. Long-term use may lead to significantly reduced bone density.[10]

How to Use Depo-Provera. Women must receive an injection of Depo-Provera once every 12 weeks, ideally within five days of the beginning of menstruation.

Barrier Contraceptives

As their name implies, **barrier contraceptives** block the meeting of egg and sperm by means of a physical barrier (a condom, diaphragm, or a cervical cap), or a chemical one (vaginal spermicide in jellies, foams, creams, suppositories, or film). These forms of birth control have become increasingly popular because they can do more than prevent conception; they can also help reduce the risk of STDs. However, fewer than one-

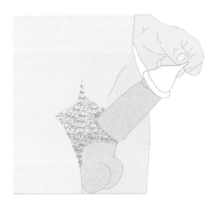

Pinch or twist the tip of the condom, leaving one-half inch at the tip to catch the semen.

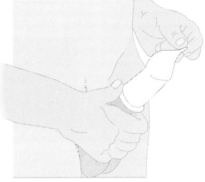

Holding the tip, unroll the condom.

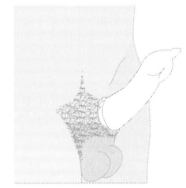

Unroll the condom until it reaches the pubic hairs.

■ Figure 10-3 **The Male Condom**
Condoms effectively reduce the risk of pregnancy as well as STDs. Using them consistently and correctly are important factors.

fourth of those needed to prevent STDs are being used worldwide.[11]

Condoms

The male **condom** covers the erect penis and catches the ejaculate, thus preventing sperm from entering the woman's reproductive tract (see Figure 10-3). Most are made of thin surgical latex or sheep membrane; a new type is made of polyurethane, which is thinner, stronger, more heat-sensitive, and more comfortable than latex. Condoms with a spermicidal lubricant (nonoxynol-9) kill most sperm on contact and are thus more effective than other brands.

Although the theoretical effectiveness rate for condoms is 97 percent, the actual rate is only 80 to 85 percent. The condom can be torn during the manufacturing process or during its use; testing by the manufacturer may not be as strenuous as it could or should be. Careless removal can also decrease the effectiveness of condoms. However, the major reason that condoms have such a low actual effectiveness rate is that couples don't use them each and every time they have sex.

Condoms are second only to the pill in popularity among college-age adults. However, men and women's attitudes toward them often differ. (See The X & Y Files: "Men, Women and Condoms.")

Advantages. Condoms made of latex or polyurethane, especially when used with spermicides containing nonoxynol-9, can help reduce the risk of certain STDs, including syphilis, gonorrhea, chlamydia, and herpes. They appear to lower a woman's risk of pelvic inflammatory disease (PID) and may protect against some parasites that cause urinary tract and genital infections. Public health officials view condoms as the best available defense against HIV infection.[12] They are available without a prescription or medical appointment, and their use does not cause harmful side effects. Some men appreciate the slight blunting of sensation they experience when using a condom because it helps prolong the duration of intercourse before ejaculation.

The X&Y Files

Men, Women, and Condoms

men purchase about half of the traditional, male condoms sold in the United States. However, purchases of male condoms by never-married women have tripled in the last decade. Although both men and women are buying more condoms, their attitudes toward them vary.

In one recent survey, men complained that condoms can be too loose, too tight, too short, difficult to apply, and susceptible to breaking. However, as the researchers noted, many of these complaints can be overcome with improvements in condom design and manufacture. Male objections to condom use often go beyond technical problems. Men may assume that even mentioning condoms decreases the likelihood of having sex with a partner.

In one experiment, researchers showed college students a videotape in which men used different ways to suggest condom use. The male viewers thought that bringing up use of a condom in any way diminished the chance of sexual intercourse; female viewers did not. In fact, women gave their highest ratings to men who talked about using a condom, describing them as nicer, more mature, and less promiscuous.

In surveys the great majority of women say they are likely to insist on condom use with their next partner, and would refuse to have sex with a man who would not use one. However, young women admit that their partners often try to talk their way out of using a condom.

The Cornell Women's Handbook has published some "condom comebacks" suggested by college women:

He: "It doesn't feel good."
She: "If you're uncomfortable using condoms, fine. Let's try something other than intercourse."

He: "It spoils the mood."
She: "So does your attitude."

He: "It takes too long."
She: "What's the rush? It's worth the wait."

He: "You won't catch anything from me."
She: "I know I won't, because we use a condom or we're not having intercourse. Besides, you might catch something from me."

He: "Just this once won't matter."
She: "Then just this once I'll have to say, 'no.'"

Sources: "Closing the Condom Gap." *Population Reports,* Vol. 27, Issue 1, April 1999. Bryan, Angela, et al. "The Impact of Males Proposing Condom Use on Perceptions of an Initial Sexual Encounter." *Personality & Social Psychology Bulletin,* Vol. 25, No. 3, March 1999. *The Cornell Women's Handbook* (www.rso.cornell.edu).

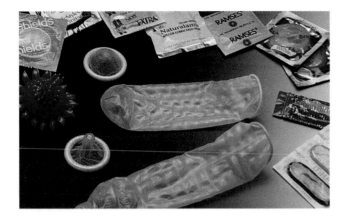

genital contact occurs (Figure 10-3). There should be a little space at the top of the condom to catch the semen. Wait until just before intercourse to apply spermicide. Any vaginal lubricant should be water-based. Petroleum based creams or jellies (such as Vaseline, baby oil, massage oil, vegetable oils, or oil-based hand lotions) can deteriorate the latex. After ejaculation, the condom should be held firmly against the penis so that it doesn't slip off or leak during withdrawal. Couples engaging in anal intercourse should use a water-based lubricant as well as a condom, but should never assume the condom will protect them from HIV infection or other STDS.

Disadvantages. Condoms are not 100 percent effective in preventing pregnancy or STDs, including infection with HIV or HPV (human papilloma virus, discussed in Chapter 12). For anyone not in a monogamous relationship with a mutually exclusive, healthy partner—heterosexual or homosexual—condoms can reduce the risks of sexual involvement, but they cannot eliminate them. Condoms may have manufacturing defects, such as pinsize holes, or they may break or slip off during intercourse.[13] Some couples feel that putting on a condom interferes with sexual spontaneity; others incorporate it into their sex play. Some men dislike the reduced penile sensitivity or will not use them because they believe they interfere with sexual pleasure. Others cannot sustain an erection while putting on a condom. A small number are allergic to latex condoms.

How to Use a Condom. Most physicians recommend prelubricated, spermicide-treated American-made latex or polyurethane condoms, not membrane condoms ("natural" or "sheepskin"). Before using a condom, check the expiration date, and make sure it's soft and pliable. If it's yellow or sticky, throw it out. Don't check for leaks by blowing up a condom before using it; you may weaken or tear it.

The condom should be put on at the beginning of sexual activity, before

The Female Condom

The female condom, made of polyurethane, consists of two rings and a polyurethane sheath, and is inserted into the vagina with a tampon-like applicator (see Figure 10-4). Once in place, the device loosely lines the walls of the vagina. Internally, a thickened rubber ring keeps it anchored near the cervix. Externally, another rubber ring, two inches in diameter, rests on the labia and resists slippage.

Although not widely used in the West, the female condom is gaining acceptance in Africa, Asia, and Latin America. Properly used, it is believed to be as good or better than the male condom for preventing infections because it is stronger and covers a slightly larger area. However, it is slightly less effective at preventing pregnancy.[14]

■ Figure 10-4 **The Female Condom**
This method is less effective than the male condom for preventing pregnancy and STDs (since no spermicide is used). Women may prefer the female condom as a way to control their risk of pregnancy and STDs. Like the male condom, this method does not require a prescription.

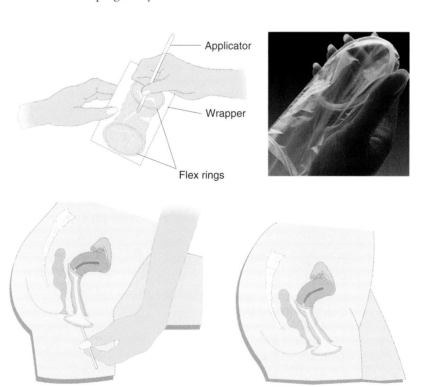

Applicator

Wrapper

Flex rings

Advantages. The female condom gives women more control in reducing their risk of pregnancy and STDS. It does not require a prescription or medical appointment. One size fits all.

Disadvantages. The failure rate for the female condom is higher than for other contraceptives. The statistical failure rate is 12.2 percent, which means that 12 of every 100 women using the device could expect to get pregnant during a six-month period. In clinical trials, the actual failure rate was even higher—20.6 percent. Since it does not have spermicide on it, the female condom does not provide as much risk-reduction against STDs as male condoms with spermicide.

How to Use the Female Condom. As illustrated in Figure 10-4, a woman removes the condom and applicator and inserts the condom slowly by gently pushing the applicator toward the small of the back. When properly inserted, the outer ring should rest on the folds of skin around the vaginal opening, and the inner ring (the closed end) should fit against the cervix. The condom should be used with a sperimcide and a water-based lubricant.

The Diaphragm

The **diaphragm** is a bowl-like rubber cup with a flexible rim that is inserted into the vagina to cover the cervix and prevent the passage of sperm into the uterus during sexual intercourse (see Figure 10-5). When used with spermicide, the diaphragm is both a physical and a chemical barrier to sperm. The effectiveness of the diaphragm in preventing pregnancy depends on strong motivation (to use it faithfully) and a precise understanding of its use. If diaphragms with spermicide are used consistently and carefully, they can be 95 to 98 percent effective. Without a spermicide, the diaphragm is not effective.

Advantages. Diaphragms have become increasingly popular, most likely because of concern about the side effects of hormonal contraceptives. Many women feel that using a diaphragm makes them more knowledgeable and comfortable about their bodies.

Disadvantages. Some people find that the diaphragm is inconvenient and interferes with sexual spontaneity or

■ **Figure 10-5 The Diaphragm**
When used correctly and consistently and with a spermicide, the diaphragm is effective in preventing pregnancy and STDs. It must be fitted by a health-care professional.

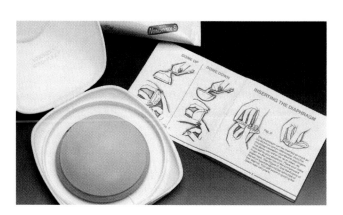

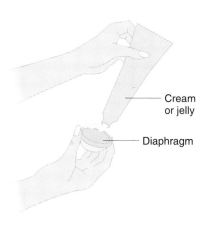

Cream or jelly

Diaphragm

Squeeze spermicide into dome of diaphragm and around the rim.

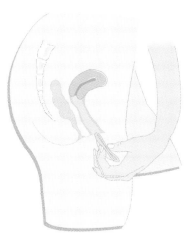

Squeeze rim together; insert jelly-side up.

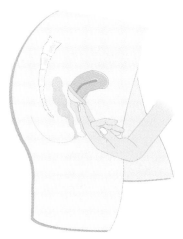

Check placement to make certain cervix is covered.

that the spermicidal cream or jelly is messy, detracts from oral-genital sex, and may cause irritation. A poorly fitted diaphragm can cause discomfort during sex; some women report bladder discomfort, urethral irritation, or recurrent cystitis as a result of diaphragm use.

How to Use a Diaphragm. Diaphragms are fitted and prescribed by a qualified health-care professional in sizes ranging from 2 to 4 inches (50–105 millimeters) in diameter. The diaphragm's main function is to serve as a container for a spermicidal (sperm-killing) foam or jelly, which is available at pharmacies without a prescription. Do not use oil-based lubricants because they will deteriorate the latex. A diaphragm should remain in the vagina for at least six hours after intercourse to assure that all sperm are killed. If intercourse occurs again during this period, additional spermicide cream or jelly must be inserted with an applicator tube.

The key to proper use of the diaphragm is having it available. A sexually active woman should keep it in the most accessible place—her purse, bedroom, bathroom. Before every use, a diaphragm should be checked for tiny leaks (hold up to the light or place water in the dome). A health-care provider should check its fit and condition every year when the woman has her annual Pap smear.

The Cervical Cap

Like the diaphragm, the **cervical cap,** combined with spermicide, serves as both a chemical and physical bar-rier blocking the path of the sperm to the uterus. The rubber or plastic cap is smaller and thicker than a diaphragm and resembles a large thimble that fits snugly around the cervix (see Figure 10-6). It is about as effective as a diaphragm.

Advantages. Women who cannot use a diaphragm because of pelvic-structure problems or loss of vaginal muscle tone can often use the cap. Also, the cervical cap does not require additional applications of spermicide if intercourse occurs more than once within several hours.

Disadvantages. Cervical caps are more difficult to insert and remove and may damage the cervix. Some women have difficulty getting a cervical cap that fits properly; others find it uncomfortable to wear.

How to Use a Cervical Cap. Like the diaphragm, the cervical cap is fitted by a qualified health-care professional. For use, the woman fills it one-third to two-thirds full with spermicide and inserts it by holding its edges together and sliding it into the vagina. The cup is then pressed onto the cervix. (Most women find it easiest to do so while squatting or in an upright sitting position.) The cap can be inserted up to 6 hours prior to intercourse and should not be removed for at least 6 hours afterward. It can be left in place up to 24 hours. Pulling on one side of the rim breaks the suction and allows easy removal. Oil-based lubricants should not be used with the cap because they can deteriorate the latex.

■ Figure 10-6 **The Cervical Cap**
This method is very similar to the diaphragm and may work better for some women. It is smaller than the diaphragm and covers only the cervix.

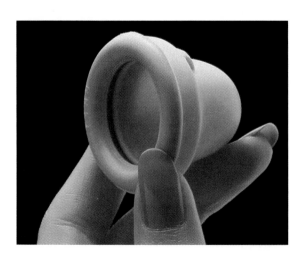

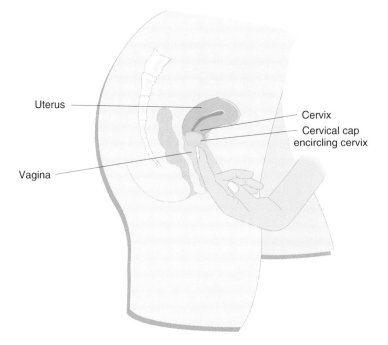

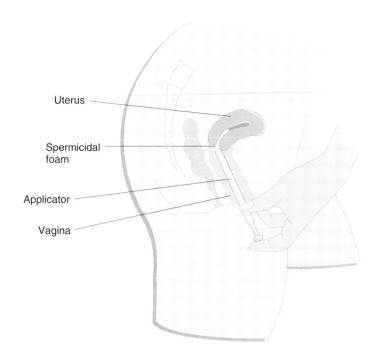

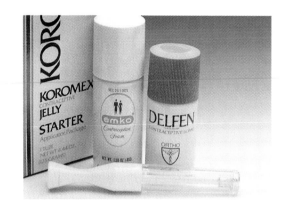

■ Figure 10-7 **Vaginal Spermicides**
These various creams and jellies are available without a prescription and have minimal side effects. They are most effective in preventing pregnancy and STDs when used together with a condom.

Vaginal Spermicides

The various forms of **vaginal spermicides** include chemical foams, creams, jellies, vaginal suppositories, and gels (see Figure 10-7). Some creams and jellies are made for use with a diaphragm; others can be used alone. Several vaginal suppositories claim high effectiveness, but no American studies have confirmed these claims. In general, failure rates for vaginal suppositories are as high as 10 to 25 percent. .

Advantages. Conscientious use of a spermicide together with another method of contraception, such as a condom, can provide safe and effective birth control and reduce the risk of some vaginal infections, pelvic inflammatory disease, and STDs. The side effects of vaginal spermicides are minimal.

Disadvantages. Even though spermicides can be applied in less than a minute, couples may feel that they interfere with sexual spontaneity. Some people are irritated by the chemicals in spermicides, but often a change of brand solves this problem. Others find foam spermicides messy or feel they interfere with oral-genital contact. Spermicidal suppositories that do not dissolve completely can feel gritty.

How to Use Vaginal Spermicides. The various types of spermicide come with instructions that should be followed carefully for maximum protection. Contraceptive vaginal suppositories take about 20 minutes to dissolve and cover the vaginal walls. Foam, inserted with an applicator, goes into place much more rapidly. You must apply additional spermicide before each additional intercourse. After sex, women should shower rather than bathe to prevent the spermicide from being rinsed out of the vagina and should not douche for at least six hours.

The Contraceptive Sponge

The nonprescription Today Sponge is a soft, disposable polyurethane sponge permeated with a spermicide. On the market from 1983 to 1995, the Today Sponge was one of the most popular contraceptive options for women. It was taken off the market because of problems at the product's sole manufacturing plant, including bacterial contamination of water and sanitizing equipment. The original manufacturer sold the manufacturing rights to American Home Products, which reintroduced the sponge.[15]

The sponge is believed to work by inactivating sperm with the spermicide, absorbing semen and thereby preventing sperm from entering the cervix, and acting as a mechanical barrier.

Advantages. The contraceptive sponge is easy to use and readily available as an over-the-counter product. It retails for $1.75 to $2.

Disadvantages. Its failure rate as a contraceptive is fairly high: about 10 percent over a year's use—comparable to that of other barrier methods. If not used properly, the failure rate rises to 15 percent. The sponge does not provide any protection against STDs.

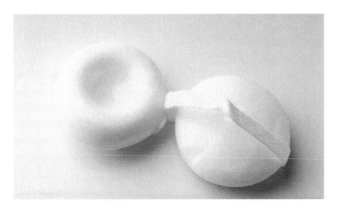

The contraceptive sponge, discontinued in 1995, will be available once more under a new manufacturer.

How to Use the Contraceptive Sponge. A woman inserts the sponge, a half-inch-thick rubbery disc with a diameter of about 1¼ inches, into her vagina before sex. It can be left there for 24 hours of protection. She removes the sponge by grasping on a ribbon-like loop attached to it.

Vaginal Contraceptive Film (VCF)

Available from pharmacies without a prescription, the 2-inch-by-2-inch thin film known as the **vaginal contraceptive film** (VCF) is laced with spermicide (Figure 10-8). Once folded and inserted into the vagina, it dissolves into a stay-in-place gel. Its theoretical effectiveness is similar to that of other forms of spermicide; paired with a condom, it is almost 100 percent effective.

Advantages. VCF film can be used by people allergic to foams and jellies. Unlike foams and jellies, it dissolves gradually and almost unnoticeably.

Disadvantages. Some people feel that insertion, even though it takes only seconds, interrupts sexual spontaneity.

How to Use VCF. A woman inserts the film by folding it and guiding it in with a finger so that it covers her cervix. VCF can be inserted from a minimum of 5 minutes to a maximum of 90 minutes before intercourse. It is effective for up to two hours and need not be removed. A new VCF must be inserted if intercourse occurs again after two hours.

The Intrauterine Device (IUD)

The **intrauterine device** (IUD) is a small piece of molded plastic, with a nylon string attached, that is inserted into the uterus through the cervix. It prevents pregnancy by interfering with implantation. Once widely used, IUDs became less popular after most brands were removed from the market because of serious complications such as pelvic infection and infertility. However, the currently

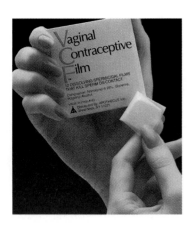

■ Figure 10-8 Vaginal Contraceptive Film (VCF)
This thin film is laced with spermicide. Its effectiveness is similar to other vaginal spermicides, and it is most effective paired with a condom.

**How to Use
Vaginal Contraceptive Film**

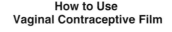

Remove the square of film from the convenient sealed envelope and fold it in half.

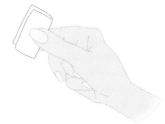

Make sure your fingers are dry. Place film on your second or third finger.

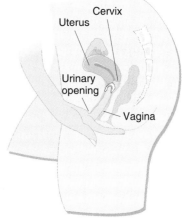

With one swift movement, place it high in your vagina against the cervix. VCF is effective for one hour. One film should be used for each act of intercourse. Follow the instructions in the product leaflet.

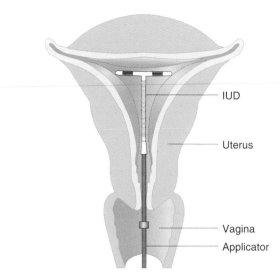

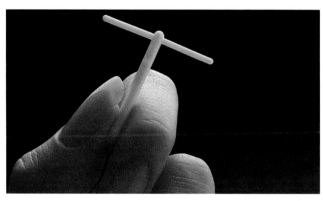

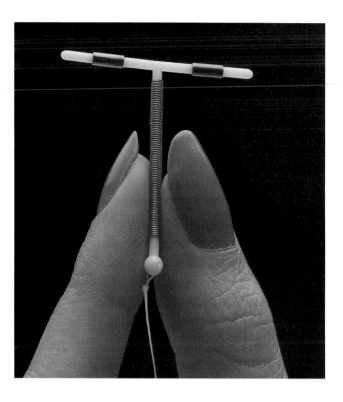

■ Figure 10-9 **The IUD**
The intrauterine device is effective and cost-efficient for preventing pregnancy, although some women may expel the device. The IUD does not offer protection against STDs, and there is increased risk of pelvic inflammatory disease (PID).

available IUDs have not been shown to increase the risk of such problems for women in mutually monogamous relationships. (See Figure 10-9.)

According to manufacturers' estimates, about 2 percent of American women using contraception currently rely on IUDs. Throughout the world more than 25 million IUDs have been distributed in 70 countries. Progestaser System is a T-shaped device containing progesterone, which prevents implantation; it must be replaced every year. The Copper T (Paragard) contains copper, which interferes with the growth of a fertilized egg by causing biochemical reactions with the uterine lining. The Copper T remains effective for ten years, making it the longest-acting reversible contraceptive available to women in the United States. Its cumulative failure rate is 2.6.

Advantages.   The IUD is highly effective and easy to reverse. According to recent analyses, the Copper T is the cheapest and most cost-effective form of birth control. Current models cause fewer complications than the pill. The IUD does not interrupt sexual activity, and 98 percent of IUD users in one survey said they are happy with this method.[16]

Disadvantages.   The most serious disadvantage is the possibility of increased risk of PID, which can lead to scarring and infertility. Many gynecologists recommend other forms of birth control for childless women who someday may want to start a family. In addition, women with many sexual partners, who are at highest risk of PID, are not good candidates for this method. During insertion of an IUD, women may experience discomfort, cramping, bleeding, or pain, which may continue for a few days or longer. The hormonal IUD causes less excess bleeding and cramping than the Copper-T. An estimated 2 to 20 percent of users expel an IUD within a year of insertion.

If a woman using an IUD does become pregnant, the IUD is removed to reduce the risk of miscarriage (which can be as high as 50 percent). Physicians generally offer therapeutic abortion to the woman because of the serious risks (including infection, premature delivery, and possibly a higher rate of birth defects) of continuing the pregnancy.

How to Use an IUD.   A physician inserts an IUD during the woman's period, when the cervix is slightly softened and dilated. Antibiotics may be prescribed to lower any risk of infection. An IUD can be removed at any time during her cycle. A woman should check regularly, particularly after each menstrual period, for the nylon string attached to the IUD, because she may not otherwise notice if an IUD has been expelled.

Sterilization

The most popular method of birth control among married couples in the United States is **sterilization** (surgery to end a person's reproductive capability). Each year an estimated 1 million men and women in the United States undergo sterilization procedures. Fewer than 25 percent ever seek reversal.[17]

Advantages. Sterilization has no effect on sex drive in either men or women. Many couples report that their sexual activity increases after sterilization, because they're free from the fear of pregnancy or the need to deal with contraceptives.

Disadvantages. Sterilization should be considered permanent and should be used only if both individuals are sure they want no more children. Although sterilization doesn't usually create psychological or sexual problems, it can worsen existing problems, particularly marital ones. Couples should discuss sterilization, together and with a physician, to understand fully the possible physical and emotional consequences. Although a link between vasectomy and an increased risk of prostate cancer was reported, the most recent research did not find a correlation.

Male Sterilization

An estimated 13 percent of married couples rely on male sterilization.[18] In men, the cutting of the *vas deferens*, the tube that carries sperm from one of the testes into the urethra for ejaculation, is called **vasectomy**. During the 15- or 20-minute office procedure, done under a local anesthetic, the doctor makes small incisions in the scrotum, lifts up each vas deferens, cuts them, and ties off the ends to block the flow of sperm (see Figure 10-10). Sperm continue to form, but they are broken down and absorbed by the body.

The man usually experiences some local pain, swelling, and discoloration for about a week after the procedure. More serious complications, including the formation of a blood clot in the scrotum (which usually disappears without treatment), infection, and an inflammatory reaction, occur in a small percentage of cases. The National Institute of Child Health and Human Development, in a 15-year follow-up study of nearly 5,000 men, found that sterilization poses no increased

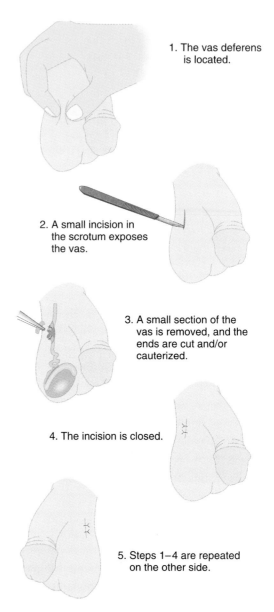

1. The vas deferens is located.

2. A small incision in the scrotum exposes the vas.

3. A small section of the vas is removed, and the ends are cut and/or cauterized.

4. The incision is closed.

5. Steps 1–4 are repeated on the other side.

■ **Figure 10-10** Male sterilization, or vasectomy.

danger of heart disease, even decades after the procedure. The pregnancy rate among the wives of men who've had vasectomies is about 15 in 10,000 women per year. Most result from a couple's failure to wait several weeks after the operation, until all sperm stored in each vas deferens have been ejaculated, before having unprotected coitus.

Sometimes men want to reverse their vasectomies, usually because they want to have children with a new spouse. Although anyone who chooses to have a vasectomy should consider it permanent, surgical reversal *(vasovasostomy)* is sometimes successful. New microsurgical techniques have led to annual pregnancy rates for the wives of men undergoing vasovasostomies of about 50 percent, depending on such factors as the doctor's expertise and the time elapsed since the vasectomy.

Female Sterilization

Female sterilization procedures modify the fallopian tubes, which each month normally carry an egg from the ovaries to the uterus. These operations may soon surpass the pill as the first contraceptive choice among women under, as well as over, age 30. The two terms used to describe female sterilization are **tubal ligation** (the cutting or tying of the fallopian tubes) and **tubal occlusion** (the blocking of the tubes). The tubes may be cut or sealed with thread, a clamp, or a clip, or by coagulation (burning) to prevent the passage of eggs from the ovaries (see Figure 10-11). They can also be blocked with bands of silicone.

The procedures used for sterilization are laparotomy, laparoscopy, and colpotomy. **Laparotomy** involves making an abdominal incision about 2 inches long and cutting the tubes. A laparotomy usually requires a hospital stay and up to several weeks of recovery. It leaves a scar and carries the same risks as all major surgical procedures: the side effects of anesthesia, potential infection, and internal scars. In a **minilaparotomy,** an incision about an inch long is made just above the pubic hairline. Most often the tubes are tied and cut. They can also be sealed by electrical coagulation, which causes extensive damage to the tubes; there is also the risk of burns to nearby organs. The operation can be performed by a skilled physician in 10 to 30 minutes, usually under local anesthesia, and the woman can generally go home the same day. The failure (pregnancy) rate is only 1 in 1,000.

Tubal ligation or occlusion can also be performed with the use of **laparoscopy,** commonly called "belly-button" or "band-aid" surgery. This procedure is done on an outpatient basis and takes 15 to 30 minutes. A lighted tube called a laparoscope is inserted through a half-inch incision made right below the navel, giving the doctor a view of the fallopian tubes. Using surgical instruments that may be inserted through the laparoscope or through other tiny incisions, the doctor then cuts or seals the tubes, most commonly by electrical coagulation. The possible complications are similar to those of minilaparotomy, as is the failure rate.

In a **colpotomy,** the fallopian tubes are reached through the vagina and cervix. This procedure leaves no external scar, but is somewhat more hazardous and less effective. A **hysterectomy** (removal of the uterus) is a major surgical procedure that is too dangerous to be used as a method of sterilization, unless there are other medically urgent reasons for removing the uterus.

Methods Based on the Menstrual Cycle (Fertility Awareness Methods)

Awareness of a woman's cyclic fertility can help in both conception and contraception. The different methods of birth control based on a woman's menstrual cycle are sometimes referred to as natural family planning or fertility awareness methods. They include the cervical mucus method, the calendar method, and the basal-body-temperature method (all described below). New fertility monitors that use saliva for testing can improve the accuracy of these methods.

Advantages. Birth control methods based on the menstrual cycle involve no expense, no side effects, and no need for prescriptions or fittings. On the days when the couple can have intercourse, there is nothing to insert, swallow, or check. In addition, abstinence during fertile periods complies with the teachings of the Roman Catholic Church.

Disadvantages. During times of possible fertility (usually eight or nine days a month), couples must abstain from vaginal intercourse—which some may find difficult—or use some form of contraception. Conscientious planning and scheduling are essential. Women with irregular cycles may not be able to rely on the calendar method. Others may find the mucus or temperature methods difficult to use. For all these reasons, this approach to birth control is less reliable than many others. In theory, the overall effectiveness rate for the various fertility awareness methods is 80 percent. In practice, of every 100 women using one of these methods for a year, 24 become pregnant. However, using a combination of the basal-body-temperature method

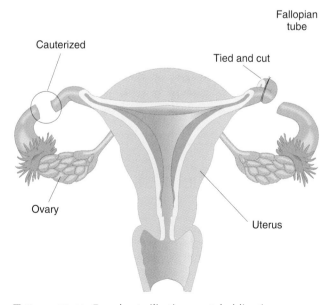

Fallopian tube

Cauterized

Tied and cut

Ovary

Uterus

■ **Figure 10-11** Female sterilization, or tubal ligation.

and the cervical mucus method may be 90 to 95 percent effective in preventing pregnancy (see Figure 10-12).

Cervical Mucus Method

This method, also called the **ovulation method,** is based on the observation of changes in the consistency of the

mucus in the vagina. In the first days after menstruation, the vagina feels dry because of a decline in hormone production, indicating a safe period for unprotected intercourse. Within a few days, estrogen levels rise, and the mucus begins to thin out and becomes less cloudy: The fertile period begins. At peak estrogen levels, the mucus is smooth, stretchable, and slippery (like raw egg white), and very clear. Mucus with these characteristics is usually observed within 24 hours of ovulation and lasts one to two days, signaling maximum fertility. The mucus becomes sticky and cloudy again three days thereafter, and the second safe period begins. Most women using this method have to refrain from unprotected intercourse for about 9 days of each 28-day menstrual cycle.

Calendar Method

This approach, often called the **rhythm method,** involves counting the days after menstruation begins to calculate the estimated day of ovulation. Ideally, a woman first keeps a chart of her monthly cycles for about a year so she knows the average length of her cycle. The first day of menstruation is day one. She counts the number of days until the last day of her cycle, which is the day before menstrual flow begins. To determine the starting point of the period during which she should avoid unprotected intercourse, she subtracts 18 from the number of days in her shortest cycle. For instance, if her shortest cycle was 28 days, day 10 would be her first high-risk day. To calculate when she can again have unprotected intercourse, she subtracts 10 from the number of days in her longest cycle. If her longest cycle is 31 days, she could resume intercourse on day 21. Other forms of sexual activity can continue from day 10 to day 21. This method requires

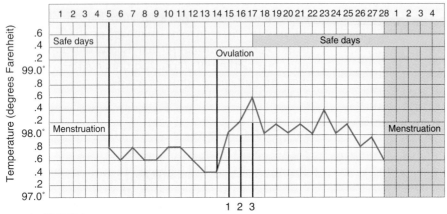

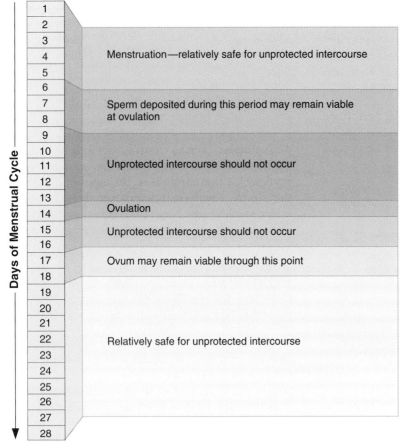

■ Figure 10-12 **Fertility Awareness Methods**
These methods are based on a woman's menstrual cycle and involve charting basal body temperature (top), careful calculation of the menstrual cycle (bottom), or careful observation of cervical mucus. Periods of abstinence are a necessary part of these methods.

careful timing to avoid the possible meeting of a ripe egg and active sperm in the woman's Fallopian tube.

Basal Body Temperature Method

In this method the woman measures her **basal body temperature,** the body temperature upon waking in the morning, using a specially calibrated rectal thermometer, which is more precise than an oral one. She records her temperature on a chart (see Figure 10-12). The basal body temperature remains relatively constant from the beginning of the menstrual cycle to ovulation. After ovulation, however, basal body temperature rises by more than 0.5 degrees F. The woman knows that her safe period has begun when her temperature has been elevated for three consecutive days. After eight to ten months, she should have a sense of her ovulatory pattern, in addition to knowing her daily readings.

 # What Is the "Morning-After" Pill?

In cases where unprotected intercourse has occurred, a condom has broken or slipped off, or another form of contraception has failed, there are **after-intercourse methods** available for preventing implantation of a fertilized egg and possible pregnancy. Emergency contraceptive pills, also known as "morning-after" pills, come in two types. One type consists of higher doses of the hormones estrogen and progestin that are found in ordinary birth control pills. Another type consists of only progestin.

National surveys indicate that a third of women and about half of men aged 18 to 44 are unaware of the availability of emergency contraception.[19] Yet some methods have been used in rape crisis centers for more than 20 years and are available from physicians, family planning clinics, and more than 80 percent of college health centers.

Some oral contraceptives, taken within 72 hours after intercourse, safely prevent pregnancy and bring on menstruation.

Researchers have been assessing various other "morning-after" methods. In one study of almost 2,000 women, the use of only levonorgestrel proved more effective than a combination approach.[20] Low doses of mifepristone (RU-486), also known as the "French abortion pill," given within five days of unprotected intercourse, also are effective for emergency contraception. In an international study of approximately 1,700 women, the women taking mifepristone reported less nausea and vomiting than those taking high doses of birth control pills.[21]

Another option for emergency contraception is the copper IUD, which may be inserted up to seven days following unprotected intercourse and left in place to provide ongoing contraception. Its failure rate is less than 1 percent, which makes the copper IUD the most effective form of emergency contraception, and, if left in place, the most cost effective.

Future Contraceptives

Other countries have taken the lead in developing new contraceptive options. These include:

- Protectaid, a contraceptive sponge that destroys sperm with three spermicides and releases a lubricating gel to decrease irritation and STD risk. It has been available in Canada since 1996.

- Mirena, an intrauterine device that delivers a progestin directly to the uterus to prevent pregnancy and is effective for up to five years. It has been available since 1990 in 14 European and Asian countries.

- Persona, a handheld computer that follows a woman's cycle and signals with a red light the days when a woman is most likely to conceive. Approved by the Roman Catholic Church, it has been available since 1996 in England, Italy, Ireland, Holland, and Germany.

- Lea contraceptive, a reusable silicone rubber device inserted like a diaphragm that allows vaginal fluids to flow out without letting sperm out. It has been available in Canada and Europe since the mid-1990s.[22]

Also on the horizon are a hormone contraceptive patch, a disposable diaphragm, a vaginal contraceptive ring, and monthly injections of low doses of the same hormones as are in the pill.[23] All are designed for exclusively female use. Despite repeated predictions that a male pill is on the horizon, there has not been a significant advance in contraception for men since the condom.

Abortion

Abortion rates vary greatly around the world. The U. S. abortion rate, which declined through most of the 1990s, still remains higher than that of many Western countries, including Canada, Great Britain, the Netherlands, and Sweden. Although there is no one single or simple explanation for this difference, researchers focus on America's high rate of unintended pregnancies. In many nations with fewer unwanted pregnancies and lower abortion rates, contraceptives are generally easier and cheaper to obtain, and early sex education strongly emphasizes their importance.

No woman in any country ever elects to be in a situation where she has to consider abortion. But if faced with an unwanted pregnancy, many women consider **elective abortion** as an option. Every year 3 out of every 100 American women between the ages of 15 and 44 choose to terminate a pregnancy. According to federal data, 43 percent of American women undergo an abortion by age 45.

These women do not fit neatly into any particular category. Most—70 percent—intend to have children, but not at this point in time. Many cannot afford a baby. Some feel unready for the responsibility; others fear that another child would jeopardize the happiness and security of their existing family.

About 55 percent of women who undergo abortion are under age 25; only 22 percent are older than age 30. Unmarried pregnant women are six times more likely to have abortions than married ones; poor women are three times more likely to abort a pregnancy than women in higher economic groups. White women account for 63 percent of abortions, yet statistically, nonwhite women (who make up a smaller proportion of the population) are twice as likely to have an abortion as white women. Catholic women are more likely than Protestant women to have abortions, but women with no religious affiliations have a higher abortion rate than those who belong to a particular religion.

Thinking Through the Options

A woman faced with an unwanted pregnancy—often alone, unwed, and desperate—can find it extremely difficult to decide what to do. The political debate over the right to life almost always is secondary to practical and emotional matters, such as the quality of her relationship to the baby's father, their capacity to provide for the child, the impact on any children she already has, and other important life issues.

Giving up her child for adoption, discussed later in this chapter, is an option for women who do not feel abortion is right for them. Because the number of would-be adoptive parents greatly exceeds the number of available newborns, some women considering adoption may feel pressured by offers of money from couples eager to adopt. Others, particularly minority women, may feel cultural pressures to keep a child—regardless of their age, economic situation, or ability to care for an infant. Advocates of adoption reform are pressing for mandatory counseling for all pregnant women considering adoption (available now in agency-arranged, but not private, adoptions) and for extending the period of time during which a new mother can change her mind about giving her child up for adoption.

In deciding whether or not to have an abortion, women report asking themselves many questions, including the following:

- How do I feel about the man with whom I conceived this baby? Do I love him? Does he love me? Is this man committed to staying with me?
- What sort of relationship, if any, have we had or might we have in the future?
- If I continue the pregnancy and give birth, could I love the baby?
- Who can help me gain perspective on this problem?
- Have I thought about adoption? Do I think I could surrender custody of my baby? Would it make a difference if the adoption process were open and I could know the adoptive parents?
- If I keep my child, can I care for him or her properly? How would the birth of another baby affect my other children?
- Do I have marketable skills, an education, an adequate income? Would I be able to go to school or keep my job if I have a child? Who would help me?
- Would this child be born with serious abnormalities? Would it suffer or thrive?
- How does each option fit with what I believe is morally correct? Could I handle each of the options emotionally?

Answering these questions honestly and objectively may help women as they think through the realities of their situation.

Medical Abortion

A hormonal compound called mifepristone (RU-486), best known as the French abortion pill, can end a pregnancy if taken within nine weeks of a woman's last menstrual period. Mifepristone, which is 96 percent effective in inducing abortion, blocks progesterone, the hormone that prepares the uterine lining for pregnancy. Two days after taking this compound, a woman takes a prostaglandin to increase uterine contractions. The uterine lining is expelled along with the fertilized egg (see Figure 10-13). Women have compared the discomfort of this experience to severe menstrual cramps. Common side effects include excessive bleeding, nausea, fatigue, abdominal pain, and dizziness. About 1 woman in 100 requires a blood transfusion.

Scientists also are testing other chemicals that could induce early abortions. These include methotrexate (a drug in use as a treatment for cancer, rheumatoid arthritis, psoriasis, and ectopic pregnancies) and misoprostol (an ulcer treatment that causes uterine contractions).

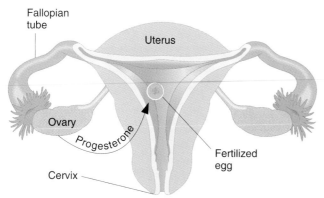

Progesterone, a hormone produced by the ovaries, is necessary for the implantation and development of a fertilized egg.

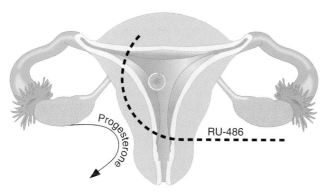

Taken early in pregnancy RU-486 blocks the action of progesterone and makes the body react as if it isn't pregnant.

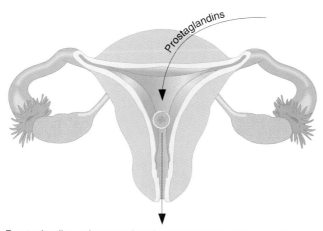

Prostaglandins, taken two days later, cause the uterus to contract and the cervix to soften and dilate. As a result, the fertilized egg is expelled in 97% of the cases.

■ **Figure 10-13** How RU-486, known as the abortion pill, works.

Reported side effects of these agents include mild diarrhea, nausea, vomiting, and severe cramping.

Although thoroughly condemned by right-to-life advocates, abortion medications may in time lower the public profile of pregnancy termination. They are not painless, cheap, or equally available to all, but they do offer women a chance to carry through on their personal choice in greater privacy and safety. This does not mean the decision to end a pregnancy is any easier.[24]

Other Abortion Methods

More than half of all abortions (54 percent) are performed within the first 8 weeks of pregnancy. Only about 1 percent of abortions occur after 20 weeks. Medically, first-trimester abortion is less risky than childbirth. However, the likelihood of complications increases when abortions are performed in the second trimester (that is, the second three-month period) of pregnancy.

Suction curettage, usually done from 7 to 13 weeks after the last menstrual period, involves the gradual dilation (opening) of the cervix, often by inserting into the cervix one or more sticks of *laminaria* (a sterilized seaweed that absorbs moisture and expands, thus gradually stretching the cervix). Some women feel pressure or cramping with the laminaria in place. Occasionally, the laminaria itself starts to bring on a miscarriage.

At the time of abortion, the laminaria is removed, and dilators are used to enlarge the cervical opening further, if needed. The physician inserts a suction tip into the cervix, and the uterine contents are drawn out via a vacuum system (see Figure 10-14). A curette (a spoon-shaped surgical instrument used for scraping) is used to check for complete removal of the contents of the uterus. With suction curettage, the risks of complication

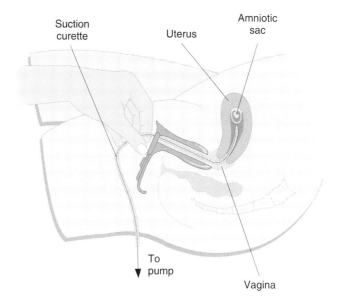

■ Figure 10-14 **Suction Curettage**
The contents of the uterus are extracted through the cervix with a vacuum apparatus.

are low. Major complications, such as perforation of the uterus, occur in fewer than 1 in 100 cases. About 90 percent of the abortions performed in this country are done by this technique.

For early-second-trimester abortions, physicians generally use a technique called **dilation and evacuation (D and E)**, in which they open the cervix and use medical instruments to remove the fetus from the uterus. D and E procedures are performed under local or general anesthesia.

To induce abortion from week 16 to week 20, prostaglandins (natural substances found in most body tissues) are administered as vaginal suppositories or injected into the amniotic sac by inserting a needle through the abdominal wall. They induce uterine contractions, and the fetus and placenta are expelled within 24 hours. Other methods for second-trimester abortions include injecting saline or urea solutions into the amniotic sac; they terminate the pregnancy by fetus-triggering contractions that expel the fetus and placenta. Sometimes vaginal suppositories or drugs that help the uterus contract are used. Complications from abortion techniques that induce labor include nausea, vomiting, diarrhea, tearing of the cervix, excessive bleeding, and possible shock and death.

Hysterotomy involves surgically opening the uterus and removing the fetus. It is generally done from week 16 to week 24 of the pregnancy, primarily in emergency situations when the woman's life is in danger, or when other methods of abortion are considered too risky. However, late pregnancy abortions increase the risk of spontaneous abortion or premature labor in subsequent pregnancies and should be avoided if possible.

Psychological Responses After Abortion

Many assume that abortion must be psychologically devastating, that women who abort a fetus sooner or later develop what some have termed "post-abortion trauma syndrome." In her studies at the University of Chicago, psychiatrist Nada Stotland found that there is no such thing. The primary emotion of women who have just had an abortion, she discovered, is relief. Although many women also express feelings of sadness or guilt, their anxiety levels eventually drop until they are lower than they were immediately before the abortion. Even highly religious women are not at greater risk of long-term psychological distress.[25]

Nonetheless, although psychologists consider the mental health risks "minimal" compared to those of bearing an unwanted child, this does not mean women who have abortions never have regrets. As Stotland notes, women have many feelings before, during, and after abortions. But a feeling—even one as painful as loss, sadness, or guilt—is not a syndrome, and a woman's responses to abortion often change with passing days, weeks, months, or years. Anniversaries—of conception, of the date a woman found out she was pregnant, of the abortion, of the delivery date—can trigger memories and a sense of loss, but most women deal with these and move on with their lives.

The best predictor of psychological well-being after abortion is a woman's emotional well-being prior to pregnancy. At highest risk are women who have had a psychiatric illness, such as an anxiety disorder or clinical depression, prior to an abortion, and those whose abortions occurred among complicated circumstances (such as a rape, or coercion by parents or a partner). The vast majority of women manage to put the abortion into perspective as one of many life events.

The Politics of Abortion

Abortion is one of the most controversial political, religious, and ethical issues of our time. The issues of when life begins, a woman's right to choose, and an unborn child's right to survival are among the most divisive Americans have ever faced. Abortions were legal in the United States until the 1860s. For decades after that, women who decided to terminate unwanted pregnancies did so by attempting to abort themselves or by obtaining illegal abortions—often performed by untrained individuals using unsanitary and unsafe procedures. In the late 1960s, some states began to change their laws to make abortions legal. In 1973, the U.S. Supreme Court, following a 1970 ruling on the case of *Roe v. Wade* by the New York Supreme Court, said that

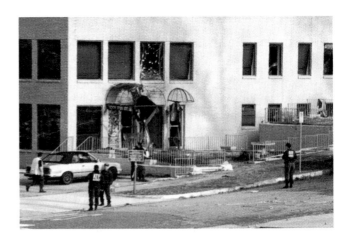

Opposition to legal abortions has often become violent. A security guard was killed and a nurse severely injured when a Birmingham, Alabama, abortion clinic was bombed several years ago.

an abortion in the first trimester of pregnancy was a decision between a woman and her physician and was protected by privacy laws. The Court further ruled that abortion during the second trimester could be performed on the basis of health risks and that abortion during the final trimester could be performed only for the sake of the mother's health.

Since then, several laws have restricted the availability of legal abortions for low-income women. In 1989, the U.S. Supreme Court narrowed the interpretation of *Roe v. Wade* by upholding a law that sharply restricted publicly funded abortions and required doctors to test if a fetus could survive if they suspected a woman was more than 20 weeks pregnant. In 1992, in *Planned Parenthood v. Casey*, the Court upheld the right to legalized abortion but gave states the right to restrict abortion as long as they did not place an "undue burden" on a woman. This has limited the availability of abortion to young, rural, or low-income women.

The Abortion Horizon

The debate over abortion continues to stir passionate emotion, with pro-life supporters arguing that life begins at conception and that abortion is therefore immoral, and pro-choice advocates countering that an individual woman should have the right to make decisions about her body and health. The controversy over abortion has at times become violent: Physicians who performed abortions have been shot and killed; abortion clinics have been bombed, wounding and killing patients and staff members.

The number of abortions performed in the United States declined in the 1990s, and the death rate from abortions has plummeted. More than half of all abortions (54 percent) are performed within the first 8 weeks of pregnancy. Only about 1 percent of abortions occur after 20 weeks, but Congress considered a ban on late abortions—or, as some labeled them, "partial birth abortions." In this procedure, the woman is sedated and her cervix dilated; the fetus is removed from her vagina. It is most often performed in cases when the fetus has life-threatening defects or if carrying the baby to term would seriously endanger the health of the mother.

Since *Roe v. Wade,* technology has had a major impact on abortion procedures as well as politics. Because of home pregnancy tests, women can detect pregnancy sooner. A new surgical procedure, called early manual vacuum aspiration, enables women to have an abortion as early as eight days after conception. And the new medicines including mifepristone (RU-486), available for abortion, also offer new options for early termination of a pregnancy. In nations where RU-486 has been available, 60 percent of the women who choose abortion choose the pill, which must be used in the first seven weeks of pregnancy.

Although the majority of Americans continue to support abortion, many feel that it should be more restricted and difficult to obtain. While 61 percent of Americans say abortion should be permitted during the first three months of pregnancy, only 15 percent support second-trimester abortions and 7 percent feel that abortions in the last trimester should be legal.

A Cross-Cultural Perspective

Throughout the world an estimated 10 to 20 million illegal abortions are performed each year. About 1 in 100 women dies as a result. Women who survive illegal abortions may suffer chronic health problems related to the lack of adequate medical care.

In other countries, abortion laws vary greatly. In Eastern Europe, where abortions were once legal and common, the collapse of communism has led to new restrictions on abortion. By contrast, Spain's supreme court has relaxed legal restrictions on abortions performed on social grounds. In Pakistan, new, more liberal rules on abortion state that abortion is no longer a crime if carried out to provide "necessary treatment." In Latin America, where anti-abortion laws are very strict, Cuba is the only country in which abortion on request is legal in early pregnancy. In other nations of Central and South America, women obtaining abortions and those performing them face criminal penalties, including imprisonment.

Childfree by Choice

In Europe, fertility rates in many nations are at an all-time low. In the United States, one in five women in the post-war baby boom generation has not given birth—many because of a decision not to. More women and men are deliberately choosing to remain "childfree."

According to the limited data available, single childfree women tend to be better educated, more cosmopolitan, less religious, and more professional than those in the general population. In general, childfree women are high achievers, often in demanding careers, who describe their work as exciting and satisfying. Childless couples are predominantly urban, well-educated, and upper middle class, with egalitarian and long-running marriages.

Their reasons for not having children are diverse: a desire to maintain their freedom, more time with their partners, career ambitions, genuine concern about overpopulation and the fate of the earth. Some women cite the hostile work environment for mothers and the inadequacy of day care. Others say they're disillusioned with the have-it-all hopes of baby boomers and believe in a have-most-of-it philosophy.

Some observers theorize that childfree women will regret their choice after it's too late to do anything about it. However, this doesn't seem to be the case. In a study of 90 childless women over age 60, a Philadelphia anthropologist found that, while the women who believed that a female's primary duty is to have children did express some regret, most women had come up with satisfying alternative ways of living. In another study of nearly 700 Canadian women and men over age 55, those who chose childlessness were just as happy as parents who had good relationships with their children—and happier than parents who described their relationships with their children as distant.[26] "Not everybody needs children to have a full life," says Leslie Lafayette, who founded the ChildFree Network (CFN) to create a sense of belonging among people without children.[27]

Pregnancy

After an upswing in the 1980s, the U. S. birth rate declined through most of the 1990s. The average age of mothers has risen, but about 70 percent of babies are still born to women in their twenties. Mothers are now averaging slightly fewer than two children each. Not every married couple is opting for parenthood.

Of course, you don't have to be part of a couple to want or to conceive a child. The number of never-married college-educated and career women who are becoming single parents has risen dramatically. They want children—with or without an ongoing relationship with a man—and may feel that, because of their age, they can't delay getting pregnant any longer.

Preconception Care: A Preventive Approach

The time *before* a child is conceived can be crucial in assuring that an infant is born healthy, full-size, and full-term. Women who smoke, drink alcohol, take drugs, eat poorly, are too thin or too heavy, suffer from unrecognized infections or illnesses, or are exposed to toxins at work or home may start pregnancy with one or more strikes against them and their unborn babies. The best chance for lowering the infant mortality rate and preventing birth defects is before pregnancy. **Preconception care**—the enhancement of a woman's health and well-being prior to con-

ception in order to ensure a healthy pregnancy and baby—includes risk assessment (including evaluation of medical, genetic, and lifestyle risks), health promotion (such as teaching good nutrition guidelines), and interventions to reduce risk (such as treatment of infections and other diseases or assistance in quitting smoking or drug use.

To determine whether you might benefit from preconception counseling, ask yourself the following questions:

- Do you have a major medical problem, such as diabetes, asthma, anemia, or high blood pressure?
- Do you know of any family members who have had a child with a birth defect or mental retardation?
- Have you had a child with a birth defect or mental retardation?
- Are you concerned about inherited diseases, such as Tay-Sachs disease, sickle-cell anemia, hemophilia, or thalassemia?
- Are you 35 years of age or older?
- Do you smoke, drink alcohol, or take illegal drugs?
- Do you take prescription or over-the-counter medications regularly?
- Do you use birth control pills?
- Do you have a cat?
- Are you a strict vegetarian?
- Are you dieting or fasting for any reason?
- Do you run long distances or exercise strenuously?
- Do you work with chemicals, toxic substances, radiation, or anesthesia?
- Do you suspect that you or your partner may have a sexually transmitted disease?
- Have you had German measles (rubella) or a German measles vaccination?
- Have you ever had a miscarriage, ectopic pregnancy, stillbirth, or complicated pregnancy?
- Have you recently traveled outside the United States?

If your answer to any of these questions is yes, you definitely should seek counseling from an obstetrician, nurse-midwife, or family practitioner three to six months before you hope to conceive a child.

How a Woman's Body Changes During Pregnancy

The 40 weeks of pregnancy transform a woman's body. At the beginning of pregnancy, the woman's uterus becomes slightly larger, and the cervix, softer and bluish due to increased blood flow. Progesterone and estrogen trigger changes in the milk glands and ducts in the breasts, which increase in size and feel somewhat tender. The pressure of the growing uterus against the bladder causes a more frequent need to urinate. As the pregnancy progresses, the woman's skin stretches as her body shape changes, her center of gravity changes as her abdomen protrudes, and her internal organs shift as the baby grows (see Figure 10-15). Pregnancy is typically divided into three-month periods called trimesters.

How a Baby Grows

Silently and invisibly, over a nine-month period, a fertilized egg develops into a human being. When the zygote reaches the uterus, it's still smaller than the head of a pin. Once nestled into the spongy uterine lining, it becomes an **embryo.** The embryo takes on an elongated shape, rounded at one end. A sac called the **amnion** envelopes it (see photo, p. 316). As water and other small molecules cross the amniotic membrane, the embryo floats freely in the absorbed fluid, cushioned from shocks and bumps. At nine weeks the embryo is called a **fetus.**

A special organ, the **placenta,** forms. Attached to the embryo by the umbilical cord, it supplies the growing baby with fluid and nutrients from the maternal bloodstream and carries waste back to the mother's body for disposal (see Figure 10-16).

Emotional Aspects of Pregnancy

Almost all prospective parents worry about their ability to care for a helpless newborn. By talking openly about their feelings and fears, however, they can strengthen the bonds between them, so that they can work together as parents as well as partners. Psychological problems, such as depression, can occur during pregnancy. The availability of social support and other resources for coping with stress can make a great difference in the potential impact of emotional difficulties.[28]

The physiological changes of pregnancy can affect a woman's mood. In early pregnancy, she may feel weepy, irritable, or emotional. As the pregnancy continues, she may become calmer and more energetic. Men, too, feel a range of intense emotions about the prospect of having a child: pride, anxiety, hope, fears for their unseen child and for the woman they love. Although many men want to be as supportive as possible, they may think that they have to be strong and calm—and may therefore pull away from their wives. The more involved fathers become in preparing for birth, the closer they feel to their partners and babies afterward.

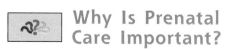

Why Is Prenatal Care Important?

A pregnant woman has to take good care of herself to provide good care for her unborn child. This means regular medical and dental checkups. A woman should have her first prenatal visit as soon as she discovers that she's pregnant. A study group of the American College of Obstetricians and Gynecologists (ACOG) has recommended seven or eight prenatal visits for women with low-risk pregnancies; women at higher risk require more frequent checkups. Many teenage and unmarried pregnant women don't get adequate prenatal care, and some don't see a health-care professional until late in their pregnancy, because they can't afford or don't have access to medical services.

Age

The risk of a poor pregnancy outcome increases with age. Women 30 or older face a 40 percent greater risk of late fetal death, compared with women ages 20 to 24. Women over 35 also face an increased risk of very low birth weight, preterm delivery, and small-for-gestational-age (SGA) infants. Preconception and prenatal care, including good nutrition and careful monitoring, increase the chances of a healthy baby for older mothers.

Nutrition

A well-balanced diet throughout pregnancy is critical for a mother and her fetus both before and at birth. If a woman—regardless of her prepregnancy weight—gains too little weight, the risk to the growing fetus is high.[29] ACOG recommends a weight gain of 22 to 27 pounds during pregnancy. The National Academy of Sciences' Food and Nutrition Board advises a maximum weight gain of 35 pounds, based on findings that weight gain aids fetal growth and lowers the risk of infant mortality and mental retardation.

No vitamin supplement can replace a well-balanced diet, but a multivitamin can help reduce or avoid deficiencies. According to the CDC, women who take a simple daily multivitamin containing a B vitamin called folate (or folic acid) before conception can cut in half the risk that their children will suffer neural tube defects, which stem from faulty development of the spinal column. These conditions include spina bifida, a defect in which the bones of the spine, the vertebrae, are incompletely formed.

Activity and Rest

Almost all pregnant women can benefit from exercise throughout pregnancy—as long as they don't push too

■ Figure 10-15
Physiological Changes of Pregnancy

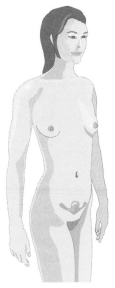

Before conception

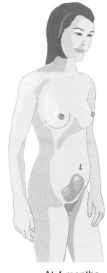

At 4 months

First Trimester

Increased urination because of hormonal changes and the pressure of the enlarging uterus on the bladder.

Enlarged breasts as milk glands develop.

Darkening of the nipples and the area around them.

Nausea or vomiting, particularly in the morning.

Fatigue.

Increased vaginal secretions.

Pinching of the sciatic nerve, which runs from the buttocks down through the back of the legs, as the pelvic bones widen and begin to separate.

Irregular bowel movements.

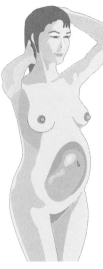

At 7 months

Second Trimester

Thickening of the waist as the uterus grows.

Weight gain.

Increase in total blood volume.

Slight increase in size and change in position of the heart.

Darkening of the pigment around the nipple and from the navel to the pubic region.

Darkening of the face.

Increased salivation and perspiration.

Secretion of colostrum from the breasts.

Indigestion, constipation, and hemorrhoids.

Varicose veins.

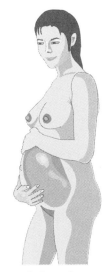

At 9 months

Third Trimester

Increased urination because of pressure from the uterus.

Tightening of the uterine muscles (called Braxton-Hicks contractions).

Shortness of breath because of increased pressure by the uterus on the lungs and diaphragm.

Heartburn and indigestion.

Trouble sleeping because of the baby's movements or the need to urinate.

Descending ("dropping") of the baby's head into the pelvis about two to four weeks before birth.

Navel pushed out.

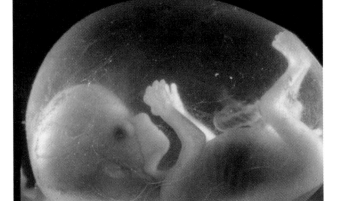

The amnion, or amniotic sac, surrounds and cushions the fetus.

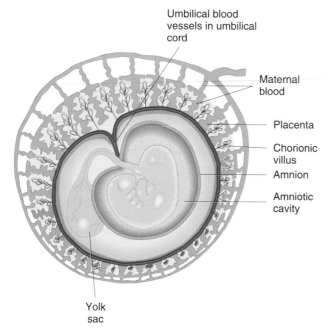

Umbilical blood
vessels in umbilical
cord

Maternal
blood

Placenta

Chorionic
villus

Amnion

Amniotic
cavity

Yolk
sac

■ Figure 10-16 **The Placenta**
The placenta supplies the growing embryo with fluid and
nutrients from the maternal bloodstream and carries waste
back for disposal.

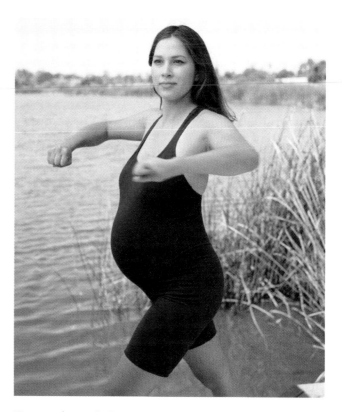

How much exercise? Most pregnant women benefit from regular, moderate exercise. For women who were very active before their pregnancies, a higher level of activity is probably fine.

hard or too far. Regular exercise (three times a week) is better, safer, and more effective than occasional workouts. While women who were athletic prior to pregnancy generally can continue their physical activity, they should be aware of warning signs that could indicate a potential problem, such as faintness, dizziness, pain, or vaginal bleeding. Recent research has found that regular, sustained exercise during pregnancy did not affect infants' physical growth or mental development at age 1.[30]

Rest is as important as exercise; the pregnant woman who's not used to taking naps may have to make time in her schedule for rest periods. If insomnia or the frequent need to urinate during the night becomes a problem, she may have to rely on catnaps during the day. She should *not* take sleeping pills.

Substance Use

Smoking endangers two lives: the mother's and the fetus's. The sooner a mother-to-be stops smoking, the better the chances that the fetus will develop normally. Smoking increases the risk of miscarriage, stillbirth, low birth weight, heart defects, and premature birth, and also impairs growth.[31] The fetus's oxygen supply is impaired by the increased levels of carbon monoxide in the smoking mother's bloodstream. Passive smoking (inhaling other people's smoke) can be hazardous for the mother and fetus as well. (See Chapter 17.) Mothers who quit smoking in the first trimester have

fewer preterm deliveries and low-birth-weight infants than those who continue smoking.

Approximately 16 percent of pregnant women report drinking in the previous month.[32] According to the CDC, more than 8,000 alcohol-damaged babies are born every year. One out of every 750 newborns has a cluster of physical and mental defects called **fetal alcohol syndrome (FAS)**: low birth weight, smaller-than-normal head circumference, smaller and shorter size, irritability as newborns, and permanent mental impairment as a result of their mothers' alcohol consumption. The milder forms of these problems, particularly impaired intellectual ability and school performance, are called fetal alcohol effects (FAE). (See Chapter 16.)

The risk of fetal alcohol syndrome is greatest if a mother drinks 3 ounces or more of pure alcohol (the equivalent of six or seven cocktails) a day. However, moderate drinking—one or two cocktails daily—may also have an effect. Even one drink a day has been associated with birth defects; binge drinking (five or more drinks on one occasion) is most toxic. The National Institute on Alcohol Abuse and Alcoholism and the Surgeon General advise pregnant women—and those trying to become pregnant—to abstain from drinking alcohol.

Moderate to heavy caffeine users are at greater risk of miscarriage than women who use little or no caffeine. Even more than one cup of coffee a day is linked with low birth weight. The FDA's advice is for pregnant women to "avoid caffeine containing products or use them sparingly."

At least one out of every ten newborns is exposed to illegal drugs before birth. The consequences of drug use during pregnancy include severe damage to the child's brain and nervous system and birth defects. Marijuana smokers have smaller, sicker babies and a higher risk of stillbirths, according to some research. Drug use also may lead to "neurochemical" birth defects by disrupting normal development of the brain. Cocaine use increases the risk of premature birth, stillbirths, and malformations.

Environmental Risks

According to a study of over 23,000 pregnant women, exposure to heat from a hot tub, sauna, or fever during the first trimester of pregnancy increases the risk of neural tube defects. Hot tubs presented the greatest single danger, while exposure to heat from multiple sources led to even greater risk. Electric blankets were not associated with increased risk.

High levels of radiation of the type used for cancer therapy have been associated with birth defects. Diagnostic X rays should be avoided during pregnancy if possible, but they're not a significant threat, particularly after the first trimester. At least in theory, the rapidly developing fetus is especially vulnerable to pollutants, toxic wastes, heavy metals, pesticides, gases, and other hazardous compounds in the environment.

Prenatal Testing

All parents worry that their unborn baby might not be normal and healthy. Sophisticated new tests can answer some, but not all, of their questions and can identify more than 250 diseases and defects. Prenatal tests are being performed earlier and with less risk to a fetus than ever before. The most common prenatal tests include the following:

- *Ultrasonography* uses high-frequency sound waves to produce an image of the fetus on a video screen and as a photographic picture. Ultrasound can check fetal age and spot certain birth defects.

- *Alpha-fetoprotein (AFP) screening,* performed from the 13th to 20th week of pregnancy, measures a substance produced by the baby's kidneys in the mother's blood. Levels that are too high could indicate a neural tube defect; levels that are too low may signal Down syndrome.

Strategies *for* Prevention

A Mother-to-Be's Guide to a Healthy Pregnancy

✓ ACOG recommends consuming about 300 more calories a day than before pregnancy and concentrating on eating the right foods, not on watching your weight. Never diet during pregnancy. Don't restrict salt intake either, unless specifically directed to by your doctor.

✓ Drink six to eight glasses of liquids each day, including water, fruit and vegetable juices, and milk.

✓ Don't exercise strenuously for more than 15 minutes, ACOG advises. Avoid vigorous exercise in hot, humid weather. Never let your body temperature rise above 100°F or your heart rate climb above 140 beats per minute.

✓ Stretch and flex carefully because the joints and connective tissue soften and loosen during pregnancy. After the fourth month of pregnancy, don't do any exercises while lying on your back, as this could impair blood flow to the placenta.

✓ Walk, swim, and jog in moderation; play tennis only if you played before pregnancy. Ski only if you're experienced, and stick to low altitudes and safe slopes. Do not water-ski, surf, or ride a horse.

- *Amniocentesis,* performed from the 14th to 16th week of pregnancy, consists of removing a small amount of the amniotic fluid surrounding the fetus. This fluid contains cells shed by the fetus, which can be grown in tissue culture and then checked for any chromosomal or genetic defects (see Figure 10-17).

- *Chorionic villi sampling (CVS),* performed from the eighth to tenth week of pregnancy, involves suctioning a small sample of the chorionic villi, the tissue surrounding the fetus, for laboratory analysis (see Figure 10-17). Results are generally available within a week.[33]

There are no known risks for ultrasonography and AFP screening. For both amniocentesis and CVS, there is about a 1 percent risk of miscarriage. Some testing centers have reported a higher incidence of both limb defects and miscarriage following CVS than others using this technique. Before choosing a facility for testing, pregnant women should inquire about that facility's experience and complication rate. Prenatal tests are usually recommended only if the mother is over age 35, has had a child with a genetic disorder, or is a known carrier of a detectable genetic disorder.

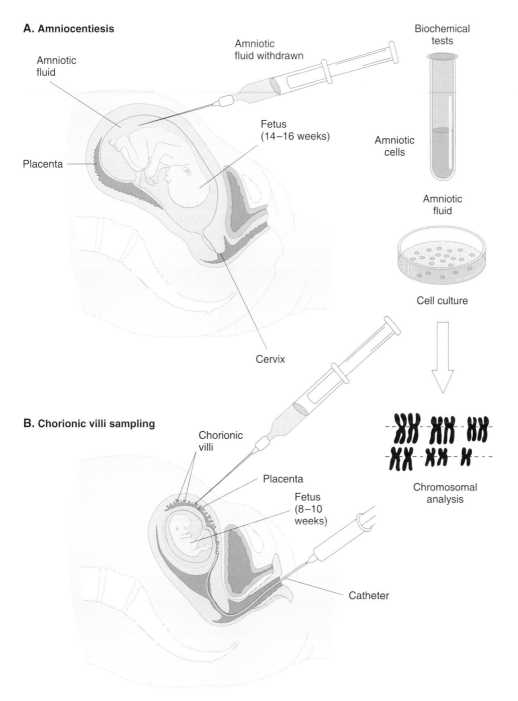

A. Amniocentiesis

Amniotic fluid

Amniotic fluid withdrawn

Amniotic fluid

Fetus (14–16 weeks)

Placenta

Cervix

B. Chorionic villi sampling

Chorionic villi

Placenta

Fetus (8–10 weeks)

Catheter

Biochemical tests

Amniotic cells

Amniotic fluid

Cell culture

Chromosomal analysis

■ **Figure 10-17 Prenatal Testing**
(A) In amniocentesis, a sample of the amniotic fluid is withdrawn; fetal cells found in that fluid can then be grown in tissue culture and checked for chromosomal defects.
(B) In chorionic villi sampling (CVS), a tissue sample of the villi is removed from the uterus and analyzed for chromosomal defects.

Ectopic Pregnancy

Any woman who is of childbearing age, has had intercourse, and feels abdominal pain with no reasonable cause may have an **ectopic pregnancy.** In this type of pregnancy, the fertilized egg remains in the fallopian tube instead of traveling to the uterus. Ectopic, or tubal, pregnancies have increased dramatically in recent years, now accounting for 2 percent of all reported pregnancies. STDs, particularly chlamydia infections (discussed in Chapter 12), have become a major cause of ectopic pregnancy. Other risk factors include previous pelvic surgery, particularly involving the fallopian tubes; pelvic inflammatory disease; infertility; and use of an IUD.

In an ectopic pregnancy, a misplaced egg develops normally, producing the usual signs of pregnancy, until the cramped amniotic sac bursts, damaging the fallopian tube. The woman will bleed internally and feel lower abdominal pains; or she may feel an aching in her shoulders, as the blood flows upward toward the diaphragm. If the bleeding is substantial, the woman can go into shock, with low blood pressure and a high pulse rate. Symptoms are hot and cold flashes, nausea, dizziness, fainting, pelvic pain, and irregular bleeding.

Treatment for the damaged fallopian tube is usually removal, but microsurgery can often repair the damage.

Complications of Pregnancy

In about 10 to 15 percent of all pregnancies, there is increased risk of some problem, such as a baby's failure to grow normally. **Perinatology,** or maternal-fetal medicine, focuses on the special needs of high-risk mothers and their unborn babies. Perinatal centers, with state-of-the-art equipment and 24-hour staffs of specialists in this field, have been set up around the country. Several of the most frequent potential complications of pregnancy are discussed below.

About 50 percent of the women who have had an ectopic pregnancy conceive again; 10 percent have another ectopic pregnancy. Ectopic pregnancies can lead to permanent infertility.

Miscarriage

About 10 to 20 percent of pregnancies end in **miscarriage,** or spontaneous abortion, before the 20th week of gestation. Major genetic disorders may be responsible for 33 to 50 percent of pregnancy losses. About 0.5 to 1 percent of women suffer three or more miscarriages, possibly because of genetic, anatomic, hormonal, infectious, or autoimmune factors.[34] An estimated 70 to 90 percent of women who miscarry eventually become pregnant again.

Physicians typically recommend bed rest if a woman begins bleeding or cramping early in pregnancy. In some cases, the cramping stops, and the pregnancy continues normally. In others, the bleeding becomes intense, the cervix widens, and the embryo is expelled. If the miscarriage is complete, the bleeding stops and the uterus returns to its normal state and shape. If it is incomplete, a physician has to remove any bits of tissue remaining in the uterus by performing a D and C.

Few medical events are more emotionally devastating than a pregnancy loss. Women often feel the loss in an extremely intense, almost physical way. Many who miscarry had not reached the point in pregnancy where the fetus seems separate from them. Typically, women feel both vulnerable and responsible, as if they did something to cause the loss or should have, could have, done something to prevent it. They try to identify what they did wrong: exercising or not exercising, working or not working; eating too much or not enough. Some women interpret a loss as a punishment for past sins, imagined or real. Such self-inflicted guilt, allowed to fester, can lead to major depression.

Infections

The infectious disease most clearly linked to birth defects is **rubella** (German measles). All women should be vaccinated against this disease at least three months prior to conception, to protect themselves and any children they may bear. (See Chapter 12 for more on immunization.) The most common prenatal infection today is *cytomegalovirus.* This infection produces mild flulike symptoms in adults but can cause brain damage, retardation, liver disease, cerebral palsy, hearing problems, and other malformations in unborn babies.

STDs, such as syphilis, gonorrhea, and genital herpes, can be particularly dangerous during pregnancy if not recognized and treated. If a woman has a herpes outbreak around the date her baby is due, her physician will deliver the baby by caesarean section to prevent infecting the baby. HIV infection endangers both a pregnant woman and her unborn baby, and all pregnant women and new mothers should be aware of the HIV epidemic, the risks to them and their babies, and the availability of anonymous testing.

Premature Labor

Approximately 10 percent of all babies are born too soon (before the 37th week of pregnancy). According to researchers, prematurity is the main underlying cause of stillbirth and infant deaths within the first few weeks after birth.[35] Bed rest, close monitoring, and, if necessary, medications for at-risk women can buy more time in the womb for their babies. But women must recognize the warning signs of **premature labor**—dull, low backache; a feeling of tightness or pressure on the lower abdomen; and intestinal cramps, sometimes with diarrhea—early enough. Low-birthweight premature babies face the highest risks, but comprehensive, enriched programs can reduce developmental and health problems.

Pregnancy and Age

Teen pregnancy and birth rates dropped throughout the 1990s.[36] Every year approximately 1 million American girls become pregnant. Most have not been using contraceptives consistently or correctly. Of those who carry to term, 90 percent keep their babies.[37]

Most teen pregnancies (85 to 95 percent, compared with 55 percent for older women) are unplanned. And a sexually active teenager is actually less likely to get pregnant today than in the 1950s (when teen pregnancy rates reached an all-time high). Largely because of increased use of contraceptives, the odds of a sexually active girl getting pregnant have fallen to one in five, down from the one-in-four odds faced by teens in the 1970s. Yet the pregnancy rate among American teenagers remains two to eight times higher than rates in other Western countries such as The Netherlands, Great Britain, and Scandinavia.

In the past, most teenage mothers married the fathers of their unborn children. Today most do not. Many teenage girls who become pregnant have partners who are aged 20 or older. However, according to a government analysis, the role of older men may have been overestimated. Many of the teen mothers involved with men over age 20 are themselves aged 18 or 19. Nearly one-quarter of minors who have had a child with an older partner are married at the time of the infant's birth; only 21 percent of births to unmarried teens are fathered by substantially older men.[38]

Why do so many teens in the United States become pregnant? When surveyed, girls themselves cite various reasons, including lack of attention and love from their parents and lack of access to contraceptives. Many, as one girl poignantly put it, "are looking for someone to love them back."

New Research

As teen births have begun to decline, the number of women deciding to have children later in life has increased. One of every five women in the United States now has her first baby after age 35; first births among women older than 40 have increased 50 percent in the last 15 years.

There are greater risks to the fetus when mothers are older than 35, primarily an increase in fetal birth defects due to chromosomal abnormalities, such as Down syndrome. At age 30, the estimated risk is 2.6 per thousand; the incidence rises to 5.6 per thousand at age 35; 15.8 at age 40; and 53.7 at age 45. However, pregnancy itself for healthy women over age 35 is safe. As discussed later in this chapter, assisted reproductive technologies have enabled women in their forties, fifties, and even sixties to have successful pregnancies.

Childbirth

A generation ago, delivering a baby was something a doctor did in a hospital. Today parents can choose from an almost bewildering array of birthing options. The first decision parents-to-be face is choosing a birth attendant, who can be a physician or a nurse-midwife. Certified nurse-midwives in the United States deliver more than 90,000 babies a year, mostly in hospitals and birth centers. Their approach is based on the belief that the typical pregnant woman can deliver her baby naturally without technological intervention. Lay midwives have a similar orientation but less formal training; only a handful of states permit lay midwives to deliver babies.

When interviewing physicians or midwives, look for the following:

- Experience in handling various complications.
- Extensive prenatal care.
- A commitment to be at the mother's side for the entire labor in order to spot complications quickly and provide assistance.
- A compatible philosophy toward childbirth and medical interventions.

Where to Have Your Baby

A hospital with trained specialists and a nursery for newborns is recommended for high-risk women. However, if their pregnancies are normal and uncomplicated, mothers-to-be have alternatives almost unheard of a generation ago. A woman at low risk for complications may consider having her baby in an independent birth center, which offers a homelike setting. If a couple chooses to have their baby in a hospital, they may do so in a birthing room decorated to look like a comfortable bedroom. In many facilities, specially shaped birthing chairs are available, so a woman can stay in an upright position to push her baby into the world.

Only about 1 percent of American babies are born at home. ACOG opposes home births because of potential hazards to mother and child. But the safety of a home birth can be maximized if the pregnant woman has been carefully screened and a skilled doctor or nurse-midwife is attending.

Preparing for Childbirth

The most widespread method of childbirth preparation is **psychoprophylaxis,** or the **Lamaze method.** Fernand Lamaze, a French doctor, instructed women to respond to labor contractions with prelearned, controlled breathing techniques. As the intensity of each contraction increases, the laboring woman concentrates on increasing her breathing rate in a prescribed way. Her partner coaches her during each contraction and helps her cope with discomfort.

Women who have had childbirth preparation training tend to have fewer complications and require fewer medications. However, painkillers or anesthesia are always an option if labor is longer or more painful than expected. The lower body can be numbed with an **epidural block,** which involves injecting an anesthetic into the membrane around the spinal cord, or a **spinal block,** in which the injection goes directly into the spinal canal. General anesthesia is usually used only for emergency caesarean births.

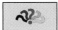 ## What Is Childbirth Like?

There are three stages of **labor.** The first starts with *effacement* (thinning) and *dilation* (opening up) of the cervix. Effacement is measured in percentages, and dilation in centimeters (cm) or finger-widths. Around this time, the amniotic sac of fluids usually breaks, a sign that the woman should call her doctor or midwife.

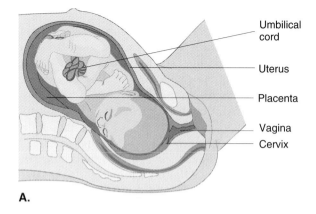

Umbilical cord

Uterus

Placenta

Vagina

Cervix

A.

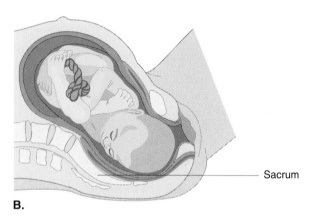

Sacrum

B.

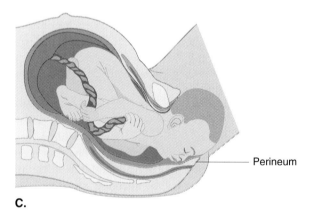

Perineum

C.

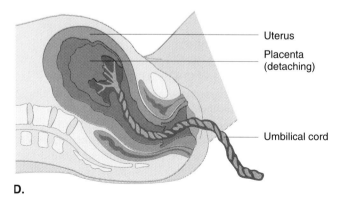

Uterus

Placenta (detaching)

Umbilical cord

D.

■ **Figure 10-18 Birth**

(A) The cervix is partially dilated, and the baby's head has entered the birth canal. (B) The cervix is nearly completely dilated. The baby's head rotates so that it can move through the birth canal. (C) The baby's head extends as it reaches the vaginal opening, and the head and the rest of the body pass through the birth canal. (D) After the baby is born, the placenta detaches from the uterus and is expelled from the woman's body.

The first contractions of the early, or *latent*, phase of labor are usually not uncomfortable; they last 15 to 30 seconds, occur every 15 to 30 minutes, and gradually increase in intensity and frequency. The most difficult contractions come after the cervix is dilated to about 8 cm, as the woman feels greater pressure from the fetus. The first stage ends when the cervix is completely dilated to a diameter of 10 cm (or five finger-widths) and the baby is ready to come down the birth canal (see Figure 10-18). For women having their first baby, this first stage of labor averages 12 to 13 hours. Women having another child often experience shorter first-stage labor.

When the cervix is completely dilated, the second stage of labor occurs, during which the baby moves into the vagina, or birth canal, and out of the mother's body. As this stage begins, women who have gone through childbirth preparation training often feel a sense of relief from the acute pain of the transition phase and at the prospect of giving birth.

This second stage can take up to an hour or more. Strong contractions may last 60 to 90 seconds and occur every two to three minutes. As the baby's head descends, the mother feels an urge to push. By bearing down, she helps the baby complete its passage to the outside.

As the baby's head appears, or *crowns*, the doctor may perform an *episiotomy*—an incision from the lower end of the vagina toward the anus to enlarge the vaginal opening. The purpose of the episiotomy is to prevent the baby's head from causing an irregular tear in the vagina, but routine episiotomies have been criticized as unnecessary. Women may be able to avoid this procedure by trying different birthing positions or having an attendant massage the perineal tissue.

Usually the baby's head emerges first, then its shoulders, then its body. With each contraction, a new part is born. However, the baby can be in a more difficult position, facing up rather than down, or with the feet or buttocks first (a **breech birth**), and a caesarean birth may then be necessary.

In the third stage of labor, the uterus contracts firmly after the birth of the baby; and, usually within five minutes, the placenta separates from the uterine wall. The woman may bear down to help expel the placenta, or the doctor may exert gentle external pressure.

If an episiotomy has been performed, the doctor sews up the incision. To help the uterus contract and return to its normal size, it may be massaged manually, or the baby may be put to the mother's breast to stimulate contraction of the uterus.

Caesarean Birth

In a **caesarean delivery** (also referred to as a caesarean section), the doctor lifts the baby out of the woman's body through an incision made in the lower abdomen and uterus. The most common reason for caesarean birth is "failure to progress," a vague term indicating that labor has gone on too long and may put the baby or mother at risk. Other reasons include the baby's position (if feet or buttocks are first) and signs that the fetus is in danger. Thirty years ago, only 5 percent of babies born in America were delivered by caesarean birth; the current rate is 22.6 percent—substantially higher than in most other industrialized countries.

About 36 percent of caesarean sections are performed because the woman has had a previous caesarean birth. Yet research indicates that more than two-thirds of women who undergo caesarean births because of failure to progress in labor, and approximately four of every five women who have had caesarean births for other reasons, can have successful vaginal deliveries in subsequent pregnancies.

Caesarean birth involves abdominal surgery, so many women feel more physical discomforts after a caesarean than a vaginal birth. These discomforts include nausea, pain, and abdominal gas. Women who have had a caesarean section must refrain from strenuous activity, such as heavy lifting, for several weeks.

The Days and Weeks Following Birth

Hospital stays for new mothers have gotten shorter. The average length of stay is now only 2.6 days for a vaginal delivery and 4.1 days after a caesarean birth. A primary reason has been pressure to reduce medical costs. Obstetricians have voiced concern that the rush to release new mothers may jeopardize their well-being and the health of their babies, who are more likely to require emergency care for problems such as jaundice. The American College of Obstetricians and Gynecologists and the American Academy of Pediatrics recommend that women remain in the hospital two days after a vaginal delivery and four days after a caesarean birth.

For the new mother, the high of delivery may be followed by a low known as **postpartum depression.** This time of fatigue, anxiety, and fluctuating moods is so common that it is listed in obstetrics texts as a normal consequence of delivery. For most women, it is a tem-

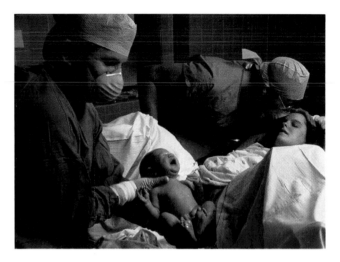

Family time. Fathers are routinely present at the birth of their children and often act as breathing coaches after both parents train in Lamaze techniques.

porary feeling. For others, the depression, combined with fatigue and the new demands of the newborn, can persist and deepen. If postpartum depression lasts more than three or four weeks, the woman should seek help from a qualified psychotherapist.

It takes a while for the mother's body to return to normal after having given birth. The woman usually loses about 11 pounds at delivery and an additional 4 to 5 pounds in the following weeks. Usually four to eight weeks are required for the woman's reproductive organs, especially the uterus, to return to normal. Breast-feeding hastens this process, and exercises help restore the abdomen's size, shape, and tone. For three to six weeks after birth, there is a vaginal discharge called **lochia,** a mixture of blood from the site in the uterus where the placenta was attached, and tissue from the uterine lining. If the mother doesn't breast-feed her infant, menstruation typically resumes about four to ten weeks after giving birth.

Breast-Feeding Versus Bottle-Feeding

A generation ago, most middle- and upper-class women bottle-fed their babies. Today, an increasing number of mothers and medical professionals feel that breast milk is best. Breast-fed babies have fewer illnesses and a much lower hospitalization rate. Their mortality rate is also lower. Breast milk seems not only to prevent disease, but also to help bring infection under control. When breast-fed babies do get sick, they recover more quickly.[39]

Despite the benefits of breast-feeding, there are valid reasons to choose bottle-feeding. According to the

American Council on Science and Health, at least 20 percent of women are unable to breast-feed after their first deliveries, and 50 percent of new mothers encounter significant difficulties nursing. Sometimes the woman's breasts become inflamed, or she must take medications that would endanger her infant; sometimes the infant is unable to suckle vigorously enough to get an adequate milk supply. Another problem is that in certain areas of the country, the levels of pesticides and other chemical contaminants in mother's milk can be high.

Babies at Risk

According to the National Center for Health Statistics, a record percentage of U. S. newborns are surviving to their first birthday. The infant mortality rate, as reported in 1999, is a record low of 7.9 deaths per 1,000 live births—a continued decline that puts the nation on track to reach its goal of no more than 7 infant deaths per 1,000 births by the year 2000. However, African-American babies are not faring as well. Their mortality rate was 16.5 in 1992—making them 2.4 times more likely to die, primarily because of prematurity and dangerously low birth weight, before their first birthday. This gap has widened from just a 60 percent greater risk in 1950. Babies of Chinese and Japanese descent have the lowest mortality rates.

In all, more than 1.3 million newborns each year require special care after birth because of prematurity, low birth weight, birth defects, jaundice, respiratory difficulties, or other problems. About 6 percent of newborns—more than 200,000 babies a year—require immediate intensive care for potentially life-threatening problems that developed before, during, or after birth.

Genetic Disorders

Two to 4 percent of babies are born with a genetic abnormality. While the overall infant mortality rate has declined, the proportion of infant deaths due to birth defects has increased.[40] However, the most common birth defects are not fatal. They include:

* *Cystic fibrosis.* The most common genetic problem among white Americans, this is a disabling abnormality of the respiratory system and sweat and mucous glands.
* *Down syndrome.* This disorder is caused by an extra number 21 chromosome and occurs in one out of every 600 to 1,000 births. Infants are born with varying degrees of physical and mental retardation. The chances of a woman delivering an infant with Down syndrome increase with her age. At age 25, the

chances are 1 in 1,200; at age 35, they rise to 1 in 365; and at age 40, they are 1 in 100.

* *Sickle-cell anemia.* About 8 to 10 percent of North America's 25 million African Americans carry a gene for sickle-cell anemia, a blood disorder that occurs when hemoglobin, the oxygen-carrying protein of red blood cells, is abnormal and causes red blood cells to assume a crescent (sickle) shape. Unable to provide adequate oxygen to vital organs of the body, sickled cells cause fatigue, loss of interest and appetite, pain, and a host of other symptoms. Blood transfusions can prolong a victim's life, but there's no cure for sickle-cell anemia. About half the victims die before age 20.
* *Phenylketonuria (PKU).* This disease occurs when the liver enzyme needed by the body for the metabolism of the amino acid phenylalanine is absent. If both parents are carriers, there's a one-in-four chance that the child will develop phenylketonuria (PKU). In most states, the law requires testing newborns for PKU. If PKU is detected, an immediate, long-term phenylalanine-free diet can reduce the effects of the disorder. If untreated, the victim becomes severely mentally retarded.
* *Tay-Sachs disease.* Occurring almost exclusively among young children of Eastern European Jewish ancestry, Tay-Sachs disease is caused by an enzyme deficiency. Infants with this disorder appear normal for perhaps nine months, but then gradually deteriorate physically and mentally. Death usually occurs before the fifth birthday. Carriers can be identified by a blood test.

The Littlest Addicts

Cocaine and crack babies suffer major complications, including withdrawal and permanent disabilities. (See Chapter 15 for a discussion of these drugs.) They have higher-than-normal incidences of respiratory and kidney troubles, premature birth, and low birth weight, and may be at greater risk of sudden infant death syndrome. Visual problems, lack of coordination, and developmental retardation are also common.

Crib Death: Sudden Infant Death Syndrome (SIDS)

SIDS, or **crib death**—the unexplained death of an apparently healthy baby under one year of age—is the second-leading cause of infant mortality in the United States. About 900 infants die of crib death each year, a significant decrease from the past.[41] Typically, a seemingly healthy infant, usually 1 to 7 months old, is put to bed according to the daily routine. The baby may have some signs of a cold or cough. When the parents return to the crib, they find the child dead. There is no sign of a struggle, nor does the baby suffocate in the blankets. Determining the cause of death often proves impossible. Premature and very small babies are the most vulnerable. A newly recognized risk factor, based on studies of 20,000 infants during the first week of life, is the "resonance frequency" of each cry—an acoustic measure of a child's cry that cannot be easily determined by listening. Computer analysis found that infants with a high-resonance frequency were more likely to die of SIDS. A screening test based on this factor may be developed to detect newborns at risk.

Based on a review of studies on SIDS from around the world, health professionals have found that sleeping on its stomach increases a baby's risk of SIDS. As a result, pediatricians now recommend that normal, full-term infants be placed on their backs for the first six months. Parents should remove pillows, quilts, comforters, stuffed toys, and other soft products from the crib.

Infertility

The World Health Organization defines infertility as the failure to conceive after one year of unprotected intercourse. About 85 percent of couples will conceive during one year, rising to almost 90 percent by two years. The main causes of infertility are ovulation problems, tubal damage, or sperm dysfunction. Less common causes are endometriosis, cervical factors, or coital difficulties. Even after intensive investigation, 10 to 20 percent of couples have "unexplained infertility" in which no cause can be demonstrated.

Of the couples who marry this year, 1 in 12 won't be able to conceive a child, and 10 percent of couples already married won't be able to have additional children. About 6.1 million women reported impaired fertility in 1995, compared with 4.9 million in 1988. **Infertility** is a problem of the couple, not of the individual man or woman. In 40 percent of cases, infertility is caused by female problems; in 40 percent by male problems; in 10% by a combination of male and female problems; and in 10 percent by unexplained causes. A thorough diagnostic workup can reveal a cause for infertility in 90 percent of cases.

In women, the most common causes of subfertility or infertility are age, abnormal menstrual patterns, suppression of ovulation, and blocked fallopian tubes. Other gynecologic disorders that can lead to infertility include endometriosis, in which cells from the endometrium (the lining of the uterus) migrate to other locations within the pelvic cavity; fibroids, benign growths of tissue within the uterus that can interfere with conception; uterine defects; problems with the cervical mucus; and an immunological reaction to a man's sperm. The prevention of STDs can help prevent some cases of infertiltiy in women.[42]

Male subfertility or infertility is usually linked to either the quantity or the quality of sperm, which may be inactive, misshapen, or insufficient (less than 20 million sperm per milliliter of semen in an ejaculation of 3 to 5 ml). Sometimes the problem is hormonal or a blockage of a sperm duct. Some men suffer from the inability to ejaculate normally, or from retrograde ejaculation, in which some of the semen travels in the wrong direction, back into the body of the male. Another problem is a *varicocele*, an enlarged vein that carries too much blood and makes the testicle too warm. An undergarment that uses a small amount of water to cool the testicles may help overcome this problem; some men require surgery to eliminate the varicocele. The use of drugs such as cocaine and marijuana can also interfere with the creation of sperm.

The treatment of infertility has become a $2 billion a year enterprise in the United States.[43] Medical treatment can identify the cause of infertility in about 90 percent of affected couples. The odds of successful pregnancy range from 30 to 70 percent, depending on the specific cause of infertility. One result of successful infertility treatments has been a boom in multiple births, including quintuplets and sextuplets. Some obstetricians have urged less aggressive treatment for infertility to avoid such high-risk multiple births.

Infertility can have an enormous emotional impact. Often, the wife begins to worry first because infertility touches on a core aspect of femininity. Many women long to experience pregnancy and childbirth and feel great loss if they cannot conceive. Their self-esteem may be diminished, and they may become obsessed with success and outcome. Women in their thirties and forties fear that their "biological clock" is running out of time. Men may be confused and surprised by the intensity of their partners' emotions. Most are more concerned about their wives than about having a baby, but they feel helpless and frustrated in their husbandly role of fixing matters for the wife. Although they both need each other's support more than ever, they may pull away because of their sadness and a sense of losing control over their lives.[44]

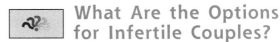

What Are the Options for Infertile Couples?

Artificial Insemination

Since the 1960s, **artificial insemination**—the introduction of viable sperm into the vagina by artificial means—

has led to an estimated 250,000 births in the United States, primarily in couples in which the husband was infertile. However, some states do not recognize such children as legitimate; others do, but only if the woman's husband gave his consent for the insemination.

There have been complaints about unethical treatment in infertility centers. Fertility specialists and government licensing agencies have been working together to set uniform standards for licensing. Infertile couples should carefully obtain as much information as possible, including the credentials of any fertility specialists, who should be board-certified in obstetrics and gynecology, with additional training in reproductive endocrinology and infertility. Those performing surgery should be members of the Society of Reproductive Surgeons; centers offering in vitro fertilization or alternative techniques should be staffed by members of the Society of Assisted Reproductive Technology.

Assisted Reproductive Technology

New approaches to infertility include microsurgery, sometimes with lasers, to open destroyed or blocked egg and sperm ducts; new hormone preparations to induce ovulation; and the use of balloons, inserted through the cervix and inflated, to open blocked fallopian tubes (a procedure called *balloon tuboplasty*). However, less than 2 percent of infertile women undergo assisted reproductive technologies in order to conceive.

Among the most promising techniques that can help couples overcome fertility problems is *in vitro fertilization,* which involves removing the ova, often with a long needle, from a woman's ovary just before normal ovulation would occur. The woman's egg and her mate's sperm are placed in a special fertilization medium (a substance that encourages fertilization) for a specific period of time, and are then transferred to another medium to continue developing. If the fertilized egg cell shows signs of development, within several days it is returned to the woman's uterus by means of a hollow tube placed through the vagina and cervix. The egg cell implants itself in the lining of the uterus, and the pregnancy continues as normal. The success rate varies from center to center but is generally less than 20 percent, and the costs are high.

Less time-consuming and less expensive than in vitro fertilization, *gamete intrafallopian transfer (GIFT)* involves placing sperm and eggs into the fallopian tubes. GIFT mimics nature by allowing fertilized eggs to develop in the fallopian tubes according to a normal timetable. The success rate is about 20 percent. In *zygote intrafallopian transfer (ZIFT),* eggs are collected from the mother-to-be and combined with the father's sperm in a laboratory dish. One day after fertilization occurs, the single-celled zygote that forms is placed in the fallopian tube. In a variation called *intracytoplasmic sperm injection (ICSI),* several eggs are harvested, and each is injected with a single sperm by means of a fine hollow needle. (This overcomes problems related to the inability of sperm to penetrate the egg.) The fertilized eggs are then placed in the fallopian tube.[45]

Fertilization rates are comparable to in vitro fertilization with sperm from normal ejaculation.[46] There is also a new technique called *gestational surrogacy,* in which an embryo is conceived in a laboratory dish using a woman's egg and her partner's sperm and then implanted into another woman's (the surrogate's) uterus. Alternatively, the fertilized donor egg can later be transferred to the uterus of the infertile woman, who carries and delivers the developing embryo. Embryos may be frozen for later implantation in a process (called *cryopreservation*) that is highly controversial because of legal issues concerning the "ownership" of the unborn. Some women are considering an experimental technique to freeze some of their eggs at a young age for later use.[47]

Older women are just as likely as younger women to have a successful pregnancy after implantation of a donor embryo. In some experimental and controversial cases, donor eggs and embryos have been successfully implanted in women in their forties, fifties, and (in at least two cases) sixties. The use of a donor egg from a younger woman eliminates the risk of increased genetic problems. There are ethical questions about using expensive assisted reproductive technologies for the sake of enabling older women to become mothers or of allowing creation of "designer" babies of a certain

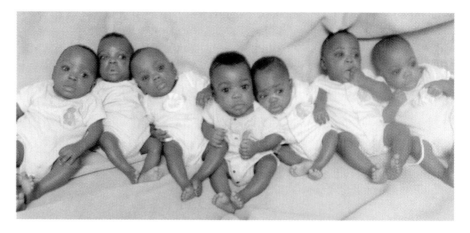

Fertility drugs can increase the chances of multiple births.

racial or ethnic identity or with certain attributes, such as sex, height, or intelligence.

Fertility drugs and assisted reproduction techniques have extended the limits of motherhood. In 1996 Arceli Keh, a 63-year-old bank teller in southern California, became the oldest mother on record when she gave birth to a baby girl. She had lied about her age to qualify for infertility treatments. In 1997 Bobbi McCaughey in Des Moines, Iowa, after treatment with fertility drugs, gave birth to seven babies—and earned her own place in the annals of reproduction as the mother of the only surviving set of septuplets.

These births set off both a media frenzy and a firestorm of controversy. Many questioned the ethics of a woman becoming a mother at over age 60. In Bobbi McCaughey's case, doctors pointed out that the chance of miscarrying and losing all the babies was greater than 50 percent.[48] Assisted reproductive techniques involve some problems, including high costs and a low success rate. One attempt at in vitro fertilization ranges from $6,000 to $10,000 and insurance rarely covers these expenses. The overall success rate for any form of assisted pregnancy is about 25 percent.

Of the pregnancies achieved by fertility treatments, 20 to 30 percent result in multiple births. As a result of hormonal stimulation, the woman's ovaries usually release several eggs; often more than one is fertilized. To increase the chances of conception, fertility specialists usually implant more than one embryo. The more that survive, the greater the risk of prematurity, low birth weight, birth defects, and death in the womb or after birth. In some cases, one or more fetuses are aborted to increase the likelihood that at least one other will survive.

There also has been controversy over whether the hormones used to stimulate the ovaries in infertility treatment may increase the risk of ovarian cancer. However, an analysis of all the research on this topic concluded that, as currently used, ovarian-stimulating drugs do not increase this risk.[49]

Adoption

Men and women who cannot conceive children biologically can still become parents. **Adoption** matches would-be parents yearning for youngsters to love with infants or children who need loving. Couples interested in adoption can work with either public agencies or private counselors who contact obstetricians directly. Or they can contact organizations that arrange adoptions of children in need from other countries.

Approximately 1 percent of the U. S. population are adopted; among children under age 18, 3 to 4 percent are adopted.[50] Each year some 50,000 U.S. children become available for adoption—far fewer than the number of would-be parents looking for youngsters to love. By some estimates, only 1 in 30 couples receive the child they want—and they spend an average of two years and as much as $100,000 on the adoption process.

Not only are the stakes high, but adoption arrangements often are chaotic. Private adoptions are legal in some states, banned in others. In some places, birth mothers sign over all claims to a child within 72 hours of giving birth; in others they have up to a year to change their minds. Sometimes foster parents are encouraged to adopt—particularly if they're African Americans caring for an African-American child. In others, they face a daunting series of bureaucratic barriers. What's needed most, say experts on every side of the issue, are uniform adoption laws in all fifty states.

An increasing number of people support *open adoptions*, which allow for visiting and communication with the biological parents even though the adoptive parents retain legal custody. Even after a *closed adoption*, the biological (or birth) parents may at some point search for their children, if only to explain why they chose to give them up for adoption.

Although fewer than 2 percent of each year's 50,000 adoptions of American children are contested, adoptive parents are nervous and confused.

"Adoptive or foster parents have no rights whatsoever until the rights of the biological parents are legally terminated," says Mary Beth Style, Vice President for policy and practice for the National Council on Adoption[51]—even when they have nurtured a child for months or years, as often happens in foster care. Although mental health professionals contend that the courts should recognize the rights of a child's "psychological" parents, most rulings have placed little importance on such bonds. Political pressure for reform has

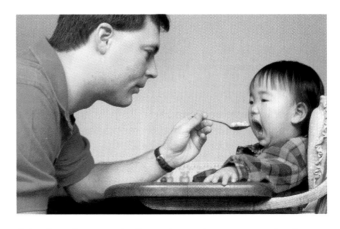

Adoption gives people the option to become parents when they would not otherwise be able to have children.

increased, which makes birthparent support groups fearful. "There's a rush to sever quickly and permanently the biological bonds between parents and their children," says Janet Fenton, President of Concerned United Birthparents. "The focus in adoption is shifting from finding homes for children who need them to finding babies for couples who can't have them."[52]

The best advice for prospective adoptive parents is to learn as much as they can about their state's adoption laws and to prepare for the reality that their plans might not work out.

Making This Chapter Work for You

Responsible Reproductive Choices

- Simply not wanting to conceive is never enough to prevent conception. Before you become sexually active, you have to decide about birth control. The fact that women bear children does not mean that men aren't equally responsible for birth control.

- A sexually active couple that doesn't use contraception has an 80 percent chance of conceiving a child within a year. If you decide to take that gamble, the stakes are your future, your partner's future, and the future of the child you may conceive.

- To prevent conception, you can make the survival of sperm in the vagina more difficult, or you can block the sperm's path into the vagina, uterus, and fallopian tubes. By preventing ovulation, you can make sure that the sperm doesn't find a ready, ripe egg; or you can prevent the fertilized egg from implanting itself in the uterine wall.

- Abstinence and sexual activities that do not involve vaginal intercourse ("outercourse") are completely safe and 100 percent effective—as long as couples are committed to this practice and make sure that sperm is never ejaculated near the vaginal opening.

- Hormonally based birth control methods include oral contraceptives (the pill); hormone implants (Norplant), which inhibit ovulation and alter the cervical mucus so that sperm are prevented from entering the uterus; and Depo-Provera, an injectable hormone that provides three months of contraceptive protection.

- The barrier contraceptives provide a physical or chemical barrier that prevents sperm from reaching an egg. They include the condom, diaphragm, cervical cap, and spermicidal foam, jelly, suppositories, and film. Use of condoms with spermicides containing nonoxynol-9 can also reduce the risk of pregnancy and some sexually transmitted diseases.

- Intrauterine devices (IUDs), made with a hormonal compound or copper, prevent implantation of a fertilized egg. They are highly effective and long-acting but are recommended only for women in monogamous relationships.

- Couples using natural family planning or fertility awareness methods refrain from unprotected vaginal intercourse during the days just preceding and just following ovulation. They may use cervical mucus, a monthly calendar, or body temperature changes to determine a woman's period of greatest fertility.

- The most popular and effective, but permanent, birth control method among married couples is sterilization: vasectomy in a man and tubal ligation or occlusion in a woman.

- After-intercourse methods of birth control include higher doses of oral contraceptives; the so-called morning-after pill, which prevents implantation of a fertilized egg; insertion of an IUD; and menstrual extraction, in which the uterine lining is suctioned out.

- One of the most controversial and divisive issues today is legalized induced abortion, the termination of pregnancy by the removal of the uterine contents. A hormonal compound, mifepristone (RU-486), often called the French abortion pill and available only at research centers, can terminate a pregnancy in its first weeks. Commonly used abortion methods in the United States are suction curettage, dilation and evacuation (D and E), prostaglandin injection, and hysterotomy.

- Good prenatal care includes good nutrition; adequate rest and exercise; and avoiding risks, such as smoking, alcohol, caffeine, harmful drugs, and exposure to radiation. Among the serious complications of pregnancy are ectopic pregnancy, in which the fertilized egg implants itself at sites other than in the uterus; miscarriages, which usually occur before the sixteenth week of pregnancy; infections, which may cause disease, brain damage, and malformations of the fetus; and premature labor, which occurs after week 20 and before week 37 of the pregnancy.

- Labor and delivery consists of three stages. During the first stage, the cervix thins and dilates to a diameter of 10 centimeters. In the next stage, the baby passes through the birth canal. The placenta is expelled during the third stage. A caesarean, or surgical, birth may be necessary to overcome certain risks. After birth, the woman's body begins to return to its prepregnant state. The woman may choose to breast-feed, which can help protect the newborn from various illnesses, or bottle-feed her baby.

■ Infertile couples may decide to attempt to have a child by such medical procedures as in vitro fertilization or other assisted forms of birth technology. Another alternative is adoption, although the number of available babies is far fewer than the number of would-be parents hoping to adopt.

Choices about sexual behavior invariably lead to choices about reproduction. Sexual responsibility means recognizing that fact and acting with full awareness of the consequences of sexual activity. You must think not just of yourself, but also of your partner, because your decisions and actions may affect both of you, now and in the future. You must also consider the baby you might conceive if you don't use contraception. If you should decide to have a child, your responsibilities extend to the new life you helped to create.

 Birth Control Pill Study. What is known about the long term effects of pill use?

health / ONLINE

Planned Parenthood
http://www.plannedparenthood.org
This site includes news, updates, articles, and detailed information about birth control, abortion, pregnancy, sexually transmitted diseases, and political action.

Harvard University Global Reproductive Health Forum
http://www.hsph.harvard.edu/Organizations/healthnet/index.html
Includes an online research library, discussion lists, and forums for discussing reproductive health topics.

Reproductive Health Online
http://www.reproline.jhu.edu/
Provides information about the latest developments in reproductive health technologies; an online library of family planning and reproductive health-related documents; and more. Affiliated with Johns Hopkins University.

Please note that links are subject to change. If you find a broken link, use a search engine like http://www.yahoo.com *and search for the web site by typing in key words.*

 Campus Chat: Do you plan on having children? If so, at what age and why? If not, why not? Share your thoughts on our online discussion forum at **http://health.wadsworth.com**

Find It On InfoTrac: You can find additional readings related to health via InfoTrac College Edition, an online library of more than 900 journals and publications. Follow the instructions for accessing InfoTrac that came packaged with your textbook; then search for articles using a key word search.

• **Suggested reading:** "Contraceptive Failure Rates: New Estimates From the 1995 National Survey of Family Growth," by Haishan Fu; Jacqueline E. Darroch; Taylor Haas; Nalini Ranjit. *Family Planning Perspectives,* March 1999, Vol. 31, Issue 2, p. 56(1).

(1) Which contraceptives had the highest failure rates, according to the study reported in this article?

(2) What kind of personal and background factors are correlated with high risks of contraceptive failure?

For additional links, resources, and suggested readings on InfoTrac, visit our Health & Wellness Resource Center at http://health.wadsworth.com

Key Terms

The terms listed here are used within the chapter. Page numbers are included for each term. A definition of each term is given in the Glossary pages at the end of this book.

Critical Thinking Questions

1. After reading about the various methods of contraception, which do you feel would be most effective for you? What factors enter into your decision (convenience, risks, effectiveness, etc.)?

2. In Wyoming, a pregnant woman went to the police station to report that her husband had beaten her. Instead of charges being brought against him, she was arrested for intoxication and charged with abusing her fetus by drinking. Across the country, other women who use hard drugs or alcohol while pregnant or whose newborns test positive for drugs have been arrested and put on trial for abusing their unborn children. Prosecutors argue that they are defending the innocent victims of substance abuse. Some health officials, on the other hand, argue that addicted women need help, not punishment. What do you think? Why?

3. If you or your partner took fertility drugs and then became pregnant with seven fetuses, would you carry them all to term? What if you knew that the chances of them all surviving were very slim and that eliminating some of them would improve the odds for the others? What ethical issues do cases like these raise?

References

1. "Family Planning Saves Millions of Women and Children's Lives." *WIN News,* Vol. 23, No. 2, Spring 1997.
2. Steinhauer, Jennifer. "Men Avoiding Obligation for Birth Control." *New York Times,* May 25, 1995.
3. Sawyer, Robin, et al. "Pregnancy Testing And Counseling: A University Health Center's 5-Year Experience." *Journal of American College Health,* Vol. 46, No. 5, March 1998.
4. Glei, Dana. "Measuring Contraceptive Use Patterns Among Teenage and Adult Women." *Family Planning Perspectives,* Vol. 31, No. 2, March 1999.
5. Fu, Haishan, et al. "Contraceptive Failure Rates." *Family Planning Perspectives,* Vol. 31, No. 2, March 1999.
6. Glei. "Measuring Contraceptive Use Patterns Among Teenage and Adult Women."

7. Fu, et al. "Contraceptive Failure Rates."

8. Walling, Anne. "Health Effects of Oral Contraceptive Use." *American Family Physician,* Vol. 59, Issue 5, March 1, 1999.

9. McCoy, Norma. Personal Interview.

10. Mahler, K. "Long-Term Users of Injectable Contraceptives May Experience Substantially Diminished Bone Density." *Family Planning Perspectives,* Vol. 31, No. 2, March 1999.

11. "Closing The Condom Gap." *Population Reports,* Vol. 27, Issue 1, April 1999.

12. Pinkerton, Steven, and Paul Abrahamson. "Condoms and the Prevention of AIDS." *American Scientist,* Vol. 85, No. 4, July–August 1997.

13. Lindberg, Laura Duberstein, et al. "Young Men's Experience with Condom Breakage." *Family Planning Perspectives,* Vol. 29, No. 3, May–June 1997.

14. McNeil, Donal. "Condoms for Women Gain Approval Among Africans." *New York Times,* July 24, 1999.

15. Leary, Warren. "A Contraceptive Returns to the Market." *New York Times,* March 30, 1999.

16. Hatcher, Robert, et al. *Contraceptive Technology.* New York: Irvington, 1994. Colditz, G. "Oral Contraceptive Use and Mortality During 12 Years of Follow-Up: The Nurses' Health Study." *Annals of Internal Medicine,* Vol. 120, 1994.

17. Moore, M. "Most U. S. Couples Who Seek Surgical Sterilization Do So for Contraception; Fewer Than 25% Desire Reversal." *Family Planning Perspectives,* Vol. 31, No. 2, March 1999.

18. Lancashire, Jeff. "New Report Documents Trends in Childbearing, Reproductive Health." National Center for Health Statistics, June 5, 1997.

19. Glei, "Measuring Contraceptive Use Patterns Among Teenage and Adult Women."

20. Dienick, I. "Levonorgestrel Is a Better Emergency Contraceptive than the Combination Pill." *Family Planning Perspectives,* Vol. 31, No. 2, March 1999.

21. Walling, Anne. "Low Doses of Mifepristone for Emergency Contraception." *American Family Physician,* Vol. 59, No. 10, May 15, 1999.

22. Cariati, Sophia. "The Battle for Birth Control." *American Health,* January 1999.

23. "A New Generation of Contraception." *New York Times,* July 6, 1999.

24. Talbot, Margaret. "The Little White Bombshell." *New York Times,* July 6, 1999, July 11, 1999.

25. Stotland, Nada. *Abortion: Facts and Feelings.* Washington, D.C.: American Psychiatric Press, 1998.

26. Hales, Dianne. *Just Like a Woman.* New York: Bantam Books, 1999.

27. Lafayette, Leslie. Personal Interview.

28. Seguin, Louise, et al. "Chronic Stressors, Social Support and Depression During Pregnancy." *Obstetrics & Gynecology,* Vol. 85, No. 4, April 1995.

29. Copper, Rachel, et al. "The Relationship of Maternal Attitude Toward Weight Gain During Pregnancy and Low Birth Weight." *Obstetrics & Gynecology,* Vol. 85, No. 4, April 1995.

30. Clapp, J. F., III, et al. "Does Regular Exercise During Pregnancy Affect the Physical Growth or Mental Development of Infants?" *Western Journal of Medicine,* Vol. 170, Issue 5, May 1999.

31. "Medical-Care Expenditures Attributable to Cigarette Smoking During Pregnancy—United States, 1995." *Journal of the American Medical Association,* Vol. 278, No. 23, December 17, 1997.

32. "Drinking in Pregnancy." *Morbidity and Mortality Weekly Report,* U.S. Centers for Disease Control, April 1997.

33. Williams, Rebecca. "Healthy Pregnancy, Healthy Baby." *FDA Consumer,* Vol. 33, Issue 2, March 1999.

34. Moore, Peter. "Tackling Autoantibody-linked Pregnancy Loss." *Lancet,* Vol. 350, No. 9073, July 26, 1997. Cowchock, Susan. "Autoantibodies and Pregnancy Loss." *New England Journal of Medicine,* Vol. 337, No. 3, July 17, 1997.

35. Wilcox, Allen, et al. "Birthweight and Perinatal Mortality." *Journal of the American Medical Association,* Vol. 273, No. 9, March 1, 1995.

36. "Low Teen Birth Rate in 1997 Drives National Birth Rate to Record Low." *School Health Opportunities and Progress (Shop) Bulletin,* Vol. 4, Issue 5, May 14, 1999.

37. "Programs Help Prevent Teen Pregnancy." *State Legislatures,* Vol. 25, Issue 1, January 1999.

38. Lindberg, Laura, et al. "Age Differences Between Minors Who Give Birth and Their Adult Partners." *Family Planning Perspectives,* Vol. 29, No. 2, March–April 1997.

39. Brody, Jane. "Breast Is Best for Babies, but Sometimes Mom Needs Help." *New York Times,* March 30, 1999.

40. "Infant Deaths from Birth Defects." *Pediatrics for Parents,* February 1999.

41. "Preventing Sudden Infant Death Syndrome." *Child Health Alert,* May 1999.

42. DeLisle, Susan. "Preserving Reproductive Choice: Preventing STD-Related Infertility in Women." *SIECUS Report,* Vol. 25, No. 3, February–March 1997.

43. "Infertility Treatments: Weighing the Risks and Benefits." *Health Facts,* February 1999.

44. Schreiber, Pamela. "From Your Patient's Perspective: The Emotional Impact of Infertility." *Focus on Fertility,* Vol. 1, No. 2, Spring 1995.

45. Huffman, Grace Brooke. "Intracytoplasmic Sperm Injection and Genetic Risk." *American Family Physician,* Vol. 55, No. 5, April 1997.

46. Crooks and Baur, *Our Sexuality.*

47. Richardson, Sarah. "Thirteen Ways of Looking At A Baby." In *Perspectives: Women's Health,* Carol Sample (ed.). St. Paul: Coursewise, 1999.

48. Kolata, Gina. "Many Specialists Are Left in No Mood for Celebration." *New York Times,* November 21, 1997.

49. Mosgaard, Berit Jul. "Infertility, Fertility Drugs, and Invasive Ovarian Cancer: A Case-Control Study." *Journal of the American Medical Association,* Vol. 278, No. 12, September 24, 1997.

50. Mulcare, S. Lynn. "Effects of Adoptive Status on Evaluations of Children." *Journal of Social Psychology,* Vol. 139, Issue 2, April 1999.

51. Style, Mary Beth. Personal interview.

52. Fenton, Janet. Personal interview.

IV

Personal Health Risks

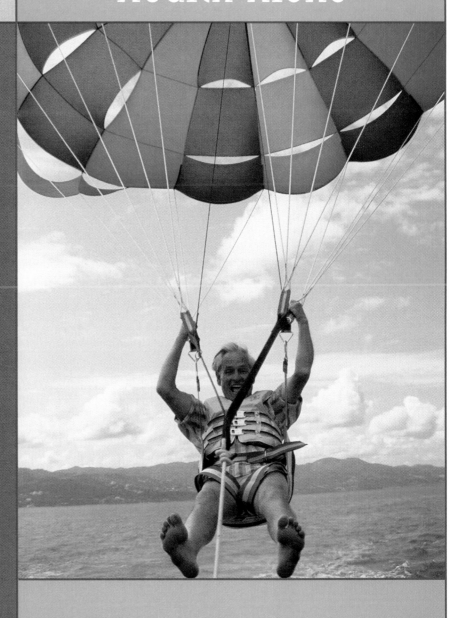

E very day you make choices that affect both the quantity and the quality of your life. The right choices aren't always easy to make or to sustain. The chapters in this section can help by providing information you can use in making and implementing healthful decisions. By understanding the risks to your health, you can prepare to overcome them—and not simply live life, but celebrate it every day.

11

Consumerism, Complementary/Alternative Medicine, and the Health Care System

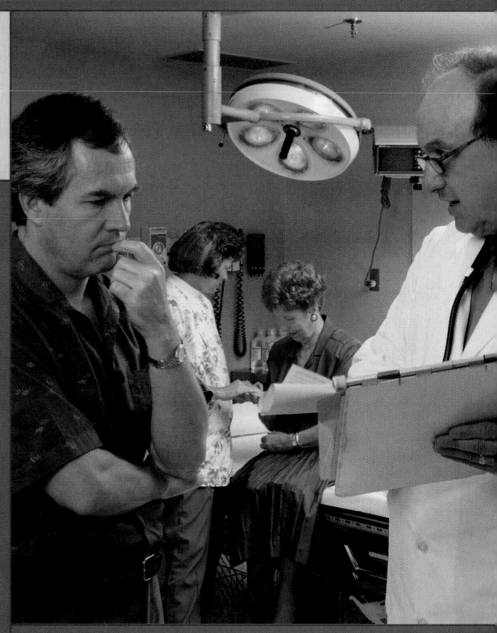

After studying the material in this chapter, you should be able to:

- **List** ways of evaluating health news and online medical advice.
- **Explain** strategies for self-care, as well as how to get the best possible health care.
- **List** your rights as a medical consumer.
- **Discuss** complementary and alternative medicine and **explain** what research has shown about its effectiveness.
- **List** at least five kinds of health-care practitioners and five kinds of health-care facilities.
- **Explain** what managed care is.

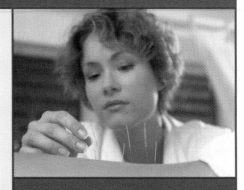

At the beginning of a new millennium, you have more health-care options than previous generations could have imagined. Americans already use more health-care services, see more health practitioners, undergo more surgery, take more prescription drugs, and spend more time in hospitals than the citizens of any other nation. We make 762 million visits to physicians and spend 539 million days in hospitals. Not surprisingly, our medical costs also are higher than in any other country: an estimated $1 trillion a year, 13.6 percent of the Gross National Product.[1] National health expenditures are expected to reach $2.2 trillion in 2008 and are likely to account for 16.2 percent of the gross domestic product.

Despite such enormous expense, not every American receives good, or even adequate, medical care. Consumers have long complained about insensitive treatment, lack of comprehensive care, and far too little emphasis on the prevention of disease. Because of recent efforts to curb spending, health-care providers may now seem to pay greater attention to cost than caring. And because of a lack of insurance, millions of people have limited access, or no access at all, to needed health services.

In part because of their disenchantment with traditional health care, many consumers are turning to complementary and alternative medicine (CAM), a term that includes a broad range of healing philosophies, approaches, and therapies not generally taught in medical schools or provided in hospitals. For the first time, vigorous scientific studies are investigating the safety and efficacy of these treatments, and more health-care providers are integrating traditional and untraditional approaches in their practices.

With so many health-care choices, you face a greater responsibility for your personal well-being. Whether you are monitoring your blood pressure, considering elective surgery, or deciding whether to try an alternative therapy, you need to gather information, ask questions, weigh advantages and disadvantages, and take charge of your health. The reason: No one cares more about your health than you do, and no one will do more to promote your well-being than you. ❖

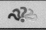 **FREQUENTLY ASKED QUESTIONS**

FAQ: **How can I evaluate online health advice? p. 336**

FAQ: **How should I choose my primary care physician? p. 342**

FAQ: **What should I expect in a medical exam? p. 344**

FAQ: **Is alternative medicine effective? p. 352**

FAQ: **What is managed care? p. 361**

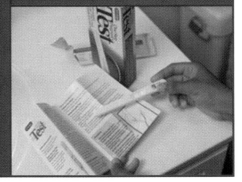

Becoming a Savvy Health-Care Consumer

Knowing how to spot health problems, how to evaluate health news, what to expect from health-care professionals, and where to turn for appropriate treatment can help you keep your own costs down while ensuring the best possible care.

Self-Care

Most people do treat themselves. You probably prescribe aspirin for a headache, chicken soup or orange juice for a cold, or a weekend trip to unwind from stress. At the very least, you should know what your **vital signs** are and how they compare against normal readings. (See Figure 11-1.)

Once a thermometer was the only self-testing equipment found in most American homes. Now an estimated 300 home tests are available to help consumers monitor everything from fertility to blood pressure to cholesterol levels. (See Table 11-1.) More convenient and less expensive than a visit to a clinic or doctor's office, the new tests are generally as accurate as those administered by a professional. Always follow directions precisely, and if your concerns persist, see your doctor.[2]

Self-care also can mean getting involved in the self-help movement, which has grown into a major national trend involving an estimated 25 million Americans. Initially criticized for implicitly blaming victims rather than changing society, many self-help groups have become more politicized and are working not just to address specific needs of individuals, but to transform social structures. The American Self-Help Clearinghouse has an information hotline and a directory of more than 700 self-help groups; the Clearinghouse and many of the groups are listed in the Your Health Directory at the back of this book.

How Can I Evaluate Online Medical Advice?

The Internet has become a major source of health information—and misinformation. There are more than 10,000 health-related sites, and an estimated 33 million Americans go online for medical information every year.[3] Many people want to learn more about medications and treatments; others share experiences with people with similar problems via chat rooms and bulletin boards.

The Internet permits ease of access to cutting-edge medical knowledge and bridges the communication gap created by high-tech medicine. However, there also are

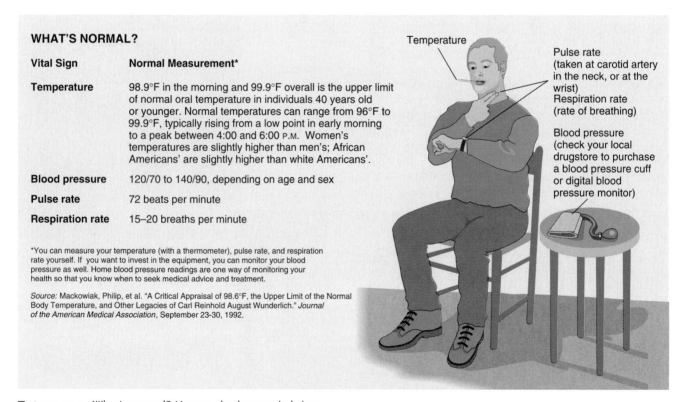

WHAT'S NORMAL?

Vital Sign	Normal Measurement*
Temperature	98.9°F in the morning and 99.9°F overall is the upper limit of normal oral temperature in individuals 40 years old or younger. Normal temperatures can range from 96°F to 99.9°F, typically rising from a low point in early morning to a peak between 4:00 and 6:00 P.M. Women's temperatures are slightly higher than men's; African Americans' are slightly higher than white Americans'.
Blood pressure	120/70 to 140/90, depending on age and sex
Pulse rate	72 beats per minute
Respiration rate	15–20 breaths per minute

*You can measure your temperature (with a thermometer), pulse rate, and respiration rate yourself. If you want to invest in the equipment, you can monitor your blood pressure as well. Home blood pressure readings are one way of monitoring your health so that you know when to seek medical advice and treatment.

Source: Mackowiak, Philip, et al. "A Critical Appraisal of 98.6°F, the Upper Limit of the Normal Body Temperature, and Other Legacies of Carl Reinhold August Wunderlich." *Journal of the American Medical Association*, September 23-30, 1992.

Temperature

Pulse rate (taken at carotid artery in the neck, or at the wrist)
Respiration rate (rate of breathing)

Blood pressure (check your local drugstore to purchase a blood pressure cuff or digital blood pressure monitor)

■ Figure 11-1 What's normal? How to check your vital signs.

■ **Table 11-1** Home Health Tests: A Consumer's Guide

Type of Test	What It Does
Pregnancy	Determines if a woman is pregnant by detecting the presence of human chorionic gonadotropin in urine. Considered 99 percent accurate.
Fertility	Measures levels of luteinizing hormone (LH), which rise 24 to 36 hours before a woman conceives. Can help women increase their odds of conceiving.
High blood pressure	Measures blood pressure by means of automatically inflating armbands or cuffs for the finger or wrist; helps people taking hypertension medication or suffering from high blood pressure monitor their condition.
Cholesterol	Checks blood cholesterol in blood from a finger prick; good for anyone concerned about cholesterol.
Colon cancer	Screening test to detect hidden blood in stool; recommended for anyone over 40 or concerned about colorectal disease.
Urinary tract infection	Diagnoses infection by screening for certain white blood cells in urine; advised for women who get frequent UTIs and whose doctors will prescribe antibiotics without a visit.
HIV	Detects antibodies to HIV in a blood sample sent anonymously to a lab. Controversial because no face-to-face counseling is available for those who test positive.

serious drawbacks. Because information on web sites is unregulated, there is no regulation of accuracy or reliability. Many sites are used to promote products or people. Some chat rooms can lead to encounters with unpleasant people. Even when information is technically precise, laypeople may not know how to interpret it properly.

Some doctors have set up web sites for the sole purpose of selling drugs such as Viagra—a practice that state and federal regulators have deemed unethical, though not illegal. The AMA has called for disciplinary action for doctors who prescribe drugs to people they have never met or examined. Other "cyberdocs" offer "virtual house calls" with board-certified physicians who engage in private chat sessions on minor illnesses and prescribe medicine (except controlled drugs like narcotics). In the future, video-conferencing may allow doctors to examine patients in cyberspace. However, there are no professional standards for doctors on the web, and experts advise caution. The "doctor" who treats your allergies may be a urologist or pathologist who is not up-to-date on new therapies or is unaware of potential side effects.

Here are some specific guidelines for evaluating online health sites:

• Check the creator. Web sites may come from health agencies, health support groups, school health programs, health-product advertisers, health educators, and health-education organizations. It is often difficult to distinguish biased commercial advertisements from unbiased sites created by scientists and health agencies. Read site headers and footers carefully.

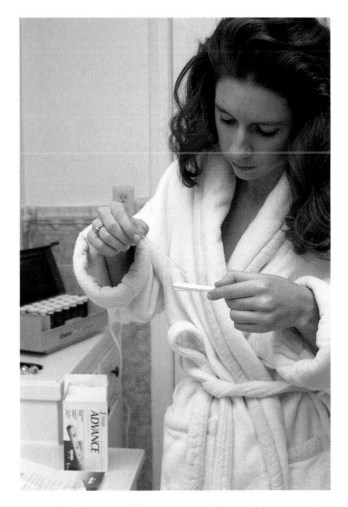

Home health tests can be more convenient and less expensive than a trip to a clinic or doctor's office.

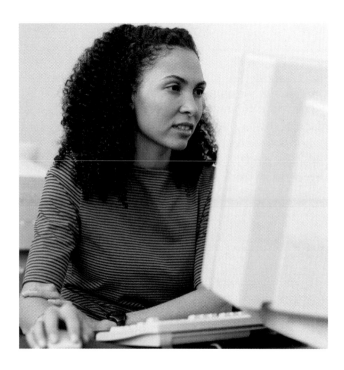

- If you are looking for the most recent research, check the date the page was created and last updated.

- Check the references. As with other health-education materials, web documents should provide the reader with complete references. Unreferenced suggestions may be unwarranted, scientifically unsound, and possibly unsafe.

- Consider the author. Is he or she recognized in the field of health education or otherwise qualified to publish a health-information web document? Does the author list his or her occupation, experience, and education?

- Look for possible bias. Web page authors may be attempting to provide healthful information to consumers, but they also may be attempting to sell a product. Many pages are merely disguised advertisements.

Evaluating Health News

Cure! Breakthrough! Medical miracle! These are the words headlines are made of. Remember that although medical breakthroughs and cures do occur, most scientific progress is made one small step at a time. Even though medicine is considered a science, some experts estimate that no more than 15 percent of medical interventions can be supported by reliable scientific evidence.

Medical opinions invariably change over time, sometimes going from one extreme to another. For instance, several decades ago the treatment of choice for breast cancer was radical mastectomy—removal of the woman's breast, lymph nodes, and chest wall. Since then much less extensive surgery (lumpectomy), coupled with chemotherapy or radiation, or both, has proven equally effective. Once individuals who'd suffered heart attacks were advised to limit all physical activity. Today a progressive exercise program is a standard component of rehabilitation.

Health researchers are struggling to find better ways of assessing what they know and need to know in order to offer more complete and balanced information to consumers. However, sometimes the only certainty is uncertainty. Rather than putting your faith in the most recent report or the hottest trend, try to gather as much background information and as many opinions as you can. Weigh them carefully—ideally with a trusted physician—and make the decision that seems best for you.

When reading a newspaper or magazine story or listening to a radio or television report about a medical advance, look for answers to the following questions:

- Who are the scientists involved? Are they recognized, legitimate health professionals? What are their credentials? Are they affiliated with respected medical or scientific institutions? Be wary of individuals whose degrees or affiliations are from institutions you've never heard of, and be sure that the person's educational background is in a discipline related to the area of research reported.

- Where did the scientists report their findings? The best research is published in peer-reviewed professional journals, such as the *New England Journal of Medicine*. Research developments also may be reported at meetings of professional societies.

- Is the information based on personal observations? Does the report include testimonials from cured patients or satisfied customers? If the answer to either question is yes, be wary.

- Does the article, report, or advertisement include words like *amazing, secret,* or *quick*? Does it claim to be something the public has never seen or been offered before? Such sensationalized language is often a tip-off to a dubious treatment.

- Is someone trying to sell you something? Manufacturers who cite studies to sell a product have been known to embellish the truth.

- Does the information defy all common sense? Be skeptical. If something sounds too good to be true, it probably is.

Making Sense of Medical Research

Medical research is the only way that anyone, physician or consumer, can assess the quality of diagnostic methods, medications, or surgical treatments. The principal rule of science is that nothing works until it's been proven.

Researchers rely on a variety of studies to determine whether a new approach to prevention, diagnosis, or treatment works. These include:

- *Epidemiological studies,* in which scientists assess the health status of a large, defined group of people, such as the population of a country or region. They may look at various health habits, such as alcohol consumption, to determine whether those who practice these habits have a higher likelihood of developing certain diseases.

- *Animal studies,* or *preclinical trials,* in which scientists administer a drug or try a procedure on various laboratory animals to assess its safety and determine its effects.

- *Clinical trials,* in which volunteers agree to act as test subjects—"human guinea pigs," as it were. Patients must give written permission in order to participate. Clinical trials generate data for the purpose of evaluating one or more diagnostic or therapeutic approaches in a population. Well-designed clinical trials, which must have strict eligibility criteria, a standardized intervention, follow-up, and measures of outcome, set the "gold standard" for new diagnostic tests or medical or surgical treatments.

In *controlled studies,* the group receiving an experimental drug or treatment is compared with a group receiving no treatment or standard therapy. In *single-blind studies,* the subjects don't know whether they're receiving the experimental drug or treatment, or an inactive substance. In *double-blind studies,* neither the subjects nor the researchers have this information. In *prospective studies,* patients are selected, assessed, participate in the trial, and are then followed for a preset period. In *retrospective studies,* investigators look back at their past experiences with a certain group of patients.

The results of even the most careful studies aren't considered conclusive in and of themselves. The FDA reviews every new drug, as well as the research methods used to test it, before it's allowed on the market. And a new therapy is widely accepted (or rejected) only after publication of study results in a *peer-reviewed* journal (one in which scientists in the same field critique the research methods before accepting the paper) and *replication* (the repetition of the same investigation by other researchers with similar results). In recent years, a technique called **meta-analysis,** which summarizes and reviews research in a particular area, has been used to evaluate the results of several large trials in a uniform manner.

One reason why study results must be confirmed is that, no matter what treatment patients receive, one-third to one-half of all patients improve temporarily. This well-documented but little-understood phenomenon is called the *placebo effect.* Scientific trials of a new treatment must show that the patients receiving the experimental medication or therapy improve *more* than those receiving a sugar pill or mock procedure (the placebo).

As part of the nationwide effort to cut costs while maintaining quality care, more research has focused on **outcomes**—the ultimate impact of treatment. The questions that outcomes research is designed to answer include: Is treatment better or worse than no treatment? Is one treatment better than another? If a treatment is effective, is a little just as good as a lot? Does quality of life change because of treatment? Are the benefits of treatment worth the cost or the risks to the patient?

Studies of outcomes look at how patients fared with or without a specific treatment, the costs involved, and the impact of undergoing or not undergoing treatment on the patients' quality of life. Outcomes research can help determine which of several therapies or approaches provides the best results at the most reasonable costs.

Dental Care

Thanks to fluoridated water and toothpaste, and improved dental care, Americans' teeth are healthier than in the past. Today's children have far less tooth decay than their parents had, and adults are keeping their teeth longer. However, as many as 32 percent of Americans are left with none of their own teeth by age 70.[4] Without good self-care, you, too, can—and probably will—lose some teeth to decay and gum disease. The best way to prevent such problems is through proper and regular brushing and flossing.

Gum, or periodontal, **disease,** is an inflammation that attacks the gum and bone that hold your teeth in place. The culprit is **plaque,** the sticky film of bacteria that forms on teeth. More than 300 species of bacteria live under the gum-line, and about half a dozen have been linked to serious gum problems. The early stage of gum disease is called **gingivitis.** If untreated, it develops into a more serious form known as **periodontitis,** in which plaque moves down the tooth to the roots, which then become infected. In advanced periodontitis, the infection destroys the bone and fibers that hold teeth in place.

Symptoms of gum disease include bleeding during brushing or flossing, redness and puffiness of gums,

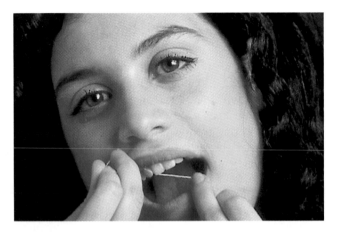

Flossing every day helps prevent gum disease and other health problems. Using a gentle sawing motion, work the floss down to your gum-line. Move the floss up and down to scrape the sides of each tooth. In this way, clean between all your teeth, using a fresh section of floss for each tooth.

tenderness or pain, persistent bad breath or a bad taste in the mouth, receding gums, shifted or loosened teeth, and changes in the way your teeth fit together when you bite. New treatments, which offer an alternative to traditional gum surgery, include a single antibiotic injection or the implant of a small antibiotic chip in the periodontal pockets to promote healing.

Taking care of your mouth isn't important only for dental health: It may affect how long you live. In one study at Emory University, people with gingivitis and periodontitis have a mortality rate that is 23 to 46 percent higher than those with healthy mouths. The reason may be that these diseases trigger an inflammatory response that causes the arteries to swell, which leads to a constriction of blood flow that can increase the incidence of cardiovascular disease. Periodontal disease also leads to a higher white blood cell count, an indicator that the immune system is under increased stress. The good news: You can prevent these problems by flossing daily and brushing your teeth and your tongue (to get rid of bacteria that can cause gum disease and bad breath).[5]

Many Americans favor dental implants, artificial teeth attached to full or partial dentures, as an option for replacing missing teeth. According to an American Dental Association (ADA), implant procedures nearly tripled in the last ten years. Tooth brighteners also have grown in popularity, but the ADA cautions against over-the-counter whitening products. Safer and more effective are in-office "power" bleaches, in which an oxidizing agent is painted onto the teeth and activated by a special light, and nightguard bleaching, which uses a bleaching gel placed in a custom-made mold and worn at night for about two weeks. Dentists often combine

these two approaches. Some dentists are using lasers to whiten teeth, but the ADA has not yet evaluated or endorsed this new approach.

Strategies *for* Prevention

Taking Care of Your Mouth

✔ Brush your teeth every morning and every night. Oral bacteria reach their highest count during sleep because fluids in the mouth accumulate. Nighttime cleaning reduces the bacterial population; morning cleaning lets you reduce the buildup.

✔ Use a toothpaste that has the American Dental Association (ADA) seal of acceptance and a toothbrush with soft, rounded bristles. Replace your toothbrush every three months.

✔ Hold the brush at a 45-degree angle from your gums. Pay particular attention to the space between your teeth and gums, especially on the inside, toward your tongue. Brush for two to five minutes. Don't brush too vigorously. If you scrub as hard as you can, you may cause damage to teeth and gums. Abrasion—a problem for more than half of American adults—erodes tooth surfaces, weakens teeth, and increases sensitivity to hot and cold foods.

✔ Because brushing can't reach plaque and food trapped between teeth, daily flossing is essential. Using waxed or unwaxed floss, start behind the upper and lower molars at one side of your mouth and work toward the other side.

✔ See your dentist twice a year for routine cleaning and examination. To find a dentist, call a local dental school, which may have a public clinic, or check with your county dental society. Ask for information regarding fees, hours, and after-hour emergency service. Your dentist should take a complete **medical history** from you and update it every six months, examine your mouth for signs of cancer, and thoroughly outline all treatment options.

✔ Make sure that everyone who works on the inside of your mouth wears a mask and rubber gloves to reduce the risk of disease transmission (that is, bacterial and viral infections, such as hepatitis, herpes, and HIV).

✔ Check out your family's dental insurance coverage. Many dental plans cover all costs for regular six-month checkups and cleanings and a percentage of the costs for fillings, gum treatment, root canals, and so on.

Getting the Best Health Care

Although considered the best in the world, the American health-care system is complex. Simply gaining access to a health-care provider can be difficult, and you may have to struggle through mountains of red tape in order to get a particular test or treatment. As discussed later in this chapter, many aspects of our health-care system are changing. However, some things remain the same, including the importance of a good doctor-patient relationship and of doing your part to get quality health care. (See Pulsepoints: "Ten Ways to Get Good Health Care.")

You and Your Doctor

Once the family doctor was indeed part of the family. The family doctor brought babies into the world, shepherded them through childhood, comforted and counseled them, stood by their bedside in their darkest hours. Patients entrusted the doctor with their cares, their confidences, their very lives. In the twentieth century, with dramatic breakthroughs in diagnosing and treating illness, the focus in medicine shifted from the family physician to the specialist, from basic caring to high-tech medical care. Patients today are more likely to be cured of a vast array of illnesses than were patients of a century ago. However, they often complain of insensitive, uncaring physicians who focus on their diseases rather than on them as individuals.

As more physicians have joined managed-care organizations (discussed later in this chapter), which emphasize efficiency, they sometimes feel pressure to see more patients a day, to spend less time with each, and to discourage expensive tests and treatments. Because physicians have less time and less autonomy, patients today must do more. Your first step should be learning more about your body, any medical conditions or problems you develop, and your options for treatment. You can find a great deal of information available via

---

PULSE *points*

Ten Ways to Get Good Health Care

1. **Trust your instincts.** You know your body better than anyone else. If something is bothering you, it deserves medical attention. Don't let your health-care provider—or your health plan administrator—dismiss it without a thorough evaluation.

2. **Inform yourself.** Go to the library or an online information service and find articles that describe what you're experiencing. The more you know about possible causes of your symptoms, the more likely you are to be taken seriously.

3. **Find a good primary care physician who listens carefully and responds to your concerns.** Look for a family doctor or general internist who takes a careful history, performs a thorough exam, and listens and responds to your concerns.

4. **See your doctor regularly.** If you're in your twenties or thir-

ties, you may not need an annual exam, but it's important to get checkups at least every two or three years, not so much for the sake of finding hidden disease, but so you and your doctor can get to know each other and develop a trusting, mutually respectful relationship.

5. **Get a second opinion.** If you are uncertain of whether to undergo treatment or which therapy is best, see another physician and listen carefully for any doubts or hesitation about what you're considering.

6. **Challenge medical judgments based on personal circumstances.** Insist that your doctor base any diagnosis on a thorough medical evaluation, not on a value judgment about you or your lifestyle.

7. **Seek support.** Patient support and advocacy groups can offer emotional support, information on many common problems, and referral to knowledgeable physi-

cians. (See the Hales Health Directory at the back of the book for numbers and addresses.)

8. **If your doctor cannot or will not respond to your concerns, get another one.** Regardless of your health coverage, you have the right to replace a physician who is not meeting your health-care needs.

9. **Speak up.** If you don't understand, ask. If you feel that you're not being taken seriously or being treated with respect, say so. Sometimes the only difference between being a patient or becoming a victim is making sure your needs and rights are not forgotten or overlooked.

10. **Bring your own advocate.** If you become intimidated or anxious talking to physicians, ask a friend to accompany you, to ask questions on your behalf, and to take notes.

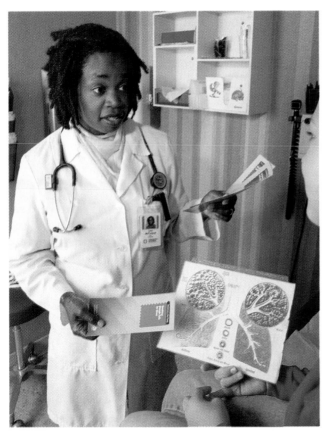

Take charge of your health—educate yourself and don't be afraid to ask your doctor questions about your care.

computer online services, patient advocacy and support organizations (see the Health Directory at the end of this book for listings), and libraries.

This information can help you know what questions to ask and how to evaluate what your doctor says. But you have to be willing to speak up. According to recent surveys, doctors give patients only 23 seconds on average during a routine visit to say what's bothering them before they interrupt.[6] This doesn't mean your doctor isn't interested, but it does mean that you have to develop good communication skills so you can tell physicians what they need to know to help you.

 ## How Should I Choose My "Primary" Care Physician?

The primary care physicians who are playing increasingly important roles in American health care include family practitioners, general internists, and pediatricians. Obstetrician-gynecologists serve as the primary providers of health care for more than half of all women. If you're a woman and your gynecologist is the only physician you see, make sure that he or she performs other tests, such as measuring your blood pressure, in addition to a pelvic and breast exam. If you develop other symptoms or health concerns, ask for an appropriate referral.

At college health centers, clinics, and some health-care organizations, consumers may be assigned to a primary physician or restricted to certain doctors. Even if your choices are limited, don't suspend your critical judgment. If you feel that your assigned physician does not listen to your concerns or is not providing adequate care, you can—and should—request another physician. Your rapport with your primary physician and the feelings of mutual trust and respect that develop between you can have as much of an impact on your well-being as your doctor's technical expertise.

When consumers can freely choose their physicians, they often do so, not just on the basis of qualifications, but also because of the physician's gender, race, or ethnic background. Frustrated by what they see as insensitive treatment by male physicians, many women are turning to female physicians—especially for gynecologic care. For other health services, women say that what matters most is having a caring physician who makes them feel comfortable and secure and invites them to participate in treatment decisions.

As the number of minority physicians has increased (up 124 percent for African-American physicians and 335 percent for Asian-American physicians from 1970 to 1980), more racial and ethnic minority group members are seeking out physicians with similar backgrounds. Often they see them as role models for their children. They may also feel that these professionals will have a natural empathy for their needs and concerns. There also are gender differences in health-care utilization. (See The X & Y Files: "Men and Women as Health-Care Consumers.") Language also affects patient choices. Some individuals, such as Mexican-American and Puerto Rican patients, find it easier to communicate with Spanish-speaking physicians.

One key to making the health-care system work for you lies in choosing a good physician. After seeing your primary care physician, ask yourself the following questions to evaluate the quality of care you are getting.

- Did your physician take a comprehensive history? Was the physical examination thorough?

- Did your physician explain what he or she was doing during the exam?

- Did he or she spend enough time with you?

- Did you feel free to ask questions? Did your physician give you straight answers? Did he or she reassure you when you were worried?

- Does your physician seem willing to admit that he or she doesn't know the answers to some questions?

- Does your physician hesitate to refer you to a specialist even when you have a complex problem that warrants such care?

Look back at your answers. If they make you feel uneasy, have a talk with your physician. Or, find a physician or a health plan that provides better service.

The X&Y Files

Men and Women as Health-Care Consumers

There are significant differences in the way the sexes use health-care services in the United States. Women see more doctors than men, take more prescription drugs, are hospitalized more, and control the spending of three of every four health-care dollars. In a national telephone poll, 76 percent of American women—but only 60 percent of men—said they had had a health exam in the last 12 months.

Many experts believe that the need for birth control and reproductive health services gets women into the habit of making regular visits to health-care professionals, primarily gynecologists. There are no comparable specialists for men, who tend to visit urologists, specialists in male reproductive organs, only when they develop problems. Men also are conditioned to take a stoic, tough-it-out attitude to early symptoms of a disease.

Men feel they are not allowed to manifest illness unless it's overt, says family practitioner Martin Miner, M.D., who has conducted research on men and health care. One reason why men die earlier than women is because of the length of time they wait to go for treatment.

The sexes also differ in the symptoms and syndromes they develop. For instance, men are more prone to back problems, muscle sprains and strains, allergies, insomnia, and digestive problems. As noted in Chapter 13, they develop heart disease about a decade earlier in life than women. More men develop ulcers and hernias; women are more likely to get gallbladder disease and irritable bowel syndrome. An estimated 3 to 6 percent of men suffer from migraines, compared with 15 to 17 percent of women. Yet women and men spend similar proportions of their lifetimes—about 81 percent—free of disability. For men, whose life spans are shorter, this translates into an average of 58.8 years; for women, 63.9 years.

There also are sex differences in access to health services. Women are more likely than men to lack health insurance, and the lower a woman's income and education, the less her likelihood of getting important preventive services, such as an annual Pap smear or prenatal care. Men and women also have different attitudes toward conventional and complementary/alternative medicine (CAM).

Women older than age 50 tend to be more satisfied with and trusting of conventional medicine than men, while younger women have less unquestioning faith in traditional medicine. Women and men are about equally likely to use complementary and alternative medicine—but different types. Men outnumber women in use of chiropractic services and acupuncture, while women are more likely to try herbal medicine, mind-body remedies, folk remedies, movement and exercise techniques, and prayer or spiritual practices. However, both sexes turn to alternative treatments for the same reason: a desire for greater control over their health

Sources: Green, Carla, and Pope, Clyde. Gender, Psychosocial Factors and the Use of Medical Services: A Longitudinal Analysis. *Social Science & Medicine,* Vol. 48, No. 10, May 15, 1999. Astin, John. Attitudes Toward Conventional Medicine and CAM: Are There Sex Differences? Presentation, Task Force on Integrative Medicine meeting, Tucson, Arizona, May 1999. Lipsyte, Robert. "Don't Take Your Medicine Like a Man," *New York Times,* February 17, 1999.

What Should I Expect in a Medical Exam?

Most physicians believe that you don't need annual checkups if you're young and feel well. However, certain types of screening tests should be performed periodically, particularly if you're 45 or older, or if you are at a higher-than-average risk of developing a particular disease, such as high blood pressure (discussed in Chapter 13) or colon cancer (discussed in Chapter 14).

Your physician will want a past medical history, including major illnesses, surgery, and treatments. Report any allergies you have, particularly to drugs, and the medications you take, including aspirin, antacids, sleeping pills, oral contraceptives, and recreational drugs, even if illegal. Your physician may also want to know about topics you consider private, such as sexually transmitted diseases. Remember that he or she is attempting to gather all the information needed to provide you with comprehensive treatment. Note, too, that a physician must report certain information—for example, certain sexually transmitted diseases—to health authorities.

After the physician has asked you questions about your complaints, medical history, and lifestyle, he or she will probably perform the standard tests described below. (See Figure 11-2.) During the examination, point out any pains, lumps, or skin growths you've noticed. If you feel pain when the physician palpates (feels) any part of your body, say so.

- *Head.* Using a flashlightlike instrument called an *ophthalmoscope*, the physician will look at the lens, retina, and blood vessels of your eyes. For patients over 40, he or she may test for a treatable eye disease called *glaucoma* (a disorder characterized by increased pressure within the eye), which can cause blindness if not detected early. The physician simply presses against the surface of each eye a soft instrument that measures the pressure within the eye and checks to see if the reading is normal. He or she will also examine your ears, mouth, tongue, teeth, and gums.

- *Neck.* Feeling around your neck, the physician will check for enlarged lymph glands (a sign of infection), for lumps in the thyroid gland, and for warning signs of stroke in the neck arteries.

- *Chest.* With a *stethoscope*, the physician will listen to the sounds made by your heart, to detect heart murmurs and irregular contractions, and by your lungs, to detect asthma or emphysema. By tapping on your chest and back with his or her fingers, the physician

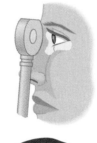
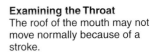
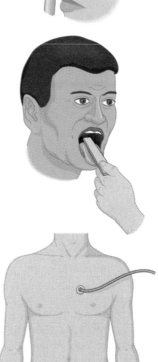
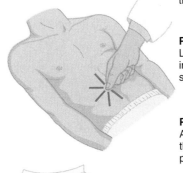
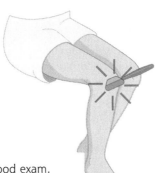

Looking into the Eyes
Changes in eye's blood vessels or the optic nerve can signal severe diabetes, high blood pressure, or a tumor in the brain.

Examining the Throat
The roof of the mouth may not move normally because of a stroke.

Listening to the Lungs
Wheezing or crackling sounds may mean asthma, bronchitis, or pneumonia.

Listening to the Heart
A "whooshing" sound, or heart murmur, means that one of the valves in the heart is not opening or closing properly.

Listening to the Abdomen
If gurgling sounds are not heard, it may mean the bowels are not working properly.

Probing the Abdomen, Right
Hepatitis or cirrhosis of the liver may change the size of the liver.

Probing the Abdomen, Left
Leukemia or a serious infection may enlarge the spleen.

Pushing on the Back
A kidney infection may make the back extremely sore to pressure.

Tapping on the Knees
Abnormal reflexes may mean problems with the brain, spinal cord, nerves, or thyroid.

Scratching the Soles of the Feet
Another reflex—the toes should curl downward in response to this. If they curl upward instead, it may be a sign of brain or spinal cord disease.

■ Figure 11-2 The basics of a good exam.

Source: Jim McManus/The *New York Times*.

can tell the size and shape of your heart, which may reveal some forms of heart disease, and whether any fluid has collected in your lungs. The physician will also check for abnormal lumps in a woman's breasts.

- *Abdomen.* Here the physician uses his or her fingers to probe for tender spots and malformations of the liver and other organs, that may reveal signs of alcoholism, hepatitis, or hernias.

- *Rectum and genitals.* With a gloved hand, the physician can feel in the rectum for growths and hemorrhoids. A rectal examination can also reveal enlargement of the male's prostate gland. The physician will check male testicles and spermatic cords for abnormalities.

- *Pelvic examination.* During a pelvic examination, a woman lies on her back, with her heels in stirrups at the end of the examining table and her legs spread out to the sides. The physician inspects the labia, clitoris, and vaginal opening. Using two gloved, lubricated fingers, the physician will check for abnormalities in the vagina, uterus, fallopian tubes, and ovaries. Many physicians will also perform a rectal or rectovaginal (one finger in the rectum and one in the vagina) examination. A nurse or other health-care worker should be present throughout the exam.

The *speculum* is a medical instrument that's used to spread the walls of the vagina so that the inside may be seen. The physician will gently scrape cells from the cervix for a **Pap smear,** a procedure that identifies abnormal cells, that may indicate an infection or, more seriously, cervical cancer, a slow-growing cancer that's usually curable if detected early (see Chapter 14). All women should start having regular Pap smears once they begin having intercourse, or at age 18. While there has been debate about how often women should have Pap smears, many health-care providers recommend Pap smears every year for women who are sexually active or have other risk factors, such as infection with the human papilloma virus (see Chapter 12).

- *Extremities.* The physician may check your knees and other joints for reflexes, which may indicate nerve disorders, and look for tremors in outstretched hands or in the face. The color, elasticity, and wetness or dryness of your skin may alert him or her to nutritional problems, or may indicate diabetes, skin cancer, and the like. Hair and nails may give indications of internal health, such as blood disorders. Swelling of the ankles can be an indication of heart, kidney, or liver disease.

- *Pulse and blood pressure.* Your physician may check your pulse in various places, looking for signs of poor circulation. The rhythm and speed of the heart may also signal diseases of the heart or thyroid gland. High blood pressure can be an early warning sign of possible heart attack, stroke, or kidney damage.

Medical Tests

Besides all the diagnostic tests listed above, the physician may order some laboratory and other tests, including the following: (See also the Hales Health Almanac at the back of this book for a comprehensive guide to medical tests.)

- *Chest X ray.* A chest X ray can reveal abnormalities of the heart and lungs; if you're a smoker, the physician may insist on one.

- *Electrocardiogram.* The *electrocardiogram* is a test performed while you're at rest that records the electrical activity of your heart. It can show irregularities in heart rhythm or muscle damage, as well as hardening of the arteries.

- *Urinalysis.* Your urine may be analyzed by a medical laboratory. If sugar (glucose) is found in your urine, your physician may order a separate blood test to check for diabetes. The presence of blood cells may indicate infection of the bladder or kidneys. Abnormal amounts of albumin (protein) in the urine may also suggest kidney disease.

- *Blood tests.* The physician or laboratory technician may draw blood to do a blood cell count. An excess of white blood cells may be an indication of infection or, occasionally, leukemia. A deficiency of red blood cells may indicate anemia. A sample of your blood may also be analyzed to measure the levels of its various components. High levels of glucose may indicate

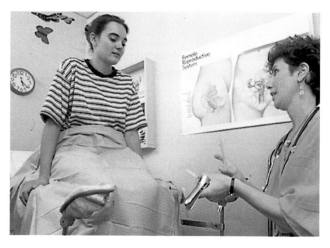

Many women choose female health-care practitioners to provide gynecologic services.

diabetes, and high levels of uric acid may mean gout or kidney stones. A high cholesterol level may indicate cardiac risk (see Chapter 13).

Strategies *for* Prevention

The Whats, Whys, and Hows of Testing

✔ Before undergoing any test, find out why you need it. Get a specific answer, not a "just in case" or "for your peace of mind." If you've had the test before, could the earlier results be used? Would a follow-up exam be just as helpful?

✔ Get some practical information as well: Are there specific things you should do before the test (such as not eat for a specified period)? How long will the test take? What will the test feel like? Will you need help getting home afterward?

✔ Check out the risks. Any invasive test—one that penetrates the body with a needle, tube, or viewing instrument—involves some risk of infection, bleeding, or tissue damage. Tests involving radiation also present risks. In addition, some people develop allergic reactions to the materials used in testing.

✔ Get information on the laboratory that will be evaluating the test. Ask how often **false positives** or **false negatives** occur. (False positives are abnormal results indicating that you have a particular condition when you really don't; false negatives indicate that you don't have a particular condition when you really do.) Find out about civil or criminal **negligence** suits filed against the laboratory on charges such as failing to diagnose cervical cancer because of incorrect reading of Pap smears.

✔ You'll also want to know what happens when the test indicates a problem: Will the test be repeated? Will a different test be performed? Will treatment begin immediately? Could any medications you're taking (including nonprescription drugs, like aspirin) affect the testing procedures or results?

Developing a Treatment Plan

After your exam, the physician will report his or her findings about your health and complaints, and advise you as to treatment. Depending on your problem, your physician may recommend an **over-the-counter (OTC)** drug, such as aspirin or an antihistamine; prescribe a medication; or recommend more invasive treatment, such as surgery. Medications are discussed in Chapter 19 on drug use.

Once a treatment recommendation has been made, you face a decision: Do you follow the advice? Be sure you understand fully the consequences of what you do—or don't do. You may be risking harm if, for instance, you don't take the antibiotics prescribed for your strep throat, or if you stop taking them in midtreatment (strep throat can lead to heart damage). For major nonemergency procedures, get more than one physician's opinion. Eight out of ten operations are elective, meaning that they don't have to be performed to save the patient's life.

Elective Treatments

As medical technology has developed new options, millions of Americans are trying elective procedures and products that are not medically necessary, but that promise to enhance health or appearance. Some are new alternatives for correcting common problems, such as poor vision, while others offer the promise of looking younger or more attractive.

Laser Vision Surgery

Each year as many as 500,000 Americans opt for an alternative to corrective lenses: laser vision surgery. Two techniques—photorefractive keratotomy (PRK) and Lasik—reshape the cornea to correct nearsightedness (myopia), farsightedness (hyperopia), and astigmatism. According to follow-up data, the vision of more than 90 percent of patients improved to 20/40 or better. Complications of laser surgery include glare, sensitivity to bright lights, and poor night vision. Costs run as high as $5,000; most health insurance plans do not cover the procedure.[7]

Cosmetic Surgery

An ever-growing number of Americans are undergoing cosmetic surgery to change the way they look—and the way they feel about themselves. Since 1992, cosmetic surgery has risen a dramatic 153 percent, and plastic surgeons perform an estimated 2.2 million procedures a year. According to the American Society of Plastic and Reconstructive Surgeons (ASPRS), 90 percent of patients are women, but more men are also undergoing cosmetic treatments. The number of men having liposuction (removal of fatty tissue) has tripled since 1992, while those having face-lifts almost doubled. Men and women between ages 35 and 50 account for 46 percent of cosmetic procedures. Health insurance rarely covers cosmetic procedures, which range in cost from $300 to upwards of $10,000.

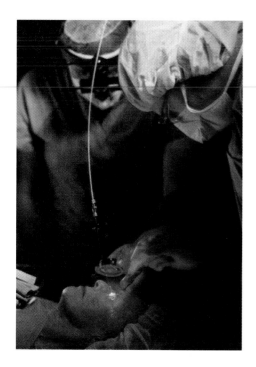 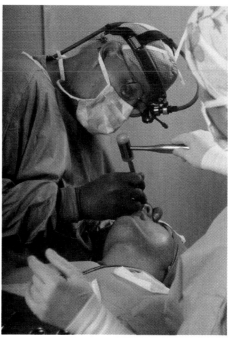

Elective treatments like laser vision surgery and cosmetic surgery can help some, but are not without risk and are generally not covered by health insurance plans.

The most commonly performed operation is liposuction, the removal of fatty tissue by means of a vacuum device. It can be performed on many areas of the body, from sagging jowls to midsection "love handles." Risks and complications include infection, numbness, bleeding, discoloration, lumpiness, and, if too much tissue is removed without proper cautions, potentially fatal complications. The ASPRS estimates that the mortality rate is one in 5,000 liposuction patients. Several states are considering legislation to tighten restrictions on training and credentialing doctors who perform liposuction.

Breast augmentation is the second most common cosmetic procedure, and surgeons report a 300 percent increase in demand in the last six years. In 1999 the Institute of Medicine, after reviewing all available evidence, reported that there appears to be no link between breast implants and autoimmune disease, connective tissue disorders, or cancer. However, today's surgeons use implants filled with a saltwater solution. Patients still face possible complications, including rupture, scarring, infection, and leaking or hardening of their implants.[8]

Your Medical Rights

As a consumer, you have basic rights that help ensure that you know about any potential dangers, receive competent diagnosis and treatment, and retain control and dignity in your interactions with health-care professionals. Many hospitals publish a patient's bill of rights, including your rights to know whether a procedure is experimental; to refuse to undergo a specific treatment; to designate someone else to make decisions about your care if and when you cannot; and to leave the hospital, even against your physician's advice. (See the Self-Survey: "Are You a Savvy Health-Care Consumer?")

You have the right to be treated with respect and dignity, including being called "Mr." or "Ms." or whatever you wish, rather than by your first name. Make clear your preferences. If you feel that health-care professionals are being condescending or inconsiderate in any way, say so—in the same tone and manner that you would like others to use with you. If you're hospitalized, find out if there's a patient advocate or representative at your hospital. These individuals can help you communicate with physicians, make any special arrangements, and get answers to questions or complaints.

You have the right to give consent to donate an organ while alive, or have your organs removed in the event of an accident, injury, or illness that leaves you brain-dead. (See Chapter 19 for definitions of death.) However, you cannot agree to donate a body part for money or other compensation. Congress has prohibited the marketing of organs; any attempt to do so is a felony punishable by up to five years in jail and a $50,000 fine.

Your Right to Information

By law, a patient must give consent for hospitalization, surgery, and other major treatments. **Informed consent** is a right, not a privilege. Use this right to its fullest. Ask questions. Seek other opinions. Make sure that your

Self-*Survey* Are You a Savvy Health-Care Consumer?

1. You want a second opinion, but your doctor dismisses your request for other physicians' names as unnecessary. Do you:
   a. Assume that he or she is right and you would merely be wasting time
   b. Suspect that your physician has something to hide and immediately switch doctors
   c. Contact your health plan and request a second opinion

2. As soon as you enter your doctor's office, you get tongue-tied. When you try to find the words to describe what's wrong, your physician keeps interrupting. When giving advice, your doctor uses such technical language that you can't understand what it means. Do you:
   a. Prepare better for your next appointment
   b. Pretend that you understand what your doctor is talking about
   c. Decide you'd be better off with someone who specializes in complementary/alternative therapies and seems less intimidating

3. You feel like you're running on empty, tired all the time, worn to the bone. A friend suggests some herbal supplements that promise to boost energy and restore vitality. Do you:
   a. Immediately start taking them
   b. Say that you think herbs are for cooking
   c. Find out as much as you can about the herbal compounds and ask your doctor if they're safe and effective

4. Your hometown physician's office won't give you a copy of your medical records to take with you to college. Do you:
   a. Hope you won't need them and head off without your records
   b. Threaten to sue
   c. Politely ask the office administrator to tell you the particular law or statute that bars you from your records

5. Your doctor has been treating you for an infection for three weeks, and you don't seem to be getting any better. Do you:
   a. Talk to your doctor, by phone or in person, and say, "This doesn't seem to be working. Is there anything else we can try?"
   b. Stop taking the antibiotic
   c. Try an herbal remedy that your roommate recommends

6. Your doctor suggests a cutting-edge treatment for your condition, but your health plan or HMO refuses to pay for it. Do you:
   a. Try to get a loan to cover the costs
   b. Settle for whatever treatment options are covered
   c. Challenge your health plan

7. You call for an appointment with your doctor and are told nothing is available for four months. Do you:
   a. Take whatever time you can get whenever you can get it
   b. Explain your condition to the nurse or receptionist, detailing any symptoms and pain you're experiencing
   c. Give up and decide you don't need to see a doctor at all

8. Even though you've been doing sit-ups faithfully, your waist still looks flabby. When you see an ad for waist-whittling liposuction, do you:
   a. Call for an appointment
   b. Talk to a health-care professional about a total fitness program that may help you lose excess pounds
   c. Carefully research the risks and costs of the procedure

9. You have a condition that you do not want anyone to know about, including your health insurer and any potential employer. Do you:
   a. Use a false name
   b. Give your physician a written request for confidentiality about this condition
   c. Seek help outside the health-care system

10. Your doctor suggests a biopsy of a funny-looking mole that's sprouted on your nose. Rather than using a laboratory that specializes in skin analysis, your HMO requires that all samples be sent to a general lab, where results may not be as precise. Do you:
    a. Ask your doctor to request that a specialty pathologist at the general lab perform the analysis
    b. Hope that in your case, the general lab will do a good-enough job
    c. Threaten to change HMOs

Answers:
1) c; 2) a; 3) c; 4) c; 5) a; 6) c; 7) b; 8) b and c; 9) b; 10) a

expectations are realistic and that you understand the potential risks, as well as the possible benefits, of a prospective treatment. Informed consent is required for research studies, but patients often don't realize that they have the right not to participate and to get complete information on the purpose and nature of the study.

Your Medical Records

You have a right to know what is in your medical records. Some states have laws assuring patient access to records. Consumer advocates advise that you routinely request records from physicians, hospitals, and laboratories—first verbally, then in writing. Privacy has become an increasing concern as patients' records have been computerized in large databases. The Medical Information Bureau (MIB) (see the Health Directory for its address and number) obtains information on individuals' medical claims and conditions from about 750 life insurance companies and combines it into the equivalent of a credit report. Anytime you fill out an application for insurance or file a claim for disability or reimbursement, your insurance company or health-care plan can contact MIB to review every medical claim you've made in the previous seven years.

To protect your privacy, don't routinely fill out medical questionnaires or histories. Always ask the purpose and find out who will have access to it. Specifically ask if your history may be entered into a computer database.[9] Tell your physician or health-care group that you do not want your records to leave their offices without your approval. Put it in writing. When you do have to authorize the release of your records, limit the information to a specific condition, physician, and hospital rather than authorizing release of all your records. Contact the MIB to find out if there is a file on you and ask to review it. Be sure to correct any inaccuracies.[10]

Your Right to Good, Safe, Care

Concern about **malpractice** suits provides an incentive for physicians to provide high-quality care. The essence of a malpractice suit is the claim that the physician failed to meet the standard of care required of a reasonably skilled and careful medical doctor. Although physicians don't have to guarantee good results to their patients and aren't held liable for unavoidable errors, they are required to use the same care and judgment in treatment that other physicians in the same specialty would use under similar circumstances. To protect themselves financially, physicians, particularly those in surgical specialties who are most likely to be sued, pay tens of thousands of dollars a year in malpractice-

insurance premiums. Some of this cost is passed on to patients.

Most lawsuits are based on negligence and assert that a physician failed to render diagnosis and treatment with appropriate professional knowledge and skill. Other cases are brought for failure to provide information, obtain consent, or respect a patient's confidentiality. However, analysis of malpractice cases has shown that, in 70 to 80 percent, a doctor's attitude and inability to communicate effectively—by devaluing patients' views, delivering information poorly, failing to understand patients' perspectives, or displaying an air of superiority—also played a role.

The Public Citizen Health Research Group has compiled a national directory of "questionable physicians," which lists physicians disciplined by state medical boards or the federal government for offenses ranging from overprescribing drugs to sexual misconduct to negligent or substandard care. Some of these physicians committed minor misdeeds, such as failing to complete continuing medical education requirements. Consumer advocates urge patients to find out why a particular name appears on the list by calling the state licensing board. At the federal level, the agencies most involved in ensuring quality health care are the Food and Drug Administration (FDA), which approves the production and labeling of drugs; and the Federal Trade Commission (FTC), which oversees advertising and prohibits deceptive or false claims.

Quackery

Every year millions of Americans go searching for medical miracles that never happen. In all, they spend more than $10 billion on medical **quackery,** unproven health products and services. Those who lose only money are the lucky ones. Many also waste precious time, during which their conditions worsen. Some suffer needless pain, along with crushed expectations. Far too many risk their lives on a false hope—and lose.

The peddlers of such false hopes are quacks, who, by definition, promote for profit worthless or unproven treatments. The Internet has become a popular method for quacks to promote themselves and their wares."[11] A quack's greatest skill is telling people what they want to hear. Quackery's most recent disguise has been in the form of untested treatments for cancer, HIV infection and AIDS, and other life-threatening conditions.

Many men and women who aren't ill or in pain take various powders and extracts to enhance their health or delay aging. Some see lifestyle or self-care approaches, such as taking megadoses of vitamins or eating special foods, as a means of staying in control of their bodies and preventing disease or deterioration.

Strategies *for* Prevention

Protecting Yourself Against Quackery

✔ Arm yourself with up-to-date information about your condition or disease from appropriate organizations, such as the American Cancer Society or the Arthritis Foundation, which keep track of unproven and ineffective methods of treatment.

✔ Ask for a written explanation of what a treatment does and why it works, evidence supporting all claims (not just testimonials), and published reports of the studies that have been done, including specifics on numbers treated, doses, and side effects. Be skeptical of self-styled "holistic practitioners," treatments supported by crusading groups, and endorsements from so-called experts or authorities.

✔ Don't part with your money quickly. You need to be especially careful because insurance companies won't reimburse for unproven therapies.

✔ Don't discontinue your current treatment without your physician's approval. Many physicians encourage supportive therapies—such as relaxation exercises, meditation, or visualization—as a supplement to standard treatments.

Sometimes individuals with certain diseases, such as arthritis or multiple sclerosis, who try unproven remedies do indeed improve. "If someone with arthritis starts feeling better the day after getting a copper bracelet, the bracelet will get the credit," says one physician. "Yet it's just coincidence." This is one reason scientists put little stock in enthusiastic testimonials from people who genuinely believe they have been helped by a new drug or treatment. Their heartfelt stories can be persuasive but are scientifically meaningless. The satisfied patient may not actually have had the disease in the first place, may have gotten other treatments too, or may be responding to a remedy that masks the symptoms without treating the disease.

Complementary and Alternative Medicine

The last decade has seen an enormous increase in interest in and use of a broad range of therapies sometimes called "alternative," "unconventional," or "holistic." The medical research community uses the term **complementary and alternative medicine**"(CAM) to apply to all health-care approaches, practices, and treatments not widely taught in medical schools, not generally used in hospitals, and not usually reimbursed by medical insurance companies.[12]

CAM includes many healing philosophies, approaches, and therapies, including preventive techniques designed to delay or prevent serious health problems before they start and **holistic** methods that focus on the whole person and the physical, mental, emotional, and spiritual aspects of well-being. Some approaches are based on the same physiological principles as traditional Western methods; others, such as acupuncture, are based on different healing systems.

According to national surveys, 40 to 45 percent of Americans say they have tried at least one nontraditional treatment.[13] Americans make more visits (an estimated 629 million) to alternative practitioners than they do to primary care physicians and spend a total of $27 billion in annual out-of-pocket expenditures—close to the $29 billion in out-of-pocket payments spent on all physician services. This figure includes money for practitioners, herbal remedies, megavitamins, diet products, and books, classes, and equipment. Most people use CAM along with their traditional medical care. (See Figure 11-3.)

Integrative medicine, which brings together both traditional and CAM, is gaining greater acceptance within the medical community. More medical schools are teaching courses in CAM,[14] and more than 60 percent of physicians say they've recommended alternative therapies to their patients at least once in the preceding year. In one study, 47 percent of physicians said they had used alternative therapies themselves; 23 percent incorporated them into their practices.[15] More than 70 percent of university-affiliated pediatrics programs use biofeedback, imagery, massage, acupuncture, art and music therapy, and other alternative therapies to manage pain in chronically ill children. More than two-thirds of health maintenance organizations cover at least one form of CAM, but the majority of people pay with their own funds.[16]

Why People Use Complementary and Alternative Therapies

People seek out CAM for various reasons, including dissatisfaction with or skepticism about conventional medicine and a desire for greater personal control over their health. Many see alternative therapies as more compatible with their worldview, values, and beliefs regarding nature and the meaning of health and illness. People who use CAM tend to have more education and believe that body, mind, and spirit are all involved in health. (See Campus Focus: "Education and Use of Complementary/Alternative Medicine.") They also have poorer health and report more anxiety, back problems, chronic pain, or urinary tract conditions.[17]

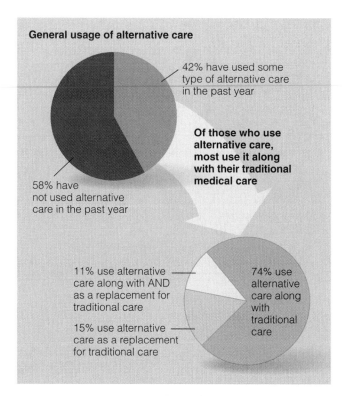

General usage of alternative care

42% have used some type of alternative care in the past year

58% have not used alternative care in the past year

Of those who use alternative care, most use it along with their traditional medical care

74% use alternative care along with traditional care

11% use alternative care along with AND as a replacement for traditional care

15% use alternative care as a replacement for traditional care

■ Figure 11-3 Americans and complementary/alternative medicine.

Source: "The Landmark Report II on HMOs and Alternative Care." Sacramento, Ca.: Landmark Healthcare, 1999.

An estimated 10 to 50 percent of cancer patients try alternative treatments. The American Cancer Society and the National Cancer Institute have cosponsored conferences on integrating conventional and CAM therapies. They also are supporting research into various alternative approaches in cancer care, such as the use of vitamin A derivatives, green tea, melatonin, and shark cartilage.[18]

Cancer patients seek out alternatives as way of taking an active role in their treatment and to be sure that "everything possible is being done," according to one survey of 164 patients. In this group, 24 percent tried nontraditional therapies. They were more likely to be young and employed and to have already undergone conventional radiation and chemotherapy.[19] Other research suggests that cancer patients in the greatest emotional distress may seek out alternative treatments. In a study of 480 women newly diagnosed with early-stage breast cancer, 28 percent began using CAM after surgery. Three months later these women had higher ratings of depression, fear of recurrence, and physical symptoms and lower scores for mental health and sexual satisfaction.[20]

"These results contrast starkly with the widely held image of the woman who seeks help from alternative medicine as self-assertive, psychologically strong, and well adjusted—a woman who likes the sense of control and empowerment she gains from finding products used in alternative medicine on the Internet, in online chat rooms, and in health food stores," commented noted cancer specialist Jimmie Holland, M.D., who speculated that physicians may not recognize patients' psychological problems or may fail to refer them for psychological counseling. They may turn to alternative medicine, in her view, "because they believe it is natural, harmless, and psychologically supportive."[21] (One year after their surgery, all of the women in the study reported similar levels of psychological well-being and quality of life, regardless of whether they had tried CAM.)

Others have criticized health-care providers for giving alternative therapies "a free ride" by not demanding the same proof and regulation required of traditional treatments.[22] Under current FDA regulations, testing required of natural health products is the same as required for food, not drugs, which allows them to be marketed without proof of purity, standardization of ingredients, or proof of medicinal efficacy. "There cannot be two kinds of medicine," the editors of the prestigious *New England Journal of Medicine* have written, "There is only medicine that has been adequately tested and medicine that has not, medicine that works and medicine that may or may not work."[23]

Many doctors are calling upon their colleagues, not to dismiss or embrace CAM, but to consider each approach thoroughly and evaluate its potential to benefit patients. "In the future, the terms *alternative* and *complementary* may well be passé, and research will have integrated what works into our everyday practices," one primary care physician observes. "Then we won't have to draw a line in the sand, saying that one treatment is **allopathic** or **osteopathic** and another is alternative."

 ## Is Alternative Medicine Effective?

In 1998, Congress created the National Center for Complementary and Alternative Medicine (NCCAM), formerly the Office of Alternative Medicine, as part of NIH. With a research budget of $50 million, NCCAM conducts and supports studies using the same rigorous standards applied to conventional medicine and disseminates information to patients and health-care consumers. Current studies are investigating shark cartilage as a cancer treatment, St. John's Wort for depression, and a complex nutritional approach to pancreatic cancer. "There's a lot to learn," one NIH official comments. "There's probably also a lot to debunk."[24]

As more studies are conducted, some alternative therapies are indeed gaining acceptance, while others

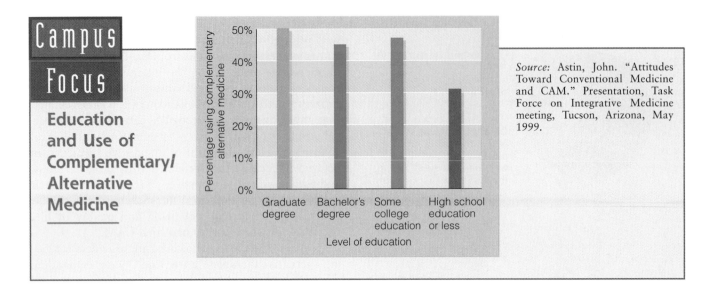

Campus Focus

Education and Use of Complementary/Alternative Medicine

Source: Astin, John. "Attitudes Toward Conventional Medicine and CAM." Presentation, Task Force on Integrative Medicine meeting, Tucson, Arizona, May 1999.

have shown little or no demonstrable benefits.[25] Among the forms of CAM that have proven effective are:

- *Moxibustion* (burning of Chinese herbs) directly over a specific acupuncture point to help breech fetuses turn around in the womb. A study of 260 pregnant women found that 98 of the 130 babies in the moxibustion group were born head-first (the preferred way), compared to 62 of the 130 babies whose mothers were not treated.[26]

- *Chinese herbs* for irritable bowel syndrome. Chinese herbs (including Dang Shen, Huo Xiang and Wu Wei Zi) proved more effective than placebo in relieving diarrhea, abdominal pain, and other symptoms.[27]

- *Saw palmetto* for enlarged prostate gland. Men with benign prostatic hyperplasia who took this herbal remedy were twice as likely to report improvement as those taking a placebo.[28]

Other treatments have not proven useful or may be dangerous for certain people. For instance, St. John's wort, a popular mood elevator, in combination with antidepressant medications such as Prozac and Paxil, can be risky, because all of these medicines boost levels of the brain chemical serotonin.[29] (See Chapter 4 for more discussion of St. John's wort.) Research has shown that engaging in yoga after open heart surgery can be hazardous.[30]

NCCAM has classified CAM practices into seven categories (see Table 11-2). The three most widely used approaches are chiropractic, herbal medicine, and acupuncture.

Chiropractic

Chiropractic is a treatment method based on the theory that many human diseases are caused by misalignment of the bones (subluxation). Chiropractors are licensed in all 50 states, but chiropractic is considered a mainstream therapy by some and a form of CAM by others. Significant research in the last ten years has demonstrated its efficacy for acute lower-back pain. NIH is funding research on other potential benefits, including headaches, asthma, middle ear inflammation, menstrual cramps, and arthritis.[31]

Chiropractors, who emphasize wellness and healing without drugs or surgery, may use X rays and magnetic

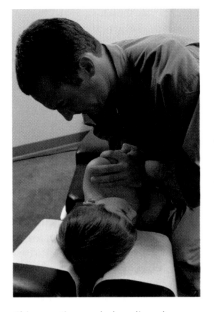

Chiropractic may help relieve lower-back pain.

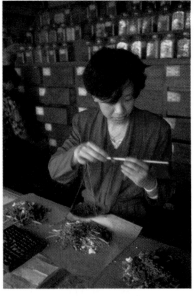

Herbal medicines are a popular form of alternative medicine.

■ Table 11-2 Complementary and Alternative Medicine Practices

The National Center for Complementary and Alternative Medicine (NCCAM) developed the following categories of classifications.

Mind-Body Medicine

These approaches include many behavioral medicine techniques, such as journaling, as well as hypnosis, yoga, meditation, biofeedback, imagery, music, art and dance therapy, spiritual healing, and community-based approaches (for example, Alcoholics Anonymous and Native American "sweat" rituals).

Alternative Medical Systems

These include acupuncture, Oriental medicine, tai chi, external and internal Qi, Ayurvedic medicine, naturopathy, and unconventional Western systems, such as homeopathy and orthomolecular medicine.

Lifestyle and Disease Prevention

Approaches include health promotion, medical intuition, and behavioral changes, such as exercise and stress management.

Biologically Based Therapies

These include botanical medicine or phytotherapy, the use of individual herbs or combinations; special diet therapies, such as macrobiotics, Ornish, McDougall, and high fiber; Mediterranean orthomolecular medicine

(use of nutritional and food supplements for preventive or therapeutic purposes); and use of other products (such as shark cartilage) and procedures applied in an unconventional manner not covered in other categories.

Manipulative and Body-Based Systems

These are systems based on manipulation and/or movement of the body, divided into three subcategories: chiropractic medicine; massage and body work (including osteopathic manipulation, Swedish massage, Alexander technique, reflexology, Pilates, acupressure, and rolfing); and unconventional physical therapies (including colonics, hydrotherapy, and light and color therapies).

Biofield

These systems use subtle energy fields in and around the body for medical purposes. They include therapeutic touch, SHEN, and biorelax methods.

Bioelectromagnetics

Bioelectromagnetics refers to the unconventional use of electromagnetic fields for medical purposes.

Source: NCCAM. For more information on complementary/alternative treatment, visit http://nccam.nih.gov

---

resonance imaging (MRI) as well as orthopedic, neurological, and manual examinations in making diagnoses. However, chiropractic treatment consists solely of the manipulation of misaligned bones that may be putting pressure on nerve tissue and affecting other parts of the body. About 65 percent of HMOs offer chiropractic services, which are the most widely used alternative treatment among managed care patients.[32]

Herbal/ Botanical Medicine

The **herbal medicine** and natural products market grew dramatically in the 1990s, to an estimated $12 billion in annual sales in 1999 (approaching the $17 billion that Americans spend each year on over-the-counter drugs).[33] In 1991 just three percent of Americans reported using herbal medicine; by 1998 37 percent had tried an herbal remedy at least once.[34] (See Table 11-3.)

An estimated 15 million adults take prescription medications along with herbal remedies and/or high-dose vitamins. However, there are dangers in doing so. When dextromethorphan, an ingredient in cough syrup, is taken with St. John's wort, it can cause sero-

tonin syndrome, a potentially fatal condition characterized by rapid pulse, high fever, and convulsions. Other herbs, such as ginkgo biloba, should not be taken with blood thinners. The American Society of Anesthesiologists has issued a warning to consumers using herbal medicines to stop taking them at least two to three weeks before surgery because they may deepen the effects of anesthesia and cause problems with blood pressure and bleeding.[35]

Even when used alone, herbs and natural substances, just like synthetic drugs, can have side effects and risks. Some users experience allergic reactions. Recent studies have connected some herbs, including St. John's wort, echinacea, and ginkgo, with blocking contraception and, in other cases, with infertility. St. John's wort has also been linked to high blood pressure. Echinacea, used for fighting off cold and flu symptoms, may exacerbate autoimmune disorders, such as lupus, rheumatoid arthritis, and multiple sclerosis. There also are suggestions of genetic damage to sperm with several popular herbs.[36]

Unlike over-the-counter and prescription drugs, "natural" remedies have not been subject to rigorous testing. The FDA categorizes herbs as "dietary supplements," which are not subject to the same efficacy and safety trials that all new drugs must undergo. Under the provisions of the 1994 Dietary Supplement Health and Education Act,

■ **Table 11-3** Popular Herbal Remedies

Herb	Used For	Does It Work?	Warning
Acidophilus	Diarrhea, digestive problems, upset stomach, or yeast infections caused by use of antibiotics.	Acidophilus, either in live lactobacillus acidophilus cultures in yogurt or in capsules, can restore the body's normal bacterial balance.	Refrigerate to preserve potency.
Aloe vera	Sunburn, cuts, burns, eczema, psoriasis.	In studies on both humans and animals, aloe vera applied directly to the skin has been shown to speed healing and have antibacterial, anti-inflammatory, and mild anesthetic effects.	Refrigerate gel to extend its shelf life.
Chamomile	Relaxation, better sleep, stomach aches, menstrual cramps.	Laboratory and animal studies indicate that chamomile's active compounds have properties that combat inflammation, bacterial infection, and spasms.	People allergic to plants in the daisy family, such as ragweed, may have an allergic reaction.
Echinacea	Colds and flu.	Inconsistent findings, although one study found that flu sufferers who used echinacea extract recovered more quickly than others.	Use for more than eight weeks at a time may lessen its effectiveness and suppress immunity. Should not be taken by pregnant women and those with diabetes, tuberculosis, or autoimmune disorders.
Evening Primrose Oil	PMS, endometriosis, eczema.	Although at least one clinical trial found that evening primrose oil does relieve endometriosis symptoms, the research on its effects on PMS and eczema has been inconclusive.	Some users report nausea or headache.
Garlic	Fighting infection, preventing heart disease and cancer, stimulating the immune system.	Extensive laboratory and animal studies and a review of clinical trials have shown that the active ingredient in garlic has anti-infective and anti-tumor properties and lowers cholesterol.	Check with your doctor if you take blood-thinning medication, including aspirin or ibuprofen, because garlic also is an anticoagulant.
Ginkgo Biloba	Improving memory, cognition, and circulation.	There is some evidence that ginkgo biloba can help stabilize mental deterioration in patients with early Alzheimer's disease or stroke-related dementia. One study found that healthy seniors who took ginkgo performed mental tasks better.	Do not take with aspirin because of risk of excessive bleeding. Should not be used during pregnancy. Side effects include upset stomach, headache, and an allergic skin reaction.
Ginseng	Improving mental and physical energy and stamina.	Small studies have shown that ginseng can help improve mental performance and respiratory function during exercise.	If used for more than two weeks, ginseng can cause nervousness and heart palpitations, especially in those with high blood pressure.
Goldenseal	Colds, allergies, upper respiratory tract infections.	Little research has been done, but some laboratory and animal studies suggest that one of goldenseal's components may have some antibiotic and antihistamine effects.	Goldsenseal should not be used instead of traditional antibiotics and should never be used for more than ten days at a time. Long-term use may interfere with the normal bacterial balance in the digestive system.

■ **Table 11-3** Popular Herbal Remedies (continued)

Herb	Used For	Does It Work?	Warning
Valerian	Anxiety, insomnia.	People who take valerian at bedtime report that they fall asleep more quickly and wake without morning drowsiness.	Some users have experienced agitation.

herbal medicine manufacturers can advertise the supposed benefits of their wares as long as they don't claim that the products affect a specific illness.[37]

Some botanicals, such as an amphetamine-like herb called ephedra, or Ma huang, sold as an energy booster and weight loss aid, can cause dangerous rises in blood pressure and speed up the heart rate. More than 800 injuries and 17 deaths have been linked to this herb. The FDA has proposed a limit on the amount of ephedra that can be added to supplements and has issued warnings on other potentially dangerous herbs, including chaparral, comfrey, yohimbe, Lobelia, germander, willow bark, Jin Bu Huan, and products containing Magnolia or Stephania.

Another problem with using herbal preparations wisely is that potency varies greatly, depending on the form in which they're used. The U. S. Pharmacopeia, a nonprofit organization that sets strength and purity standards for prescription and over-the-counter drugs, has published standards for some popular botanicals. Those that meet these standards have "NF" (for National Formulary) on the package. The FDA also now requires a "supplements facts" panel on the label, similar to the nutritional facts panel on most foods. It contains information on which part of the plant was used to make the product and how much is an appropriate amount to use.[38]

Acupuncture

An ancient Chinese form of medicine, **acupuncture** is based on the philosophy that a cycle of energy circulating through the body controls health. Pain and disease are the result of a disturbance in the energy flow, which can be corrected by inserting long, thin needles at specific points along longitudinal lines, or *meridians*, throughout the body. Each point controls a different corresponding part of the body. Once inserted, the needles are rotated gently back and forth or charged with a small electric current for a short time. Western scientists aren't sure exactly how acupuncture works, but some believe that the needles alter the functioning of the nervous system.

In *acupressure*, the therapist uses his or her finger and thumb to stimulate certain points, relieve pain, and relax muscles. **Reflexology** is based on the theory that massaging certain points on the foot or hand relieves stress or pain in corresponding parts of the body. These methods seem most effective in easing chronic pain, arthritis, and withdrawal from nicotine, alcohol, or drugs.

An NIH consensus development panel that evaluated current research into acupuncture concluded that there is "clear evidence" that acupuncture can control nausea and vomiting in patients after surgery or while undergoing chemotherapy and relieve postoperative dental pain. The panel said that acupuncture is "probably" also effective in the control of nausea in early pregnancy and that there were "reasonable" studies showing that the use of acupuncture, by itself or as an adjunct to other therapies, resulted in satisfactory treatment of a number of other conditions, even though there was not "firm evidence of efficacy at this time." These conditions include addiction to illicit drugs and alcohol (but not to tobacco), stroke rehabilitation, headache, menstrual cramps, tennis elbow, general muscle pain, low back pain, carpal tunnel syndrome, and asthma.[39]

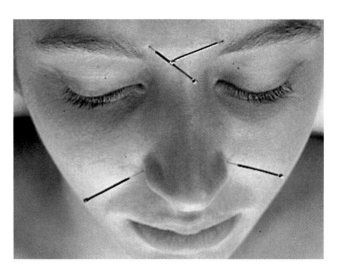

The ancient Chinese practice of acupuncture produces healing through the insertion and manipulation of needles at specific points throughout the body. The procedures are not painful.

Other Alternative Treatments

Considered alternative here, **ayurveda** is a traditional form of medical treatment in India, where it has evolved over thousands of years. Its basic premise is that illness stems from incorrect mental attitudes, diet, and posture. Practitioners use a discipline of exercise, meditation, herbal medication, and proper nutrition to cope with such stress-induced conditions as hypertension, the desire to smoke, and obesity. The best known advocate of ayurvedic medicine is Deepak Chopra, M.D., an endocrinologist (specialist in hormone-related disorders) who has written several books on ayurveda and the intimate relationship between consciousness and health.

Biofeedback uses machines that measure temperature or skin responses and then relays this information to the subject. In this way, people can learn to control usually involuntary functions, such as circulation to the hands and feet, tension in the jaws, and heartbeat rates. Biofeedback has been used to treat dozens of ailments, including asthma, epilepsy, pain, and Reynaud's disease (a condition in which the fingers become painful and white when exposed to cold). Many health insurers now cover biofeedback treatments.

Homeopathy is based on three fundamental principles: "like cures like"; treatment must always be individualized; and less is more—the idea that increasing dilution (and lowering the dosage) can increase efficacy. By administering doses of animal, vegetable, or mineral substances to a large number of healthy people to see if they all develop the same symptoms, homeopaths determine which substances may be given, in small quantities, to alleviate the symptoms. Some of these substances are the same as those used in conventional medicine: nitroglycerin for certain heart conditions, for example, although the dose is minuscule.

Naturopathy emphasizes natural remedies, such as sun, water, heat, and air, as the best treatments for disease. Therapies might include dietary changes (such as more vegetables and no salt or stimulants), steam baths, and exercise. Some naturopathic physicians (who are not M.D.s) work closely with medical doctors in helping patients.

Carl Simonton, M.D., a cancer specialist, developed the technique of creative **visualization**, or imaging, to help heal cancer patients, including some diagnosed as terminally ill. On the premise that positive and negative beliefs and attitudes have a great deal to do with whether people get well or die of disease, patients imagine themselves getting well— they "see," for instance, their immune-system cells marching to conquer the cancer cells. Others use visualization in different ways—for example, to create a clear idea of what they want to achieve, whether the goal is weight loss or relaxation.

Evaluating Complementary and Alternative Medicine

You should never decide on any treatment—traditional or complementary/alternative medicine (CAM)—without fully evaluating it. Here are some key questions to ask:

- **Is it safe?** The fact that a substance is "natural" or that a treatment does not require hospitalization or surgery doesn't mean it is safe. Talk to your medical doctor so you understand any particular risks to your overall health or any unknown long-term effects. Be particularly wary of unregulated products. In one report from the California Department of Health Services, 32 percent of Asian patent medicines tested contained undeclared heavy metals or pharmaceuticals.

- **Is it effective?** We know far less about the efficacy of many alternative treatments than we do about many traditional therapies. You can obtain information on what is known about the effectiveness of specific treatments from the NCCAM through its web site and information clearinghouse (http://nccam.nih.gov).

- **Is the practitioner qualified?** Many states license practitioners who provide acupuncture, chiropractic services, naturopathy, herbal medicine, homeopathy, and other treatments. Find out if yours does, and always choose a licensed professional. You also can contact medical regulatory agencies and consumer affairs departments, which provide information about a specific practitioner's license, education, and accreditation and will let you know if any complaints have been filed against him or her. Another source of information is the Internet. Many organizations of specific types of practitioners have web sites. However, remember that they are presenting information from an advocate's point of view.

- **How will a form of CAM affect any conventional treatments I am undergoing?** This is an important question for you to discuss with your doctor and to investigate by doing research online or in the library. Some combinations—such as the use of a prescription sleeping pill and sleep-inducing melatonin—can be dangerous, and some herbal remedies can interfere with hypertension drugs and increase the risks of anesthesia.

- **What has been the experience of others?** Talk to people who have used CAM for a similar problem, both recently and in the past. Keep in mind that their perspectives—positive or negative—are subjective and should not be your only criterion for selecting a therapy. Also try to find people who have been cared for by the practitioner you are considering.

- **What do you know about the practitioner?** Check out alternative health-care providers carefully: Did they complete professional affiliations? What is their educational background? What are their principles and beliefs?

- **Can you talk openly and easily with the practitioner?** Your relationship with your CAM practitioner is as important as your relationship with your medical doctor. You should feel comfortable asking questions and confident in the answers you receive.

- **Are you comfortable with the CAM care setting?** Visit the practitioner's office, clinic, or hospital. Does it put you at ease or make you feel out-of-place or anxious? How do conditions such as cleanliness and staff professionalism compare with the health-care settings you are more familiar with? Find out how many clients a practitioner sees every week and how much time is spent with each one.

- **What are the costs?** Many CAM services are not covered by HMOs or health insurers. Find out if your plan will cover any treatments. Also check what other practitioners charge for the same service so you can decide if a fee is appropriate. Regulatory agencies and professional associations often provide cost information.

Health-Care System

In the past, getting health care was fairly simple. When people were sick, they went to their family physician and paid in cash. If they didn't have enough money, the physician would still provide care. Today health care involves many more people, places, and processes. As a college student, you can turn to the student health service if you get sick. There, a nurse, nurse practitioner, physician's assistant, or medical doctor may evaluate your symptoms and provide basic care. However, you may rely on a primary care physician in your hometown to perform regular checkups or manage a chronic condition like asthma. If you're injured in an accident, you probably will be treated at the nearest emergency room. If you become seriously ill and require highly specialized care, you may have to go to a university-affiliated medical center to receive a state-of-the-art treatment.

Health-Care Practitioners

Fewer than 10 percent of health-care practitioners are physicians; other types of health professionals are assuming more important roles in delivering primary, or basic, health services. As a consumer, you should be aware of the range and special skills of the most common types of health-care providers.

Physicians

A medical doctor (M.D.) trained in American medical schools usually takes at least three years of premedical college courses (with an emphasis on biology, chemistry, and physics) and then completes four (but sometimes three or five) years of medical school. The first two years of medical school are devoted to the study of human anatomy, embryology, pharmacology, and similar basic subjects. During the last two years, students work directly with physicians in hospitals. Medical students who pass a series of national board examinations then enter a one-year internship in a hospital, followed by another two to five years of residency (depending on their specialty), which leads to certification in a particular field, or specialty.

About 500,000 of the nation's 700,000 physicians are specialists or subspecialists, who focus on a specific part of the body, organ system, type of disease, or type of treatment. Traditionally, they have had greater status and earned much larger incomes than primary care physicians—family practitioners, pediatricians, and internists—who provide preventive care, regular checkups, and routine treatments of uncomplicated medical conditions. However, in recent years, changes in health policy (such as increases in Medicare payments to primary care physicians) and in the delivery of services have given a more prominent role to primary care physicians. They now often function as "gatekeepers" who decide whether a patient needs to see a medical specialist.

Nurses

A registered nurse (R.N.) graduates from a school of nursing approved by a state board and passes a state board examination. R.N.s may have a bachelor's or an associate degree and may specialize in certain areas, such as intensive care or nurse-midwifery. Nurse practitioners, R.N.s with advanced training and experience, may run community clinics or provide screening and preventive care at group medical practices. Some have independent practices.

Licensed practical nurses (L.P.N.s), also called licensed vocational nurses, are licensed by the state. After graduating from state-approved schools of practical nursing, they must take a board exam. They work under the supervision of R.N.s or physicians. Nursing aides and orderlies assist registered and practical nurses in providing services directly related to the comfort and well-being of hospitalized patients.

Specialized and Allied-Health Practitioners

More than 60 different types of health practitioners work with physicians and nurses in providing medical services. Some, such as *occupational therapists*, have at least a bachelor's degree. Allied-health professionals may specialize in a variety of fields. *Clinical psychologists*, for example, have graduate degrees and provide a wide range of mental health services but don't prescribe medications—as do *psychiatrists*. *Optometrists*, trained in special schools of optometry, diagnose visual abnormalities and prescribe lenses or visual aids; however, they don't prescribe drugs, diagnose or treat eye diseases, or perform surgery—functions performed by *ophthalmologists*. *Podiatrists* are specially trained, licensed health-care professionals who specialize in problems of the feet.

Dentists

Most dental students earn a bachelor's degree and then complete two more years of training in the basic sciences and two years of clinical work before graduating with a degree of D.D.S. or D.M.D. (Doctor of Dental Surgery or Doctor of Medical Dentistry). To qualify for a license, graduates must pass both a written and a clinical examination. Dentists may work in general practice or choose a specialty, such as *orthodontics* (straightening teeth).

Chiropractors

Chiropractors hold the degree of Doctor of Chiropractic (D.C.), which signifies that they have had two years of college-level training, plus four years in a health-care school specializing in chiropractic, described earlier in this chapter.

Health-Care Facilities

As a prospective patient, you can choose from various options: a physician's office, a clinic, an emergency room, or a hospital. Most **primary care**—also referred to as ambulatory or outpatient care—is provided by a physician in an office, emergency room, or clinic. *Secondary care* usually is provided by specialists or subspecialists in either an outpatient or inpatient (hospital) setting. *Tertiary care*, available at university-affiliated hospitals and regional referral centers, includes special procedures such as kidney dialysis, open-heart surgery, and organ transplants.

College Health Centers

The American College Health Association estimates that about 1,500 institutions of higher learning provide direct health services. Student health centers

range in size from small dispensaries staffed by nurses to large-scale, multispecialty clinics that provide both inpatient and outpatient care and are fully accredited by the Joint Commission on Accreditation of Healthcare Organizations. Some serve only students; others provide services for faculty, staff, and family members.

On some campuses, health educators work with the student health centers to provide counseling on such topics as nutrition; tobacco, drug, and alcohol abuse; exercise and fitness; sexuality; and contraception. Some college health centers provide psychological counseling, as well as dental, pharmacy, and optometric services. Some campuses also provide sports-medicine services for student athletes. Services are paid for by various combinations of prepaid health fees, general university funds, fee-for-service charges, and health-insurance reimbursements.

Outpatient Treatment Centers

Increasingly, procedures that once required hospitalization, such as simple surgery, are being performed at outpatient centers, which may be freestanding or affiliated with a medical center. Patients have any necessary tests performed beforehand, undergo surgery or receive treatment, and return home after a few hours to recuperate. Outpatient centers can handle many common surgical procedures, including cataract removal, tonsillectomy, breast biopsy, dilation and curettage (D and C), vasectomy, and face-lifts.

Without the high overhead costs of a hospital, outpatient surgery costs run only about 30 to 50 percent of standard hospital fees. Today, 70 percent of hospitals do outpatient, or "in-and-out," surgery. To cut health-care costs, insurance companies are encouraging, or in some cases requiring, their policyholders to choose outpatient surgery. However, operations requiring prolonged general anesthesia (such as abdominal surgery) or extensive postoperative care (such as heart surgery) must still be performed on an inpatient basis.

Freestanding emergency centers (those not part of a hospital) claim that they deliver high-quality medical treatment with maximum convenience in minimal time. Critics dismiss them as impersonal and mechanized, and refer to them as "Big Mac" medicine. Nevertheless, many customers seem pleased. Rather than going to crowded hospital emergency rooms when they slice a finger in the kitchen, they can go to a freestanding emergency center and receive prompt attention.

Hospitals and Medical Centers

Different types of hospitals offer different types of care. The most common type of hospital is the *private*, or community, *hospital,* which may be run on a profit or a nonprofit basis, generally contains 50 to 400 beds, and provides more personalized care than public hospitals do. The quality of care individual patients receive depends mostly on the physicians themselves. *Public hospitals* include city, county, public health service, military, and Veterans Administration hospitals. The quality of patient care depends on the overall quality of the institution.

Of the more than 6,500 hospitals nationwide, about 300 are major *academic medical centers* or teaching hospitals. Affiliated with medical schools, they generally provide the most up-to-date and experienced care, because staff physicians must stay current in order to teach their students. These centers, with the best equipment, researchers, and resources, offer high-technology care—at a price. The cost of treatment at all teaching hospitals averages approximately 20 percent higher than at nonteaching hospitals. At major teaching hospitals with large graduate training programs for physicians and other health providers, the costs are as much as 45 percent higher than those at nonteaching hospitals. Faced with declining revenues as a result of the advent of managed care (discussed later in this chapter), teaching hospitals have been forced to make major cutbacks in personnel and patient services. Many are forming networks with other hospitals and developing less costly methods (such as home health services) to deliver health care.

The Joint Commission on the Accreditation of Healthcare Organizations (JCAH) reviews all hospitals every three years. Eighty percent of hospitals qualify for JCAH accreditation. If you have to enter a hospital and your health insurance or plan allows a choice, try to find out as much as you can about the alternatives available to you:

- Talk to your physician about a hospital and why he or she recommends it.

- As a cost-cutting strategy, many hospitals have cut back on the use of registered nurses. Check with the local nursing association about the ratio of patients to nurses, and the ratio of R.N.s to licensed practical, or vocational, nurses.

- Find out room rates and charges for ancillary services, including tests, lab work, X rays, and medications. Check with your health plan to see whether you need preapproval for any of these costs and ask what you will be expected to pay.

- Ask how many times in the past year the hospital has performed the procedure recommended for you, and what the success and complication rates have been. Ask about the hospital's nosocomial (hospital-caused) infection rate and accident rate. You also have the right to information on the number and types of malpractice claims filed against a hospital.

- If possible, go on a tour of the hospital. Does the setting seem comfortable? Is the staff courteous? Does the hospital seem clean and efficiently run?

Emergency Services. Hospital emergency rooms should be used only in a true emergency. Most are overwhelmed, understaffed, and underfinanced—particularly in big cities. Patients usually see a different physician each time; he or she deals with their main complaints but doesn't have time for a full examination. Extensive tests and procedures are difficult to arrange in an emergency room, and patients who don't have truly urgent problems may have to wait for a long time. Emergency-room fees are higher than those for standard office visits and are not always covered by medical insurance.

Inpatient Care. Inpatient hospital care remains the most expensive form of health care. Health-insurance companies and health-care plans (described below) often demand a second opinion or make their own evaluation before approving coverage of an elective, or nonemergency, hospital admission. As another means of controlling costs, health insurers (including Medicare) may limit hospital stays or pay for hospital care on the basis of **diagnostic-related groups,** or **DRGs.** Under this system, hospitals are paid according to a patient's diagnosis—for example, a set number of dollars for every appendectomy. If the hospital can treat and discharge patients more quickly than the national average for that DRG, it makes money. On the other hand, if a patient develops unexpected complications or is slow to recover, the hospital loses money.

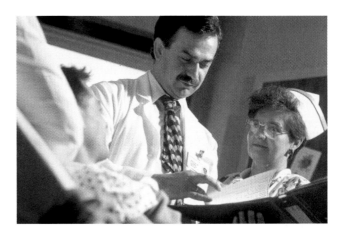

A healthy hospital stay. Read consent forms carefully and ask for more information if you don't understand. Talk to the staff and pay attention to your care routine.

Because hospital stays are shorter than in the past, patients often leave "quicker and sicker"—after a shorter stay and not as far along in their recovery. Nevertheless, the benefits of shorter hospital stays, including reduced complications and more rapid resumption of normal life activities, may outweigh the slightly increased risks associated with early discharge.

The Risks of a Hospital Stay

Hospitals are places where lives are both saved and lost, and the quality of care varies greatly. Large hospitals in big cities tend to provide better care and have lower death rates than small, rural hospitals with fewer than 100 beds.

The risks associated with hospitalization include what health workers call the "terrible I's": infection; inactivity; incorrect actions; and the inherent risks of drugs, X rays, and false lab tests. The simplest method for preventing hospital-acquired infection—handwashing—is often ignored by health-care providers.

Surgical and medication mistakes are another hazard. In highly publicized cases, hospital physicians have amputated a patient's healthy leg, operated on the wrong side of a woman's brain, and administered deadly doses of cancer drugs. As hospitals cut back on staff and services in order to control costs, the likelihood of such errors may increase.

Home Health Care

With hospitals discharging patients sooner, **home health care**—the provision of equipment and services to patients in the home to restore or maintain comfort, function, and health—has become a major industry. Advances in technology have made it possible for treatments once administered only in hospitals—such as kidney dialysis, chemotherapy, and traction—to be performed at home at 10 to 40 percent of the cost. The physician's house call, once considered an anachronism, has also come back in fashion. According to various surveys, the majority of primary care physicians see patients in their homes.

Hospital discharge planners usually arrange home health care for patients who've been hospitalized. Families can also contact health aides, nurses, and other needed professionals on their own. According to the Health Insurance Association of America, most private insurance policies offer some coverage for these home health-care costs.

Paying for Health Care

Health insurance did not become common as a standard benefit until World War II, when the government im-

posed wage controls and businesses offered free health-insurance policies to lure prospective employees. For the next 50 years, patients went to the physicians of their choice, with insurance companies usually paying part or all of their fees.

As technological breakthroughs, such as new imaging techniques and bone-marrow transplants, transformed modern medicine, subspecialists multiplied, and medical costs spiraled upward. Finally, in the 1990s, health policymakers and the employers that had footed the bills agreed that health costs, which had grown to almost 14 percent of the gross domestic product, had to be controlled. This led to the emergence of **managed care,** a new way of delivering and paying for health-care services. Managed care organizations provide health-care or health-care insurance at lower costs to employers. The tradeoff for such savings is that a third party makes the final decision on when or if a medical visit or treatment is necessary. This differs from traditional *fee-for-service* medicine, in which patients decide when to seek care and choose which physician to see. (See Figure 11-4.)

Both fee-for-service and managed-care systems have drawbacks. Fee-for-service medicine errs on the side of doing too much and providing unneeded tests and therapies. Managed-care organizations are more likely to do too little so they can keep costs low.

Traditional Health Insurance

In the past, most working Americans relied on conventional **indemnity** insurance policies to pay major medical expenses. Policyholders paid a percentage (generally 20 percent) of hospitalization costs and a deductible (a minimum paid out each year before the insurance company pays anything). While indemnity insurance gave patients freedom to choose physicians and hospitals, it often failed to cover routine physical exams and screening tests. Individuals with "preexisting" conditions often could not qualify for coverage or were not reimbursed for treatments related to these conditions. In the last decade, as health-care costs skyrocketed, insurers increasingly refused to pay claims, canceled groups with high medical bills, or denied coverage to people in high-risk occupations.

 ## What Is Managed Care?

Managed care has become the predominant form of health care in the United States. Managed-care organizations, which take various forms, deliver care through a network of physicians, hospitals, and other health-

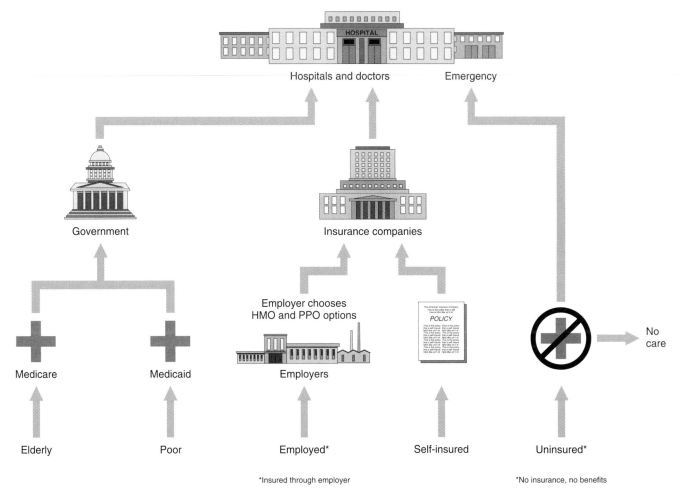

■ **Figure 11-4** Medical coverage in the United States is complex; you and your doctor are connected through a bureaucracy of policies and agencies.

care professionals who agree to provide their services at fixed or discounted rates.

Consumers in a managed-care group must follow certain procedures in advance of seeking care (for example, getting prior approval for a test or treatment) and must abide by a limit on reimbursement for certain services. Some procedures may be deemed unnecessary and not be covered at all. Patients who choose to see a physician who is not a participating member of the medical-insurance coverage group may have to pay the entire fee themselves.

Managed-care plans have been criticized for pressuring providers to "undertreat" patients—for example, sending them home from the hospital too soon or denying them costly tests or treatments. Members have complained of long waits, the need to switch primary physicians if their doctor leaves the plan, difficulty getting approval for needed services, and a sense that providers pay more attention to the bottom line than to their health needs.

As dissatisfaction with managed care has grown, consumers have demanded more choice of physicians, direct access to specialists, and the ability to go "out of network."[40] In response to consumer complaints, 39 states have approved "patient protection acts" or "comprehensive consumer bills of rights," while a total of nearly 900 laws affecting managed care have been passed by state legislators.[41] Their provisions vary, but their goal is the same: to ensure that patients get the care they need when they need it.[42] Typical provisions in these bills:

• Allow any pharmacy to provide medications for enrollees.

• Ban any limit on doctors' ability to inform patients of treatment options, especially if some choices cost more.

• Outlaw rewards to physicians for performing a less costly procedure or prescribing a less costly drug.

• Guarantee direct access to women's health specialist without referral from a primary care provider.

- Ensure a minimum 48-hour maternity stay.
- Establish a "prudent layperson" standard for emergencies. This requires insurance coverage for emergency medical conditions if they are of sufficient severity, in a nonprofessional's judgment, to place the person's health in jeopardy
- Require annual report cards on how well plans are complying with state laws and regulations.[43]

Medical professionals, particularly in academic centers, have even more negative attitudes toward managed care than their patients. In one national survey, medical students, residents, faculty members, and deans felt that managed care led to poorer access to care and harmed the doctor-patient relationship.[44] They also reported negative effects on the time they dedicate to research and teaching as well as on their incomes, job security, and relationships with colleagues.[45] In 1999 the American Medical Association voted to form a union for doctors who are salaried employees to increase their clout in dealing with managed-care organizations.[46]

Presidential order has defined a set of standards for treating individuals in federal health plans. The U. S. Congress is considering ways to reform managed care, including a new patients' bill of rights and an option for external review of cases in which managed care organizations refused to offer or reimburse for specific treatments. The government is still seeking ways in which it can hold down costs while guaranteeing high-quality health care. However, despite widespread criticisms, recent polls have found that most Americans, including those in managed care plans, are satisfied with their health care coverage.[47]

Health Maintenance Organizations (HMOs)

Health maintenance organizations, or **HMOs,** are managed-care plans that emphasize routine care and prevention by providing complete medical services in exchange for a predetermined monthly payment. (See Figure 11-5.) In a *group-model* HMO, physicians provide care in offices at a clinic run by the HMO. In an *individual practice association (IPA),* or network HMO, independent physicians provide services in their own offices. HMOs generally pay a fixed amount per patient to a physician or hospital, regardless of the type and number of services actually provided. This is called *capitation.*

Members of HMOs pay a regular, preset fee that usually includes diagnostic tests, routine physical exams, and vaccinations as well as treatment of illnesses. HMOs usually do not require a deductible, and copayments for medications or services are small. The primary draw-

back of standard HMOs is that the consumer is limited to a particular health-care facility and staff. *Open-ended* or *point-of-service* HMOs charge more but let members seek treatment elsewhere if they prefer. These "hybrid" plans have proven the most popular.

Although HMOs have been accused of undermining the quality of patient care, recent studies of the outcomes of cancer patients in HMOs and in traditional fee-for-service practices have found little difference. HMOs are, on average, more likely to detect breast cancer early and just as likely to offer breast-saving lumpectomies rather than mastectomy.[48] Prostate cancer patients treated in HMOs also had similar ten-year survival rates as those receiving fee-for-service care.[49]

One remaining difficulty in HMOs is getting a specific prescription drug. Because costs of new medications have skyrocketed, some health plans restrict their "formulary" of available drugs to older, cheaper medications or require a higher copayment for a brand-name drug or one outside the formulary.[50]

As noted earlier, most HMOs now offer at least one form of complementary or alternative care, and about 50 percent of plans report that such benefits produce cost savings. Among senior HMO executives interviewed, 85 percent expect the relationship between traditional and alternative medical care will grow closer and consumer demand for CAM will grow stronger.[51]

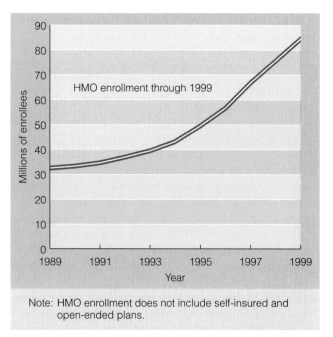

Note: HMO enrollment does not include self-insured and open-ended plans.

■ **Figure 11-5** HMOs are becoming a primary source of medical care, with membership doubling in the last decade.

Preferred Provider Organizations (PPOs)

In a **preferred provider organization (PPO)**, a third party—a union, an insurance company, or a self-insured business—contracts with a group of physicians and hospitals to treat members at a discount. PPO members may choose any physician within the network, and usually pay a 10 percent copayment for care within the system and a higher percentage (20 to 30 percent) for care elsewhere. PPOs generally require prior approval for expensive tests or major procedures.

A *point-of-service (POS)* plan is a PPO that permits patients to use physicians outside the network. Consumers pay the difference between the preferred provider's discounted fee and the outside physician's fee. A *gatekeeper* plan requires members to choose a primary physician, as in an HMO, who must approve all referrals to specialists.

Government-Financed Insurance Plans

The government provides two major forms of health financing: Medicare and Medicaid. Under Medicare, the federal government pays 80 percent of most medical bills, after a deductible fee, for people over age 65. Medicare doesn't cover drugs, eyeglasses, or dental work.

Medicaid, a federal and state insurance plan that protects people with very low or no incomes, is the chief source of coverage for the unemployed. However, many unemployed Americans don't qualify because their family incomes are above the poverty line. Publicly insured patients are more likely than those with private insurance to receive inadequate care and to experience adverse health outcomes.

The Uninsured

As many as 44 million Americans lack health insurance; many others are underinsured, meaning that they don't have adequate coverage. Eleven million children under age 19 do not have insurance coverage. (See Figure 11-6.) Uninsured patients have shorter hospital stays, cannot undergo costly therapies, and have a greater risk of dying in the hospital than insured patients. About 85 percent of uninsured Americans are from families in which the head of the family works but can't get insurance through his or her employer.[52] Some of these people work part-time and do not qualify for insurance. Others work for businesses too small to qualify for group insurance. The availability

of insurance affects both access to care and the way care is delivered.

Making This Chapter Work for You

Smart Health-Care Decisions

- The American health-care system, though considered among the best in the world, is complex and changing, and people must become savvy consumers in order to ensure that they get the best possible care.

- Self-care is an important aspect of maintaining good health and preventing disease. Home tests and equipment can identify any suspicious signs that require professional care.

- Proper dental care includes regular brushing and flossing, which can reduce the risk of cavities and of gum or periodontal disease.

- Quackery is worthless, fraudulent, or unproven treatment for incurable diseases, longer life, better health, or delayed aging.

- The term "complementary and alternative medicine" (CAM) applies to all health-care approaches, practices, and treatments not widely taught in medical schools, not generally used in hospitals, and not usually reimbursed by medical insurance companies. According to national surveys, 40 to 45 percent of

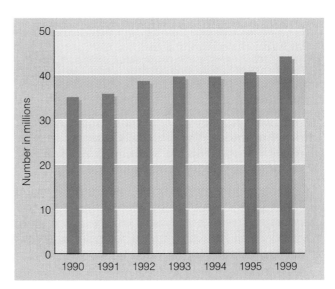

■ Figure 11-6 **The Growing Number of Uninsured in the United States**
The number of uninsured Americans grew steadily through the 1990s to 44 million.

health **/ ONLINE**

National Center for Complementary and Alternative Medicine
http://nccam.nih.gov/
Provides answers to frequently asked questions about complementary and alternative medicine; classifications of alternative therapies; an overview of six fields of practice; information on using MEDLINE (the National Library of Medicine's database) and CCI (a citation index) to research alternative medicine topics; information about CAM news and events, and more.

Agency for Health Care Policy and Research: Consumer Health
http://www.ahcpr.gov/consumer/
Provides extensive information on consumer health topics, including choosing a health plan, preventive self-care, preventive child health care, managing/treating/understanding health conditions, and more.

Consumer Information Center
http://www.pueblo.gsa.gov/health.htm
Download full-text versions of federal consumer information publications. Topics include mammography, suntanning, talking to your doctor, quitting smoking, selecting over-the-counter medicines, quackery, laser eye surgery, and much more.

Please note that links are subject to change. If you find a broken link, use a search engine like http://www.yahoo.com *and search for the web site by typing in key words.*

Campus Chat: Have you ever tried a nontraditional therapy? What did you try, what led you to try it, and what were the results? Share your thoughts on our online discussion forum at **http://health.wadsworth.com**

Find It On InfoTrac: You can find additional readings related to health via InfoTrac College Edition, an online library of more than 900 journals and publications. Follow the instructions for accessing InfoTrac that came packaged with your textbook; then search for articles using a key word search.

- **Suggested reading:** "Western Medicine Opens the Door to Alternative Medicine," by Kathleen M. Boozang. *American Journal of Law & Medicine,* Summer-Fall 1998, Vol. 24, No. 2–3, pp. 185–212.

  (1) Why do Western physicians tend to shun away from advocating alternative therapies to their patients?

  (2) Why is it difficult to subject some forms of alternative therapies to traditional scientific inquiry?

For additional links, resources, and suggested readings on InfoTrac, visit our Health & Wellness Resource Center at **http://health.wadsworth.com**

Americans say they have tried at least one nontraditional treatment. The National Center for Complementary and Alternative Medicine is evaluating the safety and efficacy of various approaches.

- As a consumer, you have the right of information about possible treatments, access to your records, respectful treatment, and safe, quality care. A health professional also can be sued for malpractice if a patient believes that the care received was substandard or that the health-care provider was negligent.

- As a consumer, you may turn to physicians, nurses, and any number of specialists and allied-health professionals.

- Health-care facilities include student health centers, clinics, hospitals, outpatient surgery centers, and freestanding emergency centers.

- Most primary care is provided by a physician in an office, emergency room, or clinic. Secondary care usually is provided by specialists or subspecialists in either an outpatient or inpatient, or hospital, setting. Tertiary care, available at university-affiliated hospitals and regional referral centers, includes special procedures such as kidney dialysis, open-heart surgery, and organ transplants.

- Increasingly, primary care physicians are playing an important role in providing basic care and serving as "gatekeepers" who determine if a patient should see a specialist.

- A thorough medical evaluation includes a medical history and a physical examination that evaluates all systems of the body and includes appropriate screening and medical tests.

■ The effort to control health-care costs has led to dramatic changes in how we pay for health care. Fewer Americans now have conventional indemnity health insurance policies, which pay physicians and hospitals for the services they perform.

■ Managed-care plans, which now dominate the health-care system, offer lower costs by providing services through an organized network of providers, who receive a fixed or discounted rate for their services.

■ Health maintenance organizations, or HMOs, are managed-care groups that emphasize preventive health care. Preferred provider organizations, or PPOs, allow consumers to choose from a preselected list of physicians and facilities.

■ The government helps defray medical expenses through two programs: Medicare, for people over age 65, and Medicaid, for people unable themselves to pay for health care.

The more you know about your body and your health, the better decisions you can make about health care. Here are a few simple steps you can take to form a partnership with the health-care professionals you see:

■ Realize that what you have to say is worth the health expert's time. Think of each professional as a highly paid consultant who's there to perform a service for you. Don't be intimidated if a health-care worker seems busy or restless. If you don't understand his or her explanations, say something like, "Please tell me about the procedure again. I'm not sure I understood everything you said."

■ Be as specific as possible in describing symptoms. Ask questions whenever you're doubtful. Try not to be rude or disagreeable. Physicians, nurses, dentists, and other health-care workers are human beings. Just like the rest of us, they pull away from confrontations with unpleasant people.

■ Inform your primary care physician about what everyone else is doing as part of your treatment. Don't assume specialists, hospital nurses, physical therapists, and others are all in contact.

■ Never leave a physician's office uncertain about the diagnosis or recommended treatment. Ask about anything that's unclear, and repeat the answers in your own words. If your physician is unwilling to talk with you or is incapable of communicating clearly, find another.

■ Your health is your most important asset. Consider the time and effort you spend learning about your body and caring for your health an investment in your future.

 Health Info on the Net. What strategies can help you find accurate online information?

Key Terms

The terms listed here are used within the chapter. Page numbers are included for each term. A definition of each term is given in the Glossary pages at the end of this book.

Critical Thinking Questions

1. Think about an experience you've had with a medical practitioner. How did you feel during the physical examination? Did you trust the practitioner? Were you comfortable with the level of communication? Evaluate your experience and give your opinion of the value of the checkup.

2. What complementary or alternative approaches to health care are you aware of? How do you feel about alternative care? Do you feel confident in knowing the difference between alternative care and quackery?

3. If you're young and healthy, you'll have little problem getting health insurance. However, if you develop a chronic illness, sustain serious injuries in an accident, or simply get older, you may find insurance harder to get and more expensive to keep. What is your insurance coverage? Do you believe insurance companies have the right to turn down applicants with preexisting conditions, such as high blood pressure? Do they have the right to require screening for potentially serious health problems, such as HIV infection, or to cancel the policies of individuals who have run up high medical bills in the past?

References

1. Weiss, Stefan. "Defining a 'Patients' Bill of Rights' for the Next Century." *JAMA*, Vol. 281, No. 9, March 3, 1999.
2. Parch, Lorie. "Do-It-Yourself Diagnoses." *American Health*, March 1999.
3. Stolberg, Sheyrl. "From M.D. to I.P.O., Chasing Virtual Fortunes." *New York Times*, July 4, 1999.
4. Graham, Janis. "What Dentists Wish You Knew." *American Health*, July-August 1999.
5. Roizen, Michael. *RealAge*. New York: HarperCollins, 1999.
6. Boland, Maureen. "Don't Be a Wimp in the Doctor's Office." *American Health*, April 1999.
7. Hales, Dianne. "Looking Your Best at Any Age." *Parade*, March 20, 1999.
8. Hales, Dianne. "If You Want a Tuck or a Lift . . . ." *Parade*, June 20, 1999.
9. Turkington, Richard. "Medical Record Confidentiality Law, Scientific Research, and Data Collection in the Information Age." *Journal of Law, Medicine & Ethics*, Vol. 25, No. 2–3, Summer–Fall 1997.
10. Woodward, Beverly. "Medical Record Confidentiality and Data Collection: Current Dilemmas." *Journal of Law, Medicine & Ethics*, Vol. 25, No. 2–3, Summer–Fall 1997.
11. Larkin, Marilynn. "Internet Accelerates Spread of Bogus Cancer Cure." *Lancet*, Vol. 353, No. 9149, Jan. 23, 1999.
12. NCCAM website: http://nccam.nih.gov
13. Eisenberg, David, et al. "Trends in Alternative Medicine Use in the United States, 1990–1997." *JAMA*, Vol. 280, No. 18, November 11, 1998.
14. Carlston, Michael, et al. "Medical School Courses in Alternative Medicine." *JAMA*, Vol. 281, No. 7, February 17, 1999. Wetzel, Miriam, et al. "Courses Involving Complementary and Alternative Medicine at U.S. Medical Schools." *JAMA*, Vol. 280, No. 9, September 2, 1998.
15. Astin, John. "Why Patients Use Alternative Medicine: Results of a National Study." *JAMA*, Vol. 280, No. 19, November 18, 1998.
16. "The Landmark Report on Public Perceptions of Alternative Care." Sacramento, Ca.: Landmark Healthcare, 1998. "The Landmark Report II on HMOs and Alternative Care." Sacramento, Ca.: Landmark Healthcare, 1999.
17. Astin, John. "Attitudes Toward Conventional Medicine and CAM." Presentation, Task Force on Integrative Medicine meeting, Tucson, Arizona, May 1999.
18. Judge, Gillian. "Alternative Cancer Treatments: Hope or Hype?" *American Health*, April 1999.
19. Henderson, Charles. "Patients Desire Active Role in Treatment." *Cancer Weekly Plus*, February 22, 1999.
20. Burstein, Harold, et al. "Use of Alternative Medicine by Women with Early-Stage Breast Cancer." *New England Journal of Medicine*, Vol. 340, No. 22, June 3, 1999.
21. Holland, Jimmie. "Use of Alternative Medicine—A Marker for Distress?" *New England Journal of Medicine*, Vol. 340, No. 22, June 3, 1999.
22. "Are 'Natural' Remedies Getting a Free Ride?" *Nursing*, Vol. 29, No. 5, May 1999.
23. Angell, Marcia, and J. Kassirer. "Alternative Medicine: The Risks of Untested and Unregulated Remedies." *New England Journal of Medicine*, September 17, 1998.
24. Couzin, Jennifer. "Beefed-Up NIH Center Probes Unconventional Therapies." *Science*, Vol. 282, No. 5397, December 18, 1998.
25. Cassileth, Carrie. *The Alternative Medicine Handbook: The Complete Reference Guide to Alternative and Complementary Therapies*. New York: W. W. Norton & Co., 1999.
26. Cardini, F, and H. Weixe. "Moxibustion for Correction of Breech Presentation." *JAMA*, Vol. 280, November 1998.
27. Bensoussan, A., et al. "Treatment of Irritable Bowel Syndrome with Chinese Herbal Medicine." *JAMA*, Vol. 280, November 1998.
28. Wilt, T. J., et al. "Saw Palmetto Extracts for Treatment of Benign Prostatic Hyperplasia." *JAMA*, Vol. 280, November 1998.
29. Hales, Robert, and Dianne Hales. *The Mind-Mood Pill Book*. New York: Bantam Books, 2000.
30. Lin, Jonathan. "Evaluating the Alternatives." *JAMA—Pulse*, Vol. 279, March 4, 1998.
31. Onderko, Patty. "Chiropractic: Beyond Back Pain." *American Health*, November/December 1998.
32. "The Landmark Report on Public Perceptions of Alternative Care." Sacramento, Ca.: Landmark Healthcare, 1998. "The Landmark Report II on HMOs and Alternative Care." Sacramento, Ca.: Landmark Healthcare, 1999.
33. Abate, Tom. "Herbal Remedies Can't Make Claims." *San Francisco Chronicle*, June 16, 1999.
34. Brevoort, Peggy. "The Booming U.S. Botanical Market: A New Overview." *HerbalGram No. 44*, 1999.

35. Nagourney, Eric. "A Warning Not to Mix Surgery and Herbs." *New York Times,* July 6, 1999.

36. Irwin, Scott, and Mary Luftus. "Add a Dose of Caution to Herbal Remedies." *New York Times,* July 13, 1999.

37. Bilger, Burkhard. "Nature's Pharmacy." *The Essential 1999 Women's Health Guide.* New York: Time, Inc., 1999.

38. Dickstein, Leslie. "Nature's Pharmacy Is Full of Surprises." *Psychology Today,* Vol. 32, No. 2, March 1999.

39. Morey, Sharon Scott. "NIH Issues Consensus Statement on Acupuncture." *American Family Physician,* Vol. 57, No. 10, May 15, 1998.

40. Kahn, Charles. "Patients' Rights Proposals: The Insurers' Perspective." *JAMA,* Vol. 281, No. 9, March 3, 1999.

41. Cauchi, Richard. "Managed Care: Where Do We Go from Here?" *State Legislatures,* Vol. 25, No. 3, March 1999.

42. Mariner, Wendy. "Going Hollywood with Patient Rights in Managed Care." *JAMA,* Vol. 281, No. 9, March 3, 1999.

43. Volpp, Kevin. "Consumer Protection and the HMO Backlash." *Inquiry,* Vol. 36, No. 1, Spring 1999.

44. Shalala, Donna. "A Patients' Bill of Rights: The Medical Student's Role." *JAMA,* Vol. 281, No. 9, March 3, 1999.

45. Westphal, Sylvia. "Academic Medicine May Lean Against Managed Care." *Focus: News from Harvard Medical, Dental and Public Health Schools,* April 2, 1999.

46. Greenhouse, Steven. "AMA's Delegates Decide to Create a Union of Doctors." *New York Times,* June 24, 1999.

47. Gold, Marsha. "The Changing U. S. Health Care Systems." *Milbank Quarterly,* Vol. 77, No. 1, Spring 1999.

48. Riley, Gerald, et al. "Stage at Diagnosis and Treatment Patterns Among Older Women with Breast Cancer: An HMO and Fee-for-Service Comparison." *JAMA,* Vol. 281, No. 8, February 24, 1999.

49. Potosky, Arnold, et al. "Prostate Cancer Treatment and Ten-Year Survival Among Group/Staff HMO and Fee-for-Service Medicare Patients." *Health Services Research,* Vol. 34, No. 2, June 1999.

50. Spragins, Ellyn. "Getting the Drug You Need." *Newsweek,* April 26, 1999.

51. "Study Finds Most HMOs Offer Alternative Care." *Best's Review—Life-Health Insurance Edition,* Vol. 99, No. 12, April 1999.

52. Jefferson, Thomas. "Care Gap 'Unconscionable': Universal Coverage AAP Aim." *JAMA,* Vol. 281, No. 22, June 9, 1999.

CHAPTER

12

Defending Yourself from Infectious Diseases

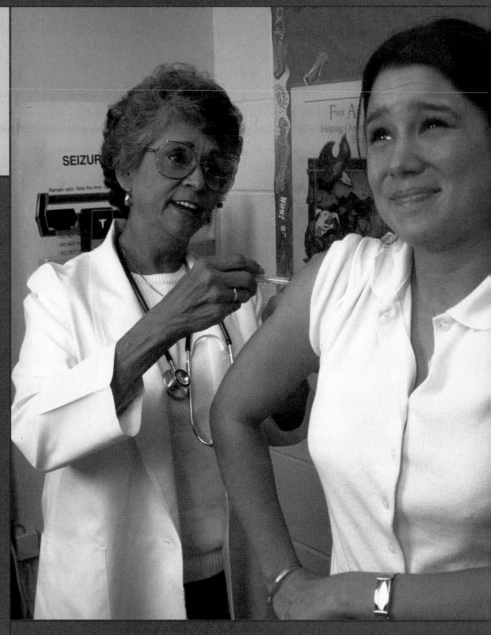

After studying the material in this chapter, you should be able to:

- **Explain** how the different agents of infection spread disease.
- **Describe** how your body protects itself from infectious disease.
- **List** and **describe** some common infectious diseases.
- **List** the sexually transmitted diseases and the symptoms and treatment for each.
- **Define** HIV infection, and **describe** its symptoms.
- **List** the methods of HIV transmission.
- **Explain** some practical methods for preventing HIV infection and other sexually transmitted diseases.

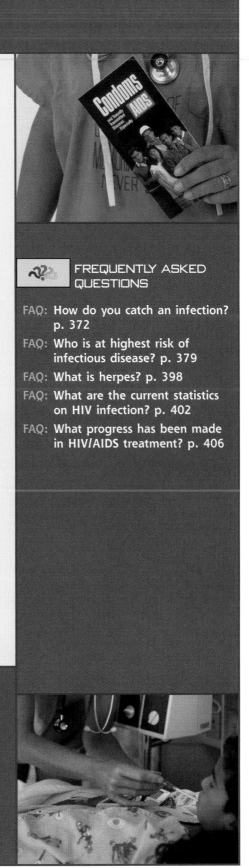

e live in a sea of microbes. Most of them don't threaten our health or survival; some, such as the bacteria that inhabit our intestines, are actually beneficial. Yet in the course of history, disease-causing microorganisms have claimed millions of lives. The twentieth century brought the conquest of infectious killers such as cholera and scarlet fever.[1] However, although modern science has won many victories against the agents of infection, infectious illnesses remain a serious health threat. Drug-resistant strains of tuberculosis and staphylococcus bacteria challenge current therapies. And scientists warn of the potential danger of new "emerging" viruses.

Some of today's most common and dangerous infectious illnesses spread primarily through sexual contact, and their incidence has skyrocketed. Every day brings 16,000 new cases of infection with human immunodeficiency virus (HIV).[2] To date, Acquired Immune Deficiency Syndrome (AIDS) has claimed the lives of 14 million adults and children worldwide.[3]

Sexually transmitted diseases (STDs) cannot be prevented in the laboratory. Only you, by your behavior, can prevent and control them.

This chapter is a lesson in self-defense against all forms of infection. The information it provides can help you boost your defenses, recognize and avoid enemies, protect yourself from STDs, and realize when to seek help. ❖

FREQUENTLY ASKED QUESTIONS

FAQ: **How do you catch an infection? p. 372**

FAQ: **Who is at highest risk of infectious disease? p. 379**

FAQ: **What is herpes? p. 398**

FAQ: **What are the current statistics on HIV infection? p. 402**

FAQ: **What progress has been made in HIV/AIDS treatment? p. 406**

Understanding Infection

Infection is a complex process, triggered by various **pathogens** (disease-causing organisms) and countered by the body's own defenders. Physicians explain infection in terms of a **host** (either a person or a population) that contacts one or more agents in an environment. A **vector**—a biological or physical vehicle that carries the agent to the host— provides the means of transmission.

Agents of Infection

The types of microbes that can cause infection are viruses, bacteria, fungi, protozoa, and helminths (parasitic worms) (see photos below).

Viruses

The tiniest pathogens—**viruses**—are also the toughest; they consist of a bit of nucleic acid (DNA or RNA, but never both) within a protein coat. Unable to reproduce on its own, a virus takes over a body cell's reproductive machinery and instructs it to produce new viral particles, which are then released to enter other cells.

Among the most common viruses are the following:

- *Rhinoviruses and adenoviruses,* which get into the mucous membranes and cause upper-respiratory tract infections and colds.
- *Influenza viruses,* which can change their outer protein coats so dramatically that individuals resistant to one strain cannot fight off a new one.
- *Herpes viruses,* which take up permanent residence in the cells and flare up periodically.
- *Papilloma viruses,* which cause few symptoms in women and almost none in men, but may be responsible, at least in part, for a rise in the incidence of cervical cancer among younger women.
- *Hepatitis viruses,* which cause several forms of liver infection, ranging from mild to potentially life threatening.
- *Slow viruses,* which give no early indication of their presence but can produce fatal illnesses within a few years.

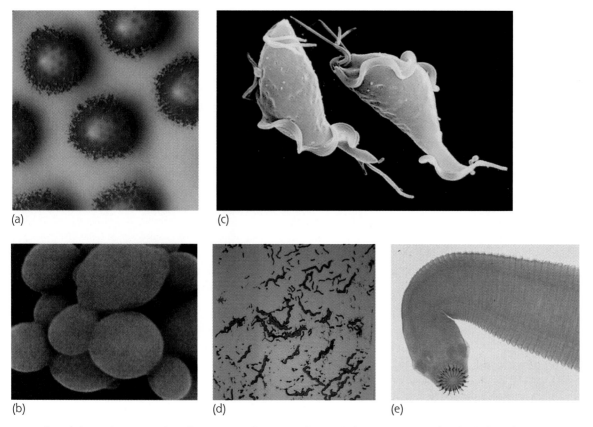

(a)

(b)

(c)

(d)

(e)

Examples of the major categories of organisms that cause disease in humans. Except for the helminths (parasitic worms), pathogens are microorganisms that can be seen only with the aid of a microscope. (a) Viruses: common cold, (b) Fungi: yeast, (c) Protozoa: trichomonas, (d) Bacteria: syphilis, (e) Helminths: tapeworm.

- *Retroviruses,* which are named for their backward ("retro") sequence of genetic replication compared to other viruses. One retrovirus, human immunodeficiency virus (HIV), causes acquired immune deficiency syndrome (AIDS). Scientists have identified different retroviruses that have been linked to several diseases, including some forms of leukemia and lymphoma (cancers of the blood and lymph glands, respectively).

- *Filoviruses,* which are newly identified viruses that resemble threads and are extremely lethal. Most of those infected with the two known filoviruses, Marburg and Ebola, develop *viral hemorrhagic fever,* which causes uncontrollable bleeding and usually proves fatal.

The problem in fighting viruses is that it's difficult to find drugs that harm the virus and not the cell it has commandeered. **Antibiotics** (drugs that inhibit or kill bacteria) have no effect on viruses. **Antiviral drugs** (such as amantadine for influenza and acyclovir for herpes simplex) don't completely eradicate a viral infection, although they can decrease its severity and duration. Because viruses multiply very quickly, antiviral drugs are most effective when taken before an infection develops or in its early stages.

Bacteria

Simple one-celled organisms, **bacteria** are the most plentiful microorganisms as well as the most pathogenic. Most kinds of bacteria don't cause disease; some, like the *Escherichia coli* that aid in digestion, play important roles within our bodies. Even friendly bacteria, however, can get out of hand and cause acne, urinary tract infections, vaginal infections, and other problems.

Bacteria harm the body by releasing enzymes that digest body cells or toxins that produce the specific effects of such diseases as diphtheria or toxic shock. In self-defense the body produces specific proteins (called *antibodies*) that attack and inactivate the invaders. Tuberculosis, tetanus, gonorrhea, scarlet fever, and diphtheria are examples of bacterial diseases.

Because bacteria are sufficiently different from the cells that make up our bodies, antibiotics can kill them without harming our cells. Some of these drugs are produced by microorganisms; others are synthetic agents. Antibiotics work only against specific types of bacteria. If your doctor thinks you have a bacterial infection, tests of your blood, pus, sputum, urine, or stool can identify the particular bacterial strain. Antibiotic medication is prescribed after determination of the bacteria.

Antibiotics may cause undesirable and sometimes serious side effects, including allergic reactions. Furthermore, frequent exposure of bacteria to a partic-ular antibiotic may cause the bacteria to become resistant to that drug so that the antibiotic loses its effectiveness. As a result, in recent years, more virulent treatment-resistant forms of bacterial infections (discussed later in this chapter) have developed.[4]

Fungi

Single-celled or multicelled organisms, **fungi** consist of threadlike fibers and reproductive spores. These plants, lacking chlorophyll, must obtain their food from organic material, which may include human tissue. Fungi release enzymes that digest cells, and are most likely to attack hair-covered areas of the body, including the scalp, beard, groin, and external ear canals. They also cause athlete's foot. Treatment consists of antifungal drugs.

Protozoa

These single-celled, microscopic animals release enzymes and toxins that destroy cells or interfere with their function. Diseases caused by **protozoa** are not a major health problem in this country, primarily because of public health measures. Around the world, however, some 2.24 billion people (more than 40 percent of the world's population) are at risk for acquiring one protozoa-caused disease—malaria—every year. Up to 3 million die of this disease annually. Many more come down with amoebic dysentery. Treatment for protozoa-caused diseases consists of general medical care to relieve the symptoms, replacement of lost blood or fluids, and drugs that kill the specific protozoa.

The most common disease caused by protozoa in the United States is *giardiasis,* an intestinal infection caused by microorganisms in human and animal feces. It has become a threat at day-care centers, as well as among campers and hikers who drink contaminated water. Once ingested, giardia organisms use an adhesive sucker to stick to the intestinal walls, where they multiply and absorb nutrients from their host. Symptoms include nausea, lack of appetite, gas, diarrhea, fatigue, abdominal cramps, and bloating. Many people recover in a month or two even without treatment. However, in some cases, the microbe causes recurring attacks over many years. Giardiasis can be life-threatening in small children and the elderly, who are especially prone to severe dehydration from diarrhea. Treatment usually consists of antibiotics.

Helminths (Parasitic Worms)

Small parasitic worms that attack specific tissues or organs and compete with the host for nutrients are called **helminths.** One major worldwide health problem is *shistosomiasis,* a disease caused by a parasitic worm, the fluke, that burrows through the skin and enters the circulatory system. Infection with another helminth, the tapeworm, may be contracted from eating undercooked beef, pork, or fish containing larval forms of the tapeworm. Helminthic diseases are treated with appropriate medications.

 ## How Do You Catch an Infection?

The major vectors, or means of transmission, for infectious disease are animals/insects, person-to-person, food, water, and airborne.

Animals/Insects

Disease may be transmitted by house pets, livestock, or wild animals. Insects also spread a variety of diseases. The housefly may spread dysentery, diarrhea, typhoid fever, or trachoma (an eye disease rare in the United States but common in other parts of the world). Other insects, including mosquitoes, ticks, mites, fleas, and lice, can transmit such diseases as malaria, yellow fever, encephalitis, dengue fever (a growing threat in Mexico), and Lyme disease (discussed later in this chapter).

Person-to-Person

The people you're closest to can transmit pathogens by coughing, sneezing, kissing, or sharing food or dishes with you. To avoid infection, stay out of range of anyone who's coughing, sniffling, or sneezing. Carefully wash your dishes, utensils, and hands, and abstain from sex or make self-protective decisions about sexual partners. (See the sections on STDs later in this chapter.)

Food

Every year foodborne illnesses strike millions of Americans, sometimes with fatal consequences. Bacteria account for two-thirds of foodborne infections, and thousands of suspected cases of infection with *Escherichia coli* bacteria in undercooked or inadequately washed food have been reported. (See Chapter 6 for a discussion of food safety.)

Every year as many as 4 million Americans have a bout with *salmonella* bacteria, which have been found in about a third of all poultry sold in the United States. These infections can be serious enough to require hospitalization, and can lead to arthritis, neurological problems, and even death. Consumers can greatly reduce the number of salmonella infections by following proper handling, cooking, and refrigeration.

A deadly food disease, *botulism,* is caused by certain bacteria that grow in improperly canned foods. Although its occurrence is rare in commercial products, botulism is a danger in home canning. Another uncommon threat is *trichinosis,* caused by the larvae of a parasitic roundworm in uncooked meat. This infection, which causes nausea, vomiting, diarrhea, fever, thirst, profuse sweating, weakness, and pain, can be avoided by thoroughly cooking meat.

Water

Waterborne diseases, such as typhoid fever and cholera, are still widespread in less developed areas of the world. They have been rare in the United States, although outbreaks caused by inadequate water purification have occurred.

The Process of Infection

If someone infected with the flu sits next to you on a bus and coughs or sneezes, tiny viral particles may travel into your nose and mouth. Immediately the virus finds or creates an opening in the wall of a cell, and the process of infection begins. During the **incubation period,** the time between invasion and the first symptom, you're unaware of the pathogen multiplying inside you. In some diseases, incubation may go on for months, even years; for most, it lasts several days or weeks.

The early stage of the battle between your body and the invaders is called the *prodromal* period. As infected cells die, they release chemicals that help block the invasion. Other chemicals, such as *histamines,* cause blood vessels to dilate, thus allowing more blood to reach the battleground. During all of this, you feel mild, generalized symptoms, such as headache, irritability, and discomfort. You're also highly contagious. At the height of the battle—the typical illness period—you cough, sneeze, sniffle, ache, feel feverish, and lose your appetite.

Recovery begins when the body's forces gain the advantage. With time, the body destroys the last of the invaders and heals itself. However, the body is not able to develop long-lasting immunity to certain viruses, such as colds, flu, or HIV.

How Your Body Protects Itself

Various parts of your body safeguard you against infectious diseases and provide **immunity,** or protection, from these health threats. Your skin, when unbroken, keeps out most potential invaders. Your tears, sweat, skin oils, saliva, and mucus contain chemicals that can kill bacteria. Cilia, the tiny hairs lining your respiratory passages, move mucus, which traps inhaled bacteria, viruses, dust, and foreign matter, to the back of the throat, where it is swallowed; the digestive system then destroys the invaders.

When these protective mechanisms can't keep you infection-free, your body's immune system, which is on constant alert for foreign substances that might threaten the body, swings into action. The immune system includes structures of the lymphatic system, which includes the spleen, thymus gland, lymph nodes, and vessels called lymphatics that help filter impurities from the body (see Figure 12-1). More than a dozen different types of white blood cells are concentrated in the organs of the lymphatic system or, by way of the blood and lymph vessels, patrol the entire body. The two basic types of immune mechanisms are humoral and cell-mediated.

Humoral immunity refers to the protection provided by antibodies, proteins derived from white blood cells called B lymphocytes or B cells (see photos, p. 374). Humoral immunity is most effective during bacterial or viral infections. An *antigen* is any substance that enters the body and triggers production of an antibody. Once the body produces antibodies against a specific antigen—the mumps virus, for instance—you're protected against that antigen for life. If you're again exposed to mumps, the antibodies previously produced prevent another episode of the disease.

But you don't have to suffer through an illness to acquire immunity. Inoculation with a vaccine containing synthetic or weakened antigens can give you the same protection. The type of long-lasting immunity in which the body makes its own antibodies to a pathogen is called *active* immunity. Immunity produced by the injection of **gamma globulin**, the antibody-containing part of the

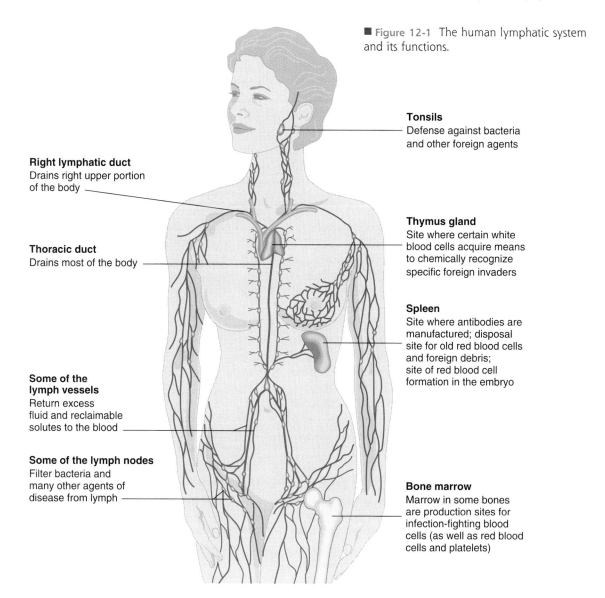

■ Figure 12-1 The human lymphatic system and its functions.

Tonsils
Defense against bacteria and other foreign agents

Right lymphatic duct
Drains right upper portion of the body

Thoracic duct
Drains most of the body

Thymus gland
Site where certain white blood cells acquire means to chemically recognize specific foreign invaders

Spleen
Site where antibodies are manufactured; disposal site for old red blood cells and foreign debris; site of red blood cell formation in the embryo

Some of the lymph vessels
Return excess fluid and reclaimable solutes to the blood

Some of the lymph nodes
Filter bacteria and many other agents of disease from lymph

Bone marrow
Marrow in some bones are production sites for infection-fighting blood cells (as well as red blood cells and platelets)

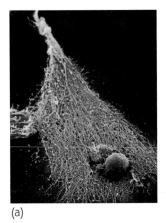 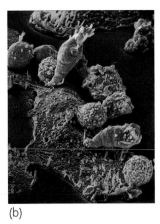

(a)   (b)

Types of lymphocytes. (a) B cell covered with bacteria. The B cells function in humoral immunity by producing antibodies. (b) T cells attack a cancer cell. The T cells function in cell-mediated immunity.

blood, from another person or animal that has developed antibodies to a disease, is called *passive* immunity.

The various types of T cells are responsible for cellular, or **cell-mediated,** immunity. These lymphocytes are manufactured in the bone marrow and carried to the thymus for maturation. Cell-mediated immunity mainly protects against parasites, fungi, cancer cells, and foreign tissue (see photos above). Thousands of different T cells work together to ward off disease. Some T cells activate other immune cells; others help in antibody-mediated responses; and still others suppress lymphocyte activity while others carry out different functions.

Immune Response

Attacked by pathogens, the body musters its forces and fights. Sometimes the invasion is handled like a minor border skirmish; other times a full-scale battle is waged throughout the body. Together, the immune cells work like an internal police force. When an antigen enters the body, the T cells aided by *macrophages* (large scavenger cells with insatiable appetites for foreign cells, diseased and run-down red blood cells, and other biological debris) engage in combat with the invader. Meanwhile, the B cells churn out antibodies, which rush to the scene and join in the fray. Also busy at surveillance are natural killer cells that, like the elite forces of a SWAT team, seek out and destroy viruses and cancer cells.

The **lymph nodes,** or glands, are small tissue masses in which some protective cells are stored. If pathogens invade your body, many of them are carried to the lymph nodes, where they are then destroyed. This is why the lymph nodes often feel swollen when you have a cold or the flu.

If the microbes establish a foothold, the blood supply to the area increases, bringing oxygen and nutrients to the fighting cells. Tissue fluids, as well as antibacterial and antitoxic proteins, accumulate. You may develop redness, swelling, local warmth, and pain—the signs of **inflammation.** As more tissue is destroyed, a cavity, or **abscess,** forms, and fills with fluid, battling cells, and dead white blood cells (pus). If the invaders aren't killed or inactivated, the pathogens are able to spread into the bloodstream and cause what is known as **systemic disease.** The toxins released by the pathogens cause fever, and the infection becomes more dangerous.

Strategies *for* Prevention

Natural Ways to Bolster Immunity

✓ *Eat a balanced diet* to be sure you get essential vitamins and minerals. Severe deficiencies in vitamins B-6, B-12, and folic acid impair immunity. Keep up your iron and zinc intake. Iron influences the number and vigor of certain immune cells, whereas zinc is crucial for cell repair. Too little vitamin C may also increase susceptibility to infectious diseases.

✓ *Avoid fatty foods.* A low-fat diet can increase the activity of immune cells that hunt down and knock out cells infected with viruses.

✓ *Get enough sleep.* Without adequate rest, your immune system cannot maintain and renew itself.

✓ *Exercise regularly.* Aerobic exercise stimulates the production of an immune-system booster called interleukin-2.

✓ *Don't smoke.* Smoking decreases the levels of some immune cells.

✓ *Control your alcohol intake.* Heavy drinking interferes with normal immune responses and lowers the number of defender cells.

Immunity and Stress

Whenever we confront a crisis, large or small, our bodies produce powerful hormones that provide extra energy. However, this stress response dampens immunity, reducing the number of some key immune cells and the responsiveness of others. (See Chapter 2 for more on how our bodies respond to stress.)

A study of male students aged 18 to 28 found that the body's immune system is affected in different ways by two factors: the controllability or uncontrollability of the stressor, and the mental effort required to cope with the stress. An uncontrollable stressor that lasts longer than 15 minutes may interfere with cytokine interleukin-6, which plays an essential role in activating the immune defenses. Uncontrollable stressors also produce high levels of cortisol, which suppresses immune system functioning. The mental efforts required to cope with high-level stressors produce only brief immune changes that appear to have little consequence for health.[5] However, stress has been shown to slow pro-inflammatory cytokine production, which is essential for wound-healing. In a study of post-menopausal women, those who reported more stress produced significantly lower levels of two crucial cytokines.[6]

Immune Disorders

Sometimes our immune system overreacts to certain substances, or mistakes the body's own tissues for enemies, or doesn't react adequately. The result is an immune disorder. The most common are **allergies,** which essentially represent a hypersensitivity to a substance in one's environment or diet.

According to a 1999 survey by the American College of Allergy, Asthma and Immunology, allergies affect about 38 percent of all Americans—almost twice as many as allergy experts have believed—and millions of them suffer unnecessarily or rely on medications they don't want to take because they don't know about effective treatment options, such as allergy shots (immunotherapy).[7] Allergy sufferers run up annual tabs of $1.8 to $2 billion in doctor visits, diagnostic tests, prescriptions, and decreased productivity. Every year they account for more than 10 million workdays missed; every day they keep 10,000 children out of school.

"Allergies may seem trivial to people who don't have them, but they have an enormous effect on a person's quality of life," says Robert Miles, M.D., of the American College of Allergy, Asthma and Immunology.[8] Their symptoms are many and miserable: itching, nasal congestion, eye irritation, coughing, wheezing, hives, vomiting, and diarrhea (from food allergies), even sudden, life-threatening collapse (from anaphylaxis, the most extreme allergic reaction). While victims seldom die of allergies, they just as rarely recover. And when individuals try to outrun allergies by moving away from one region's irritants, they often end up acquiring new sensitivities on their new home ground.

A list of allergic triggers, or allergens, reads like an inventory of creation, including life's pleasures (such as foods and flowers), perils (insect stings and poison ivy), and inescapable realities (like mold and dust). The very air we breathe can be a danger. The symptoms of allergy and of its more sinister sister-disease, asthma, increase along with pollutants, such as diesel fumes, and the number of small particles in the environment.

But breakthroughs in treatments are helping many allergy sufferers breathe more easily. "In the past, allergy symptoms and medications both made people so drowsy that they often couldn't concentrate or function at their best," says Miles, who notes that today's allergy sufferers no longer have to choose between feeling better or feeling alert.

In 1999, for the first time ever, experts from 21 major health care and medical organizations developed physician guidelines for diagnosing and treating allergies.[9] Treatment options include oral medications, nasal sprays, and immunotherapy, which consists of a series of injections of small but increasing doses of an allergen.

Immunotherapy has proven to have long-term, perhaps permanent, benefits. In one recent study, traditional allergen immunotherapy with a grass-pollen extract, administered for three to four years, induced a clinical remission that persisted for at least three years after treatment. Immunotherapy in patients allergic to insect stings also induces long-lasting immunologic changes and reduces their risk of potentially fatal reactions. Immunotherapy has the greatest benefit, relative to the investment of time and cost, for allergies that persist for more than one season or throughout the year.[10]

Strategies *for* Prevention

Fighting Hidden Allergens

✓ *Switch to feather pillows.* Researchers in the United Kingdom found significantly higher levels of house dust mite allergens in synthetic pillows.

✓ *Use bleach rather than detergent.* Very low concentrations of bleach are more effective in removing allergens from various surfaces around the house than other common cleaners.

✓ *Cover mattresses and pillows with tightly woven fabrics.* These materials, compared with non-woven or semi-permeable synthetic fabrics, effectively block cat and dust allergens even after repeated washings.

✓ *Use multilayer vacuum bags.* To prevent allergens from "leaking" into the air, choose bags that have two to three layers.

✓ *Store clothing in sealed containers with moth-killing products.* Products such as moth balls or crystals and lavandin oil packets also kill house dust mites and their eggs.

✓ *Put comforters in the clothes dryer.* An hour of dry heat in a home dryer dramatically reduces the number of house dust mites in comforters and duvets filled with synthetic materials.[11]

Autoimmune disorders result when the immune system fails to recognize body tissue as self and attacks it. Many of these severely disabling diseases, such as myasthenia gravis, rheumatoid arthritis, and systemic lupus erythematosus, primarily strike women systematically in their childbearing years. (See The X and Y Files: "Sex Differences in Susceptibility.") These diseases, which often worsen with time, may be treated with drugs that suppress the immune system.[12]

Some people have an **immune deficiency**—either inborn or acquired. A very few children are born without an effective immune system; their lives can be endangered by any infection. Although still experimental, genetic therapy to implant a missing or healthy gene may offer new hope for a normal life.

Immunization: The Key to Prevention

One of the great success stories of American medicine has been the development of vaccines that provide protection against many infectious diseases. Unfortunately, many Americans, including large numbers of children in urban centers, haven't been properly immunized. Nearly a quarter of youngsters lack complete protection against polio, tetanus, and other illnesses, according to the National Vaccine Advisory Committee. While there has been progress in protecting most American children against diphtheria, whooping cough, tetanus, Haemophilus influenzae type B (HIB),

---

The **Files**

Sex Differences in Susceptibility

When the flu hits a household, the last one left standing is likely to be Mom. The female immune system responds more vigorously to common infections, offering extra protection against viruses, bacteria, and parasites. But this enhanced immunity doesn't apply to sexually transmitted diseases (STDs). A woman who has unprotected sex with an infected man is more likely to contract an STD than a man who has sex with an infected woman. Symptoms of STDs also tend to be more "silent" in women, so they often go undetected and untreated, leading to potentially serious complications.

The sexes also differ in their vulnerability to allergic and autoimmune disorders. Although both men and women frequently develop allergies, allergic women are twice as likely to experience potentially fatal anaphylactic shock. A woman's "robust" immune system also is more likely to overreact and turn on her own organs and tissues. On average, three of four people with autoimmune disorders, such as multiple sclerosis, Hashimoto's thyroiditis, and scleroderma, are women. Of the 8.5 million people in the United States with rheumatoid arthritis, about 6.7 million are women. Another autoimmune disease, lupus, affects nine times as many women as men.

Autoimmune disorders often follow a different course in men and women. Women with multiple sclerosis develop symptoms earlier than men, but the disease tends to progress more quickly and be more severe in men. In lupus, women first show symptoms during their childbearing years, while men develop the illness later in life.

Why are there such large sex differences in susceptibility? Scientists believe that the sex hormones have a great impact on immunity. Estrogen, which protects heart, bone, brain, and blood vessels, also bolsters the immune system's response to certain infectious agents. Women produce greater numbers of antibodies when exposed to an antigen; after immunization, they show increased cell-mediated immunity.

In contrast, testosterone may dampen this response—possibly to prevent attacks on sperm cells, which might otherwise be mistaken as alien invaders. When the testes are removed from mice and guinea pigs, their immune systems become more active. Pregnancy dampens a woman's immune response, probably to ensure that her natural protectors don't attack the fetus as a "foreign" invader. This impact is so great that pregnant women with transplanted kidneys may require lower doses of drugs to prevent organ rejection. Pregnant women with multiple sclerosis and rheumatoid arthritis typically experience decreased symptoms during the nine months of gestation, then return to their prepregnancy state after giving birth. Oral contraceptives also can diminish symptoms of multiple sclerosis and rheumatoid arthritis. Neither pregnancy nor birth control pills has such an impact on lupus.

Other hormones, such as prolactin and growth hormone, may affect autoimmune disease. Women have higher levels of these hormones, which may act directly on immune cells through interactions with receptors on the surface of cells. These hormones also may affect the complex interworkings of the hypothalamus, pituitary, and adrenal glands.

Sources: Whitacre, Caroline, et al. "A Gender Gap in Autoimmunity." *Science,* Vol. 283, Issue 5406, February 26, 1999. The full report of the Task Force on Gender, Multiple Sclerosis and Autoimmunity is available at www.sciencemag/feature/data/98319.shl

polio, and measles, some children are going without the "booster" shots necessary for complete immunization.[13]

As shown in Figure 12-2, the American Academy of Pediatrics recommends that all children be immunized against measles, mumps, German measles (rubella), diphtheria, tetanus, chickenpox, and hepatitis B. Although some vaccines confer lifelong protection, others do not. The protection provided by diphtheria and tetanus vaccinations, for example, diminishes over time, so booster vaccinations are required every ten years. Health officials also recommend measles booster shots for students entering college, and suggest that people born after 1956 be revaccinated for polio, measles, and other infectious diseases before visiting developing countries. In the future "designer" vaccines may be individualized to protect recipients from the diseases for which they are at highest risk.[14]

If you're uncertain about your past immunizations, check with family members or your doctor. If you can't find answers, a blood test can show whether you carry antibodies to specific illnesses.

If you're pregnant or planning to get pregnant within the next three months, do not get a measles, mumps, rubella, or oral polio vaccination. If you're allergic to neomycin, consult your doctor before getting a measles, mumps, rubella, or intramuscular polio vac-

cination. Those with egg allergies should also check with a doctor before getting a measles, mumps, or flu vaccination. Also, never get a vaccination when you have a high fever.

Poliomyelitis

Immunization has greatly reduced the incidence of polio in the United States. The American Academy of Pediatrics recommends two doses of inactivated polio virus at 2 months and 4 months, followed by oral polio vaccine at 12 to 18 months and 4 to 6 years.[15] Additional boosters for polio aren't necessary, except when traveling to an area where the disease is common.

Tetanus (Lockjaw)

Tetanus is an uncommon disease transmitted via a variety of injuries. Since the tetanus germ cannot grow in the presence of air, puncture wounds, such as those caused by stepping on a nail or gardening rake, pose the greatest danger. Tetanus is often called "lockjaw," because the characteristic symptom is a stiffening of the jaws so severe that the patient is unable to open his or

Vaccines are listed under routinely recommended ages.

Bars indicate range of recommended ages for immunization. Any dose not given at the recommended age should be given as a "catch-up" immunization at any subsequent visit when indicated and feasible.

Ovals indicate vaccines to be given if previously recommended doses were missed or given earlier than the recommended minimum age.

Vaccine	Birth	1 month	2 months	4 months	6 months	12 months	15 months	18 months	4–6 years	11–12 years	14–16 years
Hepatitis B	Hep B		Hep B			Hep B				Hep B	
Diphtheria, Tetanus, Pertussis			DTaP	DTaP	DTaP		DTaP		DTaP	Td	
H. influenzae type b			Hib	Hib	Hib	Hib					
Polio			IVP	IVP		Polio			Polio		
Rotavirus			*Rv*	*Rv*	*Rv*						
Measles, Mumps, Rubella						MMR			MMR	MMR	
Varicella						Var				Var	

Approved by the Advisory Committee on Immunization Practices (ACIP), the American Academy of Pediatrics (AAP), and the American Academy of Family Physicians (AAFP). For detailed information, please contact your pediatrician or local health clinic.

■ **Figure 12-2** Recommended childhood immunization schedule, United States, January–December 1999

Source: http://www.aap.org/family/parents/immunize.htm.

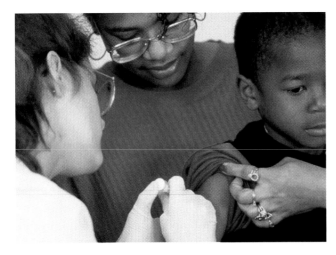

Immunizations are an important protection against childhood diseases. Neighborhood clinics in urban centers offer immunizations to those children at particular risk.

her mouth. Everyone should get booster inoculations for tetanus at least once every ten years.

Diphtheria

Diphtheria, a dangerous disease, is rare because of immunization. An average of fewer than three cases per year have been reported in the last decade. Diphtheria and tetanus vaccinations (toxoids) are usually given in combination with the pertussis (whooping cough) vaccine-part of the DTP shot. The schedule for these consists of a basic series and two boosters prior to entering school. Older children and adults receive only diphtheria and tetanus toxoid (DT) in a more dilute form. Adults as well as children should get booster shots every ten years.

Pertussis

Pertussis (whooping cough), a bacterial infection that can develop into pneumonia, is potentially fatal. Until recently, the pertussis vaccine was made with killed whole pertussis cells and mixed with diphtheria and tetanus vaccines to make the whole cell DTP shot. For years parents have been concerned about its safety because of reports of permanent brain damage and even death. Careful analysis by many investigators found that any increased risk of permanent neurological damage was so small as to be virtually unmeasurable. However, new *acellular* pertussis vaccines, made of only a few parts of the pertussis cell, have proven effective against pertussis and produce fewer side effects. An esti-

mated 95 percent of two-year-olds have been vaccinated against pertussis.[16]

Measles

The number of cases of measles has fallen to an all-time low. However, the Centers for Disease Control (CDC) recommends continued vigilance and immunizations.[17]

Symptoms include a rash on the face and body, runny nose, high fever, cough, eye inflammation, and fatigue. Ten to 15 percent of measles patients develop serious complications, such as ear infections, diarrhea, or pneumonia. One out of every 1,000 develops encephalomyelitis, an inflammation of the brain that can be fatal or lead to mental retardation, or to movement, behavioral, or neurological disorders.

CDC officials estimate that 5 to 15 percent of college students are susceptible to measles because they were vaccinated at 12 months of age rather than the currently recommended 15 months, or did not receive a second dose of the vaccine between ages 4 and 12. Others were given immune globulin, which was intended to lower the risk of reaction but which also reduced the vaccine's effectiveness. Many colleges are requiring students to submit proof of measles immunization before allowing them to enroll. In all, some 3 million Americans, aged 20 to 37, are at risk.

Rubella (German Measles)

About 85 percent of adults are immune to rubella, even if they have no history of the disease. The most serious result of this mild disease is the destructive effect it has on an unborn baby—including blindness—if the mother is infected in early pregnancy. All children should be immunized against rubella at 1 year of age or later.[18]

Adults who are not immune may be immunized at any age, but women should not receive the vaccine during pregnancy or during the two to three months immediately preceding pregnancy. All unimmunized children in a pregnant woman's household should be immunized against rubella, for they are the most likely potential carriers. Recent outbreaks of rubella among newborns have been blamed on the lack of routine rubella screening and followup vaccination of susceptible women of childbearing age.

Varicella (Chickenpox)

A vaccine against chickenpox, a common childhood disease that causes itchy red pustules, was approved by the FDA and became available in 1995. The vaccine seems more effective when given alone rather than in combination with MMR vaccine.[19]

Hepatitis B

The U. S. Public Health Service recommends immunization against hepatitis B for infants as a way of preventing a disease (discussed later in this chapter) that infects an estimated 200,000 people in the United States and kills 4,000 to 5,000 Americans each year. However, some object to hepatitis B vaccinations for children, because the potential risks associated with the vaccine are greater than the odds of a child contracting what is primarily an adult disease.[20] They argue that children younger than 14 are three times more likely to die or suffer adverse reactions after receiving hepatitis B vaccines than they are to catch the disease.[21] Public health professionals counter by saying that children under age 5, although they constitute a small minority of those with hepatitis B, face the highest risk of death from cirrhosis and liver cancer.

HIB Infection

In the United States, *Hemophilus* influenza type B, or HIB, was once a cause of bacterial *meningitis*, a life-threatening infection of the lining of the brain and spinal cord. A vaccine that protects children has nearly eliminated this potentially deadly disease. The frequency of HIB infection dropped by 99 percent in the 1990s.[22]

Infectious Diseases

An estimated 500 microorganisms cause disease; no effective treatment exists for about 200 of these illnesses. Although infections can be unavoidable at times, the more you know about their causes, the more you can do to protect yourself.

Who Is at Highest Risk of Infectious Disease?

Like human bullies, the viruses responsible for the most common infectious illnesses tend to pick on those least capable of fighting back. Among the most vulnerable are the following groups:

- *Children and their families.* Youngsters get up to a dozen colds annually; adults average two a year. When a flu epidemic hits a community, about 40 per-

cent of school-age boys and girls get sick, compared with only 5 to 10 percent of adults. But their parents get up to six times as many colds as other adults.

- *The elderly.* Statistically, fewer older men and women are likely to catch a cold or flu, yet when they do, they face greater danger than the rest of the population. People over 65 who get the flu have a one in ten chance of being hospitalized for pneumonia or other respiratory problems, and a one in fifty chance of dying from the disease.

- *The chronically ill.* Lifelong diseases, such as diabetes, kidney disease, or sickle cell anemia, decrease an individual's ability to fend off infections. Individuals taking medications that suppress the immune system, such as steroids, are more vulnerable to infections, as are those with medical conditions that impair immunity, such as infection with HIV, the virus that causes AIDS.

- *Smokers and those with respiratory problems.* Smokers are a high-risk group for respiratory infections and serious complications, such as pneumonia. Chronic breathing disorders, such as asthma and emphysema, also greatly increase the risk of respiratory infections.

- *Those who live or work in close contact with someone sick.* Health-care workers who treat high-risk patients, nursing home residents, and others living in close quarters—such as students in dormitories—face greater odds of catching others' colds and flus.

- *Residents or workers in poorly ventilated buildings.* The technology of the twentieth century has helped spread certain airborne illnesses, such as tuberculosis, via recirculated air. Indoor air quality may be closely linked with disease transmission in winter, when people spend a great deal of time in tightly sealed rooms.

The Common Cold

There are more than 200 distinct cold viruses, or rhinoviruses. Although in a single season you may develop a temporary immunity to one or two, you may then be hit by a third. Americans come down with 66 million colds a year.[23] Colds can strike in any season, but different cold viruses are more common at different times of years. Rhinoviruses cause most spring, summer, and early fall colds, and tend to cause more symptoms above the neck (stuffy nose, headache, runny eyes). Adenoviruses, parainfluenza viruses, corona viruses, influenza viruses, and others that strike in the winter are more likely to get into the bronchi and trachea (the breathing passages) and cause more fever and bronchitis. Cold viruses spread by coughs, sneezes, and touch. Cold-sufferers who sneeze and then touch a doorknob or countertop leave a trail of highly contagious viruses behind them.

Scientists are making progress in the endless pursuit of a cure for the common cold. "If you define 'cure' as an effective therapy that helps you recover faster and gets at the root cause of an illness, then it's not unrealistic to expect one for the common cold in three to five years," predicts the nation's premier cold expert, Jack Gwaltney, M.D., of the University of Virginia, "Even though human beings have been getting colds for five million years, we didn't know much about them until the twentieth century. Now we're entering a new era of treating the virus that causes colds and not just the symptoms."[24]

Among the most promising approaches are a protease inhibitor, similar to those used against HIV, that disrupts viral reproduction, a capsid binder that slots into the protective outer shell of a rhinovirus and changes its shape so it can't attach to cells within the nose, a nasal spray containing interferon, the body's natural virus fighter, and e tremacara, an antiviral nasal spray that blocks rhinovirus "receptors" or binding sites. Which will ultimately prove best? No one yet knows. Despite the enthusiasm—and fierce competition—in the $2 billion cold remedy market, consumers face at least a few more seasons of sniffles before experimental cold treatments reach pharmacy shelves.[25]

Until effective cold treatments are available, experts advise against taking aspirin and acetaminophen (Tylenol), which may suppress the antibodies the body produces to fight cold viruses and increase symptoms such as nasal stuffiness. A better alternative for achiness is ibuprofen (brand names include Motrin, Advil, and Nuprin), which doesn't seem to affect immune response. Children, teenagers, and young adults should never take aspirin for a cold or flu because of the danger of Reye's syndrome, a potentially deadly disorder that can cause convulsions, coma, swelling of the brain, and kidney damage.

Fluids (especially chicken soup) help, but dairy products contribute to congestion. Mild exercise boosts immunity, but once you're sick, it's better not to work out strenuously. In general, doctors recommend treating specific symptoms—headache, cough, chest congestion, sore throat, and so on—rather than taking a multi-symptom medication.[26]

The best preventive tactics are frequent hand-washing, replacing tooth brushes regularly, and avoiding stress overload. High levels of stress increase the risk of becoming infected by respiratory viruses and developing cold symptoms. New research shows that people who feel unable to deal with everyday stresses have an exaggerated immune reaction that may intensify cold or flu symptoms once they've contracted a virus.[27]

The main drawback of antihistamines, the most widely used cold remedy, is drowsiness, which can impair a person's ability to drive or operate machinery safely. Another ingredient, pseudoephedrine, can open and drain sinus passages without drowsiness but can speed up heart rate and cause complications for individuals with high blood pressure, diabetes, heart disease, or thyroid disorders. Nasal sprays can clear a stuffy nose, but they invariably cause a rebound effect.

For a cough, the ingredient to look for in any suppressant is dextromethrophan, which turns down the brain's cough reflex. In expectorants, the only medicine the FDA has deemed effective is guaifenesin, which helps liquefy secretions so you can bring up mucus from the chest. Unless you're coughing up green or foul yellow mucus—signs of a "secondary" bacterial infection—antibiotics won't help. They have no effect against viruses and may make your body more resistant to such medications when you develop a bacterial infection in the future.

Your own immune system can do something modern science cannot: cure a cold. All that it needs is time, rest, and plenty of fluids. Warmth also is important, because the aptly named "cold" viruses replicate at lower temperatures. Hot soups and drinks (particularly those with a touch of something pungent, like lemon or ginger) both raise body temperature and help clear the nose. Even more important is getting off your feet. Taking it easy reduces demands on the body, which helps speed recovery.

Strategies *for* Prevention

Taking Care of Your Cold

✓ Drink plenty of liquids (except alcohol) to liquify mucus, replace lost fluids, and prevent complications such as ear infections and bronchitis.

✓ If you have a sore throat, gargle with warm, salty water. While sprays or lozenges can relieve the pain of a sore throat, none cures the inflammation causing the discomfort.

✓ If you have a cough, a cold-mist humidifier or steam vaporizer will liquefy secretions and help more than expectorants (drugs that bring up the mucus in your chest). If you do use an expectorant, make sure it contains guaifenesin, the only ingredient the FDA has found effective. The primary benefit of cough suppressants is that they allow a person with a dry, hacking cough to sleep through the night.

✓ Symptoms requiring medical attention include: fever lasting more than four or five days, or rising over 104°F; yellow-green or rust-colored discharge from the nose or throat; significant pain in the throat, sinuses, eyes, or chest; or a cough that persists.

Influenza

Although similar to a cold, **influenza**—or the flu—causes more severe symptoms that last longer (see Table 12-1). Every year an estimated 65 million Americans develop influenza, 30 million seek medical care, 300,000 are hospitalized, and 25,000 die.[28]

Flu viruses, transmitted by coughs, sneezes, laughs, and even normal conversation, are extraordinarily contagious, particularly in the first three days of the disease. The usual incubation period is two days, but symptoms can hit hard and fast. Two varieties of viruses—influenza A and influenza B—cause most flus. In recent years, the deadliest flu epidemics have been caused by various forms of influenza A viruses.

A vaccine against the flu is available, but it is not foolproof. "Because the flu virus is constantly changing, you need a new shot every year," explains Edwin Kilbourne, M.D., of New York Medical College, who has decided the components of each year's flu shots for 22 years. "And because it takes the body time to manufacture antibodies to the new viruses, you should get a vaccination at least 10 to 14 days before an outbreak hits your area."[29]

Long recommended for high-risk individuals, such as the elderly or chronically ill, flu shots now are advised for almost everyone. "The vaccine is so very safe, and the effects of the flu can be so serious that the only people we advise against it are those who are allergic to eggs. Doctors now recommend flu shots for pregnant women, particularly those who will be in the latter stages of pregnancy because flu could endanger an unborn child. "The vaccine is well proven to be safe and effective—providing 70 to 80 percent protection against flu," says Kilbourne. The only individuals who should steer clear, as already noted, are those allergic to eggs, since the inactivated flu viruses are grown in chick embryos.

A new alternative to flu "shots" is an intrasal spray containing a live, attenuated influenza virus (LAIV) vaccine. Researchers have found that the aerosol vaccine significantly reduces flu severity, days lost from work, health-care visits, and the use of over-the-counter medication. The spray represents a particular advantage for children since more than 30 percent of youngsters get the flu, but most don't receive a "flu shot." In tests of the inhaled vaccine, slightly over 1 percent of the children who received it developed the flu while 18 percent of those receiving a placebo became ill with the flu. Children who received the vaccine and still got the flu had milder symptoms, were less likely to have a fever, and recovered faster than the children given the placebo. An unexpected benefit of the nasal flu vaccine was a 30 percent reduction in ear infections in youngsters.[30]

For those who don't get vaccinated this year, Relenza (zanamivir) and Tamiflu (oseltamivir) are the next best line of defense. Both are "neuraminidase inhibitors," drugs designed to block a protein (neuraminidase) that allows the flu virus to escape from one cell and infect others. A small handheld oral inhaler, used twice a day for five days, delivers Relenza to the surface of the lungs, the primary site of flu infection. Tamiflu, taken twice a day for five days, comes in pill form. Unlike earlier antiviral flu drugs, these agents act against both Type A and Type B flu viruses and cause few side effects. In research trials, they shortened the duration of flu by up to two days and

■ Table 12-1 Is It a Cold or the Flu?

Symptoms	Cold	Flu
Fever	Rare	Characteristic, high (102°F–104°F); lasts 3–4 days
Headache	Rare	Prominent
General aches, pains	Slight	Usual; often severe
Fatigue, weakness	Quite mild	Can last up to 2–3 weeks
Prostration (extreme exhaustion)	Never	Early and prominent
Stuffy nose	Common	Sometimes
Sneezing	Usual	Sometimes
Sore throat	Common	Sometimes
Chest discomfort, cough	Mild to moderate; hacking cough	Common; can become severe
Complications	Sinus congestion or earache	Bronchitis, pneumonia; can be life-threatening
Prevention	None	Annual vaccination)
Treatment	Only temporary relief of symptoms	Relenza or Tamiflu within 36 hours after onset of symptoms

Source: National Institutes of Health.

decreased the likelihood of complications such as bronchitis, sinusitis, and ear infections. However, in order to be effective, treatment with either medication must begin within 36 to 48 hours of the first flu symptom. Although approved only for use as a treatment, Relenza and Tamiflu also can prevent flu from spreading through a family, workplace, or school.[31]

Meningitis

Meningococcal disease or miningitis, caused by the bacterium *Neisseria meningitis,* which attacks a person's spinal fluid as well as the fluid that surrounds the brain, is an extremely serious, potentially fatal illness that can result in hearing loss, kidney failure, and permanent brain injury. This illness, spread through coughing, kissing or prolonged exposure to infected persons, strikes about 3,000 Americans a year and kills about 10 percent of these individuals. College students, particularly those who live in close quarters in dormitories and residence halls, are at increased risk. An estimated 100 to 150 cases occur annually among undergraduates, and 5 to 15 students die as a result. The CDC's Advisory Committee on Immunization Practices has recommended that all college freshmen be informed that a safe and effective vaccine is available. There is a viral form of meningitis, but it is typically less severe and does not require specific treatment.

Strategies *for* Prevention

Protecting Yourself from Colds and Flus

✔ Wash your hands frequently with hot water and soap. In a public restroom, use a paper towel to turn off the faucet after you wash your hands, and avoid touching the doorknob. Wash objects used by someone contagious with a cold.

✔ Take good care of yourself: Make sure you're getting adequate sleep. Eat a balanced diet. Exercise regularly. Don't share food or drinks.

✔ Spend as little time as possible in crowds, especially in closed places, such as elevators and airplanes. When out, keep your distance from sneezers and coughers. Don't touch your eyes, mouth, and nose after being with someone who has cold symptoms.

✔ Use tissues rather than cloth handkerchiefs, which may harbor viruses for hours or days.

✔ Try to avoid irritating air pollutants. Don't smoke, which destroys protective cells in the airways and worsens any cough. Limit your intake of alcohol, which depresses white blood cells and increases the risk of bacterial pneumonia in flu sufferers.

Mononucleosis

You can get **mononucleosis** through kissing—or any other form of close contact. "Mono" is a viral disease that's most common among people 15 to 24 years old; its symptoms include a sore throat, headache, fever, nausea, and prolonged weakness. The spleen is swollen, and the lymph nodes are enlarged. You may also develop jaundice or a skin rash similar to German measles.

The major symptoms usually disappear within two to three weeks, but weakness, fatigue, and often depression may linger for at least two more weeks. The greatest danger is from physical activity that might rupture the spleen, resulting in internal bleeding. The liver may also become inflamed. A blood test can determine whether you have mono. However, there's no specific treatment for it, other than rest.

Chronic Fatigue Syndrome (CFS)

An estimated 200,000 to 500,000 Americans have the array of symptoms known as **chronic fatigue syndrome (CFS)**. According to the CDC, symptoms of chronic fatigue syndrome include chills or low grade fever, sore throat, tender lymph nodes, muscle pain, muscle weakness, extreme fatigue that doesn't improve with rest, headaches, joint pain (without swelling), neurological problems (confusion, memory loss, visual disturbances), and sleep disorders. Symptoms may begin suddenly and persist for six months to several years. Depression and anxiety attacks generally develop after ten months of illness.

Once dismissed as the yuppie flu, CFS has long baffled scientists. Some researchers contend that a single agent, perhaps a retrovirus, triggers the collapse of the immune system. Others think that repeated, undetected infections by bacteria, viruses, fungi, and parasites may lead to a gradual decline, while another theory blames symptoms on chronic low blood pressure.

Diagnosis of CFS remains difficult, although numerous studies have found significant immune abnormalities, such as high levels of certain immune cells (B lymphocytes and cytokines) that act as if they were constantly battling a viral infection. Researchers are working to develop a blood test that will definitively diagnose CFS. No specific treatments have proven effective for all patients, although some have responded to nicotinamide adenine dinucleotide (NADH), a coenzyme that plays a role in cellular energy production.[32]

Hepatitis

At least five different viruses, referred to as **hepatitis** A, B, C, Delta, and E, can cause this inflammation of the liver. Newly identified viruses also may be responsible for some causes of what is called "non-A, non-B" hepatitis. An estimated 500,000 Americans contract hepatitis each year; about 6,000 people die as a result.

All forms of hepatitis target the liver, the body's largest internal organ. Symptoms include headaches, fever, fatigue, stiff or aching joints, nausea, vomiting, and diarrhea. The liver becomes enlarged and tender to the touch; sometimes the yellowish tinge of jaundice develops. Treatment consists of rest, a high-protein diet, and the avoidance of alcohol and drugs that may stress the liver until the disease runs its course. Alpha interferon, a protein that boosts immunity and prevents viruses from replicating, may be used for some forms.

Most people begin to feel better after two or three weeks of rest, although fatigue and other symptoms can linger. As many as 10 percent of those infected with hepatitis B and up to two-thirds of those with hepatitis C become carriers of the virus for several years or even life. Some have persistent inflammation of the liver, which may cause mild or severe symptoms and increase the risk of liver cancer.

Hepatitis A, a less serious form, is generally transmitted by poor sanitation, primarily fecal contamination of food or water, and is less common in industrialized nations than in developing countries. Among those at highest risk in the United States are children and staff at day-care centers, residents of institutions for the mentally handicapped, sanitation workers, and workers who handle primates such as monkeys. Gamma globulin can provide short-term immunity; vaccines against hepatitis A have been approved by the FDA. The CDC is calling for routine immunization against hepatitis A in 11 Western states with high rates.[33]

Hepatitis B, a potentially fatal disease transmitted through the blood and other bodily fluids, infects an estimated 350,000 people around the world each year. Once spread mainly by contaminated tattoo needles, needles shared by drug addicts, or transfusions of contaminated blood, hepatitis B is now transmitted mostly through sexual contact. It can cause chronic liver infection, cirrhosis, and liver cancer.

Hepatitis B is a particular threat to young people, because 75 percent of new cases are diagnosed in those between ages 15 to 39. They usually contract hepatitis B through high-risk behaviors such as multiple sex partners and use of injected drugs. Individuals who have tattoos or body piercing may also be at risk if procedures are not done under regulated conditions.[34] At highest risk are male homosexuals, heterosexuals with multiple sex partners, health-care workers with frequent contact with blood, IV-drug abusers, and infants born to infected mothers. Vaccination can prevent hepatitis B and is recommended for children, teens, and adults at high risk.

As many as 4 million people in the United States and 200 million people worldwide harbor the hepatitis C virus (HCV). Hepatitis C, which can lead to chronic liver disease, cirrhosis, and liver cancer, is the leading reason for liver transplantation in the United States.

The number of new cases has fallen dramatically in the last decade because of improved blood screening for transfusions and a decrease in the number of injection drug users.[35] However, because infected individuals are typically asymptomatic for years—and even decades—after becoming infected, many are unaware they have contracted the virus until they sustain irreparable liver damage. The number of deaths from hepatitis C-related liver disease is expected to triple in the next 10 to 20 years.[36]

Viewed as the most serious of the five types of hepatitis, HCV is spread primarily through contact with infected blood. High-risk activities include injection of illegal drugs, getting pricked with a needle with infected blood, exposure to contaminated blood products, a tattoo or body piercing with nonsterile instruments used on someone infected with HCV, use of an infected person's toothbrush or razor, and engaging in high-risk sexual behavior, such as having multiple partners or failing to use condoms.

Federal health officials have approved the first at-home test kit for hepatitis C (HCV) .The kit, called the Hepatitis C Check, can be purchased without a prescription and includes a lancet for drawing a drop of blood, filter paper, and a mailer. The user collects a blood sample through a finger stick, then mails it to a testing laboratory, where the blood can be analyzed to see if a person has been exposed to the virus. The test detects antibodies to HCV but cannot pick up infections that have occurred in the past six months. Results are made available in about four to ten days through an automated phone system, coded by an anonymous identification number.

There is no vaccine for hepatitis C, but there are drug treatments, such as interferon alpha or a combination of interferon with ribavirin. The CDC also recommends that infected individuals stop using alcohol, see a doctor regularly, not start any new herbals, over-the-counter preparations, or drugs without consulting a physician, and get vaccinated against hepatitis A.[37]

Hepatitis D, sometimes called the delta virus, can only infect individuals already suffering from hepatitis B. Because it is incomplete, this virus needs to borrow some proteins from the B virus in order to replicate. Like hepatitis B and C, it is spread by blood and bodily fluids. In the United States, it is most common among individuals who are in frequent contact with blood and among users of IV drugs. Hepatitis E is transmitted primarily through water contaminated by sewage. Although rare in the United States, this potentially deadly virus has caused epidemics in Africa and Asia.

Pneumonia

An inflammation of the lungs, **pneumonia** fills the fine, spongy networks of the lungs' tiny air chambers with fluid. It can be caused by bacteria, viruses (including flu), or foreign material in the lungs (such as smoke). The symptoms of classic bacterial pneumonia are fever, shortness of breath, and general weakness. Along with influenza, pneumonia is the fifth-leading killer of Americans and the most common infectious cause of death.

The typical signs of pneumonia include cough, a fever of more than 101°F, difficulty breathing, chills, and excessive yellow green phlegm. Symptoms of pneumonia can develop either gradually or else so quickly that a person's life is in danger within hours. Antibiotics can control bacterial pneumonia, but they must be given before microbes erode local tissues and spread through the blood elsewhere in the body, causing a condition known as septicemia, or blood poisoning. Because of the dangers of pneumonia, you should see a doctor if there's any chance you have it. Severe cases may require hospitalization and high doses of antibiotics.

Vaccination against pneumonia is recommended for those who've had pneumonia in the past, those with impaired immune function, and those over age 50. The pneumonia vaccine greatly reduces the risk of this disease, especially for women and those with impaired immunity.

Tuberculosis

A bacterial infection of the lungs that was once the nation's leading killer, **tuberculosis (TB)** claims the lives of more people than any acute infectious disease other than pneumonia (Figure 12-3). One-third of the world's population is infected with the TB organism, although not all develop active disease. Each year the infection spreads to another 8 million people. In the United States, TB cases, after declining for decades, increased from the mid-1980s to the early 1990s. The reasons include immigration from countries where TB is common, poverty, homelessness, alcoholism and drug abuse, the HIV/AIDS epidemic, and the emergence of resistant strains of TB.[38] By the late 1990s, some cities reported a decline in TB, thanks to better infection control and greater monitoring to ensure completion of treatment.

Although TB is most prevalent among high-risk groups, the overall danger increases as more people develop active disease because TB is highly contagious. TB outbreaks have occurred throughout the country in hospitals, nursing homes, prisons, and office buildings, where inadequate ventilation increases the risk of infection.

Most TB patients recover completely after six months of taking a combination of three different medicines. Drug-resistant forms of the tuberculosis microor-

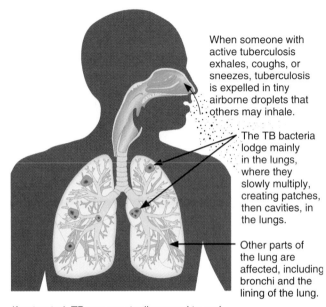

When someone with active tuberculosis exhales, coughs, or sneezes, tuberculosis is expelled in tiny airborne droplets that others may inhale.

The TB bacteria lodge mainly in the lungs, where they slowly multiply, creating patches, then cavities, in the lungs.

Other parts of the lung are affected, including bronchi and the lining of the lung.

If untreated, TB can eventually spread to and damage the brain, bone, eyes, liver and kidneys, spine, and skin.

■ **Figure 12-3** How tuberculosis spreads.

ganism strike mostly patients who start drug treatment but don't follow through with it. Because they don't take enough of the medication to kill all the TB bacteria in their system, those that survive become resistant. Even with full treatment, the risk of dying from drug-resistant tuberculosis is 50 percent. HIV infection greatly increases susceptibility to infection with TB and the risk of dying if infected with treatment-resistant forms.

If you think you may have been exposed to TB or if you develop suspicious symptoms (loss of appetite and weight, low-grade fever, fatigue, chills, night sweats, coughing), see your doctor for a TB test. This consists of an injection just under the skin. The area of the arm where the test was administered should be checked by a health-care professional. The test results help to determine the presence of the TB bacteria; further tests confirm the diagnosis. If the skin test is positive, indicating that TB is present, you'll be monitored with yearly chest X rays. You may also require treatment with a drug such as refampin or isoniazid (also called INH).

Group A and Group B Strep Infection

Sore throats are common winter complaints, but those caused by group A streptococcus bacteria—"strep throats"—are more than a trivial threat. If not treated promptly with antibiotics, strep bacteria can travel to the kidneys, the liver, or the heart, where they can cause rheumatic fever—an inflammation of the heart that can cause weakness, shortness of breath, joint pain, and an abnormal heartbeat. In recent years clusters of rheumatic fever have sprung up in several major cities. Pediatricians are urging parents to consult their doctors if a youngster complains of a sore throat or if strep is widespread in the community. Rapid new diagnostic tests can identify strep within minutes. If the test is positive, treatment with penicillin or a similar antibiotic is indicated. Brief treatment (five days) with Omnicef, a new antibiotic, has proven as effective as ten days of oral penicillin.[39]

A new danger linked with group A strep is toxic streptococcal shock syndrome, or toxic strep. This is an invasive form of the disease in which strep gains access to the blood and causes a drop in blood pressure, a very high fever, and the production of exotoxins (substances that can attack various organs, such as the kidneys, heart or, in rare cases, flesh). Toxic strep is rather rare and usually doesn't occur with strep throats. Prompt treatment is critical.

Group B streptococcus (GBS), the leading cause of life-threatening perinatal infections in the United States, is primarily a threat to newborns. Because some 15 to 40 percent of pregnant women carry GBS but have no symptoms, the American Academy of Pediatrics has called for universal screening of expectant mothers. Each year 12,000 newborns are infected, most of them during childbirth; more than 1,600 die, and another 1,600 suffer permanent brain damage from meningitis. Women at high risk of infecting their newborns with GBS are those who have premature labor, early rupture of their amniotic membranes, fever, and a high group B strep count before or during pregnancy, or who have previously borne an infant infected with GBS. Also at risk are diabetics, poor women, and those under age 20. Treating all high-risk pregnant women could prevent most GBS infections in newborns.

Toxic Shock Syndrome

As discussed in Chapter 9, **toxic shock syndrome (TSS)** is a potentially deadly disease associated with the use of tampons, particularly high-absorbency types. It is caused by *Staphylococcus aureus* and group A *Streptococcus pyogenes* bacteria that release toxins (poisonous waste products) into the bloodstream. Symptoms include a high fever; a rash that leads to peeling of the skin on the fingers, toes, palms, and soles; dizziness; dangerously low blood pressure; and abnormalities in several organ systems (the digestive tract and the kidneys) and in the muscles and blood.

In addition to women who use high-absorbency tampons, or leave their tampons in too long, those who

have given birth within the preceding six to eight weeks are at greater risk. Children (including newborns), men, and postmenopausal women also have developed TSS, which usually has been traced to bacteria in skin abscesses, boils, cuts, or postsurgical wounds.

Without prompt treatment, TSS can cause severe and permanent damage, including muscle weakness, partial paralysis, amnesia, disorientation, an inability to concentrate, and impaired lung and kidney function. Sometimes toxic shock weakens the blood vessels, increasing the risk of heart problems. Victims can enter the state of life-threatening crisis called shock, in which blood flow throughout the body is inadequate to sustain life. Treatment usually consists of immediate hospitalization, intravenous administration of fluids, medications to raise blood pressure, and powerful antibiotics; intravenous administration of immunoglobins that attack the toxins produced by these bacteria may also be beneficial.

Lyme Disease

Lyme disease, a bacterial infection, is spread by ticks carrying a kind of bacterium, the spirochete *Borrelia burgdorferi*. An infected person may have various symptoms, including joint inflammation, heart arrhythmias, blinding headaches, and memory lapses. The disease can also cause miscarriages and birth defects. Lyme disease is by far the most commonly reported vector-borne infectious disease in the United States. The vast majority of all reported cases have occurred in just ten states; those leading the list are New York, New Jersey, Connecticut, Pennsylvania, and Wisconsin. Nationwide cases of Lyme disease have been dropping throughout the 1990s.[40] (See Figure 12-4.)

The FDA has licensed a vaccine to prevent Lyme disease in individuals 15 to 70 years old. LYMErix, like

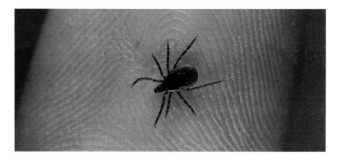

Ticks are responsible for the spread of Lyme disease. If you spot a tick, remove it as soon as possible with tweezers or small forceps. Put it in a plastic bag or sealed bottle and save it. If you develop a rash or other symptoms, take it with you to the doctor.

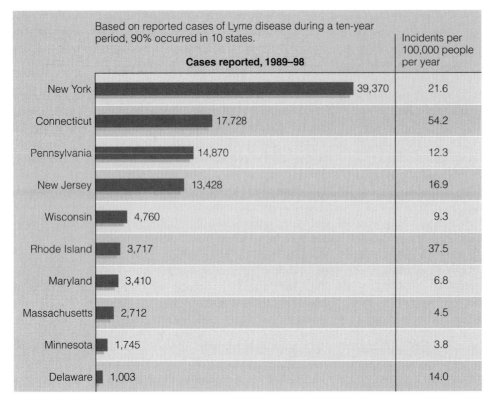

Based on reported cases of Lyme disease during a ten-year period, 90% occurred in 10 states.

Cases reported, 1989–98		Incidents per 100,000 people per year
New York	39,370	21.6
Connecticut	17,728	54.2
Pennsylvania	14,870	12.3
New Jersey	13,428	16.9
Wisconsin	4,760	9.3
Rhode Island	3,717	37.5
Maryland	3,410	6.8
Massachusetts	2,712	4.5
Minnesota	1,745	3.8
Delaware	1,003	14.0

■ **Figure 12-4** Regional risk of Lyme disease.

Source: Centers for Disease Control and Prevention. © 1999, *USA Today*. Reprinted with permission.

most vaccines, stimulates the immune system to produce antibodies, in this case against the bacteria that cause Lyme disease. But the vaccine, administered in three doses over a one-year period, is not 100 percent effective and should not be considered a substitute for protective clothing and tick repellent. Administration must be timed so the second and third doses are given at the beginning of the tick transmission season, usually April in the Northeastern United States. It is not known how long protection against Lyme disease lasts after vaccination.[41]

The primary culprit in most cases of Lyme disease is the deer tick, although other ticks, including the Western black-legged tick, the dog tick, and the Lone Star tick, also may transmit the bacterium that causes Lyme disease as well as organisms that transmit other diseases, such as Rocky Mountain spotted fever and babesiosis.

Hunters and campers are more likely to test positive for Lyme disease. Pet owners are not at additional risk. The most important preventive step is to check yourself for ticks whenever you come in from the outdoors. However, detecting some types of ticks can be difficult. In their nymphal stage, when they're most likely to bite, ticks are about the size of a poppyseed. Even as adults, some ticks are no bigger than a sesame seed.

Regardless of whether or not they've spotted a tick, residents of infested areas should check regularly for signs of a bite. About two-thirds of those bitten develop some skin changes from two days to four weeks afterward. The classic skin lesion is a small, clear-centered red doughnut that expands, but most people simply have a red blotch or two blotches. However, the rash always expands, usually to about 2 inches in diameter. In some cases, it may cover a person's entire chest or thigh; others develop rashes far from the bite, caused by spirochetes that travel through the bloodstream. More sensitive diagnostic tests allow detection of extremely low numbers of spirochetes and make earlier diagnosis possible. However, they should be used only to support a clinical diagnosis of Lyme disease.[42]

Strategies *for* Prevention

Protecting Yourself

✓ If you live in the North Atlantic states, the north central Midwest, or along the Pacific coast, wear long pants rather than shorts, and tuck your pants into your socks when walking through woods or fields of high grass.

✓ Stick to the center of trails when hiking, and avoid piles of leaves and branches.

✓ In tick-infested areas, use insect repellents. People who use insect repellents are half as likely to get Lyme disease as those who don't.

✓ After spending time outdoors, examine yourself for ticks or bites every day. Check less obvious places, such as the scalp and behind the ears.

✓ If you do spot a tick, remove it right away. Using tweezers or forceps, grasp the tick firmly as close to its head and as near to your skin as possible. Gently pull backward, without squeezing the tick's body, until its hold is released. Wash your hands thoroughly. Treat the wound with rubbing alcohol.

The Threat of Emerging and Re-Emerging Infectious Diseases

As defined by the National Institute of Allergy and Infectious Diseases (NIAID), emerging infections are those that have been recently recognized, are increasing in humans, or threaten to spread to new areas in the near future. The most widespread is HIV, which is believed to have emerged from Central Africa less than 30 years ago. (See Figure 12-5.) Other emerging viruses, such as Hantavirus, Ebola, dengue, Lassa, and Marburg, have been responsible for deadly outbreaks around the globe.[43] The most well-known may be Ebola, a particularly virulent virus that is transmitted by direct contact with blood or bodily fluids. In several outbreaks in Africa, this filovirus has resisted all medication and killed up to 90 percent of its victims.

Another threat comes from mutated, or changed, forms of familiar microbes (such as those that cause tuberculosis) that have become resistant to standard medications. Why, despite enormous scientific progress, do emerging and resistant microbes remain such a formidable foe? "Viruses and bacteria have the capacity to reinvent themselves rapidly," says John La Montagne of NIAID. "Because they have few genes compared to people, one mutation can change an organism's ability to infect, spread, or cause disease." There are other reasons why deadly infections are becoming a greater threat. As civilization spreads into previously undeveloped areas, such as the rainforests of Central Africa, and goods and animals are imported from distant lands, more human beings are encountering microbes that were once confined to very remote regions.[44]

Reproductive and Urinary Tract Infections

Reproductive and urinary tract infections are very common. Many are not spread exclusively by sexual contact, and so they are not classified as sexually transmitted diseases (STDs), discussed later in this chapter.

Vaginal Infections

The most common vaginal infections are **trichomoniasis, candidiasis,** and **bacterial vaginosis.**

Protozoa *(Trichomonas vaginalis)* that live in the vagina can multiply rapidly, causing itching, burning, and discharge—all symptoms of trichomoniasis. Male carriers usually have no symptoms, although some may develop urethritis or an inflammation of the prostate and seminal vesicles. All patients with this infection should be screened for syphilis, gonorrhea, chlamydia, and HIV. Sexual partners must be treated with oral medication (metronidazol; trade name Flagyl), even if they have no symptoms, to prevent reinfection.

Populations of a yeast called *Candida albicans*—normal inhabitants of the mouth, digestive tract, and vagina—are usually held in

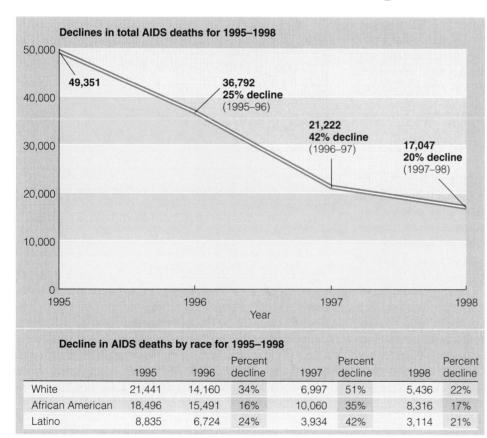

Declines in total AIDS deaths for 1995–1998

49,351

36,792
25% decline
(1995–96)

21,222
42% decline
(1996–97)

17,047
20% decline
(1997–98)

Year

Decline in AIDS deaths by race for 1995–1998

	1995	1996	Percent decline	1997	Percent decline	1998	Percent decline
White	21,441	14,160	34%	6,997	51%	5,436	22%
African American	18,496	15,491	16%	10,060	35%	8,316	17%
Latino	8,835	6,724	24%	3,934	42%	3,114	21%

■ Figure 12-5 The latest trends in AIDs deaths.

Source: Centers for Disease Control and Prevention. From *The New York Times,* 9/10/99. Reprinted by permission.

check. Under certain conditions, however (such as poor nutrition, stress, or antibiotic use), the microbes multiply, causing burning, itching, and a whitish discharge, and producing what is commonly known as a yeast infection. Common sites for candidiasis, which is also called moniliasis, are the vagina, vulva, penis, and mouth. The women most likely to test positive for candidiasis have never been pregnant, use condoms for birth control, have sexual intercourse more than four times a month, and have taken antibiotics in the previous 15 to 30 days.[45] Vaginal medications, such as GyneLotrimin and Monistat, available as OTC drugs for women with recurrent infections, provide effective treatment. Male sexual partners may be advised to wear condoms during outbreaks of candidiasis. Women should keep the genital area dry and wear cotton underwear.

Bacterial vaginosis is characterized by alterations in the microorganisms that live in the vagina, including depletion of certain bacteria and overgrowth of others. It typically causes a white or gray vaginal discharge with a distinctive fishy odor similar to that of trichomoniasis. Its underlying cause is unknown, although it occurs most frequently in women with multiple sex partners. Long-term dangers include pelvic inflammatory disease (PID), (discussed later in this chapter) and pregnancy complications. Metronidazole, either in the form of a pill or a vaginal gel, is the primary treatment. According to CDC guidelines, treatment for male sex partners appears to be of little benefit, but some health practitioners recommend treatment for both partners in cases of recurrent infections.

Urinary Tract Infections (UTIs)

A urinary tract infection (UTI) can be present in any of the three parts of the urinary tract: the urethra, bladder, or kidney. An infection involving the urethra is known as **urethritis.** If the bladder is also infected, it's called **cystitis.** If it reaches the kidneys, it's called **pyelonephritis.**

An estimated 40 percent of women report having had a UTI at some point in their lives. Three times as many women as men develop UTIs, probably for anatomical reasons. A woman's urethra is only 1.5 inches long; a man's is 6 inches. Therefore bacteria, the major cause of UTIs, have a shorter distance to travel to infect a woman's bladder and kidneys. About one-fourth to one-third of all women between ages 20 and 40 develop UTIs, and 80 percent of those who experience one infection develop recurrences.[46]

Conditions that can set the stage for UTIs include irritation and swelling of the urethra or bladder as a result of pregnancy, bike riding, irritants (such as bubble bath, douches, or a diaphragm), urinary stones, enlargement in men of the prostate gland, vaginitis, and

stress. Early diagnosis is critical, because infection can spread to the kidneys and, if unchecked, result in kidney failure. Symptoms include frequent burning, painful urination, chills, fever, fatigue, and blood in the urine.[47]

Recurrent UTIs, a frequent problem among young women, have been linked with a genetic predisposition, sexual intercourse, and the use of diaphragms. Postintercourse treatment with antibiotics can lower the risk. Frequent recurrence of symptoms may not be caused by infection but by interstitial cystitis, a little-understood bladder inflammation that affects an estimated 450,000 Americans, almost all of them women.

Strategies *for* Prevention

How to Prevent UTIs

✔ Be conscientious about general cleanliness. Since a major cause of UTIs is the bacteria normally found in stools, be sure to wipe from front to back after bowel movements.

✔ Drink five to six glasses of water a day.

✔ Don't wait when you feel the urge to urinate.

✔ Don't use chemical irritants, such as perfumed hygiene sprays or bubble bath.

✔ If you use a diaphragm, have the fit checked regularly, especially after giving birth.

✔ If UTIs seem to follow sex, ask about prophylactic medication. Urinate immediately after intercourse.

✔ If you have a relapse after treatment or have recurrent infections, ask your partner to get a checkup too.

Sexually Transmitted Diseases (STDs)

Venereal diseases (from the Latin *venus*, meaning "love" or "lust") are more accurately called **sexually transmitted diseases (STDs).** Around the world, more than 250 million cases of STDs are diagnosed each year (more than a million are of HIV). Almost 700,000 people are infected every day with one of the over 20 STDs tracked by world health officials. STDs are much more widespread (or "prevalent") in developing nations because of lack of adequate health standards, prevention practices, and access to treatment.

More Americans are infected with STDs now than at any other time in history. According to the Institute of Medicine, the odds of acquiring an STD during a lifetime are one in four.[48] STDs are among the top ten most frequently reported diseases in the United States, and their annual economic cost is $17 billion. The major cause of preventable sterility in America, STDs have tripled the rate of ectopic (tubal) pregnancies, which can be fatal if not detected early. STD complications, including miscarriage, premature delivery, and uterine infections after delivery, affect more than 100,000 women annually. Moreover, infection with an STD greatly increases the risk of HIV transmission (discussed later in this chapter). The incidence of STDs is highest in young adults and homosexual men. Others affected by STDs include unborn and newborn children who can "catch" potentially life-threatening infections in the womb or during birth.

Although each STD is a distinct disease, all STD pathogens like dark, warm, moist body surfaces, particularly the mucous membranes that line the reproductive organs; they hate light, cold, and dryness. It is possible to catch or have more than one STD at a time. Curing one doesn't necessarily cure another, and treatments don't prevent another bout with the same STD. (See Table 12-2.)

Many STDs, including early HIV infection and gonorrhea in women, may not cause any symptoms. As a result, infected individuals can continue their usual sexual activity without realizing that they're jeopardizing others' well-being. (See the Self-Survey: "STD Attitude Scale.")

STDs, Adolescents, and Young Adults

Nearly two-thirds of people who acquire STDs in the United States are under age 25. The most common bacterial STD is chlamydia, with two of the highest rates of chlamydia occurring among adolescents in general and among young adult women. Cases of genital herpes among white adolescents have increased five times, and cases among white people in their twenties have doubled over the past few years. Among college-age women in one study, cases of human papillomavirus (HPV) infections increased from 26 percent to 43 percent over a three-year period. Contracting STDs may increase the risk of being infected with HIV, and as many as half of new HIV infections may be among people under age 25. Because college students have more opportunities to have different sex partners and may use drugs and alcohol more often before sex, they are at greater risk. More than half of 13-to-24-year-old women with HIV are infected heterosexually.[49]

Even when high school and college students have generally accurate knowledge about STDs, they don't necessarily practice safe sex. According to research, those students with the greatest number of sexual partners are least likely to use condoms. Other studies have shown that proximity to a high-density AIDS epicenter (such as San Francisco) has no impact on HIV/AIDS knowledge and attitudes, and that religious affiliation does not decrease risky sexual behavior, at least among religious students who are sexually active. As shown in the Campus Focus: "College Students and Safer Sex Precautions," students say they're comfortable asking about sexual history and HIV testing, but most have never been tested.[50]

Various factors put young people at risk of STDs, including:

- *Feelings of invulnerability,* which lead to risk-taking behavior. Even when they are well-informed of the risks, adolescents may remain unconvinced that anything bad can or will happen to them.

- *Multiple partners.* In student surveys, a significant minority report having had four or more sex partners during their lifetime.

- *Failure to use condoms.* Among those who reported having had sexual intercourse in the previous three months, fewer than half reported condom use. Students who'd had four or more sex partners were significantly *less* likely to use condoms than those who'd had fewer partners.

- *Widespread substance abuse.* Teenagers who drink or use drugs are more likely to engage in sexually risky behaviors, including sex with partners whose health status and history they do not know and unprotected intercourse.

The college years are a prime time for contracting sexually transmitted diseases. According to the American College Health Association, chlamydia and human papilloma virus (HPV) have reached epidemic levels at many schools—although many of those infected aren't even aware of it.

Educators and health officials have struggled to find ways to bridge the gap between what college students know about the threat of STDs and what they do to protect themselves. Some universities are experimenting with alternatives to workshops or traditional informational materials, such as peer counseling. Others have invited individuals who are HIV-positive or who have AIDS to meet with students and talk about their experiences. In a study of psychology students, those who listened to a lecturer with HIV had significantly higher scores in terms of knowledge and behavioral intent to practice safer sex, compared with their scores before the lecture and with students who had no AIDS education. Many health professionals believe that education must begin much earlier and so are endeavoring to introduce HIV/AIDS education programs at the elementary school level.

■ **Table 12-2** Common Sexually Transmitted Diseases (STDs): Mode of Transmission, Symptoms, and Treatment

STD	Transmission	Symptoms	Treatment
Chlamydial infection	The *Chlamydia trachomatis* bacterium is transmitted primarily through sexual contact. It may also be spread by fingers from one body site to another.	In women, PID (pelvic inflammatory disease) caused by *Chlamydia* may include disrupted menstrual periods, pelvic pain, elevated temperature, nausea, vomiting, headache, infertility, and ectopic pregnancy. In men, chlamydial infection of the urethra may cause a discharge and burning during urination. *Chlamydia*-caused epididymitis may produce a sense of heaviness in the affected testicle(s), inflammation of the scrotal skin, and painful swelling at the bottom of the testicle.	Doxycycline, azithromycin, or ofloxacin
Gonorrhea ("clap")	The *Neisseria gonorrhoeae* bacterium ("gonococcus") is spread through genital, oral–genital, or genital–anal contact.	The most common symptoms in men are a cloudy discharge from the penis and burning sensations during urination. If disease is untreated, complications may include inflammation of scrotal skin and swelling at base of the testicle. In women, some green or yellowish discharge is produced but commonly remains undetected. Later, PID (pelvic inflammatory disease) may develop.	Dual therapy of a single dose of ceftriaxone, cefixime, ciprofloxacin, or ofloxacin plus doxycycline for seven days
Non-gonococcal urethritis (NGU)	Primary causes are believed to be the bacteria *Chlamydia trachomatis* and *Ureaplasma urealyticum*, most commonly transmitted through coitus. Some NGU may result from allergic reactions or from *Trichomonas* infection.	Inflammation of the urethral tube. A man has a discharge from the penis and irritation during urination. A woman may have a mild discharge of pus from the vagina but often shows no symptoms.	Doxycycline or erythromycin
Syphilis	The *Treponema pallidum* bacterium ("spirochete") is transmitted from open lesions during genital, oral–genital, or genital–anal contact.	*Primary stage:* A painless chancre appears at the site where the spirochetes entered the body. *Secondary stage:* The chancre disappears and a generalized skin rash develops. *Latent stage:* There may be no visible symptoms. *Tertiary stage:* Heart failure, blindness, mental disturbance, and many other symptoms occur. Death may result.	Benzathine penicillin G, doxycycline, tetracycline, or erythromycin
Chancroid	The *Haemophilus ducreyi* bacterium is usually transmitted by sexual interaction.	Small bumps (papules) in genital regions eventually rupture and form painful, soft, craterlike ulcers that emit a foul-smelling discharge.	Single doses of either ceftriaxone or azithromycin or seven days of erythromycin
Herpes	The genital herpes virus (HSV-2) seems to be transmitted primarily by vaginal, anal, or oral–genital intercourse. The oral herpes virus (HSV-1) is transmitted primarily by kissing.	Small, painful red bumps (papules) appear in the genital region (genital herpes) or mouth (oral herpes). The papules become painful blisters that eventually rupture to form wet, open sores.	No known cure; a variety of treatments may reduce symptoms; oral or intravenous acyclovir (Zovirax) promotes healing and suppresses recurrent outbreaks.

■ Table 12-2 Continued

STD	Transmission	Symptoms	Treatment
Genital warts (condylomata acuminata)	The virus is spread primarily through vaginal, anal, or oral-genital sexual interaction.	Hard and yellow-gray on dry skin areas; soft, pinkish-red, and cauliflowerlike on moist areas.	Freezing, application of topical agents like trichloroacetic acid or podofilox, cauterization, surgical removal, or vaporization by carbon dioxide laser
Viral hepatitis	The hepatitis B virus may be transmitted by blood, semen, vaginal secretions, and saliva. Manual, oral, or penile stimulation of the anus are strongly associated with the spread of this virus. Hepatitis A seems to be primarily spread via the fecal–oral route. Oral–anal sexual contact is a common mode for sexual transmission of hepatitis A.	Vary from nonexistent to mild, flulike symptoms to an incapacitating illness characterized by high fever, vomiting, and severe abdominal pain.	No specific therapy; treatment generally consists of bed rest and adequate fluid intake.
Bacterial vaginosis	The most common causative agent, the *Gardnerella vaginalis* bacterium, is sometimes transmitted through coitus.	In women, a fishy- or musty-smelling, thin discharge, like flour paste in consistency and usually gray. Most men are asymptomatic.	Metronidazole (Flagyl) by mouth or intra-vaginal applications of topical metronidazole gel or clindamycin cream
Candidiasis (yeast infection)	The *Candida albicans* fungus may accelerate growth when the chemical balance of the vagina is disturbed; it may also be transmitted through sexual interaction.	White, "cheesy" discharge; irritation of vaginal and vulval tissues.	Vaginal suppositories or topical cream, such as clotrimazole and miconazole, or oral fluconazole
Trichomoniasis	The protozoan parasite *Trichomonas vaginalis* is usually passed through genital sexual contact.	White or yellow vaginal discharge with an unpleasant odor; vulva is sore and irritated.	Metronidazole (Flagyl) for both women and men
Pubic lice ("crabs")	*Phthirus pubis,* the pubic louse, is spread easily through body contact or through shared clothing or bedding.	Persistent itching. Lice are visible and may often be located in pubic hair or other body hair.	Preparations such as A-200 pyrinate or Kwell (gamma benzene hexachloride)
Scabies	*Sarcoptes scabiei* is highly contagious and may be transmitted by close physical contact, sexual and nonsexual.	Small bumps and a red rash that itch intensely, especially at night.	5% permethrin lotion or cream
Acquired immuno-deficiency syndrome (AIDS)	Blood and semen are the major vehicles for transmitting HIV, which attacks the immune system. It appears to be passed primarily through sexual contact, or needle sharing among injecting drug users.	Vary with the type of cancer or opportunistic infections that afflict an infected person. Common symptoms include fevers, night sweats, weight loss, chronic fatigue, swollen lymph nodes, diarrhea and/or bloody stools, atypical bruising or bleeding, skin rashes, headache, chronic cough, and a whitish coating on the tongue or throat.	Commence treatment early after seroconversion with a combination of three antiviral drugs ("triple drug therapy") plus other specific treatment(s), if necessary, of opportunistic infections and tumors.

Source: Crooks, Robert, and Baur, Karla. *Our Sexuality,* 7th ed. Pacific Grove, CA: Brooks Cole, 1999.

Self-*Survey* | STD Attitude Scale

Directions: Please read each statement carefully: STD means sexually transmitted diseases, once called venereal diseases. Record your first reaction by marking an "X" through the letter that best describes how much you agree or disagree with the idea.

1. How one uses his/her sexuality has nothing to do with STDs.

   SA   A   U   D   SD

2. It is easy to use the prevention methods that reduce one's chances of getting an STD.

   SA   A   U   D   SD

3. Responsible sex is one of the best ways of reducing the risk of STDs.

   SA   A   U   D   SD

4. Getting early medical care is the main key to preventing harmful effects of STDs.

   SA   A   U   D   SD

5. Choosing the right partner is important in reducing the risk of getting an STD.

   SA   A   U   D   SD

6. A high rate of STDs should be a concern for all people.

   SA   A   U   D   SD

7. People with an STD have a duty to get their sex partners to seek medical care.

   SA   A   U   D   SD

8. The best way to get a sex partner to STD treatment is to take him/her to the doctor with you.

   SA   A   U   D   SD

9. Changing one's sex habits is necessary once the presence of an STD is known.

   SA   A   U   D   SD

10. I would dislike having to follow the medical steps for treating an STD.

    SA   A   U   D   SD

11. If I were sexually active, I would feel uneasy doing things before and after sex to prevent getting an STD.

    SA   A   U   D   SD

12. If I were sexually active, it would be insulting if a sex partner suggested we use a condom to avoid STDs.

    SA   A   U   D   SD

13. I dislike talking about STDs with my peers.

    SA   A   U   D   SD

14. I would be uncertain about going to the doctor unless I was sure I really had an STD.

    SA   A   U   D   SD

15. I would feel that I should take my sex partner with me to a clinic if I thought I had an STD.

Use This Key: SA = Strongly agree; A = Agree; U = Undecided; D = Disagree; SD = Strongly disagree.
Remember: STD means sexually transmitted disease, such as gonorrhea, syphilis, genital herpes, and AIDS.

         SA   A   U   D   SD

16. It would be embarrassing to discuss STDs with one's partner if one were sexually active.

    SA   A   U   D   SD

17. If I were to have sex, the chance of getting an STD makes me uneasy about having sex with more than one person.

    SA   A   U   D   SD

18. I like the idea of sexual abstinence (not having sex) as the best way to avoid STDs.

    SA   A   U   D   SD

19. If I had an STD, I would cooperate with public health persons to find the sources of the STD.

    SA   A   U   D   SD

20. If I had an STD, I would avoid exposing others while I was being treated.

    SA   A   U   D   SD

21. I would have regular STD checkups if I were having sex with more than one partner.

    SA   A   U   D   SD

22. I intend to look for STD signs before deciding to have sex with anyone.

    SA   A   U   D   SD

23. I will limit my sex activity to just one partner because of the chances I might get an STD.

    SA   A   U   D   SD

24. I will avoid sex contact anytime I think there is even a slight chance of getting an STD.

    SA   A   U   D   SD

25. The chance of getting an STD would not stop me from having sex.

    SA   A   U   D   SD

26. If I had a chance, I would support community efforts toward controlling STDs.

    SA   A   U   D   SD

27. I would be willing to work with others to make people aware of STD problems in my town.

    SA   A   U   D   SD

Scoring: Calculate total points for each subscale and total scale, using the point values below.

For items 1, 10–14, 16, 25:
Strongly agree = 5 points; Disagree = 2 points; and Agree = 4 points; Strongly disagree = 1 point.
Undecided = 3 points;

For items 2–9, 15, 17–24, 26, 27:
Strongly agree = 1 point;   Disagree = 4 points; and
Agree = 2 points;   Strongly disagree = 5 points.
Undecided = 3 points;

Total scale: items 1–27
Belief Subscale: items 1–9
Feeling Subscale: items 10–18
Intention to Act Subscale: items 19–27

Interpretation

High score predisposes one toward high-risk STD behavior. Low score predisposes one toward low-risk STD behavior.

Yarber, Torabi, and Veenker (1989) developed the STD Attitude Scale by administering three experimental forms of 45 items each. Respondents were 2,980 students in six secondary school districts in the Midwest and East. Based on statistical analysis, the scale was reduced to the final 27 items. Reliability coefficients for the entire scale and the three subscales ranged from .48 to .73. The developers reported evidence of construct validity in that the scale was sensitive to positive attitude changes resulting from STD education.

Reference: Yarber, W. L., Torabi, M. R., and Veneer, C. H. Development of a Three-Component STD Attitude Scale. *Journal of Sex Education and Therapy,* Vol. 15, 1989, pp. 36–39. Used by permission.

Prevention and Protection

Abstinence is the only guarantee of sexual safety—and one that more and more young people are choosing. As discussed in Chapter 9, the choice of an abstinent (or celibate) lifestyle offers many advantages, both in the present and the future. By choosing not to be sexually active with a partner, individuals can safeguard their physical health, their fertility, and their future.

For men and women who are sexually active, a mutually faithful sexual relationship with just one healthy partner is the safest option. For those not in such relationships, safer-sex practices are essential for reducing risks [see Pulsepoints: "Ten Ways to Prevent Sexually Transmitted Diseases (STDs)"]. Some experts believe that condom use may be a more effective tactic than any drug or vaccine in preventing STDs and are focusing their efforts on increasing condom use among sexually active adolescents.[51]

How can you tell if someone you're dating or hope to date has been exposed to an STD? The bad news is, you can't. But the good news is, it doesn't matter—as long as you avoid sexual activity that could put you at risk of infection. Ideally, before engaging in any such behavior, both of you should talk about your prior sexual history (including number of partners and sexually transmitted diseases) and other high-risk behavior, such as the use of injection drugs. If you know someone well enough to consider having sex with that person, you should be able to talk about STDs. If the person is unwilling to talk, you shouldn't have sex.

Even if you do talk openly, you can't be sure a potential partner is telling you the truth. In various surveys of college students, a significant proportion of the men and women said they would lie to a potential partner about having an STD or testing positive for HIV. The only way of knowing for certain that a prospective partner is safe is through laboratory testing. Sex educators and health professionals strongly encourage couples to abstain from any sexual activity that puts them at risk for STDs until they both undergo medical examinations and laboratory testing to rule out STDs. This process greatly reduces the danger of disease transmission and can also help foster a deep sense of mutual trust and commitment. Many campus and public health clinics provide exams or laboratory testing either free of charge or on a sliding scale determined by your income.

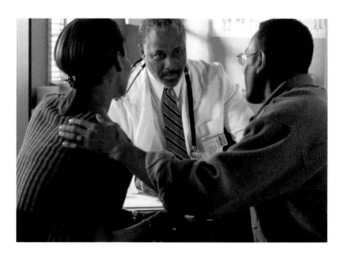

Talking openly about STDs and being tested with your partner protects your health and can foster a sense of trust and commitment.

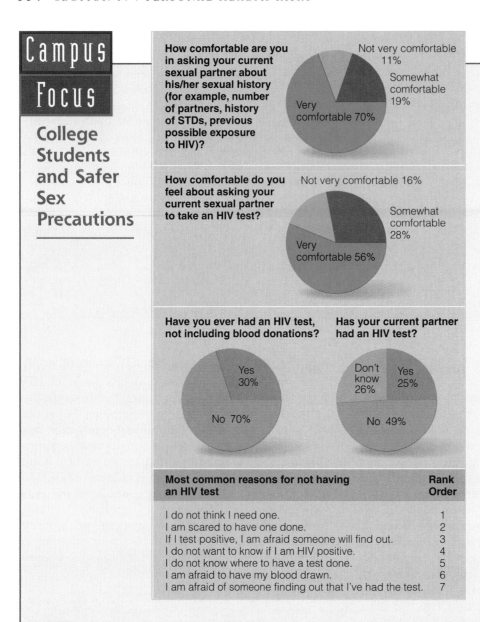

Most common reasons for not having an HIV test	Rank Order
I do not think I need one.	1
I am scared to have one done.	2
If I test positive, I am afraid someone will find out.	3
I do not want to know if I am HIV positive.	4
I do not know where to have a test done.	5
I am afraid to have my blood drawn.	6
I am afraid of someone finding out that I've had the test.	7

Source: These data come from a random survey of 319 students attending four community colleges in Southern California. Shapiro, Johanna, et al. "Sexual Behavior and AIDS-Related Knowledge Among Community College Students in Orange County, California." *Journal of Community Health,* Vol. 24, Issue 1, February 1999.

Chlamydia

The most widespread sexually transmitted bacterium in the United States is *Chlamydia trachomatis,* which causes 3 to 5 million **chlamydial infections** each year. *Chlamydia trachomatis* infections are more common in younger than in older women, in African-American than in white women, and in unmarried than in married pregnant women. They also occur more often in both men and women with gonorrhea.

Those at greatest risk of chlamydial infection are individuals 25 years old or younger who engage in sex with more than one new partner within a two-month period and women who use birth control pills or other nonbarrier contraceptive methods. Many physicians recommend testing for any woman who has more than one sexual partner in a year; for anyone who seeks medical treatment for an STD; for those seeking health care at adolescent or family planning clinics where chlamydia is seen often; and for young individuals, particularly in urban settings, with multiple sexual partners.[52]

As many as 75 percent of women and 50 percent of men with chlamydia have no symptoms or symptoms so mild that they don't seek medical attention. Without treatment, up to 40 percent of cases of chlamydia can lead to pelvic inflammatory disease, a serious infection of the woman's fallopian tubes that can also damage the ovaries and uterus. Also, women infected with chlamydia may have three to five times the risk of getting infected with HIV if exposed. Babies exposed to

PULSE *points*

Ten Ways to Prevent Sexually Transmitted Diseases (STDs)

1. **Abstain from sexual intercourse.** You don't have to abstain from all sexual activity. Fantasizing, masturbating, touching, hugging, and petting are all safe and pleasurable.

2. **Don't rush into a sexual relationship.** Get to know a potential partner well over a period of several months or more. Share your sexual histories, and build an honest, mutually caring, and trusting relationship.

3. **Get checked out.** The only accurate way to assess the risks of STDs is a thorough medical examination, including laboratory testing.

4. **Maintain a mutually faithful sexual relationship with just one** uninfected partner. An exclusive sexual relationship with a person who has never been exposed to any STD is safe, regardless of what type of sexual activity you engage in.

5. **Always use condoms and spermicides.** Although their use reduces your risk, keep in mind that doing so does not guarantee protection.

6. **Don't have sex with multiple partners.** The risk of STDs increases along with the number of sexual partners. Also avoid sexual contact with individuals who've had multiple or anonymous sexual partners.

7. **Inspect your partner's genitals before sex.** Although some STDs produce no visible signs, it is possible to see herpes blisters, chancres, rashes, genital warts, and the like.

8. **Wash your own—and your partner's—genitals before and after sex.** Although it's not clear how effective soap and water are, washing—especially of the penis—is generally believed to have some benefits.

9. **Don't have sexual contact with individuals who use injection drugs.** Regardless of the type of drug—anabolic steroids, cocaine, heroin, and so on—users are at higher risk for several STDs, including hepatitis and HIV infection.

10. **Keep a clear head.** Don't make decisions about sexual activity while under the influence of alcohol or drugs that could affect your judgment.

---

chlamydia in the birth canal during delivery can be born with pneumonia or with an eye infection called conjunctivitis, both of which can be dangerous unless treated early with antibiotics. Symptomless women who are screened and treated for chlamydial infection are almost 60 percent less likely than unscreened women to develop pelvic inflammatory disease.[53]

Traditional methods of screening require a health professional to collect a swab sample of genital secretions. In the past, the sample had to be "cultured" in a laboratory to look for *C. trachomatis,* and it could take three days or more for results to become available. Today, a number of tests are available to supplement or sometimes replace the relatively expensive and slow traditional culture. The three major types of nonculture tests are:

- Direct fluorescent antibody test, which uses a scientific method called staining to make chlamydia easier to spot under a microscope. DFA can give quicker results than culture and can be performed on specimens taken from the eye, cervix, or penis.

- Enzyme immunoassays, available in some forms that don't require special lab equipment. Results are more rapid than with culture, and costs can be lower.

- Tests to detect the genes of *C. trachomatis* in urine, as well as genital, samples, which can accurately identify even very small numbers of genes in a specimen. While expensive, they are easy to perform and have a high level of accuracy

According to CDC guidelines, the treatment of choice for uncomplicated chlamydia infections is a seven-day regimen of doxycycline or a single, 1-gram dose of azithromycin (Zithromax). Because chlamydia often occurs along with gonorrhea, some health practitioners prescribe seven days of ofloxacin, a drug effective against both chlamydial and gonorrheal infections. The use of condoms with spermicide can reduce, but not eliminate, the risk of chlamydial infection. Sexual partners should be examined and treated if necessary.

Pelvic Inflammatory Disease (PID)

Infection of a woman's fallopian tubes or uterus, called **pelvic inflammatory disease (PID)**, is not actually an STD, but rather a complication of STDs. About one in every seven women of reproductive age has PID; by the year 2000, half of all adult women may have had it. Each year, about 1 million new cases are reported.

Ten to 20 percent of initial episodes of PID lead to scarring and obstruction of the fallopian tubes severe enough to cause infertility. Other long-term complications are ectopic pregnancy and chronic pelvic pain. The risk of these complications rises with subsequent PID episodes, bacterial vaginosis (discussed earlier in this chapter), and use of IUDs. Smoking also may increase the likelihood of PID. Two bacteria—gonococcus (the culprit in gonorrhea) and chlamydia—are responsible for one-half to one-third of all cases of PID. Other organisms are responsible for the remaining cases.

Most cases of PID occur among women under age 25 who are sexually active. Gonococcus-caused cases tend to affect poor women; those caused by chlamydia range across all income levels. One-half to one-third of all cases are transmitted sexually, and others have been traced to some IUDs that are no longer on the market. Several studies have shown that women with PID are more likely to have used douches than those without the disease.

PID is a silent disease that, in half of all cases, often produces no noticeable symptoms as it progresses and causes scarring of the fallopian tubes. Experts are encouraging women with mild symptoms, such as abdominal pain or tenderness, to seek medical evaluation and physicians to test these patients for infections. Urine testing is a cost-effective method of detecting gonorrhea and chlamydia in young women and can prevent development of PID.[54] For women with symptoms, magnetic resonance imaging (MRI) is highly accurate in establishing a diagnosis of PID and detecting other processes responsible for the symptoms.[55]

Women may learn that they have PID only after discovering that they cannot conceive, or after they develop an ectopic pregnancy (see Chapter 10). PID causes an estimated 15 to 30 percent of all cases of infertility every year, and about half of all cases of ectopic pregnancy. Most women do not experience any symptoms, but some may develop abdominal pain, tenderness in certain sites during pelvic exams, or vaginal discharge. Treatment may require hospitalization and intensive antibiotics therapy.

Gonorrhea

Gonorrhea (sometimes called "the clap" in street language) is one of the most common STDs in the United States and is increasing in occurrence. By some estimates, there may be approximately 1 million new cases every year. The incidence is highest among teenagers and young adults. Sexual contact, including oral-genital sex, is the primary means of transmission.

Most men who have gonorrhea know it. Thick, yellow-white pus oozes from the penis, and urination

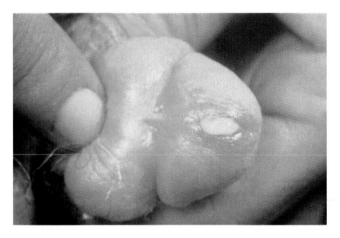

A cloudy discharge is symptomatic of gonorrhea.

causes a burning sensation. These symptoms usually develop two to nine days after the sexual contact that infected them. Men have a good reason to seek help: It hurts too much not to. Women also may experience discharge and burning on urination. However, as many as eight out of ten infected women have no symptoms.

Gonococcus, the bacterium that causes gonorrhea, can live in the vagina, cervix, and fallopian tubes for months, even years, and continue to infect the woman's sexual partners. Approximately 5 percent of sexually active American women have positive gonorrhea cultures but are unaware that they are silent carriers.

If left untreated in men or women, gonorrhea spreads through the urinary-genital tract. In women, the inflammation travels from the vagina and cervix, through the uterus, to the fallopian tubes and ovaries. The pain and fever are similar to those caused by stomach upset, so a woman may dismiss the symptoms. Eventually these symptoms diminish, even though the disease spreads to the entire pelvis. Pus may ooze from the fallopian tubes or ovaries into the peritoneum (the lining of the abdominal cavity), sometimes causing serious inflammation. However, this, too, can subside in a few weeks. Gonorrhea, the leading cause of sterility in women, can cause PID. In pregnant women, gonorrhea becomes a threat to the newborn. It can infect the infant's external genitals and cause a serious form of conjunctivitis, an inflammation of the eye that may lead to blindness. As a preventive step, newborns may have penicillin dropped into their eyes at birth.

In men, untreated gonorrhea can spread to the prostate gland, testicles, bladder, and kidneys. Among the serious complications are urinary obstruction and sterility caused by blockage of the vas deferens (the excretory duct of the testis). In both sexes, gonorrhea can develop into a serious, even fatal, bloodborne infection that can cause arthritis in the joints, attack the heart muscle and lining, cause meningitis, and attack the skin and other organs.

Although a blood test has been developed for detecting gonorrhea, the tried-and-true method of diagnosis is still a microscopic study and analysis of cultures from the male's urethra, the female's cervix, and the throat and anus of both sexes.

In the last decade, antibiotic-resistant strains of gonorrhea have emerged, and the current CDC treatment guidelines suggest the use of drugs effective against both resistant and nonresistant strains of *Neisseria gonorrhoeae.* Because gonorrhea often occurs along with chlamydia, practitioners often use an agent effective against both, such as ofloxacin. Antibiotics taken for other reasons may not affect or cure the gonorrhea because of their dosage or type. And you can't develop immunity to gonorrhea; within days of recovering from one case, you can catch another.

Nongonococcal Urethritis (NGU)

The term **nongonococcal urethritis (NGU)** refers to any inflammation of the urethra that is not caused by gonorrhea. NGU is the most common STD in men, accounting for 4 million to 6 million visits to a physician every year. Two separate microorganisms, *Chlamydia trachomatis* and *Ureaplasma urealyticum,* are the primary causes; the usual means of transmission is sexual intercourse. Other infectious agents, such as fungi or bacteria, allergic reactions to vaginal secretions, or irritation by soaps or contraceptive foams or gels may also lead to NGU.

In the United States, NGU is more common in men than gonoccocal urethritis. The symptoms in men are similar to those of gonorrhea, including discharge from the penis (usually less than with gonorrhea) and mild burning during urination. Women frequently develop no symptoms or very mild itching, burning during urination, or discharge. Symptoms usually disappear after two or three weeks, but the infection may persist and causes cervicitis or PID in women and, in men, may spread to the prostate, epididymis, or both. Treatment usually consists of doxycline or erythromycin and should be given to both sexual partners after testing. For men, a single oral dose of azithromycin has proven as effective as a standard seven-day course of doxycycline.

Syphilis

A corkscrew-shaped, spiral bacterium called *Treponema pallidum* causes **syphilis.** This frail germ dies in seconds if dried or chilled, but grows quickly in the warm, moist tissues of the body, particularly in the mucous membranes of the genital tract. Entering the body through any tiny break in the skin, the germ burrows its way into the bloodstream. Sexual contact, including oral sex or intercourse, is a primary means of transmission. Genital ulcers caused by syphilis may increase the risk of HIV infection, while individuals with HIV may be more likely to develop syphilis.

The incidence of syphilis has increased and decreased several times over recent decades, rising in the 1970s and early 1980s, declining in the mid-1980s and rising again in the closing years of the 1980s, mostly among the urban poor. Several studies have shown a link between increases in syphilis, gonorrhea, AIDS, and other STDs and the use of crack cocaine, along with the exchange of sex for drugs or money.[56] Other influences include unemployment, poverty, poor education, and inadequate health care, which in turn can lead to crime, prostitution, substance abuse, family disruption, and despair. Public education programs, expanded screening and surveillance, increased tracing of contacts, and condom promotion have helped to control the spread of syphilis in some areas.

There are clearly identifiable stages of syphilis:

* *Primary syphilis.* The first sign of syphilis is a lesion, or chancre (pronounced "shanker"), an open lump or crater the size of a dime or smaller, teeming with bacteria. The incubation period before its appearance ranges from 10 to 90 days; three to four weeks is average. The chancre appears exactly where the bacteria entered the body: in the mouth, throat, vagina, rectum, or penis. Any contact with the chancre is likely to result in infection.

* *Secondary syphilis.* Anywhere from one to twelve months after the chancre's appearance, secondary-stage symptoms may appear. Some people have no symptoms. Others develop a skin rash or a small, flat rash in moist regions on the skin; whitish patches on the mucous membranes of the mouth or throat; temporary baldness; low-grade fever; headache; swollen glands; or large, moist sores around the mouth and genitals. These are loaded with bacteria; contact with them, through kissing or intercourse, may transmit the infection. Symptoms may last for several days or several months. Even without treatment, they eventually disappear as the syphilis microbes go into hiding.

* *Latent syphilis.* Although there are no signs or symptoms, no sores or rashes at this stage, the bacteria are invading various organs inside the body, including the heart and brain. For two to four years, there may be recurring infectious and highly contagious lesions of the skin or mucous membranes. However, syphilis loses its infectiousness as it progresses: After the first two years, a person rarely transmits syphilis through intercourse.

After four years, even congenital syphilis is rarely transmitted. Until this stage of the disease, however, a pregnant woman can pass syphilis to her unborn child. If the fetus is infected in its fourth month or earlier, it may be disfigured or may even die. If infected late in pregnancy, the child may show no signs of infection for months or years after birth, but may then become disabled with the symptoms of tertiary syphilis.

- *Tertiary syphilis.* Ten to twenty years after the beginning of the latent stage, the most serious symptoms of syphilis emerge, generally in the organs in which the bacteria settled during latency. Syphilis that has progressed to this stage has become increasingly rare. Victims of tertiary syphilis may die of a ruptured aorta or of other heart damage, or may have progressive brain or spinal cord damage, eventually leading to blindness, insanity, or paralysis. About a third of those who are not treated during the first three stages of syphilis enter the tertiary stage later in life.

Health experts are urging screening for syphilis for everyone who seeks treatment for an STD, especially adolescents; for everyone using illegal drugs; and for the partners of these two groups. They also recommend that anyone diagnosed with syphilis be screened for other STDs and be counseled about voluntary testing for HIV.

Early diagnosis of syphilis can lead to a complete cure. The most widely used diagnostic techniques are the Venereal Disease Research Laboratory (VDRL) test or the rapid-plasma-reagin (RPR) test. However, these may be positive only during the secondary stage of the disease, when the bacteria have reached the bloodstream. A positive finding always requires additional information, including a physical exam and other laboratory tests, to confirm the diagnosis and help in planning treatment.

Penicillin is the drug of choice for treating primary, secondary, or latent syphilis. The earlier treatment begins, the more effective it is. Those allergic to penicillin may be treated with doxycycline, tetracycline, or erythromycin. An added danger of not getting treatment for syphilis is an increased risk of HIV transmission.

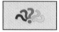 ## What Is Herpes?

Herpes (from the Greek word that means "to creep") collectively describes some of the most common viral infections in humans. Characteristically, **herpes simplex** causes blisters on the skin or mucous membranes. Herpes simplex exists in several varieties. Herpes simplex virus 1 (HSV-1) generally causes cold sores and fever blisters around the mouth. Herpes simplex virus 2

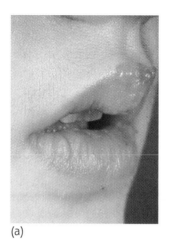 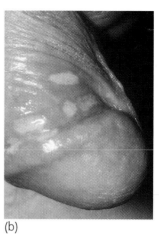

(a)   (b)

Herpes. (a) Herpes simplex virus 1, or HSV-1, as a mouth sore. (b) Herpes simplex virus 2, or HSV-2, usually causes genital sores.

(HSV-2) may cause blisters on the penis, inside the vagina, on the cervix, in the pubic area, on the buttocks, or on the thighs. With the increase of oral-genital sex, some doctors report finding Type 2 herpes lesions in the mouth and throat.

The incidence of herpes infection has soared. Since the late 1970s, the proportion of Americans with herpes simplex type 2 virus has increased by almost one-third. One in five women and one in seven men over age 12— some 45 million people—carry this virus. Two out of three people with the virus do not know they are infected and potentially contagious. Recent research with a new, more sensitive test reveals that individuals without any obvious symptoms shed the virus "subclinically" whether or not they have lesions. Most people with herpes contract it from partners who were not aware of any symptoms or of their own contagiousness.[57] Standard methods of diagnosing genital herpes in women, which rely primarily on physical examination and viral cultures, may miss as many as two-thirds of all cases. Newly developed blood tests are more effective in detecting unrecognized and subclinical infections with HSV-2.

HSV transmission occurs through close contact with mucous membranes or abraded skin. Condoms help prevent infection but aren't foolproof. When herpes sores are present, the infected person is highly contagious and should avoid bringing the lesions into contact with someone else's body through touching, sexual interaction, or kissing. However, HSV also can be transmitted when there are no signs or symptoms of the disease.

A newborn can be infected with genital herpes while passing through the birth canal, and the frequency of mother-to-infant transmission seems to be increasing.

Most infected infants develop typical skin sores, which should be cultured to confirm a herpes diagnosis. Some physicians recommend treatment with acyclovir. Because there is a risk of severe damage and possible death, caesarean delivery may be advised for a woman with active herpes lesions.

The virus that causes herpes never entirely goes away; it retreats to nerves near the lower spinal cord, where it remains for the life of the host. Herpes sores can return without warning weeks, months, or even years after their first occurrence, often during menstruation or times of stress, or with sudden changes in body temperature. Of those who experience HSV recurrence, 10 to 35 percent do so frequently— that is, about six or more times a year. In most people, attacks diminish in frequency and severity over time. Herpes, like other STDS, can trigger feelings of shame, guilt, and depression.

Acyclovir (Zovirax), a prescription drug, has proven effective in treating and controlling herpes. Available as an ointment, in capsules, and in injection form, it relieves the symptoms but doesn't kill the virus. Whereas the ointment works only for the initial bout with herpes, acyclovir in injectable and pill form dramatically reduces the length and severity of herpes outbreaks. Continuing daily oral acylcovir can reduce recurrences by about 80 percent. However, its safety in pregnant women has not been established. Infection with herpes viruses resistant to acyclovir is a growing problem, especially in individuals with immune-suppressing disorders.

Various treatments—compresses made with cold water, skim milk, or warm salt water, ice packs, or a mild anesthetic cream—can relieve discomfort. Herpes sufferers should avoid heat, hot baths, or nylon underwear. In recent years physicians have tried a host of therapies, including topical ointments, various vaccines, exposure to light, and ultrasonic waves—all with little success. Some physicians have used laser therapy to vaporize the lesions. Clinical trials of an experimental vaccine to protect people from herpes infections are underway.

Human Papilloma Virus Infection (Genital Warts)

Infection with **human papilloma virus (HPV)**, a pathogen that can cause genital warts, is the most common viral STD. By some estimates, 20 million or more women in the United States are infected with HPV, as are three out of four of their male sexual partners. College-age women are among those at greatest risk of acquiring HPV infection. In various studies conducted

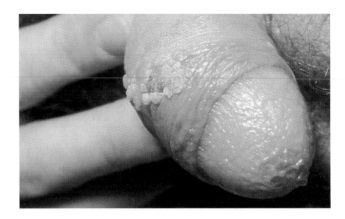

Human papilloma virus, which causes genital warts, is the most common viral STD.

in college health centers, 10 to 46 percent of female students (mean age 20 to 22) had a cervical HPV infection—and increased risk of precancerous cell changes. Risk factors include smoking, use of oral contraceptives, multiple sex partners, anal as well as vaginal intercourse, alcohol consumption at the time of engaging in vaginal intercourse, and sex partners with a history of HPV. Many women often believe they are at low risk for HPV, even if they engage in unprotected sexual activity.[58]

HPV infections in young women tend to be of short duration. In a three-year study, 60 percent of 608 college women became infected with the virus; the average duration of infection was eight months. According to the researchers, many young women who get HPV may not require treatment because the condition often regresses on its own.[59]

HPV is transmitted primarily through vaginal, anal, or oral-genital sex. More than half of HPV-infected individuals do not develop any symptoms. Genital warts may appear from three weeks to eighteen months after contact, with an average period of about three months after contact with an infected individual. These are treated by freezing, cauterization, chemicals, or surgical removal. Recurrences are common, for the virus remains in the body.

HPV infection may invade the urethra and cause urinary obstruction and bleeding. It greatly increases a woman's risk of developing a precancerous condition called cervical intraepithelial neoplasia, which can lead to cervical cancer. There also is a strong association between HPV infections and cancer of the vagina, vulva, urethra, penis, and anus.[60]

HPV may be the single most important risk factor in 95 percent of all cases of cervical cancer.[61] Adolescent girls infected with HPV appear to be particularly vulnerable to developing cervical cancer. It is not known if HPV itself causes cancer or acts in conjunction with cofactors (such as other infections, smoking, or suppressed immunity). HPV transmission may be the reason women are five to eleven times as likely to get cervical cancer if their steady sexual partner has had 20 or more previous partners.

Women who have had an HPV infection should examine their genitals regularly and get an annual Pap smear. However, this standard diagnostic test for cervical cancer doesn't identify HPV infection. A newer, more specific test can recognize HPV soon after it enters the body. Women who test positive should undergo checkups for cervical changes every six to twelve months. If precancerous cells develop, surgery or laser treatment can prevent further growth. Smoking may interact with HPV to increase the risk of cancer.

HPV may also cause genital warts in men and increase the risk of cancer of the penis. HPV-infected men, who may not develop any symptoms, can spread the infection to their partners. People with visible genital warts also may have asymptomatic or subclinical HPV infections that are extremely difficult to treat.

No form of therapy has been shown to eradicate HPV completely, nor has any single treatment been uniformly effective in removing warts or preventing their recurrence. CDC guidelines suggest treatments that focus on the removal of visible warts—cryotherapy (freezing) and topical applications of podofilox, pdophyllin, or trichloroacetic acid—and then eradication of the virus. At least 20 to 30 percent of treated individuals experience recurrence. In experimental studies, interferon—a biologic substance produced by virus-infected cells that inhibits viral replication—has proven helpful.

Chancroid

A **chancroid** is a soft, painful sore or localized infection caused by the bacterium *Haemophilus ducrevi* and usually acquired through sexual contact. Half of the cases heal by themselves. In other cases, the infection may spread to the lymph glands near the chancroid, where large amounts of pus can accumulate and destroy much of the local tissue. The incidence of this STD, widely prevalent in Africa and tropical and semitropical regions, is rapidly increasing in the United States, with outbreaks in several states, including Louisiana, Texas, and New York. Chancroids, which may increase susceptibility to HIV infection, are believed to be a major factor in the heterosexual spread of HIV. This infection is treated with antibiotics (ceftriaxone, azithromycin, or erythromycin) and can be prevented by keeping the genitals clean and washing them with soap and water in case of possible exposure.

Strategies *for* Change

What to Do If You Have an STD

✔ If you suspect that you have an STD, don't feel too embarrassed to get help through a physician's office or a clinic. Treatment relieves discomfort, prevents complications, and halts the spread of the disease.

✔ Following diagnosis, take oral medication (which may be given instead of or in addition to shots) exactly as prescribed.

✔ Try to figure out from whom you got the STD. Be sure to inform that person, who may not be aware of the problem.

✔ If you have an STD, never deceive a prospective partner about it. Tell the truth—simply and clearly. Be sure your partner understands exactly what you have and what the risks are.

Pubic Lice and Scabies

These infections are sometimes, but not always, transmitted sexually. Pubic lice (or "crabs") are usually found in the pubic hairs, although they may migrate to any hairy areas of the body. Lice lay eggs called nits that attach to the base of the hair shaft. Irritation from the lice may produce intense itching. Scratching to relieve the itching can produce sores. Scabies is caused by a mite that burrows under the skin and lays eggs that hatch and undergo many changes in the course of their life cycle, producing great discomfort, including intense itching.

Lice and scabies are treated with applications of Kwell or A-200 pyrinate shampoo (which kills the adult lice but not always the nits) to all the areas of the body where there are concentrations of body hair (genitals,

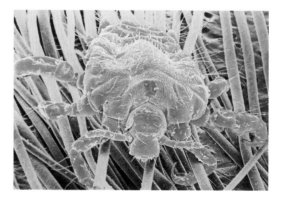
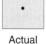

Actual size

A pubic louse, or "crab."

armpits, scalp). You must repeat treatment in seven days to kill any newly developed adults. Wash or dry-clean clothing, and bedding.

HIV/AIDS

Thirty years ago, no one knew what the **human immu-nodeficiency virus (HIV)** was. No one had ever heard of **acquired immunodeficiency syndrome (AIDS)**. Globally, HIV, once seen as an epidemic affecting primarily gay men and injection drug users, has taken on a very different form. Today, heterosexuals in developing countries have the highest rates of infection and mortality. And the HIV epidemic continues to spread, doubling at an estimated rate of every ten years.[62] The United Nations AIDS Program estimates that about 47 million people have been infected with HIV since the start of the global epidemic. An estimated 14 million children and adults have died, while 33.4 million are living with HIV and AIDS.[63]

AIDS has surpassed tuberculosis and malaria as the leading infectious cause of death and has become the fourth-largest killer worldwide.[64] The cumulative death toll for AIDS exceeds 14 million. The region that has been hardest hit is sub-Saharan Africa, the site of seven out of every ten of the world's cases of HIV infection and nine of every ten deaths due to AIDS. In the two hardest-hit countries, Zimbabwe and Botswana, one of every four adults is infected, and AIDS has cut the average life expectancy by nearly 20 years.[65]

In the United States, the CDC estimates that between 650,000 and 900,000 people are living with HIV. The mortality rate for AIDS is declining, but HIV infection rates are increasing in certain groups, including women and racial and ethnic minorities.[66] Almost two-thirds of new infections occur in blacks and Hispanics, who account for just 24 percent of the population. About 40,000 Americans become infected with HIV every year.[67] In Asia, the total number of people infected is expanding rapidly, even though the rate of new infection remains relatively low. Since 1994, the number of people living with HIV in Eastern Europe has surged nearly sevenfold.[68]

There has been progress in lowering the rates of HIV transmission through measures such as reducing the incidence of unprotected intercourse and the number of sex partners, delaying sexual initiation, decreasing the incidence of other STDs, directing injection drug users into drug treatment programs, and reducing needle sharing. Screening the blood supply has reduced the rate of transfusion-associated HIV transmission by 99.9 percent.

Treatment with anti-retroviral drugs during pregnancy and birth has reduced transmission by about 90 percent in optimal conditions. Among some groups of gay men in the United States, safer sex practices have reduced the annual incidence of HIV infection from about 15 percent to 5 percent. Among drug users in some settings, programs that combine addiction treatment and needle exchange reduced the incidence of HIV infection by 30 percent. Even in developing nations, such as Thailand and Uganda, national prevention programs, such as free distribution of condoms and needle-exchange programs, have reduced HIV prevalence by as much as 50 percent.

The Spread of HIV

HIV came to the United States in the late 1970s. Several factors—including frequent sexual activity with multiple, anonymous partners and high-risk sexual practices, such as anal intercourse—may have caused its quick spread through gay communities in the 1980s. As more became known about HIV transmission, many homosexual men adopted safer ways of sexual expression, reduced their number of sexual partners, or entered into monogamous relationships. As a result, the spread of HIV among gay men—especially older men in metropolitan areas—slowed. However, the incidence of AIDS in young gay men and homosexual men in rural or suburban areas increased steadily in the 1990s.

In the 1980s, HIV also spread among injecting drug users, who, by sharing contaminated needles, injected the virus directly into their bloodstream. Injection drug use has been the number-one source of HIV infection in heterosexual men and women in this country. Sex with an infected injecting drug user is also a major cause of HIV infection. (See Chapter 14 for further discussion of drug use.) Almost one-third of reported cases of AIDS have been directly or indirectly related to injection drug use. CDC-sponsored studies indicate that needle exchange programs that provide drug users with sterile needles could significantly reduce HIV transmission.

HIV also spread through blood transfusions, blood products, and organ transplants from HIV-positive individuals during the period between 1978 and 1985, before testing to identify contaminated blood became routine. Today's blood and organ supply is much safer, primarily because of more sophisticated testing of donated blood, blood products used for hemophiliacs, and donated organs, tissues, and sperm. There have been several documented cases of HIV infection through artificial insemination performed prior to 1986. Even today, women who use semen from men who have not been tested for HIV are at risk of infection.

How Widespread is HIV Infection?

The rate of infection with HIV, which had been declining in the mid-1990s, has stabilized. Health officials describe new infections with HIV as "dangerously high" among some groups, including gay young men, heterosexual women, and blacks and other minorities.

As many as half of new infections occur among people under age 25; a quarter may be among individuals younger than age 22. Individuals with other sexually transmitted diseases are especially susceptible. One in three people with HIV do not yet know they are infected. An estimated 650,000 to 900,000 Americans are living with HIV—approximately one in every 300 persons of all ages. Of these, more than 270,000 have the symptoms and syndromes characteristic of AIDS.[69]

Men are more likely to be infected through sex with other men, which accounts for almost half of new cases of HIV/AIDS in adult men. Injection drug use accounts for one-fifth of new cases. Women are most likely to be infected with HIV through heterosexual contact, which accounts for 38 percent of new cases. Of these, 29 percent come from partners who are injection drug users. (See Figures 12-6 and 12-7.)

Although the majority of new AIDs cases are among men, almost one-quarter are among women. Among the youngest, women account for an even higher proportion of reported cases—including about half of 13-to-19 year-olds with AIDS and 40 percent of 20 to 24 year-olds. The proportion of new AIDS cases among women rose significantly through the 1990s, from 11 percent in 1990 to 23 percent in 1998.

HIV infection and AIDS also have been increasing among people of color. (See Figure 12-8.) African Americans, who make up only 12 percent of the U. S. population, represented 45 percent of new AIDS cases in 1998, compared with 30 percent in 1990. Since 1996

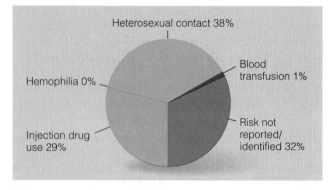

■ **Figure 12-6** Reported AIDS cases among women age 13 and older, by means of infection.

Source: "The HIV/AIDS Epidemic in the U.S." Kaiser Family Foundation, June 1999.

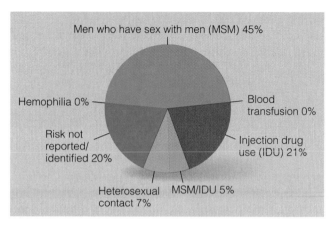

■ **Figure 12-7** Reported AIDS cases among men age 13 and older, by means of infection.

Source: "The HIV/AIDS Epidemic in the U.S." Kaiser Family Foundation, June 1999.

African Americans have accounted for more AIDS diagnoses annually than whites. Latinos accounted for 20 percent of new AIDS cases in 1998, compared to 17 percent in 1990. Men of all races are most likely to be infected with HIV through sex with other men. Injection drug use accounts for a greater proportion of cases among Latino and African-American men than among white men.

HIV is transmitted to infants by HIV-positive mothers in three possible ways: before birth via circulation; during labor and birth; or after birth, through infected breast milk. Every year about 7,000 HIV-infected women give birth. The risk is highest in women with high levels of HIV.[70] Experts advise HIV screening for all pregnant women.[71] Treatment of both mothers and newborns with zidovudine (AZT) can reduce the risk of HIV transmission from mother to child from one in four to less than one in ten—a 67.5 percent reduction.[72]

Accidental contact with HIV-contaminated blood or bodily fluids has led to some cases of HIV infection and AIDS. According to the CDC, HIV is transmitted among health-care workers in about 1 per 250 instances of their accidental injection with needles containing HIV-positive blood.

The threat of transmission from infected health-care professionals to patients has proven to be very low. To protect both health-care workers and their patients, the CDC requires all professionals to follow basic precautions, such as wearing protective gloves while performing medical procedures. The CDC has also issued guidelines urging health-care workers to inform patients if they are infected with HIV and to stop performing surgery or any procedure in which bleeding might occur.

A small number of cases of HIV infection in heterosexual men in the United States have been traced to prostitutes. However, in big cities, as many as half the prostitutes tested have been exposed to HIV, almost all through injection drug use or sex with injecting drug users.

Race/Ethnicity	Number of New AIDS Cases	Percent of New AIDS Cases	Percent of Population
White, non-Hispanic	16,116	34%	73%
Black, non-Hispanic	21,752	45%	12%
Hispanic	9,650	20%	11%
Asian/Pacific Islander	390	<1%	4%
American Indian/Alaskan Native	147	<1%	<1%
TOTAL	48,055	100%	100%

Note: Cases do not include those reported for whom race/ethnicity was unknown.

■ **Figure 12-8** New AIDS cases by race and ethnicity.

Source: "The HIV/AIDS Epidemic in the U.S.," Kaiser Family Foundation, June 1999.

Reducing the Risk of HIV Transmission

HIV/AIDS can be so frightening that some people have exaggerated its dangers, whereas others understate them. The fact is that although no one is immune to HIV, you can reduce the risk if you abstain from sexual activity, remain in a monogamous relationship with an uninfected partner, and do not inject drugs. If you're not in a long-term monogamous relationship with a partner you're sure is safe, and you're not willing to abstain from sex, there are things you can do to lower your risk of HIV infection. Remember that the risk of HIV transmission depends on sexual behavior, not sexual orientation. Among young men, the prevalence and frequency of sexual risk behaviors are similar regardless of sexual orientation, ethnicity, or age.[73] Homosexual, heterosexual, and bisexual individuals all need to know about the kinds of sexual activity that increase their risk.

Here's what you should know about HIV transmission (see Figure 12-9):

- Casual contact does *not* spread HIV infection. Compared to other viruses, HIV is extremely difficult to get. HIV can live in blood, semen, vaginal fluids, and breast milk. Many chemicals, including household bleach, alcohol, and hydrogen peroxide, can inactivate it. In studies of family members sharing dishes, food, clothing, and frequent hugs with people with HIV infection or AIDS, those who have contracted the virus have shared razor blades, toothbrushes, or had other means of blood contact.
- You cannot tell visually whether a potential sexual partner has HIV. A blood test is needed to detect the antibodies that the body produces to fight HIV, thus indicating infection.

- HIV can be spread in semen and vaginal fluids during a single instance of anal, vaginal, or oral sexual contact between heterosexuals, bisexuals, or homosexuals. The risk increases with the number of sexual encounters with an infected partner.
- Teenage girls may be particularly vulnerable to HIV infection because the immature cervix is easily infected.
- Anal intercourse is an extremely high-risk behavior because HIV may enter the bloodstream through tiny breaks in the lining of the rectum. HIV transmission is much more likely to occur during unprotected anal intercourse than vaginal intercourse.
- Other behaviors that increase the risk of HIV infection include having multiple sex partners, engaging in sex without condoms or virus-killing spermicides, sexual contact with persons known to be at high risk (for example, prostitutes or injecting drug users), and sharing injection equipment for drugs.
- Individuals are at greater risk if they have an active sexual infection. Sexually transmitted diseases, such as herpes, gonorrhea, and syphilis, facilitate transmission of HIV during vaginal or rectal intercourse.
- No cases of HIV transmission by deep kissing have been reported, but it could happen. Studies have found blood in the saliva of healthy people after kissing; other lab studies have found HIV in saliva. Social (dry) kissing is safe.
- Oral sex can lead to HIV transmission. The virus in any semen that enters the mouth could make its way into the bloodstream through tiny nicks or sores in the mouth. A man's risk in performing oral sex on a woman is smaller because an infected woman's genital fluids have much lower concentrations of HIV than does semen.
- HIV infection is not widespread among lesbians, although there have been documented cases of possible female-to-female HIV transmission. In each instance, one partner had had sex with a bisexual man or male injecting drug user or had injected drugs herself.

HIV Infection

HIV infection refers to a spectrum of health problems that result from immunologic abnormalities caused by the virus when it enters the bloodstream. In theory, the body may be able to resist infection by HIV. In reality, in almost all cases, HIV destroys the cell-mediated immune system, particularly the CD4+ T-lymphocytes (also called T4 helper cells). The result is greatly increased susceptibility to various cancers and opportunistic infections (infections that take hold because of the reduced effectiveness of the immune system).

According to new insights into the pathogenesis of HIV—the way in which HIV attacks the immune

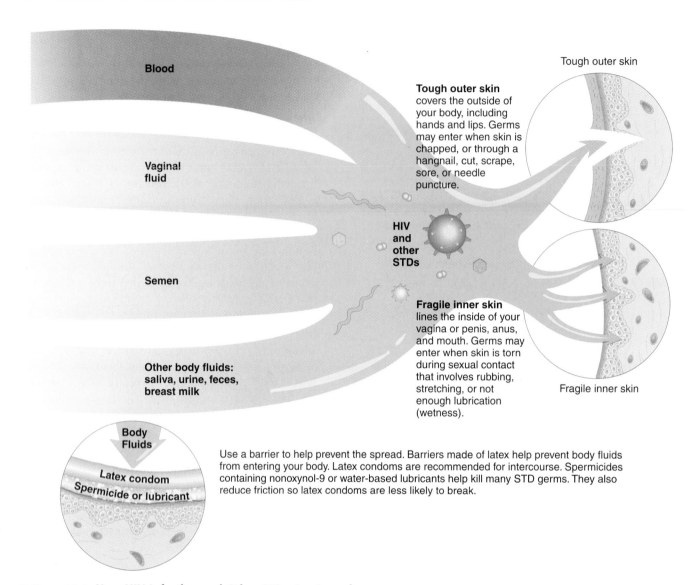

■ Figure 12-9 **How HIV Infection and Other STDs Are Spread**
Most STDs are spread by viruses, such as HIV, or bacteria carried in certain body fluids.

system—researchers now know that HIV triggers a state of all-out war within the immune system. Almost immediately following infection with HIV, the immune system responds aggressively by manufacturing enormous numbers of CD4 cells. However, it eventually is overwhelmed as the viral particles continue to replicate, or multiply. The intense war between HIV and the immune system indicates that the virus itself, not a breakdown in the immune system, is responsible for disease progression.

Shortly after becoming infected with HIV, individuals may experience a few days of flulike symptoms, which most ignore or attribute to other viruses. Some people develop a more severe mononucleosis-type syndrome. After this stage, individuals may not develop any signs or symptoms of disease for a period ranging from weeks to more than 12 years.

HIV infection can itself be a serious illness and is associated with a variety of HIV-related diseases,

including different cancers and dangerous infections. HIV-infected individuals may develop persistent generalized lymphadenopathy, enlargement of the lymph nodes at two or more different sites in the body. This condition typically persists for more than three months without any other illness to explain its occurrence. Diminished mental function may appear before other symptoms. Tests conducted on infected, but apparently healthy, men have revealed impaired coordination, problems in thinking, or abnormal brain scans.

HIV Testing

Every year approximately 25 million people in the United States are tested for HIV. About 10,000 facilities provide publicly funded HIV testing and counseling in the United States; approximately 2.6 million tests are performed annually at these sites. As shown in Figure 12-10, men

Strategies *for* Prevention

Lowering Your Risk of Exposure to HIV

✔ Abstain from sexual contact with anyone who is infected with HIV, whether or not he or she has symptoms, or with anyone who is at high risk of HIV infection because of his or her behavior or sexual history.

✔ Avoid sexual contact with anyone who has had sex with people at risk of HIV infection. Avoid multiple or anonymous sex partners. Avoid sex with anyone who has had multiple or anonymous sex partners, or with anyone who has had a sex partner infected with HIV.

✔ Use a condom during every sexual act, including oral sex, from start to finish. Also use a spermicide that provides extra protection against STDS.

✔ Don't have sexual contact with individuals who use injection drugs.

✔ Avoid receptive anal intercourse, as well as the insertion of fingers or objects into your anus, because these acts could tear your rectal tissues, allowing direct access to your bloodstream. Avoid contact with your partner's blood, semen, urine, and feces.

✔ Don't use amyl nitrite (poppers), a sexual stimulant that may be associated with the development of a cancer characteristic of AIDS.

✔ Don't have sex with prostitutes.

✔ Don't share needles (or other injection drug equipment), razor blades, or toothbrushes.

✔ In addition to their partner's use of a condom, women should use a diaphragm with a spermicide for extra protection.

and women between the ages of 18 and 29 are most likely to report that they've been tested for HIV.[74]

One in four sexually experienced 15-to-17-year-olds report undergoing HIV testing. The most common reasons that young people give for not having HIV tests include not thinking they are at risk, lack of awareness of HIV infection rates in their communities, fear of being stigmatized by family and friends, apprehension of the conse-

quences of testing positive, and lack of knowledge about testing facilities where they would be treated with professionalism and respect.[75]

All HIV tests measure antibodies, cells produced by the body to fight HIV infection. A negative test indicates no exposure to HIV. However, since it can take three to six months for the body to produce the telltale antibodies, a negative result may not be accurate, depending on the timing of the test.

HIV testing can be either confidential or anonymous. In confidential testing, a person's name is recorded along with the test results, which are made available to medical personnel and, in 32 states, the state health department. In anonymous testing, no name is associated with the test results. Anonymous testing is available in 39 states. The CDC reported a decline of 26.6 percent and an increase of 2.9 percent in confidential testing from 1995 to 1997. Different groups of individuals at risk prefer different tests. Asian-Pacific Islander and white men who have sex with men are most likely to choose anonymous testings; African-American men who have sex with men are much more likely to choose confidential testing. [76]

The HIV tests currently available in the United States are:

• *ELISA (Enzyme-Linked ImmunoSorbent Assay).* This is the most commonly used HIV test. A health-care provider draws a blood sample, which is analyzed for antibodies produced to fight against HIV particles. Results are generally available within a few days to two weeks.

• *Oral HIV tests.* These tests have become available in some doctors' offices and health clinics. A health-care worker swabs a tissue sample from the inside of the mouth. The only FDA-approved oral test is the OraSure.

• *HomeAccess.* This test—the only home HIV test approved by the FDA—is available in drug stores for about $40. An individual draws a blood sample by pricking a finger and sends it to a laboratory along

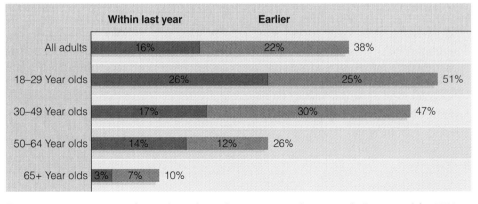

■ **Figure 12-10** Percent of Americans in each age group who report being tested for HIV.

Source: "HIV Testing." Fact Sheet, Kaiser Family Foundation, June 1999.

with a personal identification number. Results are given over the phone by a trained counselor, usually within several days. (See Consumer Health Watch: "Bogus HIV Tests on the Internet.")

- *A rapid HIV Test.* This test, which is currently being tested, can provide results in as little as ten minutes. A health-care provider draws a blood sample for immediate analysis. A "reactive" test (one that detects antibodies) should be repeated and, if still reactive, requires confirmation with the more definitive Western blot.

- *The Western blot.* This is a more accurate and expensive test used to confirm the results of a positive HIV test.

Newly developed blood tests can determine how recently a person was infected with HIV and distinguish between long-standing infections and those contracted within the previous four to six months. Health officials recommend HIV testing for the following individuals:

- Men who have had sex with other men, regardless of whether they consider themselves homosexual.

- Anyone who uses injection drugs and has shared needles, or has had sex with someone who has done so.

- Women who have had sex with bisexual men.

- Anyone who has had sex with someone from an area with a high incidence of HIV infection.

- Individuals who have had sex with people they do not know well.

- Anyone who received blood transfusions or blood products between 1978 and 1985. (Their sexual partners, or, if they are new mothers, their infants may also be at risk.)

AIDS

A diagnosis of AIDS applies to anyone with HIV whose immune system is severely impaired, as indicated by a CD4 count of less than 200 cells per cubic millimeter of blood, compared to normal CD4 cell counts in healthy people not infected with HIV of 800 to 1,200 per cubic millimeter of blood. In addition, AIDS is diagnosed in persons with HIV infection who experience recurrent pneumonia, invasive cervical cancer, or pulmonary tuberculosis.

People with AIDS also may experience persistent fever, diarrhea that persists for more than one month, or involuntary weight loss of more than 10 percent of normal body weight. Generalized lymphadenopathy may persist. Neurological disease—including dementia (confusion and impaired thinking) and other problems with thinking, speaking, movement, or sensation—may occur. Secondary infectious diseases that may develop in people with AIDS include *Pneumocystis carinii* pneumonia, tuberculosis, or oral candidiasis (thrush). Secondary cancers associated with HIV infection include Kaposi's sarcoma and cancer of the cervix.

What Progress Has Been Made in HIV/AIDS Treatments?

New forms of therapy have been remarkably effective in boosting levels of protective T cells and reducing "viral

Consumer Health Watch

Bogus HIV Tests on the Internet

The Internet has been used as a tool for marketing unscientific HIV self-diagnostic tests. The Federal Trade Commission (FTC) has issued a warning that home test kits for HIV that are advertised and sold over the Internet—some of which claim or imply that they are approved by the FDA or the World Health Organization—are unreliable. After testing a variety of such kits, the FTC found that in every case, the kits yielded false negatives. In other words, they showed a negative result when they should have shown a positive one. This means that a person who might be infected with HIV would get the false impression that he or she is HIV-negative.

In several cases, businessmen have been found guilty of fraud for selling medically useless HIV test kits for home use via the Internet. In one case, the tests were represented as "confidential, safe, accurate, and easy to use," although they lacked any scientific or factual basis. As part of the scheme, the marketer provided bogus test results to purchasers.

The FTC suggests that anyone who has used such a kit be retested for HIV. The only kit approved by the FDA for self-diagnosis is the Home Access Express HIV-1 Test System, which allows a person to collect a blood sample at home and ship it to a laboratory for analysis.

load"—the amount of HIV virus in the bloodstream. Since 1995, there has been a reduction in hospitalization for AIDS patients and a dramatic 62 percent decline in the AIDS death rate.[77] However, the rate of decline in AIDS deaths slowed by the end of the 1990s. According to the CDC, AIDS deaths dropped 42 percent from 1996 to 1997, but only 20 percent from 1997 to 1998. The slowing rate of decline may mean that the impact of promising drug therapies is wearing off or that new HIV strains are resistant to these treatments.[78]

Stress accelerates the progression from HIV to AIDS. In a five-and-a-half year study of HIV-infected men, those with more than average stress or less than average support were two to three times more likely to progress to AIDS. Every increase in cumulative average stressful life events—either one severe stressor or two moderate stressors—doubled the likelihood of AIDS.[79]

People with high viral loads are more likely to progress rapidly to AIDS than people with low levels of the virus. Current HIV therapy involves the use of antiretroviral drugs to slow viral replication (that is, the virus making copies of itself). The three classes of antiviral that are most widely used today include:

- NRTIs (Nucleoside Reverse Transcriptase Inhibitors), such as zidovudine (AZT), zalcitabine (ddC), didanosine (ddI), stavudine (D4T), lamivudine (3TC) and abacavir succinate.

- PIs (Protease Inhibitors), such as ritonavir, saquinavir, indinavir, and nelfinavir.

- NNRTIs (Non-nucleoside Reverse Transcriptase Inhibitors), such as nevirapine (Viramune) and efavirenz (Sustiva).

The preferred treatment for HIV is a triple drug combination, called HAART (Highly Active Antiretroviral Therapy), which may consist of two NRTIs and one or two NRTIs plus efavirenz or two NRTIs plus ritonavir and saquinavir. In most people who start antiretroviral therapy, the viral load drops to undetectable levels within 12 to 16 weeks.

None of the currently available drugs cures people of HIV infection or AIDS, and they all have potentially severe side effects. AZT may cause a depletion of red or white blood cells, especially in the later stages of the disease. The most common side effects associated with protease inhibitors include nausea, diarrhea, and other gastrointestinal symptoms. Protease inhibitors also can interact with other drugs and cause potentially serious side effects.

In addition to antiretroviral therapy, adults with HIV whose CD4 cell counts drop below 200 are given treatment to prevent the occurrence of PCP, which is one of the most deadly infections associated with HIV. Regardless of their CD4 cell counts, HIV-infected children and adults who have survived an episode of PCP are given drugs for the rest of their lives to prevent a recurrence of the pneumonia. HIV-infected individuals who develop Kaposi's sarcoma or other cancers are treated with radiation, chemotherapy or injections of alpha interferon, a genetically engineered naturally occurring protein.

Scientists are testing more than a dozen HIV vaccines in people, and many drugs for HIV infection or AIDS-associated infections are either in development or being tested. Researchers are investigating exactly how HIV damages the immune system and documenting how the disease progresses in different people.[80] They also are studying the small number of people (fewer than 50) initially infected with HIV ten or more years ago who have not developed symptoms of AIDS. Scientists hope that understanding the body's natural method of control may lead to ideas for new HIV vaccines to prevent disease progression.

 Meningitis on Campus. What aspects of campus life make students susceptible to meningitis?

Making This Chapter Work for You

Guarding Against Infectious Diseases

◼ Infectious illnesses remain a serious health threat. Disease-causing organisms called pathogens, carried by various vectors, can infect a host (either a person or a population) in various ways.

◼ The types of microbes that can cause infection are viruses, which invade a body cell and take over its reproductive processes; bacteria, one-celled organisms that release disease-causing toxins; fungi, microscopic plants that feed on human tissue; protozoa, one-celled organisms that release substances that destroy or damage cells; and helminths, parasitic worms that invade body tissue.

◼ During the incubation period, a pathogen is multiplying; in the prodromal period, symptoms appear; during active infection, symptoms are most intense; during recovery, symptoms subside.

◼ Antibacterial drugs, sulfa drugs, and antibiotics treat diseases caused by bacteria, but they have no effect on viruses or other pathogens. Antiviral drugs can damage cells invaded by viruses.

◼ The body's natural defenses against pathogens include the skin; antibacterial substances in tears, sweat, saliva, and mucus; and the immune system, which includes many different types of defenders. Humoral immunity involves an antigen-antibody response. Cell-mediated immunity refers to the activity of various types of protective cells. Once a person has produced antibodies to a pathogen, he or she has developed active immunity and is usually protected from that disease for life.

■ Immune system disorders include allergies, autoimmune disorders, and acquired immunodeficiency syndrome (AIDS).

■ Immunizations are the best method of prevention against infectious diseases such as polio, tetanus, diphtheria, rubella, measles, chickenpox, hepatitis B, and HIB.

■ Infectious diseases caused by viruses include the common cold, influenza, viral pneumonia, mononucleosis, and hepatitis. Bacterial infections include bacterial pneumonia, tuberculosis, group A and group B strep, toxic shock syndrome, and Lyme disease.

■ Emerging infections are those recently recognized, increasing in humans, or threatening to spread to new areas in the near future. They include HIV, Hantavirus, Ebola, dengue, Lassa, and Marburg, which have been responsible for deadly outbreaks around the globe.

■ Reproductive and urinary tract infections are very common and include trichomoniasis, candidiasis, and bacterial vaginosis, as well as infections of the urethra, bladder, or kidney.

health / ONLINE

National Center for HIV, STD and TB Prevention
http://www.cdc.gov/nchstp/od/nchstp.html
This site, from the Centers for Disease Control and Prevention, contains general information on HIV/AIDS, sexually transmitted diseases, and tuberculosis.

Cells Alive!
http://www.cellsalive.com/
This site features interactive animations, illustrations, and clear written descriptions to help explain how pathogens and the immune system work in the human body. Topics include HIV infection, making antibodies, penicillin, parasites, and streptococcus.

Journal of the American Medical Association HIV/AIDS Information Center
http://www.ama-assn.org/special/hiv/search/search.htm
From this page, you can enter key words to search for HIV/AIDS information within issues of the *Journal of the American Medical Association (JAMA)*.

Please note that links are subject to change. If you find a broken link, use a search engine like http://www.yahoo.com *and search for the web site by typing in key words.*

 Campus Chat: Now that you have read about ways to bolster your immune system, will you make any lifestyle changes to reduce your risk of contracting an infectious disease? Share your thoughts on our online discussion forum at **http://health.wadsworth.com**

Find It On InfoTrac: You can find additional readings about infectious diseases via InfoTrac College Edition, an online library of more than 900 journals and publications. Follow the instructions for accessing InfoTrac that came packaged with your textbook; then search for articles using a key word search.

• **Suggested article:** "The Cold War: How to Prevent the Flu and the Cold" by Norine Dworkin. *Vegetarian Times*, February 1999, p. 22.

(1) What are some dietary strategies that may help prevent the common cold and the flu?

(2) Based on symptoms, what is the difference between the common cold and the flu?

(3) Why should antibiotics not be used to treat a cold or the flu?

For additional links, resources, and suggested readings on InfoTrac, visit our Health & Wellness Resource Center at **http://health.wadsworth.com**

■ The incidence of sexually transmitted diseases (STDs) is increasing. Because many STDs do not cause any symptoms in their initial stages, infected individuals may continue their usual sexual activity without realizing that they're jeopardizing others' well-being.

■ While STDs strike both sexes, all classes, and all ages, young Americans are at greatest risk. According to the CDC, as many as half of all young people may develop an STD by age 30.

■ The most widespread sexually transmitted bacterium in the United States is *Chlamydia trachomatis,* which causes 3 to 5 million infections each year, most in individuals 25 years old or younger.

■ Infection of a woman's fallopian tubes or uterus, called pelvic inflammatory disease (PID), is the second-most serious STD affecting women (after HIV infection). About one in every seven women of reproductive age has PID.

■ One of the most common and dangerous STDs in the United States is gonorrhea, which is caused by the gonococcus bacterium and is diagnosed with a blood test or a culture. The incidence is highest among teenagers and young adults.

■ Nongonoccal urethritis (NGU) refers to any inflammation of the urethra that is not caused by gonorrhea. Two separate microorganisms, *Chlamydia trachomatis* and *Ureaplasma urealyticum,* are the primary causes.

■ Syphilis, caused by a bacterium, is easily treated in its stages but can progress and, over time, invade various organs inside the body, including the heart and brain.

■ Herpes simplex virus causes painful blisters during flareups and never entirely leaves the body. Human papilloma virus (HPV) and chancroid infections are other STDs that are spreading rapidly.

■ Human immunodeficiency virus (HIV) is a retrovirus that attacks the body's immune system and causes various problems, ranging from symptomatic infection to generalized swelling of the lymph glands. It is spread through anal, vaginal, and oral sexual contact; contaminated needles of drug abusers; blood transfusions, blood products, and organ transplants from HIV-positive individuals; from HIV-positive mothers to their babies before, during, or after birth; and accidental contact with HIV-contaminated blood or bodily fluids.

■ Acquired immunodeficiency syndrome (AIDS) is diagnosed when HIV severely impairs a person's immune system, as indicated by a CD4 count of less than 200 cells per cubic millimeter of blood. People with AIDS also may experience persistent fever, diarrhea, involuntary weight loss, neurological disease, and secondary infectious diseases and cancers.

■ HIV is transmitted through sexual contact, blood transfusions, organ transplants, and sharing contaminated needles.

Key Terms

The terms listed here are used within the chapter. Page numbers are included for each term. A definition of each term is given in the Glossary pages at the end of this book.

abscess   374
acquired immunodeficiency
   syndrome (AIDS)   401
allergy   375
antibiotics   371
antiviral drug   371
autoimmune   376
bacteria   371
bacterial vaginosis   387
candidiasis   387
cell-mediated   374
chanchroid   400
chlamydial infections   394
chronic fatigue syndrome
   (CFS)   382
cystitis   388
fungi   371
gamma globulin   373
gonorrhea   396
helminth   371

hepatitis   382
herpes simplex   398
host   370
human immunodeficiency
   virus (HIV)   401
human papilloma virus
   (HPV)   399
humoral   373
immune deficiency   376
immunity   372
immunotherapy   375
incubation period   372
inflammation   374
influenza   381
Lyme disease   385
lymph nodes   374
mononucleosis   382
nongonococcal urethritis
   (NGU)   397
pathogen   370

pelvic inflammatory disease (PID)
   395
pneumonia   383
protozoa   371
pyelonephritis   388
sexually transmitted diseases
   (STDs)   388
syphilis   397
systemic disease   374
toxic shock syndrome (TSS)   385
trichomoniasis   387
tuberculosis   384
urethritis   388
vector   370
virus   370

Critical Thinking Questions

1. What are several practices that you know of or use to avoid contracting infectious diseases? Briefly explain the convenience, advantages, and disadvantages of each practice.

2. The U.S. military and some employers routinely screen personnel for HIV. Some hospitals test patients and note their HIV status on their charts. Some insurance companies test for HIV before selling a policy. Do you believe that an individual has the right to refuse to be tested for HIV? Should a physician be able to order an HIV test without a patient's consent? Can a surgeon refuse to operate on an HIV-infected patient or one who refuses HIV testing? Do patients have the right to know if their doctors, dentists, or nurses are HIV-positive?

3. A man who developed herpes sued his former girlfriend. A woman who became sterile as a result of pelvic inflammatory disease (PID) took her ex-husband to court. A woman who contracted HIV infection from her dentist, who had died of AIDS, filed suit against his estate. Do you think that anyone who knowingly transmits a sexually transmitted disease should be held legally responsible? Do you think such an act should be a criminal offense?

References

1. CDC. *Morbidity and Mortality Weekly Report,* July 30, 1999.
2. "AIDS Is World's Fourth-Largest Killer." *AIDS Weekly Plus,* May 24, 1999.
3. "How Many People Have HIV and AIDS?" *CDC Update,* May 13, 1999.
4. Goff, Karen Goldberg. "Germ Wars." *Insight on the News,* Vol. 15, Issue 22, June 14, 1999.
5. Peters, Madelon, et al. "Immune System Responds Greater to Uncontrollable Stresses." *Psychosomatic Medicine* news release, August 2, 1999.
6. "Mechanism of Stress Revealed." *World Disease Weekly Plus,* June 28, 1999.
7. Blum, Caroline. "Allergies Nearly Twice as Common as Believed." American College of Allergy, Asthma and Immunology news release, August 11, 1999.
8. Miles, Robert. Personal interview.
9. Derebery, M. Jennifer. "Allergy and Health-Related Quality of Life." Presentation, American Academy of Otolaryngic Allergy Foundation, April 1999, Palm Desert, Ca.
10. Adkinson, N. Franklin. "Immunotherapy for Allergic Rhinitis." *New England Journal of Medicine,* Vol. 341, No. 7, August 12, 1999.
11. Judge, Gillian. "Breathe Easier." *American Health,* January 1999. Langer, Stephen, and Andersen-Parrado, Patricia. "Stifling Allergies." *Better Nutrition,* Vol. 61, No. 4, April 1999.
12. Whitacre, Caroline, et al. "A Gender Gap in Autoimmunity." *Science,* Vol. 283, Issue 5406, February 26, 1999.
13. National Vaccine Advisory Committee. "Strategies to Sustain Success in Childhood Immunizations." *Journal of American Medical Association,* Vol. 281, July 28, 1999.
14. Seder, Robert, and Sanjay Gurunathan. "DNA Vaccines— Designer Vaccines for the 21st Century." *New England Journal of Medicine,* Vol. 341, No. 4, July 22, 1999.
15. "Polio Vaccination Schedule." *The Lancet,* Vol. 353, Issue 9160, April 10, 1999.
16. "Whooping Cough—Still Around." *Pediatrics for Parents,* Vol. 18, Issue 4, April 1999.
17. "Measles on the Run." *Pediatrics for Parents,* Vol. 18, Issue 3, March 1999.
18. Liesegang, Thomas. "The Ocular Manifestation of Congenital Infection: A Study of the Early Effect and Long-Term Outcome of Maternally Transmitted Rubella and Toxoplasmosis." *American Journal of Ophthalmology,* Vol. 127, Issue 4, April 1999.
19. Sadovsky, Richard. "Varicella Vaccine: Alone or With MMR and DTP/HbOC?" *American Family Physician,* Vol. 59, Issue 6, March 15, 1999.
20. Marwick, Charles K., and Mike Mitka. "Debate Revived on Hepatitis B Vaccine Value." *Journal of American Medical Association,* Vol. 281, July 7, 1999.
21. "Adverse Events Reported for Hepatitis B Vaccine." *Health Facts,* February 1999.
22. "Decrease in Incidence of HIB Disease." *American Family Physician,* February 15, 1999.
23. Taubes, Gary. "The Cold Warrior." *Discover,* February 1999.
24. Gwaltney, Jack. Personal interview.
25. Hales, Dianne. "Is a Cure in Sight?" *Parade,* January 23, 2000.
26. "What To Do About a Cold or Flu." *Consumer Reports,* January 1999.
27. Cohen, Sheldon, et al. "Susceptibility to the Common Cold." *Psychosomatic Medicine,* March 1999.
28. Poland, Gregory, and Robert Crouch. "Intranasal Influenza Vaccine: Adding to the Armamentarium for Influenza Control." *New England Journal of Medicine,* July 14, 1999.
29. Kilbourne, Edwin. Personal interview.
30. Sagall, Rich. "Flu Vaccine & Kids." *Pediatrics for Parents,* November 1998.
31. Hales. "Is a Cure in Sight?"
32. Anderson-Parrado, Patricia. "Beating Chronic Fatigue Syndrome." *Better Nutrition,* Vol. 61, Issue 5, May 1999.
33. "More Hepatitis Shots Loom for Many Kids." *U.S. News & World Report,* Vol. 126, Issue 8, March 1, 1999.
34. Abramovitz, Melissa. "How to Avoid Hepatitis B & C." *Current Health,* Vol. 25, Issue 6, February 1999.
35. Friedrich, M. J. "Third Millennium Challenge: Hepatitis C." *JAMA,* Vol. 282, July 21, 1999.
36. "Shedding Light on the Shadow Epidemic." *Harvard Health Letter,* Vol. 24, Issue 10, July 1999.
37. Henkel, John. "Hepatitis C: New Treatment Helps Some, but Cure Remains Elusive." *FDA Consumer,* Vol. 33, Issue 2, March 1999.
38. "Evolutionary Bottleneck May Explain TB Persistence." *World Disease Weekly Plus,* June 28, 1999.
39. Sagall, Rich. "Short Treatment for Strep Throat." *Pediatrics for Parents,* Vol. 18, Issue 3, March 1999.

40. Chang, Maria. "Ticked Off!" *Science World*, Vol. 55, Issue 14, May 10, 1999.

41. Lewis, Carol. "New Vaccine Targets Lyme Disease." *FDA Consumer*, Vol. 33, Issue 3, May 1999.

42. Brown, S. Lori, et al. "Role of Serology in the Diagnosis of Lyme Disease." *JAMA*, Vol. 282, July 7, 1999.

43. DeNoon, Daniel. "CDC's 21st Century Plan: Repair, Prepare." *World Disease Weekly Plus*, June 28, 1999.

44. Rose, Verna. "Special Medical Reports: CDC Releases Updated Plan for Emerging Infectious Diseases." *American Family Physician*, Vol. 59, Issue 8, April 15, 1999.

45. Walling, Anne. "A Cost-Effective Strategy for Diagnosing Vaginal Candidiasis." *American Family Physician*, Vol. 59, Issue 5, March 1, 1999.

46. Orenstein, Robert, and Edward Wong. "Urinary Tract Infections in Adults." *American Family Physician*, Vol. 59, Issue 5, March 1, 1999.

47. Ibid.

48. "Sexual Health." *Newsletter—People's Medical Society*, Vol. 18, Issue 1, February 1999.

49. Staton, Michele, et al. "Risky Sex Behavior and Substance Use Among Young Adults." *Health and Social Work*, Vol. 24, No. 2, May, 1999.

50. Shapiro, Johanna, et al. "Sexual Behavior and AIDS-Related Knowledge Among Community College Students in Orange County, California." *Journal of Community Health*, Vol. 24, Issue 1, February 1999.

51. Christ, M. J., et al. "Prioritizing Education About Condom Use Among Sexually Active Adolescent Females." *AIDS Weekly Plus*, February 15, 1999.

52. Duncan, Barbara, and Graham Hart. "Sexuality and Health: The Hidden Costs of Screening for Chlamydia Trachomatis." *British Medical Journal*, Vol. 316, Issue 7188, April 3, 1999.

53. Nordenberg, Tamar. "Chlamydia's Quick Cure." *FDA Consumer*, Vol. 33, No. 4, July 1999.

54. "What's New in Research." *Brown University Child and Adolescent Behavior Letter*, Vol. 15, Issue 6, June 1999.

55. Apgar, Barbara. "Diagnosing PID: Comparing Ultrasound, MRI, Laparoscopy." *American Family Physician*, Vol. 59, March 15, 1999.

56. Crooks, Robert, and Karla Baur. *Your Sexuality*, 6th ed. Pacific Grove, CA: Brooks Cole, 1999.

57. Arvin, Ann, and Charles Prober. "Herpes Simplex Virus Type 2— A Persistent Problem." *New England Journal of Medicine*, Vol. 337, No. 16, October 16, 1997.

58. Linnehan, Mary Jane, and Nora Ellen Groce. "Psychosocial and Educational Services for Female College Students with Genital Human Papillomavirus Infection." *Family Planning Perspectives*, Vol. 31, Issue 3, May 1999.

59. Ho, Gloria, et al. "Natural History of Cervicovaginal Papillomavirus Infection in Young Women." *New England Journal of Medicine*, Vol. 338, No. 7, February 12, 1998.

60. "HPV Test, Education and Early Detection Recommended." *Cancer Weekly Plus*, February 22, 1999.

61. "Unprotected Sex Can Lead to Cancer." *Cancer Weekly Plus*, April 19, 1999.

62. "AIDS Is World's Fourth-Largest Killer."

63. "The HIV/AIDS Epidemic in the U.S." Kaiser Family Foundation Fact Sheet, June 1999.

64. "HIV Infection and AIDS." NAIAD Fact Sheet, March 1999.

65. Halweil, Brian. "HIV/AIDS Pandemic Is Worsening." *World Watch*, Vol. 12, Issue 2, March–April 1999.

66. Nathanson, Neal, and Judith Auerbach. "Confronting the HIV Pandemic." *Science*, Vol. 284, Issue 5420, June 4, 1999.

67. Altman, Lawrence. "Focusing on Prevention in Fight against AIDS." *New York Times*, August 31, 1999.

68. Halweil. "HIV/AIDS Pandemic Is Worsening."

69. "The HIV/AIDS Epidemic in the U.S." Kaiser Family Foundation Fact Sheet, June 1999.

70. Garcia, Patricia, et al. "Maternal Levels of Plasma Human Immunodeficiency Virus Type 1 RNA and the Risk of Perinatal Transmission." *New England Journal of Medicine*, Vol. 341, No. 6, August 5, 1999.

71. Monaco, John. "HIV Testing during Pregnancy." *Pediatrics for Parents*, Vol. 18, Issue 3, March 1999.

72. Mofenson, Lynne, et al. "Risk Factors for Perinatal Transmission of Human Immunodeficiency Virus Type 1 in Women Treated with Zidovudine." *New England Journal of Medicine*, Vol. 341, No. 6, August 5, 1999.

73. Rotheram-Borus, Mary Jane, et al. "HIV Risk among Homosexual, Bisexual, and Heterosexual Male and Female Youths." *Archives of Sexual Behavior*, Vol. 28, Issue 2, April 1999.

74. "HIV Testing." Kaiser Family Foundation Fact Sheet, June 1999.

75. "New Study Examines Teens Attitudes toward HIV Testing." *SHOP Talk (School Health Opportunities and Progress) Bulletin*, Vol. 4, Issue 9, July 9, 1999.

76. CDC. "Anonymous or Confidential HIV Counseling and Voluntary Testing in Federally Funded Testing Sites." *JAMA*, Vol. 282, No. 4, July 28, 1999.

77. "New Data Show AIDS Patients Less Likely to Be Hospitalized." CDC Press release, June 8, 1999.

78. Altman, Lawrence. "Focusing on Prevention in Fight against AIDS." *New York Times*, August 31, 1999.

79. "Stress Speeds Passage from HIV to AIDS, Support Slows It." *AIDS Weekly Plus*, June 14, 1999.

80. "HIV Infection and AIDS." NAIAD Fact Sheet, March 1999.

CHAPTER

13

Keeping Your Heart Healthy

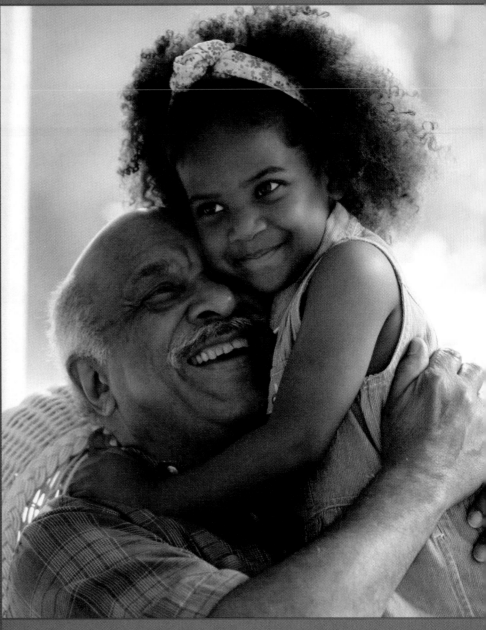

After studying the material in this chapter, you should be able to:

- **Describe** how the heart functions.
- **List** and **explain** the risk factors for cardiovascular disease.
- **Explain** the relationship of cholesterol to the risk of heart attack.
- **Define** hypertension, and **list** its common risk factors.
- **Define** atherosclerosis, and **list** effective treatments for it.
- **Explain** what happens during a myocardial infarction (MI) (heart attack) and what can be done to prevent and treat such attacks.
- **Define** stroke and transient ischemic attacks (TIAs), and **explain** their cause, prevention, and treatment.

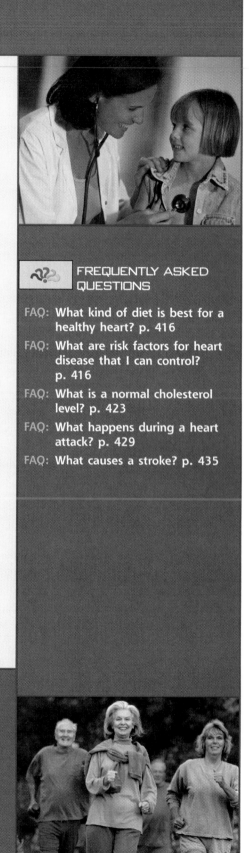

The news about cardiovascular disease—disorders of the heart and blood vessels—is heartwarming. Although cardiovascular disease is still the nation's top killer, death rates have dropped by 60 percent since 1950, a decline that many consider to be one of the major health achievements of the twentieth century.[1] The medical advances described in this chapter have contributed to the decline, but much of the credit goes to lifestyle changes, such as quitting smoking and making dietary changes that lower blood pressure and cholesterol levels.

Yet we still have a long way to go to keep the hearts of all Americans healthy. One of every two men and one of every three women in the United States will develop some form of cardiovascular illness.[2] Heart-related disorders account for almost as many deaths as the *combined* total for cancer, accidents, influenza, pneumonia, AIDS, and all other causes.

The time to start protecting your heart is now. Many people mistakenly think of cardiovascular disorders as illnesses of middle and old age. However, the events leading up to heart disease often begin in childhood, develop more rapidly throughout adolescence, and become a serious health threat to men in their thirties and forties and to women in their forties and fifties. It's never too soon to start being heart smart. This chapter provides the information you need about risk factors, silent dangers such as high blood pressure and cholesterol, and medical advances that can help your chances to have a healthier heart and a longer life. ❖

FREQUENTLY ASKED QUESTIONS

FAQ: **What kind of diet is best for a healthy heart? p. 416**

FAQ: **What are risk factors for heart disease that I can control? p. 416**

FAQ: **What is a normal cholesterol level? p. 423**

FAQ: **What happens during a heart attack? p. 429**

FAQ: **What causes a stroke? p. 435**

How the Heart Works

The heart is a hollow, muscular organ with four chambers that serve as two pumps (see Figure 13-1). It is about the size of a clenched fist. Each pump consists of a pair of chambers formed of muscles. The upper two—each called an **atrium**—receive blood, which then flows through valves into the lower two chambers, the **ventricles,** which contract to pump blood out into the arteries through a second set of valves. A thick wall divides the right side of the heart from the left side; but even though the two sides are separated, they contract at almost the same time. Contraction of the ventricles is called **systole;** the period of relaxation between contractions is called **diastole.** The heart valves, located at the entrance and exit of the ventricular chambers, have flaps that open and close to allow blood to flow through the chambers of the heart.

The myocardium (heart muscle) consists of branching fibers that enable the heart to contract or beat between 60 and 80 times per minute, or about 100,000 times a day. With each beat, it pumps about 2 ounces of blood. This may not sound like much, but it adds up to nearly 5 quarts of blood pumped by the heart in one minute, or about 75 gallons per hour.

The heart is surrounded by the pericardium, which consists of two layers of a tough membrane. The space between the two contains a lubricating fluid that allows the heart muscle to move freely. The endocardium is a smooth membrane lining the inside of the heart and its valves.

Blood circulates through the body by means of the pumping action of the heart, as shown in Figure 13-2. The right ventricle (on your own right side) pumps blood, via the *pulmonary arteries,* to the lungs, where it picks up oxygen (a gas essential to the body's cells) and gives off carbon dioxide (a waste product of metabolism). The blood returns from the lungs via the *pulmonary veins* to the left side of the heart, which pumps it, via the **aorta,** to the arteries in the rest of the body.

The arteries divide into smaller and smaller branches, and finally into **capillaries,** the smallest blood vessels of all (only slightly larger in diameter than a single red blood cell). The blood within the capillaries supplies oxygen and nutrients to the cells of the tissues, and takes up various waste products. Blood returns to the heart via the veins: The blood from the upper body (except the lungs) drains into the heart through the *superior vena cava,* while blood from the lower body returns via the *inferior vena cava.*

The workings of this remarkable pump affect your entire body. If the flow of blood to or through the heart or to the rest of the body is reduced, or if a disturbance occurs in the small bundle of highly specialized cells in the heart that generate electrical impulses to control heartbeats, the result may at first be too subtle to notice. However, without diagnosis and treatment, these changes could develop into a life-threatening problem.

Perhaps the biggest breakthrough in the field of cardiology has been not a test or a treatment, but a realization: Heart disease is not inevitable. We can keep our hearts healthy for as long as we live, but the process of doing so must start early and continue throughout life.

Trends in Cardiovascular Disease: Good News/Bad News

In the last half-century, death rates from cardiovascular disease have dropped by 60 percent. (See Figure 13-3.)

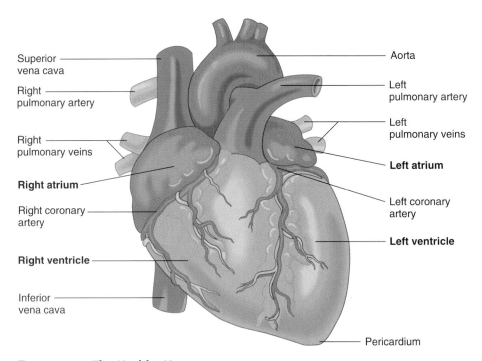

Superior vena cava
Right pulmonary artery
Right pulmonary veins
Right atrium
Right coronary artery
Right ventricle
Inferior vena cava

Aorta
Left pulmonary artery
Left pulmonary veins
Left atrium
Left coronary artery
Left ventricle
Pericardium

■ Figure 13-1 **The Healthy Heart**
The heart muscle is nourished by blood from the coronary arteries, which arise from the aorta. The pericardium is the outer covering of the heart.

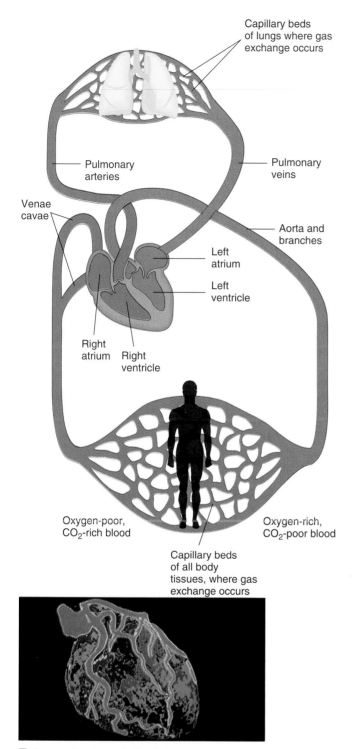

Capillary beds
of lungs where gas
exchange occurs

Pulmonary
arteries

Pulmonary
veins

Venae
cavae

Aorta and
branches

Left
atrium

Left
ventricle

Right
atrium   Right
ventricle

Oxygen-poor,
CO_2-rich blood

Oxygen-rich,
CO_2-poor blood

Capillary beds
of all body
tissues, where gas
exchange occurs

■ Figure 13-2 **The Path of Blood Flow**
Blood is pumped from the right ventricle into the pulmonary
arteries, which lead to the lungs, where gas exchange
(oxygen for carbon dioxide) occurs. Oxygenated blood
returning from the lungs drains into the left atrium and is
then pumped into the left ventricle, which sends the blood
into the aorta and its branches. The oxygenated blood flows
through the arteries, which extend to all parts of the body.
Again, gas exchange occurs in the body tissues; this time
oxygen is "dropped off" and carbon dioxide "picked up."
Photo depicts a computer-enhanced image of a healthy heart.

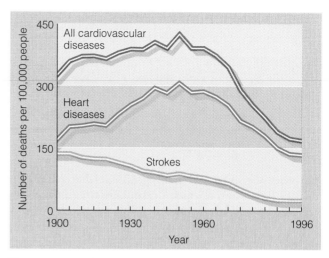

■ Figure 13-3 The decline in cardiovascular deaths.

Source: National Heart, Lung and Blood Institute and Centers for
Disease Control and Prevention, August 1999.

A reduction in the number of heart attacks is responsible for about two-thirds of this decline; the other third
is due to an increase in the number of people surviving
heart attacks.

Are fewer Americans suffering heart attacks because
of lifestyle changes that lower their risk or because of
improved medical treatment for many risk factors? No
one knows for sure. However, we may get answers and
insights from a World Health Organization-sponsored
project called MONICA (monitoring trends and determinants in cardiovascular disease), the largest collabora-
tive study of heart disease ever undertaken, which is
tracking heart attack rates, risk factors, and heart disease treatment in 37 medical centers, in 21 countries, on
4 continents.[3]

In the meantime, health officials stress that heart
disease remains public health enemy number-one. An
estimated 58,800,000 Americans have some form of
cardiovascular disease. As the American Heart
Association reports, the actual number of people
dying from cardiovascular illnesses has risen by 37
percent since 1950. This translates into 200,000
deaths each year.[4]

Many more people also are living with heart disease: Some 50 million have high blood pressure; 12
million suffer from coronary heart disease; 7 million
have had a heart attack; more than 6 million experience chest pain; more than 4 million have had strokes.
In all, one of every five Americans has some form of
heart disease. By age 50, one in three men and one in
10.5 women can expect to develop some major cardiovascular disease.[5]

Preventing Heart Problems

In order to continue making progress and saving lives, cardiologists stress the need for preventive measures, including lifestyle changes.

Physical Activity

For years we've known that regular exercise reduces the risk of heart attack, helps maintain a healthy body weight, lowers blood pressure, and improves metabolism. If rigorous and frequent enough, it also may increase longevity. But you don't have to head to a gym or hit the bike path to keep your heart healthy. As recent studies have confirmed, "lifestyle" activities, such as walking, housecleaning, and gardening, are as effective as a structured exercise program in improving heart function, lowering blood pressure, and maintaining or losing weight.[6] (See Chapter 5 for a complete discussion of physical activity.)

The federal government recommends that adults try to get at least 30 minutes of moderate-intensity physical activity on most and preferably all days of the week. In one study, those who added simple lifestyle changes, such as taking longer walks on the way to office meetings, or walking around airports instead of sitting while waiting for a plane, improved their cardiorespiratory fitness and blood pressure as much as those in structured programs.

Walking, in particular, has proven an excellent way of keeping the heart healthy throughout life. In a study of 2,678 men aged 71 to 93, those who walked about two miles a day had half the risk of heart attack of males who walked a quarter mile. These findings may extend to younger men as well as to women, and similar studies have found that walking can reduce a person's risk of heart disease.[7]

What Kind of Diet Is Best for a Healthy Heart?

A balanced, low-fat diet is the best recipe for a healthy heart. In particular, foods rich in cell-protecting antioxidants, folic acid, and vitamin E supplements have all been linked with a lower risk of heart disease.

As described in Chapter 6, free radicals—rogue molecules of oxygen—in the cardiovascular system combine with cholesterol and dangerous low-density lipoprotein to damage the inner lining of blood vessels. Vitamin E, a fat-soluble vitamin found in wheat germ, vegetable oils and nuts, short-circuits this process. In various clinical studies, it has lowered the risk of heart attacks and strokes by 40 to 60 percent. Because it is difficult to get adequate levels of vitamin E in a daily diet, some experts recommend supplements of 100 to 400 IU a day.[8]

Other antioxidants, particularly vitamin C and beta-carotene, have not proved as helpful in protecting the heart. In one study of 22,000 male physicians, 20 milligrams of beta-carotene, either alone or combined with vitamin E, did not reduce the risk of heart attacks. However, in epidemiological studies, individuals eating lots of dark green, yellow, and orange fruits and vegetables (good sources of vitamin C and beta-carotene) consistently have lower rates of coronary disease.

Increased intake of the B vitamins, particularly folate, can lower elevated levels of homocysteine, a naturally occurring amino acid and a recently identified risk factor for heart disease (discussed later in this chapter). The recommended daily dietary intake is 400 micrograms a day.[9]

Risk Factors for Cardiovascular Disease

Several major risk factors contribute to disorders of the heart and blood vessels. The greater the number or severity of these risk factors, the greater your overall risk. (See Self-Survey: "What's Your Risk of Heart Disease?")

What Are Risk Factors for Heart Disease That I Can Control?

The choices individuals make and the habits they follow can have a significant impact on whether or not their hearts remain healthy. The following are potential risks that you can avoid for the sake of your heart's health.

Physical Inactivity

Most Americans get too little physical activity. About one in four U. S. adults are sedentary and another third are not active enough to reach a healthy level of fitness.[10] People who are not even somewhat physically active face a much greater risk of fatal heart attack than those who engage in some form of exercise or activity. Individuals who work out rigorously and regularly have the healthiest hearts and the lowest risks of heart disease.

Self-*Survey*   What's Your Risk of Heart Disease?

Take this test developed by doctors at Washington Hospital Center. Answer the following questions, total your score, then see "What Your Score Means" below for advice.

Risk Factors You Can't Control

1. Family History
Do you have a parent, sibling, or grandparent who developed heart disease

at age 59 or younger?	3
at age 60 or older?	1
I don't have any close relatives with heart disease	0 _____

2. Personal Medical History
Were you diagnosed with heart disease

at age 49 or younger?	6
at age 50 or older?	3
I have never been diagnosed with heart disease.	0 _____

Has your menstrual cycle stopped completely?

Yes	1
No	0 _____

3. Race
Are you black?

Yes	1
No	0 _____

4. Diabetes
Do you have diabetes?

Yes	1
No	0 _____

Risk Factors You Can Control

5. Weight
Are you

40 pounds overweight or more?	5
20 to 39 pounds overweight?	1
fewer than 20 pounds overweight or at ideal weight?	0 _____

6. Exercise
Do you exercise and reach your target heart rate less

than once a week or never?	2
twice a week?	1
three or more times a week?	0 _____

7. Cholesterol
Is your cholesterol level

300 or above?	4
250 to 299?	2
200 to 249?	1
199 or below?	0 _____

If you know your cholesterol level, proceed to question 8. If you don't know your cholesterol level, answer the next question.

Do you eat red meat, eggs, whole milk, cheese and/or butter at least five times a week?

Yes	2
No	0 _____

8. High Blood Pressure
Is your blood pressure

above 160/100?	3
140/90 to 160/100?	2
below 140/90?	0 _____

9. Cigarette Smoking

I smoke two or more packs a day.	6
I smoke one to two packs a day.	4
I smoke up to half a pack a day.	2
I've been a nonsmoker for less than one year.	2
I've been a nonsmoker for one year or more.	0
I've never smoked.	0 _____

If you smoke, do you also take birth control pills?

Yes	1
No	0 _____

10. Stress
Are you frequently tense, angry, irritable, or rushed?

Yes	1
No	0 _____

11. Alcohol Use
Do you consumer more than three drinks a day?*

Yes	2
No	0 _____

Total Score: _____

What Your Score Means

0 to 5 points: Congratulations! This is the lowest-risk category. If you scored points for questions 5 through 11, however, you may still want to make changes in your lifestyle to lower these risk factors.

6 to 10 points: You're at moderate risk and should consider changing your lifestyle. Look over the categories in which you scored the most points in order to pinpoint problem areas. Do you need to lose weight? Start exercising? Cut the fat in your diet?

11 points or higher: You are at high risk and should talk to your doctor right away. You'll probably need to make several changes in your lifestyle. But a lower risk of heart attack and an improved sense of well-being will be worth it.

*Experts generally advise women to limit alcohol consumption to one drink per day.

Cigarette Smoking

Each year smoking causes more than 250,000 deaths from cardiovascular disease—far more than it causes from cancer and lung disease. Smokers who have heart attacks are more likely to die from them than are nonsmokers. Smoking is the major risk factor for *peripheral vascular disease,* in which the blood vessels that carry blood to the leg and arm muscles get hardened and clogged. Cigar smoking causes a moderate, but significant increase in an individual's risk for coronary artery disease, as well as for cancers of the upper digestive tract and chronic obstructive pulmonary disease. Men who smoke five or more cigars per day have the highest risk, compared with those who do not smoke cigars at all.[11] Both active and passive smoking accelerate the process by which arteries become clogged and increase the risk of heart attacks and strokes.[12]

The American Heart Association estimates that 37,000 to 40,000 nonsmokers die each year from cardiovascular diseases as a result of exposure to environmental tobacco smoke.[13] Overall, nonsmokers exposed to environmental tobacco smoke are at a 25 percent higher relative risk of developing coronary heart disease than nonsmokers not exposed to environmental tobacco smoke.[14] Cigarette smoking and secondhand smoke may damage the heart in several ways:

- The nicotine may repeatedly overstimulate the heart.
- Carbon monoxide may take the place of some of the oxygen in the blood, which reduces the oxygen supply to the heart muscle.
- The tars and other smoke residues may damage the lining of the coronary arteries, making it easier for cholesterol to build up and narrow the passageways.
- Smoking also increases blood clotting, leading to a higher incidence of clotting in the coronary arteries and subsequent heart attack. Clotting in the peripheral arteries is also increased, which can cause leg pain with walking and, ultimately, stroke.
- Even ex-smokers may have irreversible damage to their arteries.

High Blood Pressure (Hypertension)

Blood pressure is a result of the contractions of the heart muscle, which pumps blood through your body, and the resistance of the walls of the vessels through which the blood flows. Each time your heart beats, your blood pressure goes up and down within a certain range. It's highest when the heart contracts; this is called *systolic blood pressure.* It's lowest between contractions; this is called *diastolic blood pressure.* A blood pressure reading consists of the systolic measurement "over" the diastolic measurement, recorded in millimeters of mercury (mmHg) by a sphygmomanometer (see Figure 13-4).

High blood pressure, or **hypertension,** occurs when the artery walls become constricted so that the force exerted as the blood flows through them is greater than it should be. Physicians see blood pressure as a continuum: the higher the reading, the greater the risk of stroke and heart disease. (See also the further discussion of high blood pressure later in this chapter.)

As a result of the increased work in pumping blood, the heart muscle of a person with hypertension can become stronger and also stiffer. This stiffness increases resistance to filling up with blood between beats, which can cause shortness of breath with exertion. Hypertension can also act on the kidney arteries, which can lead to kidney failure in some cases. In addition, hypertension accelerates the development of plaque buildup within the arteries. Especially when combined with obesity, smoking, high cholesterol levels, or diabetes, hypertension increases the risks of cardiovascular problems several times. However, you can control high blood pressure through diet, exercise, and medication (if necessary).

Blood Fats

Cholesterol is a fatty substance found in certain foods and also manufactured by the body (see Chapter 6). The measurement of cholesterol in the blood is one of the most reliable indicators of the formation of plaque, the sludgelike substance that builds up on the inner walls of arteries. You can lower blood cholesterol levels by cutting back on high-fat foods and exercising more, thereby reducing the risk of a heart attack. According to the National Heart, Lung, and Blood Institute (NHLBI), for every 1 percent drop in blood cholesterol, studies show a 2 percent decrease in the likelihood of a heart attack. (See The Cholesterol Connection, later in this chapter.)

Triglycerides

These fats, which flow through the blood after meals, have been linked to increased risk of coronary artery disease, especially in women. **Triglyceride** levels tend to be highest in those whose diets are high in calories, sugar, alcohol, and refined starches. High levels of these fats may increase the risk of obesity, but cutting back on these foods can reduce high triglyceride levels.

According to the NHLBI, triglyceride levels should be between 30 and 150 milligrams per decaliter (mg/dL) of blood. Triglyceride levels in the range of 250–500 mg/dL are a danger sign of an increased risk of heart disease. Higher levels, especially over 1,000 mg/dL, also

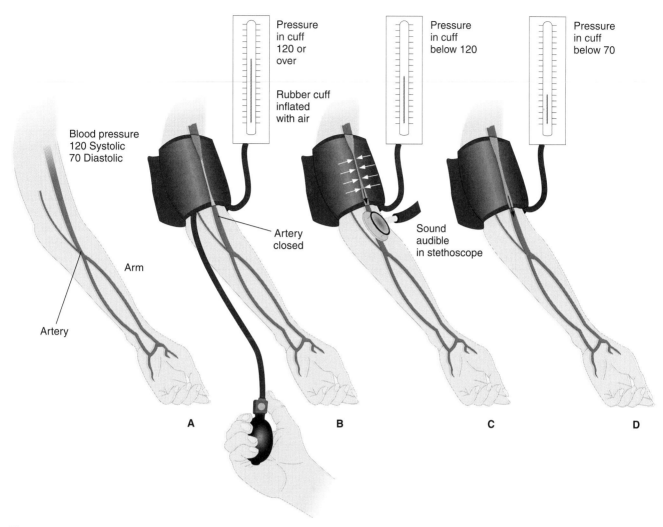

Pressure
in cuff
120 or
over

Rubber cuff
inflated
with air

Pressure
in cuff
below 120

Pressure
in cuff
below 70

Blood pressure
120 Systolic
70 Diastolic

Arm

Artery

Artery
closed

Sound
audible
in stethoscope

A   B   C   D

■ Figure 13-4 **Measurement of Blood Pressure**
Assume a blood pressure of 120/70 in a young, healthy individual. (A) The brachial artery of the arm is used to measure blood pressure. (B) The cuff of the sphygmomanometer (blood pressure cuff) is wrapped snugly around the arm just above the elbow and infalted until the blood flow into the brachial artery is stopped. This stoppage is detected with a stethoscope. (C) The cuff is gradually loosened, while the examiner listens carefully for pulse sounds with the stethoscope. The pressure reading as the first soft tapping sounds are heard (as a small amount of blood spurts through the constricted artery) is the systolic pressure. (D) As the cuff is loosened still further, the sounds become louder and more distinct. When the artery is no longer constricted and blood flows freely, however, the pulse sounds can no longer be heard. The reading at which the sounds disappear is recorded as the diastolic pressure.

increase the risk of pancreatitis, an inflammation of the pancreas requiring immediate medical attention.

Lipoproteins

Lipoproteins are compounds in the blood that are made up of proteins and fat. The different types are classified by their size or density. The heaviest are *high-density lipoproteins,* or HDLs, which have the highest portion of protein. These "good guys," as some cardiologists refer to them, pick up excess cholesterol in the blood and carry it back to the liver for removal from the body. *Low-density lipoproteins,* or LDLs, and very-low-density lipoproteins

(VLDLs) carry more cholesterol than HDLs and deposit it on the walls of arteries—they're the bad guys.

HDLs are most plentiful in the people least likely to get cardiovascular disease, such as young women and athletes. The higher the level of HDL and the higher the ratio of HDL to total cholesterol (HDL plus other blood fats), the lower the likelihood of heart disease. An HDL level of less than 45 mg/dL and an HDL-cholesterol ratio of less than 1 to 5 increase a man's risk of coronary artery disease. Women should have an HDL level above 55 mg/dL and an HDL-cholesterol ratio of more than 1 to 4.10. (See The Cholesterol Connection for ways to lower elevated levels.)

Diabetes Mellitus

Diabetes mellitus, a disorder of the endocrine system, increases the likelihood of hypertension and atherosclerosis, thereby increasing the risk of heart attack and stroke. Cardiovascular disease is the leading cause of death among all diabetics. A physician can detect diabetes and prescribe a diet, exercise program, and, if necessary, medication to keep it in check. Even before developing diabetes, individuals at high risk for this disease—those who are overweight, have a family history of the disease, have mildly elevated blood pressure and blood sugar levels, and above-ideal levels of harmful blood fats—may already be at increased risk of heart disease. Up to one-half of diabetics also have hypertension, another risk factor.[15] Diabetics who develop heart disease are more likely to die if they suffer a heart attack or develop heart failure.[16]

Weight

According to the National Heart, Lung, and Blood Institute, losing weight at any age can help reduce the risk of heart problems. For women, obesity is as great a cause of excess death and disability from heart disease as smoking and heavy drinking. Even mild to moderately obese women are more likely to suffer chest pain or a heart attack than thinner women. Weight loss significantly reduces high blood pressure, another risk factor for heart disease.[17] (See Chapter 7 for a discussion of weight control.)

Psychosocial Factors

As discussed in Chapter 2, the way we respond to everyday sources of stress can affect our hearts as well as our overall health. While we may not be able to control the sources of stress, we can change how we habitually respond to it. Various psychological and social influences may affect vulnerability to heart disease. The most widely studied are Type A traits, particularly anger and hostility; depression and anxiety; work characteristics; and social supports. These factors may act alone or combine and may exert different effects at different ages and stages of life. They may influence behaviors such as smoking, diet, alcohol consumption, and physical activity, and they also may directly cause changes in physiology.[18]

Although Type A behavior—especially anger—has long been linked with heart disease, a recent review of all prospective studies of its effects found no increased risk for Type A patients with coronary heart disease. However, women who bottle up their anger may be more likely to have a heart attack by age 60 than other women. According to a ten-year study of 200 women, those who conceal their anger or are concerned about their public appearance may have rising heart rates, elevated stress hormones, and high blood pressure—all associated with thickening of the carotid arteries.[19]

Depression takes a heavy toll on heart disease patients, making it more difficult for them to work, socialize, and perform other daily activities. Regardless of whether it's mild or severe, depression decreases ability to function on a daily basis by amplifying heart disease symptoms and reducing patients' interest in daily activities.[20]

Job stress also can be hard on the heart, particularly for employees who have little control over their work. A lack of social supports also seems to increase risk, possibly because intimate, caring relationships may buffer the effect of other stressors in life.[21]

Risks You Can't Control

Heredity

Anyone whose parents, siblings, or other close relatives suffered heart attacks before age 50 is at increased risk of developing heart disease. Certain risk factors, such as abnormally high blood levels of lipids, can be passed down from generation to generation. Although you can't rewrite your family history, individuals with an inherited vulnerability to cardiovascular disease can lower the danger by changing the risk factors within their control. Your heart's health depends to a great extent on your behavior, including the decisions you make about the foods you eat, or the decision not to smoke. As an added preventive step, cardiologists may prescribe a small daily dose of aspirin to individuals with a history of coronary artery disease who are at risk of forming clots that could block blood supplies to the heart, brain, and other organs. (*Note:* Daily aspirin is not advised for individuals who are not at risk because of their age or health history.)

Race and Ethnicity

African Americans are twice as likely to develop high blood pressure as are whites. African Americans also suffer strokes at an earlier age and of greater severity. Poverty may be an unrecognized risk factor for members of this minority group, who are less likely to receive medical treatments or undergo corrective surgery. Family history, lifestyle, diet, and stress may also play a role, starting early in life. However, researchers have found no single explanation for why African-American youngsters, like their parents, tend to have higher blood pressure than white children.

Age

Almost four out of five people who die of heart attacks are over age 65. Heart disease accounts for more than 40 percent of deaths among people between 65 and 74 and almost 60 percent at age 85 and above. However, the risk factors that are likely to cause heart disease later in life, including high blood pressure and cholesterol levels, may begin to develop in childhood. Nevertheless, although cardiovascular function declines with age, heart disease is not an inevitable consequence of aging. Many 80- and 90-year-olds have strong, healthy hearts.

Gender

Men have a higher incidence of cardiovascular problems than women, particularly before age 40. The incidence of coronary artery disease in women remains lower than in men until the sixth and seventh decades of life, but heart disease often takes a greater toll on women. The major risk factors for heart disease in women are diabetes and menopause without hormone replacement; hypertension, smoking, and abnormal blood fats (lipids) are intermediate risks; sedentary lifestyle, obesity, age, and family history are relatively minor risk factors.[22]

The female sex hormone estrogen may have a protective effect by increasing HDL levels and decreasing harmful LDL levels. After menopause or surgical removal of the ovaries, women's estrogen levels drop and their LDL levels tend to go up. Postmenopausal hormone replacement therapy (HRT) can protect women against heart disease by keeping their HDL levels up and their LDL levels down. However, the question of which women should take estrogen remains controversial (see Chapter 9).

Because heart disease has been perceived as a man's problem, research on women's hearts has lagged behind. The current recommendations for blood pressure, cholesterol levels, and prevention are based almost entirely on research on men. However, heart disease is the fourth-leading cause of death among women aged 30 to 34, third among women aged 35 to 39, second among women aged 40 to 64, and first among women over age 65. Although heart disease causes greater disability in women, it is routinely treated less aggressively than in men.[23] (See The X & Y Files: "The Hearts of Men and Women.")

Heart disease takes different forms in men and women. Middle-aged men are more likely to have a heart attack or sudden heart stoppage, while women in their middle years are more likely to suffer angina or chest pain (discussed later in this chapter). However, the rate of heart attacks increases in women in their sixties or older. As discussed later in this chapter, a woman's risk of dying within a month of a heart attack is much higher than for a man.[24]

Male Pattern Baldness

Male pattern baldness (the loss of hair at the vertex, or top, of the head) is associated with increased risk of heart attack in men under age 55. A study of 1,437 men showed a "modest" increased risk for those men who'd lost hair at the top of their heads but not for those with receding hairlines. The speed at which men lose their hair also may be an indicator of risk. Scientists speculate that men with male pattern baldness who lose their hair quickly may metabolize male sex hormones differently than others, thereby increasing the likelihood of heart disease.

Although it's premature to say that baldness is definitely "bad news for the heart," health experts advise bald men to follow basic guidelines, such as not smoking and controlling their cholesterol levels, to lower any possible risk.

Other Risk Factors

Researchers continue to investigate other possible factors that may increase the risk of heart disease, including some that were not even recognized a few years ago.

Homocysteine

Several long-term studies, including the Physicians' Health Study at Harvard University and the Framingham Heart Study, have found that people with high levels of the amino acid **homocysteine** are more likely to have narrowed carotid arteries (those leading to the brain) and to be at increased risk of heart attacks. About one in five Americans may have homocysteine levels high enough to increase their chances of developing heart disease.

Scientists are investigating the possible role of the B vitamins, particularly folate and vitamins B-6 and B-12, on reducing homocysteine levels. Others are not sure whether homocysteine or B-6 levels actually predict heart-disease risk. Until final results are in, many physicians recommend a multivitamin that includes 400 micrograms of folate as well as the recommended daily intakes of the other B vitamins. Researchers also are studying the impact on homocysteine and heart health of the federal government's requirement that bread and other grain food products be supplemented with the vitamin folate.[25]

Bacterial Infection

Unlike the illnesses discussed in Chapter 12, heart disease was never viewed as an illness caused by an infectious agent. However, recent investigations suggest that certain bacteria may indeed put the heart at risk. *Streptococcus*

<table>
<tr><td>

The   X&Y   **Files**

</td><td>

The Hearts of Men and Women

</td></tr>
</table>

m any people still think of heart disease as a "guy problem." However, in every year since 1984, heart disease has claimed the lives of more females than males. Cardiovascular diseases are the number-one killer of women as well as men. Yet most women are far more afraid of breast cancer (the cause of 1 in 27 female deaths) than heart disease (which is responsible for almost 1 in 2 female deaths).

The same risk factors—high cholesterol, high blood pressure, and obesity—endanger both sexes, but they play out differently in women than in men. A healthy norm for a woman's cholesterol is ten points higher than a man's—210 versus 200 milligrams per deciliter—but this figure matters less than HDL. Women with an HDL under 45 mg/dl are at greater risk, while men don't seem to be at risk unless their HDL dips below 35.

High blood pressure is more common in older women, but treating it may not be as beneficial for women as it is for men. In men, reducing blood pressure by any means reduces the mortality risk by 15 percent. The use of blood pressure medications to lower mild to moderate hypertension actually increases women's overall risk of dying.

For women, extra pounds spell extra danger. Even those who are moderately overweight (10 to 20 percent above their ideal weight) may have twice the risk of leaner women—particularly if they put on weight after age eighteen. In both men and women, the risk of heart disease increases if their extra pounds lodge around the waist rather than in the hips and thighs. Mid-torso fat seems more likely to move to the bloodstream, where it can build up and clog arteries.

Standard diagnostic tests are less precise in detecting heart disease in women. The traditional treadmill or exercise stress test, the gold standard for evaluating men, produces a high rate of false positive results in women. A thallium stress test also is less accurate than in men. Cardiologists recommend evaluation of a the female heart with an "echo stress test," an echocardiogram that uses sound waves to create a 3-D image of the heart at work.

If tests indicate a problem, the next step is an "invasive" diagnostic procedure called angiography or cardiac catheterization. But as recently as a decade ago, ten times as many men as women (40 percent versus 4 percent) were referred for this definitive test. Women still remain much less likely to undergo angiography—a critical prerequisite for angioplasty (balloon surgery to unclog arteries) or coronary bypass surgery.

Women who have heart attacks are less likely than men to survive over both the short and the long term. A woman's risk of dying within a month of a heart attack is 75 percent higher than a man's, in part because women typically take an hour longer to get to the hospital than men. Women also have more complications than men during hospitalization and a higher death rate after 30 days. Among patients under age 50, when heart attacks are especially rare among women, just 3 percent of male victims died, compared with 6 percent of females. By age 75, the death rate for both sexes is about equal, at 19 percent.

However, some advances are offering more hope for both male and female hearts. Vitamin E intake, according to research in both sexes, can reduce the risk of coronary artery disease in women and men. Both men and women benefit from cardiac rehabilitation—an option that cardiologists often didn't even suggest for women in the past. Given the same opportunity to strengthen their hearts, women continue to show improvements for three years after they start an exercise program; men reach a certain performance plateau within months.

Sources: "Women and Cardiovascular Disease," American Heart Association; "Men and Cardiovascular Disease," American Heart Association; Wexler, Laura. "Studies of Acute Coronary Syndromes in Women," *New England Journal of Medicine,* Vol. 341, No. 4, July 22, 1999; Vaccarino, Viola, et al. "Sex Based Differences in Early Mortality after Myocardial Infarction," *New England Journal of Medicine,* Vol. 341, No. 4, July 22, 1999; Hochman, Judith, et al. "Sex, Clinical Presentation and Outcome in Patients with Acute Coronary Syndromes," *New England Journal of Medicine,* Vol. 341, No. 4, July 22, 1999.

sanguis, the bacteria found in dental plaque, has been implicated in the buildup of atherosclerotic plaque. Individuals with periodontal disease are at increased risk of heart disease and stroke. Regular brushing, flossing, and dental visits can reduce this danger.

Another common bacteria, *Chlamydia pneumoniae,* long linked to respiratory infections, also may threaten the heart. Individuals with high levels of antibodies to this bacteria are more likely to suffer a heart-related problem. Researchers have reported that

antibiotics, taken to treat common infections, may protect against first-time heart attacks.[26] A national clinical trial to determine whether antibiotics can reduce the risk of heart attack and stroke is underway.[27]

Cocaine

More than 30 million Americans are believed to have tried cocaine, and an estimated 5 million are regular users. According to the first large study of the long-suspected relationship between cocaine and heart disease, cocaine significantly increases the risk of heart attack in individuals who are otherwise at low risk. During the first hour after using cocaine, the risk of heart attack increases nearly 24 times.

The average age of people in the study who suffered heart attacks soon after using cocaine was 44, about 17 years younger than the average heart attack patient. Of the 38 cocaine users who had heart attacks, 29 had no prior symptoms of heart disease.[28]

Cocaine may trigger a heart attack in several ways. The drug can cause a sudden rise in blood pressure, heart rate, and contractions of the left ventricle (or pumping chamber) of the heart. These effects can increase the risk of a heart attack. Cocaine also tightly squeezes, or constricts, the coronary arteries that feed blood to the heart. If the artery constricts, blood flow to the heart and brain can be obstructed, causing a heart attack or stroke.

The Cholesterol Connection

Cholesterol levels have dropped steadily among Americans since 1980; this change alone may account for an 8 to 17 percent decline in the incidence of heart disease.[29] For the sake of a healthy heart, all adults should know what their cholesterol level is, whether it's too high and if it is, what they can do to lower cholesterol.

What Is a Normal Cholesterol Level?

When it comes to cholesterol, "normal" isn't good enough. The average cholesterol level for middle-aged men and women in the United States is about 215 mg/dL of blood—more than the recommended desirable limit set by the NHLBI. Adults with a cholesterol level of 220 mg/dL may be more than twice as likely to get heart disease as those with a level of 180 mg/dL; for those with levels of 300 mg/dL or higher, the risk is four times greater.

According to the NHLBI:

- Total cholesterol should be below 200 mg/dL of blood for men and below 210 mg/dL for women.
- A total cholesterol reading of 201–239 mg/dL is considered borderline and presents a moderate to high risk for heart disease. Americans with cholesterol levels below 240 mg/dL account for more than 60 percent of the cases of coronary heart disease in this country.
- Total cholesterol levels of 240 or more mg/dL are dangerously high.

- LDL levels should be less than 130 mg/dL: a level of 160 mg/dL or more is high.
- HDL levels should be at least 35 mg/dL.

Persons in the moderate- to high-risk categories (as many as half of all adults, according to some estimates) should undergo a test of the concentrations of the different types of lipoproteins (HDLs and LDLs), the protein-fat complexes that carry cholesterol in the blood. (See Consumer Health Watch: "What You Need to Know About Cholesterol Testing.")

Cholesterol in the Young

Watching cholesterol levels isn't just for grown-ups anymore. In its guidelines for children, the National Cholesterol Education Program recommends cholesterol testing for youngsters at possible risk of heart disease, including those who have any of the following risk factors:

- A parent or grandparent who developed atherosclerosis (narrowing of the arteries due to plaque buildup) at or before age 55.
- A parent or grandparent who suffered a heart attack at or before age 55.
- A parent whose blood cholesterol level is over 240 mg/dL.

Federal health officials aren't advising cholesterol screening for all youngsters, in part because children with high cholesterol levels don't necessarily end up with high blood cholesterol as adults. For those with moderately elevated cholesterol levels, the suggested treatment is a low-fat, high-fiber diet, identical to the one most beneficial for adults' hearts. For children whose blood cholesterol is within normal ranges,

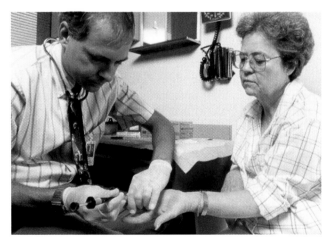
Getting a cholesterol test is a quick, simple, and relatively painless procedure.

Consumer Health Watch

What You Need to Know About Cholesterol Testing

- Go to your usual primary health-care provider to have your cholesterol level checked. Although cholesterol tests at shopping malls or health fairs can help identify people at risk, the analyzers are often not certified technicians, and the readings may occasionally be inaccurate. In addition, without a health expert to counsel them, some people may be unnecessarily frightened by a high reading—or falsely reassured by a low one.

- Ask about accuracy. Even at first-rate laboratories, cholesterol readings are often inaccurate. Find out if the lab is using the National Institutes of Health (NIH) standards, and ask about the lab's margin for error (which should be less than 5 percent).

- Think about timing. A cholesterol test is most accurate after a 12- to 14-hour fast. Schedule the test before breakfast if you can, or at least two hours after eating. Women may not want to get tested at the end of their menstrual cycles, when minor elevations in cholesterol levels occur because of lower estrogen levels. Cholesterol levels can also rise 5 to 10 percent during periods of stress. Reschedule the test if you come down with an intestinal flu, because the viral

infection could interfere with the absorption of food and thus with cholesterol levels. Let your doctor know if you're taking any drugs. Common medications, including birth control pills and hypertension drugs, can affect cholesterol levels.

- Sit down before allowing blood to be drawn or your finger to be pricked, because fluids pool differently in the body when you're standing than when you're sitting. Don't let a technician squeeze blood from your finger, because that forces fluid from cells, diluting the blood sample and possibly leading to a falsely low reading.

- Get real numbers. Don't settle for "normal" or "high," because laboratories can label results inaccurately. Find out exactly what your reading is. Find out your HDL/LDL ratio. If your cholesterol level is high, have it retested; ask to find out HDL and LDL levels as well.

- Some physicians advise getting two or three tests in the same month and averaging the result. A person's cholesterol levels vary so much from day to day that a single measurement may be meaningless.

doctors advise a balanced diet, with moderate amounts of a full range of nutrients.[30]

Across the Lifespan: Cholesterol and the Elderly

After age 70, elevated cholesterol levels seem less of a threat—at least in men. In a study of nearly 1,000 people at Yale University, high cholesterol did not increase the risk of heart disease in those over age 70. This study suggests that the 2 million elderly people taking cholesterol-lowering drugs may be receiving little, if any benefit and may even be risking some harm. However, another report concluded that, in older women, elevated cholesterol may indeed predict a greater risk of potentially fatal heart disease.

Lowering Cholesterol

There are various ways to reduce cholesterol levels and the risk of heart disease, including changes in diet and lifestyle and medications to bring down high levels of cholesterol in the blood.

Diet and Lifestyle

The National Cholesterol Education program recommends gradual dietary changes as part of its "Step I" Diet. According to its guidelines, individuals should get 8 to 10 percent of their daily total calories from saturated fat, 30 percent or less from fat, less than 300 milligrams of dietary cholesterol, and just enough total calories to achieve and maintain a healthy weight. If the Step I diet doesn't lower cholesterol, doctors may recommend the Step II diet, which calls for no more than 7 percent of daily calories from saturated fat and no more than 200 milligrams of dietary cholesterol. In many people, cholesterol levels begin to drop a few weeks after starting on the Step I or Step II diet. With time, these diets can reduce cholesterol levels by 10 to 50 mg/dl or more—a clinically significant amount.[31] Some researchers have found that patients who were highly motivated to reduce cholesterol and who worked closely with dietitians, were able to bring down their cholesterol levels by as much as 22 percent.[32]

Fruits, vegetables, and whole-grain products that contain fiber, particularly soluble fiber, also can help lower cholesterol levels and the risk of heart disease. (See Chapter 6.) Controlling weight and increasing physical activity also can help.

Cholesterol-Lowering Medications

Sometimes dietary changes are not enough to cut cholesterol levels. As many as nine million Americans take medications to reduce cholesterol.[33] Most of these treatments primarily lower elevated LDL levels, but medications that raise HDL and lower triglycerides without affecting LDL, such as the fibric acid derivative gemfibrozil (Lopid), also have proven beneficial.[34] Cholesterol-lowering drugs also may have anti-inflammatory effects that increase their potential to reduce a person's risk of heart disease.[35]

The most commonly used medications are:

- **Statins.** When combined with a low-fat diet, these cholesterol-lowering medications reduce the risk of death from heart disease by as much as 40 percent. They work by interfering with the liver's ability to make cholesterol, thereby lowering LDL and raising HDL. Three of the drugs—simvastatin (Zocor), lovastatin (Mevacor), and pravastatin (Pravachol)—have proven effective in long-term controlled trials.[36]

- **Nicotinic acid (niacin).** This is a B vitamin that, in large doses, reduces LDL and triglycerides and boosts HDL. Side effects include flushing, panic attacks, and itching. Because of its potential toxicity, this drug should be taken only under a doctor's care.

- **Resins.** A standard part of treatment for more than 20 years, resins such as cholestryramine (Questran) and colestipol (Colestid) bind bile acids in the intestine to prevent their recycling through the liver, which then increases its update of cholesterol from the blood.

- **Fibric acid derivatives.** Mainly used to lower triglycerides, gemfibrozil (Lopid), and fenofibrate (Tricor) also can increase HDL levels.

- **Aspirin.** Physicians often prescribe this medication because of its protective effects against heart attacks.

- **Alternative remedies.** Although they have not been rigorously tested, many people have tried to lower their cholesterol levels with arginine, an amino acid that may act as an antioxidant, and coenzyme Q10, an antioxidant widely used to prevent heart disease in Japan and Europe.

There is some question about whether too-low cholesterol levels might cause different health problems over time. Numerous reports have linked total blood cholesterol levels of 160 or lower with greater mortality from liver cancer, lung disease, hemorrhagic stroke, suicide, and alcoholism. There are many reasons why a person's cholesterol levels may be low—genetics, an extremely rigorous diet and exercise regimen, or illness, including anemia and diseases of the lungs or liver.

The Silent Killers

The two most common forms of cardiovascular disease in this country are high blood pressure (hypertension) and coronary artery disease, the gradual narrowing of the blood vessels of the heart. Often these two problems go together.

High Blood Pressure

Hypertension forces the heart to pump harder than is healthy. Because the heart must force blood into arteries that are offering increased resistance to blood flow, the left side of the heart often becomes enlarged (see Figure 13-5). The term *essential hypertension* indicates that the cause is unknown, as is usually the case. Occasionally, abnormalities of the kidneys or the blood vessels feeding them, or certain substances in the bloodstream, are identified as the culprits. Whatever its cause, hypertension is dangerous because excessive pressure can wear out arteries, leading to serious cardiovascular diseases, vision problems, and kidney disease.

More than 40 million Americans have high blood pressure that requires monitoring or treatment. While most are under age 65, hypertension has become increasingly common among people in their twenties and thirties. Physicians urge all adults to have their blood pressure checked at least once a year.

A blood pressure reading that's slightly above normal isn't necessarily proof of a blood pressure problem. Due to nervousness, blood pressure may shoot up when anxious individuals enter a medical office, causing what's known as *white coat hypertension*. Other factors, such as warm weather or variations in how healthcare practitioners do the test, also can cause elevated readings. It can help to take blood pressure readings at home and compare them with your physician's readings. (Equipment for measuring blood pressure is sold at most pharmacies.)

Normal blood pressure in most young adults is 120/80 mmHg (120 systolic pressure, 80 diastolic pressure) under relaxed conditions. Borderline hypertension is 140/90 to 160/95; definite hypertension is 160/95 and above. The lower, or diastolic, number has increasingly been used in categorizing high blood pressure, with 90 to

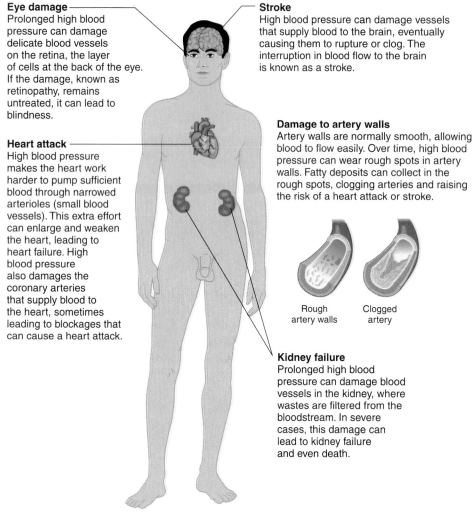

Eye damage
Prolonged high blood pressure can damage delicate blood vessels on the retina, the layer of cells at the back of the eye. If the damage, known as retinopathy, remains untreated, it can lead to blindness.

Heart attack
High blood pressure makes the heart work harder to pump sufficient blood through narrowed arterioles (small blood vessels). This extra effort can enlarge and weaken the heart, leading to heart failure. High blood pressure also damages the coronary arteries that supply blood to the heart, sometimes leading to blockages that can cause a heart attack.

Stroke
High blood pressure can damage vessels that supply blood to the brain, eventually causing them to rupture or clog. The interruption in blood flow to the brain is known as a stroke.

Damage to artery walls
Artery walls are normally smooth, allowing blood to flow easily. Over time, high blood pressure can wear rough spots in artery walls. Fatty deposits can collect in the rough spots, clogging arteries and raising the risk of a heart attack or stroke.

Rough artery walls

Clogged artery

Kidney failure
Prolonged high blood pressure can damage blood vessels in the kidney, where wastes are filtered from the bloodstream. In severe cases, this damage can lead to kidney failure and even death.

■ Figure 13-5 **The Consequences of High Blood Pressure**
If left untreated, elevated blood pressure can damage blood vessels in several areas of the body and lead to serious health problems.

104 indicating mild hypertension; 105 to 114, moderate; and 115 and over, severe. A high diastolic reading indicates an increased risk of heart disease, even if the systolic pressure is normal (see Table 13-1). People whose systolic blood pressure is slightly above normal also face increased health risks of heart disease and stroke, compared with those whose blood pressure is under 140. The World Health Organization (WHO) recommends a target blood pressure below 130/85 mmHg.[37]

In evaluating individual patients, most health-care professionals look not just at the numbers but also at other risk factors, such as cholesterol levels and family history. Physicians have warned that people with borderline hypertension may sustain damage to their heart and blood vessels and should seek more aggressive treatment for their high blood pressure. Even people with blood pressure of 130/93 may show early signs of cardiovascu-

lar problems, such as changes in the heart muscle such that it cannot relax completely between contractions.

Prevention pays off when it comes to high blood pressure. The most effective preventive measures involve lifestyle changes. Losing weight is the best approach for individuals with high normal values. Exercise may be effective in lowering mildly elevated blood pressure. Restriction of sodium intake also helps. There are no data showing an association between individuals with normal blood pressure, salt intake, and the risk of heart attack. However, individuals with hypertension who are sensitive to sodium are at about twice the risk of heart attack and stroke as others. Among the approaches that have not proven effective are dietary supplements, such as calcium, magnesium, potassium, and fish oil.

The same lifestyle changes that work as preventive measures are the best forms of nondrug (or nonpharmacologic) treatment for hypertension (see Pulsepoints: "Ten Keys to a Healthy Heart"). However, there is no single ideal prescription for reducing high blood pressure in all patients.

If exercise, dietary changes, and restriction of salt intake fail to bring down blood pressure, some health experts argue that even those with mild hypertension should take drugs to prevent damage to the heart and blood vessels. There is controversy about the best medications for treating hypertension. Medications called beta-blockers and diuretics are recommended as the first-line treatment for hypertension, but newer drugs such as angiotensin-converting enzyme (ACE) inhibitors and calcium channel blockers are becoming increasingly popular. They account for 55 percent of prescriptions for antihypertensives in the United States. However, there is no conclusive evidence that they are more effec-

■ **Table 13-1** Classification of High Blood Pressure

Category	Systolic Reading	Diastolic Reading	Followup Recommended
Normal	Less than 130	Less than 85	Check again in two years.
High normal	130–139	85–89	Check in one year. Many physicians recommend lifestyle modifications at this stage.
Hypertension			
Stage 1	140–159	90–99	Modify lifestyle. Begin drug treatment if lifestyle modifications are not effective within six months.
Stage 2	160–179	100–109	Begin drug treatment and modify lifestyle.
Stage 3	180–209	110–119	Begin drug treatment and modify lifestyle.
Stage 4	More than 210	More than 120	Immediate medical evaluation and treatment with drugs. Modify lifestyle.

Source: Joint National Committee on Detection, Evaluation, Treatment of High Blood Pressure.

tive or better tolerated.[38] No single drug works well in everyone, so physicians have to rely on clinical judgment and trial and error to find the best possible medication for an individual patient.

Across the Lifespan: Treating Hypertension in the Elderly

Traditionally physicians viewed a rise in blood pressure as a normal age-related change and usually did not prescribe medications for hypertension in older men and women, particular if only their systolic blood pressure (the first and higher blood pressure reading) was elevated. However, clinical trials have clearly shown that treating hypertension in the elderly can significantly reduce their risk of heart disease.[39]

"We've found that treating high systolic pressure with diuretics (water pills), a simple, inexpensive treatment, dramatically reduces the risk of heart attack, stroke and congestive heart failure," says Richard Hodes, M.D., director of the National Institute on Aging. But even though we have a well-demonstrated therapy that can prevent terrible long-term consequences, a lot of people don't have their blood pressures checked or their doctors don't realize the importance of keeping systolic pressures low."[40]

PULSE points

Ten Keys to a Healthy Heart

1. **Don't smoke.** There's no bigger favor you can do your heart—and lungs!
2. **Watch your weight.** Even relatively modest gains can have a big effect on your risk of heart disease.
3. **Cut down on saturated fats and cholesterol.** This could help prevent high blood cholesterol levels, obesity, and heart disease.
4. **Get moving.** Engage in regular physical activity. A little is better than none; more is even better.
5. **Lower your stress levels.** If too much stress is a problem in your life, try the relaxation techniques described in Chapter 2.
6. **Know your family history.** Inheriting a predispositon to high blood pressure or heart disease means that your heart needs extra preventive care.
7. **Get your blood pressure checked regularly.** Knowing your numbers can alert you to a potential problem long before you develop any symptoms.
8. **Tame your temper.** Hostility can be hazardous to the heart. Look for other ways of releasing anger and frustration.
9. **Find out your cholesterol levels.** You can't know if your heart is in danger unless you know if your cholesterol is too high. Get a blood test at your next physical, and discuss the results with your physician.
10. **Take appropriate medications.** Those with high cholesterol or high blood pressure should seek their physicians' advice.

In general, older patients take their medications as reliably as younger ones and tolerate them well, although they may experience dizziness if they suddenly rise to their feet. The most effective medications are diuretics or a combination of small doses of two different drugs, such as a diuretic and a beta blocker.[41]

Coronary Artery Disease

The general term for any impairment of blood flow through the blood vessels, often referred to as "hardening of the arteries," is **arteriosclerosis.** The most common form is **atherosclerosis,** a disease of the lining of the arteries in which plaque—deposits of fat, fibrin (a clotting material), cholesterol, other cell parts, and calcium—narrows the artery channels.

Clogging the Arteries

Atherosclerosis, which may begin in childhood, worsens with the continued buildup of plaque on the arterial lining (see photos on this page). The arteries lose their ability to expand and contract. Blood moves with increasing difficulty through the narrowed channels, making it easier for a clot (thrombus) to form, perhaps blocking the channel and depriving vital organs of blood. When such a blockage is in a coronary artery, the result is coronary thrombosis, one form of heart attack. When the clot occurs in the brain, the result is cerebral thrombosis, one form of stroke (discussed later in this chapter).

Unclogging the Arteries

For years, heart specialists said that, once clogged, arteries couldn't be unclogged. However, recent research has shown that it is possible to reverse the buildup of plaque inside the arteries by means of cholesterol-lowering drugs and a low-fat diet. A strict program of dietary and lifestyle change without any medication, developed by Dean Ornish, M.D., of the University of California, San Francisco, also has proven effective in reversing coronary artery disease. The following are the key elements of this approach:

- A very low-fat, vegetarian diet, including nonfat dairy products and egg whites, keeping fat intake to below 8 percent of total calories consumed. Ornish's recommended diet allows no meat, poultry, fish, butter, cheese, ice cream, or any form of oil.
- Moderate exercise, consisting of an hour of aerobic activity three times a week. Walking is recommended because more rigorous exercise might be dangerous for heart patients, who may develop increased risk of

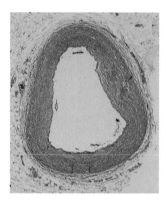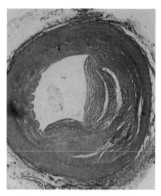

(A) A healthy coronary artery. (B) An artery partially blocked by the buildup of atherosclerotic plaque.

blood clots, irregular heartbeats, or coronary artery spasms during exertion.

- Stress counseling. Ornish's patients learn how the body's stress response can cause a rapid heartbeat and narrowing of the arteries, and how stress reduction can reduce cholesterol levels.
- An hour a day of yoga, meditation, breathing, and progressive relaxation. Some patients use visualization, for instance, imagining their arteries being cleared by a tunneling machine.[42]

Crises of the Heart

For many people, the first sign of heart disease is pain, ranging from mild to excruciating. They may be experiencing angina pectoris, spasms of the coronary artery, or myocardial infarction (heart attack). According to the American Heart Association (AHA), as many as 1.5 million men and women have heart attacks each year; almost 5 million Americans alive today have had a heart attack, chest pain, or both.

Angina Pectoris

A temporary drop in the supply of oxygen to the heart tissue causes feelings of pain or discomfort in the chest known as **angina pectoris.** Some people suffer angina only when the demands on their hearts increase, such as during exercise or when under stress. Many people have angina for years and yet never suffer a heart attack; in some, the angina even disappears. However, angina should be considered a warning of danger if it becomes more severe or more frequent, occurs with less activity or exertion, begins to waken a person from a sound sleep at night, persists for more than ten to fifteen minutes, or causes unusual perspiration.

Angina is most commonly treated with beta blockers, calcium channel blockers, or nitrates. The American College of Cardiology, the American Heart Association and the American College of Physicians have issued guidelines that call for daily aspirin, sublingual (under the tongue) nitroglycerine, and appropriate medications for lowering of cholesterol and control of diabetes.[43]

Coronary Artery Spasms

Sometimes the arteries tighten suddenly or go into a spasm, cutting off or reducing blood flow. Spasms can produce heart attacks, as well as angina, and can be fatal. Several factors may trigger spasms in the heart, including the following:

- *Clumping of platelets.* When *platelets* (a type of blood cell) clump together, they produce a substance called thromboxane A-2, which causes the narrowing of a blood vessel.

- *Smoking.* When some angina victims stop smoking, their chest pain declines or disappears.

- *Stress.* No one knows exactly how stress may lead to spasms, but many heart specialists believe that it's a culprit.

- *Increased calcium flow.* Calcium regularly flows into smooth muscle cells; too much calcium, however, may lead to a spasm. (This calcium flow is not regulated by the amount of calcium in your diet.)

What Happens During a Heart Attack?

According to the AHA, one person in the United States has a heart attack every 20 seconds, while one person dies of a heart attack every 60 seconds.[44] The medical name for a heart attack, or coronary, is **myocardial infarction (MI)**. The *myocardium* is the cardiac muscle layer of the wall of the heart. It receives its blood supply, and thus its oxygen and other nutrients, from the coronary arteries. If an artery is blocked by a clot or plaque, or by a spasm, the myocardial cells do not get sufficient oxygen, and the portion of the myocardium deprived of its blood supply begins to die (see Figure 13-6). Although such an attack may seem sudden, usually it has been building up for years, particularly if the person has ignored risk factors and early warning signs.

Individuals should seek immediate medical care if they experience the following symptoms:

- A tight ache, heavy, squeezing pain or discomfort in the center of the chest, which may last for 30 minutes or more and is not relieved by rest.

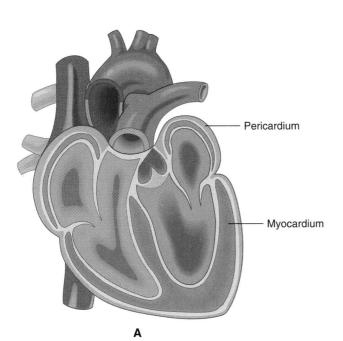

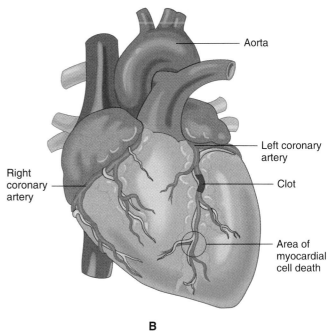

■ Figure 13-6 **The Making of a Heart Attack**
(A) The bulk of the heart is composed mainly of the myocardium, the muscle layer that contracts. (B) A clot in one of the arteries that feeds into the myocardium can cut off the blood supply to part of the myocardium, causing cells in that area to die. This is called a myocardial infarction, or heart attack.

- A pain that may radiate to the shoulder, arm, neck, back, or jaw.
- Anxiety.
- Sweating or cold, clammy skin.
- Nausea and vomiting.
- Shortness of breath.
- Dizziness, fainting, or loss of consciousness.[45]

The two hours immediately following the onset of such symptoms is the most crucial period. About 40 percent of those who suffer an MI die within this time. According to the American Heart Association, most patients wait three hours after the initial symptoms begin before seeking help. By that time, half of the affected heart muscle may already be lost.

Heart attacks in the United States may be becoming less severe, as measured by the average size of myocardial infarcts. Prompt treatment may be one reason.[46] However, this is not true for women.

Women's heart attacks are more likely to be fatal than men's. Heart attacks are twice as likely to kill women under age 50 than men in the same age range. A review of the records of 384,878 heart attack victims found that 17 percent of female heart attack victims die while still in the hospital, compared with 12 percent of males. The difference results entirely from a much higher death rate among the younger victims.[47]

Women wait hours longer after a heart attack before going to the hospital, then are treated less aggressively than men. This delay, which allows further damage to the oxygen-starved heart, results partly because women tend to experience less painful heart attack symptoms. Sometimes they feel only pressure or a burning feeling, not crushing pain. Younger female victims are more likely than men to have other health problems, such as diabetes, high blood pressure, and heart failure.[48]

In another study of 12,142 men and women who had bad heart attacks, milder ones, or severe chest pain, women were up to twice as likely to suffer serious complications. Among those who had heart attacks, the women were 50 percent more likely to die within 30 days.[49]

More doctors' offices, airlines, and public meeting places, such as casinos, are purchasing heart defibrillators. This life-saving equipment may seem expensive, at an estimated $3,500, but the cost of defibrillators and training teams of nurses in their use comes to only about a nickel per paying patient. State-of the-art treatments for heart attacks include clot-dissolving drugs, early administration of medications to thin the blood, intravenous nitroglycerin, and, in some cases, a beta blocker (which blocks many of the effects of adrenaline in the body, particularly its stimulating impact on the heart).

Clot-dissolving drugs called thrombolytic agents are the treatment of choice for acute myocardial infarction in most clinical settings. Administered through a *catheter* (flexible tube) threaded through the arteries to the site of the blockage (the more effective method of delivery) or injected intravenously (the faster, cheaper method of delivery), these agents can save lives and dissolve clots, but don't remove the underlying atherosclerotic plaque.

Two clot-thinning drugs may be better than one for treating heart attacks. One drug, called a thrombolytic, dissolves blood clots. The second drug, a platelet receptor blocker, keeps platelets from clumping and forming the blood clots that can obstruct blood flow and thereby trigger a heart attack or stroke. The platelet blockers, sometimes called "super aspirin," are more potent than aspirin. They are also administered through an intravenous drip or infusion.[50] Patients receiving such therapy may require further procedures, such as bypass surgery or **angioplasty,** which can reduce their risk of another heart attack or death.

Emergency balloon angioplasty has shown greater effectiveness than clot-dissolving medication in restoring blood flow in arteries immediately after an attack. With this approach, arteries are less likely to close down again and patients have shorter hospital stays and fewer hospital readmissions. Angioplasty patients also are less likely to die of the heart attack or to experience repeat attacks. However, most American hospitals do not perform angioplasty, and not all can do it on an emergency basis.

Strategies *for* Prevention

What to Do If a Heart Attack Strikes

✓ If you develop chest discomfort that lasts for two minutes or more, call the local emergency rescue service immediately.

✓ If you're with someone who's exhibiting the classic signs of heart attack, and if they last for two minutes or more, act at once. Expect the person to deny the possibility of anything as serious as a heart attack, but insist on taking prompt action.

✓ Call for help. Bystanders should call the emergency medical system (available by dialing 911 in many places) immediately. The odds of survival are greatest if emergency teams get to a heart attack victim quickly and administer advanced cardiac life support. Individuals trained in **cardiopulmonary resuscitation (CPR),** a combination of mouth-to-mouth breathing and chest compression for victims of cardiac arrest, should use this technique only after calling or having someone else call for emergency help.

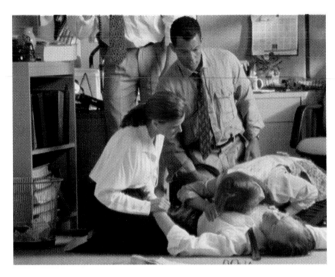

If you witness someone who appears to be experiencing a heart attack, the best thing you can do is call for emergency help immediately. Only after medical emergency personnel are called should you begin any CPR efforts.

Arrhythmias (Heart Rate Abnormalities)

The heart has its own electrical system, which produces an evenly timed, regular beat. When relaxed, most adults have a heart rate of between 60 and 80 beats per minute—slower if they're in good physical condition. During strenuous activity or stress, the heart beats faster. Sometimes the heart seems to skip a beat or experience premature (or early) heartbeats. In many cases, these irregularities are no cause for alarm; but they can be dangerous in an MI victim. Caffeine, long suspected of triggering irregular heartbeats, doesn't seem to be a culprit.

A very fast heart rate (over 100 beats per minute) is known as **tachycardia;** a very slow one (under 60 beats per minute) is **bradycardia.** Resting heart rates of under 60 beats per minute aren't necessarily signs of illness, even though they meet the definition of bradycardia; in fact, they may reflect excellent physical condition. Portable monitors that patients wear around the clock are most likely to catch the heart in an irregular pattern. One, the Holter monitor, provides a continuous 24-hour record of the heart rate. Another is a "loop" recorder or event monitor that "lies in ambush" for an attack.

Treatment options include medications, an artificial pacemaker about the size of a small beeper (to ensure that the heart keeps beating regularly), and radiofrequency ablation, a nonsurgical procedure that has revolutionized arrhythmia therapy. In this treatment, cardiologists thread a catheter with an electrode at its tip into the blood vessels of the heart. Using drugs to

trigger an irregular heart beat, they pinpoint its source and administer pulses of radiofrequency energy (similar to microwave heat) that destroy the cells sending errant signals. The risks are low, and more than 90 percent of patients report a complete cure.

As both sexes age, other arrhythmias, often linked with coronary artery disease, increase—and become increasingly perilous. Half of all deaths associated with coronary artery disease are due to arrhythmias. The most common such arrhythmia, affecting two million middle-aged and elderly Americans, is **atrial fibrillation** (AF), in which the upper chambers of the heart quiver rather than working together so blood pools in the heart rather than flowing through it. This greatly increases the risk of clotting, strokes, and death.

Mitral-Valve Prolapse

Mitral-valve prolapse (MVP) is a condition in which a valve in the heart is abnormally long and floppy. Normally, after blood rushes from the left atrium to the left ventricle, the valve between the two chambers slaps shut. But in some people, the closed valve bulges or prolapses back into the atrium. This often occurs because the leaflets are too large to fit snugly or the leaflets don't close completely and blood leaks back into the atrium. This leakage, also called regurgitation, is what doctors may hear as a murmur when listening to your heart.

In the past doctors calculated that up to 30 percent of otherwise healthy young people had MVP. However, this problem is substantially less common and less serious than previously believed. According to recent estimates, MVP affects about 2 percent of the population rather than the 5 to 35 percent of the population previously believed. MVP, once thought to be more common in women, affects men and women equally.[51]

In addition to being thought to have a high prevalence rate, MVP was seen as a disease with frequent and serious complications, including stroke and heart failure. New data show that these complications do not occur at higher rates among patients with mitral-valve prolapse compared to those patients without prolapse. MVP also is no more common among young people (45 years old or younger) with stroke or transient ischemic stroke (TIA or "little" stroke).[52]

Congestive Heart Failure

When the heart's pumping power is well below normal capacity, fluid begins to collect in the lungs, hands, and feet. The heart is then said to be in failure. As blood fluids accumulate in the lungs, pulmonary congestion occurs, causing shortness of breath. In other parts of the body, fluid seeps through the thin capillary walls and causes swelling (edema), especially in the ankles and legs. **Congestive heart failure** usually results from myocardial infarction, but can also be the result of rheumatic fever, birth defects, hypertension, or atherosclerosis. As many as 4.7 million Americans develop congestive heart failure, which causes 250,000 deaths a year.[53] It is treated by reducing the workload on the heart, modifying salt intake, administering drugs that rid the body of excess fluid, and using medications (such as digitalis) to improve the heart's pumping efficiency. Adding the medication spironolactone, a standard diuretic, can reduce heart failure deaths by 30 percent.

Rheumatic Fever

Rheumatic fever, which strikes most often between the ages of 5 and 15, is a disease that causes painful, swollen joints; skin rashes; and heart damage in half its victims. It is always preceded by a streptococcal infection (see Chapter 11 on infectious diseases). A new strain of streptococcal bacteria has caused a resurfacing of rheumatic fever, which had been considered a disease of the past. The first step to prevention is early identifi-

cation of the streptococcal infection; the second is treatment with antibiotics to avoid permanent scarring of the heart valves.

Congenital Defects

As noted in Campus Focus: "Young at Heart?" heart disease can occur very early in life. Approximately 8 out of every 1,000 children born in the United States have congenital heart disease. The most common defects are holes in the ventricular septum, the wall dividing the lower chambers of the heart. Holes may also occur in the atrial septum, the wall between the upper chambers. Sometimes the arteries delivering blood to the body and lungs are transposed and thus attached to the wrong ventricles. Such babies have a bluish color because their blood isn't carrying sufficient oxygen.

Heart Savers

A generation ago physicians had no way of detecting problems before the symptoms of heart disease began

---

Campus Focus

Young at Heart?

Many college students think of cardiovascular diseases as a problem only for older men and women. As the following statistics from the American Heart Association show, this isn't so:

- **Congenital heart defects.** About 32,000 babies are born each year with congenital heart defects; 58 percent of deaths from these problems occur in boys and girls under age 15.

- **Mitral valve prolapse.** This defect is diagnosed most often in young women ages 14 to 30.

- **Cardiomyopathy.** This serious disease, characterized by deterioration of the heart muscle, kills 36 percent of young athletes who die suddenly.

- **Stroke.** Young African Americans have a two- to three-fold greater risk of ischemic stroke when compared with whites.

- **Heart Surgery.** An estimated 164,000 cardiovascular procedures are performed annually on children age 15 and younger.

- **Heart disease risk factors:** Nearly half of American youth ages 12 to 21 are not vigorously active on a regular basis. Physical activity declines dramatically from early to late adolescence. Among white American adolescents ages 12 to 17, 11.1 percent of boys and 8.5 percent of girls are overweight (with BMIs above the 95th percentile), as are 10.7 percent of African-American boys and 15.7 percent of girls, and 14.6 percent of Mexican-American boys and 13.7 percent of girls.

Source: American Heart Association.

and could offer little more than bed rest as a therapy after they struck. The last decade, however, has brought tremendous progress in the diagnosis and treatment of heart problems. Today men and women with heart problems can learn of possible dangers much earlier than in the past and undergo treatments that may add years to their lives.

Diagnostic Tests

The **electrocardiogram (ECG, EKG),** a recording of the electrical activity of the heart, is the traditional method of evaluating the heart's health (see Figure 13-7). An exercise ECG—or *stress test*—is one method of finding out whether an area of the heart begins to run out of blood during the stress of an athletic workout. The subject walks or jogs on a treadmill while the ECG monitors the heart's response. This test is less accurate in women because of a high rate of false positives.

Thallium scintigraphy uses radioactive isotopes that are injected into the bloodstream. A special imaging device called a *scintillation,* or gamma camera, picks up the rays emitted by the isotopes; a computer translates these signals into images of the heart as it pumps. The test can be performed while the patient is either resting or exercising on a treadmill or bicycle. Adding a thallium scan to an exercise ECG increases the probability of detecting existing heart disease by 70 to 90 percent. A stress echocardiogram uses ultrasound to study the heart.

In **coronary angiography,** the most complete and accurate diagnostic test for heart problems, a thin tube is threaded through the blood vessels of the heart, a radiopaque dye is injected, and X rays are taken to detect any blockage of the arteries. Angiography is extremely precise, but it's also costly and risky: About one out of every 1,500 patients dies as a result of the test. New methods of diagnosing the heart include "ultra-fast" scans that can capture the heart as it beats.

Treatments

Most people with heart disease can be treated successfully with medications. Other alternatives are bypass surgery, balloon angioplasty, heart transplants, and external and implanted mechanical devices. Patients who respond positively, remain optimistic, and are conscientious in taking prescribed medications significantly reduce their risk of death, a subsequent heart attack, or another coronary event.[54]

Medications

The main types of drugs used to treat high blood pressure and heart disease include diuretics; beta blockers; calcium channel blockers; and angiotensin converting enzyme (ACE) inhibitors, which block a hormone known as angiotensin that strongly influences blood pressure. Side effects range from lethargy and fatigue to an increased risk of chest pain and heart attack if certain drugs are discontinued abruptly. Calcium channel blockers and ACE inhibitors have become more popular, even though they have not proved more effective than older medications such as diuretics and beta blockers. Unlike the older drugs, the new ones are less likely to cause side effects such as impotence, insomnia, lethargy, and depression. The newer drugs can be taken in lower doses with negligible side effects.

Recent reports have found dangers associated with several widely used heart medications, including a modestly increased risk of heart attack in patients taking some calcium channel blockers, which are used to lower

■ Figure 13-7 **ECG Readings**
(A) A recording of normal electrical activity in the heart. (B) Grossly irregular activity seen in an acute heart attack.

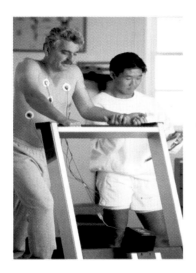

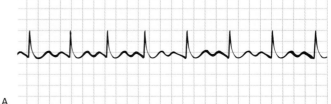

A

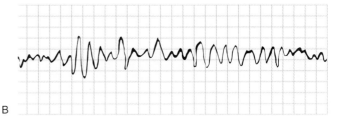

B

blood pressure, raise cardiac output in heart failure, relieve various forms of angina, and control arrhythmias. They work by countering the flow of calcium ions into the heart muscle cells; calcium is believed to stimulate and contract heart muscle, occasionally causing a sudden spasm that can completely close an artery.

Beta blockers lower the heart's demand for blood by producing changes in the autonomic (involuntary) nervous system. A variety of beta blockers are widely used for medical problems, including migraine headaches and glaucoma (a serious eye disease), as well as heart disease. Other cardiac medications include thrombolytic drugs and antiarrythmics. These drugs are not risk-free, and there have been recent reports that some may actually increase the likelihood of a heart attack.

Surgical Procedures and Mechanical Aids

A **coronary bypass** is a procedure in which an artery from the patient's leg or chest wall is grafted onto a coronary artery to detour blood around the blocked area. Each year hundreds of thousands of coronary bypasses are performed in the United States; about 1 to 5 percent of these patients die as a result of surgical complications.

For many patients, the results of bypass surgery are positive. But about one out of five patients suffers subtle, long-lasting impairment of mental performance, including problems concentrating and learning, remembering new information, and performing mental tasks as quickly as before the surgery. About 20 percent remain depressed a year after their operations; their mood changes may stem from damage sustained in the surgery.

Coronary bypasses do not extend life for individuals with mild to moderate angina unless the left main coronary artery was the one that was blocked. If drugs fail to control angina, a coronary bypass can eliminate pain. But surgery is not a cure for the atherosclerotic process that caused the blockage; indeed, in as many as 80 percent of bypass patients, the grafts themselves develop blockages within ten years.

Percutaneous transluminal coronary angioplasty (PTCA), also called balloon angioplasty, is the most often performed heart operation. Less costly and less risky than bypass surgery, PTCA opens blood vessels in the heart that are narrowed but not completely blocked. PTCA involves a precise, time-consuming technique called *cardiac catheterization*—the threading of a narrow tube or catheter through an artery to the heart. An X ray taken with a special dye injected into the arteries reveals the location and extent of a blockage. By inflating a tiny balloon at the tip of the catheter, physicians can break up the clog and widen the narrowed artery. When they deflate the balloon, circulation is restored. Balloon angioplasties are not without risks, however; and balloon-opened arteries can clog up again.

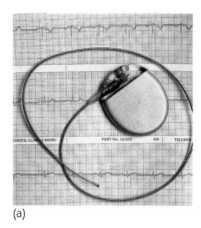 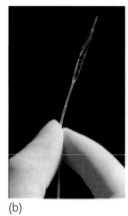

(a)   (b)

Medical technology has more options now for treating heart disorders. (a) The pacemaker can be surgically implanted in the chest to deliver electrical impulses that normalize a weak or irregular heartbeat. (b) A catheter with a tiny balloon is used in balloon angioplasty to widen a clogged artery.

In the near future, heart specialists may be able to sand plaque off artery walls with a tiny rotating sander, although this method has risks similar to those of balloon angioplasty. The most promising and commonly used nonballoon method is coronary stents, which can reduce complications and the risk of later renarrowing.

For a variety of heart disorders in which the heart muscle has become so damaged that it can no longer effectively pump blood throughout the body, the only hope is a heart transplant. In recent years the survival rates for transplant recipients have improved dramatically. *Left-ventricular-assist devices (LVADs)* enhance the pumping action of the heart. Used as external, temporary measures until a donor heart becomes available, fully implantable models may someday serve as permanent blood-pumping devices.

Gene Therapy

The first human test of a gene therapy that is injected directly into the oxygen-starved heart muscle has shown the technique to be safe, opening the door to promising new treatments for heart disease. The small, preliminary study of 21 heart patients was not designed to prove gene therapy's effectiveness. That will require further research, including clinical trials with large numbers of patients.

Stroke: From No Hope to New Hope

When the blood supply to a portion of the brain is blocked, a cerebrovascular accident, or **stroke,** occurs.

About 500,000 people suffer strokes each year, and strokes rank third, after heart disease and cancer, as a cause of death in this country. After decades of steady decline, the number of strokes per year has begun to rise. The main reasons seem to be that more Americans are living longer, advanced medical care is allowing more people to survive heart disease, and doctors are better able to diagnose and detect strokes. Yet 80 percent of strokes are preventable, and key risk factors can be modified through either lifestyle changes or drugs. The most important steps are treating hypertension, not smoking, managing diabetes, lowering cholesterol, and taking aspirin.[55]

Strategies *for* Prevention

How to Prevent a Stroke

✔ Quit smoking. Smokers have twice the risk of stroke that nonsmokers have. When they quit, their risk drops 50 percent in two years. Within five years after quitting, their risk is nearly the same as nonsmokers.

✔ Keep blood pressure under control. Treating hypertension with medication can lead to a 40 percent reduction in fatal and nonfatal strokes.

✔ Eat a low-fat, low-cholesterol diet, which reduces your risk of fatty buildup in blood vessels.

✔ Avoid obesity, which burdens the blood vessels as well as the heart.

✔ Exercise. Moderate amounts of exercise improve circulation and may help dissolve deposits in the blood vessels that can lead to stroke.

 ## What Causes a Stroke?

There are two types of stroke: ischemic stroke, which is the result of a blockage that disrupts blood flow to the brain, and hemorrhagic stroke, which occurs when blood vessels rupture.[56] One of the most common causes of ischemic stroke is the blockage of a brain artery by a thrombus, or blood clot—a *cerebral thrombosis.* Clots generally form around deposits sticking out from the arterial wall. Sometimes a wandering blood clot (embolus), carried in the bloodstream, becomes wedged in one of the cerebral arteries. This is called a *cerebral embolism,* and it can completely plug up a cerebral artery (see Figure 13-8a).

In hemorrhagic stroke, a diseased artery in the brain floods the surrounding tissue with blood. The cells nourished by the artery are deprived of blood and can't function, and the blood from the artery forms a clot that may interfere with brain function. This is most likely to occur if the patient suffers from a combination of hypertension and atherosclerosis. Hemorrhage (bleeding) may also be caused by a head injury or by the bursting of an aneurysm, a blood-filled pouch that balloons out from a weak spot in the wall of an artery (see Figure 13-8b).

Brain tissue, like heart muscle, begins to die if deprived of oxygen, which may then cause difficulty speaking and walking, and loss of memory. These effects may be slight or severe, temporary or permanent, depending on how widespread the damage is and whether other areas of the brain can take over the function of the damaged area. About 30 percent of stroke survivors develop dementia, a disorder that robs a person of memory and other intellectual abilities.[57]

The following symptoms should alert you to the possibility that you or someone with you has suffered a stroke:

- Sudden weakness, loss of strength, or numbness of face, arm, or leg.
- Loss of speech, or difficulty speaking or understanding speech.
- Dimness or loss of vision, particularly double vision in one eye.
- Unexplained dizziness.
- Change in personality.
- Change in pattern of headaches.

Transient Ischemic Attacks (TIAs)

Sometimes a person will suffer **transient ischemic attacks (TIAs),** "little strokes" that cause minimal damage but serve as warning signs of a potentially more severe stroke. One out of three people who suffer TIAs will have a stroke during the following five years if they don't get treatment. The two major types of TIAs are:

- *Transient monocular blindness.* Blurring, a blackout or whiteout of vision, a sense of a shade coming down, or another visual disturbance in one eye.
- *Transient hemispheral attack.* Diminished blood flow to one side of the brain, causing numbness or weakness of one arm, leg, or side of the face, or problems speaking or thinking.

Many TIAs are caused by a narrowing of blood vessels in the neck (carotid arteries) because of a buildup of plaque. Specialists can diagnose this problem by feeling and listening to the arteries, by ultrasound, by measuring the pressure or circulation rate from the carotid arteries to the eyes, or by arterial angiography (injection of a dye into the arteries as X rays are taken), a procedure that can be dangerous, even deadly, or lifesaving.

Surgery to widen the carotid arteries may be recommended for individuals under age 60 with significant narrowing (50 to 80 percent or more). However, this is a risky procedure, and often physicians advise it only when clearly necessary. For other patients, aspirin and other drugs that make platelets less sticky and interfere with clotting may be effective.

Risk Factors for Strokes

People who've experienced TIAs are at the highest risk for stroke. Other risk factors, like those for heart disease, include some that can't be changed (such as gender and race) and some that can be controlled:

* *Gender.* Men have a greater risk of stroke than women do. However, women are at increased risk at times of marked hormonal changes, particularly pregnancy and childbirth. Past studies have shown an association between oral contraceptive use and stroke, particularly in women over age 35 who smoke. The newer low-dose oral contraceptives have not shown an increased stroke risk among women ages 18 to 44. A woman's stroke risk may increase markedly at menopause.[58]

* *Race.* African Americans have a much greater risk of stroke than whites do. Hispanics also are more likely to develop hemorrhagic strokes than whites.[59]

* *Age.* A person's risk of stroke more than doubles every decade after age 55.

* *Hypertension.* Detection and treatment of high blood pressure are the best means of stroke prevention.

* *High red blood cell count.* A moderate to marked increase in the number of a person's red blood cells increases the risk of stroke.

* *Heart disease.* Heart problems can interfere with the flow of blood to the brain; clots that form in the heart can travel to the brain, where they may clog an artery.

* *Blood fats.* Although the standard advice from cardiologists is to lower harmful LDL levels, what may be more important for stroke risk is a drop in the levels of protective HDL.

* *Diabetes mellitus.* Diabetics have a higher incidence of stroke than nondiabetics.

Treatments for Strokes

A small ("baby") aspirin a day cuts in half the risk of strokes caused by abnormal heartbeats, which strike 75,000 Americans each year. Extremely rapid beating of the heart's upper chambers causes blood clots to form; they may enter the bloodstream and travel to the brain, where they can get stuck and choke off the blood supply. In the past, the only way to prevent such strokes was regular use of a medication called warfarin, which inhibits blood clotting and therefore increases the risk of severe bleeding. However, aspirin proved as

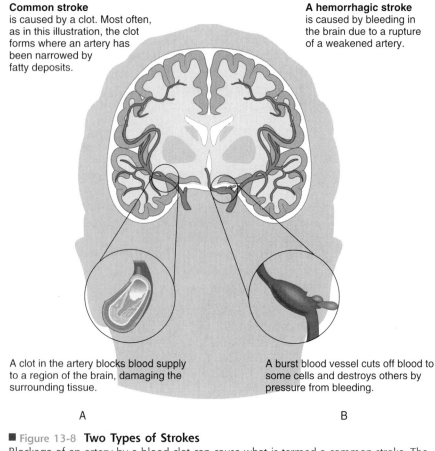

Common stroke is caused by a clot. Most often, as in this illustration, the clot forms where an artery has been narrowed by fatty deposits.

A hemorrhagic stroke is caused by bleeding in the brain due to a rupture of a weakened artery.

A clot in the artery blocks blood supply to a region of the brain, damaging the surrounding tissue.

A burst blood vessel cuts off blood to some cells and destroys others by pressure from bleeding.

A   B

■ Figure 13-8 **Two Types of Strokes**
Blockage of an artery by a blood clot can cause what is termed a common stroke. The bursting of an artery in the brain is called a hemorrhagic stroke, or cerebral hemorrhage.

effective as warfarin—without that dangerous side effect.

Increasingly, surgeons are operating on carotid arteries that may have been narrowed by a buildup of atherosclerotic plaque—a condition that contributes to 20 to 30 percent of strokes, some in individuals with no symptoms—by cleaning them out in a procedure called *carotid endartectomy*. This procedure has been shown to be effective in preventing stroke in patients with and without early symptoms of stroke. A new alternative is brain angioplasty, in which surgeons thread a catheter tipped with a tiny inflatable balloon into an artery and gently inflate it to restore blood flow.[60]

It now seems possible to save brain cells for a brief time after a thrombotic stroke occurs. Thrombolytic drugs, used for heart attack victims, can restore brain blood flow after a thrombotic stroke; other medications called heparinoids can reduce the blood's tendency to clot. In order for thrombolytic drugs to be effective, they must be administered within 90 minutes after the stroke; heparinoids must be given within 24 hours. However, many stroke victims do not seek help for 24 hours or longer.

In addition, drugs such as nimodipine and other agents undergoing clinical testing at major medical centers, are being used to protect brain cells from damage. Clinicians also are experimenting with ways to tie off tiny, bleeding, cranial arteries with tiny clothespins or to suction off blood that is exerting pressure on the brain. Using stereotactic radioimagery, which relies on a three-dimensional imaging system, surgeons can focus an X-ray beam on a clot or hemorrhage and destroy it.

Making This Chapter Work for You

Becoming Heart Smart

- Heart disease develops over time; the processes leading to heart disease often begin in childhood. Early recognition of risks and lifestyle changes to reduce them can have a dramatic impact in lowering the likelihood of heart-related problems in middle and old age.

- Factors predisposing an individual to heart disease or stroke include risks you can control, such as lack of exercise, cigarette smoking, obesity, high blood pressure, and high cholesterol levels. Other predisposing factors include diabetes mellitus, a family history of heart disease, age, race, and, to a certain degree, gender.

- Men tend to develop heart disease about a decade earlier in life than women, but women are less likely to respond as well to various treatments and are more likely to die as the result of a heart attack.

- Individuals with high cholesterol levels are at risk of developing atherosclerosis and having a heart attack. Federal health officials, supported by dozens of medical organizations, have called upon all Americans to lower their cholesterol levels by reducing their intake of saturated fats and cholesterol-rich foods. All adults should undergo cholesterol testing every five years. Dietary changes and exercise can lower cholesterol readings. Treatment with cholesterol-lowering drugs has proven effective in reducing and reversing coronary artery disease.

- Hypertension, or high blood pressure, occurs when the arterial walls offer too much resistance to blood flow. Health officials have recently learned that even borderline or mildly elevated blood pressure can be dangerous. Treatment of mild hypertension includes diet modification, exercise, and restriction of salt intake. For more severe hypertension, medication to widen the blood vessels or to decrease cardiac output may be necessary.

- The most common form of coronary artery disease is atherosclerosis, in which blood flow is impaired as the arteries narrow and lose their ability to dilate and contract because of plaque deposits inside the arteries. Thrombosis, or blockage of an artery by a thrombus, is the major danger of atherosclerosis, because a blocked artery can cause a heart attack or stroke.

- Some people suffer from chest pains, or angina pectoris, caused by periodic and temporary inadequate blood flow to the heart. Chest pain may also be a result of coronary artery spasms caused by the clumping of platelets, which results in a narrowing of the blood vessel.

- Myocardial infarction, or heart attack, occurs when heart muscle tissue in the myocardium begins to die because its supply of oxygen and other nutrients has been cut off by a blocked artery. The damage caused by a heart attack can be reduced with early treatment, including the use of clot-dissolving drugs or tiny balloons to unclog arteries (a procedure called angioplasty).

- Other heart problems include heartbeat irregularities, or arrhythmias; mitral-valve prolapse; congestive heart failure, which occurs when the heart is unable to pump at its normal capacity; heart damage from rheumatic fever; and congenital heart defects.

- Doctors can evaluate the heart's condition through such procedures as electrocardiography, angiography, and various types of imaging procedures. Hypertension, heart failure, angina, and arrhythmias can be treated with drugs. Surgical treatments for heart disease include the coronary bypass operation, balloon angioplasty, pacemaker implantation, heart transplants, and external and implanted mechanical devices.

- A stroke, or cerebrovascular accident, occurs when the blood supply to the brain is restricted or blocked, and can be caused by a cerebral thrombosis, cerebral embolism, or cerebral hemorrhage. Transient ischemic attacks (TIAs) may precede a serious stroke.

- Surgery to unclog the carotid arteries carrying blood to the brain can reduce the risk of stroke.

- In the past, physicians believed that little could be done once a stroke occurred. However, speedy treatment with clot-dissolving drugs can limit braincell damage and prevent death.

 Vitamin E and Fish Oil. What has research shown about the heart benefits of vitamin E and fish oil?

health / ONLINE

American Heart Association
http://www.americanheart.org/
This site includes an interactive risk assessment for heart disease, a reference guide to heart-related topics, information about common heart conditions and treatments, and more.

The Virtual Body: The Human Heart
http://www.medtropolis.com/vbody/heart.html
This site takes you on a narrated, interactive tour of an animated human heart.

National Heart, Lung and Blood Institute Cholesterol Education Program
http://rover.nhlbi.nih.gov/chd/
This site focuses on how to control your cholesterol intake and prevent heart disease.

Please note that links are subject to change. If you find a broken link, use a search engine like http://www.yahoo.com *and search for the web site by typing in key words.*

 Campus Chat: What actions are you taking now that can help you prevent heart disease in the future? Share your thoughts on our online discussion forum at **http://health.wadsworth.com**

Find It On InfoTrac: You can find additional readings related to heart health via InfoTrac College Edition, an online library of more than 900 journals and publications. Follow the instructions for accessing InfoTrac that came packaged with your textbook; then search for articles using a key word search.

- **Suggested article:** "Beer, Wine or Liquor and the Risk of Myocardial Infarction" by Richard Sadovsky, M.D., *American Family Physician,* April 1, 1999, Vol. 59, Issue 7, p. 1923.

  (1) What ingredient in alcoholic drinks is responsible for the lower risk of heart attacks?

  (2) How do the HDL cholesterol levels of regular beer/wine/liquor drinkers compare to those of nondrinkers, when adjusted for age and gender?

For additional links, resources, and suggested readings on InfoTrac, visit our Health & Wellness Resource Center at http://health.wadsworth.com

Key Terms

The terms listed here are used within the chapter. Page numbers are included for each term. A definition of each term is given in the Glossary pages at the end of this book.

angina pectoris   428
angioplasty   430
aorta   414
arrhythmia   431
arteriosclerosis   428
atherosclerosis   428
atrial fibrillation   431
atrium   414
bradycardia   431
capillary   414
cardiopulmonary
   resuscitation (CPR)   430
cholesterol   418
congestive heart failure   432

coronary angiography   433
coronary bypass   434
diastole   414
electrocardiogram (ECG, EKG)   433
hymocysteine   421
hypertension   418
lipoprotein   419
male pattern baldness   421
mitral-valve prolapse   431
myocardial infarction (MI)   429
percutaneous transluminal coronary
   angioplasty (PTCA)   434
stroke   434

systole   414
tachycardia   431
thallium scintigraphy   433
transient ischemic attacks
   (TIAs)   435
triglyceride   418
ventricle   414

Critical Thinking Questions

1. Have you had your blood pressure checked lately? If your reading was high, what steps are you now taking to help reduce your blood pressure?

2. Have you had a cholesterol reading lately? Do you think it's necessary for you to obtain one? If your reading was/is borderline or high, what lifestyle changes can you make to help control your cholesterol level?

3. The costs for a heart transplant are over $100,000. The annual price tag for a year's worth of cyclosporine, the drug that prevents rejection and must be taken for

the rest of a transplant recipient's life, is about $5,000. The total medical bill can come to hundreds of thousands of dollars—enough to fund programs to improve the nutrition of poor pregnant women, to treat alcoholism, or to provide regular preventive care. Does treatment of any single individual justify such huge costs? Should our society try to balance the costs versus the benefits of such heroic measures as heart transplants? How would you go about making such decisions?

References

1. Centers for Disease Control and Prevention. Kolata, Gina. "Vast Advance Is Reported in Preventing Heart Illnesses." *New York Times*, August 6, 1999.
2. "Researchers Pinning Down Risk of Heart Disease, Stroke." *FDA Consumer*, Vol. 33, Issue 3, May 1999.
3. American Heart Association Comment. "Contributions of Trends in Survival and Coronary Event Rates to Changes in Coronary Heart Disease Mortality: 10-Year Results from 37 WHO MONICA Project Populations." *Lancet*, May 8, 1999.
4. "Figures on Diseases of the Heart Don't Tell the Whole Story: American Heart Association Says Deaths Up 37 Percent." American Heart Association Comment, August 6, 1999.
5. American Heart Association. For most recent statistics, check www.americanheart.org
6. "Moderate Activity Keeps Heart, Waistline in Shape." *Harvard Health Letter*, Vol. 24, No. 7, April 1999.
7. Bullock, Carole. "Walking Cuts Heart Attack Risk." Press release, American Heart Association, June 30, 1999.
8. "Antioxidants: Separating Hope from Hype." *Harvard Health Letter*, Vol. 24, Issue 5, February 1999.
9. Havranek, Edward. "Primary Prevention of CHD: Nine Ways to Reduce Risk." *American Family Physician*, Vol. 59, Issue 6, March 15, 1999.
10. Centers for Disease Control and Prevention.
11. Iribarren, Carlos. "The Effect of Cigar Smoking on the Risk of Cardiovascular Disease, Chronic Obstructive Pulmonary Disease, and Cancer in Men." *New England Journal of Medicine*, June 10, 1999.
12. Gottlieb, Scott. "Study Confirms Passive Smoking Increases Coronary Heart Disease." *British Medical Journal*, Vol. 318, Issue 1888, April 3, 1999.
13. American Heart Association Comment: "Passive Smoking and the Risk of Coronary Heart Disease—A Meta-Analysis of Epidemiologic Studies." *New England Journal of Medicine*, March 25, 1999.
14. Jiang, He, et al. "Passive Smoking and the Risk of Coronary Heart Disease—A Meta-Analysis of Epidemiologic Studies." *New England Journal of Medicine*, March 25, 1999.
15. Walling, Anne. "Hypertension in Diabetic Patients." *American Family Physician*, February 15, 1999.

16. Cooper, Stephanie, and James Caldwell. "Coronary Artery Disease in People with Diabetes." *Clinical Diabetes,* Vol. 17, Issue 2, April 1999.

17. "Effects of Weight Loss on Cardiac Function." *Nutrition Research Newsletter,* Vol. 18, Issue 2, February 1999.

18. Hemingway, Harry, and Michael Marmot. "Psychosocial Factors in the Etiology and Prognosis of Coronary Heart Disease: Systematic Review of Prospective Cohort Studies." *British Medical Journal,* Vol. 318, Issue 7196, May 29, 1999.

19. Preboth, Monica, and Shyla Wright. "Women and Anger." *American Family Physician,* Vol. 59, Issue 6, March 15, 1999.

20. Sullivan, Mark. "For Heart Disease Patients, Depression Takes Heavy Toll." *Psychosomatics,* July 1999.

21. Hemingway Marmot. "Psychosocial Factors in the Etiology and Prognosis of Coronary Heart Disease: Systematic Review of Prospective Cohort Studies."

22. "Coronary Artery Disease and Women." American Heart Association.

23. Wexler, Laura. "Studies of Acute Coronary Syndromes in Women." *New England Journal of Medicine,* Vol. 341, No. 4, July 22, 1999.

24. Vaccarino, Viola, et al. "Sex Based Differences in Early Mortality After Myocardial Infarction." *New England Journal of Medicine,* Vol. 341, No. 4, July 22, 1999.

25. Eckel, Robert. Personal Interview.

26. Tanne, Janice Hopkins. "Antibiotics May Prevent Heart Attacks." *British Medical Journal,* Vol. 318, Issue 7181, February 13, 1999.

27. "Can Antibiotics Reduce Heart Disease Risk?" Wake Forest University School of Medicine press release, August 10, 1999.

28. Mittleman, Murray, et al. "Cocaine and Heart Attack Risk." *The Journal of the American Heart Association,* May 31, 1999.

29. National Cholesterol Education Program.

30. Comarow, Avery. "Not Too Young for Heart Disease." *U.S. News and World Report,* Vol. 126, Issue 9, March 8, 1999.

31. Henkel, John. "Food for Thought." *FDA Consumer,* Vol. 33, Issue 1, January 1999.

32. Evans, David. "Cholesterol-Lowering Diets And Coronary Heart Disease." *British Medical Journal,* Vol. 318, Issue 7188, April 3, 1999.

33. Henkel, John. "Keeping Cholesterol Under Control." *FDA Consumer,* Vol. 33, Issue 1, January 1999.

34. Rubins, Hanna, et al. "Gemfibrozil for the Secondary Prevention of Coronary Heart Disease in Men with Low Levels of High-Density Lipoprotein Cholesterol." *New England Journal of Medicine,* Vol. 341, No. 6, August 5, 1999.

35. "Cholesterol-Lowering Drugs Provide Double Protection Against Heart Disease." Press release, American Heart Association, July 12, 1999.

36. Lindbloom, Erik. "Treating Average Cholesterol Levels in Patients with Coronary Artery Disease." *Journal of Family Practice,* Vol. 49, Issue 2, February 1999.

37. Dinsdale, Paul. "New Guidelines for Mild Hypertension." *British Medical Journal,* Vol. 318, Issue 7183, February 27, 1999.

38. Pickering, Thomas, and Jefferson, Thomas. "Advances in the Treatment of Hypertension." *JAMA,* Vol. 281, No. 2, January 13, 1999.

39. Moser, Marvin. "Hypertension Treatment and the Prevention of Coronary Heart Disease in the Elderly." *American Family Physician,* Vol. 59, Issue 5, March 1, 1999.

40. Hodes, Richard. Personal interview.

41. Moser. "Hypertension Treatment and the Prevention of Coronary Heart Disease in the Elderly."

42. Ornish, Dean, et al. "Intensive Lifestyle Changes for Reversal of Coronary Heart Disease." *JAMA,* Vol. 280, No. 23, December 16, 1998.

43. Napoli, Maryann. "Angina Treatments Often Inappropriate." *HealthFacts,* July 1999.

44. American Heart Association.

45. "JAMA Patient Page: Heart Attack." *JAMA,* July 28, 1999.

46. Charatan, Fred. "Severity of Heart Attacks in U.S. May be Declining." *British Medical Journal,* Vol. 318, Issue 7188, April 3, 1999.

47. Vaccarino, Viola, et al. "Sex-Based Differences in Early Mortality after Myocardial Infarction." *New England Journal of Medicine,* Vol. 341, No. 4, July 22, 1999.

48. Wexler, Laura. "Studies of Acute Coronary Syndromes in Women." *New England Journal of Medicine,* Vol. 341, No. 4, July 22, 1999.

49. Hochman, Judith, et al. "Sex, Clinical Presentation and Outcome in Patients with Acute Coronary Syndromes." *New England Journal of Medicine,* Vol. 341, No. 4, July 22, 1999.

50. Antman, Elliott. "'Super' Aspirin and Clot Buster Drug Therapy." *Circulation: The Journal of the American Heart Association,* May 31, 1999

51. Freed, Lisa, et al. "Prevalence and Clinical Outcome of Mitral-Valve Prolapse." *New England Journal of Medicine,* Vol. 341, No. 1, July 1, 1999.

52. Gilon, Dan, et al. "Lack of Evidence of an Association Between Mitral-Valve Prolapse and Stroke in Young Patients." *New England Journal of Medicine,* Vol. 341, No. 1, July 1, 1999.

53. Gavin, Kara. "Heart Failure Deaths Reduced by 30 Percent with New Drug Regimen." University of Michigan School of Medicine press release, July 20, 1999.

54. Helgeson, Vicki, et al. "Reacting Well to Heart Disease Can Help Avoid Future Attacks." *Psychosomatic Medicine,* August 1999. Irvine, Jane, et al. "Conscientious Patients Less Likely to Die." *Psychosomatic Medicine,* August 1999.

55. Barnett, Henry, et al. "Prevention of Ischemic Stroke." *British Medical Journal,* Vol. 318, Issue 7197, June 5, 1999.

56. "Stroke." *Harvard Women's Health Watch,* Vol. 6, Issue 11, July 1999.

57. Henry, Brian. "Memory-Robbing Disorder Detected in One in Three Stroke Survivors." American Heart Association, December 1997.

58. "Stroke." *Harvard Women's Health Watch.*

59. Henry, Brian. "Hispanics Face Higher Risk for Bleeding Strokes Than Whites, Native Americans." American Heart Association, December 1997.

60. "Brain Angioplasty May Prevent Strokes." *Science News,* Vol. 155, Issue 25, June 19, 1999.

V

Avoiding Health Risks

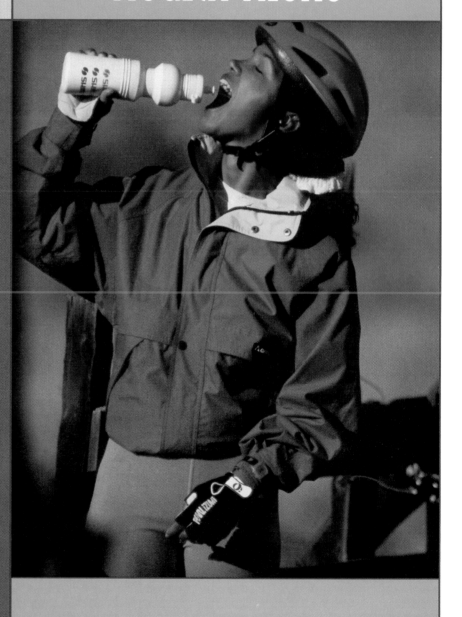

We constantly hear messages encouraging us to take risks with our health, to try drugs, to have a drink, to smoke cigarettes. We also live with the consequences of others' drug abuse, alcoholism, and smoking. That's why it's important to know about potentially harmful habits—even if you never rely on drugs to pick you up or bring you down, never smoke, and never drink to excess. This section provides information you can use to avoid or overcome habits that could destroy your health, happiness, and life.

14

Lowering Your Risk of Cancer and Other Major Diseases

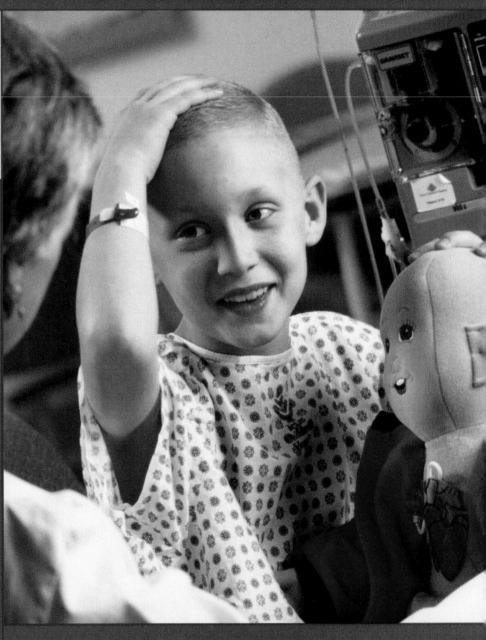

After studying the material in this chapter, you should be able to:

- **Define** cancer, and **list** the seven warning signs.
- **List** and **explain** the risk factors for cancer.
- **Describe** practical behaviors to reduce the risk.
- **Describe** appropriate treatment for cancer.
- **Define** *diabetes mellitus*, and **describe** the early symptoms and treatment for this disease.
- **List** and **explain** other major noninfectious illnesses.

W hether or not you will get a serious disease at some time in your life may seem to be a matter of odds. Genetic tendencies, environmental factors, and luck affect your chances of having to face many health threats. However, you do have some control over such risks, and even if a major illness may be inevitable, you can often prevent or delay it for years, even decades.

Cancer is an excellent example. For the first time since 1900, the overall cancer death rates in the United States are coming down. More people survive cancer than ever. An estimated 8.4 million Americans—nearly 1 in 30—have a history of cancer.[1] Some experts predict that within 20 years, cancer deaths could be cut an additional 25 percent.

Prevention and health promotion hold great promise for the other noninfectious illnesses discussed in this chapter: diabetes mellitus; epilepsy; respiratory diseases; anemias; liver disorders; kidney problems; digestive diseases; disorders of the muscles, joints, and bones; and skin disorders. This chapter also explains the causes, risk factors, development, diagnosis, and treatment of these disorders and discusses special needs related to differences in physical and mental abilities. ❖

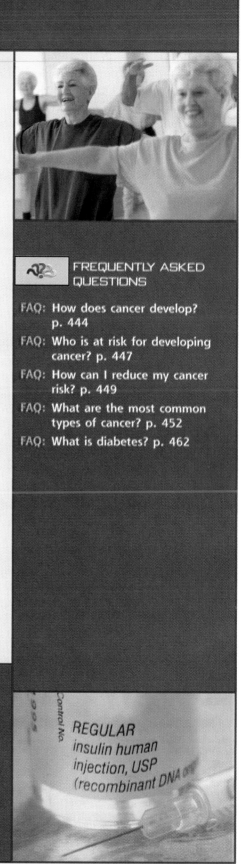

FREQUENTLY ASKED QUESTIONS

FAQ: **How does cancer develop?** p. 444

FAQ: **Who is at risk for developing cancer?** p. 447

FAQ: **How can I reduce my cancer risk?** p. 449

FAQ: **What are the most common types of cancer?** p. 452

FAQ: **What is diabetes?** p. 462

REGULAR
insulin human
injection, USP
(recombinant DNA o

Understanding Cancer

The uncontrolled growth and spread of abnormal cells causes cancer. Normal cells follow the code of instructions embedded in DNA (the body's genetic material); cancer cells do not. Think of the DNA within the nucleus of a cell as a computer program that controls the cell's functioning, including its ability to grow and reproduce itself. If this program or its operation is altered, the cell goes out of control. The nucleus no longer regulates growth. The abnormal cell divides to create other abnormal cells, which again divide, eventually forming **neoplasms** (new formations), or tumors.

Tumors can be either *benign* (slightly abnormal, not considered life-threatening) or *malignant* (cancerous). The only way to determine whether a tumor is benign is by microscopic examination of its cells. Cancer cells have larger nuclei than the cells in benign tumors, they vary more in shape and size, and they divide more often.

At one time cancer was thought to be a single disease that attacked different parts of the body. Now scientists believe that cancer comes in countless forms, each with a genetically determined molecular "fingerprint" that indicates how deadly it is. With this understanding, doctors can identify how aggressively a tumor should be treated.[2]

Without treatment, cancer cells continue to grow, crowding out and replacing healthy cells. This process is called **infiltration,** or invasion. They may also **metastasize,** or spread to other parts of the body via the bloodstream or lymphatic system (see Figure 14-1). For many cancers, as many as 60 percent of patients may have metastases (which may be too small to be felt or seen without a microscope) at the time of diagnosis.

Although all cancers have similar characteristics, each is distinct. Some cancers are relatively simple to cure, whereas others are more threatening and mysterious. The earlier any cancer is found, the easier it is to treat and the better the patient's chances of survival. Cancers are classified according to the type of cell and the organ in which they originate, such as the following:

- *Carcinoma,* the most common kind, which starts in the epithelium, the layers of cells that cover the body's surface or line internal organs and glands.
- *Sarcomas,* which form in the supporting, or connective, tissues of the body: bones, muscles, blood vessels.
- *Leukemias,* which begin in the blood-forming tissues (bone marrow, lymph nodes, and the spleen).
- *Lymphomas,* which arise in the cells of the lymph system, the network that filters out impurities.

 ## How Does Cancer Develop?

For decades researchers have tried to figure out exactly how a normal cell turns into a cancer cell. In the last few years, they've made dramatic progress in unraveling this mystery by studying **oncogenes,** normal genes that control growth but have gone awry. For reasons that scientists don't yet understand, the DNA in these genes changes and cells proliferate at a very rapid rate. In addition, other genes, called **tumor suppressor genes,** which normally control cell growth, fail to stop cells from dividing before they become cancerous. More than half of all known types of cancer, including those of the colon, brain, lung, breast, bone, and blood, have been linked to defects in one particular tumor suppressor gene: *p53.* Mismatch/repair genes correct mistakes in a cell's DNA when it is copied. If they do not function properly, mutations can occur in other genes, including oncogenes and tumor suppressor genes. (See Figure 14-2.)

In this sense, all cancers are genetic. However, scientists have linked several cancers—including cancers of

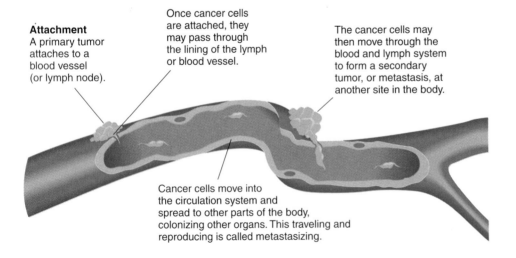

Attachment
A primary tumor attaches to a blood vessel (or lymph node).

Once cancer cells are attached, they may pass through the lining of the lymph or blood vessel.

The cancer cells may then move through the blood and lymph system to form a secondary tumor, or metastasis, at another site in the body.

Cancer cells move into the circulation system and spread to other parts of the body, colonizing other organs. This traveling and reproducing is called metastasizing.

■ Figure 14-1 **Metastasis, or Spread of Cancer**
Cancer cells can travel through the blood vessels to spread to other organs, or through the lymphatic system to form secondary tumors.

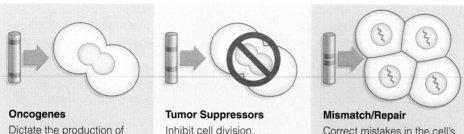

■ Figure 14-2 Looking at Cancer on the Genetic Level
Three different gene types are linked to the development of cancer cells.

Source: The New York Times, September 10, 1999. Reprinted by permission.

Oncogenes

Dictate the production of proteins that stimulate normal cell growth.

When mutations occur, cells multiply at an accelerated rate.

Tumor Suppressors

Inhibit cell division.

When mutations deactivate the gene, cell multiplication can continue unchecked.

Mismatch/Repair

Correct mistakes in the cell's DNA when the cell replicates.

When they function improperly, mutations of other genes are passed from one generation to the next.

the ovaries, prostate, pancreas, gall bladder, bile duct, colon, and stomach, as well as malignant melanoma, the deadliest skin cancer—to two tumor suppressor genes, BRCA-1 and BRCA-2, initially linked only with breast cancer.[3] Mutations in these genes, which are carried by 1 in 400 Americans, can be passed from a mother or father and can put both sons and daughters at increased cancer risk.[4]

At any time during a person's lifetime, a genetic mutation that allows uncontrolled cell growth may be triggered, directly or indirectly, by environmental risk factors, such as tobacco smoke or toxic chemicals. Mutations also can occur spontaneously when the body's self-monitoring systems do not detect an error made during cell division.

Often genetic and environmental risk factors interact. In colon cancer, for instance, an individual may inherent a gene that has been linked to colon cancer and develop hundreds to thousands of benign adenomatous polyps, which can progress to cancer if not treated. However, the trigger for polyp growth may be in a gene involved in fat metabolism; therefore, eating a high-fat diet increases any inherited vulnerability.

Most cancers develop over a period of many years. Once detected, cancers are classified in terms of how far they've spread and to which organs. An *in situ* cancer is contained in the place where it originated. An invasive cancer has spread to surrounding tissues. A metastasized cancer has traveled to distant sites in the body.

Cancer Staging

Once they diagnose a cancer, oncologists (specialists in cancer care) calculate the extent of the disease or the spread of cancer from the site of origin. This process, called staging, is essential in determining therapy and assessing prognosis. A cancer's stage is based on the primary tumor's size and location and whether it has spread to other areas of the body. According to one

staging system, if cancer cells have not spread to other parts of the affected organ or elsewhere in the body, the stage is "in situ." If cancer cells have spread beyond the original layer of tissue, then the cancer is considered invasive. If it has traveled to distant parts of the body, it has metastasized.[5]

Strategies *for* Prevention

The Seven Warning Signs of Cancer

If you note any of the following seven warning signs, immediately schedule an appointment with your doctor:

✔ Change in bowel or bladder habits.

✔ A sore that doesn't heal.

✔ Unusual bleeding or discharge.

✔ Thickening or lump in the breast, testis, or elsewhere.

✔ Indigestion or difficulty swallowing.

✔ Obvious change in a wart or mole.

✔ Nagging cough or hoarseness.

Cancer Trends

According to the American Cancer Society (ACS), the number of new cases of cancer peaked in the early 1990s, and the overall rate of new cancers in the United States has been falling ever since. About 1,221,800 new cancer cases were diagnosed in 1999. Since 1990, approximately 12 million new cancer cases have been diagnosed.[6] (See Figures 14-3 and 14-4.)

In 1999 about 563,100 Americans died of cancer—more than 1,500 people a day. Cancer is the second leading cause of death in the United States, exceeded only by heart disease, and is responsible for one of every

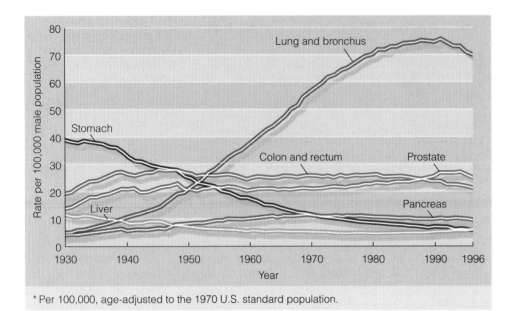

■ **Figure 14-3** Age-adjusted cancer death rates,* males.

Source: American Cancer Society, Surveillance Research, 1999. Data source: *Vital Statistics of the United States.*

* Per 100,000, age-adjusted to the 1970 U.S. standard population.

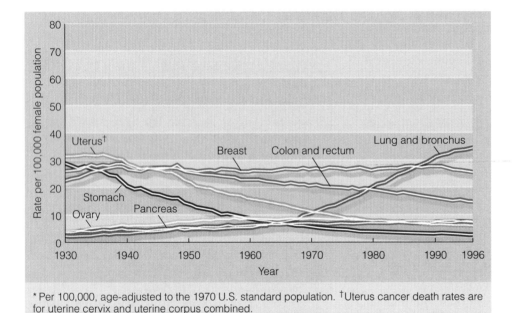

■ **Figure 14-4** Age-adjusted cancer death rates,* females.

Source: American Cancer Society, Surveillance Research, 1999. Data source: *Vital Statistics of the United States.*

* Per 100,000, age-adjusted to the 1970 U.S. standard population. †Uterus cancer death rates are for uterine cervix and uterine corpus combined.

four deaths. Since 1990, approximately 5 million people have died of cancer. However, death rates for most major cancers are declining. The five-year survival rate for all cancers improved from 51 percent in the 1980s to almost 60 percent in the 1990s; for children, it went from 65 percent to 74 percent. Of the ten most life-threatening cancers, only the mortality rates for non-Hodgkin's lymphoma and melanoma have continued to rise, although the rates of increase were lower than they were in the 1970s.[7]

Two million women are breast cancer survivors; one million men are prostate cancer survivors.[8] Rates of new cases of prostate cancer, and deaths from this cancer have fallen, as have rates of new cases and deaths due to colorectal cancer. Breast cancer incidence has remained about the same, but the number of deaths from breast cancer has fallen by about 2 percent. Lung cancer incidence and death rates fell in most men (except those of American Indian or Alaska native ethnic backgrounds); however, these rates increased among women.[9]

The Potential of Prevention

Prevention is the key to greater reductions in cancer rates and mortality. According to ACS estimates, tobacco use causes about 173,000 cancer deaths each year. Excessive alcohol use claims another 20,000 lives.

Researchers believe that up to one-third of the 563,100 cancer deaths that occurred in 1999 were related to nutrition and could also have been prevented. Adequate sun protection also may have prevented many of the more than 1 million skin cancers diagnosed in 1999.

 ## Who Is at Risk for Developing Cancer?

Everyone and anyone can develop cancer. However, since the occurrence of cancer increases over time, most cases affect adults who are middle-aged or older. In the United States, men have a one in two lifetime risk of developing cancer; for women, the risk is one in three.

(See The X and Y Files: "Sex Differences in Cancer Sites and Deaths.")

The term **relative risk** compares the risk of developing cancer in persons with a certain exposure or trait to the risk in persons who do not have this exposure or trait. Smokers, for instance, have a ten-times-greater relative risk of developing lung cancer than nonsmokers. This means that smokers have a 900 percent increased risk of lung cancer. Most relative risks are smaller. For example, women who have a first-degree (mother, sister, or daughter) family history of breast cancer have about a twofold increased risk of developing breast cancer compared with women who do not have a family history of the disease. This means that they are about twice as likely to develop breast cancer. (To assess your risk of developing cancer, see the Self-Survey: "Are You at Risk of Cancer?")

The X&Y Files

Sex Differences in Cancer Sites and Deaths

Cancer Cases by Site and Sex

Male	Female
Prostate 180,400	Breast 182,800
Lung and bronchus 89,500	Lung and bronchus 74,600
Colon and rectum 63,600	Colon and rectum 66,600
Urinary bladder 38,300	Uterine Corpus 36,100
Non-Hodgkin's lymphoma 31,700	Non-Hodgkin's lymphoma 23,200
Melanoma of the skin 27,300	Ovary 23,100
Oral cavity 20,200	Melanoma of the skin 20,400
Kidney 18,800	Urinary bladder 14,900
Leukemia 16,900	Pancreas 14,600
Pancreas 13,700	Thyroid 13,700
All sites 619,700	All sites 600,400

Cancer Deaths by Site and Sex

Male	Female
Lung and bronchus 89,300	Lung and bronchus 67,600
Prostate 31,900	Breast 40,800
Colon and rectum 27,800	Colon and rectum 28,500
Pancreas 13,700	Pancreas 14,500
Non-Hodgkin's lymphoma 13,700	Ovary 14,000
Leukemia 12,100	Non-Hodgkin's lymphoma 12,400
Esophagus 9,200	Leukemia 9,600
Liver 8,500	Uterine Corpus 6,500
Urinary bladder 8,100	Brain 5,900
Stomach 7,600	Stomach 5,400
All sites 284,100	All sites 268,100

Source: American Cancer Society, Surveillance Research, 2000.

Self-*Survey*   Are You at Risk of Cancer?

Answer the following questions:

1. Do you protect your skin from overexposure to the sun? _____
2. Do you abstain from smoking or using tobacco in any form? _____
3. If you're over 40 or if family members have had colon cancer, do you get routine digital rectal exams? _____
4. Do you eat a balanced diet that includes the RDA for vitamins A, B, and C? _____
5. If you're a woman, do you have regular Pap tests and pelvic exams? _____
6. If you're a man over 40, do you get regular prostate exams? _____
7. If you have burn scars or a history of chronic skin infections, do you get regular checkups? _____
8. Do you avoid smoked, salted, pickled, and high-nitrite foods? _____
9. If your job exposes you to asbestos, radiation, cadmium, or other environmental hazards, do you get regular checkups?
10. Do you limit your consumption of alcohol? _____
11. Do you avoid using tanning salons or home sunlamps? _____
12. If you're a woman, do you examine your breasts every month for lumps? _____
13. Do you eat plenty of vegetables and other sources of fiber? _____
14. If you're a man, do you perform regular testicular self-exams? _____
15. Do you wear protective sunglasses in sunlight?
16. Do you follow a low-fat diet? _____
17. Do you know the cancer warning signs? _____

Scoring:

If you answered no to any of the questions, your risk for developing various kinds of cancer may be increased.

Making Changes

Cutting Your Cancer Risk

You may not be able to control every risk factor in your life or environment, but you can protect yourself from the obvious ones.

- *Avoid excessive exposure to ultraviolet light.* If you spend a lot of time outside, you can protect your skin by using sunscreen and wearing long-sleeve shirts and a hat. Also, wear sunglasses to protect your eyes. Don't purposely put yourself at risk by binge-sunbathing or by using sunlamps.
- *Avoid obvious cancer risks.* Besides ultraviolet light, other environmental factors that have been linked with cancer include tobacco, asbestos, and radiation.
- *Keep yourself as healthy as possible.* The healthier you are, the better able your body is to ward off diseases that can predispose you to cancer. Get regular exercise; eat a balanced, high-fiber, low-fat diet; and avoid excessive alcohol use.
- *Be alert to changes in your body.* You know your body's rhythms and appearance better than anyone else, and only you will know if certain things aren't right. Changes in bowel habits, skin changes, unusual lumps or discharges—anything out of the ordinary may be clues that require further medical investigation.
- *Don't put off seeing your doctor if you detect any changes.* Procrastination can't hurt anyone but you.

Heredity

Heredity may account for about 10 percent of all cancers, and an estimated 13 to 14 million Americans may be at risk. Yet most people—and many physicians who haven't kept up with the dramatic breakthroughs in cancer genetics in recent years—don't realize that a person's genetic legacy can be a significant risk factor. Genetic tests can identify carriers of BRCA-1 and BRCA-2 mutations, but the results are often difficult to interpret.[10]

In hereditary cancers, such as retinoblastoma (an eye cancer that strikes young children) or certain colon cancers, a specific cancer-causing gene is passed down from generation to generation. The odds of any child with one affected parent inheriting this gene and developing the cancer are fifty-fifty. In familial cancers, close relatives develop the same types of cancer, but no one knows exactly how the disease is transmitted. In the future, genetic tests may be able to identify individuals who are born with an increased susceptibility. Tracing cancers through a family tree is one simple way of checking your own risk.

The most likely sites for inherited cancers to develop are the breast, brain, blood, muscles, bones, and adrenal gland. The telltale signs of inherited cancers include the following:

- *Early development.* Genetic forms of certain diseases strike earlier than noninherited cancers. For example, the average age of women diagnosed with breast cancer is 62. But if breast cancer is inherited, the average age at diagnosis is 44, an 18-year difference.

- *Family history.* Anyone with a close relative (mother, father, sibling, child) with cancer has about three times the usual chance of getting the same type of cancer.
- *Multiple targets.* The same type of hereditary cancer often strikes more than once—in both breasts or both kidneys, for instance, or in two separate parts of the same organ.
- *Unusual gender pattern.* Genes may be responsible for cancers that generally don't strike a certain gender—for example, breast cancer in a man.
- *Cancer family syndrome.* Some families, with unusually large numbers of relatives affected by cancer, seem clearly cancer-prone. For instance, in Lynch syndrome (a form of colon cancer), more than 20 percent of the family members in at least two generations develop cancer of both the colon and endometrium.

Cancer and Minorities

African Americans are more likely to develop cancer than any other racial or ethnic group. In the first half of the 1990s, cancer incidence rates were 445.8 per 100,000 among African Americans, 405.2 per 100,000 among whites, 278.1 per 100,000 among Hispanics, 277.9 per 100,000 among Asian/Pacific Islanders, and 153.8 per 100,000 among American Indians. During these same years, cancer incidence rates decreased among whites and Hispanics but remained relatively stable among other racial and ethnic groups.

The incidence of female breast cancer is highest among white women and lowest among American-Indian women. African-American women have the highest rates of colorectal and lung and bronchial cancer, followed by whites, Asian/Pacific Islanders, Hispanics, and American Indians. African-American men have the highest incidence of prostate, colorectal, and lung and bronchial cancer. African-American men are at least 50 percent more likely to develop prostate cancer than men of any other racial or ethnic group. They are about 34 percent more likely to die of cancer than whites and twice as likely to die of cancer as Asian/Pacific Islanders, American Indians, and Hispanics.[11]

Viruses

Researchers have long known that viruses can cause tumors in animals, but only recently have they shown a connection between several different viruses and cancer in humans. Viruses have been implicated in certain leukemias (cancers of the blood system) and lymphomas (cancers of the lymphatic system), cancers of the nose and pharynx, liver cancer, and cervical cancer. Human immunodeficiency virus (HIV) can lead to certain lymphomas and leukemias and to a type of cancer called Kaposi's sarcoma. Human papilloma virus (HPV) has been linked to an increased risk of cervical cancer and cancer of the penis.[12] (See Chapter 12 on infectious diseases.)

Environmental Risks

Many chemicals used in industry today are carcinogens, and employees as well as people living near a factory that creates smoke, dust, or gases are at risk. Among the known dangers are nickel, chromate, asbestos, and vinyl chloride. (See Chapter 20 for more information on environmental risks.)

Three to 5 percent of all cancers might be caused by radiation, including medical, occupational, and environmental exposures. Large doses clearly cause cancer; the effects of lower doses are not as clear. Among those at greater risk are workers at and residents near nuclear facilities, pregnant women and their fetuses, and children exposed to nuclear fallout. Clinical studies have revealed a long latent period before a radiation-induced cancer appears (usually a minimum of five years).

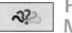 ## How Can I Reduce My Cancer Risk?

Environmental factors may cause between 80 and 90 percent of cancers and, at least in theory, can be prevented by avoiding cancer-causing substances (such as tobacco and sunlight) or using substances that protect against cancer-causing factors (such as antioxidants and vitamin D). How do you start protecting yourself? Simple changes in lifestyle—not smoking, protecting yourself from the sun, exercising regularly—are essential (see Pulsepoints: "Ten Ways to Protect Yourself from Cancer" for practical guidelines).

Cancer-Smart Nutrition

Diets high in antioxidant-rich fruits and vegetables have long been linked with lower rates of esophageal, lung, colon, and stomach cancer. At least in theory, antioxidants can block genetic damage induced by free radicals that could lead to some cancers (see Chapter 6 on nutrition). However, scientific studies have not proven conclusively that any specific antioxidant, particularly in supplement form, can prevent cancer.[13]

In studies of beta-carotene, this carotenoid did not reduce overall cancer rates or mortality. In two studies of smokers, beta-carotene actually was associated with increased mortality from lung cancer. Researchers are

PULSE *points*

Ten Ways to Protect Yourself from Cancer

1. **Don't smoke.** Cigarette smoke is the number-one carcinogen in this country, responsible for one in every three cancers.

2. **Stay out of the sun.** Wearing sunscreen (with a Sun Protection Factor of at least 15) is better than not using any, but protective clothing is better—and staying in the shade is best.

3. **Limit your intake of alcohol.** Heavy drinkers are more likely to develop oral cancer and cancers of the larynx, throat, esophagus, liver, and breast.

4. **Watch your weight.** Obesity increases the risks of several cancers, including endometrial cancer and, particularly among postmenopausal women, breast cancer.

5. **Get moving.** Exercise—the heart strengthener and stamina build-er—also can reduce the risk of colon cancer. Women who exercised early in life are less likely to develop breast cancer as adults.

6. **Be sexually cautious.** Cervical cancer has been linked with intercourse at an early age, multiple sex partners, and infection with the human papilloma virus (HPV), the virus that causes genital warts. The incidence of prostate cancer in men increases with multiple sexual partners and a history of frequent sexually transmitted diseases.

7. **Check yourself out.** Scan your skin for suspicious moles every month. If you're a woman, examine your breasts. If you're a man, check your testicles. Follow ACS recommendations for other cancer checkups.

8. **Protect yourself from possible environmental carcinogens.** Many chemicals used in industry can increase the risk to employees and people living near a factory that creates smoke, dust, or gases. Follow safety precautions at work, and check with local environmental protection officials about possible hazards in your community.

9. **Watch what you eat.** Cut down on fat; eat more fruits, vegetables and whole grains. High-fat foods have been linked to several cancers, including breast, prostate, colon. Fruits, vegetables, and grains are rich in potentially protective antioxidants.

10. **Inform yourself.** Know the warning signs of cancer (see page 445), and see a physician if you develop any of them. Find out about any history of cancer in your family. Even though heredity accounts for a relatively small percentage of cancer cases, the more you know about potential risks, the more you can do to protect yours.

---

continuing to investigate a variety of antioxidants that have shown promise as cancer-fighters.[14] The mineral selenium, which promotes antioxidant activity, may protect against prostate cancer and possibly also lower the risk of cancer of the lung, colon, and esophagus. Diets rich in vitamin C and folate also may have some specific benefits against breast cancer.[15] The role of dietary fat in breast and other cancers remains controversial, as discussed in Chapter 6.[16] Your best bet is eating as many different types of fruits and vegetables as possible—for a total of five to nine servings a day.

Another way to lower your cancer risk is to reduce the fat in your diet. There is solid evidence that cutting back on fat can lower the risks of colon, ovarian, and pancreatic cancer. However, recent research suggests that a low-fat diet does not protect women from breast cancer.

It's also important to pay attention to food processing and preparation. Whenever possible, select foods close to their natural state, grown locally and without pesticides. Avoid cured, pickled, or smoked meats. When cooking, try not to fry or barbecue often; these cooking methods can produce mutagens that induce cancer in animals. The process of smoking or charcoal-grilling releases carcinogenic tar that may increase the risk of cancer of the stomach and esophagus.

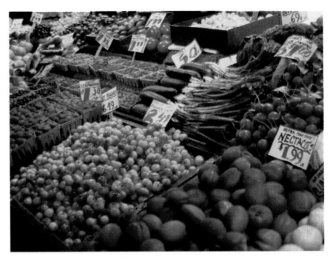

Eating at least five servings of fruits and vegetables a day can help reduce your cancer risk.

Strategies *for* Prevention

Eating to Reduce Your Cancer Risk

✓ Eat at least five servings of fruits and vegetables a day: at least one rich in vitamin A (e.g., cantaloupe, carrots, spinach, or sweet potatoes), at least one high in vitamin C (for example, grapefruit, oranges, cauliflower, or green peppers), at least one high-fiber selection (for example, winter squash, corn, figs, or apples).

✓ Have cabbage family (cruciferous) vegetables such as cabbage, brussels sprouts, and cauliflower several times a week.

✓ Don't fry or barbecue often. Safer cooking methods are baking, boiling, steaming, microwaving, poaching, and roasting.

✓ Choose foods without added chemicals or pesticides. Whenever possible, select foods that are close to their natural state, grown locally, and freshly picked.

Cigarette Smoke and Environmental Tobacco Smoke

Cigarette smoking is the single most devastating and preventable cause of cancer deaths in the United States. People who smoke two or more packs of cigarettes a day are 15 to 25 times more likely to die of cancer than are nonsmokers. Cigarettes cause most cases of lung cancer and increase the risk of cancer of the mouth, pharynx, larynx, esophagus, pancreas, and bladder. Pipes, cigars, and smokeless tobacco also increase the danger of cancers of the mouth and throat.[17]

Environmental tobacco smoke can increase the risk of cancer even among those who've never smoked. For example, researchers have found that exposure to others' tobacco smoke for as little as three hours a day can increase the risk of developing cancer threefold.[18] (See the discussion of passive smoking in Chapter 17.)

Possible Carcinogens

Although it may not be possible to avoid all possible **carcinogens** (cancer-causing chemicals), you can take steps to minimize your danger. Many chemicals used in industry, including nickel, chromate, asbestos, and vinyl chloride, are carcinogens, and employees as well as people living near a factory that creates smoke, dust, or gases are at risk. If your job involves their use, follow safety precautions at work. If you are concerned about possible hazards in your community, check with local

environmental protection officials (see Chapter 20 on environmental health).

Women and men who dye their hair frequently, particularly with very dark shades of permanent coloring, may be at increased risk for leukemia (cancer of blood-forming cells), non-Hodgkin's lymphoma (cancer of the lymph system), multiple myeloma (cancer of the bone marrow) and, in women, ovarian cancer. Lighter shades and less permanent tints do not seem to be a danger.

Chemoprevention

In recent years scientists have focused on what has long seemed revolutionary: **chemoprevention,** the use of natural or laboratory-made substances to reduce the risk of developing cancer. They are believed to work by halting or reversing the process by which a cell becomes cancerous.

The first medication that has proved effective in preventing a major cancer is **tamoxifen,** a modified or "designer" estrogen. In 1998 the landmark Breast Cancer Prevention Trial showed that women at high risk of breast cancer who took tamoxifen for an average of four years reduced their chance of developing breast cancer by 45 percent. Subsequently, the FDA approved tamoxifen to reduce the likelihood of breast cancer in high-risk women.

Tamoxifen belongs to a group of medications called selective estrogen receptor modulators (SERMs), which have different effects in various parts of the body. In the breast, they block estrogen's harmful effects and lower cancer risk; in the skeleton, they mimic estrogen's beneficial impact and maintain bone density. Tamoxifen's primary disadvantage is an increased risk of three rare but potentially life-threatening problems: endometrial cancer, deep vein thrombosis (a blood clot in a large vein), and pulmonary embolism (a clot in the lung) in women over age 50. A second SERM—raloxifene (Evista), FDA-approved to prevent osteoporosis—also may lower breast cancer risk without such serious side effects. In a recent study of 7,705 postmenopausal women at risk for osteoporosis, those taking raloxifene reduced their risk of developing breast cancer by approximately 66 percent. Which SERM is better for women at high risk for breast cancer? NCI's ongoing STAR (Study of Tamoxifen and Raloxifene) trial aims to find the answer. However, there is considerable debate over giving any drug that can cause significant side effects to healthy women.[19]

NCI also is investigating the possible chemopreventive benefits of finasteride (Proscar), a drug used to treat benign swelling of the prostate, a common problem in older men. Unlike tamoxifen, it does not increase the risk of other cancers, but it does have side effects, including sexual dysfunction.

Another approach to prevention is vaccination, and investigators currently are studying vaccines for colon cancer and melanoma.[20] Vaccines targeted against the human papilloma virus, both to prevent and to treat cervical cancer, are undergoing clinical trials.

Early Detection

Cancers that can be detected by screening account for approximately half of all new cancer cases. Screening examinations, conducted regularly by a health-care professional, can lead to early diagnosis of cancers of the breast, colon, rectum, cervix, prostate, testicles, and oral cavity and can improve the odds of successful treatment. Self-examinations for cancers of the breast, testicles, and skin may also result in detection of tumors at earlier stages. The five-year relative survival rate for all these cancers is about 81 percent. If all Americans participated in regular cancer screenings, this rate could increase to more than 95 percent.[21]

Studies of chemoprevention with dietary supplements have produced contradictory—and confusing—results. In research sponsored by the National Cancer Institute (NCI) in China, daily vitamin and mineral supplements reduced the risk of dying of cancer in a population whose diet is very low in fresh fruits and vegetables. But another study of Finnish men, all smokers over age 50, found that beta-carotene and vitamin E supplements provided no benefit and may have somewhat increased their risk of dying of lung cancer. Ongoing NCI studies are investigating possible benefits from vitamin-A related compounds, folic acid, selenium, and calcium.

 ## What Are the Most Common Types of Cancer?

Cancer refers to a group of more than a hundred diseases characterized by abnormal cell growth. The most common are discussed in the following sections.

Skin Cancer

Sunlight is the primary culprit in the 1 million new cases of skin cancer that develop every year. Most damage is caused by exposure to the B range of ultraviolet light (UVB); the longer wavelength of light known as UVA also may be damaging to the skin. An estimated 80 percent of total lifetime sun exposure occurs during childhood, so sun protection is especially important in youngsters.[22] Tanning salons or sunlamps also increase the risk of skin cancer because they produce ultraviolet radiation. A half-hour dose of radiation from a sunlamp

can be equivalent to the amount you'd get from an entire day in the sun.

The most common skin cancers are basal-cell (involving the base of the epidermis, the top level of the skin) and squamous-cell (involving cells in the epidermis). (See Figure 14-5.) Every year more than 5 million Americans develop skin lesions known as actinic keratoses (AKs), rough red or brown scaly patches that develop in the upper layer of the skin, usually on the face, lower lip, bald scalp, neck, and back of the hands and forearms. Forty percent of squamous cell carcino-

Strategies *for* Prevention

Scanning Your Skin

Here's how to screen yourself for possible changes that may indicate skin cancer:

✔ Once a month, stand in front of a full-length mirror to examine your front and back, and your left and right sides with your arms raised. Check the backs of your legs, the tops and soles of your feet, and the surfaces between your toes. Use a hand mirror to check the back of your neck, behind your ears, and your scalp.

✔ Watch for changes in the size, color, number, and thickness of moles. Suspicious moles are likely to be asymmetrical (one half doesn't match the other), with ragged, notched, or blurred edges. Also look for any signs of darkly pigmented growth, oozing, scaliness, bleeding, or a change in sensation, itchiness, tenderness, or pain.

✔ Don't put too much faith in sunscreens. Wearing sunscreen (with a Sun Protection Factor, or SPF, of at least 15) is good, but protective clothing is better—and staying in the shade is best.[23]

✔ Check your shadow. One simple guideline for reducing the risk of skin cancer risk is avoiding the sun anytime your shadow is shorter than you are. According to NCI, this shadow method—based on the principle that the closer the sun comes to being directly overhead, the stronger its ultraviolet rays—works for any location and at any time of year.

✔ Check for photosensitivity. If you are taking any drugs, ask your doctor or pharmacist to see if the medication could make you more sensitive to sun damage. Be especially cautious about sun exposure if you have been using a synthetic preparation derived from vitamin A (Retin A) as an acne or anti-wrinkle treatment; it can increase your susceptibility.

■ Figure 14-5 **Three Types of Skin Cancer**
Squamous-cell cancer; malignant melanoma, the deadliest form of cancer; and basal-cell cancer.

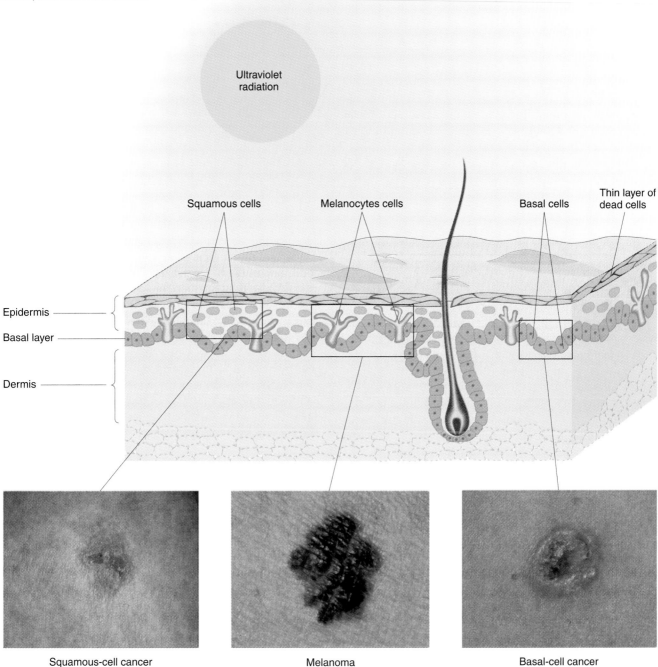

Squamous-cell cancer   Melanoma   Basal-cell cancer

mas, the second leading cause of skin cancer deaths, begin as AKs. Treatments include surgical removal, cryosurgery (freezing the skin), electrodesiccation (heat generated by an electric current), topical chemotherapy, and removal with lasers, chemical peels, or dermabrasion.[24]

Smoking and exposure to certain hydrocarbons in asphalt, coal tar, and pitch may increase the risk of squamous-cell skin cancer.

The incidence of the deadliest type of skin cancer, malignant melanoma, is rising by 4 to 5 percent per year. The overall risk of getting melanoma for Americans is about 1 in 120, but increases for individuals with any of the following characteristics:

- Blond or red hair.
- Marked freckling of the upper back.
- Rough red bumps on the skin called actinic keratoses.
- A family history of melanoma.
- Three or more blistering sunburns in the teenage years.
- Three or more years at an outdoor summer job as a teenager.

Any one or two of these factors increases a person's risk of melanoma three or four times. A combination of three or more factors increases the risk 20 to 25 times. Other risk factors include occupational exposure to carcinogens and inherited skin disorders, such as xeroderma pigmentosum and familial atypical multiple-mole melanoma.[25]

Across the Life Span: How the Risk of Melanoma Increases with Age

The incidence of melanoma is increasing faster than any other cancer in the United States, with more than 41,000 new cases diagnosed each year. While dermatology textbooks often report that crude rates of melanoma increase into middle age and then level off, cumulative damage to the immune system from exposure to ultraviolet light is expected to increase melanoma rates throughout the life span among aging baby boomers, as indicated by the adjusted rates depicted in Figure 14-6.[26]

If detected early, melanoma is highly curable. However, once a tumor is thicker than an eighth of an inch—about the thickness of a dime—it probably has metastasized. Treatment may consist of surgery, radiation, electrodesiccation (tissue

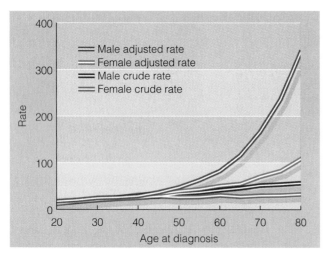

■ Figure 14-6 How the risk of melanoma increases with age.

destruction by heat), cryosurgery (tissue destruction by cold), or a combination of these therapies. Individuals who've had melanoma may be at high risk for developing this cancer again.

Breast Cancer

Every 3 minutes a woman in the United States learns that she has breast cancer. Every 12 minutes a woman dies of breast cancer. But a new word has entered medical discussions about breast cancer: hope. "Death and incidence rates for breast cancer are heading down," says Harmon Eyre, M.D., chief medical officer of the American Cancer Society. "In 30 years in the field, this is the most optimistic time I have seen."[27]

Despite these encouraging trends, breast cancer remains the illness women worry about most—even though they are ten times more likely to die of heart disease.[28] Many women misjudge their own likelihood of developing breast cancer, either overestimating or underestimating their susceptibility. In a recent national poll, one in every ten surveyed considered herself at no risk at all. This is never the case. "Every woman is at risk for breast cancer simply because she's female," says Leslie Ford, M.D., associate director for early detection at NCI.[29]

However, not all women's risks are equal. NCI has developed a computerized Breast Cancer Risk Assessment Tool, based on data from more than 280,000 women, that allows a woman to sit down with her doctor and discuss her own odds of developing breast cancer within the next five years and over her entire lifetime. These calculations include a variety of risk factors, including the following:

- **Age.** As shown in Figure 14-7, at 25, a woman's chance of developing breast cancer is 1 in 19,608; at 45, 1 in 93; at 65, 1 in 17; at 85, 1 in 9. By age 90 to 95, 1 in 8 women will have developed breast cancer. The mean age at which women are diagnosed is 63.
- **Family history.** "The overwhelming majority of breast cancers—90 to 95 percent—are not due to strong genetic factors," says Barnett Kramer, M.D., deputy director for cancer prevention at NCI.[30] "However, having a first-degree relative—mother, sister or daughter—with breast cancer does increase risk. And if the relative developed breast cancer before menopause, the cancer is more likely to be hereditary." As noted earlier, genetic testing, controversial but sometimes recommended for women in cancer-prone families, can identify these defects. However, it's not yet clear how many women with a defective gene actually will develop breast cancer; estimates range from 50 to 80 percent —or higher in families with many affected members.

By age 25	1 in 19,608	By age 60	1 in 24
By age 30	1 in 2,525	By age 65	1 in 17
By age 35	1 in 622	By age 70	1 in 14
By age 40	1 in 217	By age 75	1 in 11
By age 45	1 in 93	By age 80	1 in 10
By age 50	1 in 50	By age 85	1 in 9
By age 55	1 in 33	Ever	1 in 8

■ **Figure 14-7** A woman's risk of developing breast cancer.

Source: NCI Surveillance Program.

- **Age at menarche.** Women who got their first period before age 12 are at greater risk than women who began menstruating later. The reason is that the more menstrual cycles a woman has, the longer her exposure to estrogen, a hormone known to increase breast cancer danger. For similar reasons, childless women, who menstruate continuously for several decades, are also at greater risk.

- **Age at birth of first child.** An early pregnancy—in a woman's teens or twenties—changes the actual maturation of breast cells and decreases risk. But if a woman has her first child in her forties, precancerous cells may actually flourish with the high hormone levels of the pregnancy.

- **Breast biopsies.** Even if laboratory analysis finds no precancerous abnormalities, women who require such tests are more likely to develop breast cancer. Fibrocystic breast disease, a term often used for "lumpy" breasts, is not a risk factor.

- **Race.** Breast cancer rates are lower in Hispanic and Asian populations than in whites, but higher in African-American women up to age 50. In postmenopausal African-American women, rates are lower. Nonetheless, African-American women are still more likely to die of breast cancer than whites. Scientists don't know if that's because they don't have equal access to care, if they don't get optimal care, or if the disease itself is more aggressive in black women.

- **Occupation.** Based on two decades of following more than a million women, Swedish researchers have developed a list of jobs linked with a high risk of breast cancer. These include pharmacists, certain types of teachers, school masters, systems analysts and programmers, telephone operators, telegraph and radio operators, metal platers and coaters, and beauticians.[31]

- **Estrogen.** The role of estrogen replacement as a cancer risk factor remains controversial.[32] Some studies have documented an increase in certain types of breast cancer in women who have used hormone replacement therapy (HRT) for more than five years.[33] Some experts feel that HRT's other benefits in protecting women from heart disease and osteo-

porosis outweigh these risks and that the failure of well-designed epidemiological studies conducted over the last 25 years to confirm a risk indicates that the dangers, if they exist, are not great.[34]

The development of selective estrogen receptor modulators (SERMs) has revolutionized the medical view of hormones and their role in breast cancer. As noted earlier, the "designer estrogens" tamoxifen and raloxifene may prevent breast cancer in healthy women at increased risk for the disease. However, recent studies have shown that after five years, women develop a resistance to tamoxifen's effect. Some women at especially high risk for breast cancer have undergone mastectomy to remove the breast tissue at risk for developing cancer. Most of these women say they are satisfied that they took this radical step.[35]

Detection. To detect lumps or changes that could signal breast cancer, all women should perform monthly breast self-exams seven to ten days after their periods (see Figure 14-8) and have a professional breast exam yearly if over 40 and every three years if between ages 20 and 40.

The best tool for early detection is the diagnostic X-ray exam called **mammography.** Overall, screening mammograms could reduce breast cancer deaths by 25 percent. Mammograms can detect a tumor two to three years before it can be detected by manual exam (see Figure 14-9). According to a recent report, annual mammography for women in their forties is more cost-effective than Pap smear tests for cervical cancer and installation of airbags and seat belts in vehicles. The annual cost of mammography screening for women aged 40 to 49 is $9,000 per year of life saved, compared with $12,000 for cervical cancer screening, is $12,000 and $32,000 for seat belt and airbag installation.[36] The ACS, AMA, and the National Cancer Society recommend that all women begin routine mammographic screening by age 40. Other new diagnostic methods, including digital ultrasound (computerized enhancement of images created with high-frequency sound waves), magnetic resonance imaging, and minimally invasive biopsy technique, are improving the odds of early detection.[37]

Treatments. Breast cancer can be treated with surgery, radiation, and drugs (chemotherapy and hormonal therapy). Doctors may use one of these options or a combination, depending on the type and location of the cancer and whether the disease has spread.

Most women undergo some type of surgery. **Lumpectomy** or breast-conserving surgery removes only the cancerous tissue and a surrounding margin of normal tissue. A modified radical mastectomy includes the entire breast and some of the underarm lymph

Looking

Stand in front of a mirror with your upper body unclothed. Look for changes in the shape and size of the breast, and for dimpling of the skin or "pulling in" of the nipples. Any changes in the breast may be made more noticeable by a change in position of the body or arms. Look for any of the above signs or for changes in shape from one breast to the other.

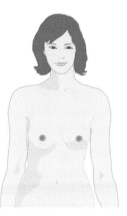
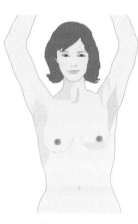
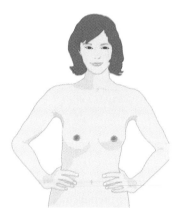

1. Stand with your arms down.

2. Raise your arms overhead.

3. Place your hands on your hips and tighten your chest and arm muscles by pressing firmly.

Feeling

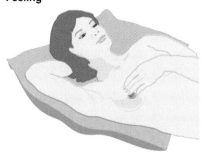
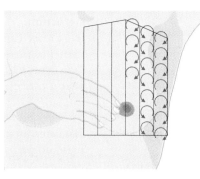
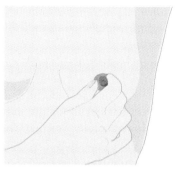

1. Lie flat on your back. Place a pillow or towel under one shoulder, and raise that arm over your head. With the opposite hand, you'll feel with the pads, not the fingertips, of the three middle fingers, for lumps or any change in the texture of the breast or skin.

2. The area you'll examine is from your collarbone to your bra line and from your breastbone to the center of your armpit. Imagine the area divided into vertical strips. Using small circular motions (the size of a dime), move your fingers up and down the strips. Apply light, medium, and deep pressure to examine each spot. Repeat this same process for your other breast.

3. Gently squeeze the nipple of each breast between your thumb and index finger. Any discharge, clear or bloody, should be reported to your doctor immediately.

■ Figure 14-8 **Breast Self-Exam**
The best time to examine your breasts is after your menstrual period every month.

nodes. Radical **mastectomy,** in which the breast, lymph nodes, and chest wall muscles under the breast are removed, is rarely performed today because modified radical mastectomy has proven just as effective. Removing underarm lymph nodes is important to determine if the cancer has spread, but a new method, sentinel node biopsy, allows physicians to pinpoint the first lymph node into which a tumor drains (the sentinel node), and remove only the nodes most likely to contain cancer cells.

Radiation therapy is treatment with high-energy rays or particles given to destroy cancer. In almost all cases, lumpectomy is followed by six to seven weeks of radiation. Chemotherapy is used to reach cancer cells that may have spread beyond the breast—in many cases even if no cancer is detected in the lymph nodes after surgery.

The use of the drugs paclitaxe (Taxol) or docetaxel (Taxotere), which inhibit cell division, in addition to standard chemotherapy, can significantly lower the risk of recurrence. A new "biotherapy"—a monoclonal antibody that zeros in on cancer cells like a miniature guided missile—also has shown promise against some aggressive breast tumors. The drug Herceptin targets a defective growth-promoting gene known as HER-2/neu, found in about 30 percent of women with breast cancer. The combination of Herceptin and standard chemotherapy has significantly improved survival rates in women with this gene.

Preliminary finding of studies of bone marrow transplantation for women with breast cancer indicate that this treatment may not improve survival odds any more than traditional therapy.[38] More than 12,000

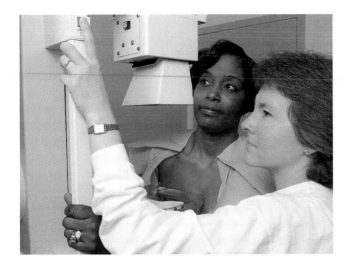

■ **Figure 14-9** This comparison of cancer sizes found by various breast-cancer detection methods shows the difference between mammography and other methods. Mammography, a diagnostic X-ray technique, is able to detect a lump that is much smaller than what a woman can find with regular breast self-exams.

Cancer calcifications of this size and smaller can be seen on mammograms.

Average-size lump found by mammogram.

Average-size lump found by women practicing frequent breast self-exam.

Smallest-size cancer that can be felt by physician's palpation exam.

Average-size lump found by women practicing occasional breast self-exam.

women have had bone marrow transplants; many have had to battle their insurance companies to pay for this costly therapy.

Although treatment is initially successful for many women, breast cancer returns in about 50 percent of cases. The "SERMs" tamoxifen and raloxifene, as discussed earlier, can lower the recurrence rate in women with early breast cancer by 50 to 66 percent.

Cervical Cancer

An estimated 12,800 cases of invasive cervical cancer are diagnosed in the United States every year, with about 4,800 annual deaths from this disease. The highest incidence rate occurs among Vietnamese women; Alaska Native, Korean, and Hispanic women also have higher rates than the national average. The mortality rate for African-American women is more than twice that of whites, largely because of a high number of deaths among older black women.

The primary risk factor for cervical cancer is infection with certain types of the human papillomavirus (HPV), discussed in Chapter 12. However, not every HPV infection becomes cervical cancer, and while HPV infection is very common, cervical cancer is not.

Other risk factors for cervical cancer include early age of first intercourse, multiple sex partners, genital herpes, and significant exposure to passive smoking. The standard screening test for cervical cancer is the Pap smear (described in Chapter 11). Each year this test detects about 1.2 million cases of abnormal cell growth. Since Pap tests were introduced, the death rate from cervical cancer has decreased by 70 percent. However, they can fail to detect cancerous cells in as many as 20 to 40 percent of the women tested.[39] An estimated 5 to 10 percent of Pap smears require some follow-up.[40]

Warning signs for cervical cancer include irregular bleeding or unusual vaginal discharge. In precancerous stages, cervical cells may be destroyed by laser surgery or freezing in a doctor's office.

In 1999 the National Cancer Institute called for a change in the way physicians treat invasive cervical cancer and recommended a combination of chemotherapy and radiation rather than the standard use of radiation alone. In clinical studies, women with moderately advanced disease who simultaneously received chemotherapy and radiation reduced their risk of dying of these tumors by 30 to 50 percent. For women whose cervical cancer is detected early, a biopsy or hysterectomy remains the standard treatment.[41]

Ovarian Cancer

Ovarian cancer is the leading cause of death from gynecological cancers, with 25,200 new cases diagnosed and 14,500 deaths each year. Risk factors include a family history of ovarian cancer; personal history of breast cancer; obesity; infertility (because the abnormality that interferes with conception may also play a role in cancer development); and low levels of transferase, an enzyme involved in the metabolism of dairy foods. Often women develop no obvious symptoms until the advanced stages, although they may experience painless swelling of the abdomen; irregular bleeding; lower abdominal pain; digestive and urinary abnormalities; fatigue; backache; bloating; and weight gain.

The lifetime risk of ovarian cancer in a woman with no affected relatives is 1 in 70. The risk for a woman with one first-degree relative with ovarian cancer is 1 in 20, and the risk increases with additional affected relatives. For women who may have a hereditary ovarian cancer syndrome and have mutations in BRCA-1 or BRCA-2, the lifetime risk may be as high as 1 in 2. Routine screening is not recommended for women who are not at known risk. For those at increased risk, an NIH consensus panel has recommended annual pelvic and rectal exams, and ultrasound imaging of the pelvic region and a blood test for a substance called CA125 every six months. In cases of very high risk, some oncologists (cancer specialists) recommend prophylactic removal of the ovaries when childbearing is completed or by no later than age 35. Treatment involves surgery, radiation therapy, and chemotherapy.

Colon and Rectal Cancer

Colon and rectal cancer accounts for 10 percent of cancer deaths. Most cases occur after age 50; African Americans and men are more likely to develop and die of colon cancer.[42] Risk factors include a personal or family history of colon and rectal cancer, polyps (growths) in the colon or rectum, and ulcerative colitis (described later in this chapter). Early signs of colorectal cancer are bleeding from the rectum, blood in the stool, or a change in bowel habits.

The simplest test for this common cancer—the Fecal Occult Blood Test—detects blood in a person's stool. According to the Congressional Office of Technology Assessment, such tests, which cost only about $4, could prevent 23,000 cancers a year among those aged 65 or older.[43] The other standard screening tests for colon cancer are a digital rectal exam, which should be performed annually after age 40, a stool blood slide test that detects blood in feces (recommended every year after age 50), proctosigmoidoscopy, which involves inserting a fiber-optic tube for visual inspection of the colon and rectum (recommended every three to five years after age 50) and colonoscopy, a similar test that uses a longer tube to visualize the entire colon.

Treatment may involve surgery, radiation therapy, or chemotherapy. Regular exercise can lower the risk of colon and rectal cancer in both men and women. Hormone replacement after menopause may significantly reduce women's risk of colon cancer.

Prostate Cancer

Prostate cancer is the most frequently diagnosed nonskin cancer among American men, with an estimated 179,000 new cases each year. African-American men have the highest rate of prostate cancer in the world; their death rate from this cancer is twice that of white men.[44]

The risk of prostate cancer increases with age, family history, exposure to the heavy metal cadmium, high number of sexual partners, and history of frequent sexually transmitted diseases. An inherited predisposition may account for 5 to 10 percent of cases.[45]

Several studies exploring a link between vasectomy and prostate cancer have produced conflicting results. In a recent investigation, men over age 55 who had had a vasectomy were at no greater risk for prostate cancer than men who had not had one. Men under age 55 who had prostate cancer were nearly twice as likely to have had a vasectomy as men under 55 who did not have cancer. However, researchers speculate that this finding may have been a statistical fluke, since it seems unlikely that vasectomy, a surgical procedure with permanent effects, would increase the risk only in younger men.

The development of a simple screening test that measures levels of a protein called prostate-specific antigen (PSA) in the blood has revolutionized the diagnosis of prostate cancer. Although PSA testing has proven more accurate than previous methods in detecting prostate cancers at early stages, it has created an ethical dilemma for physicians. Because PSA also can be elevated in men with a benign condition called prostatic hyperplasia, the test can indicate cancer where none exists.

In addition, there seem to be different forms of the cancer—some aggressive and deadly, some "low grade" and slow moving. Among men older than age 70, life expectancy without treatment is nearly identical to survival following definitive treatments. Many older men with low-grade prostate cancer may expect a normal life span without undergoing potentially debilitating surgery or radiation.

Men whose brothers or fathers had the disease and African Americans should begin getting tested at age 40. All men over age 50 should also undergo an annual rectal examination, in which a doctor inserts a gloved finger into the rectum and feels the prostate for abnormal growths that may indicate cancer. As noted above, a chemoprevention trial is looking at the possible preventive benefits of Proscar (finasteride), a drug used to treat benign swelling of the prostate, a common problem in aging men.

Early warning signs of prostate cancer are frequent or difficult urination, blood in the urine, painful ejaculation, or constant lower-back pain. Treatments include surgical removal of the prostate, conventional radiation, implanting "seeds" of radioactive iodine in the prostate, and hormone therapy to suppress testosterone. Recent studies have shown that, in most men, prostate cancer does not progress after surgery.[46] Another treatment, cryosurgery, has been used for men with prostate cancer who are not helped by radiation therapy. Its long-term effects are unclear. Short-term postoperative complications include incontinence, impotence, and obstructive urinary symptoms.[47]

Testicular Cancer

In the last 20 years the incidence of testicular cancer has risen 51 percent in the United States—from 3.61 to 5.44 per 100,000. About 7,400 men were diagnosed with the disease in 1999. It is not clear why testicular cancer may be on the rise, although researchers speculate that changing environmental or socioeconomic risk factors could have a role.[48] Testicular cancer occurs mostly among young men between the ages of 18 and 35, who are not normally at risk of cancer. At highest risk are men with an undescended testicle (a condition that is almost always corrected in childhood to prevent this danger). To detect possibly cancerous growths, men should perform monthly testicular self-exams, as shown in Figure 14-10.

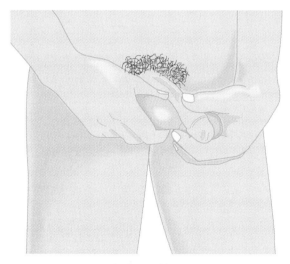

■ **Figure 14-10** **Testicular Self-Exam**
The best time to examine your testicles is after a hot bath or shower, when the scrotum is most relaxed. Place your index and middle fingers under each testicle and the thumb on top, and roll the testicle between the thumb and fingers. If you feel a small, hard, usually painless lump or swelling, or anything unusual, consult a urologist.

Often the first sign of this cancer is a slight enlargement of one testicle. There also may be a change in the way it feels when touched. Sometimes men with testicular cancer report a dull ache in the lower abdomen or groin, along with a sense of heaviness or sluggishness. Lumps on the testicles also may indicate cancer.

A man who notices any abnormality should consult a physician. If a lump is indeed present, a surgical biopsy is necessary to find out if it is cancerous. If the biopsy is positive, a series of tests generally is needed to determine whether the disease has spread. Treatment for testicular cancer generally involves surgical removal of the diseased testis, sometimes along with radiation therapy, chemotherapy, and the removal of nearby lymph nodes. The remaining testicle is capable of maintaining a man's sexual potency and fertility. Only in rare cases is removal of both testicles necessary. Testosterone injections following such surgery can maintain potency. The chance for a cure is very high if testicular cancer is spotted early.

Leukemia

Risk factors for this cancer of the blood include Down syndrome and other inherited abnormalities and excessive exposure to radiation or certain chemicals, such as benzene. Leukemia can be difficult to detect early because its symptoms are often similar to those of less serious conditions, such as influenza. Diagnosis is based on blood tests and a bone-marrow biopsy. Treatment may involve chemotherapy, drugs, blood transfusions, and bone-marrow transplants.

Lung Cancer

Cigarettes cause most cases of lung cancer, which is the leading cause of cancer deaths in women and the second leading cause in men. Risk factors include smoking for 20 or more years; exposure to certain industrial substances, particularly asbestos; passive smoking; radiation or radon exposure, and environmental tobacco smoke. A smoker's risk of developing lung cancer drops almost to that of a nonsmoker within ten years after his or her last cigarette, although the lungs may still be damaged.

Warning signs include a persistent cough, sputum streaked with blood, chest pain, recurring bronchitis, or pneumonia. Diagnosis is based on a chest X-ray, sputum cytology (cell) testing, and fiber-optic bronchoscopy (direct examination of the lungs by means of a specially lighted tube). The use of CT scans, which can detect tiny tumors, can lead to earlier diagnosis and might improve survival rates from 15 percent to up to 80 percent.[49] Treatment generally involves surgery, chemotherapy, and/radiation.

Oral Cancer

Heavy smoking of cigarettes, cigars, or pipes; excessive drinking; and the use of chewing tobacco increase the risk of oral cancer. Those who drink as well as smoke are particularly vulnerable. Early signs include a mouth sore that bleeds easily and doesn't heal; a lump or thickening; a reddish or whitish patch; and difficulty chewing, swallowing, or moving the tongue or jaws. Regular exams by your dentist or primary care physician can detect oral cancers. Surgery and radiation are the standard treatments.

New Hope Against Cancer

A variety of treatments, described below, have had a dramatic effect on improving the prognosis and decreasing mortality rates for most major cancers. However, cancer therapy remains a challenging experience for patients and their families, and many turn to unproven alternative therapies. (See Consumer Health Watch: "Alternative Cancer Treatments.") Conventional cancer therapies now include:

- *Surgery* to remove a tumor and surrounding cells. The oldest and most widely used approach, surgery is most effective for small, localized cancers.
- *Radiation therapy,* which exposes the involved area of the body to powerful radiation, which destroys cancer cells. Radiation therapy is sometimes used as an adjuvant, or supplementary, treatment along with surgery or chemotherapy.
- *Chemotherapy,* which uses powerful drugs or hormones, taken orally or through injection, to interfere with the reproduction of fast-multiplying cancer cells.
- *Angiogenesis Inhibitors,* Angiogenesis is the process by which new blood vessels form. Solid tumors cannot grow beyond the size of a pinhead without new blood vessels to supply their nutritional needs. By using drugs that inhibit or block the development of new blood vessels, researchers are hoping to cut off a tumor's supply of oxygen and nutrients, and therefore its ability to grow and spread to other parts of the body. About 20 angiogenesis inhibitors are currently being tested in human trials.[50]
- *Immunotherapy,* which stimulates the body's own immune system to attack cancer cells. One approach uses biological response modifiers (BRMs), substances normally produced by the immune system in small amounts to fight infection. The most commonly used BRMs include interferons (proteins produced by cells to resist viruses) and interleukins (proteins released by certain white blood cells to support the growth of others). A related approach uses monoclonal antibodies (made by combining a cancer cell with an antibody forming cell) that can target and kill cancer cells without damaging healthy cells.[51]

Consumer Health Watch

Alternative Cancer Treatments

About one-third of cancer patients use alternative medicine, such as meditation, reflexology, herbal medicine, food supplements, or homeopathy. None of these can cure cancer, but some may help ease patient suffering when used to complement mainstream treatments. Nonetheless, alternative therapies that are overused or used in lieu of mainstream treatments may be dangerous to a patient's health. Here's what to keep in mind when evaluating unconventional treatments for cancer:

- Special diets, especially those rich in high-antioxidant foods, may help prevent cancer. No diet can cure cancer.
- Vitamins, even in very high doses, cannot cure cancer. Excessive amounts of vitamins and minerals can be harmful and may even speed tumor growth.
- Over-the-counter herbal remedies for cancer can be contaminated or diluted with useless leaves.

- Detoxification regimens, such as high colonic irrigation to remove toxins thought to cause cancer, can be dangerous and have resulted in infection and death.
- Among the alternative therapies that can decrease pain and improve the quality of a cancer patient's life are relaxation techniques, massage, and aromatherapy.
- Patients should never put their trust in an alternative practitioner who encourages them to avoid or stop conventional cancer therapy.
- Many web sites offering cancer information, particularly about unproven or alternative therapies, are unreliable. Always check to be sure the web site creators are clearly identified, that their credential are reputable, and that the posting date is recent.

Bone-marrow transplantation involves extremely high doses of radiation or, increasingly, chemotherapy to kill cancer cells; however, the marrow in the patient's body is also destroyed. The patient then receives healthy bone-marrow cells, either his or her own (which may have undergone treatment in a laboratory) or a carefully matched donor's. *Autologous* transplants (those using the person's own blood) have produced long-term survival rates of more than 50 percent for certain leukemias and lymphomas (cancer of the immune system). They're also being used experimentally in treating other cancers, including breast and ovarian tumors. Most patients with leukemia and other life-threatening cancers who survive the initial recovery period following bone marrow transplants have survival rates that approach that of the general population.[52]

Cancer treatments affect normal, healthy cells as well as cancerous ones. Most vulnerable to radiation and chemotherapy are the fastest-growing body cells: hair cells, cells of the gastrointestinal tract, cells in the reproductive organs, and cells of the blood-producing tissue, the bone marrow.

Promising advances in cancer treatment that may save lives in the future include new and more powerful forms of chemotherapy and adding immunotherapy agents to standard anticancer drugs to make chemotherapy more effective. Researchers are also experimenting with **gene therapy,** the insertion of genes into a patient, as a possible cancer treatment, and with the development of cancer vaccines.

About 30 to 50 percent of those undergoing treatment for a tumor and 70 to 90 percent of those with advanced cancer suffer chronic pain. Here, too, there has been great progress. The World Health Organization and national and international medical organizations have launched campaigns to educate doctors so they can assess pain more precisely and provide much greater pain relief to cancer patients.[53]

Using the Mind to Help the Body

The powers of the mind can be a powerful resource for cancer patients. In fact, knowledge itself can be powerful. According to recent studies, cancer patients who participate in educational programs that explain their disease and treatment have significantly higher survival rates. Support groups also affect both the quality and quantity of life. Patients with melanoma who attended support groups did much better both on psychological tests and on measures of tumor-fighting immune cells. Melanoma patients with strong religious and spiritual beliefs also were able to cope with their illness better and to view it in a positive, meaningful way.[54]

In another landmark study, women with metastatic breast cancer who participated in weekly support groups reported less depression, anxiety, fatigue, and pain and greater self-esteem than women who received standard medical care. Participation in the groups, which focused on the psychological impact of cancer, doctor-patient issues, and pain control, also doubled their survival times. Average survival time for group members was 36.6 months from diagnosis, compared to 18.9 months for those in the control group.

Cancer Survivorship

Cancer survivors make up one of the fastest growing groups in the American population. Many have had no evidence of cancer for years; others are in remission, a state in which the spread of cancerous cells is presumed to be temporarily stopped. But for millions of men, women, and children who "win" their battle against cancer, survival, even when they live past the milestone five-year mark, does not mark the end of their cancer experience.

Many cancer survivors encounter difficulties that often persist for years after initial diagnosis and treatment. These include physical problems, such as pain and fatigue, that can stem from the cancer itself or from cancer treatments. Sexual problems are a common consequence, affecting as many as 50 percent of women surviving breast and gynecologic cancers and as many as 70 percent of men surviving prostate cancer. Coping with cancer also causes psychological and emotional difficulties that can lead to depression, posttraumatic stress disorder, and profound fear of recurrence. Another source of anxiety is the cost of medical treatments, which, along with the loss of wages or a job, can be financially devastating.

Cancer survivors also are at risk of another bout with cancer. Of the 1.4 million new cancer cases diagnosed each year, almost 100,000 are second cancers. Patients surviving one cancer have almost twice the risk of developing a second cancer as the general population has of developing an initial cancer. Children under age 15 who have survived cancer have eight times the risk.[55]

Diabetes Mellitus

About 100 million people around the world—including an estimated 14 million people in the United States—have **diabetes mellitus,** a disease in which the body doesn't produce or respond properly to insulin, a hormone essential for daily life. In those who have diabetes, the pancreas, which produces insulin (the hormone that regulates carbohydrate and fat metabolism) doesn't function as it should. When the pancreas either stops producing insulin or doesn't produce sufficient insulin to meet the body's needs, almost every body system can be damaged.

 ## What Is Diabetes?

Glucose is the primary form of sugar that the body cells use for energy. When a healthy person eats a meal, the level of glucose in the blood rises, triggering the production and release of insulin by special cell clusters in the pancreas called the islets of Langerhans. Insulin enhances the movement of glucose into various body cells, bringing down the level of glucose in the blood. In those who have diabetes, however, insulin secretion is either nonexistent (referred to as Type 1 or *insulin-dependent diabetes*) or deficient (referred to as Type 2 or *non-insulin-dependent diabetes*). Without sufficient insulin, the glucose in the blood is unable to enter most body cells, so the cells' energy needs aren't met. The levels of glucose in the blood rise higher and higher after each meal. This unused glucose eventually passes through the kidneys, which are unable to process the excessive glucose, and out of the body in urine.

Deprived of the fuel it needs, the body begins to break down stored fat as a source of energy. This process produces weak acids, called ketones. A buildup of ketones leads to ketoacidosis, an upheaval in the body's chemical balance that brings on nausea, vomiting, abdominal pain, lethargy, and drowsiness. Severe ketoacidosis can lead to coma and eventual death.

An estimated 5.4 million adults in the United States have undiagnosed diabetes. Type 2 diabetes, the most prevalent form of the disease, often causes no symptoms for many years. In order to identify individuals with this disease as early as possible, the American Diabetes Association now recommends screening every three years for all men and women beginning at age 45. Those at highest risk include relatives of diabetics (whose risk is two and a half times that of others); obese persons (85 percent of diabetics are or were obese); older persons (four out of five diabetics are over age 45); and mothers of large babies, because this is an indication of maternal prediabetes. A child of two parents with Type 2 diabetes faces an 80 percent likelihood of also becoming diabetic.

The prevalence of Type 2 diabetes has been increasing steadily in the United States, along with a nationwide increase in obesity. While obesity in middle age is a well-known risk factor for the development of Type 2 diabetes, recent studies in men have shown that being overweight at age 25 also is a strong predictor of diabetes risk in middle age.[56]

The early signs of diabetes are frequent urination, excessive thirst, a craving for sweets and starches, and weakness. Diagnosis is based on tests of the sugar level in the blood. Researchers are working to develop a test that would help identify telltale antibodies in the blood which could indicate that pancreas cells are being destroyed years before the first signs of diabetes.

The Dangers of Diabetes

Before the development of insulin injections, diabetes was a fatal illness. Today diabetics may have normal life spans. However, both types of diabetes can lead to devastating complications, including increased risk of heart attack or stroke, kidney failure, blindness, and loss of circulation to the extremities. Although few people realize it, diabetes claims more than 100,000 women's lives a year—more than the number who succumb to breast cancer.

Diabetic women who become pregnant face higher risks of miscarriage and serious birth defects; however, precise control of blood sugar levels before conception and in early pregnancy can lower the likelihood of these problems. The development of diabetes during pregnancy—called gestational diabetes—may pose potentially serious health threats to mother and child years later. Women who develop gestational diabetes are more than three times as likely to develop Type II diabetes if they have a second pregnancy; their infants may be at increased risk of cardiovascular disease later in life.

Strategies *for* Prevention

Lowering the Risk of Diabetes

✓ Eat a diet rich in complex carbohydrates (bread and other starches) and high-fiber foods, and low in sodium and fat.

✓ Eat fruits and vegetables that are rich in antioxidants, substances that prevent oxygen damage to cells.

✓ Avoid alcohol.

✓ Keep your weight down. Weight loss for those who are overweight can sometimes decrease or eliminate the need for insulin or oral drugs. For individuals at high risk of developing non-insulin-dependent diabetes, losing just half the pounds needed to reach their ideal weight can prevent the onset of the disease.

✓ Exercise regularly. Regular, vigorous aerobic activity reduces the risk of non-insulin-dependent diabetes in men and women.

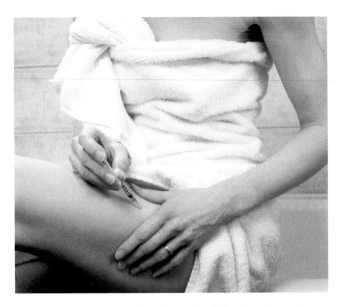

Many diabetics control their disease by injecting themselves with insulin.

Diabetes and Ethnic Minorities

Several minority groups, especially African Americans, Native Americans, and Latinos, are at high risk of developing diabetes. One in every ten African Americans and Latinos has this disease. And the members of some Native-American tribes are 300 percent more likely to develop diabetes than the general population. For many, obesity and unhealthy food choices increase the risk. Researchers now believe that the interaction of environmental factors and genes varies among different racial and ethnic groups.

Treatments for Diabetes

There's no cure for diabetes at this time. The best treatment option is to keep blood sugar levels as stable as possible to prevent complications, such as kidney damage. Home glucose monitoring allows diabetics to check their blood sugar levels as many times a day as necessary and to adjust their diet or insulin doses as appropriate.

Those with insulin-dependent diabetes require daily doses of insulin via injections, an insulin infusion pump, or oral medication. Those with non-insulin-dependent diabetes can control their disease through a well-balanced diet, exercise, and weight management. However, insulin therapy may be needed to keep blood glucose levels near normal or normal, thereby reducing the risk of damage to the eyes, nerves, and kidneys.

Medical advances hold out bright hopes for diabetics. Laser surgery, for instance, is saving eyesight. By-

pass operations are helping restore blood flow to the heart and feet. Dialysis machines and kidney and pancreas transplants save many lives. Researchers are exploring various approaches to prevention, including early low-dose insulin therapy, oral insulin to correct immune intolerance, and immunosuppressive drugs. Still on the horizon is the promise of a true cure through transplanting insulin-producing cells from healthy pancreases. In very preliminary trials, this procedure has helped patients become insulin-independent, at least temporarily.

Other Major Illnesses

Other noninfectious diseases besides cancer and diabetes have a debilitating effect on many people. But most of the diseases discussed in this section can be controlled, if not cured.

Epilepsy and Seizure Disorders

About 10 percent of all Americans will have at least one seizure at some time. Between 0.5 and 1 percent of all Americans have recurrent seizures. Derived from the Greek word for seizure, **epilepsy** is the term used to refer to a variety of neurological disorders characterized by sudden attacks (seizures) of violent muscle contractions and unconsciousness. Epilepsy is rarely fatal; the primary danger to life is to suffer an attack while driving or swimming.

Seizures can be major, referred to as *grand mal;* minor, referred to as *petit mal;* or psychomotor. In a grand-mal seizure, the person loses consciousness, falls to the ground, and experiences convulsive body movements. Petit-mal seizures are brief, characterized by a loss of consciousness for 10 to 30 seconds, by eye or muscle flutterings, and occasionally by a loss of muscle tone. About 90 percent of all epileptics have grand-mal seizures; 40 percent suffer both petit-mal and grand-mal seizures. The frequency of attacks defines the severity of the epilepsy. Diagnosis is based on a history of recurring attacks and a study of the brain's electrical activity, called an electroencephalogram (EEG).

About half of all cases of epilepsy have no known cause and are therefore classified as *idiopathic.* All others stem from conditions that affect the brain, such as trauma, tumors, congenital malformations, or inflammation of the membranes covering the brain. Idiopathic epilepsy usually begins between the ages of 2 and 14. Seizures before age 2 are usually related to developmental defects, birth injuries, or a metabolic disease affecting the brain. (Fever-induced convulsions are not related to epilepsy.) Seizures after age 14 are generally symptoms of brain disease or injury.

Seizure disorders don't reflect or affect intellectual or psychological soundness; people who suffer from them have normal intelligence. Therapy with anticonvulsant drugs can control seizures in most people, and once seizures are under control, epileptics can live full, normal lives by continuing to take their medications. However, about 10 to 20 percent of the 120,000 people who develop epilepsy every year continue to have seizures despite medical therapy. Technological advances have allowed doctors to identify more accurately where seizures originate in the brain; and surgery, though risky and expensive, is offering new hope to many epileptics.

If you're with a person who suffers a grand-mal seizure, make sure he or she isn't injured during the attack. Don't try to restrain the person or interfere with his or her movements, and don't try to force anything into the person's mouth. Medical treatment usually isn't needed unless the seizure lasts more than a couple of minutes or is almost immediately followed by another.

Respiratory Diseases

Asthma

Asthma is a disease characterized by constriction of the breathing passages. As with allergy, asthma rates have skyrocketed in the last two decades. Since 1980 U.S. mortality rates have doubled, with asthma claiming the lives of 5,000 Americans every year. The problem is especially severe in inner cities, where emergency room visits and asthma mortality rates run as high as eight times the national average.

The Centers for Disease Control and Prevention (CDC) estimates that approximately 17 million people in the United States, or 6.4 percent of the population, say they have asthma. Between 1980 and 1994, the number of people self-reporting asthma grew 75 percent. Asthma prevalence is also increasing in many of the richer industrialized countries.[57]

While asthma is not always linked to allergy, the two are related. Among people with asthma, 90 percent of the children, 70 percent of young adults, and 50 percent of older adults also have allergies. According to epidemiologic research, 23 percent of youngsters diagnosed with allergies by age 1 develop asthma by age 6. Of those diagnosed after age 1, 13 percent eventually become asthmatic. Symptoms include wheezing, coughing, shortness of breath, and chest tightness. If the symptoms are untreated or undertreated, they can worsen and damage the lungs.[58]

The two main approaches to asthma treatment are control of the underlying inflammation by means of anti-inflammatory drugs, such as corticosteroids, cromolyn sodium, and neodocromil, and short-term relief of symptoms with bronchodilators, such as albuterol, which expand the breathing passages. In its most recent official guidelines, the National Heart, Lung and Blood Institute encouraged more frequent use of inhaled steroids and less reliance on bronchodilators, which have little effect on the underlying inflammation. In one major study, the use of inhaled steroids decreased the risk of hospitalization by 50 percent.[59]

Some new asthma medications, such as Accolate and Zyflo, directly target leukotriene, one of the chemicals involved in an inflammatory response. These drugs seem useful in cases of mild to moderate asthma, but specialists are still uncertain of exactly how they'll fit into long-term asthma management. Standard bronchodilator inhalers are being removed from the market because of the global ban on chlorofluorocarbons (CFCs), and new "environmentally friendly" inhalers are available.

Chronic Obstructive Lung Disease (COLD)

Chronic obstructive lung disease (COLD), also called chronic obstructive pulmonary disease (COPD), is characterized by progressively more limited flow of air into, and out of, the lungs. COLD consists of two separate but closely related conditions: chronic bronchitis and emphysema. Most COLD patients develop both forms. The major cause is cigarette smoking, although air pollution may also play a role. (See also Chapter 17.)

In chronic bronchitis, the bronchial passageways are constantly inflamed, and individuals develop a persistent, sputum-producing cough; shortness of breath; and wheezing. They must stop smoking, lose excess weight, exercise, and avoid or reduce contact with air pollutants.

Chronic bronchitis can lead to emphysema, a deterioration of the lungs that may begin in adolescence. Eventually, the alveoli, tiny air sacs in the lungs, tear, reducing the lungs' ability to exhale. This condition can lead to heart failure.

Anemias

The **anemias** are diseases affecting the oxygen-carrying capacity of the blood. Usually there's a reduced number of red blood cells or a reduced amount of hemoglobin, the oxygen-carrying component of red blood cells. Anemia can be caused by nutritional inadequacies; loss of blood, including heavy menstrual bleeding; deficiencies in red-cell production; or genetic disorders. Iron-deficiency anemia is a form of anemia caused by a lack of dietary iron, an essential component of the hemoglobin molecule that carries oxygen. It's the most common form of anemia and often goes undiagnosed in women.

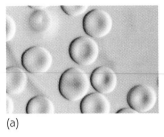 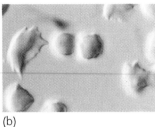

(a)   (b)

Sickle-cell anemia. (a) Normal mature red blood cells are disk-shaped and concave. (b) In sickle-cell anemia, the red blood cells are crescent-shaped and jagged, causing them to pile up and obstruct small blood vessels. Areas of the body are thus deprived of oxygen and nutrients.

- *Sickle-cell anemia* is a genetic blood disorder that occurs when the hemoglobin contained in the red blood cells is abnormal. The red blood cells become crescent or sickle-shaped and unable to supply oxygen to body tissues (see photos above). This disease causes crippling, severe pain, and premature death. About 8 to 10 percent of African Americans carry the gene for sickle-cell anemia.

- *Pernicious anemia* results from a lack of vitamin B-12 (cobalamine), which causes a deficiency in the formation of red blood cells. Although B-12 is usually present in the diet, some people lack a substance needed to absorb it into their blood. Injections of B-12 can control this condition.

- *Aplastic anemia,* most common in young adults and adolescents, interferes with the bone marrow's ability to form blood. Usually it results from ingesting a toxic agent, often a medication; symptoms include multiple internal hemorrhages. Whole-blood transfusions are the primary therapy, but the condition is usually fatal.

Noninfectious diseases of the respiratory system, including chronic bronchitis and emphysema, can also be causes of disability and death. (See Chapter 12 for the major infectious respiratory diseases, and Chapter 17 for smoking-induced problems.)

Liver Disorders

Cirrhosis is characterized by significant loss of liver cells and the formation of scar tissue that can interfere with circulation in the liver. The major cause of one of the most common forms of cirrhosis, Laennec's cirrhosis, is chronic alcoholism. Each year, about 30,000 Americans die of alcohol-related liver disorders. (See also Chapter 16.)

Early signs of liver damage include an enlarged liver (which your doctor can feel during a physical exam) and tiny, spiderlike blood vessels on the surface of the skin. Blood tests may show abnormal levels of certain enzymes, or enlarged red blood cells. Even people with advanced liver disease feel better and live longer once they've stopped drinking alcohol. Cirrhosis symptoms, which occur only in the advanced stages of the disease, include yellow discoloration of the skin and eyes (jaundice), accumulation of fluid in the abdomen, and mental confusion.

Liver transplants are the only hope for those with advanced liver disease. With improvements in surgical techniques and the use of antirejection drugs (including cyclosporin, a combination of cyclosporin and an antifungal medication, and a new drug called FK-506), 70 percent or more of liver-transplant recipients—including some in their sixties and seventies—now live for at least a year. Some liver transplant recipients have lived longer than 20 years.

Kidney Diseases

A wide range of diseases can affect the kidneys and their ability to process fluids and waste. Some are acute, temporary problems; others are chronic, progressive illnesses that permanently impair kidney function. (See Chapter 12 for a description of kidney infections.)

Nephrosis refers to a cluster of symptoms indicating chronic damage to the kidneys, including chronic proteinuria (the loss of more than one gram of protein a day in the urine), hypercholesteremia (high levels of fats in the blood), and edema (fluid retention). The kidney damage can be the result of diabetes, heavy metal poisoning, allergic reactions to insect stings, or other disorders.

Kidney stones may form either from calcium salts or from minerals (the causes are unknown). Most stones eventually pass out of the body in urine, which can be extremely painful. They don't usually obstruct the flow of urine or interfere with kidney function. However, infection can develop behind a stone. Larger stones can be surgically removed or painlessly shattered into harmless fragments by high-frequency sound waves.

The various chronic and inflammatory diseases of the kidney can all lead to kidney failure. A mechanical process of clearing waste fluids from the body, called *dialysis,* can do the kidneys' job temporarily. Another alternative is a kidney transplant, either from a living, related donor or from a cadaver whose kidney has been carefully tissue-matched to the recipient to minimize the risk of rejection. On average, a transplanted kidney continues to function for only nine years. Kidneys that came from cadaver donors are especially likely to deteriorate slowly but steadily. The anti-rejection drugs that transplant recipients must take may themselves cause side effects and impair the functioning of the new kidney over time. High blood pressure and high glucose and cholesterol levels also can be harmful.[60] A lack of organ donors remains a critical obstacle to performing more of these lifesaving operations.

Digestive Diseases

Most disorders of the digestive tract affect only one section: either the esophagus, the stomach and duodenum, the small intestine, the large intestine, the liver, the pancreas, the gallbladder, or the rectum. The most dangerous are Crohn's disease and ulcerative colitis. According to the National Digestive Diseases Advisory Board, almost half of the U.S. population will suffer a digestive problem at some time in their lives.

Ulcers

Open sores, often more than an inch wide, that develop in the lining of the stomach or the duodenum (the first part of the small intestine) are called **ulcers.** They are caused by excessive acidic digestive juices. The major symptom is a burning pain felt throughout the upper abdomen. The pain may come and go, lasting up to three hours. It may begin either right after eating or several hours later.

One in five men and one in ten women get ulcers of the stomach or duodenum, but the number of ulcers is declining. Risk factors include heavy use of cigarettes, alcohol, or caffeine; the ingestion of large amounts of painkillers that contain aspirin or ibuprofen; and advanced age. Bleeding is not common but may be dangerous, even life-threatening. An untreated stomach ulcer can lead to serious weight loss and anemia.

Researchers have identified a bacterium, *Helicobacter pylori,* or *H. pylori* (formerly named *Campylobacter*), that may infect the digestive system and set the stage for ulcers. According to various studies, most ulcer patients carry this organism. One theory is that infection leads to an inflammation of the stomach lining called gastritis, which increases vulnerability to other stressors, such as smoking, alcohol, or anxiety.

H. pylori can be detected in several ways. A blood test can reveal the presence of infection by detecting antibodies against *H. pylori.* However, a blood test can be positive even if someone has long been free of the bacteria. The most definitive test requires endoscopy, a procedure in which a physician examines the lining of the stomach or duodenum by passing a thin flexible tube (an endoscope) down the patient's throat and snips a small bit of tissue for laboratory analysis to detect bacteria. Researchers are experimenting with a simpler diagnostic breath test in which patients drink a special liquid that triggers a response by *H. pylori* bacteria in the stomach. Treatment with antibiotics leads to improvement in most patients.

Conventional therapy for ulcers includes self-help measures, such as avoiding aspirin; eating small, frequent meals; taking antacids; and not smoking or drinking alcohol or caffeine. Drugs such as cimetidine, ranitidine, and sucralfate can reduce the amount of acid produced by the stomach and relieve ulcer symptoms. If a stomach ulcer doesn't heal after six to eight weeks of drug treatment, physicians may recommend surgery to remove the ulcer.

Inflammatory Bowel Disease (IBD)

As many as 2 million Americans—many in the prime of life—suffer from one of the two forms of **inflammatory bowel disease (IBD):** *Crohn's disease,* which causes inflammation anywhere in the digestive tract, and *ulcerative colitis,* which creates severe ulcers in the inner lining of the colon and rectum. Both illnesses can trigger frequent and intense diarrhea, abdominal pain, gas, fever, and rectal bleeding.

The specific causes of IBD remain unknown, but scientists speculate that some irritating substance—perhaps a bacterium, virus, or chemical or environmental agent—somehow leaks through the intestine's thin lining into the bowel's deep inner wall. Inflammation develops, setting into motion a chain of harmful reactions by the body's protective immune system and causing swelling, pain, and damage to the intestinal wall. Ulcers (small perforations or holes) may form, exposing cells and tissues to destructive intestinal bacteria and enzymes. Blood and fluid from body tissues may leak into the intestines, showing up as diarrhea or blood in the stool. Twenty percent of cases involve a genetic or familial predisposition.

Treatment for IBD consists primarily of drugs, including powerful steroids, antibiotics, and medications that fight inflammation. Dietary changes can also help. Crohn's patients who don't improve on medication or who develop life-threatening complications, such as a severe intestinal blockage, may undergo surgery to remove or bypass the diseased part of the intestine and reconnect two healthy segments. However, the disease very often recurs in another part of the intestinal tract. For those with ulcerative colitis, removal of the entire colon brings an end to troubling symptoms—and to the increased risk of colon cancer that these individuals face. Most gastroenterologists advise patients with ulcerative colitis to undergo annual examinations of the colon (colonoscopies) to detect precancerous changes in cells.

Irritable Bowel Syndrome

Irritable bowel syndrome (also called irritable colon or spastic colon) is a common problem caused by intestinal spasms. The muscular contractions that move waste material through the intestines become irregular and uncoordinated, causing frequent feelings of a need to defecate, nausea, cramping, pain, gas, and a sensation that the rectum is never emptied.

Diagnostic tests, including X rays, stool samples, and examination of the colon with a sigmoidoscope, can rule out colon cancer and other problems. Travel, stress, changes in diet, and smoking often worsen these symptoms. Many people respond well to a high-fiber diet; others prefer a bland diet. There's no standard medical treatment for irritable bowel syndrome; some physicians prescribe stool softeners, laxatives, or drugs to reduce intestinal spasms.

Gallstones

An estimated 25 million Americans—about 10 percent of the population—have **gallstones:** clumps of solid material, usually cholesterol, that form in bile stored in the gallbladder. One-third to one-half of all gallstones produce no symptoms. However, some gallstones, carried out of the liver with bile, get stuck in the bile duct and cause intense pain that lasts for several hours. Ultrasound and special X rays called cholecystograms can detect gallstones.

During an attack of gallstone pain, a physician may recommend a painkiller. Some gallstones can be dissolved by long-term drug treatment. Another alternative to traditional gallbladder surgery is laparoscopic surgery, in which gallstones are removed without having to cut through the major abdominal muscles.

Disorders of the Muscles, Joints, and Bones

Because they're constantly being used, muscles, joints, and bones are more susceptible to damage from injury than are most other parts of the body.

Arthritis

More than 17 million people suffer from some form of **arthritis,** an inflammatory disease of the joints that takes over a hundred forms. Rheumatoid arthritis is an autoimmune disease in which the body attacks its own connective tissue; it's fairly common among younger people. Degenerative arthritis, or osteoarthritis, characterized by changes in bone tissue and cartilage, primarily at the joints, seems to be the result of normal wear and tear. Women are generally affected by arthritis three times more often than are men, until the seventh or eighth decade of life. Race and occupation don't seem to be factors; climate affects symptoms but not causes.

Aggressive treatment of arthritis pays off, but to be successful, early diagnosis before cartilage destruction

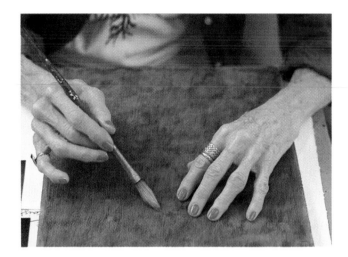

Those who suffer arthritis pain may tend to minimize movement in their joints, but moderate activity will help keep muscles functioning that stabilize the joints.

occurs is critical.[61] The most effective therapies include methotrexate and anti-inflammatory agents, which prevent or delay joint destruction. An educational arthritis self-help course can reduce physician visits by 40 percent and pain perception by about 20 percent. Relaxation training and cognitive-behavioral techniques also have proven highly effective in controlling arthritis pain.[62]

The goal of all treatments for arthritis is to maintain the patient's ability to function. Drugs can relieve pain and reduce inflammation; surgical treatments, including total joint replacement, and physical therapy are also used to maintain motion and strength, and to correct deformities.

Hernias

A **hernia** is a bulge of soft tissue that forces its way through or between strained or weakened muscles. Hernias can occur in many parts of the body, but they're most common in the abdominal wall. A surgeon can push the protruding tissue back into place and tighten or sew together the loose muscles.

Backaches

Back woes, which rank second only to headaches among modern miseries, eventually afflict seven of every ten adults. Anyone from a college athlete to a retired grandparent can suffer a back injury, but the risks increase with time as the deeper muscles and tendons surrounding the spine become less resilient. Yet age itself is rarely the only factor in a disabling back attack; almost always tense, injured, or weak muscles are to blame. Other risk factors include extra pounds, particularly if stuffed into a pot belly; lack of exercise;

Preventing Back Problems

✓ When standing, shift your weight from one foot to the other. If possible, place one foot on a stool, step, or railing 4 to 6 inches off the ground. Hold in your stomach, tilt your pelvis toward your back, and tuck in your buttocks to provide crucial support for the lower back.

✓ Because sitting places more stress on the lower back than standing, try to get up from your seat at least once an hour to stretch or walk around. Whenever possible, sit in a straight chair with a firm back. Avoid slouching in overstuffed chairs or dangling your legs in midair. When driving, keep the seat forward so that your knees are raised to hip level; your right leg should not be fully extended. A small pillow or towel can help support your lower back.

✓ Sleep on a flat, firm mattress. The best sleep position is on your side, with one or both knees bent at right angles to your torso. The pillow should keep your head in line with your body so that your neck isn't bent forward or to the side.

✓ When lifting, bend at the knees, not from the waist. Get close to the load. Tighten your stomach muscles, but don't hold your breath. Let your leg muscles do the work.

✓ Don't smoke. Smoking may interfere with circulation to the lower back; and a chronic smoker's cough can be so irritating that it provokes a back spasm.

poor posture; and bending from the waist to hoist a heavy load.

Strain from use or abuse accounts for 80 percent of back ailments. Most vulnerable is the lower, or lumbar, part of the spine, which bears the greatest pressure when bending and lifting. Five to 10 percent of back problems involve the discs between the vertebrae. Most common is the protrusion (or herniation) of the soft center of a disc through the casing so that it presses on spinal nerves. Another 10 percent of back problems involve structural defects, which may be the result of injuries, tumors, arthritis, congenital malformations, osteoporosis (the weakening of the bones), or scoliosis (side-to-side curving of the spine). Sometimes a sore back is a symptom of diseases of other organs, such as the kidneys, gallbladder, or stomach. A physical exam and various tests, including electrodiagnostic studies, X rays, CT scans, and MRIs (magnetic resonance imaging), may be necessary to pinpoint the problem.

Bed rest, supplemented by moist heat or other muscle relaxants and anti-inflammatory drugs, eases most backaches. However, the days when doctors advised two weeks of bed rest for a bad back are gone. After two or three days, most back patients are urged to get up, start walking, and resume light activity.

Back specialists tailor treatment programs to an individual's needs. Different forms of physical therapy—including specific exercises, massage, heat, ultrasound, and electrical stimulation—often relieve pain and speed recovery. Some people successfully use chiropractic, acupuncture, hypnosis, biofeedback, or relaxation techniques to cope with back pain. Regardless of treatment, more than 85 percent of back-injury patients get well within two weeks. Fewer than 2 percent eventually require surgery to repair a herniated disc.

Skin Disorders

Your skin is the largest organ of your body. Because of its visibility, none of its problems may seem trivial. The more serious skin diseases are discussed below. (See also the "A-to-Z Self-Care Guide" at the back of this book for a discussion of more common problems, such as acne and athlete's foot.)

Eczema and Dermatitis

Dermatitis is any inflammation of the skin. *Eczema*, a specific type of dermatitis usually caused by allergies, is a skin inflammation that results from internal processes. Symptoms of eczema include redness, flaking, blistering, and thickening of the skin. Self-help treatments include avoiding irritants, such as dishwater, and using steroid creams containing 0.5 percent hydrocortisone.

Psoriasis

In **psoriasis,** the rate of skin cell production is speeded up. As skin cells pile up faster than they can be shed, they produce scaly, deep-pink, raised patches on the skin. Triggers of psoriasis are stress, skin damage, and illness. Self-help measures include sunbathing or using ultraviolet light to clear up the psoriasis. Physicians usually prescribe ointments, creams, or pastes, including some steroid preparations, or ultraviolet treatment.

Special Needs for Different Abilities

About 49 million Americans have physical or mental impairments, including blindness, deafness, disorders of

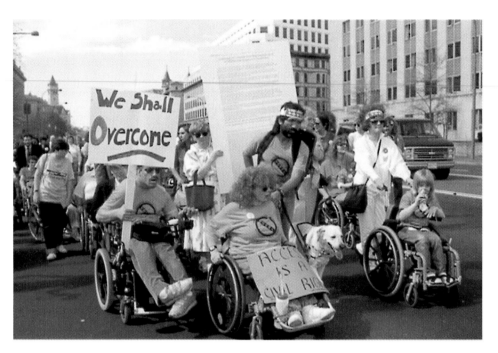

Disabled Americans have lobbied for changes in attitudes and for legislation that enables them to participate more fully in society.

Individuals with special needs face special challenges in their daily lives. Some are primarily physical, such as difficulty bathing, lifting groceries, opening cans and bottles, or going someplace. They also face many social and economic challenges. Because some people feel uncomfortable about disabilities, they may not treat individuals with special needs with the same acceptance and respect that they show to others. This can lead to discrimination from employers.

The Americans with Disabilities Act protects disabled people from discrimination by private employers, requires wheelchair access to public buildings and mass transportation, and orders telephone companies to provide telephone relay services that allow people with impaired speech or hearing to make and receive calls. Many states require insurers to provide coverage for high-risk individuals such as cancer survivors. The names of many of the organizations that help the disabled, such as the National Coalition for Cancer Survivorship and the National Council on Independent Living, are in "Your Health Directory" at the back of the book.

the muscles or nerves, paralysis, loss of limbs, or mental retardation, that substantially limit one or more major life activities. Most are the result of illnesses, such as strokes, arthritis, or heart disease, and affect the ability to walk, speak, or live independently. Some congenital disorders, such as cerebral palsy, cause speech problems, muscular weakness, and mental retardation. Accidents are responsible for other disabilities, including paralysis (see Chapter 18).

Individuals with special needs and abilities can live full, happy, and productive lives. Famous people who've made major contributions to the world despite disabilities include the composer Ludwig van Beethoven, who wrote some of his most famous music after becoming deaf; the inventor Thomas A. Edison, who was deaf throughout much of his life; and President Franklin D. Roosevelt, who became paralyzed in both legs at the age of 39.

Few such problems can be cured, but a great deal can be done to overcome them. **Rehabilitation medicine,** the specialty dedicated to improving the condition of the disabled, can provide treatments such as surgery for certain types of blindness or deafness, medications to ease the crippling pain of arthritis, and physical therapy, including special exercises to build up endurance and muscle strength. Mechanical devices, such as electric wheelchairs, artificial limbs, and hearing aids, can open up wider worlds to the disabled. Occupational therapy teaches skills to help the disabled gain confidence. Vocational training prepares them to find employment.

Making This Chapter Work for You

Staying Alive and Healthy

■ You can do a great deal to prevent or delay many serious illnesses, including the one we fear most: cancer. In all types of cancer, changes in the genetic material in the cells cause normal cells to turn into abnormal cells and multiply to form malignant tumors, or neoplasms. Benign tumors are not normally life-threatening. Hereditary, viral, chemical, and physical factors can cause malignant, or cancerous, tumors.

■ Prevention is the best approach to cancer. Lifestyle changes—including not smoking; limiting sun exposure; restricting alcohol intake; eating a high-fiber, low-fat diet; and exercising—can reduce the risk of developing cancer. Tamoxifen is the first "chemo-preventive" agent that has proven effective in lowering the risk of cancer in healthy people. Having regular cancer checkups, knowing the warning signs of cancer, and performing periodic self-exams can help identify potentially cancerous changes so that treatment can begin as early as possible.

■ Traditionally, cancer treatment includes some form or combination of chemotherapy (drug treatment), surgery, and radiation. Promising new developments in fighting cancer include more effective forms of treatment, such as powerful drug combinations, immunotherapy, and gene therapy. Psychological support can make a big difference in enhancing the quality and extending the quantity of life for cancer patients.

■ Diabetes mellitus is a serious medical problem in which the pancreas produces an insufficient amount of insulin, a hormone needed by the body's cells to metabolize glucose. Treatment for milder cases of diabetes is a carefully controlled diet; insulin is necessary in more severe cases.

■ Other major illnesses include epilepsy and seizure disorders, which can usually be controlled by medication or surgery.

■ A growing problem is asthma, which can be triggered by allergens, pollution, respiratory infections,

health / ONLINE

American Cancer Society
http://www.cancer.org/
This comprehensive site includes information about different types of cancer, treatments, prevention, and patient services.

Oncolink: University of Pennsylvania Cancer Center
http://www.oncolink.upenn.edu/
This site provides information about specific types of cancer, support for those living with cancer, answers to frequently asked questions, cancer prevention, and new treatments under evaluation.

Ask Noah: Health Topics and Resources
http://www.noah.cuny.edu/qksearch.html
ASK NOAH provides reliable information on a wide variety of health topics, including cancer, diabetes, arthritis, and asthma.

Please note that links are subject to change. If you find a broken link, use a search engine like http://www.yahoo.com *and search for the web site by typing in key words.*

 Campus Chat: In California, smoking is banned in all public places due to the health risks posed by secondhand smoke. Do you agree or disagree with this policy? Share your thoughts on our online discussion forum at **http://health.wadsworth.com**

Find It On InfoTrac: You can find additional readings related to cancer and other major diseases via InfoTrac College Edition, an online library of more than 900 journals and publications. Follow the instructions for accessing InfoTrac that came packaged with your textbook; then search for articles using a key word search.

• **Suggested reading:** "Cancer Cure is Elusive, but Therapies Hold Hope," by Ruth Larson. *Insight on the News*, August 16, 1999, Vol. 15, Issue 130, p. 26.

  (1) What is CGAP, and what is its goal?

  (2) List at least three different avenues researchers are exploring in the search for a cancer cure.

For additional links, resources, and suggested readings on InfoTrac, visit our Health & Wellness Resource Center at **http://health.wadsworth.com**

and stress; complications and death rates for asthma are rising. The symptoms of chronic bronchitis, a common disorder among smokers, include a persistent cough, shortness of breath, and wheezing. In emphysema, the air sacs in the lungs lose their elasticity, and the lungs become enlarged.

■ Other major diseases include anemia, liver disease, kidney disorders, digestive diseases, and disorders of the muscles, joints, and bones.

■ Physical and mental impairments, whether caused by congenital disorders, illnesses, or accidents, affect millions of Americans; but a great deal can often be done to overcome their effects.

 New Sunscreen Ratings. What are the new standards for sunscreen labels?

Key Terms

The terms listed here are used within the chapter. Page numbers are included for each term. A definition of each term is given in the Glossary pages at the end of this book.

anemia   464
arthritis   467
asthma   464
bone-marrow transplantation   461
carcinogen   451
chemoprevention   451
chronic obstructive lung disease
   (COLD)   464
cirrhosis   465
dermatitis   468
diabetes mellitus   461
epilepsy   463

gallstones   467
gene therapy   461
hernia   467
infiltration   444
inflammatory bowel disease (IBD)
   466
irritable bowel syndrome   466
kidney stones   465
lumpectomy   455
mammography   455
mastectomy   456
metastasize   444

neoplasm   444
nephrosis   465
oncogene   444
psoriasis   468
rehabilitation medicine   469
relative risk   447
tamoxifen   451
tumor suppressor genes   444
ulcer   466

Critical Thinking Questions

1. A friend of yours, Karen, discovered a small lump in her breast during a routine self-examination. When she mentions it, you ask if she has seen a doctor. She tells you that she hasn't had time to schedule an appointment; besides, she says she's not sure it's really the kind of lump one has to worry about. It's clear to you that Karen is in denial and procrastinating about seeing a doctor. What advice would you give her?

2. Do you know someone who is disabled? How do their lifestyle practices differ from your own? What is the effect of their health-care practices and behaviors on your own behavior?

3. Because of advances in antirejection treatment, organ transplants have proven highly successful in helping many people who otherwise might have died. Even elderly patients have clearly benefited from donated kidneys and livers. However, because the demand for organs to transplant greatly exceeds the supply, health experts have debated setting priorities. Should a 30-year-old be placed higher on the waiting list for a particular organ than a 70-year-old? Should a nurse who needs a liver because she contracted hepatitis on the job get priority over an alcoholic whose liver has been destroyed by cirrhosis? Who, if anyone, should make such decisions? Would a lottery be more fair?

References

1. "Cancer Survivorship." NCI Press Office, August 10, 1999.
2. "Cancer's Many Faces." *FDA Consumer,* Vol. 33, No. 4, July 1999.
3. "Gene Family May Regulate Important Biological Processes." *Cancer Weekly Plus,* July 12, 1999.
4. Brody, Jane. "Cancer Genes Tests Turn Out to Be Far from Simple." *New York Times,* August 17, 1999.
5. American Cancer Society.
6. Ibid.
7. "Cancer Rates and Mortality." *Journal of the National Cancer Institute,* Vol. 91, 1999.
8. "Cancer Survivorship."
9. "Cancer Facts and Figures—1999." American Cancer Society, 1999.
10. Brody, Jane. "Choosing to Test for Cancer's Genetic Link." *New York Times,* August 17, 1999.
11. "Cancer Facts and Figures—1999."
12. National Cancer Institute. "Human Papillomavirus." *Cancer Facts.* Bethesda, MD: National Institutes of Health.
13. Cooper, Dale, et al. "Dietary Carotenoids and Lung Cancer: A Review of Recent Research." *Nutrition Reviews,,* Vol. 57, No. 5, May 1999.
14. "Antioxidants: Separating Hope from Hype." *Harvard Health Letter,* Vol. 24, Issue 5, February 1999.
15. "A Prospective Study of Folate Intake and the Risk of Breast Cancer." *Cancer Weekly Plus,* June 14, 1999.
16. Holmes, Michelle, et al. "Association of Dietary Intake of Fat and Fatty Acids With Risk of Breast Cancer." *JAMA,* Vol. 281, No. 10, March 10, 1999.
17. Iribarren, Carlos. "The Effect of Cigar Smoking on the Risk of Cardiovascular Disease, Chronic Obstructive Pulmonary Disease, and Cancer in Men." *New England Journal of Medicine,* June 10, 1999.
18. "Cancer Facts and Figures—1999."
19. Stephenson, Joan. "Experts Debate Drugs for Healthy Women With Breast Cancer Risk." *JAMA,* Vol. 282, No. 2, July 14, 1999.
20. "Polynucleotide Vaccines for Colon Cancer and Melanoma." *Cancer Weekly Plus,* July 26, 1999.
21. American Cancer Society.
22. Glanz, Karen. "Children Benefit Most from Sun Safety Interventions." *Health Education & Behavior,* May 1999.
23. Dennis, Leslie. "Increasing Risk of Melanoma with Increasing Age." *JAMA,* September 15, 1999.
24. Callen, Jeffrey. "Acetinic Keratoses." Presentation, American Academy of Dermatology Press Conference, April 28, 1999.
25. "10 Rules to Save Your Skin." University of California, *Berkeley Wellness Letter,* Vol. 15, No. 9, June, 1999.
26. Leslie. "Increasing Risk of Melanoma with Increasing Age."
27. Eyre, Harmon. Personal interview.
28. Pettibone, Deborah. "Global Progress: Breast Cancer Mortality Rates." Roswell Park Institute, May 11, 1999.
29. Ford, Leslie. Personal interview.
30. Kramer, Barnett. Personal interview.
31. Voelker, Rebecca. "Jobs and Breast Cancer Risk." *JAMA,* Vol. 282, No. 2, July 14, 1999. "High-Risk Occupations for Breast Cancer." *Cancer Weekly Plus,* July 26, 1999.
32. "Reexamining Breast Cancer Link to Hormone Use." *Cancer Weekly Plus,* July 26, 1999.
33. Gapstur, Susan, et al. "Hormone Replacement Therapy and Risk of Breast Cancer With a Favorable Histology: Results of the Iowa Women's Health Study." *JAMA,* Vol. 281, No. 22, June 9, 1999.
34. Bush, Trudy, and Maura Whiteman. "Hormone Replacement Therapy and Risk of Breast Cancer." *JAMA,* June 9, 1999.
35. Lewis, Carol. "Breast Cancer." *FDA Consumer,* Vol. 33, No. 4, July 1999.
36. "FDA Sets Higher Standards for Mammography." *FDA Consumer,* January–February 1999.
37. Marsa, Linda. "Better Breast Tests." *American Health,* May 1999.
38. Stephenson, Joan. "Opinions Divided on High-Dose Chemotherapy for Breast Cancer." *JAMA,* Vol. 282, No. 2, July 14, 1999.
39. "Evaluation of Cervical Cytology." Agency for Health Care Policy Research, January 1999.
40. "Contending with the Abnormal Pap Test." *Patient Care,* Vol. 33, No. 12, July 15, 1999.
41. Cervical Cancer, National Cancer Institute Statement, April 15, 1999.
42. Slattery, Martha, et al. "An Assessment of Factors Associated with Risk of Colon Cancer." *American Journal of Epidemiology,* Vol. 150, No. 8, Oct. 15, 1999.
43. O'Leary, Timothy J. "Molecular Diagnosis of Hereditary Nonpolyposis Colorectal Cancer." *JAMA,* Vol. 282, No. 3, July 21, 1999.
44. "Cancer Facts and Figures—1999."
45. "Links Between Genetic and Environmental Factors and Prostate Cancer Risk." *Impotence & Male Health Weekly Plus,* July 26, 1999.
46. Pound, Charles, et al. "Natural History of Progression After PSA Elevation Following Radical Prostatectomy." *JAMA,* Vol. 281, No. 17, May 5, 1999.
47. "Prostate Cancer Patients Get Second Chance with Cryo-surgery." *Cancer Weekly,* Jan. 25, 2000.
48. Fisch, Harry, et al. "Incidence of Testicular Cancer." *Journal of Urology,* August 1999.
49. Sone, Shusuke, et al. "Mass Screening for Lung Cancer with Mobile Spiral Computed Tomography Scanner." *Lancet,* Vol. 351, No. 9111, April 25, 1999.
50. "Angiogenesis Inhibitors in Cancer Research." National Institutes of Health press release, April 2, 1999.
51. Wakeling, Kate Sandstrom. "The Latest Weapon in the War Against Cancer." *RN,* Vol. 62, No. 7, July 1999.
52. Socie, Gerard, et al. "Long-Term Survival and Late Deaths after Allogeneic Bone Marrow Transplantation." *Lancet,* Vol. 353, No. 9163, May 1, 1999. "Does Bone Marrow Transplantation Confer a Normal Life Span?" *New England Journal of Medicine,* Vol. 341, No. 1, July 1, 1999.
53. Portenoy, R.K., and P. Lesage. "Management of Cancer Pain." *Lancet,* May 15, 1999.
54. Holland, J.C., et al. "The Role of Religious and Spiritual Beliefs in Coping with Malignant Melanoma." *Psycho-Oncology,* Vol. 8, 1999.
55. "Cancer Survivorship."
56. Brancati, Frederick, et al. "Body Weight Patterns from 20 to 49 Years of Age and Subsequent Risk for Diabetes Mellitus." *Archives of Internal Medicine,* July 26, 1999.

57. Mitka, Mike. "Why the Rise in Asthma? New Insight, Few Answers." *JAMA,* Vol. 281, 1999.

58. "NAEPP Guidelines: Progress in Asthma Management." *American Family Physician,* Vol. 56, No. 2, August 1997.

59. "NHLBI Issues Updated Guidelines for the Diagnosis and Management of Asthma." *American Family Physician,* Vol. 56, No. 2, August 1997.

60. "New Strategy May Succeed at Extending Life of Transplanted Kidneys." Abstracts, *Archives of Internal Medicine,* April 26, 1999.

61. Marwick, Charles. "Treat Arthritis Earlier, Better." *JAMA,* July 12, 1999.

62. "Treating Arthritis with More than Pain-Killers." *Facts of Life,* Vol. 4, No. 5, June–July 1999.

15

Drug Use, Misuse, and Abuse

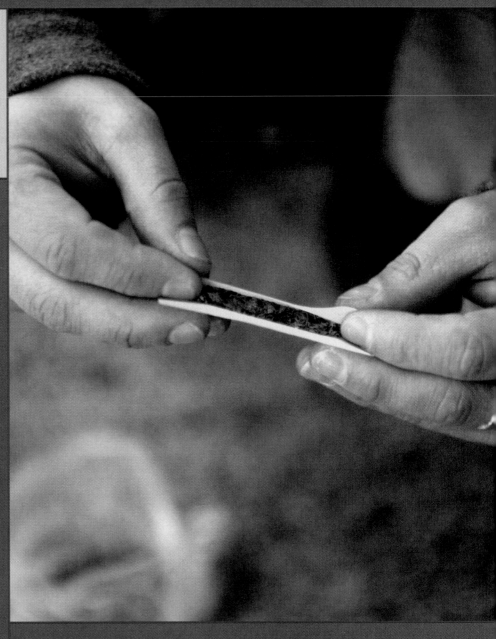

After studying the material in this chapter, you should be able to:

- **Explain** factors affecting drug dependence.
- **Describe** the methods of use and effects of cocaine and crack abuse.
- **Describe** the common forms and effects of amphetamines, depressants, cannabis products, psychedelics and hallucinogens, and narcotic drugs.
- **Discuss** the issues affecting the treatment of drug dependence.
- **Define** addiction, and **explain** the addictive process.
- **Explain** codependency and some ways that a codependent person can enable another to continue an addictive behavior.
- **Describe** the 12-step plan for recovery from addiction.

At a concert on campus, students pass around a marijuana joint while listening to the music. A bored teenager in an affluent suburb swallows a tab of LSD. At a party, a group of 20-something singles snort lines of cocaine. A middle-aged woman, troubled by worries and unable to relax, starts taking more and more of the medications she's gotten from various physicians to relieve her anxiety.

These people may not fit the image of a desperate addict that many conjure up when they think about drug users. Yet drugs are a fact of life for each of them, and each faces a risk of developing a substance abuse disorder. Although drug use has declined in the last two decades, the rates of drug abuse and drug-related problems remain high. About half of American adults surveyed report having used an illicit drug at some time in their lives. The typical drug user is not poor or unemployed; seven in ten people who use illegal drugs have full-time jobs.[1]

No one who uses illicit drugs expects to lose control. Even regular drug users believe they are smart enough, strong enough, or lucky enough not to get hooked. But after continued use, a person's need for a drug can outweigh everything else, including the values, people, and relationships he or she once held dearest.

This chapter provides information on the nature and effects of drugs, the impact of drugs on individuals and society, and the drugs Americans most commonly use, misuse, and abuse. ❖

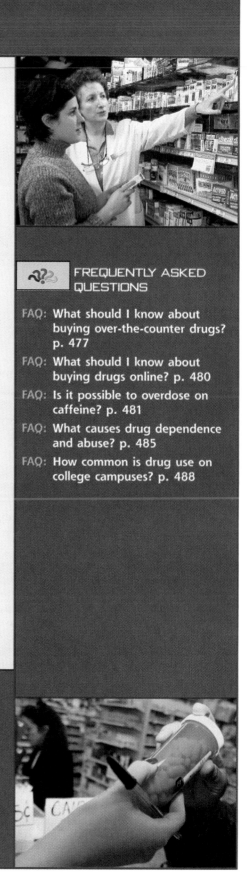

FREQUENTLY ASKED QUESTIONS

FAQ: **What should I know about buying over-the-counter drugs?** p. 477

FAQ: **What should I know about buying drugs online?** p. 480

FAQ: **Is it possible to overdose on caffeine?** p. 481

FAQ: **What causes drug dependence and abuse?** p. 485

FAQ: **How common is drug use on college campuses?** p. 488

Understanding Drugs and Their Effects

A **drug** is a chemical substance that affects the way you feel and function. In some circumstances, taking a drug can help the body heal or relieve physical and mental distress. In other circumstances, taking a drug can distort reality, undermine well-being, and threaten survival. No drug is completely safe; all drugs have multiple effects that vary greatly in different people at different times. Knowing how drugs affect the brain, body, and behavior is crucial to understanding their impact and making responsible decisions about their use.

Drug misuse is the taking of a drug for a purpose or by a person other than that for which it was medically intended. Borrowing a friend's prescription for penicillin when your throat feels scratchy is an example of drug misuse. The World Health Organization defines **drug abuse** as excessive drug use that's inconsistent with accepted medical practice. Taking anabolic steroids, discussed later in this chapter, to look more muscular is an example of drug abuse.

There are risks involved with all forms of drug use. Even medications that help cure illnesses or soothe symptoms have side effects and can be misused. Some substances that millions of people use every day, such as caffeine, pose some health risks. Others—like the most commonly used drugs in our society, alcohol and tobacco—can lead to potentially life-threatening problems. With some illicit drugs, any form of use can be dangerous.

Many factors determine the effects a drug has on an individual. These include how the drug enters the body, the dosage, drug action, and presence of other drugs in the body—as well as the physical and psychological make-up of the person taking the drug and the setting in which the drug is used.

Routes of Administration

Drugs can enter the body in a number of ways (see Figure 15-1). The most common way of taking a drug is by swallowing a tablet, capsule, or liquid. However, drugs taken orally don't reach the bloodstream as quickly as drugs introduced into the body by other means. A drug taken orally may not have any effect for 30 minutes or more.

Drugs can enter the body through the lungs either by inhaling smoke, for example, from marijuana, or by inhaling gases, aerosol sprays, or fumes from solvents or other compounds that evaporate quickly. Young users of such **inhalants,** discussed later in this chapter, often soak a rag with fluid and press it over their noses. Or they may place inhalants in a plastic bag, put the bag

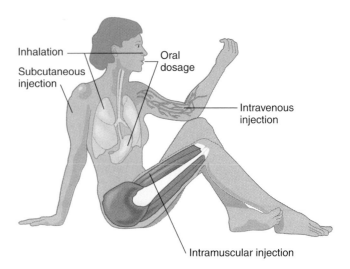

■ **Figure 15-1** Routes of administration of drugs.

over their noses and mouths, and take deep breaths—a practice called *huffing* and one that can produce serious, even fatal consequences.

Drugs can also be injected with a syringe subcutaneously (beneath the skin), intramuscularly (into muscle tissue, which is richly supplied with blood vessels), or intravenously (directly into a vein). **Intravenous** (IV) injection gets the drug into the bloodstream immediately (within seconds in most cases); **intramuscular** injection, moderately fast (within a few minutes); and **subcutaneous** injection, more slowly (within ten minutes).

Approximately 1.5 million Americans use illegal IV drugs. This practice is extremely dangerous because many diseases, including hepatitis and infection with human immunodeficiency virus (HIV), can be transmitted by sharing contaminated needles. Indeed, an estimated 250,000 to 300,000 of the nation's injection-drug users are HIV-positive; they are the chief source of transmission of HIV among heterosexuals. (See Chapter 12 for more on HIV infection and AIDS.)

Dosage

The effects of any drug depend on the amount an individual takes. Increasing the dose usually intensifies the effects produced by smaller doses. Also, there may be a change in the kind of effect at different dose levels. For example, low doses of barbiturates may relieve anxiety, while higher doses can induce sleep, loss of sensation, even coma and death.

Individual Differences

Each person responds differently to different drugs, depending on circumstances or setting. The enzymes in our bodies reduce the levels of drugs in our bloodstream; because there can be 80 variants of each enzyme, every person's body may react differently.

Often drugs intensify the emotional state a person is in. If you're feeling depressed, a drug may make you feel more depressed. A generalized physical problem, such as having the flu, may make your body more vulnerable to the effects of a drug. Genetic differences among individuals also may account for varying reactions.

Personality and psychological attitude also play a role in drug effects, so that one person may have a frighteningly bad trip on the same LSD dosage on which another person has a positive experience. To a certain extent, this depends on each user's **set** (or mind-set)—his or her expectations or preconceptions about using the drug. Someone who snorts cocaine to enhance sexual pleasure may feel more stimulated simply because that's what he or she expects.

Setting

The setting for drug use also influences its effects. Passing around a joint of marijuana at a friend's is not a healthy or safe behavior, but the experience of going to a crack house is very different—and entails greater dangers.

Toxicity

The dosage level at which a drug becomes poisonous to the body, causing either temporary or permanent damage, is called its **toxicity**. In most cases, drugs are eventually broken down in the liver by special body chemicals called *detoxification enzymes*.

Types of Action

A drug can act *locally,* as novocaine does to deaden pain in a tooth; *generally,* throughout a body system, as barbiturates do on the central nervous system; or *selectively,* as a drug does when it has a greater effect on one specific organ or system than on others, such as a spinal anesthetic. A drug that accumulates in the body because it's taken in faster than it can be metabolized and excreted is called *cumulative;* alcohol is such a drug.

Interaction with Other Drugs or Alcohol

A drug can interact with other drugs in four different ways:

- An **additive** interaction is one in which the resulting effect is equal to the sum of the effects of the different drugs used.

- A **synergistic** interaction is one in which the total effect of the two drugs taken together is greater than the sum of the effects the two drugs would have had if taken by themselves on separate occasions. Mixing barbiturates and alcohol, for example, has up to four times the depressant effect than either drug has alone.

- A drug can be **potentiating**—that is, one drug can increase the effect of another. Alcohol, for instance, can increase the drowsiness caused by antihistamines (antiallergy medications).

- Drugs can interact in an **antagonistic** fashion—that is, one drug can neutralize or block another drug with opposite effects. Tranquilizers, for example, may counter some of the nervousness and anxiety produced by cocaine.

The danger of mixing alcohol with other drugs cannot be emphasized too strongly. Alcohol and marijuana intensify each other's effects, making driving and many other activities extremely dangerous. Some people have mixed sedatives or tranquilizers with alcohol and never regained consciousness.

Medications

Many of the medications and pharmaceutical products available in this country do indeed relieve symptoms and help cure various illnesses. However, improper use of medications leads to more than 170,000 hospitalizations and costs of about $750 million every year.[2] Because drugs are powerful, it's important to know how to use them appropriately.

What Should I Know About Buying Over-the-Counter Drugs?

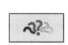

More than half a million health products—remedies for everything from bad breath to bunions—are readily available without a doctor's prescription. This doesn't mean that they're necessarily safe or effective. Indeed, many widely used **over-the-counter** (OTC) **drugs** pose unsuspected hazards. Among the most potentially dangerous is aspirin, the "wonder drug" in practically everyone's home pharmacy. When taken by someone who's been drinking (often to prevent or relieve hangover symptoms), for instance, aspirin increases blood-alcohol concentrations (see Chapter 16). Along with other nonsteroidal anti-inflammatory drugs, such as ibuprofen (brand names include Advil and Nuprin), aspirin can damage the lining of the stomach and lead to ulcers in those who take large daily doses for arthritis or other problems. Kidney problems have also been traced to some pain relievers.

Some health products that aren't even considered true drugs can also cause problems. As noted in Chapter 6, many Americans take food supplements, even though the FDA has never approved their use for any medical disorder. OTC supplements of niacin, a vitamin that can help lower cholesterol levels, have produced liver damage in some people for reasons that doctors have not yet determined.

A growing number of drugs that once were available only with a doctor's prescription can now be bought over the counter. These include Gyne-Lotrimin and Monistat, which combat vaginal yeast infections, and famotidine (sold as Pepcid AC) and cimetidine (sold as Tagamet), which offer an alternative to antacids for people suffering from heartburn and acid indigestion. For consumers, the advantages of this greater availability include lower prices and fewer visits to the doctor. The disadvantages, however, are the risks of misdiagnosing a problem and misusing or overusing medications.

Like other drugs, OTC medications can be used improperly, often simply because of a lack of education about proper use. Among those most often misused are the following:

- *Nasal sprays.* Nasal sprays relieve congestion by shrinking blood vessels in the nose. If they are used too often or for too many days in a row, however, the blood vessels widen instead of contracting, and the surrounding tissues become swollen, causing more congestion. To make the vessels shrink again, many people use more spray more often. The result can be permanent damage to nasal membranes, bleeding, infection, and partial or complete loss of smell.

- *Laxatives.* Believing that they must have one bowel movement a day (a common misconception), many people rely on laxatives. Brands that contain phenolphthalein imitate the lining of the intestines and cause muscles to contract or tighten, often making constipation worse rather than better. Bulk laxatives are less dangerous, but regular use is not advised. A high-fiber diet and more exercise are safer and more effective remedies for constipation.

- *Eye drops.* Eye drops make the blood vessels of the eye contract. However, as in the case of nasal sprays, with overuse (several times a day for several weeks), the blood vessels expand, making the eye look redder than before.

- *Sleep aids.* Although over-the-counter sleeping pills are widely used, there has been little research on their use and possible risks.

Prescription Drugs

Medications are a big business in this country. (See Table 15-1.) However, the latest, most expensive drugs aren't necessarily the best. Each year the Food and Drug Administration (FDA) approves about 20 new drugs, yet no more than four are rated as truly meaningful advances. The others often are no better or worse than what's already on the market. (For tips on using prescription drugs, see Consumer Health Watch: "Getting the Most Out of Medications.")

Both doctors and patients make mistakes when it comes to prescription drugs. The most frequent mistakes doctors make are over- or underdosing, omitting information from prescriptions, ordering the wrong dosage form (a pill instead of a liquid, for example), and not recognizing a patient's allergy to a drug.

Drug Nonadherence

Many prescribed medications aren't taken the way they should be; millions simply aren't taken at all. As many as 70 percent of adults have trouble understanding dosage information and 30 percent of people can't read standard labels, according to the FDA, which has called for larger, clearer drug labeling.[3] The dangers of nonadherence (not taking prescription drugs properly) include recurrent infections, serious medical complications, and emergency hospital treatment.[4] The drugs most likely to be taken incorrectly are those that treat problems with no obvious symptoms (such as high blood pressure), that require complex dosage schedules, that treat psychiatric disorders, or that have unpleasant side effects.

Some people skip or stop taking medications because they fear that any drug can cause tolerance and eventual dependence. Others fail to let doctors know about side effects. For instance, patients may stop taking anti-inflammatory drugs because they irritate their

■ **Table 15-1** Top-Selling Prescription Drugs

Type of Drug	Application
1. Premarin Tabs	hormone replacement therapy
2. Synthroid	hypothyroid treatment
3. Prilosec	ulcer treatment
4. Prozac	antidepressant
5. Lipitor	cholesterol-lowering treatment
6. Norvasc	heart, blood pressure treatment
7. Claritin	antihistamine
8. Lanoxin	heart treatment
9. Zoloft	antidepressant
10. Paxil	antidepressant

Source: Drug Topics, March 1, 1999.

Consumer Health Watch

Getting the Most Out of Medications

Before you leave with a prescription, be sure to ask the following:

- What is the name of the drug? What's it supposed to do? How and when do I take it? For how long? What foods, drinks, other medications, or activities should I avoid while taking this drug? Are there any side effects? What do I do if they occur? What written information is available on this drug? Are there other, possibly cheaper alternatives? Why do you recommend this particular drug? Are there nondrug alternatives, such as using a vaporizer, gargling with salt water, and drinking plenty of liquids for a viral infection; or losing weight and exercising to lower blood pressure?

- If you're taking a medication, tell your doctor if you plan to change your diet significantly—cutting calories or fat, stopping or starting vitamin supplements, or changing the amount of fiber you consume.

- Don't keep old medications around, and don't take drugs prescribed for someone else unless your doctor tells you to. Keep medications out of reach of small children.

- Ask your pharmacist how best to store your prescriptions. (A hot, damp bathroom medicine chest is often the worst place.) Have all prescriptions filled at the same pharmacy, and ask your pharmacist to keep a record of your medications to avoid hazardous interactions.

stomachs. However, taking the drugs with food can eliminate this problem. The side effects of other drugs may disappear as the person's body becomes accustomed to the drug.

Physical Side Effects

Most medications, taken correctly, cause only minor complications. However, no drug is entirely without side effects for all individuals taking it. Serious complications that may occur include heart failure, heart attack, seizures, kidney and liver failure, severe blood disorders, birth defects, blindness, memory problems, and allergic reactions.

Allergic reactions to drugs are common. The drugs that most often provoke allergic responses are penicillin and other antibiotics (drugs used to treat infection). Aspirin, sulfa drugs, barbiturates, anticonvulsants, insulin, and local anesthetics can also provoke allergic responses. Allergic reactions range from mild rashes to hives to anaphylaxis—a life-threatening constriction of the airways and sudden drop of blood pressure that causes rapid pulse, weakness, paleness, confusion, nausea, vomiting, unconsciousness, and collapse. This extreme response, which is rare, requires immediate treatment with an injection of epinephrine (adrenaline) to open the airways and blood vessels.

Psychological Side Effects

Dozens of drugs—both over-the-counter and prescription—can cause changes in the way people think, feel, and behave. Unfortunately, neither patients nor their physicians usually connect such symptoms with medications. Doctors may not even mention potential mental and emotional problems because they don't want to scare patients away from what otherwise may be a very effective treatment. But what you don't know about a drug's effects on your mind can hurt you.

Among the medications most likely to cause psychiatric side effects are drugs for high blood pressure, heart disease, asthma, epilepsy, arthritis, Parkinson's disease, anxiety, insomnia, and depression. Some drugs—such as the powerful hormones called corticosteroids, used for asthma, autoimmune diseases, and cancer—can cause different psychiatric symptoms, depending on dosage and other factors. Other drugs, such as ulcer medications, can cause delirium and disorientation, especially when given in high doses or to elderly patients. More subtle problems, such as forgetfulness or irritability, are common reactions to many drugs—but also are more likely to be ignored or dismissed.

The older you are, the sicker you are, and the more medications you're taking, the greater your risk of developing some psychiatric side effects. "Even medications that don't usually cause problems, such as antibiotics, can cause psychiatric side effects in some individuals," says Jack Gorman, M.D., a professor of clinical psychiatry at Columbia University School of Medicine. "Whenever you sense a change in yourself, always ask, 'Could a drug be causing this?'"[5]

Any medication that slows down bodily systems—as many high blood pressure and cardiac drugs do—can cause depressive symptoms. Estrogen in birth control pills can cause mood changes. As many as 15 percent of women using oral contraceptives have reported feeling depressed or moody. For many people, switching to another medication quickly lifts a drug-induced depression.

All drugs that stimulate or speed up the central nervous system can cause agitation and anxiety—including the almost 200 allergy, cold, and congestion remedies containing pseudoephedrine hydrochloride (Sudafed). Other common culprits in inducing anxiety are caffeine and theophylline, a chemical relative of caffeine found in many medications for asthma and other respiratory problems. These drugs act like mild amphetamines in the body, making people feel hyper and restless.

Drug Interactions

OTC and prescription drugs can interact in a variety of ways. For example, mixing some cold medications with tranquilizers can cause drowsiness and coordination problems, thus making driving dangerous. Moreover, what you eat or drink can impair or completely wipe out the effectiveness of drugs or lead to unexpected effects on the body. For instance, aspirin takes five to ten times as long to be absorbed when taken with food or shortly after a meal than when taken on an empty stomach. Or if tetracyclines encounter calcium in the stomach, they bind together and cancel each other out.

To avoid potentially dangerous interactions, check the label(s) for any instructions on how or when to take a medication, such as "with a meal." (See Figure 15-2.) If the directions say that you should take a drug on an empty stomach, do it at least one hour before eating or two or three hours after eating. Don't drink a hot beverage with a medication, because the temperature may interfere with the effectiveness of the drug. Don't open, crush, or dissolve tablets or capsules without checking first with your physician or pharmacist.

Whenever you take a drug, be especially careful of your intake of alcohol, which can change the rate of metabolism and the effects of many different drugs.

Because it dilates the blood vessels, alcohol can add to the dizziness sometimes caused by drugs for high blood pressure, angina, or depression. Also, its irritating effects on the stomach can worsen stomach upset from aspirin, ibuprofen, and other anti-inflammatory drugs.

Generic Drugs

The **generic** name is the chemical name for a drug. A specific drug may appear on the pharmacist's shelf under a variety of brand names, which may cost more than twice the generic equivalent. About 75 percent of all prescriptions specify a brand name, but pharmacists may—and in some states must—switch to a generic drug unless the doctor specifically tells them not to. Prescriptions filled with generic drugs cost 20 to 85 percent less than their brand-name counterparts.

Generic drugs have the same active ingredients as brand-name prescriptions, but their fillers and binders, which can affect the absorption of a drug, may be different. For some serious illnesses, the generics may not be as effective; some experts recommend sticking with brand names for heart medications, psychiatric drugs, and anticonvulsant drugs (for epilepsy and other seizure disorders).

To determine whether you should buy the generic version of a drug, ask your physician whether it matters if you get a brand-name or generic drug. If it does, ask which brand name is best. Also, find out if switching to a generic or from one generic to another might harm your condition in any way.

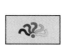

What Should I Know About Buying Drugs Online?

In the late 1990s a new phenomenon emerged: the selling of prescription medications online. Although some web

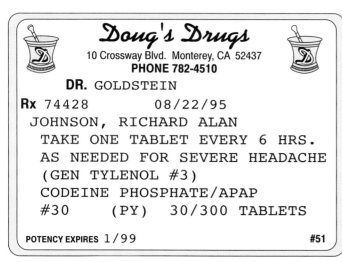

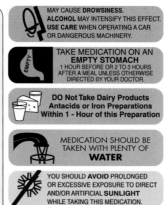

■ Figure 15-2 Drug interactions can alter the effectiveness of your medication. When you take a prescription medication, be sure to read warning labels about interactions, possible side effects, and whether the medication interacts with certain foods.

sites fill only faxed prescriptions from medical doctors, others ignore or sidestep traditional regulations and safeguards. Cyberspace distributors often ship pills across state lines without requiring a physical examination by a medical doctor. Instead, a "cyberdoc," who may or may not be qualified or up-to-date in a given specialty, reviews information submitted by a "patient." International pharmacies sometimes sell drugs that are not available or approved in the United States. And patients themselves use bulletin boards and other web areas to sell unused or unwanted medications to each other.

Many individuals turn to the Internet for "lifestyle" drugs such as Viagra, the impotence pill, and Propecia, a baldness treatment. Other medications commonly sought and bought online include Xenical, a diet pill; Zyban, an anti-smoking treatment; Celebrex, for arthritis; and Claritin, for allergies. Many customers turn to cyberspace because of the convenience and anonymity. Although many assume drugs cost less on the Internet, shipping costs tend to drive prices up to the same amount or more than they would have paid in a pharmacy.

The dangers of unregulated distribution of medications have alarmed government agencies and medical groups. The American Medical Association has declared it unethical for physicians to write prescriptions for people they've never met. The National Association of Boards of Pharmacy has developed a seal of approval to help customers determine which sites are legitimate. The FDA and other federal agencies, such as the Federal Trade Commission, which regulates advertising, are trying to find ways to impose some controls. However, the problem is so complex and pervasive that one observer compares it to "trying to nail Jello to a wall."[6]

In the meantime, consumers have to be wary. Ordering a drug like Accutane, an acne treatment, online may seem harmless. However, without close monitoring by a physician, you could develop complications, such as a bad reaction that aggravates hepatitis or inflames the pancreas. Quality control is another concern. Cyberspace pharmacies provide no information on how the drug was stored or whether its expiration date has passed. In addition, since importing medications without a prescription is against the law, you could find yourself in legal trouble.[7]

Caffeine Use and Misuse

Caffeine, which has been drunk, chewed, or swallowed since the stone age, is the most widely used **psychotropic** (mind-affecting) drug in the world. Eighty percent of Americans drink coffee, our principal caffeine source—an average of 3.5 cups a day. Coffee contains 100 to 150 milligrams of caffeine per cup; tea, 40

to 100 milligrams; cola, about 45 milligrams. Most medications that contain caffeine are one-third to one-half the strength of a cup of coffee. However, some, such as Excedrin, are very high in caffeine (Table 15-2).

The effects of caffeine vary. Because it is a **stimulant,** it relieves drowsiness, helps in the performance of repetitive tasks, and improves capacity for work.[8] Some athletes feel that caffeine gives them an extra boost that allows them to go farther and longer in endurance events. Consumption of high doses of caffeine can lead to dependence, anxiety, insomnia, faster breathing, upset stomach and bowels, and dizziness.[9]

Although there is no conclusive proof that caffeine causes birth defects, it does cross the placenta into the tissues of a growing fetus. Because of an increased risk of miscarriage, the U. S. surgeon general has recommended that pregnant women avoid or restrict their caffeine intake. Some fertility specialists also have urged couples trying to conceive to reduce caffeine to increase their chance of success. Women who are heavy caffeine users tend to have shorter menstrual cycles than nonusers.[10]

Is It Possible to Overdose on Caffeine?

It is possible to overdose on caffeine. The characteristic symptoms of caffeine intoxication are restlessness, nervousness, excitement, insomnia, flushed face, increased urination, digestive complaints, muscle twitching, rambling thoughts and speech, rapid heart rate or arrhythmias, periods of inexhaustibility, and physical restlessness. Some people develop these symptoms after as little as 250 milligrams of caffeine a day; others, only with much larger doses. Higher doses may produce ringing in the ears or flashes of light, grand mal seizures, and potentially fatal respiratory failure.

■ Table 15-2 Caffeine Counts

Substance (typical serving)	Caffeine (milligrams)
No Doz (one pill)	200
Coffee (drip), one 5-ounce cup	130
Excedrin (two pills)	130
Espresso (2-ounce cup)	100
Instant coffee (5-ounce cup)	74
Coca-Cola (12 ounces)	46
Tea (5-ounce cup)	40
Dark chocolate (1 ounce)	20
Milk chocolate	6
Cocoa (5 ounces)	4
Decaffeinated coffee	3

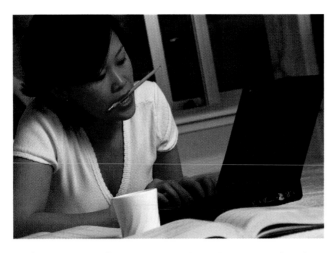

Coffee and work often go hand in hand, but too much caffeine can lead to dependence, anxiety, and other problems.

Caffeine withdrawal for those dependent on this substance can cause headaches and other neurological symptoms.[11] Those who must cut back should taper off gradually. One approach is to mix regular and decaffeinated coffee, gradually decreasing the quantity of the former.

Substance Use Disorders

People have been using mind-altering, or **psychoactive,** chemicals for centuries. Citizens of ancient Mesopotamia and Egypt used opium. More than 3,000 years ago Hindus included cannabis products in religious ceremonies. For centuries the Inca Indians in South America have chewed the leaves of the coca bush. Yet while drugs existed in most societies, their use was usually limited to small groups. Today millions of Americans regularly turn to drugs to pick them up, bring them down, alter perceptions, or ease psychological pain.

Both men and women are vulnerable to substance use disorders, although they tend to have different patterns of drug use. (See The X & Y Files: "Sex Differences in Drug Use.") The 1960s ushered in an explosive increase in drug use and in the number of drug users in our society. Marijuana use soared in the 1960s and 1970s; cocaine, in the 1980s. In 1986, crack—a cheap, smokeable form of cocaine—hit the streets and cities of America, and the number of regular cocaine users zoomed. In the years since, government officials, describing drugs as the number-one public health threat in our society, have declared war against them. Yet the abuse of both legal and illegal drugs continues to be an enormous problem. An estimated 5.5 million Americans are in need of treatment for drug abuse and dependence.

Millions more are struggling to live drug-free lives.[12] (See Self-Survey: "Is It a Substance Use Disorder?")

Understanding Substance Use Disorders

In early Roman law, *addictus* referred to someone who, because he could not pay his debts, was sentenced into slavery. Indeed, one of the meanings of addiction given by the *Oxford Latin Dictionary* is "enslavement."[13] For much of the twentieth century, addiction to drugs was viewed as a social or criminal problem, and the only people called addicts were "drug-crazed junkies" desperate for a fix. In the 1960s, however, when scientists switched to the *medical model* for understanding addictions, they began to view addictions to chemicals—such as alcohol and psychoactive drugs—as lifelong chronic diseases that affect a person's mind and body.

Today the word **addiction** has moved out of the realm of scientific terminology and into the mainstream of American life. Among laypeople, addiction refers to the habitual use of substances, such as alcohol, psychoactive drugs, and nicotine, and also to compulsive behaviors, such as overeating (discussed in Chapter 7). Like drugs, these activities can be used repeatedly to numb pain or enhance pleasure; some may alter a person's brain chemistry or create cravings; all can lead to a loss of internal control.

Chemical addiction is now viewed as a lifelong, chronic illness that affects mind, body, and spirit. Its key characteristics are repeated drug use, loss of control over how much or how often a person takes a drug, and continued use despite harmful consequences. Because addiction is considered too broad and judgmental a term for scientific use, mental health professionals describe drug-related problems in terms of dependence and abuse. However, they agree that there are four characteristic symptoms of addiction: compulsion to use the substance, loss of control, negative consequences, and denial.

Dependence

Individuals may develop **psychological dependence** and feel a strong craving for a drug because it produces pleasurable feelings or relieves stress or anxiety. **Physical dependence** occurs when a person develops *tolerance* to the effects of a drug and needs larger and larger doses to achieve intoxication or another desired effect. Individuals who are physically dependent and have a high tolerance to a drug may take amounts many times those that would produce intoxication or an overdose in someone who was not a regular user.

The X&Y Files

Sex Differences in Drug Use

Beginning at a very early age, males and females show different patterns in drug use. In the *National Household Survey on Drug Abuse,* overall a higher percentage of boys than girls reported using illicit drugs at least once during the previous year. As has been the case since 1991—the first year for which data are available— younger girls remain more likely than boys to use illicit drugs other than marijuana, primarily stimulants and tranquilizers. In the survey, 12.1 percent of eighth-grade girls and 9.6 percent of eighth-grade boys reported using drugs other than marijuana. This sex difference reversed itself in high school. Among twelfth-graders, 21.7 percent of boys and 18.0 percent of girls said they had used drugs other than marijuana.

Among college students, men are more likely than women to report using drugs, but the differences are not large. For instance, in one national survey, 30 percent of college men and 28 percent of college women said they had smoked marijuana. In another, 15 percent of male students and 14 percent of female students reported using cocaine at some time in their lives.

There also are sex-specific risks of drug use. Research suggests that women may become more quickly addicted than men to certain drugs, such as crack cocaine, even after casual or experimental use. They also are more vulnerable to poor nutrition and below-average weight, depression, physical abuse, and, if pregnant, preterm labor or early delivery. Substance abuse compounds the risk of AIDS for women, who may acquire it by sharing needles with other injection drug users and by engaging in unprotected sex with a drug user. More than 60 percent of new cases of HIV infection in women are related either to the woman's own injection drug use or to her having sex with an injection drug user. Traditional drug treatment programs, created for men, have proven to be less effective for women than programs that provide more comprehensive services, including child care, assertiveness training, and parenting training.

Sources: National Household Survey on Drug Abuse. Washington, D.C.: White House Office of Drug Control Policy, 1999. Pacula, Rosalie. "Women and Substance Use: Are Women Less Susceptible to Addiction?" *American Economic Review,* Vol. 87, No. 2, May 1997. Douglas, Kathy, et al. "Results from the 1995 National College Health Risk Behavior Survey." *Journal of American College Health,* Vol. 46, September 1997. "Treatment Methods for Women," National Institute on Drug Abuse, http://www.nida.nih.gov

Men and women with a substance dependence disorder may use a drug to avoid or relieve withdrawal symptoms or consume larger amounts of a drug or use it over a longer period than they'd originally intended. They may try repeatedly to cut down or control drug use without success; spend a great deal of time obtaining or using drugs or recovering from their effects; give up or reduce important social, occupational, or recreational activities because of their drug use; or continue to use a drug despite knowledge that the drug is likely to cause or worsen a persistent or recurring physical or psychological problem.

Specific symptoms of dependence vary with particular drugs. For instance, certain drugs, such as marijuana, hallucinogens, or phencyclidine, do not cause withdrawal symptoms. The degree of dependence also varies. In mild cases, a person may function normally most of the time. In severe cases, the person's entire life may revolve around obtaining, using, and recuperating from the effects of a drug.

Individuals with drug dependence become intoxicated or high on a regular basis—whether every day, every weekend, or several binges a year. They may try repeatedly to stop using a drug and yet fail—even though they realize that their drug use is interfering with their health, family life, relationships, and work.

Abuse

Some drug users do not develop the symptoms of tolerance and withdrawal that characterize dependence, yet they use drugs in ways that clearly have a harmful effect on them. These individuals are diagnosed as having a *psychoactive substance abuse disorder.* They continue to use drugs despite their awareness of persistent or repeated social, occupational, psychological, or physical problems related to drug use, or they use drugs in dangerous ways or situations (before driving, for instance). (See Pulsepoints: "Ten Ways to Tell If Someone Is Abusing Drugs.")

Intoxication and Withdrawal

Intoxication refers to maladaptive behavioral, psychological, and physiologic changes that occur as a result of substance use. **Withdrawal** is the development of symptoms that cause significant psychological and physical distress when an individual reduces or stops drug use.

Self-*Survey* Is It a Substance Use Disorder?

Individuals with a substance dependence or abuse disorder may

- Use more of an illegal drug or a prescription medication or use a drug for a longer period of time than they desire or intend. _____
- Try, repeatedly and unsuccessfully, to cut down or control their drug use. _____
- Spend a great deal of time doing whatever is necessary in order to get drugs, taking them, or recovering from their use._____
- Be so high or feel so bad after drug use that they often cannot do their job or fulfill other responsibilities. _____
- Give up or cut back on important social, work, or recreational activities because of drug use. _____
- Continue to use drugs even though they realize that they are causing or worsening physical or mental problems. _____
- Use a lot more of a drug in order to achieve a "high" or desired effect or feel fewer such effects than in the past. _____
- Use drugs in dangerous ways or situations. _____
- Have repeated drug-related legal problems, such as arrests for possession. _____
- Continue to use drugs, even though the drug causes or worsens social or personal problems, such as arguments with a spouse. _____
- Develop hand tremors or other withdrawal symptoms if they cut down or stop drug use. _____
- Take drugs to relieve or avoid withdrawal symptoms. _____

The more blanks that you or someone close to you checks, the more reason you have to be concerned about drug use. The most difficult step for anyone with a substance use disorder is to admit that he or she has a problem. Sometimes a drug-related crisis, such as being arrested or fired, forces individuals to acknowledge the impact of drugs. If not, those who care—family, friends, boss, physician—may have to confront them and insist that they do something about it. This confrontation, planned beforehand, is called an intervention and can be the turning point for drug users and their families.

This chapter provides information on drug dependence and abuse and specific drugs of abuse.

Making Changes

Alternatives to Drugs

If you are an addict, you must first admit that you have a problem before you can begin the process of recovery. Then you should seek help from health-care professionals. If your answers raised doubts about your drug use, try to stop using them. Consider these alternatives instead of drugs:

- If you need physical relaxation, try athletics, exercise, or outdoor hobbies. For adventure, sign up for a wilderness survival outing; or take up windsurfing or rock climbing.
- If you want to stimulate your senses, train yourself to be more sensitive to nature and beauty. Take time to appreciate the sensations you experience when you're walking in the woods or embracing a person you love.
- If you're anxious, depressed, or uptight and want relief from emotional pain, turn to people—either friends or professional counselors or support groups. If you want to find meaning in life or expand your personal awareness, explore various philosophical theories through classes, seminars, and discussion groups. Study yoga or meditation.
- If you want to enhance your creativity or appreciation of the arts, challenge your mind through reading, classes, creative games, discussion groups, memory training, or travel. Pursue training in music, art, singing, or writing. Attend more concerts, ballets, or museum shows.
- If you want to be accepted, volunteer in programs in which you can assist others and not focus solely on yourself. If you want to promote political or social change, volunteer in political campaigns, or join lobbying and political-action groups.

(Intoxication and withdrawal from specific drugs are discussed later in this chapter.)

Polyabuse

Most users prefer a certain type of drug but also use several others; this behavior is called **polyabuse.** The average user who enters treatment is on five different drugs.

The more drugs anyone uses, the greater the chance of side effects, complications, and possibly life-threatening interactions.

Comorbidity

There is a great deal of overlap between mental disorders and substance abuse disorders. "A little more than

PULSE points

Ten Ways to Tell If Someone Is Abusing Drugs

1. **An abrupt change in attitude.** Individuals may lose interest in activities they once enjoyed or in being with friends they once valued.

2. **Mood swings.** Drug users may often seem withdrawn or "out of it," or they may display unusual temper flareups.

3. **A decline in performance.** Students may start skipping classes, stop studying, or not complete assignments; their grades may plummet.

4. **Increased sensitivity.** Individuals may react intensely to any criticism or become easily frustrated or angered.

5. **Secrecy.** Drug users may make furtive telephone calls or demand greater privacy concerning their personal possessions or their whereabouts.

6. **Physical changes.** Individuals using drugs may change their pattern of sleep, spending more time in bed or sleeping at odd hours. They also may change their eating habits and lose weight.

7. **Money problems.** Drug users may constantly borrow money, seem short of cash, or begin stealing.

8. **Changes in appearance.** As they become more involved with drugs, users often lose regard for their personal appearance and look disheveled.

9. **Defiance of restrictions.** Individuals may ignore or deliberately refuse to comply with deadlines, curfews, or other regulations.

10. **Changes in relationships.** Drug users may quarrel more frequently with family members or old friends and develop new, strong allegiances with new acquaintances, including other drug users.

---

a third of those with a psychiatric disorder also have a chemical dependency problem, and a little more than a third of those with a chemical dependency problem have a psychiatric disorder," notes psychiatrist Richard Frances, M.D., the founding president of the American Association of Addiction Psychiatry.[14] Individuals with such "dual diagnoses" require careful evaluation and appropriate treatment for the complete range of complex and chronic difficulties that they face.

 ## What Causes Drug Dependence and Abuse?

No one fully understands why some people develop drug dependence or abuse disorders, while others, who may experiment briefly with drugs, do not. Inherited body chemistry, genetic factors, and sensitivity to drugs may make some individuals more susceptible. These disorders may stem from many complex causes.

The Biology of Addiction

Scientists now view addiction as a brain disease triggered by frequent use of drugs that change the biochemistry and anatomy of neurons and alter the way they work.[15] A major breakthrough in understanding the roots of addiction has been the discovery that certain mood-altering substances and experiences—a puff of marijuana, a slug of whiskey, a snort of cocaine, a big win at black jack—trigger a rise in a brain chemical called dopamine, which is associated with feelings of satisfaction and euphoria. This neurotransmitter, one of the crucial messengers that link neurons, or nerve cells, in the brain, rises during any pleasurable experience, whether it be a loving hug or a taste of chocolate.

Addictive drugs have such a powerful impact on dopamine and its receptors (its connecting cells) that they change the pathways within the brain's pleasure centers. As Figure 15-3 indicates, in different ways, different substances create a craving for more of the same.

Strategies for Prevention

Saying No to Drugs

If people offer you a drug, here are some ways to say no:

✓ Let them know you're not interested. Change the subject. If the pressure seems threatening, just walk away.

✓ Have something else to do: "No, I'm going for a walk now."

✓ Be prepared for different types of pressure. If your friends tease you, tease them back.

✓ Keep it simple. "No, thanks," "No," or "No way" all get the point across.

✓ Hang out with people who won't ask you questions you have to say no to.

According to this hypothesis, addicts do not specifically yearn for heroin, cocaine, or nicotine but for the rush of dopamine that these drugs produce. Other brain chemicals, including glutamate, GABA (gamma-amino-butyric-acid) and possibly norepinephrine, may also be involved.[16] Some individuals, born with low levels of dopamine, may be particularly susceptible to addiction.

Other Routes of Addiction

Although scientists do not believe there is an "addictive" personality, certain individuals are at greater risk of drug dependence because of psychological risk factors, including difficulty controlling impulses, a lack of values that might constrain drug use (whether based in religion, family, or society), low self-esteem, feelings of powerlessness, and depression. The one psychological trait most often linked with drug use is denial. Young people in particular are absolutely convinced that they will never lose control or suffer in any way as a result of drug use.

Many diagnosed drug users have at least one mental disorder, particularly depression or anxiety. Disorders that emerge in adolescence, such as bipolar disorder, may increase the risk of substance abuse.[17] Many people with psychiatric disorders abuse drugs. Individuals may self-administer drugs to treat psychiatric symptoms; for example, they may take sedating drugs to suppress a panic attack.

Individuals who are isolated from friends and family, or who live in communities, such as poor inner-city areas where drugs are widely used, have higher rates of drug abuse. Young people from lower socioeconomic backgrounds are more likely to use drugs than their more affluent peers, possibly because of economic disadvantage; family instability; a lack of realistic, rewarding alternatives and role models; and increased hopelessness.

Those whose companions are substance abusers are far more likely to use drugs. Peer pressure to use drugs can be a powerful factor for adolescents and young adults. Young people growing up in families in which parents or an older sibling abuse drugs tend to develop drug problems themselves. The likelihood of drug abuse is also related to family instability, parental rejection, and divorce.

Drugs that produce an intense, brief high—like crack cocaine—lead to dependence more quickly than slower-acting agents, like cocaine powder. Drugs that cause uncomfortable withdrawal symptoms, such as barbiturates, may lead to continued use to avoid such discomfort.

Drug use involves certain behaviors, situations, and settings that users may, in time, associate with getting high. Even after long periods of abstinence, some for-

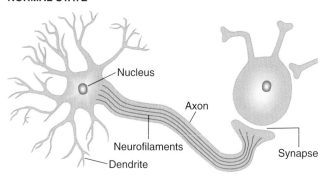

NORMAL STATE

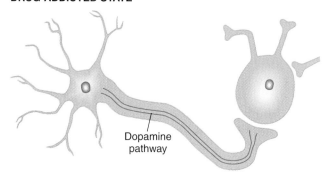

DRUG-ADDICTED STATE

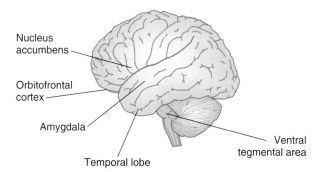

AFFECTED AREAS OF THE BRAIN

■ Figure 15-3 **The Normal vs. Drug-Addicted Nervous System**
Repeated drug doses overload normal neurotransmitter systems, and cells compensate by making dopamine less effective and becoming smaller. When doses stop, craving ensues.

Source: The Neuroscientist.

mer drug users find that they crave drugs when they return to a site of drug use or meet people with whom they used drugs. Former cocaine users report that the sight of white powder alone can serve as a cue that triggers a craving.

Most individuals who use drugs first try them as adolescents. Teens are likely to begin experimenting with tobacco, beer, wine, or hard liquor, then smoke marijuana or sniff inhalants. Teens who smoke cigarettes are 11 times as likely to use drugs and 16 times as likely to drink heavily as non-smoking youths.[18] Some then go on to try sedative-hypnotics, stimulants (including cocaine), and hallucinogens such as LSD. A much smaller percentage of teens try the opioids. Over time some individuals give up certain drugs, such as hallucinogens, and return to old favorites, such as alcohol and marijuana. A smaller number continue using several drugs, a pattern called polysubstance abuse.

The Toll of Drugs

Drugs affect a person's physical, psychological, and social health; their effects can be *acute* (resulting from a single dose or series of doses) or *chronic* (resulting from long-term use). Acute effects vary with different drugs. Stimulants may trigger unpredictable rage; an overdose of heroin may lead to respiratory depression, a breathing impairment that can be fatal.

Over time, chronic drug users may feel fatigued, cough constantly, lose weight, become malnourished, and ache from head to toe. They may suffer blackouts, flashbacks, and episodes of increasingly bizarre behavior, often triggered by escalating paranoia. Their risk of overdose rises steadily, and they must live with constant stress: the fear of getting busted for possession or of losing a job if they test positive for drugs, the worry of getting enough money for their next fix, the dangers of associating with dealers and other users.

The toll of drug use can be especially great on teenagers. Teenage drug use disrupts many critical developmental tasks of adolescence and young adulthood. Use of drugs during the teen years can lead to drug-related crime (including stealing), poor achievement in high school or college, and job instability.

Drugs in Society

Drug abuse remains a major problem even though drug use among teenagers has declined in recent years. The estimated medical and social costs of drug abuse are believed to exceed $245 billion. Addiction to drugs, alcohol, or tobacco accounts for a third of all hospital admissions and a quarter of all deaths.[19]

At the end of the twentieth century, federal officials reported good and bad news about drugs in America: Use among teens between the ages of 12 and 17 dropped to about one in ten adolescents—down 15 percent in a single year. However, drug use among young adults between the ages of 18 and 25 rose to its highest level since 1989, with 16 percent of those in this age group reporting drug use in the previous month—a 10 percent rise within a year's time.[20]

Here are the trends for specific drugs (see also Figure 15-4):

* *Marijuana.* Use has declined but remains prevalent: 22 percent of eighth graders and nearly half of twelfth graders surveyed reported that they have tried marijuana.

* *Heroin.* Use remained unchanged among all students in 1998: 1.3 percent of eighth graders, 1.4 percent of tenth graders, and 1.0 percent of twelfth graders said they had used heroin.

* *Hallucinogens.* Overall use has decreased slightly at all grade levels.

* *MDMA or ecstasy.* Decreases were recorded for the second year in a row.

* *Crack cocaine.* Among eighth graders, use of crack cocaine increased to its highest level, 2.1 percent, since 1991. Slight increases were reported for crack use by tenth graders, to 2.5 percent, and twelfth graders, to 2.5 percent.

* *Inhalants.* Use has declined among all students for three consecutive years.

As teenagers, in varying numbers, continue to experiment with drugs, experts debate the best approaches to prevention. The most popular antidrug program is DARE (for Drug Abuse Resistance Education), which is used by nearly 75% of the nation's schools. However, a ten-year follow-up study has found that DARE has no long-term effect on drug use. Most children, it turns out, do not engage in drug use, even without drug prevention programs.

America's Drug Problem

There is no typical drug user. High school students, professional athletes, business executives, inner-city teenagers, rock musicians, doctors, truckers, teachers, and many others of different ages and ethnic groups use drugs regularly. Overall an estimated 13.6 million people in the United States use illicit drugs. The most commonly used is marijuana. About 11 million people report using it in the previous month—six times the number of cocaine users.

We all pay a price for living in a drug-using society, including the costs of medical care, treatment, and imprisonment for addicts and drug traffickers. Other hidden costs include accidents caused by drug-using drivers and workers, drug-related violence and crime, and care for babies born to drug-dependent mothers.

In the last 20 years, the United States has spent nearly $70 billion fighting drugs. But victory is nowhere in sight. Criminal organizations in Latin America and

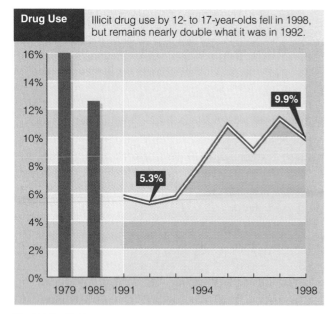

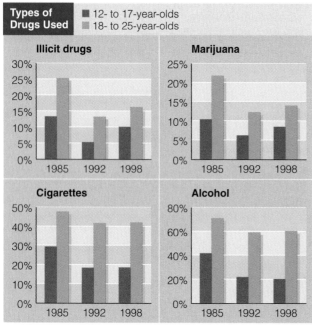

■ Figure 15-4 Trends in drug use among 12-to-25-year-olds.

Asia have increased production and become more sophisticated in distributing cocaine and heroin. Illicit drugs have become more available in more countries and at lower prices than ever before.

Critics of the nation's drug policy argue that the war is being fought on the wrong front. Currently, about two-thirds of federal spending for drug control goes toward law enforcement and only one-third toward prevention and treatment. Many contend that more should be spent on antidrug education for children, on treatment for addicts, and on researching drugs that could help in overcoming drug dependence.

There is evidence that prevention can and does work. According to the National Clearinghouse for Alcohol and Drug Information, each month prevention efforts keep approximately 3.5 million youngsters from drinking alcohol and 24 million young adults from using illicit drugs. Experts have identified a set of principles that they see as essential for the success of prevention efforts, including the following realizations:

• Drug problems are too complex to be changed significantly through individual decision making alone. Programs must be developed to help young people build skills to resist pressures to take drugs.

• Shared responsibility is more appropriate than blaming the victim of drug abuse. Families, peers, and the community have to work together, because everyone benefits when an individual avoids drug abuse.

• Education is necessary but insufficient to produce needed change in societal attitudes and values related to drugs. Millions of Americans have banded together to support antidrunk-driving and nonsmoking laws; a similar approach could be effective in getting across the message that drug use will no longer be tolerated.

How Common Is Drug Use on College Campuses?

As discussed in Chapter 16, alcohol is the number-one drug of abuse on college campuses. Marijuana remains the most commonly used illegal drug. According to a national survey, about half of college students have tried marijuana, but the percentage of current users is much lower: 11.6 percent of women and 17.1 percent of men. About 14 percent of undergraduates say they have tried cocaine.[21]

However, there is a large gap between actual drug use on campus and how prevalent students believe drug use to be. In an analysis of surveys representing 100 diverse campuses, researchers compared students' self-reports of frequency of drug use with what students perceived to be the frequency of drug use by "the average student." In general, students greatly overestimated the use of a variety of drugs.[22]

Various factors influence which students use drugs, including the following:

• *Race/ethnicity.* In general, white students have higher levels of alcohol and drug use than do African-American students. In a comparison of African-American students at predominantly white and predominantly black colleges, those at historically black colleges had lower rates of alcohol and drug use than did either white or African-American students at white schools. The reason, according to the researchers,

Campus Focus

Trends in Illicit Drug Use Over Three Years at a Large University Campus

Percentage of students reporting:	1994	1995	1996
Marijuana use in the last year			
No use	63.0%	65.7%	64.6%
Occasional use	28.3%	24.1%	23.2%
Weekly use	6.2%	8.2%	10.7%
Cocaine use in the last year			
No use	91.0%	92.3%	92.0%
Occasional use	6.4%	5.9%	6.7%
Weekly use	0.2%	0.4%	0.8%
Other illicit drug use in the last year			
No use	82.8%	82.2%	86.1%
Occasional use	13.4%	13.7%	12.0%
Weekly use	1.3%	2.5%	1.4%

Note: Occasional use is defined as use once per year to twice per month. Weekly use is defined as use once per week or more.

Source: "Drinking, Binge Drinking, and Other Drug Use Among Southwestern Undergraduates: Three-Year Trends." Melanie E. Bennett, Joseph H. Miller, W. Gill Woodall. *American Journal of Drug and Alcohol Abuse,* Vol. 25, Issue 2, p. 331, May 1999.

---

may be that these colleges provide a greater sense of self-esteem, which helps prevent alcohol and drug use.

- *Perception of risk.* Students seem most likely to try substances they perceive as being "safe," or low-risk. Of these, the top three are caffeine, alcohol, and tobacco; marijuana is listed fourth in terms of perceived safety. Other agents—barbiturates, heroin, cocaine, PCP, speed, LSD, crack, and inhalants—are viewed as about equally risky and are used much less often. Why do today's students believe that using certain types of drugs is not harmful? Researchers have identified three possible explanations: In general, less public attention is being paid to the drug problem and to educating youngsters about drugs. Second, young people have less chance to learn about the dangers of drugs because fewer fellow students and celebrities have been abusers in recent year. Thus, they have not seen, either personally or in the media, the ravages drug use can cause. Third, an increased glorification of marijuana and other drugs by rock, grunge, and rap music groups supports the notion that these drugs are safe to use.

- *Environment.* As with alcohol use, students are influenced by their friends, their residence, and the general public's attitude toward drug use. Increasingly, college health officials are realizing that, rather than simply trying to change students' substance abuse, they also must change the environment to promote healthier lifestyle choices.

Drugs on the Job

According to the National Household Survey on Drug Abuse, seven in ten illegal drug users have full-time jobs.[23] Workers of every variety—from truck drivers to stockbrokers—use drugs. However, young adults, men, whites, and those with less than a high school education are more likely to use drugs than other workers. At the very least, drug-abusing employees may affect their workplace by being unproductive, making poor decisions, and having strained relationships with coworkers.[24] Even more frightening, however, is the threat to themselves and others from accidents due to their drug use.

Along with alcohol and nicotine, cocaine and marijuana are the primary drugs of abuse on or off the job. As a result of widespread drug use, the military and a growing number of companies are requiring drug tests of job applicants and employees. However, drug testing is not 100 percent precise. For example, individuals who have recently eaten poppy seeds (as in a muffin or bagel) can test positive for opiates. Increasingly, employers are shifting from policing employees to setting up programs to help those with drug problems overcome their drug dependence.

Drug use is also common among the unemployed. According to a survey by the National Institute for Drug Abuse, of all adults between the ages of 18 and 34 who don't have jobs, 21.5 percent used illicit drugs in the prior month. Among those with full-time jobs, only

9.7 percent used drugs. In particular, unemployed young adults are much more likely to use cocaine and marijuana than those who are working full-time.

Drugs and Driving

One important impact of drugs is their effect on driving ability (see Chapter 16). Alcohol and drug use are equally common in drivers injured in traffic accidents. Often drivers using alcohol also test positive for other drugs. Different drugs affect driving ability in different ways. Here are the facts from the National Institute on Drug Abuse:

- *Alcohol* affects perception, coordination, and judgment, and increases the sedative effects of tranquilizers and barbiturates.

- *Marijuana* affects a wide range of driving skills—including the ability to track (stay in the lane) through curves, brake quickly, and maintain speed and a safe distance between cars—and slows thinking and reflexes. Normal driving skills remain impaired for four to six hours after smoking a single joint.

- *Sedatives, hypnotics, and antianxiety agents* slow reaction time, and interfere with hand–eye coordination and judgment; the greatest impairment is in the first hour after taking the drug. The effects depend on the particular drug: some build up in the body and can impair driving skills the morning after use; others make drivers very sleepy and, therefore, incapable of driving safely.

- *Amphetamines,* after repeated use, impair coordination. They can also make a driver more edgy and less coordinated, and thus more likely to be involved in an accident.

- *Hallucinogens* distort judgment and reality, and cause confusion and panic, thus making driving extremely dangerous.

Common Drugs of Abuse

The psychoactive substances most often associated with both abuse and dependence include alcohol (discussed in Chapter 16); amphetamines; cocaine; cannabis (marijuana); hallucinogens; inhalants; opioids; phencyclidine (PCP); and sedative-hypnotic or anxiolytic (antianxiety) drugs.

Amphetamines

Amphetamines, stimulants that were once widely prescribed for weight control because they suppress appetite, have emerged as a global danger. They trigger the release of epinephrine (adrenalin), which stimulates the central nervous system. Amphetamines are sold under a variety of names: amphetamine (brand name Benzedrine, street-name "bennies"), dextroamphetamine (Dexedrine, or "dex"), methamphetamine (Methedrine, or "meth" or "speed"), and Desoxyn ("copilots"). Related *uppers* include the prescription drugs methylphenidate (Ritalin), pemoline (Cylert), and phenmetrazine (Preludin).

Amphetamines are available in tablet or capsule form. Abusers may grind and sniff the capsules, or make a solution and inject the drug. "Ice" is a smokable form of methamphetamine that is highly addictive and produces an intense physical and psychological high that can last from four to fourteen hours. *Crank* is the street term for another central nervous system stimulant, propylexedrine, which is less potent than amphetamine. Abusers often extract the drug from the cotton plug of decongestant inhalants and inject it intravenously.

How Users Feel

Amphetamines produce a state of hyper-alertness and energy. Users feel confident in their ability to think clearly and to perform any task exceptionally well—although amphetamines do not, in fact, significantly boost performance or thinking. Higher doses make them feel "wired": talkative, excited, restless, irritable, anxious, moody.

If taken intravenously, amphetamines produce a characteristic "rush" of elation and confidence, as well as adverse effects, including confusion, rambling or incoherent speech, anxiety, headache, and palpitations. Individuals may become paranoid; be convinced they are having "profound" thoughts; feel increased sexual interest; and experience unusual perceptions, such as ringing in the ears, a sensation of insects crawling on their skin, or hearing their name called. Crank users may feel high and sleepy or may hallucinate and lose contact with reality. Methamphetamine, which produces a rapid high when inhaled, produces exceptionally long-lasting toxic effects, including psychosis, violence, seizures, and cardiovascular abnormalities.[25] Although methamphetamine has long been linked with violence, methamphetamine users are less likely to be charged with a violent offense than are other drug users.[26]

Risks

Dependence on amphetamines can develop with episodic or daily use. Users typically take amphetamines in large doses to prevent crashing. "Bingeing"—taking high doses over a period of several days—can lead to an extremely intense and unpleasant crash—characterized by a craving for the drug, shakiness, irritability, anxiety, and depression—that requires two or more days for recuperation.

Amphetamine intoxication may cause the following symptoms:

- Feelings of grandiosity, anxiety, tension, hypervigilance, anger, social hypersensitivity, fighting, jitteriness or agitation, paranoia, and impaired judgment in social or occupational functioning.
- Increased heart rate, dilated pupils, elevated blood pressure, perspiration or chills, and nausea or vomiting.
- Less frequent effects such as speeding up or slowing down of physical movement; muscular weakness, impaired breathing, chest pain, heart arrhythmia; confusion, seizures, impaired movements or muscle tone, or even coma.
- In high doses, a rapid or irregular heartbeat, tremors, loss of coordination, and collapse.

Smokeable methamphetamine, or "ice," also increases heart rate and blood pressure; high doses can cause permanent damage to blood vessels in the brain. Other physical effects of methamphetamine include dilated pupils, blurred vision, dry mouth, and increased breathing rate. Prolonged use can cause fatal lung and kidney disorders. Injecting propylexedrine can lead to convulsions, strokes, and respiratory and kidney failure. Abusers also may develop infected veins, and if they share needles, they risk HIV infection.[27]

The long-term effects of amphetamine abuse include malnutrition; skin disorders; ulcers; insomnia; depression; vitamin deficiencies; and, in some cases, brain damage that results in speech and thought disturbances. Sexual dysfunction and impaired concentration or memory also may occur.

Withdrawal

When the immediate effects of amphetamines wear off, users experience a "crash"—they crave the drug and become shaky, irritable, anxious, and depressed. Amphetamine withdrawal usually persists for more than 24 hours after cessation of prolonged, heavy use. Its characteristic features include fatigue, disturbing dreams, much more or less than usual sleep, increased appetite, and speeding up or slowing down of physical movements. Those who are unable to sleep despite their exhaustion often take sedative-hypnotics (discussed later in this chapter) to help them rest and may become dependent on them as well as amphetamines. Symptoms usually reach a peak in two to four days, although depression and irritability may persist for months. Suicide is a major risk.

Cannabis Products

Marijuana ("pot") and hashish—the most widely used illegal drugs—are derived from the *cannabis* plant. The major psychoactive ingredient in both is *THC (delta-9-tetrahydrocannabinol)*. Nearly one of every three Americans over age 12 has tried marijuana at least once. Some 12 million Americans use it; more than 1 million cannot control this use. Marijuana has been used therapeutically, primarily to ease the nausea of chemotherapy, and some researchers urge further study of its potential benefits. A recent report from the Institute of Medicine found "strong scientific evidence" that the active ingredients in marijuana (cannabinoids) are potentially effective in treating pain, nausea, and the severe weight loss associated with AIDS. Although the IOM found no evidence that use of marijuana leads to other drug use, it cautioned that the benefits of marijuana are limited because of the harmful effects of smoking it and that it should be recommended only for terminally ill patients or those with debilitating symptoms that do not respond to approved medications.[28] Several states—Alaska, Arizona, California, Colorado, Nevada, Oregon, and Washington—have passed referenda in support of the legal medical use of marijuana. However, "compassionate" use has been limited by law because some believe it undercuts government opposition to drug use.

Different types of marijuana have different percentages of THC. Because of careful cultivation, the strength of today's marijuana is much greater than that of the pot used in the 1970s; the physical and mental effects are therefore greater. Usually, marijuana is smoked in a cigarette ("joint") or pipe; it may also be eaten as an ingredient in other foods (as when baked in brownies), though with a less predictable effect. The drug high is enhanced by holding the marijuana smoke in the lungs, and experienced smokers learn to hold the smoke for longer periods to increase the amount of drug diffused into the bloodstream. The circumstances in which marijuana is smoked, the communal aspects of its use, and the user's experience all can affect the way a pot-induced high feels.

How Users Feel

In low to moderate doses, marijuana typically creates a mild sense of euphoria, a sense of slowed time (five minutes may feel like an hour), a dreamy sort of self-absorption, and some impairment in thinking and communicating. Users report heightened sensations of color, sound, and other stimuli, relaxation, and increased confidence. The sense of being "stoned" peaks within half an hour and usually lasts about three hours. Even when alterations in perception seem slight, as noted earlier, it is not safe to drive a car for as long as four to six hours after smoking a single joint. Some users—particularly those smoking marijuana for the first time or taking a high dose in an unpleasant or unfamiliar setting—experience acute anxiety, which may be accompanied by a panicky fear of losing control. They may believe that their companions are ridiculing or threatening them and experience a panic attack, a state of intense terror.

The immediate physical effects of marijuana include increased pulse rate, bloodshot eyes, dry mouth and throat, slowed reaction times, impaired motor skills, increased appetite, and diminished short-term memory (see Figure 15-5). High doses reduce the ability to perceive and to react; all the reactions experienced with low doses are intensified, leading to sensory distortion and—in the case of hashish—vivid hallucinations and LSD-like psychedelic reactions. The drug remains in the body's fat cells 50 hours or more after use, so people may experience psychoactive effects for several days after use. Drug tests may produce positive results for days or weeks after last use.

Risks

Dependence or abuse usually develops with repeated use over a long period of time. Typically, individuals smoke more often rather than smoking a larger amount. With chronic heavy use, users may feel a lessening or loss of the pleasurable effect and may develop lethargy, a loss of pleasure in activities, and persistent attention and memory problems. Chronic marijuana use seems to impair thinking, reading comprehension, verbal and mathematical skills, coordination, and short-term memory. Teenagers who smoke pot regularly often lose interest in school and do not remember what they learned when they were high. Some long-term regular users of marijuana may experience *burnout*, a dulling of their senses and responses termed *amotivational syndrome*.

A Harvard Medical School study that compared the cognitive functioning of college students who were heavy marijuana users (who'd smoked the drug 29 out of the previous 30 days), light users (who'd smoked marijuana once in the previous 30 days), and nonusers found significant impairments of thinking and specific cognitive abilities, such as sustained attention, in heavy users. These effects persisted even after a day of supervised abstinence from marijuana.[29] Over time, continued heavy marijuana use might interfere with students' ability to learn and perform well in school and in challenging careers.

Chronic use can also lead to bronchitis, emphysema, and lung cancer. Smoking a single "joint," or marijuana cigarette, can be as damaging to the lungs as

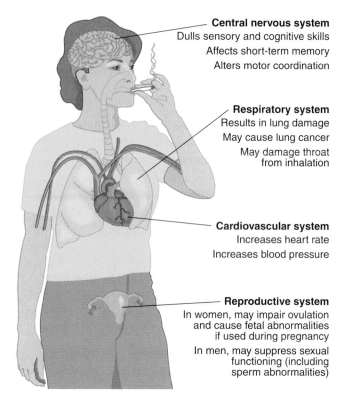

Central nervous system
Dulls sensory and cognitive skills
Affects short-term memory
Alters motor coordination

Respiratory system
Results in lung damage
May cause lung cancer
May damage throat
from inhalation

Cardiovascular system
Increases heart rate
Increases blood pressure

Reproductive system
In women, may impair ovulation
and cause fetal abnormalities
if used during pregnancy
In men, may suppress sexual
functioning (including
sperm abnormalities)

■ **Figure 15-5** Some effects of long-term marijuana use on the body.

smoking five tobacco cigarettes. Marijuana may suppress ovulation and alter hormone levels in female users and may impair the fertility of male users. Frequent use of marijuana during pregnancy can lower birth weight and cause abnormalities in the fetus similar to those of fetal alcohol syndrome. (See Figure 15-5.)

Withdrawal

Stopping after long-term marijuana use can produce what experts call "marijuana withdrawal syndrome," which is characterized by insomnia, restlessness, loss of appetite, and irritability.[30] People who smoked marijuana daily for many years also may become aggressive after they stop using it and may relapse to prevent aggression and other symptoms.[31]

Cocaine

Cocaine ("coke," "snow," "lady") is a white crystalline powder extracted from the leaves of the South American coca plant. Usually mixed with various sugars and local anesthetics like lidocaine and procaine, cocaine powder is generally inhaled. When sniffed or snorted, cocaine anesthetizes the nerve endings in the nose and relaxes the lung's bronchial muscles. Frequent snorting can irritate and damage the mucous membrane in the nose, cause sinusitis, destroy a user's sense of smell, and occasionally create a hole in the septum (the membrane between the nostrils).

Cocaine can be dissolved in water and injected intravenously. The drug is rapidly metabolized by the liver, so the high is relatively brief, typically lasting only about 20 minutes. This means that users will commonly inject the drug repeatedly, increasing the risk of infection and damage to their veins. Many intravenous cocaine users prefer the practice of *speedballing,* the intravenous administration of a combination of cocaine and heroin.

Cocaine alkaloid—or *freebase*—is obtained by removing the hydrochloride salt from cocaine powder. "Freebasing" is smoking the fumes of the alkaloid form of cocaine. *Crack,* pharmacologically identical to freebase, is a cheap, easy-to-use, widely available, smokeable and potent form of cocaine named for the popping sound it makes when burned. Because it is absorbed rapidly into the bloodstream and large doses reach the brain very quickly, it is particularly dangerous. However, its low price and easy availability have made it a common drug of abuse in poor urban areas.[32]

How Users Feel

A powerful stimulant to the central nervous system, cocaine produces feelings of soaring well-being and boundless energy. This may be because cocaine targets, not one, but several chemical sites in the brain.[33] Users feel that they have enormous physical and mental ability, yet are also restless and anxious. After a brief period of euphoria, users slump into a depression. They often go on cocaine binges, lasting from a few hours to several days, and consume large quantities of cocaine.

With crack, dependence develops quickly. As soon as crack users come down from one high, they want more crack. Whereas heroin addicts may shoot up several times a day, crack addicts need another hit within minutes. Thus, a crack habit can quickly become more expensive than heroin addiction. Some "crackheads" have $1,000-a-day habits. Police in big cities have traced many brutal crimes and murders to young crack addicts, who often are extremely paranoid and dangerous. Smoking crack doused with liquid PCP, a practice known as *space-basing,* has especially frightening effects on behavior.

With continuing use, cocaine users experience less pleasure and more unpleasant effects. Eventually they may reach a point at which they no longer experience euphoric effects and crave the drug simply to alleviate their persistent hunger for it. They think about it constantly, dream about it, spend all their money on it, and borrow, steal, or deal to pay for it. They cannot concentrate on work; they become increasingly irritable and confused. They may also become dependent on alcohol, sedatives, or opioids, which they use to calm down from cocaine's aftereffects.

Risks

Cocaine dependence is an easy habit to acquire. With repeated use, the brain becomes tolerant of the drug's stimulant effects, and users must take more of it to get high. Its grip is strong. Those who smoke or inject cocaine can develop dependence within weeks. Those who sniff cocaine may not become dependent on the drug for months or years. It is thought that 5 to 20 percent of all coke users—a group as large as the estimated total number of heroin addicts—are dependent on the drug.

The physical effects of acute cocaine intoxication include dilated pupils, elevated or lowered blood pressure, perspiration or chills, nausea or vomiting, speeding up or slowing down of physical activity, muscular weakness, impaired breathing, chest pain, and impaired movements or muscle tone.

Although some users initially try cocaine as a sexual stimulant, it does not enhance sexual performance. At low doses, it may delay ejaculation and orgasm and cause heightened sensory awareness, but men who use cocaine regularly have problems maintaining erections and ejaculating. They also tend to have low sperm counts, less active sperm, and more abnormal sperm than nonusers. Both male and female chronic cocaine users tend to lose interest in sex and have difficulty in reaching orgasm.

Cocaine use can cause blood vessels in the brain to clamp shut and can trigger a stroke, bleeding in the brain, and potentially fatal brain seizures. Cocaine users can also develop psychiatric or neurological complications (Figure 15-6). Repeated or high doses of cocaine can lead to impaired judgment, hyperactivity, nonstop babbling, feelings of suspicion and paranoia, and violent behavior. The brain never learns to tolerate cocaine's negative effects; users may become incoherent and paranoid and may experience unusual sensations, such as ringing in their ears, feeling insects crawling on the skin, or hearing their name called.

Cocaine can damage the liver and cause lung damage in freebasers. Smoking crack causes bronchitis as well as lung damage and may promote the transmission of HIV through burned and bleeding lips. Some smokers have died of respiratory complications, such as pulmonary edema (the buildup of fluid in the lungs).

Cocaine causes the heart rate to speed up and blood pressure to rise suddenly. Its use is associated with many cardiac complications, including arrhythmia (disruption of heart rhythm), angina (chest pain), and acute myocardial infarction (heart attack). These cardiac complications can lead to sudden death.

Cocaine users who inject the drug and share needles put themselves at risk for another potentially lethal problem: HIV infection. Other complications of injecting cocaine include skin infections, hepatitis, inflammation of the arteries, and infection of the lining of the heart.

The most common ways of dying from cocaine use are persistent seizures that result in respiratory collapse, cardiac arrest from arrhythmias, myocardial infarction, and intracranial hemorrhage or stroke. The combination of alcohol and cocaine is particularly lethal. Alcohol and cocaine together are second only to the combination of heroin and alcohol in causing deaths related to substance abuse.

Cocaine is dangerous for pregnant women and their babies, causing miscarriages, developmental disorders, and life-threatening complications during birth. Women who use the drug while pregnant are more likely to miscarry in the first three months of pregnancy than women who do not use drugs or who use heroin and other opioids. When used early in pregnancy, cocaine can reduce the fetal oxygen supply, possibly interfering with the development of the fetus's nervous system. Infants born to cocaine and crack users can suffer withdrawal and may have major complications, or permanent disabilities. Cocaine babies have higher-than-normal rates of respiratory and kidney troubles, visual problems, and developmental retardation and may be at greater risk of sudden infant death syndrome.

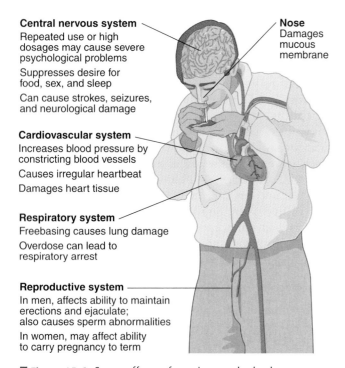

Central nervous system
Repeated use or high dosages may cause severe psychological problems
Suppresses desire for food, sex, and sleep
Can cause strokes, seizures, and neurological damage

Nose
Damages mucous membrane

Cardiovascular system
Increases blood pressure by constricting blood vessels
Causes irregular heartbeat
Damages heart tissue

Respiratory system
Freebasing causes lung damage
Overdose can lead to respiratory arrest

Reproductive system
In men, affects ability to maintain erections and ejaculate; also causes sperm abnormalities
In women, may affect ability to carry pregnancy to term

■ Figure 15-6 Some effects of cocaine on the body.

Withdrawal

The symptoms of cocaine withdrawal include fatigue, vivid and disturbing dreams, excessive or too little sleep, irritability, increased appetite, and physical slowing down or speeding up. This initial crash may last one to to three days after cutting down or stopping the heavy use of cocaine. Depression is common. Some individuals become violent, paranoid, and suicidal.

Symptoms usually reach a peak in two to four days, although depression, anxiety, irritability, lack of pleasure in usual activities, and low-level cravings may continue for weeks. As memories of the crash fade, the desire for cocaine intensifies. For many weeks after stopping, individuals may feel an intense craving for the drug. Experimental medical approaches for treating cocaine dependence include antidepressant drugs, anticonvulsant drugs, and the naturally occurring amino acids tryptophan and tryrosine. However, these have only limited benefit, and much more research into medical treatments is needed.

Prevention remains the best option. Researchers calculate that each dollar spent on a school prevention program would save an eventual $2.40 in the costs of cocaine-related crime, health care, and lost productivity.[34]

Hallucinogens

The drugs known as **hallucinogens** produce vivid and unusual changes in thought, feeling, and perception. The most widely used in the United States is *LSD* (*lysergic acid diethylamide*, or "acid"), which was initially developed as a tool to explore mental illness. It became popular in the 1960s and resurfaced among teenagers in the 1990s. LSD is taken orally, either blotted onto pieces of paper which are held in the mouth or chewed along with another substance, such as a sugar cube. Much less commonly used in this country is *peyote* (whose active ingredient is *mescaline*).

How Users Feel

LSD produces hallucinations, including bright colors and altered perceptions of reality. Effects from a single dose begin within 30 to 60 minutes and last 10 to 12 hours. During this time, there are slight increases in body temperature, heart rate, and blood pressure; sweating, chills, and goose pimples appear. Some users develop headache and nausea. Mescaline produces vivid hallucinations—including brightly colored lights, animals, and geometric designs—within 30 to 90 minutes of consumption. These effects may persist for 12 hours.

The effects of hallucinogens depend greatly on the dose, the individual's expectations and personality, and the setting for drug use. Many users report religious or mystical imagery and thoughts; some feel they are experiencing profound insights. Usually the user realizes that perceptual changes are caused by the hallucinogen, but some become convinced that they have lost their minds. Drugs sold as hallucinogens are frequently mixed with other drugs, such as PCP and amphetamines, which can produce unexpected and frightening effects.

Hallucinogens do not produce dependence in the same way as cocaine or heroin. Individuals who have an unpleasant experience after trying a hallucinogen may stop using the drugs completely without suffering withdrawal symptoms. Others continue regular or occasional use because they enjoy the effects.

Risks

Physical symptoms include dilated pupils, rapid heart rate, sweating, heart palpitations, blurring of vision, tremors, and poor coordination. These effects may last eight to twelve hours. Hallucinogen intoxication also produces changes in emotions and mood, such as anxiety, depression, fear of losing one's mind, and impaired judgment.

LSD can trigger irrational acts. LSD users have injured or killed themselves by jumping out of windows, swimming out to sea, or throwing themselves in front of cars. Some individuals develop a delusional disorder, in which they become convinced that their distorted perceptions and thoughts are real. They may experience flashbacks (reexperiencing of symptoms felt while intoxicated), which include geometric hallucinations, flashes of color, halos around objects, and other perceptual changes.

Individuals having a "bad trip" may blame themselves and feel excessively guilty, tense, and so agitated that they cannot stop talking and they have trouble sleeping. They may fear that they have destroyed their brains and will never return to normal. Someone who already is depressed may take a hallucinogen to lift his or her spirits, only to become more depressed. Suicide is a real danger.

Inhalants

Inhalants or **deleriants** are chemicals that produce vapors with psychoactive effects. The most commonly abused inhalants are solvents, aerosols, model-airplane glue, cleaning fluids, and petroleum products like kerosene and butane. Some anesthetics and nitrous oxide (laughing gas) are also abused. Almost 21 percent of eighth graders surveyed have used household products, such as glue, solvents, and aerosols, to get high.[35]

In order to inhale intoxicating vapors, individuals soak a rag in the substance, place it against the mouth and nose, and inhale; or inhale fumes from a substance placed in a paper or plastic bag; or inhale vapors directly from their containers. Young people, especially those who may not have money for or access to other drugs, are those most likely to try inhalants. Children between the ages of 9 to 13 tend to use inhalants with a group of peers who are likely to use alcohol and marijuana as well. Users are in all racial, socioeconomic, and gender groups, but the incidence of use is higher among poor minority youth than among others. Many users come from families that have separated or been affected by alcohol or drug problems; they often have school difficulties, such as truancy and poor grades, or problems adjusting to work.

How Users Feel

Inhalants reach the lungs, bloodstream, and other parts of the body very rapidly. At low doses, users may feel slightly stimulated; at higher doses, they may feel less inhibited. Intoxication often occurs within five minutes and can last more than an hour. Inhalant users do not report the intense rush associated with other drugs, nor do they experience the perceptual changes associated with LSD. However, inhalants interfere with thinking and impulse control, so users may act in dangerous or destructive ways.

Often there are visible external signs of use: a rash around the nose and mouth; breath odors; residue on face, hands and clothing; redness, swelling, and tearing of the eyes; and irritation of throat, lungs and nose that leads to coughing and gagging. Nausea and headache also may occur.

Risks

Regular use of inhalants leads to tolerance, so that the sniffer needs more and more to attain the desired effects. Younger children who use inhalants several times a week may develop dependence. Older users who become dependent may use the drugs many times a day. Those who become dependent on inhalants are likely to have used many different substances as adolescents, and to have gradually turned to inhalants as their preferred substance.

Although some young people believe inhalants are safe to use, this is far from true. Inhalation of butane from cigarette lighters displaces oxygen in the lungs, causing suffocation. Users also can suffocate while covering their heads with a plastic bag to inhale the substance, or from inhaling vomit into their lungs while high. According to the International Institute on Inhalant Abuse, the effects of inhalants are unpredictable, and even a single episode could trigger asphyxiation or cardiac arrhythmia, leading to disability or death. Abusers also can develop difficulties with memory, with abstract reasoning, problems with coordination, and with uncontrollable movements of the extremities.

Opioids

The **opioids** include *opium* and its derivatives (that is, *morphine*, *codeine*, and *heroin*) and nonopioid synthetic drugs that have similar sleep-inducing and pain-relieving properties. The opioids come from a resin taken from the seed pod of the Asian poppy. **Nonopioids,** such as *meperidine* (Demerol), *methadone*, and *propoxyphene* (Darvon), are chemically synthesized. These drugs are powerful narcotics, or painkillers.

Heroin, the most widely abused opioid, is illegal in this country. In other nations it is used as a potent painkiller for conditions such as terminal cancer. There are an estimated 600,000 heroin addicts in the United States, with men outnumbering women addicts by three to one. The number of teens using heroin rose in the 1990s, although the percentage remains low.[36] Purer forms of heroin, available in many cities, can be snorted; this has led to a surge in the drug's popularity, especially among middle- and upper-class users.[37]

Morphine, used as a painkiller and anesthetic, acts primarily on the central nervous system, eyes, and digestive tract and masks pain by producing mental clouding, drowsiness, and euphoria. It does not decrease the physical sensation of pain as much as it alters a person's awareness of the pain; in effect, he or she no longer cares about it.

Two semisynthetic derivatives of morphine are *hydromorphone* (trade name Dilaudid, or "little D"), with two to eight times the painkilling effect of morphine, and *oxycodone* (Percocet, Percodan, or "perkies"), similar to codeine but more potent. The synthetic narcotic *meperidine* (Demerol, or "demies") is now probably second only to morphine for use in relieving pain. It is also used by addicts as a substitute for morphine or heroin.

Codeine is a weaker painkiller and sedative than morphine. It is an ingredient in liquid products prescribed for relieving coughs, and in tablet and injectable form for relieving pain. The synthetic narcotic *propoxyphene* (Darvon) is a somewhat less potent painkiller than codeine; in fact, it is no more effective than aspirin in usual doses. It has been one of the most widely prescribed drugs for headaches, dental pain, and menstrual cramps. At higher doses, Darvon produces a euphoric high, which may lead to misuse.

Prescription opioids are taken orally in pill form but can also be injected intravenously. Heroin users typically inject the drug into their veins. However, individuals who experiment with whatever recreational drug is

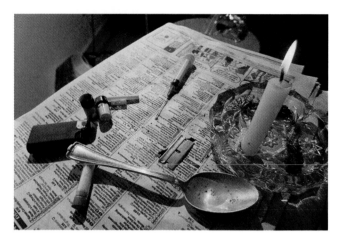

Opioid drugs, made from the Asian poppy, come in both legal and illegal forms. In any form, these substances can readily become addictive.

new and trendy often prefer *skin-popping* (subcutaneous injection) rather than *mainlining* (intravenous injection); they also may snort heroin as a powder, or dissolve it and inhale the vapors. To try to avoid addiction, some users begin by *chipping,* taking small or intermittent doses. Regardless of the method of administration, tolerance can develop rapidly.

Some individuals first take a medically prescribed opioid for pain relief or cough suppression, then gradually increase the dose and frequency of use on their own, often justifying this because of their symptoms rather than for the sensations the drug induces. They expend increasing efforts to obtain the drug, frequently seeking out several doctors to write prescriptions.

How Users Feel

All the opioids relax the user. When injected, they can produce an immediate "rush," or high, that lasts 10 to 30 minutes. For two to six hours thereafter, users may feel indifferent, lethargic, and drowsy; they may slur their speech and have problems paying attention, remembering and going about their normal routine. The primary attractions of heroin ("horse," "junk," "smack," or "downtown") are the euphoria and pain relief it produces. However, some people experience very unpleasant feelings, such as anxiety and fear. Other effects include a sensation of warmth or heaviness, dry mouth, facial flushing, and nausea and vomiting (particularly in first-time users).

Some addicts report a rush when heroin is injected directly into their veins. Since the effects of heroin do not last long—usually only two to four hours—addicts have to "shoot up" two to five times a day. With large doses, the pupils become smaller; and the skin becomes cold, moist, and bluish. Breathing slows down; the user cannot be awakened and may stop breathing completely.

Risks

Addiction is common. Almost all regular users of opioids rapidly develop drug dependence, which can lead to lethargy, weight loss, loss of sex drive, and the continual effort to avoid withdrawal symptoms through repeated drug administration. In addition, they experience anxiety; insomnia; restlessness; and craving for the drug. Users continue taking opioids as much to avoid the discomfort of withdrawal—a classic sign of addiction—as to experience pleasure.

Opioid intoxication is characterized by changes in mood and behavior, such as initial euphoria followed by apathy or discontent and impaired judgment. Physical symptoms include constricted pupils (although pupils may dilate from a severe overdose), drowsiness, slurred speech, and impaired attention or memory. Morphine affects blood pressure, heart rate, and blood circulation in the brain. Both morphine and heroin slow down—depress—the respiratory system; overdoses can cause fatal respiratory arrest.

Opioid poisoning or overdose causes shock, coma, and depressed respiration and can be fatal. Emergency medical treatment is critical, often with drugs called narcotic antagonists that rapidly reverse the effects of opioids when administered intravenously.

Over time, users who inject opioids may develop infections of the heart lining and valves, skin abscesses, and lung congestion. Infections from unsterile solutions, syringes, and shared needles can lead to hepatitis, tetanus, liver disease, and HIV transmission. Depression is common and may be both an antecedent and risk factor for needle-sharing.[38] The annual death rate among those dependent on opioids is 20 times higher than among other young people, primarily because of physical complications, overdose, suicide, and the violent lifestyle of many users.

Withdrawal

If a regular user stops taking an opioid, withdrawal begins within 6 to 12 hours. The intensity of the symptoms depends on the degree of the addiction; they may grow stronger for 24 to 72 hours and gradually subside over a period of 7 to 14 days, though some symptoms, such as insomnia, may persist for several months. Individuals may develop craving for an opioid, irritability, nausea or vomiting, muscle aches, runny nose or eyes, dilated pupils, sweating, diarrhea, yawning, fever, and insomnia. Desperately craving the drug, users may plead, demand, or manipulate others to obtain more. Opioid withdrawal usually is not life-threatening.

Methadone Maintenance

Opioid dependence is a very difficult addiction to overcome. Studies demonstrate that only 10 to 30 percent of heroin users are able to maintain abstinence. This fact contributed to the development of a unique, yet still controversial, treatment for opioid dependence: the use of methadone, a long-acting opioid that users can substitute for heroin or other opioids.

Methadone is used in two basic ways to treat opioid dependence: as an opioid substitute for detoxification, usually with a gradual tapering of methadone over a period of 21 to 180 days, and as a maintenance treatment. Methadone maintenance has been criticized by some as nothing more than the substitution of a legal opioid, methadone, for an illegal opioid, heroin. Critics charge that since methadone maintenance does not have abstinence as its goal, it contributes to continued use of other drugs, such as cocaine or alcohol. There also is concern, especially by those in law enforcement, that methadone recipients will engage in "diversion," the sale of take-home doses of methadone for profit. Despite these charges, methadone maintenance remains the mainstay of opioid dependence treatment and is the most successful treatment currently available.

Methadone maintenance may be the most thoroughly studied drug treatment. Research has clearly documented several important positive benefits, including decreased use of illicit opioids; decreased criminal behavior; decreased risk of contracting HIV infection (through sharing of infected needles); and improvements in physical health, employment, and other lifestyle factors. Individuals who have been on methadone maintenance for a long time (often years), have stable relationships and employment, have assimilated themselves into the nondrug culture, and are highly motivated to get off methadone have the best chance for successful detoxification from methadone.

A number of new drug therapies are emerging as useful agents in the treatment of opioid dependence. Naltrexone (Trexan) has been approved as medication for alcohol-dependence and opioid-dependence treatment. Temgesic (buprenorphine), a mild, nonaddicting opiate that, like heroin and methadone, bonds to certain receptors in the brain, also has proven useful. It blocks pain messages and persuades the brain that its cravings for heroin have been satisfied. As long as they take buprenorphine, even long-term junkies report they simply do not want heroin any more.[39] ORLAAU (levoacetyl methadol) also is used to treat opiate dependence.

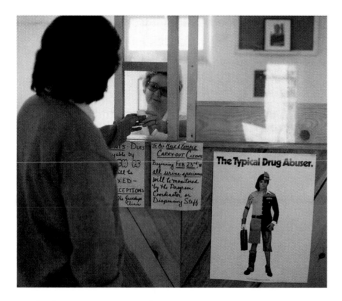

Methadone treatment has been criticized as a treatment for opioid addiction, but research clearly demonstrates positive benefits. Those who participate in long-term methadone maintenance programs usually move out of the drug culture and are candidates for eventually leaving methadone dependence behind them.

Phencyclidine (PCP)

PCP (phencyclidine—brand name Sernyl; streetnames "angel dust," "peace pill," "lovely," and "green")—is an illicit drug manufactured as a tablet, capsule, liquid, flake, spray, or crystal-like white powder that can be swallowed, smoked, sniffed, or injected. Sometimes it is sprinkled on crack, marijuana, tobacco, or parsley, and smoked. A fine-powdered form of PCP can be snorted or injected. Once PCP was thought to have medicinal value as an anesthetic, but its side effects, including delirium and hallucinations, made it unacceptable for medical use.

PCP use peaked in the 1970s, but it remains a popular drug of abuse in both inner-city ghettos and suburban high schools. Often users think that it is the PCP that they take together with another illegal psychoactive substance, such as amphetamines, coke, or hallucinogens, that is responsible for the highs they feel, so they seek it out specifically.

How Users Feel

The effects of PCP are utterly unpredictable. It may trigger violent behavior or irreversible psychosis the first time it is used, or the twentieth time, or never. In low doses, PCP produces changes—from hallucinations to euphoria to feelings of emptiness or numbness—similar to those produced by other psychoactive drugs. Higher doses may produce a stupor that lasts several days,

increased heart rate and blood pressure, flushing, sweating, dizziness, and numbness.

Risks

Some first-time users feel PCP is too unpredictable and do not try it again. Others quickly become heavy users. Many go on PCP binges or runs that can last several days. Some people use it daily, often along with alcohol and marijuana. It takes only a short period of occasional use for dependence or abuse to develop.

The behavioral changes associated with PCP intoxication, which can develop within minutes, include belligerence, aggressiveness, impulsiveness, unpredictability, agitation, poor judgment, and impaired functioning at work or in social situations. The physical symptoms of PCP intoxication include involuntary eye movements, increased blood pressure or heart rate, numbness or diminished responsiveness to pain, impaired coordination and speech, muscle rigidity, seizures, and a painful sensitivity to sound. Some people experience repetitive motor movements, such as facial grimacing, hallucinations, and paranoia. Suicide is a definite risk. Intoxication typically lasts four to six hours, but some effects can linger for several days. Delirium may occur within 24 hours of taking PCP or after recovery from an overdose and can last as much as a week.

PCP can trigger an episode of depression or anxiety that may persist for months. Some users reproach themselves constantly in the fear that they have destroyed their brains and will never return to normal. Some feel so restless that they cannot stop talking; some think they have superhuman strength. Large amounts can lead to convulsions, coma, heart and lung failure, ruptured blood vessels in the brain, and death.

Sedative-Hypnotics or Anxiolytic (Antianxiety) Drugs

These drugs depress the central nervous system, reduce activity, and induce relaxation, drowsiness, or sleep. They include the benzodiazepines and the barbiturates.

The **benzodiazepines**—the most widely used drugs in this category—are commonly prescribed for tension, muscular strain, sleep problems, anxiety, panic attacks, anesthesia, and in the treatment of alcohol withdrawal. They include such drugs as *chlordiazepoxide* (Librium), *diazepam* (Valium), *oxazepam* (Serax), *lorazepam* (Ativan), *flurazepam* (Dalmane), and *alprazolam* (Xanax). They differ widely in their mechanism of action, absorption rate, and metabolism, but all produce similar intoxication and withdrawal symptoms.

Benzodiazepine sleeping pills have largely replaced the **barbiturates,** which were used medically in the past for inducing relaxation and sleep, relieving tension, and treating epileptic seizures. These drugs are usually taken by mouth in tablet, capsule, or liquid form. When used as a general anesthetic, they are administered intravenously. Barbiturates such as *pentobarbital* (brand name Nembutal, or "yellow jackets"), *secobarbital* (Seconal, or "reds"), and *thiopental* (Pentothal) are short-acting and rapidly absorbed into the brain. The longer-acting barbiturates, such as *amobarbital* (brand name Amytal, or "blues" or "downers") and *phenobarbital* (Luminal, or "phennies"), which usually are taken orally and absorbed slowly into the bloodstream, take a while to reach the brain and have an effect for several days.

How Users Feel

The lower doses of these drugs may reduce or relieve tension, but increasing doses can cause a loosening of sexual or aggressive inhibitions. Individuals using this class of drugs may experience rapid mood changes, impaired judgment, and impaired social or occupational functioning. High doses produce slurred speech, drowsiness, and stupor.

Young people in their teens or early twenties who have used many illegal substances typically take sedative-hypnotic or anxiolytic drugs to obtain a high or a state of euphoria. Some use them in combination with other drugs. Less commonly, individuals may first obtain sedatives, hypnotics, or antianxiety medications by prescription from a physician for insomnia or anxiety and then gradually increase the dose or frequency of use on their own, often by seeking prescriptions from several physicians. While they justify this continued use because of their symptoms, the fact is that they reach a state in which they cannot function normally without the drug.

Risks

All the sedative-hypnotic and anxiolytic drugs can produce physical and psychological dependence within two to four weeks. A complication specific to sedatives is *cross-tolerance*—or cross-addiction—which occurs when users develop tolerance for one sedative or become dependent on it and develop tolerance for other sedatives as well. Individuals with a prior history of substance abuse are at greatly increased risk of abusing this class of drugs if they are prescribed by a physician. However, those who have not abused drugs or alcohol in the past rarely develop a substance-abuse problem from these medications when they are prescribed for legitimate psychiatric disorders, such as panic disorder or generalized anxiety disorder.

Intoxication with these drugs can produce changes in mood or behavior, such as inappropriate sexual or aggressive acts, mood swings, and impaired judgment. Physical signs include slurred speech, poor coordina-

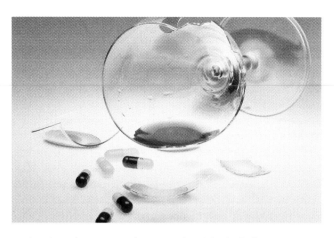

Antianxiety drugs react dangerously with alcohol.

tion, unsteady gait, involuntary eye movements, impaired attention or memory, and stupor or coma.

Taken in combination with alcohol, these drugs have a synergistic effect that can be dangerous or even lethal. For example, an individual's driving ability, already impaired by alcohol, will be made even worse, increasing the risk of an accident. Alcohol in combination with sedative-hypnotics leads to respiratory depression and may result in respiratory arrest and death. Regular users of any of these drugs who become physically dependent should not try to cut down or quit on their own. If they try to quit suddenly, they run the risk of seizures, coma, and death.

Sedative-hypnotic and anxiolytic drugs can easily cross through the placenta, and cause birth defects and behavioral problems. Babies born to women who used these drugs during pregnancy may be physically dependent on the drugs and may develop breathing problems, feeding difficulties, disturbed sleep, sweating, irritability, and fever.

Withdrawal

Withdrawal from sedative-hypnotic and anxiolytic drugs may range from relatively mild discomfort to a severe syndrome with grand mal seizures, depending on the degree of dependence. Withdrawal symptoms include malaise or weakness, sweating, rapid pulse, coarse tremor of the hands, tongue, and eyelids, insomnia, nausea or vomiting, temporary hallucinations or illusions, physical restlessness, anxiety or irritability, and grand mal seizures. Withdrawal may begin within two to three days after stopping drug use, and symptoms may persist for many weeks.

Other Drugs of Abuse

Anabolic steroids, synthetic derivatives of the male hormone testosterone, are powerful compounds prescribed for the treatment of burns and injuries. An estimated

1 million Americans, half of them adolescents (many of whom started steroid use before age 16), use black-market steroids. Nonmedical distribution of steroids is a federal offense punishable by five years in prison. (See Chapter 5 for a discussion of steroid use as a means of building muscle strength and size.)

The potential side effects of anabolic steroids include an increased risk of heart disease, stroke, or obstructed blood vessels; liver tumors and jaundice; acne; transmission, through shared needles, of HIV; breast enlargement, atrophy of the testicles, and impotence in men; and deepened voice, breast reduction, and beard growth in women. Even a brief period of use in childhood or adolescence can have lasting effects on brain and body chemistry. Steroids may increase the risk of heart disease by lowering levels of high-density lipoproteins (HDL), the "good" blood fat believed to remove deposits from artery walls.[40] Steroids can also create the same problems with dependence and withdrawal as cocaine.

Typical steroid users are male, middle-class, and white, who either want to boost their strength or look more muscular. They often take steroids in cycles of 4 to 18 weeks, followed by a break. Most "stack" the drugs, taking several pills or injectable drugs at once. Initially, they feel "juiced" or "pumped up," but they can also become irritable and aggressive. Some explode in unexpected violent outbursts, called "roid rages," or develop signs of mental illness, such as paranoia and delusions.

GHB and GBL

The brain messenger chemical called **GHB (gammahydroxybutyrate)**, stimulates the release of human growth hormone but has no known effects on muscle growth. Although this substance is banned by the FDA, users obtain it illegally either for its high, which is similar to that caused by alcohol or marijuana, or for its alleged ability to trim fat and build muscles. However, GHB can act in unpredictable ways in the body, and the Drug Enforcement Agency reports 3,500 cases of abuse, overdose, and arrests and at least 32 GHB-related deaths.

GHB, known as "blue nitro" or the "date rape drug" (discussed as such in Chapter 18), is popular at clubs and all-night dance parties called "raves." Its main ingredient is **GBL (gamma butyrolactone)**, an industrial solvent often used to strip floors. Once ingested, GBL converts into GHB, an odorless, colorless sedative that can be slipped into someone's drink to knock them out. The DEA reports at least 22 sexual assaults involving GHB. In one case, a young woman who lost consciousness after sipping a spiked Mountain Dew at a suburban party died the next day, and the teens accused of doctoring her drink were arraigned for manslaughter.[41]

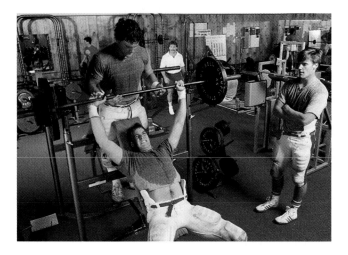

Pumping up. Steroids are an attractive—and highly dangerous—route to a muscular body. They are also illegal, and the side effects range from signs of mental illness to serious heart and liver damage.

In small doses, GHB and GBL are believed to induce euphoria and enhance sex by increasing dopamine in the brain. However, a larger dose can cause someone to pass out in 15 minutes and fall into a coma within half an hour. Other side effects include nausea, amnesia, hallucinations, decreased heart rate, and convulsions. Some users brew mixes in bathtubs and home labs, and police in several cities have reported an increase in deaths among those who drank GHB at clubs or "raves."

Similar chemicals can be found in other "party drugs," muscle builders, and sleep aids, often sold online with names such as "Thunder Nectar" and "Revitalize Plus." These products also contain 1,4 butanediol, a chemical that can cause dangerously low respiratory rates or even death.

Designer drugs are produced in chemical laboratories and sold illegally. Easy to manufacture from available raw materials, the drugs themselves were once technically legal because the law had to specify the exact chemical structure of an illicit drug. However, a law now bans all chemical "cousins" of illegal drugs.

Some of the drugs that emerged as dangers in the 1990s are legal and have legitimate medical uses (see Table 15-3). They include gamma hydroxybutyrate, or GHB or Liquid X (discussed above), a depressant with potential benefits for people with narcolepsy, and Rohypnol, a tranquilizer used overseas that also can be slipped into women's drinks to knock them out and cause short-term amnesia (see Chapter 18). Since the drugs are odorless and tasteless, a woman has no way of knowing whether her drink has been tampered with; the subsequent loss of memory leaves her with no explanation for where she's been or what's happened in the hours before she regains consciousness.

Another new drug of abuse is "K," or ketamine, an anesthetic used by veterinarians. When cooked, dried, and ground into a powder for snorting, K blocks chemical messengers in the brain that carry sensory input. As a result, the brain fills the void with hallucinations. Too much K can cause such massive sensory deprivation that researchers compare the impact to a near-death experience. Ketamine is illegal in several states, but the federal government has not yet deemed it a controlled substance—a step that would substantially increase penalties for its use.

Another synthetic, developed by college students in Pennsylvania in the early 1990s, is *methcathinone,* or "cat," a powerful synthetic stimulant that can produce a high that lasts up to six days. Cat usually contains a mix of chemicals along with small doses of Drano or battery acid, which act as a catalyst.

College and street chemists have also produced synthetic opiates that are particularly dangerous because they're far more potent than those derived from natural substances. Derivatives of *fentanyl,* an anesthetic widely used for surgery in the United States, are 20 to 2,000 times as powerful as heroin, and the risk of a fatal overdose or brain damage is much greater.

MDMA (methylene dioxymethylamphetamine, commonly called "ecstasy," Adam, or "X-TC") is somewhat related to mescaline and amphetamine. Psychiatrists once experimented with MDMA in patients because it alters a user's social and personal perceptions. However, the FDA has classified it, along with heroin and LSD, as a drug with "high potential for abuse and no medical usefulness." An estimated 500,000 to 4 million people—mostly college-age Americans—use the drug, which creates feelings of warmth and openness. The use of ecstasy has increased greatly on campus, with almost one of every four students at some universities reporting its use.

Users can develop insomnia, loss of appetite, muscle aches or stiffness, nausea, fatigue, and problems concentrating. MDMA destroys brain cells in animals; in humans it may damage the nerve cells that produce

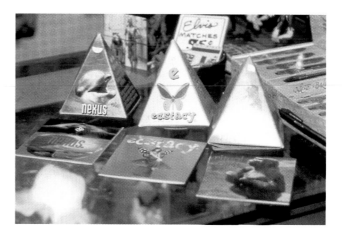

Designer drugs, made in the laboratory and sold on the street, aren't subject to quality controls and don't always contain what the buyer expects.

serotonin, a neurotransmitter involved in regulating responses to stress and pain, appetite, and sexual behavior. The damage produced by ecstasy may do lasting harm by causing key nerve cells in the brain to grow back abnormally.[42]

In Great Britain, MDMA has killed at least 15 young persons and caused serious medical complications in many others. Almost all the victims took recreational doses at a club or "rave." Usually the stricken users collapse or develop seizures while dancing. Their body temperatures soar to as high as 110°F, while their pulses race and their blood pressures plummet. Some die, generally because of the effects of *hyperthermia* (elevated body temperature), within 2 to 60 hours. Prolonged vigorous dancing, particularly in hot, poorly ventilated rooms in which dancers can become dehydrated, may compound the dangers of this drug.

"Herbal" drugs also are being marketed as substitutes for standard street drugs. With names such as "herbal ecstasy," "nexus," and "ritual spirit," these tablets and capsules are advertised as safe and potent agents that can lead to "sacred visions," "tingly happy-

■ Table 15-3	New Drugs of Abuse			
Drug	**Street Name**	**Medical Use**	**Effect**	**Cost**
Ketamine hydrochloride	K, Special K, Vitamin K	An anesthetic used in animals and frail humans	Hallucinations, sensory distortions	$40–$100 per gram of powder or 10-ml bottle of liquid
Gamma-hydroxybutyrate	Liquid X, Blue nitro, Grievous bodily harm, G	A depressant that could possibly be used to treat narcolepsy	Relaxation and temporary euphoria	$5–$20 per dose
Flunitrazepam	Roofies, Roach	A strong sedative used overseas	Alcohol-like intoxication, drowsiness	$3–$5 per pill

happy buzz," and better sex. However, critics warn that the herbal pills have dangerous and unpleasant side effects, including stroke, heart attack, and a disfiguring skin condition. They are sold at head shops, night clubs, and raves. The FDA has been investigating these agents, after receiving hundreds of complaints of strokes, seizures, and possibly even some deaths.

Treating Drug Dependence and Abuse

The most difficult step for a drug user is to admit that he or she *is* in fact an addict. If they are not forced to deal with their problem through some unexpected trauma, such as being fired or going bankrupt, those who care—family, friends, coworkers, doctors—may have to confront them and insist that they do something about their addiction. Often this intervention can be the turning point for addicts and their families.

Treatment may take place in an outpatient setting, a residential facility, or a hospital. Increasingly, treatment thereafter is tailored to address coexisting or dual diagnoses. A personal treatment plan may consist of individual psychotherapy, marital and family therapy, medication, and behavior therapy. Once an individual has made the decision to seek help for substance abuse, the first step usually is detoxification, which involves clearing the drug from the body. An exception is methadone maintenance, discussed earlier in this chapter, which does not rely on complete detoxification.

Controlled and supervised withdrawal within a medical or psychiatric hospital may be recommended if an individual has not been able to stop using drugs as an outpatient or in a residential treatment program. Detoxification is most likely to be complicated when a person is a polysubstance abuser and may require close monitoring and treatment of potentially fatal withdrawal symptoms. Other reasons for inpatient treatment include lack of psychosocial support for maintaining abstinence; the absence of a drug-free living environment; or a complicated drug history with addiction to multiple substances. However, restrictions on insurance coverage may limit the number of days of inpatient care. Increasingly, once individuals complete detoxification, they continue treatment in residential programs or as outpatients.

Medications are used in detoxification to alleviate withdrawal symptoms and prevent medical and psychiatric complications. Once withdrawal is complete, adjunctive medications are discontinued, so the individual is in a drug-free state. However, those with mental disorders may require appropriate psychiatric medication to manage their symptoms and reduce the risk of relapse. For example, a person suffering from major depression or panic disorder may require ongoing treatment with antidepressant medication.

The aim of chemical dependence treatment is to help individuals establish and maintain their recovery from alcohol and drugs of abuse. Recovery is a dynamic process of personal growth and healing that takes place as one makes the transition from a lifestyle of active substance use to drug-free recovery.

Whatever their setting, chemical dependence treatment programs initially involve some period of intensive treatment followed by one or two years of continuing aftercare. Most freestanding programs—those not affiliated with a hospital—follow what is known as the *Minnesota Model,* a treatment approach developed at Hazelden Recovery Center in Center City, Minnesota, more than 30 years ago. Its key principles include a focus on drug use as the primary problem, not as a symptom of underlying emotional problems; a multidisciplinary approach that addresses the physical, emotional, spiritual, family, and social aspects of the individual; a supportive community; and a goal of abstinence and health.

Outpatient programs for substance abuse, offered by freestanding centers, hospitals, and community mental health centers, often run four or five nights a week for four weeks to eight weeks, or in daily eight-hour sessions for seven to eight days, followed by weekly group therapy. These outpatient programs allow recovering drug users to go on with their daily lives and learn to deal with day-to-day work and family stresses. Mental health professionals in private practice also offer individually structured outpatient treatment.

Therapy groups provide an opportunity for individuals who have often been isolated by their drug use to participate in normal social settings. Small groups with other drug users can be especially valuable because they all share the experience of drug use; the members can confront one another with frankness and cut through lies and rationalizations. A professional therapist keeps members of the group from ganging up on one person. After their discharge from inpatient treatment, individuals who became involved in self-help groups were less likely to use drugs, coped better with stress, and developed richer friendship networks.[43]

12-Step Programs

Since its founding in 1935, Alcoholics Anonymous (AA)—the oldest, largest, and most successful self-help program in the world—has spawned a movement (see Chapter 16). As many as 200 different recovery programs are based on the spiritual **12-step program** of AA. Participation in 12-step programs for drug abusers, such as Substance Anonymous, Narcotics

Anonymous, and Cocaine Anonymous, is of fundamental importance in promoting and maintaining long-term abstinence.[44]

The basic precept of 12-step programs is that members have been powerless when it comes to controlling their addictive behavior on their own. These programs don't recruit members. The desire to stop must come from the individual, who can call the number of a 12-step program, listed in the telephone book, and find out when and where the next nearby meeting will be held. A representative may offer to send someone to the caller's house to talk about the problem and to escort him or her to the next meeting.

Meetings of various 12-step programs are held daily in almost every city in the country. (Some chapters, whose members often include the disabled or those in remote areas, "meet" via electronic bulletin boards on their personal computers.) There are no dues or fees for membership. Many individuals belong to several programs because they have several problems, such as alcoholism, substance abuse, and pathological gambling. All have only one requirement for membership: a desire to stop an addictive behavior.

To get the most out of a 12-step program:

- Try out different groups until you find one you like and in which you feel comfortable.

- Once you find a group in which you feel comfortable, go back several times (some recommend a minimum of six meetings) before making a final decision on whether to continue.

- Keep an open mind. Listen to other people's stories and ask yourself if you've had similar feelings or experiences.

- Accept whatever feels right to you, and ignore the rest. One common saying in 12-step programs is, "Take what you like and leave the rest."

Relapse Prevention

The most common clinical course for substance abuse disorders involves a pattern of multiple relapses over the course of a life span. It is important for individuals with these problems and their families to recognize this fact. When relapses do occur, they should be viewed as neither a mark of defeat nor evidence of moral weakness. While painful, they do not erase the progress that has been achieved and ultimately may strengthen self-understanding. They can serve as reminders of potential pitfalls to avoid in the future.

One key to preventing relapse is learning to avoid obvious cues and associations that can set off intense cravings. This means staying away from the people and places linked with past drug use. Some therapists use

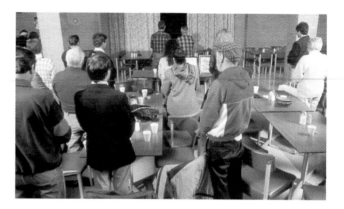

Twelve-step programs, based on the Alcoholics Anonymous model, have helped many people overcome behavioral addictions and addictions to alcohol, food, and drugs. The one requirement for membership is a desire to stop living out a pattern of addictive behavior.

conditioning techniques to give former users some sense of control over their urge to use the drug. The theory behind this approach, which is called *extinction* of conditioned behavior, is that with repeated exposure—for example, to videotapes of dealers selling crack cocaine—the arousal and craving will diminish. While this technique by itself cannot ward off relapses, it does seem to enhance the overall effectiveness of other therapies.

Another important lesson that therapists emphasize is that every "lapse" does not have to lead to a full-blown relapse. Users can turn to the skills acquired in treatment—calling people for support or going to meetings—to avoid a major relapse. Ultimately, users must learn much more than how to avoid temptation; they must examine their entire view of the world and learn new ways to live in it without turning to drugs. This is the underlying goal of the recovery process.

Outlook

Whatever the drug, recovery from dependence and abuse is a process of immense inner change that involves every aspect of a person's life. It does not follow a straight, even course, but moves back and forth between denial—of dependence, of loss of control, or of the severity of the problem—and awareness, ignorance and knowledge, craving and commitment. It often starts with a feeling of great relief, followed by a deep sense of emptiness. Individuals who have abused or become dependent on drugs must form a new identity, stop living in the past or future, give up their search for a quick fix, change the way they relate to family and old friends, find new things to do with the time they previously spent on their drug habit, learn new behaviors, and adopt new attitudes. Through treatment, education, and a reevaluation of what is meaningful in life, drug users can find a better way of living.

Strategies *for* Prevention

Relapse-Prevention Planning

The following steps, from Terence Gorski and Merlene Miller's *Staying Sober* can lower the likelihood of relapses:

✓ *Stabilization and self-assessment.* Get control of yourself. Find out what's going on in your head, heart, and life.

✓ *Education.* Learn about relapse and what to do to prevent it.

✓ *Warning-sign identification and management.* Make a list of your personal relapse warning signs. Learn how to interrupt them before you lose control.

✓ *Inventory training.* Learn how to become consciously aware of warning signs as they develop.

✓ *Review of the recovery program.* Make sure your recovery program is able to help you manage your warning signs of relapse.

✓ *Involvement of significant others.* Teach them how to help you avoid relapses.

Codependence

Codependence refers to the tendency of the spouses, partners, parents, and friends of individuals who use drugs or alcohol to allow, or *enable,* their loved ones to continue their drug use and self-destructive behavior. (Codependence is also discussed in Chapter 16.)

Codependents Anonymous, founded in 1986 for "men and women whose common problem is an inability to maintain functional relationships," sponsors support programs throughout the country. Nar-Anon provides groups for people affected by drug abuse. Both are listed in the resource directory at the back of this book; local chapters are in the white pages of the telephone directory.

If someone you love has a drug problem, get as much information as you can so that you understand what you—and your loved one—are up against. Also get some intervention training. Specially trained counselors work at most chemical-dependency units; some offer advice by phone. Here are some specific recommendations:

- Confront the user. Along with other loved ones and, if possible, a professional counselor, detail incident

after incident in which the drug abuse affected or hurt you, other members of your family, or the user.

- Don't expect a drug abuser to quit without help. Chemical dependence is a medical and psychological disorder that requires professional treatment. Offer your support, but make it clear that you expect your loved one to undergo therapy.

- If your loved one agrees to treatment, make sure that the program is based on a complete evaluation, checking for medical and emotional problems, as well as chemical dependency.

- Don't believe abusers who say they've learned to control their drug use. Abstinence is a cornerstone of any good rehabilitation program.

- Encourage a user to attend support groups, such as Cocaine Anonymous or Narcotics Anonymous, for at least one year after rehabilitation. Get help for yourself. Most hospitals and chemical-dependency programs offer educational programs for codependents.

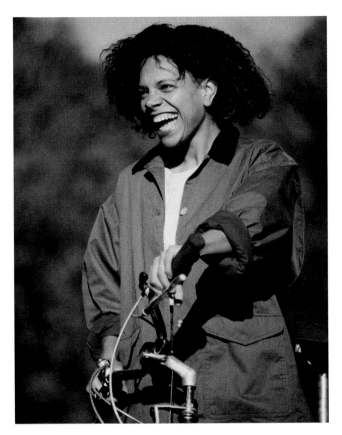

A quick fix? If drugs appear attractive as a "fix" for difficult times, try healthier remedies first, especially those that take you out-of-doors or get you active.

Making This Chapter Work for You

Working Toward a Drug-Free Future

■ Drugs—chemical substances that alter physiological or psychological processes—can be misused (used for a purpose—or person—other than that for which they were medically intended) or abused (used excessively or inappropriately). The misuse or abuse of psychoactive drugs can lead to physical and psychological dependence.

■ Physical dependence occurs when physiological changes in the body caused by a drug result in an intense need for the drug. Psychological dependence occurs when users crave a drug for the emotional or mental changes it produces.

■ Over-the-counter (OTC) drugs and prescription drugs can be misused or abused. The OTCs most often abused include painkillers and nasal inhalants. Prescription medications are often misused despite serious physical risks. The nonmedical, illegal use of anabolic steroids has become popular among young men who want to look muscular or build up their strength.

■ Caffeine, though habit-forming and implicated in various health problems, doesn't seem to present any clear health threat if used in moderation.

■ Amphetamine abusers may suffer from tremors, irregular heartbeat, loss of coordination, psychosis and paranoia, malnutrition, skin disorders, ulcers, depression, brain damage, and heart failure. A form of smokeable methamphetamine, known as ice or glass, increases heart rate and blood pressure; high doses can cause permanent damage to blood vessels in the brain. Like ice, crank (propylhexedrine) produces effects similar to those of amphetamines.

■ THC, the primary psychoactive ingredient in marijuana and hashish, can produce an increased heart rate, dry mouth and throat, and altered perception; high doses may result in distorted perception, hallucinations, and acute panic attacks. Long-term marijuana use may result in psychological dependence; lung damage; impairment of the central nervous system, reproductive system, and immune system; use of other drugs; mental and emotional dulling; loss of drive; and legal consequences.

■ Cocaine, which produces feelings of high energy, may be snorted as a powder, smoked (or freebased) in a form called crack or rock, or dissolved in a solution that's then injected. The effects of cocaine use include impaired judgment, psychological disorders (including psychosis), headache, nausea, damaged nasal membranes in snorters, weight loss, liver damage, heart attack, stroke, brain seizure or hemorrhage, complications during pregnancy, and mental and physical damage to infants born to cocaine users.

■ Sedative-hypnotics and antianxiety agents turn down the central nervous system. Barbiturate use can result in physical dependence, and because the addict needs increasingly larger doses, the risk of fatal overdose is high. Antianxiety medications, such as Valium and Xanax, can produce dependence, drowsiness, and slurred speech; withdrawal can produce coma, psychosis, and even death.

■ Hallucinogens, including peyote and its active ingredient, mescaline; lysergic acid diethylamide (LSD); psilocybin; and phencyclidine (PCP) can produce hallucinations and, in some users, panic, paranoia, and psychotic episodes. PCP is a dangerous psychoactive drug because of its effects on behavior.

■ The opiates, including opium, morphine, heroin, and codeine, may lead to infections of the heart, skin abscesses, and congested lungs, as well as tetanus, liver disease, hepatitis, and HIV infection from the use of unsterile syringes and needles. An addict who stops taking an opiate will experience withdrawal sickness—nausea, abdominal cramps, fever, sweating and chills, diarrhea, and severe aches and pains. The most abused synthetic opiates are Demerol and Darvon.

■ Inhalants, including amyl nitrite and butyl nitrite, can lead to serious complications. Designer drugs are illegally manufactured drugs that are far more potent than natural substances.

■ Treatment for drug dependence usually includes a combination of approaches, including detoxification in a hospital or as an outpatient; admission to a residential therapeutic community; or treatment in an outpatient drug-counseling program that may use behavioral, cognitive, and social-skills training techniques.

■ Codependence is an emotional and psychological behavioral pattern in which the spouses, partners, parents, and friends of individuals with addictive behaviors allow or enable their loved ones to continue their self-destructive habits. Codependents feel responsible for meeting others' needs, have low self-esteem, and frequently have compulsions of their own.

 Buying Drugs Online. What are the risks and benefits of buying prescription drugs online?

health **/ ONLINE**

Partnership for a Drug Free America
http://www.drugfreeamerica.org/
This site contains comprehensive information on commonly abused drugs, including photos and effects of use.

National Institute on Drug Abuse
http://www.nida.nih.gov/
From this site, you can access fact sheets on commonly abused drugs, view results from drug use surveys, and more.

Web of Addictions
http://www.well.com/user/woa/
From this site you can find fact sheets on drugs, information about self-help and support groups for drug addiction, and links to other resources on the web.

Please note that links are subject to change. If you find a broken link, use a search engine like http://www.yahoo.com *and search for the web site by typing in key words.*

 Campus Chat: Are campus drug prevention programs effective? Share your thoughts on our online discussion forum at **http://health.wadsworth.com**

Find It On InfoTrac: You can find additional readings related to drugs via InfoTrac College Edition, an online library of more than 900 journals and publications. Follow the instructions for accessing InfoTrac that came packaged with your textbook; then search for articles using a key word search.

- **Suggested reading:** "Early Drug Use May/May not Predict Long-term Problems" by Fruma Efreom. The Brown University Digest of Addiction Theory and Application, Vol. 18, Issue 4, p. 1, April 1999.

  (1) What are the two most important determinants for assessing one's potential risk for future drug dependency and/or abuse?

  (2) At most ages, what gender and ethnic group have the highest potential for developing drug abuse?

For additional links, resources, and suggested readings on InfoTrac, visit our Health & Wellness Resource Center at **http://health.wadsworth.com**

Key Terms

The terms listed here are used within the chapter. Page numbers are included for each term. A definition of each term is given in the Glossary pages at the end of this book.

Critical Thinking Questions

1. Some argue that marijuana should be a legalized drug like alcohol and tobacco. What is your opinion on this issue? Defend your position.

2. Some web enthusiasts oppose any kind of government regulations on the Internet. Do you agree or disagree?

How would you address the problems associated with distributing drugs online?

References

1. Department of Health and Human Services.
2. Chen, Ingfet, and Elizabeth Krieger. "Now, Fine Print You Can Read." *Health,* Vol. 13, Issue 5, June 1999.
3. Ibid.
4. "Drug Adherence." *Journal of the American Medical Association,* July 21, 1999.
5. Gorman, Jack. Personal interview.
6. Stolberg, Sheryl. "Internet Prescriptions Boom in the 'Wild West' of the Web." *New York Times,* June 27, 1999.
7. Fischmann, Joshua, and Marissa Melton. "Drug Bazaar." *U.S. News & World Report,* Vol. 126, Issue 24, June 21, 1999.
8. Herz, Rachel. "Caffeine Effects on Mood and Memory." *Behavior Research and Therapy,* Vol. 37, No. 9, September 1999.
9. Nehlig, Astrid. "Does Caffeine Lead to Psychological Dependence?" *CHEMTECH,* Vol. 29, No. 7, July 1999.
10. Fenster, Laura, et al. "Caffeine Consumption and Menstrual Function." *American Journal of Epidemiology,* Vol. 149, No. 6, March 15, 1999.
11. Dager, Stephen, et al. "Human Brain Metabolic Response to Caffeine and the Effects of Tolerance." *American Journal of Psychiatry,* Vol. 156, No. 2, February 1999.
12. Franklin, John. "Addiction Medicine." *Journal of the American Medical Association,* Vol. 273, No. 21, June 7, 1995.
13. Glare, P.G.W. *Oxford Latin Dictionary.* Oxford, England: Clarendon Press, 1985.
14. Frances, Richard. Personal interview.
15. Powledge, Tabitha. "Addiction and the Brain." *BioScience,* Vol. 49, Issue 7, July 1999.
16. Ibid.
17. Wilens, Timothy, et al. "Risk for Substance Use Disorders in Youths with Child- and Adolescent-Onset Bipolar Disorder." *Journal of the American Academy of Child and Adolescent Psychiatry,* Vol. 38, Issue 6, June 1999.
18. *National Household Survey on Drug Abuse.* Washington, D.C.: White House Office of Drug Control Policy, 1999.
19. "Costs to Society." National Institute on Drug Abuse, http://www.nida.nih.gov
20. *National Household Survey on Drug Abuse.*
21. Douglas, Kathy, et al. "Results from the 1995 National College Health Risk Behavior Survey." *Journal of American College Health,* Vol. 46, September 1997.
22. Perkins, H. Wesley, et al. "Misperceptions for the Frequency of Alcohol and Other Drug Use on College Campuses." *Journal of American College Health,* Vol. 47, No. 6, May 1999.
23. "Typical Drug User Is Profiled by the U.S." *New York Times,* September 9, 1999.
24. Bennett, Joel. "Substance Use Impacts Co-Workers." *Journal of Health and Social Behavior,* September 1999.
25. Albertson, Timothy, et al. "Methamphetamine and the Expanding Complications of Amphetamines." *Western Journal of Medicine,* Vol. 170, Issue 4, April 1999.
26. "NIJ Study Question Link Between Methamphetamine Use, Violence." *Alcoholism & Drug Abuse Weekly,* Vol. 11, Issue 20, May 17, 1999.
27. "Methamphetamine." National Institute on Drug Abuse, http://www.nida.nih.gov
28. "Marijuana and Medicine: Assessing the Science Base." Washington, D.C.: National Academy of Science, 1999.
29. Pope, Harrison, and Deborah Yurgulen-Todd. "The Residual Cognitive Effects of Heavy Marijuana Use in College Students." *Journal of the American Medical Association,* Vol. 275, No. 7, February 21, 1996.
30. "Study Finds Withdrawal Syndrome from Long-Term Marijuana Use." *Alcoholism & Drug Abuse Weekly,* Vol. 11, Issue 17, April 26, 1999.
31. "Marijuana and Medicine: Assessing the Science Base."
32. "Crack and Cocaine." National Institute on Drug Abuse, http://www.nida.nih.gov
33. Stocker, Steven. "Cocaine's Pleasurable Effects May Involve Multiple Chemical Sites." *NIDA Notes,* Vol. 14, No. 2, September 1999.
34. "Study Outlines Limited Effectiveness of Prevention on Cocaine Use." *Alcoholism & Drug Abuse Weekly,* Vol. 11, Issue 23, June 7, 1999.
35. "Inhalants." National Institute on Drug Abuse, http://www.nida.nih.gov
36. "Teen Heroin Use Continues to Rise." *Brown University Digest of Addiction Theory and Application,* Vol. 18, Issue 3, March 1999.
37. "Heroin." National Institute on Drug Abuse, http://www.nida.nih.gov
38. Mandell, Wallace, et al. "Depressive Symptoms, Drug Network, and Their Synergistic Effect on Needle-Sharing Behavior Among Street Injection Drug Users." *American Journal of Drug and Alcohol Abuse,* Vol. 25, No. 1, February 1999.
39. "Buprenorphine Update: Questions and Answers." National Institute on Drug Abuse, http://www.nida.nih.gov
40. Sachtleben, Thomas, et al. "Serum Lipoprotein Patterns in Long-term Anabolic Steroid Users." *Research Quarterly for Exercise and Sport,* Vol. 68, No. 1, March 1997.
41. Cannon, Angie. "Sex, Drugs, and Sudden Death." *U.S. News & World Report,* Vol. 126, Issue 20, May 24, 1999.
42. "Ecstasy." National Institute on Drug Abuse, http://www.nida.nih.gov
43. Humphreys, Keith. "Substance Abuse Support Groups Improve Coping, Friendships." *Annals of Behavioral Medicine,* June 1999.
44. Lurtz, Linda. "Recovery, the 12-step Movement, and Politics." *Social Work,* Vol. 42, No. 14, July 1997.

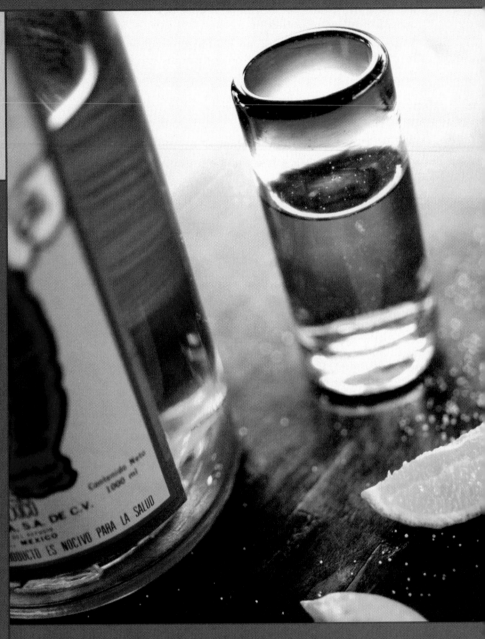

CHAPTER

16

Alcohol Use, Misuse, and Abuse

After studying the material in this chapter, you should be able to:

- **Describe** the factors affecting a drinker's response to alcohol consumption.
- **List** the effects of alcohol on the body systems.
- **Describe** the impact of alcohol misuse among women and different ethnic groups.
- **Define** alcoholism, and **list** common symptoms of this disease.
- **List** the negative consequences to individuals, and to our society, from alcohol abuse.
- **Explain** the common treatment methods for alcoholism.

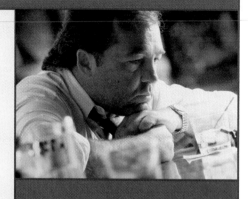

Alcohol is the most widely used mind-altering substance in the world. In the United States, about half of all adults drink, at least occasionally. Ninety percent of college students use alcohol, and dangerous practices, such as drinking binges, are common on campuses across the country.

The majority of people who use alcohol don't abuse it. The key to their responsible drinking isn't necessarily saying "No," but knowing when to say "No more." Even occasional drinkers need to learn their limits and recognize the point at which alcohol impairs their judgment or threatens their well-being. For some people in some circumstances, one drink may be too many.

When not used responsibly, alcohol can take an enormous toll. No medical conditions, other than heart disease, cause more disability and premature death than alcohol-related problems. No mental or medical disorders touch the lives of more families. No other form of disability costs individuals, employers, and the government more for treatment, injuries, reduced worker productivity, and property damage. The costs in emotional pain and in lost and shattered lives because of irresponsible drinking are beyond measure.

This chapter provides information about alcohol, its impact on the body, brain, behavior, and society, patterns of drinking, and the recognition, understanding, and treatment of drinking problems and of alcoholism. ❖

FREQUENTLY ASKED QUESTIONS

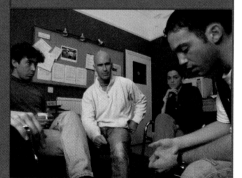

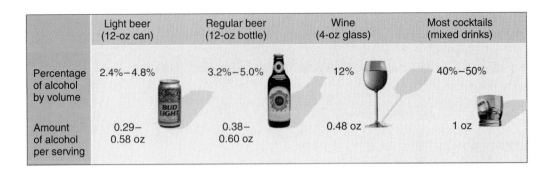

	Light beer (12-oz can)	Regular beer (12-oz bottle)	Wine (4-oz glass)	Most cocktails (mixed drinks)
Percentage of alcohol by volume	2.4%–4.8%	3.2%–5.0%	12%	40%–50%
Amount of alcohol per serving	0.29–0.58 oz	0.38–0.60 oz	0.48 oz	1 oz

Alcohol and Its Effects

Pure alcohol is a colorless liquid obtained through the fermentation of a liquid containing sugar. **Ethyl alcohol,** or *ethanol,* is the type of alcohol in alcoholic beverages. Another type—methyl, or wood, alcohol—is a poison that should never be drunk. Any liquid containing 0.5 to 80 percent ethyl alcohol by volume is an alcoholic beverage. However, different drinks contain different amounts of alcohol (see Figure 16-1).

One drink can be any of the following:

- One bottle or can (12 ounces) of beer, which is 5 percent alcohol.
- One glass (4 ounces) of table wine, such as burgundy, which is 12 percent alcohol.
- One small glass (2 1/2 ounces) of fortified wine, which is 20 percent alcohol.
- One shot (1 ounce) of distilled spirits (such as whiskey, vodka, or rum), which is 50 percent alcohol.

All of these drinks contain close to the same amount of alcohol—that is, if the number of ounces in each drink is multiplied by the percentage of alcohol, each drink contains the equivalent of approximately 1/2 ounce of 100 percent ethyl alcohol. With distilled spirits (such as bourbon, scotch, vodka, gin, and rum), alcohol content is expressed in terms of **proof,** a number that is *twice* the percentage of alcohol: 100-proof bourbon is 50 percent alcohol; 80-proof gin is 40 percent alcohol.

But the words *bottle* and *glass* can be deceiving in this context. Drinking a 16-ounce bottle of malt liquor, which is 6.4 percent alcohol, is not the same as drinking a 12-ounce glass of 3.2 percent beer. Two bottles of high-alcohol wines (such as Cisco), packaged to resemble much less powerful wine coolers, can lead to alcohol poisoning, especially in those who weigh less than 150 pounds. This is one reason why it is a serious danger for young people.

How Much Alcohol Can I Drink?

The best way to figure how much you can drink safely is to determine the amount of alcohol in your blood at any given time, or your **blood-alcohol concentration (BAC).** BAC is expressed in terms of the percentage of alcohol in the blood and is often measured from breath or urine samples. Law enforcement officers use BAC to determine whether a driver is legally drunk. The Federal Department of Transportation has called on states to set 0.08 percent—the BAC that a 150-pound man would have after consuming about three mixed drinks within an hour—as the threshold at which a person can be cited for drunk driving. In the past, 0.1 percent was often the legal limit. (See Figure 16-2.)

A BAC of 0.05 percent indicates approximately 5 parts alcohol to 10,000 parts other blood components. Most people reach this level after consuming one or two drinks and experience all the positive sensations of drinking—relaxation, euphoria, and well-being—without feeling intoxicated. If they continue to drink past the 0.05 percent BAC level, they start feeling worse rather than better, gradually losing control of speech, balance, and emotions (see Table 16-1). At a BAC of 0.2 percent, they may pass out. At a BAC of 0.3 percent, they could lapse into a coma; at 0.4 percent, they could die.

For some people, even very low blood alcohol concentrations can cause a headache, upset stomach, or dizziness. These reactions often are inborn. People who have suffered brain damage—often as a result of head trauma or encephalitis—may lose all tolerance for alcohol, either temporarily or permanently, and behave abnormally after drinking small amounts. The elderly, as well as those who are unusually fatigued or have a debilitating physical illness, may also have a low tolerance to alcohol and respond inappropriately to a small amount.

Men	Approximate blood alcohol percentage								
	Body weight in pounds								
Drinks	100	120	140	160	180	200	220	240	
0	.00	.00	.00	.00	.00	.00	.00	.00	Only safe driving limit
1	.04	.03	.03	.02	.02	.02	.02	.02	Impairment begins
2	.08	.06	.05	.05	.04	.04	.03	.03	Driving skills significantly affected
3	.11	.09	.08	.07	.06	.06	.05	.05	
4	.15	.12	.11	.09	.08	.08	.07	.06	
5	.19	.16	.13	.12	.11	.09	.09	.08	Possible criminal penalties
6	.23	.19	.16	.14	.13	.11	.10	.09	
7	.26	.22	.19	.16	.15	.13	.12	.11	
8	.30	.25	.21	.19	.17	.15	.14	.13	Legally intoxicated
9	.34	.28	.24	.21	.19	.17	.15	.14	Criminal penalties
10	.38	.31	.27	.23	.21	.19	.17	.16	

Subtract .01% for each 40 minutes of drinking.
One drink is 1.25 oz. of 80 proof liquor, 12 oz. of beer, or 5 oz. of table wine.

Women	Approximate blood alcohol percentage									
	Body weight in pounds									
Drinks	90	100	120	140	160	180	200	220	240	
0	.00	.00	.00	.00	.00	.00	.00	.00	.00	Only safe driving limit
1	.05	.05	.04	.03	.03	.03	.02	.02	.02	Impairment begins
2	.10	.09	.08	.07	.06	.05	.05	.04	.04	Driving skills significantly affected
3	.15	.14	.11	.10	.09	.08	.07	.06	.06	
4	.20	.18	.15	.13	.11	.10	.09	.08	.08	Possible criminal penalties
5	.25	.23	.19	.16	.14	.13	.11	.10	.09	
6	.30	.27	.23	.19	.17	.15	.14	.12	.11	
7	.35	.32	.27	.23	.20	.18	.16	.14	.13	Legally intoxicated
8	.40	.36	.30	.26	.23	.20	.18	.17	.15	Criminal penalties
9	.45	.41	.34	.29	.26	.23	.20	.19	.17	
10	.51	.45	.38	.32	.28	.25	.23	.21	.19	

Subtract .01% for each 40 minutes of drinking.
One drink is 1.25 oz. of 80 proof liquor, 12 oz. of beer, or 5 oz. of table wine.

■ Figure 16-2 Alcohol impairment charts.

Source: http://www.health.org/pubs/qdocs/alcohol/bac-chrt.htm. Data supplied by the Pennsylvania Liquor Control Board.

What Factors Influence the Body's Response to Alcohol?

Many factors affect an individual's BAC and response to alcohol, including the following:

- *How much and how quickly you drink.* The more alcohol you put into your body, the higher your BAC. If you chug drink after drink, your liver, which metabolizes about 1/2 ounce of alcohol an hour, won't be able to keep up—and your BAC will soar.

- *What you're drinking.* The stronger the drink, the faster and harder the alcohol hits. Straight shots of liquor and cocktails such as martinis will get alcohol into your bloodstream faster than beer or table wine. Beer and wine not only contain lower concentrations of alcohol, but they also contain nonalcoholic substances that slow the rate of **absorption** (passage of the alcohol into your body tissues). If the drink contains water, juice, or milk, the rate of absorption will be slowed. However, carbon dioxide—whether in champagne, ginger ale, or a cola—whisks alcohol into your bloodstream. Also, the alcohol in warm drinks—such as a hot rum toddy or warmed sake—moves into your bloodstream more quickly than the alcohol in chilled wine or scotch on the rocks.

- *Your size.* If you're a large person (whether due to fat or to muscle), you'll get drunk more slowly than someone smaller who's drinking the same amount of alcohol at the same rate. Heavier individuals have a larger water volume, which dilutes the alcohol they drink.

- *Your gender.* Women have lower quantities of a stomach enzyme that neutralizes alcohol, so one drink for

■ Table 16-1 Recognizing the Warning Signs of Alcoholism

- Experiencing the following symptoms after drinking: frequent headaches, nausea, stomach pain, heartburn, gas, fatigue, weakness, muscle cramps, or irregular or rapid heartbeats.
- Needing a drink in the morning to start the day.

- Denying any problem with alcohol.
- Doing things while drinking that are regretted afterward.
- Dramatic mood swings, from anger to laughter to anxiety.
- Sleep problems.

- Depression and paranoia.
- Forgetting what happened during a drinking episode.
- Changing brands or going on the wagon to control drinking.
- Having five or more drinks a day.

a woman has the impact that two drinks have for a man. Hormone levels also affect the impact of alcohol. Women are more sensitive to alcohol just before menstruation, and birth control pills and other forms of estrogen can intensify alcohol's impact. (See the section "Women and Alcohol" later in this chapter.)

- *Your age.* The same amount of alcohol produces higher BACs in older drinkers, who have lower volumes of body water to dilute the alcohol than younger drinkers do.

- *Your race.* Many members of certain ethnic groups, including Asians and Native Americans, are unable to break down alcohol as quickly as Caucasians. This can result in higher BACs, as well as uncomfortable reactions, such as flushing and nausea, when they drink.

- *Other drugs.* Some common medications—including aspirin, acetaminophen (Tylenol), and ulcer medications—can cause blood-alcohol levels to increase more rapidly. Individuals taking these drugs can be over the legal limit for blood-alcohol concentration after as little as a single drink.

- *Family history of alcoholism.* Some children of alcoholics don't develop any of the usual behavioral symptoms that indicate someone is drinking too much. It's not known whether this behavior is genetically caused or is a result of growing up with an alcoholic.

- *Eating.* Food slows the absorption of alcohol by diluting it, by covering some of the membranes through which alcohol would be absorbed, and by prolonging the time the stomach takes to empty.

- *Expectations.* In various experiments, volunteers who believed they were given alcoholic beverages but were actually given nonalcoholic drinks acted as if they were guzzling the real thing and became more talkative, relaxed, and sexually stimulated.

- *Physical tolerance.* If you drink regularly, your brain becomes accustomed to a certain level of alcohol. You may be able to look and behave in a seemingly normal fashion, even though you drink as much as

would normally intoxicate someone your size. However, your driving ability and judgment will still be impaired.

Once you develop tolerance, you may drink more to get the desired effects from alcohol. In some people, this can lead to abuse and alcoholism. On the other hand, after years of drinking, some people become exquisitely sensitive to alcohol. Such reverse tolerance means that they can become intoxicated after drinking only a small amount of alcohol.

 ## How Much Alcohol Is Too Much?

Federal health authorities at the National Institute of Alcohol and Alcohol Abuse (NIAAA) recommend that men have no more than two drinks a day and women, no more than one. The American Heart Association (AHA) advises that alcohol account for no more than 15 percent of the total calories consumed by an individual every day, up to an absolute maximum of 1.75 ounces of alcohol a day—the equivalent of three beers, two mixed drinks, or three and a half glasses of wine. Your own limit may well be less, depending on your sex, size, and weight. Some people—such as women who are pregnant or trying to conceive; individuals with problems, such as ulcers, that might be aggravated by alcohol; those taking medications such as sleeping pills or antidepressants; and those driving or operating any motorized equipment—shouldn't drink at all.

The dangers of alcohol increase along with the amount you drink. Heavy drinking destroys the liver, weakens the heart, elevates blood pressure, damages the brain, and increases the risk of cancer. Individuals who drink heavily have a higher mortality rate than those who have two or fewer drinks a day. However, the boundary between safe and dangerous drinking isn't the same for everyone. For some people, the upper limit of safety is zero: Once they start, they can't stop.

Intoxication

If you drink too much, the immediate consequence is that you get drunk—or, more precisely, intoxicated. According to the American Psychiatric Association's definition, **intoxication** consists of "clinically significant maladaptive behavioral or psychological changes," such as inappropriate sexual or aggressive behavior, mood changes, and impaired judgment and social and occupational functioning.[1] Alcohol intoxication, which can range from mild inebriation to loss of consciousness, is characterized by at least one of the following signs: slurred speech, poor coordination, unsteady gait, abnormal eye movements, impaired attention or memory, stupor, or coma. Medical risks of intoxication include falls, hypothermia in cold climates, and increased risk of infections because of suppressed immune function.

Time and a protective environment are the recommended treatments for alcohol intoxication. Anyone who passes out after drinking heavily should be monitored regularly to ensure that vomiting (the result of excess alcohol irritating the stomach) doesn't block the breathing airway. Always make sure that an unconscious drinker is lying on his or her side, with the head lower than the body. Intoxicated drinkers can slip into shock, a potentially life-threatening condition characterized by a weak pulse, irregular breathing, and skin-color changes. This is an emergency, and professional medical care should be sought immediately.

Strategies *for* Change

How to Promote Responsible Drinking

✔ When preparing drinks for guests, measure the amount of alcohol you use, and figure out how many ounces your wine and beer glasses hold. Avoid pushing drinks on guests and refilling glasses quickly. Make sure nonalcoholic alternatives are available.

✔ Always serve food when serving drinks—but not the salty nuts, chips, and pretzels bars serve to increase thirst. Stop serving alcohol one hour before the evening is to end.

✔ Never serve alcohol to a guest who seems intoxicated.

✔ Never let an intoxicated person drive home. You could be legally, as well as morally, responsible in the event of an accident. Call a taxi, or have a friend who hasn't been drinking drive the person home. As a last resort, call the police. In many communities, they'll drive an intoxicated person home as a public service.

The Impact of Alcohol

Unlike drugs in tablet form or food, alcohol is directly and quickly absorbed into the bloodstream through the stomach walls and upper intestine. The alcohol in a typical drink reaches the bloodstream in 15 minutes and rises to its peak concentration in about an hour. The bloodstream carries the alcohol to the liver, heart, and brain. (See Figure 16-3.)

Alcohol is a *diuretic*, a drug that speeds up the elimination of fluid from the body. Most of the alcohol you drink can leave your body only after metabolism by the liver, which converts about 95 percent of the alcohol to carbon dioxide and water. The other 5 percent is excreted unchanged, mainly through urination, respiration, and perspiration. Alcohol lowers body temperature, so you should never drink to get or stay warm.

Digestive System

Alcohol reaches the stomach first, where it is partially broken down. The remaining alcohol is absorbed easily through the stomach tissue into the bloodstream. When it's in the stomach, alcohol triggers the secretion of acids in the stomach, which irritate its lining. Excessive drinking at one sitting may result in nausea; chronic drinking may result in peptic ulcers (breaks in the stomach lining) and bleeding from the stomach lining.

The alcohol in the bloodstream eventually reaches the liver. The liver, which bears the major responsibility of fat metabolism in the body, converts this excess alcohol to fat. After a few weeks of four or five drinks a day, liver cells start to accumulate fat. Alcohol also stimulates liver cells to attract white blood cells, which normally travel throughout the bloodstream engulfing harmful substances and wastes. If white blood cells begin to invade body tissue, such as the liver, they can cause irreversible damage.

Cardiovascular System

Alcohol gets mixed reviews regarding its effects on the cardiovascular system. Moderate drinkers have healthier hearts, suffer fewer heart attacks, have less buildup of cholesterol in their arteries, and are less likely to die of heart disease than heavy drinkers or teetotalers. French researchers have associated moderate drinking of only wine with lower mortality, although drinking both wine and beer reduced the risk of cardiovascular death.[2]

However, heavier drinking triggers the release of harmful oxygen molecules called free radicals, which can increase the risk of heart disease, stroke, and cirrhosis of the liver.[3] Alcohol use can weaken the heart

■ Figure 16-3 The effects of alcohol abuse on the body.

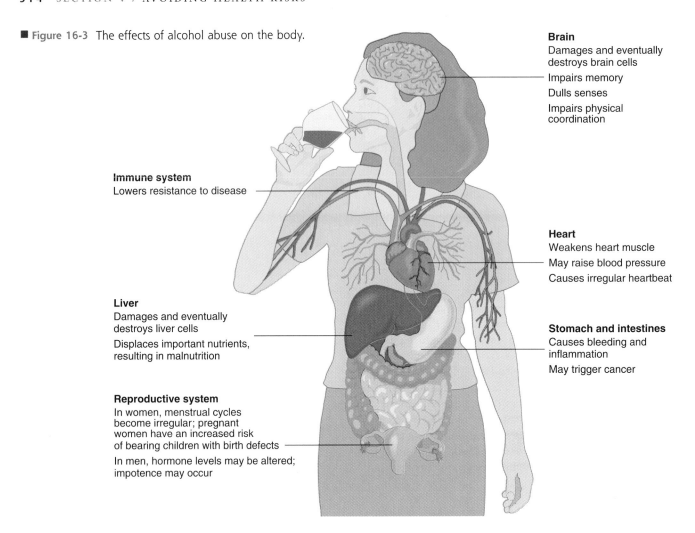

Brain
Damages and eventually destroys brain cells
Impairs memory
Dulls senses
Impairs physical coordination

Immune system
Lowers resistance to disease

Heart
Weakens heart muscle
May raise blood pressure
Causes irregular heartbeat

Liver
Damages and eventually destroys liver cells
Displaces important nutrients, resulting in malnutrition

Stomach and intestines
Causes bleeding and inflammation
May trigger cancer

Reproductive system
In women, menstrual cycles become irregular; pregnant women have an increased risk of bearing children with birth defects
In men, hormone levels may be altered; impotence may occur

muscle directly, causing a disorder called cardiomyopathy. The combined use of alcohol and other drugs, including tobacco and cocaine, greatly increases the likelihood of damage to the heart.

Immune System

Chronic alcohol use can inhibit the production of both white blood cells, which fight off infections, and red blood cells, which carry oxygen to all the organs and tissues of the body. Alcohol may increase the risk of infection with human immunodeficiency virus (HIV), by altering the judgment of users so that they more readily engage in activities, such as unsafe sexual practices, that put them in danger. If you drink when you have a cold or the flu, alcohol interferes with the body's ability to recover. It also increases the chance of bacterial pneumonia in flu-sufferers.

Brain and Behavior

At first, when you drink, you feel up. In low dosages, alcohol affects the regions of the brain that inhibit or control behavior, so you feel looser and act in ways you might not otherwise. However, you also experience losses of concentration, memory, judgment, and fine motor control; and you have mood swings and emotional outbursts. Moderate and heavy drinkers show signs of impaired intelligence, slowed-down reflexes, and difficulty remembering. As recent research has shown, heavy drinking also depletes the brain's supplies of crucial chemicals, including dopamine, gamma aminobutyric acid, opioid peptides, and serotonin, that are responsible for our feelings of pleasure and well-being. At the same time, it promotes the release of stress chemicals, such as corticotropin releasing factor (CRF), that create tension and depression.[4]

Because alcohol is a central nervous system depressant, it slows down the activity of the neurons in the brain, gradually dulling the responses of the brain and nervous system. One or two drinks act as a tranquilizer or relaxant. Additional drinks result in a progressive reduction in central nervous system activity, leading to sleep, general anesthesia, coma, and even death. Moderate amounts of alcohol can have disturbing effects on perception and judgment, including the following:

- *Impaired perceptions.* You're less able to adjust your eyes to bright lights because glare bothers you more. Although you can still hear sounds, you can't distinguish between them or judge their direction well.

- *Dulled smell and taste.* Alcohol itself may cause some vitamin deficiencies, and the poor eating habits of heavy drinkers result in further nutrition problems.

- *Diminished sensation.* You may walk outside without a coat on a freezing winter night and not feel the cold.

- *Altered sense of space.* You may not realize, for instance, that you have been in one place for several hours.

- *Impaired motor skills.* Writing, typing, driving, and other abilities involving your muscles are impaired. This is why law enforcement officers sometimes ask suspected drunk drivers to touch their nose with a finger or to walk a straight line. Drinking large amounts of alcohol impairs reaction time, speed, accuracy, and consistency, as well as judgment.

- *Impaired sexual performance.* While drinking may increase your interest in sex, it may also impair sex-

ual response, especially a man's ability to achieve or maintain an erection. As Shakespeare wrote, "It provokes the desire, but it takes away the performance."

Interaction with Other Drugs

Alcohol can interact with other drugs—prescription and nonprescription, legal and illegal. Of the 100 most frequently prescribed drugs, more than half contain at least one ingredient that interacts adversely with alcohol. Because alcohol and other psychoactive drugs may work on the same areas of the brain, their combination can produce an effect much greater than that expected of either drug by itself. The consequences of this synergistic interaction can be fatal (see Consumer Health Watch: "Alcohol and Drug Interactions"). Alcohol is particularly dangerous when combined with depressants and antianxiety medications.

Aspirin—long used to prevent or counter alcohol's effects—may actually enhance its impact by significantly lowering the body's ability to break down alcohol in the stomach. In a study of healthy men between

Consumer Health Watch

Alcohol and Drug Interactions

Drug	Possible effects of interaction
Analgesics (painkillers)	
Narcotic (Codeine, Demerol, Percodan)	Increase in central nervous system depression, possibly leading to respiratory failure and death.
Nonnarcotic (aspirin, acetaminophen)	Irritation of stomach, resulting in bleeding, and increased susceptibility to liver damage.
Antabuse	Nausea, vomiting, headache, high blood pressure, and erratic heartbeat.
Antianxiety drugs (Valium, Librium)	Increase in central nervous system depression; decreased alertness and impaired judgment.
Antidepressants	Increase in central nervous system depression; certain antidepressants in combination with red wine could cause a sudden increase in blood pressure.
Antihistamines (Actifed, Dimetap, and other cold medications)	Increase in drowsiness; driving more dangerous.
Antibiotics	Nausea, vomiting, headache; some medications rendered less effective.
Central nervous system stimulants (caffeine, Dexedrine, Ritalin)	Stimulant effects of these drugs may reverse depressant effect of alcohol but do not decrease intoxicating effects of alcohol.
Diuretics (Diuril, Lasix)	Reduction in blood pressure, resulting in dizziness upon rising.
Sedatives (Dalmane, Nembutal, Quaalude)	Increase in central nervous system depression, possibly leading to coma, respiratory failure, and death.

the ages of 30 and 45, volunteers who took two extra-strength aspirin tablets an hour before drinking a glass and a half of wine had a 30 percent higher BAC than when they drank alcohol alone. This increase could make a difference in impairment for individuals driving cars or operating machinery.

If you want to drink while taking medication, be sure you read the warnings on nonprescription-drug labels or prescription-drug containers; ask your doctor about possible alcohol–drug interactions; and check with your pharmacist if you have any questions about your medications, especially over-the-counter (OTC) products.

Increased Risk of Dying

Alcohol kills. While light alcohol intake is associated with lower mortality than either abstinence or heavy drinking, mortality risks increase with the amount of alcohol consumed.[5] The mortality rate for alcoholics is two and a half times higher that for nonalcoholics of the same age. The leading alcohol-related cause of death is injury, chiefly auto accidents involving a drunk driver. Alcohol is associated with at least half of all traffic fatalities, half of all homicides, and a quarter of all suicides.

The second leading cause of alcohol-related deaths is digestive disease, including *cirrhosis* of the liver, a chronic disease that causes extensive scarring and irreversible damage. In addition, as many as half of patients admitted to hospitals and 15 percent of those making office visits seek or need medical care because of the direct or indirect effects of alcohol.

Young drinkers—teens and those in their early twenties—are at highest risk of dying from injuries, mostly car accidents. Older drinkers over age 50 face the greatest danger of premature death from cirrhosis of the liver, hepatitis, and other alcohol-linked illnesses.

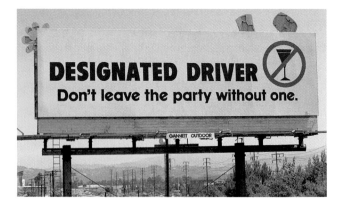

Driving and drinking don't mix! Alcohol is associated with at least half of all traffic fatalities—to the drunk driver and to others.

Drinking in America

Research has shown little variation among the races with respect to quantity, frequency, and amount of alcohol consumed, although whites are more likely to be classified as daily or nearly daily drinkers than nonwhites. A greater percentage of females than males report a lifetime pattern of infrequent drinking (less than 12 drinks a year). Men and women are most likely to drink between the ages of 21 and 34. Drinking typically declines with age.

Why People Drink

The most common reason why people drink alcohol is to relax. Because it depresses the central nervous system, alcohol can make people feel less tense. Other motivations for drinking include the following:

- *Celebration.* Unless alcohol use violates family, ethnic, or religious values, people raise their glasses together on life's important occasions—births, graduations, weddings, promotions.

- *Friendship.* When friends visit, you may have a drink, or you may meet them somewhere "for a drink." Young people are much more likely to experiment with alcohol if their friends drink.

- *Social ease.* When we use alcohol, we may seem bolder, wittier, sexier. At the same time, the people drinking with us become more relaxed and seem to enjoy our company more. Because alcohol lowers inhibitions, some people see it as a prelude to seduction.

- *Self-medication.* Like other drugs, alcohol may be the means some people use to treat—or escape from—painful feelings or bad moods.

- *Role models.* Athletes, some of the most admired celebrities in our country, have a long history of appearing in commercials for alcohol. Many advertisements feature glamorous women holding or sipping alcoholic beverages.

- *Advertising.* Brewers and beer distributors spend $15 to $20 million a year promoting the message: If you want to have fun, have a drink. Adolescents may be especially responsive to such sales pitches. Nearly two dozen national groups, including the American Medical Association, have petitioned the Federal Trade Commission to ban alcohol advertisements that link drinking to risky activities (such as driving, water skiing, and sky-diving) and that target youth.

Patterns of Alcohol Use

Because of concern about alcohol's health effects, increasing numbers of Americans are choosing not to drink at all. (See Pulsepoints: "Ten Steps to Responsible Drinking.") With alcohol consumption in the United States at its lowest level in 30 years, nonalcoholic beverages have grown in popularity. They appeal to drivers, boaters, pregnant women, individuals with health problems that could worsen with alcohol, those who are older and can't tolerate alcohol, anyone taking medicines that interact with alcohol (including antibiotics, antidepressants, and muscle relaxers), and everyone interested in limiting alcohol intake. Under federal law, these drinks can contain some alcohol, but a much smaller amount than regular beer or wine. Nonalcoholic beers and wines on the market also are lower in calories than alcoholic varieties.

Among the 52 percent of adults who drink, fewer than 10 percent ever develop drinking problems. They also vary greatly in how much and how often they drink. Although there are no standard definitions for drinking patterns, the following are generally recognized as most common:

- *Light drinking.* This is defined as having fewer than three alcoholic drinks a week. (A drink equals 1 ounce of spirits, a 4-ounce glass of table wine, or a 12-ounce can of beer, each of which contains approximately 12 grams of absolute alcohol.)
- *Infrequent drinking.* This term refers to frequency, not quantity. Infrequent drinkers have less than one drink a month but drink at least once a year. Some "low maximum" infrequent drinkers drink one to three times a month but never have five or more drinks at a sitting. "High maximum" infrequent drinkers do not drink more often, but they occasionally have five or more drinks at a sitting.

- *Moderate drinking.* Moderate drinking generally is defined as having an upper limit of four standard drinks on any day, on no more than three days a week. For women, the upper limit is three drinks a day, on no more than three days a week.
- *Social drinking.* This term—used by laypeople rather than health-care professionals or researchers—refers to drinking patterns that are accepted by friends and peers. If your friends drink only on special occasions, you may think that having one glass of wine at a party is social drinking. On the other hand, if the people you socialize with drink regularly and heavily, you may mistakenly think that having a six-pack of beer every night is social drinking.
- *Problem drinking.* Any kind of drinking that interferes with a major aspect of life, such as sleep, energy, family relationships, health, or safety, qualifies as problem drinking. Some of the problems associated with drinking—getting into fights, unwanted sexual activity, car accidents—are obvious. Others, such as alcohol-related damage to the digestive system, heart, liver or brain, may remain invisible for years.
- *Binge drinking.* When applied to alcohol, a binge consists of having five or more drinks at a single sitting for a man or four drinks at a single sitting for a

---

PULSE *points*

Ten Steps to Responsible Drinking

1. **Don't drink alone.** Cultivate friendships with nondrinkers and responsible moderate drinkers.

2. **Don't use alcohol as a medicine.** Rather than reaching for a drink to put you to sleep, help you relax, or relieve tension, develop alternative means of unwinding, such as exercise, meditation, or listening to music.

3. **Develop a party plan.** Set a limit on how many drinks you'll have before you go out—and stick to it.

4. **Alternate alcoholic and nonalcoholic drinks.** At a social occasion, have a nonalcoholic beverage to quench your thirst.

5. **Drink slowly.** Never have more than one drink an hour.

6. **Eat before and while drinking.** Choose foods high in protein (cheese, meat, eggs, or milk) rather than salty foods, like peanuts or chips, that increase thirst.

7. **Be wary of mixed drinks.** Fizzy mixers, like club soda and ginger ale, speed alcohol to the blood and brain.

8. **Don't make drinking the primary focus of any get-together.** Cultivate other interests and activities that you can enjoy on your own or with friends.

9. **Learn to say no.** A simple "Thank you, but I've had enough" will do.

10. **Stay safe.** During or after drinking, avoid any tasks, including driving, that could be affected by alcohol.

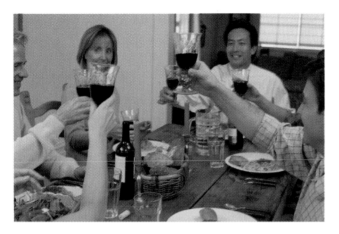

Alcohol can be part of many enjoyable social situations, as long as individuals know when to say "No more." Increasingly, many people are substituting nonalcoholic drinks.

woman. Binge drinking is most common among young men, especially those who are single, separated, or divorced, who drink beer, or who concentrate most of their drinking on weekends. Bingeing has been linked to a substantially increased risk of serious injury—especially from automobile accidents—as well as higher rates of unsafe sex, assault, and aggressive behavior. As discussed later in this chapter, binge drinking is common in college.

Underage Drinking

By age 14, over half of secondary school students drink at least occasionally and rates of drinking and heavy drinking increase steadily throughout adolescence.[6] By ages 17 and 18, more than 30 percent of males and 15 percent of females can be classified as heavy drinkers.[7] Various psychosocial factors, such as low expectations for success, academic failure, and peer models for substance abuse, increase the risk of adolescent drinking.[8]

Underage drinking is associated with use of illegal drugs and with risky behaviors. In one survey, 45 percent of teenage boys and 27 percent of girls reported they had played sports such as swimming, rollerblading, and swimming while under the influence of alcohol.[9] As shown in Figure 16-4, underage drinking also takes an enormous economic toll on our society.[10]

An estimated 30 percent of teenagers experience some negative consequences of alcohol abuse, including impaired health, poor school performance, psychosocial problems, automobile accidents, and arrests. Teenagers who begin drinking before age 15 are four times as likely to become alcohol dependent as individuals who start drinking at age 21, the legal drinking age.[11]

How Common Is Drinking on College Campuses?

Most college students use alcohol, but they vary greatly in how often and how much they drink. (See Campus Focus: "How Much Do College Students Drink?") According to a recent report on 17,592 students at colleges, undergraduates average 5.1 drinks per week. Some students—frequent binge drinkers—consume considerably more, while those who do not binge—the majority of undergraduates—consume much less.[12]

Drinking patterns vary greatly on different campuses and among different students. Heavy drinking is not typical at many colleges, and a growing number report a decline in undergraduate drinking. As shown in Figure 16-5, beer drinking has decreased on campuses nationwide in the last 20 years. In a recent analysis, 51 percent of students at four-year colleges said they consumed one drink or less in a typical week.[13] In random Breathalyzer tests on other campuses, the majority of students had no alcohol in their blood.[14]

Despite these trends, alcohol remains a major problem on many college campuses. Every year, students spend $5.5 billion on alcohol, mostly beer—more than they spend on books, soda pop, coffee, juice, and milk combined, for an average of $466 per student per year. The total amount of alcohol consumed by college students each year is 430 million gallons, enough for every college and university in the United States to fill an Olympic-size swimming pool.[15]

According to a national survey released by the Higher Education Center for Alcohol and Other Drug Prevention, 75 to 90 percent of all violence on college campuses is alcohol-related. About 300,000 of today's college students will eventually die from alcohol-related causes, including drunk driving accidents, cirrhosis of the liver, various cancers, and heart disease, estimates the Core Institute, an organization that studies college drinking.

Traffic crashes	$18,200,000,000
Violent crimes	$35,900,000,000
Burns	$315,000,000
Drownings	$532,000,000
Suicide attempts	$1,510,000,000
Fetal alcohol syndrome	$493,000,000
Alcohol poisonings	$340,000,000
Treatment	$1,008,000,000

■ **Figure 16-4** The consequences and costs of underage drinking.

Source: "MADD, OJJDP Expand Program to Combat Underage Drinking." *Alcoholism & Drug Abuse Weekly*, Vol. 11, Issue 29, July 16, 1999.

Campus Focus

How Much Do College Students Drink?

Average Number of Drinks Per Week	
All Students	5.1
Frequent Bingers	17.9
Infrequent Bingers	4.8
Non-bingers	.8
Men	
Frequent Bingers	22.6
Infrequent Bingers	5.7
Non-bingers	1
Women	
Frequent Bingers	13.3
Infrequent Bingers	3.9
Non-bingers	.7

Percentage of Frequent Bingers Who Have Experienced Problems Related to Frequent Binge Drinking

Problem	
Was injured	58.9%
Damaged property	58.8%
Had trouble with police	58.4%
Missed class	53.9%
Fell behind	53.9%
Engaged in unprotected sex	52.3%
Experienced blackouts	52.3%
Engaged in unplanned sex	49.7%
Argued with friends	49.7%
Did something later regretted	45.4%
Overdosed on alcohol	41.1%
Drove after drinking or bingeing	40.6%
Experienced 5 or more of these problems	53.9%

Source: Wechsler, Henry, et al. "College Alcohol Use: A Full or Empty Glass?" *Journal of American College Health*, Vol. 47, No. 6, May 1999.

Drinking also increases sexual risks for college students. In a sample of college students ages 17 to 24, 47 percent of the men and 57 percent of the women said that they had had sexual intercourse one to five times while under the influence of alcohol. Heavy drinking has been correlated with increased casual sex without condoms and with increased numbers of sex partners.[16] According to other research, alcohol affects the frequency and severity of sexual attacks on women.[17]

In a study of the relationships between alcohol, religious beliefs, and risky sexual behaviors at a large public university in the southeast, men had higher rates of alcohol consumption and unprotected sexual activity, but the sexes did not differ in the overall frequency of sexual activity. Women with strong religious beliefs consumed less alcohol and were less likely to engage in risky sexual behavior than females with weaker religious convictions. Among men, religious conviction was not significantly related to alcohol consumption or risky sex behavior.[18]

Why College Students Drink

Most college students drink for the same reasons undergraduates have always turned to alcohol. Away from home, often for the first time, many are both excited by and apprehensive about their newfound independence. When new pressures seem overwhelming, when they

feel awkward or insecure, when they just want to let loose and have a good time, they reach for a drink.

Students may be especially vulnerable to dangerous drinking in their freshman year as they struggle to adapt to an often bewildering new world. In a study of

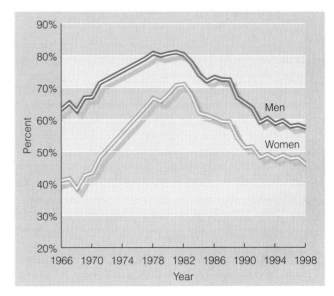

■ **Figure 16-5** Percentage of freshmen who drink beer.

Source: Sax, Linda, et al. *The American Freshman: National Norms for Fall 1998.* Los Angeles Higher Education Research Institute, UCLA, 1998.

freshmen at a medium-sized state university and at a small, predominantly African-American university who were nondrinkers as high school seniors, almost half (46.5 percent) started to drink in college. They were less likely to do so if they had friends who discouraged them from drinking.

Other studies have also linked alcohol consumption with where students live on campus and what they perceive as the norm for acceptable drinking. Stress-related drinking is common. Students in competitive academic environments may turn to alcohol to reduce their anxiety and the pressure to perform.[19] Members of sororities and fraternities rated all drinking norms as more extreme and perceived fraternity drinking as particularly heavy. Fraternity leaders are among the heaviest drinkers and most out-of-control partygoers, with the highest incidence of heavy drinking and bingeing.

The most dramatic increases in college drinking have been among women: 86 percent of female undergraduates say they drink; 37 percent—compared with only 14 percent in 1977—say they get drunk one to three times in a month. While men tend to drink as a way of partying, women on campus may drink for other reasons. (See The X & Y Files: "Men, women, and Drinking.")

Among both men and women, those with alcoholic parents and dysfunctional families are at greater risk of substance abuse. By some estimates, one of five college students comes from an alcoholic home and may be at increased risk of developing a drinking problem.

Binge Drinking

One in five college students is a frequent binge drinker. These undergraduates consume 68 percent of all the

---

The X&Y Files — Men, Women, and Drinking

According to conventional gender stereotypes, drinking is a symbol of manliness. In the past, far more men than women drank. In America today, both sexes are likely to consume alcohol. However, there are well-documented differences in how often and how much men and women drink. In general, men drink more frequently, consume a larger quantity of alcohol per drinking occasion, and report more problems related to drinking.

In recent years, researchers have been comparing and contrasting the reasons why men and women drink. An analysis of survey data on approximately 1,800 students at a New York State liberal arts college found that undergraduate women and men are equally likely to drink for stress-related reasons and that both sexes perceive alcohol as a means of tension relaxation. In another study, psychologist Susan Nolen-Hoeksema of the University of Michigan interviewed approximately 1,300 adults (631 males, 697 females) about how they coped with sadness or distress. She asked about their tendency to ruminate or stew about how bad they felt, and about the extent to which they drank to cope with negative feelings, help themselves feel better, and deal with stress.

"The gender differences in both rumination and drinking to cope were quite pronounced," Nolen-Hoeksema reports. "In general, women think and men drink. But some men are ruminators and some women drink to cope, and for both men and women, rumination and drinking to cope are related." In other words, people who do one are at increased risk of doing the other.

In men, alcohol temporarily dampens rumination, says Nolen-Hoeksema, but in women, using alcohol just gives them one more thing to ruminate about—for reasons that are cultural as well as social and personal. For both men and women, she notes, the tendency to ruminate is linked not only to depression, but also to alcohol use. Therefore, both sexes might benefit from learning more adaptive ways of coping with stress.

Other psychologists theorize that men engage in "confirmatory" drinking, that is, they drink to reinforce the image of masculinity associated with alcohol consumption. Both sexes may engage "compensatory" drinking and consume alcohol to heighten their sense of masculinity or femininity. Numerous studies in the past showed that men and women with low scores on various scales of masculinity and femininity are more vulnerable to problem drinking. High scores of masculinity have been associated with greater problem drinking by men, while high scores on femininity correlated with less problem drinking by women. However, a recent study of Australian undergraduates challenges these associations. It found that the more men and women resemble each other on various measures of masculinity and femininity, the more similar their drinking patterns appear.

Sources: Perkins, Wesley. "Stress-Motivated Drinking in Collegiate and Postcollegiate Young Adulthood: Life Course and Gender Patterns." *Journal of Studies on Alcohol,* Vol. 60, No. 2, March 1999. Nolen-Hoeksema, Susan. "Women Think, Men Drink: The Link Between Gender, Depression and Alcohol." Presentation, American Psychological Association, Boston, August 1999. Williams, Robert, and Lina Ricciardelli. "Gender Congruence in Confirmatory and Compensatory Drinking." *Journal of Psychology,* Vol. 133, Issue 3, May 1999.

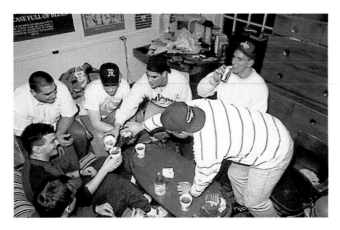

Binge drinkers can get into—and cause—trouble. Dangerously large amounts of alcohol can cause death, and heavy party drinking often results in violence.

alcohol that students report drinking, and they account for the majority of alcohol-related problems on campus. About one in four students (24 percent) are infrequent binge drinkers. Even though binge drinkers represent less than half (44 percent) of the college population, they account for almost all (91 percent) of the alcohol consumed on campus. Nonbingers—who account for the majority of students (56 percent)—drink only nine percent of the alcohol consumed on campus.[20]

The majority of college students do not engage in heavy drinking. However, because of the danger it poses to drinkers and others, bingeing has become a major public health concern, with newspaper campaigns designed to call attention to this serious threat. In recent years, several students have died after consuming numerous drinks in a short period of time, sometimes as part of hazing rituals. Binge drinking is especially common in fraternities and sororities.[21] By some estimates, more than 80 percent of "Greeks" who live in fraternity or sorority houses engage in binge drinking. The second highest rate occurs among athletes participating in intercollegiate sports.[22]

College students who binge on alcohol face other dangers: They are seven to ten times more likely to engage in unplanned or unprotected sex, to have problems with campus police, or to get hurt. Although female students drink less and less dangerously than men, female binge drinkers are more likely to engage in sexual activity, including intercourse, under the influence of alcohol than women who never binge. Binge-drinking women also report engaging in sexual behaviors when they would otherwise not have and not practicing safe sex, thereby putting themselves at greater risk. Binge drinkers create problems, not just for themselves, but for others. According to one survey, at schools where drinking was most popular, two-thirds of students reported having their sleep or studies interrupted by drunken students; more than half had been forced to care for a drunk friend; and at least a fourth had suffered an unwanted sexual advance.

The American College Health Association estimates that drinking accounts for almost two-thirds of all violence on campus and about one-third of all emotional and academic problems among students.[23] Alcohol may play a role in 90 percent of rapes and sexual assaults. Drinking also claims the lives of many students each year, sometimes because of car accidents, and sometimes because of drinking games, in which individuals consume dangerously large quantities of alcohol.

Colleges have been struggling to find ways to respond to the problems of binge drinking, underage drinking, and driving after drinking.[24] Some have set up alcohol-free dormitories, banned alcohol from fraternity and sorority events, and barred alcohol companies from sponsoring campus activities. Others are urging stricter enforcement of the legal drinking age, although there is concern that tough campus policies will drive student drinkers into the neighboring community. The most successful programs involve student leaders, who take on responsibility for educating their peers about the risks posed by alcohol.[25] There has been an increase in on-campus chapters of national support groups such as AA, Al-Anon, Adult Children of Alcoholics, and a peer-education program called BACCHUS: Boost Alcohol Consciousness Concerning the Health of University Students.

Drinking and Race

Increasingly, experts in alcohol treatment are recognizing racial and ethnic differences in risk factors for drinking problems, patterns of drinking, and most effective types of treatment. Increases in drinking have been traced to stresses related to immigration, acculturation, poverty, racial discrimination, and powerlessness. Environmental factors, such as aggressive marketing and advertising of alcoholic beverages in minority neighborhoods, also play a role.

The African-American Community

Overall, African Americans consume less alcohol per person than whites, yet twice as many blacks die of cirrhosis of the liver each year. In some cities, the rate of cirrhosis is ten times higher among African-American than white men. Alcohol also contributes to high rates of hypertension, esophageal cancer, and homicide among African-American men.

The makers of alcoholic beverages market their products aggressively to African Americans, and there are many more liquor stores (per capita) in many

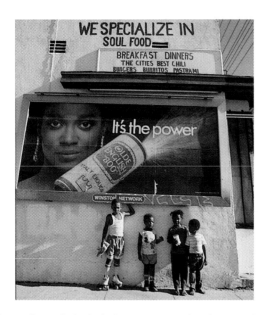

The makers of alcoholic beverages market their products aggressively in poor urban neighborhoods, where liquor stores and bars are common.

African-American neighborhoods than in white communities. Peer pressure to drink, the easy accessibility of alcohol, and socioeconomic frustrations increase the likelihood of alcohol problems among African Americans. Moreover, recovery can be especially difficult because of the lack of treatment programs and role models in the African-American community, and the ongoing pressures to resume drinking.

The Latino Community

Latino societies discourage any drinking by women but encourage heavy drinking by men as part of their machismo, or feelings of manhood. According to the Department of Health and Human Services, Latino men have higher rates of alcohol use and abuse than the general population, and suffer a high rate of cirrhosis. Moreover, American-born Latino men drink more than those born in other countries.

Few Latinos enter treatment, partly because of a lack of information, language barriers, and poor community-based services. Latino families generally try to resolve problems themselves, and their cultural values discourage the sharing of intimate personal stories, which characterizes Alcoholics Anonymous and other support groups. Churches often provide the most effective forms of help.

The Native-American Community

European settlers introduced alcohol to Native Americans. But because of the societal and physical problems resulting from excessive drinking, at the request of tribal leaders, the U.S. Congress in 1832 prohibited the use of alcohol by Native Americans. Many reservations still ban alcohol use, a policy that may force Native Americans who want to drink to travel long distances to obtain alcohol—and may contribute to the high death rate from hypothermia and pedestrian and motor-vehicle accidents among Native Americans. (Injuries are the leading cause of death among this group.)

Certainly, not all Native Americans drink, and not all who drink do so to excess. However, they have three times the general population's rate of alcohol-related injury and illness. Moreover, cirrhosis of the liver is the fourth-leading cause of death among this cultural group. While many Native-American women don't drink, those who do have high rates of alcohol-related problems, which affect both them and their children. Their rate of cirrhosis of the liver is 36 times that of white women. In some tribes, 10.5 out of every 1000 newborns have fetal alcohol syndrome, compared with 1 to 3 out of 1,000 in the general population. (See the section on fetal alcohol syndrome in this chapter.)

Both a biological predisposition and socioeconomic conditions may contribute to alcohol abuse by Native Americans. In addition, according to their cultural beliefs, alcoholism is not a physical disease but a spiritual disorder—making it less likely that they'll seek appropriate treatment.

The Asian-American Community

Asian Americans tend to drink very little or not at all, in part because of an inborn physiological reaction to alcohol that causes facial flushing, rapid heart rate, lowered blood pressure, nausea, vomiting, and other symptoms. A very high percentage of women of all Asian-American nationalities abstain completely. Some sociologists have expressed concern, however, that as Asian Americans become more assimilated into American culture, they'll drink more—and possibly suffer very adverse effects from alcohol.

Women and Alcohol

About half of women drink: of these, 45 percent are light drinkers; 3 percent, moderate drinkers; 2 percent, heavy drinkers; and 21 percent, binge drinkers.[26] According to the NIAAA, almost 4 million women suffer from alcohol abuse or dependence. But women who drink have different risk factors, potential dangers, and drinking patterns than men.

Why Women Drink

In the past, most people, including physicians and therapists, assumed that women who drank heavily did so pri-

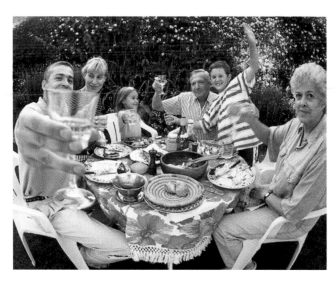

Genetics as well as life experience contribute to a woman's vulnerability to heavy drinking and alcohol dependence. Risk factors and drinking patterns are different for women and men.

marily for social and psychological reasons—because they were lonely, isolated, broken-hearted. Many of these assumptions have proven to be false. The following are more likely to lead to drinking problems in women.

- *Inherited susceptibility.* In women, as in men, genetics account for 50 to 60 percent of a person's vulnerability to a serious drinking problem. But while heredity increases the risk of alcoholism, life circumstances also play an important role in determining whether young women will have drinking problems. Female alcoholics are more likely than males to have a parent who abused drugs or alcohol, who had psychiatric problems, or who attempted suicide.

- *Childhood traumas.* Female alcoholics often report that they were physically or sexually abused as children or suffered great distress because of poverty or a parent's death.

- *Depression.* "At all stages over the life span, female problem drinking is linked to depression," Edith Gomberg reports. Women are more likely than men to be depressed prior to drinking and to suffer from both depression and a drinking problem at the same time. Even after women enter and complete treatment for their alcohol problems, depressive symptoms may persist.[27]

- *Relationship issues.* Single, separated, or divorced women drink both more and more often than married women; women with live-in male partners have the highest rates of drinking problems. "Functioning women alcoholics may be very successful in other areas of their lives but have problems in their relationships," says Sharon Wilsnack, Ph.D., a professor at the University of North Dakota School of Medicine

who studied the drinking habits of more than 1,100 women over ten years.

- *Psychological factors.* Like men, women may drink to compensate for feelings of inadequacy.[28] Women who tend to "ruminate" or mull over bad feelings may find that alcohol increases this tendency and makes them feel more distressed.[29] Women involved with heavy drinkers are at risk of drinking heavily themselves, at least as long as the relationship continues.

- *Employment.* Women who work outside the home are less likely to become problem drinkers or alcoholics than those without paying jobs. The one exception: women in occupations still dominated by men, such as engineering, science, law enforcement and top corporate management. "Often women in these fields drink as a way of fitting in," observes Wilsnack. "Drinking takes on symbolic value. It's a way of signalling power, equality, status."

- *A lack or loss of roles.* Women of all ages, regardless of marital or employment status, tend to drink more and lean on alcohol when they lose a valued role, for example, when they're laid off from a job or their marriage ends in divorce.

- *Use of alcohol to self-medicate.* "In our society, women are permitted to use medication, so they feel it's permissible to use alcohol as if it were a medicine," observes Gomberg. "As long as they're taking it for a reason, it seems acceptable to them, even if they're drifting into a drinking problem."

Alcohol's Effects on Women

Problems directly related to a woman's alcohol use range from the consequences of risky sexual behavior after alcohol consumption (such as unwanted pregnancy or STDs) to severe physiological problems related to fertility and pregnancy. Because they have far smaller quantities of a protective enzyme in the stomach to break down alcohol before it's absorbed into the bloodstream, women absorb about 30 percent more alcohol into their bloodstream than men do. The alcohol travels through the blood to the brain, so women become intoxicated much more quickly. And because there's more alcohol in the bloodstream to break down, the liver may also be adversely affected. In alcoholic women, the stomach seems to stop digesting alcohol completely, which may explain why women alcoholics are more likely to suffer liver damage than are men.

Among the other health dangers that alcohol holds for women are:

- *Gynecologic problems.* Moderate to heavy drinking may contribute to infertility, menstrual problems, sexual dysfunction, and premenstrual syndrome.

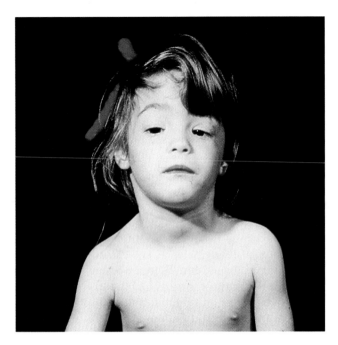

A child with fetal alcohol syndrome (FAS) has distinctive facial characteristics that vary with the severity of the disease, including droopy eyelids, a thin upper lip, and a wide space between the nose and upper lip.

- *Pregnancy and fetal alcohol syndrome (FAS).* When a woman drinks during pregnancy, her unborn child drinks, too. According to CDC estimates, more than 8,000 alcohol-damaged babies are born every year. One out of every 750 newborns has a cluster of physical and mental defects called **fetal alcohol syndrome (FAS):** small head, abnormal facial features (see photo above), jitters, poor muscle tone, sleep disorders, sluggish motor development, failure to thrive, short stature, delayed speech, mental retardation, or hyperactivity. Many more babies suffer **fetal alcohol effects (FAE)**—low birth weight, irritability as newborns, and permanent mental impairment—as a result of their mothers' alcohol consumption. (See Chapter 10 for further discussion of these conditions.)

Labels on alcoholic beverages have had a proven but modest effect on reducing drinking in pregnancy, while community-based education efforts have been much more effective. Drug and alcohol abuse also can affect the quality of a woman's mothering.

- *Breast cancer.* Numerous studies have suggested an increased risk of breast cancer among women who drink, and many physicians feel that those at high risk for breast cancer should stop, or at least reduce, their consumption of alcohol. (See Chapter 14 for more information on breast cancer risks.)

- *Osteoporosis.* As women become older, their risk of osteoporosis, a condition characterized by calcium loss and bone thinning, increases. Alcohol can block the absorption of many nutrients, including calcium, and heavy drinking may worsen the deterioration of bone tissue.

- *Heart disease.* Women who are very heavy drinkers are more at risk of developing irreversible heart disease than are men who drink even more.

Alcohol Treatments for Women

Women who abuse alcohol also face a special burden: intense social disapproval. Many become cross-addicted to prescription medicines, or they develop eating disorders or sexual dysfunctions. Women often don't get the same care men do, frequently because of financial limitations and childcare responsibilities. Also, women are more likely to blame their symptoms on depression or anxiety, whereas men attribute them directly to alcohol. As a result, women often obtain treatment later in the course of their illness, at a point when their problems are more severe. Increasingly, prevention programs are targeting high-risk women to recognize alcohol problems early and to tackle underlying problems, such as depression and low self-esteem.

One of the most effective programs for women is Women for Sobriety, founded in 1975 by sociologist Jean Kirkpatrick, Ph.D. Its meetings focus on building self-esteem, self-confidence, and responsibility. "AA was started by men, and its message is very disempowering for women," says Kirkpatrick. "We view members as competent women who are struggling with issues that all women must face. Women don't need to recall the painful process of becoming alcoholics. They need to put the past behind them and move on, upward and onward." (See "Your Health Directory" at the back of this book.)[30]

Drinking and Driving

Drunk driving is the most frequently committed crime in the United States. In the last two decades, families of the victims of drunk drivers have organized to change the way America treats its drunk drivers. Because of the efforts of MADD (Mothers Against Drunk Driving), SADD (Students Against Driving Drunk), and other lobbying groups, cities, counties, and states are cracking down on drivers who drink. Since courts have held bars liable for the consequences of allowing drunk customers to drive, many bars and restaurants have joined the campaign against drunk driving. (There's even a group called Bartenders Against Drunk Driving, or BADD.) Many communities also provide free rides home on holidays and weekends for people who've had too much to drink.

To keep drunk drivers off the road, many cities have set up checkpoints, where they stop automobiles and inspect the drivers for intoxication. The U.S. Supreme Court has ruled that a driver's refusal to submit to a blood-alcohol concentration test at such checkpoints or at any other time can be used as evidence to prosecute him or her for drunk driving. An increasing number of states have toughened their enforcement of drunk-driving penalties. Some suspend a driver's license for several months for a first offense; repeat offenders can lose their licenses for a year or more.

The National Highway Traffic Safety Administration estimates that setting the legal age limit for drinking at 21 has saved 16,500 lives in traffic crashes alone since 1975. The majority of states have made it illegal for people younger than 21 to drive with a measurable amount of alcohol in their blood. Research comparing states that adopted such zero tolerance laws to those that did not have found that zero tolerance states experienced 20 percent declines in the proportions of fatal single-vehicle, night crashes (the type most often alcohol-related) involving young drivers. Nationwide, alcohol-related traffic deaths among 15- to 20-year-olds have declined 57 percent. Raising the drinking age also has lowered the rate of pedestrian injuries.[31]

Strategies *for* Prevention

How to Prevent Drunk Driving

✓ When going out in a group, always designate one person who won't drink at all to serve as the driver.

✓ Never get behind the wheel if you've had more than two drinks within two hours, especially if you haven't eaten.

✓ Never let intoxicated friends drive home. Call a taxi, drive them yourself, or arrange for them to spend the night in a safe place.

Alcohol-Related Problems

The misuse and abuse of alcohol can lead to a range of problems, from intoxication to problem drinking to alcohol dependence or abuse. "For years, the United States lagged behind other countries in recognizing the spectrum of alcohol-related problems," says Frederick Bruhnsen, manager of DrinkWise at the University of Michigan, an innovative treatment program for problem drinkers. "Of all the people who drink, 20 to 25 percent develop some problem at some point. About four to five percent develop problems so severe as to be termed *alcoholic*."[32]

By the simplest definition, problem drinking is the use of alcohol in any way that creates difficulties or potential difficulties or health risks for an individual. Like alcoholics, problem drinkers are individuals whose lives are in some way impaired by their drinking. The only difference is one of degree. Alcohol becomes a problem, and a person becomes an alcoholic, when the drinker can't "take it or leave it." He or she spends more and more time anticipating the next drink, planning when and where to get it, buying and hiding alcohol, and covering up secret drinking.

Alcohol abuse involves continued use of alcohol despite awareness of social, occupational, psychological, or physical problems related to drinking, or drinking in dangerous ways or situations (before driving, for instance). A diagnosis of alcohol abuse is based on one or more of the following occurring at any time during a 12-month period:

• Recurrent alcohol abuse resulting in a failure to fulfill major role obligations at work, school, or home (such as missing work or school).

• Recurrent alcohol abuse in situations in which it is physically hazardous (such as before driving).

• Recurrent alcohol-related legal problems (such as drunk-driving arrests).

• Continued alcohol use despite persistent or recurring social or interpersonal problems caused or exacerbated by alcohol (such as fighting while drunk).[33]

Alcohol dependence is a separate disorder, in which individuals develop a strong craving for alcohol because it produces pleasurable feelings or relieves stress or anxiety. Over time they experience physiological changes that lead to *tolerance* of its effects; this means that they must consume larger and larger amounts to achieve intoxication. If they abruptly stop drinking, they suffer *withdrawal*, a state of acute physical and psychological discomfort. A diagnosis of alcohol dependence is based on three or more of the following symptoms occurring during any 12-month period:

• Tolerance, as defined by either a need for markedly increased amounts of alcohol to achieve intoxication or desired effect, or a markedly diminished effect with continued drinking of the same amount of alcohol as in the past.

• Withdrawal, as manifested by characteristic symptoms, including at least two of the following: sweating, rapid pulse, or other signs of autonomic hyperactivity; increased hand tremor; insomnia; nausea or vomiting; temporary hallucinations or illusions;

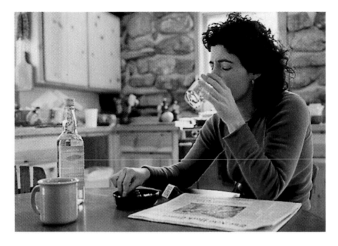

Alcohol dependence may spring from the perception that alcohol relieves stress and anxiety, or creates a pleasant feeling. Chronic drinking—especially daytime drinking and drinking alone—can be a sign of serious problems, even though the drinker may otherwise appear to be in control.

physical agitation or restlessness; anxiety; or grand mal seizures; or

- Drinking to avoid or relieve these symptoms.
- Consuming larger amounts of alcohol, or over a longer period than was intended.
- Persistent desire or unsuccessful efforts to cut down or control drinking.
- A great deal of time spent in activities necessary to obtain alcohol, drink it, or recover from its effects.
- Important social, occupational, or recreational activities given up or reduced because of alcohol use.
- Continued alcohol use despite knowledge that alcohol is likely to cause or exacerbate a persistent or recurring physical or psychological problem.

Alcoholism, as defined by the National Council on Alcoholism and Drug Dependence and the American Society of Addiction, is a primary, chronic disease in which genetic, psychosocial, and environmental factors influence its development and manifestations. The disease is often progressive and fatal. Its characteristics include impaired control of drinking, a preoccupation with alcohol, continued use of alcohol despite adverse consequences, and distorted thinking, most notably denial. Like other diseases, alcoholism is not simply a matter of insufficient willpower, but a complex problem that causes many symptoms, can have serious consequences, yet can improve with treatment.

A lack of obvious signs of alcoholism can be deceiving. If a person doesn't drink in the morning but feels that he or she must always have a drink at a certain time of the day, that may represent loss of control. If a person never drinks alone but always drinks socially with others, that can camouflage loss of control. If a person is holding a job or taking care of the family, he or she may still spend every waking hour thinking about that first drink at the end of the day (preoccupation).

How Common Are Alcohol-Related Problems?

According to the NIAAA, 9 percent of adults meet the criteria for alcohol abuse or dependence. White males 18 to 29 years old have 2.4 times greater prevalence of abuse and dependence than nonwhites. Among those over age 64, nonwhites have a prevalence rate of abuse and dependence 28.4 percent higher than whites.[34]

Probably fewer than 5 percent of alcoholics and problem drinkers are "skid-row drunks." The other 95 percent are all around us, every day. (See Self-Survey: "Do You Have a Drinking Problem?") Alcoholism generally first appears between the ages of 20 and 40, although even children and young teenagers can become alcoholics. It takes 5 to 15 years of heavy drinking for an adult to become alcoholic, but just 6 to 18 months for an adolescent to develop the disease.

According to the National Comorbidity Survey, published in 1995, 23.5 percent of Americans may become dependent on or abuse alcohol in the course of a lifetime, while 9.7 percent experience these disorders in the course of a year. At all ages, men are two to five times more likely than women to abuse alcohol. In men, drinking usually starts in the late teens or twenties. Women tend to start drinking at a later age, are less likely to stop without help, and often have a history of depression.[35]

 ## What Causes Alcohol Dependence and Abuse?

Although the exact cause of alcohol dependence and abuse is not known, certain factors—including biochemical imbalances in the brain, heredity, cultural acceptability, and stress—all seem to play a role. They include the following:

- *Genetics.* Scientists who are working toward mapping the genes responsible for addictive disorders have not yet been able to identify conclusively a specific gene that puts people at risk for alcoholism. However, epidemiological studies have shown evidence of heredity's role. An identical twin of an alcoholic is twice as likely as a fraternal twin to have an alcohol-related disorder. The incidence of alcoholism is four times higher among the sons of Caucasian alcoholic fathers, regardless of whether they grow up

Self-*Survey* Do You Have a Drinking Problem?

This self-assessment, the Michigan Alcoholism Screening Test (MAST), is widely used to identify potential problems. This test screens for the major psychological, sociological, and physiological consequences of alcoholism.

To complete it, simply answer Yes or No to the following questions, and add up the points shown in the right column for your answers.

	Yes	No	Points
1. Do you enjoy a drink now and then?			(0 for either)
2. Do you think that you're a normal drinker? (By normal, we mean that you drink less than or as much as most other people.)			(2 for no)
3. Have you ever awakened the morning after some drinking the night before and found that you couldn't remember part of the evening?			(2 for yes)
4. Does your wife, husband, a parent, or other near relative every worry or complain about your drinking?			(1 for yes)
5. Can you stop drinking without a struggle after one or two drinks?			(2 for no)
6. Do you ever feel guilty about your drinking?			(1 for yes)
7. Do friends or relatives think that you're a normal drinker?			(2 for no)
8. Do you ever try to limit your drinking to certain times of the day or to certain places?			(0 for either)
9. Have you ever attended a meeting of Alcoholics Anonymous?			(2 for yes)
10. Have you ever gotten into physical fights when drinking?			(1 for yes)
11. Has your drinking ever created problems for you and your wife, husband, a parent, or other relative?			(2 for yes)
12. Has your wife, husband, or other family members ever gone to anyone			

	Yes	No	Points
for help about your drinking?			(2 for yes)
13. Have you ever lost friends because of your drinking?			(2 for yes)
14. Have you ever gotten into trouble at work or school because of your drinking?			(2 for yes)
15. Have you ever lost a job because of your drinking?			(2 for yes)
16. Have you ever neglected your obligations, your family, or your work for two or more days in a row because of drinking?			(2 for yes)
17. Do you drink before noon fairly often?			(1 for yes)
18. Have you ever been told you have liver trouble? cirrhosis?			(2 for yes)
19. After heavy drinking, have you ever had delirium tremens (DTs) or severe shaking, or heard voices or seen things that weren't actually there?			(2 for yes*)
20. Have you ever gone to anyone for help about your drinking?			(5 for yes)
21. Have you ever been in a hospital because of your drinking?			(5 for yes)
22. Have you ever been a patient in a psychiatric hospital or on a psychiatric ward of a general hospital where drinking was part of the problem that resulted in hospitalization?			(2 for yes)

	Yes	No	Points
23. Have you ever been seen at a psychiatric or mental health clinic or gone to any doctor, social worker, or clergyman for help with any emotional problem where drinking was part of the problem?	____	____	(2 for yes)
24. Have you ever been arrested for drunk driving, driving while intoxicated, or driving under the influence of alcoholic beverages?	____	____	(2 for yes)

	Yes	No	Points
25. Have you ever been arrested, or taken into custody, even for a few hours, because of drunken behavior? (If Yes, How many times? ____**)	____	____	(2 for yes)

*Five points for delirium tremens
**Two points for each arrest

Scoring:
In general, five or more points places you in an alcoholic category; four points suggests alcoholism; while three or fewer points indicates that you're *not* alcoholic.

---

with their biological or adoptive parents. The sons of alcoholic fathers have characteristic changes in brain wave activity.

- *Stress and traumatic experiences.* Many people start drinking heavily as a way of coping with psychological problems. About half of all individuals who abuse or are dependent on alcohol also have another mental disorder. Alcohol often is linked with depressive and anxiety disorders. Men and women with these problems may start drinking in an attempt to alleviate their anxiety or depression.

- *Parental alcoholism.* According to researchers, alcoholism is four to five times more common among the children of alcoholics, who may be influenced by the behavior they see in their parents. The sons and daughters of alcoholics share certain characteristics, including early onset of problem drinking with severe social consequences, an unstable family, poor academic and social performance in school, and antisocial behavior.

- *Drug abuse.* Alcoholism is also associated with the abuse of other psychoactive drugs, including marijuana, cocaine, heroin, amphetamines, and various antianxiety medications. Adults under age 30 and adolescents are most likely to use alcohol plus several drugs of abuse, such as marijuana and cocaine. Middle-aged men and women are more likely to combine alcohol with benzodiazepines, such as antianxiety medications or sleeping pills, which may be prescribed for them by a physician. Whatever the reason they start, some people keep drinking out of habit. Once they develop physical tolerance and dependence—the two hallmarks of addiction—they may not be able to stop drinking on their own.

Types of Alcoholism

Mental health professionals have developed different theoretical models to explain alcoholism. Although these models are used mainly by researchers and clinicians, they offer individuals with drinking problems and those close to them some insight into various personality and drinking patterns.

According to one long-established model, there are two primary types of alcoholics. *Type I,* or milieu-limited, alcoholics generally start heavy drinking, often in response to setbacks, losses, or other external circumstances, after age 25. They can abstain for long periods of time and frequently feel loss of control, guilt, and fear about their alcoholism. They also have characteristic personality traits: they tend to be anxious, shy, pessimistic, sentimental, emotionally dependent, rigid, reflective, and slow to anger. Because alcohol reduces their anxiety level, it serves as a positive reinforcer for continued use and contributes to the development of alcohol dependence.

Type II alcoholics are close relatives of an alcoholic male and become heavy drinkers before age 25. They drink regardless of what is going on in their lives; have frequent fights and arrests; and do not usually experience guilt, fear, or loss of control over their drinking. Unlike Type I alcoholics, they are impulsive and aggressive risk-takers, curious, excitable, quick-tempered, optimistic, and independent. Alcohol reinforces their feelings of euphoria and pleasant excitement. Often they abuse drugs as well as alcohol.

Newer research on male and female alcoholics classifies alcoholics as *Type A* or *Type B.* Type A alcoholism is a milder form, characterized by onset later in life, fewer childhood risk factors, less severe dependence, fewer alcohol-related physical and social consequences, fewer symptoms of other mental disorders, and less interference with work and family. Type B alcoholism is linked with childhood and familial risk factors, begins at an earlier age, involves more severe dependence and abuse of other substances, leads to more serious consequences, and often occurs along with other mental disorders. Type B alcoholics are younger, more inclined to experiment with other drugs and are more anxious, and of lower occupational status than Type A alcoholics.

Medical Complications of Alcohol Abuse and Dependence

Excessive alcohol use adversely affects virtually every organ system in the body, including the brain, the digestive tract, the heart, muscles, blood, and hormones. In addition, because alcohol interacts with many drugs, it can increase the risk of potentially lethal overdoses and harmful interactions. Among the major risks and complications are:

- *Liver disease.* Because the liver is the organ that breaks down and metabolizes alcohol, it is especially vulnerable to its effects. Chronic heavy drinking can lead to alcoholic hepatitis (inflammation and destruction of liver cells) and, in the 15 percent of people who continue drinking beyond this stage, cirrhosis (irreversible scarring and destruction of liver cells). (See Figure 16-6.) The liver eventually may fail completely, resulting in coma and death.

- *Cardiovascular system.* Heavy drinking can weaken the heart muscle (causing cardiac myopathy), elevate blood pressure, and increase the risk of stroke. The combined use of alcohol and tobacco, or heavy drinking greatly increases the likelihood of damage to the heart.

- *Cancer.* Heavy alcohol use may contribute to cancer of the liver, stomach, and colon, as well as malignant melanoma, a deadly form of skin cancer. Alcohol, in combination with tobacco use, also increases the risk of cancer of the mouth, tongue, larynx, and esophagus. Several major studies have implicated alcohol as a possible risk factor in breast cancer, particularly in young women, although the degree of danger remains unclear.

- *Brain damage.* Chronic brain damage resulting from alcohol consumption is second only to Alzheimer's disease as a cause of cognitive deterioration in adults. Long-term heavy drinkers may suffer memory losses, be unable to think abstractly or recall names of common objects, and not be able to follow simple instructions.[36] Further cognitive deterioration can be stopped if drinking stops.

- *Vitamin deficiencies.* Alcoholics often tend to have very poor nutrition. Alcoholism is associated with vitamin deficiencies, especially of thiamine (B-12), which may be responsible for certain diseases of the neurological, digestive, muscular, and cardiovascular systems. Lack of thiamine, caused by alcoholism, may result in Wernicke's syndrome, a serious disease characterized by a "clouding" of consciousness and paralysis of eye nerves. Korsakoff's syndrome, a rare form of amnesia caused by alcohol-associated thiamine deficiency, is characterized by disorientation, memory failure, confabulation, and hallucinations, and can be disabling enough to require lifelong custodial care.

- *Digestive problems.* Alcohol triggers the secretion of acids in the stomach, which irritate the mucous lining and cause gastritis. Chronic drinking may result in peptic ulcers (breaks in the stomach lining) and bleeding from the stomach lining.

- *Reproductive and sexual dysfunction.* Alcohol interferes with male sexual function and fertility through direct effects on testosterone and the testicles. In half of alcoholic men, increased levels of female hormones lead to breast enlargement and a feminine pubic hair pattern. Damage to the nerves in the penis by heavy drinking can lead to impotence. In women who drink heavily, a drop in female hormone production may cause menstrual irregularity and infertility.

- *Fetal alcohol syndrome.* The risk of this condition, discussed earlier in the chapter, is greatest if a mother-to-be drinks 3 ounces or more of pure alcohol (the equivalent of six or seven cocktails) a day. Consumption of lower quantities of alcohol can lead to fetal alcohol effects, including low birth weight, irritability in a newborn, and permanent mental impairment. Because no one knows how much—if any—alcohol is safe during pregnancy, the National Institute of Alcohol Abuse and Alcoholism recommends that pregnant women not drink at all.

- *Accidents and injuries.* Alcohol may contribute to almost half of the deaths caused by car accidents,

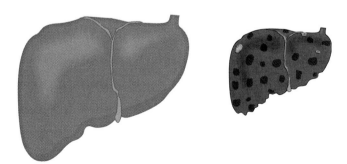

■ **Figure 16-6** A normal liver (left) compared to one with cirrhosis.

burns, falls, and choking. Nearly half of those convicted and jailed for criminal acts committed these crimes while under the influence of alcohol.

- *Higher mortality.* The mortality rate for alcoholics is two to three times higher than that for nonalcoholics of the same age. The leading alcohol-related cause of death is injury, chiefly in auto accidents involving a drunk driver. The second leading cause of alcohol-related deaths is digestive disease, most notably cirrhosis of the liver. In addition, alcohol plays a role in about 30 percent of all suicides. Alcoholics who attempt suicide may have other risk factors, including major depression, poor social support, serious medical illness, and unemployment.

- *Withdrawal dangers.* Withdrawal can be life-threatening when accompanied by medical problems, such as grand mal seizures, pneumonia, liver failure, or gastrointestinal bleeding.

Alcoholism Treatments

Almost 600,000 Americans undergo treatment for alcohol-related problems every year. Until recent years, the only options for professional alcohol treatment were, as one expert puts it, "intensive, extensive and expensive," such as residential programs at hospitals or specialized treatment centers. Today individuals whose drinking could be hazardous to their health may choose from a variety of approaches. Treatment that works well for one person may not work for another. As research into the outcomes of alcohol treatments has grown, more attempts have been made to match individuals to approaches tailored to their needs and more likely to help them overcome their alcohol problems.

Detoxification

The first phase of treatment for alcohol dependence focuses on **detoxification,** the gradual withdrawal of alcohol from the body. For 90 to 95 percent of alcoholics, withdrawal symptoms are mild to moderate. They include sweating; rapid pulse; elevated blood pressure; hand tremor; insomnia; nausea or vomiting; malaise or weakness; anxiety; depressed mood or irritability; headache; and temporary hallucinations or illusions.

Those who have drunk heavily for a prolonged period may develop more severe symptoms, including seizures or alcohol withdrawal delirium, commonly known as **delirium tremens,** or **DTs,** characterized by agitated behavior, delusions, rapid heart rate, sweating, vivid hallucinations, trembling hands, and fever. This problem is most likely to develop in chronic heavy drinkers who also suffer from a physical illness, fatigue, depression, or malnutrition. The symptoms usually appear over several days after heavy drinking stops. Individuals frequently report terrifying visual hallucinations, such as seeing insects all over their bodies. With treatment, most cases subside after several days, although delirium tremens has been known to last as long as four or five weeks. In some cases, complications such as infections or heart arrhythmias prove fatal.

 ## Are There Medications That Treat Alcoholism?

Antianxiety and antidepressive drugs are sometimes used in early treatment for alcoholism, especially for those with underlying mental disorders. Several medications, including certain antidepressant drugs that increase the neurotransmitter serotonin, are being studied as medical interventions to reduce cravings or prevent relapses.[37] Two new medications, naltrexone and acamprosate, also have shown promise.[38] Vitamin supplements, especially thiamine and folic acid, can help overcome some of the nutritional deficiencies linked with alcoholism.

The drug disulfiram (Antabuse), given to deter drinking, causes individuals to become nauseated and acutely ill when they consume alcohol. Antabuse interrupts the removal of acetaldehye by the liver, so this toxic substance accumulates and causes nausea or vomiting. If individuals taking Antabuse drink at all or consume foods with alcoholic content, they become extremely ill. They must avoid foods cooked or marinated in wine and cough syrup preparations containing alcohol. Some individuals have reactions to the alcohol in after-shave lotion. A large amount of alcohol can make them dangerously ill; fatalities have occurred. Side effects are usually mild and include drowsiness, bad breath, skin rash, and temporary impotence. Because Antabuse does not reduce cravings for alcohol, psychotherapy and support groups remain a necessary part of treatment.

Inpatient or Residential Treatment

In the past, 28-day treatment programs in a medical or psychiatric hospital or a residential facility were the cornerstone of early recovery treatment. According to outcome studies, inpatient treatment was effective, with as many as 70 percent of "graduates" remaining abstinent or stable, nonproblem drinkers for five years after. However, because of cost pressures from the insurance industry, the length of stay has been reduced, and there's been increasing emphasis on outpatient care.

Outpatient Treatment

Outpatient treatment may involve group therapy, individual supportive therapy, marital or family therapy, regular attendance at Alcoholics Anonymous (AA) or another support group, brief interventions, and relapse prevention. According to outcome studies, intensive outpatient treatment at a day hospital (with individuals returning home every evening) are as effective as inpatient care. Outpatient therapy continues for at least a year, but many individuals continue to participate in outpatient programs for the rest of their lives.

Brief Interventions

These methods include individual counseling, group therapy and training in specific skills—such as assertiveness—all packed into a six- to eight-week period. Offered at a growing number of centers, brief interventions may be most helpful for problem drinkers who are not physically dependent on alcohol. The University of Michigan's DrinkWise program offers clients the options of one-on-one therapy, group sessions, or telephone counseling. In its first year of operation, DrinkWise reported a success rate of 90 percent in helping clients quit or control their drinking.

Moderation Training

Highly controversial, this approach uses cognitive-behavioral techniques, such as keeping a diary to chart drinking patterns and learning "consumption management" techniques, such as never having more than one drink an hour. "We tell our clients that there is no such thing as no-risk drinking," says Keith Bruhnsen, manager of DrinkWise. "What we offer are guidelines for low-risk drinking."[39] The upper limits are nine drinks a week for women, with no more than three drinks on any one day, and twelve drinks a week for men, with a one-day maximum of four drinks.

Treatment programs in other countries, such as Great Britain and Canada, have long offered moderation training for problem drinkers who consume too much alcohol. However, most experts agree that the best—and perhaps only—hope for recovery for chronic alcoholics who are physically dependent on alcohol is complete abstinence. Because support is critical for maintaining moderation as well as abstinence, those trying to cut back on alcohol can turn to a new support

network called Moderation Management. Aimed at problem drinkers rather than alcoholics, it teaches members how to use alcohol responsibly. After a period of abstinence, members follow drinking guidelines that restrict the number of drinks they have per day and the number of days per week that they drink.

Self-Help Programs

The best-known and most commonly used self-help program for alcohol problems is Alcoholics Anonymous (AA), which was founded more than 60 years ago and which has grown into an international organization that includes 2 million members and 185,000 groups worldwide. Acknowledging the power of alcohol, AA offers support from others struggling with the same illness, from a sponsor available at any time of the day or night, and from fellowship meetings that are held every day of the year. Because anonymity is a key part of AA, it has been difficult for researchers to study its success, but it is generally believed to be a highly effective means of overcoming alcoholism and maintaining abstinence. Its 12 steps, which emphasize honesty, sobriety, and acknowledgment of a "higher power," have become the model for self-help groups for other addictive behaviors, including drug abuse (discussed in Chapter 15) and compulsive eating.

The average age of entry into AA is 30; about 60 percent of the members are men. Members encompass a wide range of ages, occupations, nationalities, and socioeconomic classes. People generally attend 12-step meetings every day when they first begin recovery; most programs recommend 90 meetings in 90 days. Many people taper off to one or two meetings a week as their recovery progresses. No one knows exactly how 12-step programs help people break out of addictions. Some individuals stop their drinking, or other destructive behavior, simply on the basis of the information they get at meetings. Others bond to the group and use it as a social support and refuge while they explore and release their inner feelings—a process similar to what happens in psychotherapy.

Alternatives to AA

Secular Organizations for Sobriety (SOS) was founded in 1986 as an alternative for people who couldn't accept the spirituality of AA. Like AA, SOS holds confidential meetings, celebrates sobriety anniversaries, and views recovery as a one-day-at-a-time process.

Rational Recovery, which also emphasizes anonymity and total abstinence, focuses on the self rather than spirituality. Members use reason instead of prayer and learn to control the impulse to drink by learning how to control the emotions that lead them to drink. Women for Sobriety (WFS), discussed earlier in the chapter, addresses the unique needs of women with drinking problems.

Across the Lifespan: Treating Alcohol Problems in the Elderly

Community surveys suggest that persons older than 65 years consume less alcohol and have fewer alcohol-related problems than younger drinkers. In contrast, surveys conducted in health-care settings have found increasing prevalence of alcoholism among older adults. In acute care hospitals, rates of alcohol-related admissions are similar to rates for heart attacks, and some surveys have found the prevalence of problem drinking in nursing homes to be as high as 49 percent. In addition to the direct risks of alcohol, older individuals face additional dangers when they drink, including falls, fractures, traffic crashes, medication interactions, and depression.[40]

Brief treatment can be effective in helping the elderly overcome alcohol problems, according to a University of Wisconsin study. In the study, half of 158 patients participated in an intervention program that included two visits with their primary physician, a review of problem-drinking and the adverse effects of alcohol, a discussion of the patients' reasons for drinking and drinking cues, a drinking agreement in the form of a prescription, and drinking diary cards. In addition, clinic nurses telephoned the patients regularly. The other patients received only a general health booklet. The patients in the intervention group experienced a 34 percent reduction in weekly alcohol use and a 74 percent reduction in mean number of binge-drinking episodes. There was a 62 percent reduction in the proportion of older adults who consumed more than 21 drinks a week. These data provided the first direct evidence that brief physician advice can decrease alcohol use by older adults.[41]

Recovery

Recovery from alcoholism is a lifelong process of personal growth and healing. The first two years are the most difficult, and relapses are extremely common. By some estimates, more than 90 percent of those recovering from substance use will use alcohol or drugs in any one 12-month period after treatment. However, approximately 70 percent of those who get formal treatment stop drinking for prolonged periods. Even without treatment, 30 percent of alcoholics are able to stop drinking for long periods. Those most likely to remain sober after treatment have the most to lose by continu-

ing to drink: they tend to be employed, married, and upper-middle class.

Most recovering alcoholics experience urges to drink, especially during early recovery when they are likely to feel considerable stress. These urges are a natural consequence of years of drinking and diminish with time. Mood swings are common during recovery, and individuals typically describe themselves as alternately feeling relieved or elated and then discouraged or tearful. Such disconcerting ups and downs also decrease over time. Patience—learning to take "one day at a time"—is crucial.

Increasingly, treatment programs focus on **relapse prevention,** which includes the development of coping strategies and learning techniques that make it easier to live with alcohol cravings and rehearsal of various ways of saying "no" to offers of a drink. According to outcomes research, social skills training—a combination of stress management therapy, assertiveness and communication skills training, behavioral self-control training, and behavioral marital therapy—has proven effective in decreasing the duration and severity of relapses after one year in a group of alcoholics.

A medication called nalmefene, an opioid antagonist, has proven effective in preventing relapse in alcohol-dependent individuals. In one trial, patients receiving nalmefene were 2.4 times less likely to relapse to heavy drinking than those who received a placebo.[42]

Alcoholism's Impact on Relationships

Alcoholism shatters families and creates unhealthy patterns of communicating and relating. Separation and divorce rates are high among alcoholics. Another common occurrence is **codependence,** a term used to describe the behavior of close family members or friends who act in ways that enable their spouses, parents, or friends to continue their self-destructive behavior.

Codependence and Enabling

Codependent spouses of alcoholics follow a predictable pattern of behavior: While trying to control the drinkers, they act in ways that enable the drinkers to keep drinking. If an alcoholic finds it hard to get up in the morning, his wife wakes him up, pulls him out of bed and into the shower, and drops him off at work. If he is late, she makes excuses to his boss. By helping him evade his responsibilities, his wife is helping him continue drinking. Indeed, he might not be able to keep up his habit without her cooperation.

Such behavior is harmful for individuals who are dependent on alcohol because it reinforces their denial. They do not feel out of control or powerless over alcohol because the person or persons closest to them are constantly protecting them from the consequences of their actions. Every crisis—a missed deadline, a forgotten appointment, a child's disappointment when a parent doesn't come to an important event—should be seen as a chance for the individual to recognize what alcohol is doing to the lives of all those close to him or her. If family members let their loved one experience the consequences of drinking, the person may be able to come to the moment of truth concerning alcohol.

Codependents often need help in acknowledging their own feelings and needs. National self-help organizations, such as Al-Anon, help adult family members recognize dysfunctional behaviors in their relationships and start looking at their own problems. Similar self-help groups, such as Alateen, provide support for the teenaged children of alcoholics. These organizations also help family members cope with their loved one's alcoholism—whether or not codependence is a problem.

Growing Up with an Alcoholic Parent

An estimated 7 million youngsters in the United States live with an alcoholic parent. Parental alcoholism increases the likelihood of childhood ADHD, conduct disorder, and anxiety disorders.[43] The experience often leads youngsters to play certain roles: The adjuster or "lost child" does whatever the parent says. The responsible child, or "family hero," typically takes over many household tasks and responsibilities. The acting-out child, or "scapegoat," shows his or her anger early in life by causing problems at home or in school and taking on the role of troublemaker. The "mascot" disrupts tense situations by focusing attention on himself or herself, often by clowning. Regardless of which roles they assume, the children of alcoholics are prone to learning disabilities, eating disorders, and addictive behavior.

Numerous studies have linked child abuse and neglect to parental drinking. Children of women who are problem drinkers have 2.1 times the risk of serious injury as children of mothers who don't drink. Children with two parents who are problem drinkers are at even higher risk. As teenagers, children of alcoholics are more likely to report early sexual intercourse and face a greater risk of adolescent pregnancy.

Adult Children of Alcoholics

Growing up with an alcoholic parent can have a long-lasting effect. Adult children of alcoholics are at risk for many problems. Some try to fill the emptiness inside with alcohol, drugs, or addictive habits. Others find themselves caught up in destructive relationships that repeat the patterns of their childhood. They are likely to have difficulty solving problems, identifying and expressing their feelings, trusting others, and being intimate. In addition to their own increased risk of addictive behavior, they are likely to marry individuals with some form of addiction and keep on playing out the roles of their childhood. They may feel inadequate, not know how to set limits or recognize normal behavior, be perfectionistic, and want to control all aspects of their lives. However, not all adult children are alike or necessarily suffer from psychological problems or face an increased risk of substance abuse themselves.

Because the impact of alcoholism can be so enduring, support groups—such as Adult Children of Alcoholics, Children of Alcoholics, and Adult Children of Dysfunctional Families—have spread throughout the country in the last decade. These organizations provide adult children of alcoholics a mutually supportive group setting to discuss their childhood experiences with alcoholic parents and the emotional consequences they carry into adult life. Through such groups or other forms of therapy, individuals may learn to move beyond anger and blame, see the part they themselves play in

---

Strategies *for* Change

If Someone Close to You Drinks Too Much

✔ Try to remain calm, unemotional, and factually honest in speaking about the drinker's behavior. Include the drinker in family life.

✔ Discuss the situation with someone you trust: a member of the clergy, social worker, friend, or someone who has experienced alcoholism directly.

✔ Never cover up or make excuses for the drinker, or shield him or her from the consequences of drinking. Assuming the drinker's responsibilities undermines his or her dignity and sense of importance.

✔ Refuse to ride with the drinker if he or she is driving while intoxicated.

✔ Encourage new interests and participate in leisure-time activities that the drinker enjoys.

✔ Try to accept setbacks and relapses calmly.

their current state of unhappiness, and create a future that is healthier and happier than their past.

Making This Chapter Work for You

Responsible Drinking

■ When comparing amounts and types of alcohol, assume that one drink contains the equivalent of 1/2 ounce of 100 percent ethyl alcohol. The percentage of alcohol in a person's blood, or blood-alcohol concentration, is the measurement used by law enforcement officers to determine whether someone is legally drunk.

■ The rate of alcohol absorption depends on many factors: the strength of the drink; the drinker's size, sex, age, and race; family history of alcoholism; whether there's food in the drinker's stomach; and the drinker's expectations and tolerance for alcohol.

■ Moderate amounts of alcohol may have a positive effect on the cardiovascular system. In excess, however, alcohol can weaken the heart muscle, increase blood pressure, increase the risk of stroke, and inhibit the production of white and red blood cells.

■ Alcohol, a central nervous system depressant, also impairs thinking, vision, motor skills, hearing, smell and taste, pain perception, sense of time and space, speech, and sexual response and performance. When combined with other drugs, alcohol can have serious adverse effects.

■ About half (52 percent) of American adults drink, with little variation among the races with respect to quantity, frequency, and amount of alcohol consumed. Men generally drink more, in quantity and frequency, than women. Children are beginning to experiment with alcohol at a younger age than in the past.

■ Patterns of drinking vary greatly, from complete abstinence to infrequent drinking to moderate drinking. None of these patterns poses a current or future threat to a drinker's well-being. Problem drinking refers to any kind of drinking that interferes with a major aspect of life, such as sleep, energy, family relationships, health, or safety. A drinking binge consists of having five or more drinks at a single sitting for a man and four drinks at a single sitting for women.

■ Alcohol is the substance most commonly used by college students. Alcohol abuse by students has led to violence, sexual assaults, and other dangers, which have triggered a backlash among students who drink little or no alcohol.

■ Women drink for different reasons and in different ways than men. Because of their smaller bodies and lack of a stomach enzyme that neutralizes alcohol, they feel its impact much more quickly and severely than men do. Breast cancer, infertility, and osteoporosis are among the possible special health risks that women face. Many respond best to treatments tailored to the unique needs of women, such as Women for Sobriety, a national network of self-help groups.

■ Although there has been a successful campaign against drunk driving, this dangerous crime continues to kill thousands of Americans. Families of the victims of drunk drivers continue to work to change the way America treats its drunk drivers and to keep drunk drivers off the road.

■ There is a spectrum of alcohol problems that range from problem drinking to alcohol dependence or abuse. The difference is one of degree and of loss of control over one's craving for alcohol.

■ Alcohol abuse involves continued use of alcohol despite awareness of social, occupational, psychological, or physical problems related to drinking, or to drinking in dangerous ways or situations (before driving, for instance).

■ Alcohol dependence is a distinct disorder in which individuals develop a strong craving for alcohol because it produces pleasurable feelings or relieves stress or anxiety. Over time they experience physiological changes that lead to tolerance; if they abruptly stop drinking, they suffer withdrawal, a state of acute physical and psychological discomfort.

■ Although the exact cause of alcohol dependence or abuse isn't known, certain factors—including a biochemical imbalance in the brain, heredity, cultural acceptability, and stress—may play a role in the development of this disease.

■ In the past, alcoholics were categorized as Type 1, who generally start heavy drinking, reinforced by external circumstances, after age 25; and Type 2, who typically become heavy drinkers before age 25 and drink regardless of external circumstances.

■ Newer research classifies alcoholics as Type A or Type B. Type A alcoholism develops later in life and involves less severe dependence, fewer alcohol-related problems, and less distress in the areas of work and family. Type B alcoholism, linked with childhood and familial risk factors, starts earlier and involves greater dependence and more serious complications.

■ Chronic heavy drinking can cause severe liver damage, hepatitis, or cirrhosis. Vitamin deficiencies, which commonly occur with alcoholism, can result in severe neurological, muscular, digestive, and cardiovascular diseases. Excessive alcohol consumption can damage the brain, causing mental deterioration, and is also associated with heart damage and several types of cancer.

- Treatments for alcohol problems include detoxification, medications, inpatient care, outpatient treatment, and brief interventions. Problem drinkers who have not become dependent on alcohol may be able to learn to control their alcohol intake through moderation training.

- Self-help groups, including AA, Rational Recovery, Secular Organizations for Sobriety, and Women for Sobriety, can offer ongoing support to individuals recovering from alcohol problems as they build a new alcohol-free life.

- Individuals with addictive behaviors or dependence on drugs or alcohol, and the children or partners of such people, are especially likely to find themselves in dysfunctional relationships that do not promote healthy communication, honesty, and intimacy.

- Children of an alcoholic parent are vulnerable to learning disabilities, eating disorders, and addictive behavior. Adult children of parents with addictive behaviors are more likely to have difficulty solving problems, identifying and expressing their feelings, trusting others, and being intimate. They may develop some form of addiction themselves or marry someone with addictive behavior patterns.

- Support groups, such as Al-Anon, Codependents Anonymous, and Adult Children of Dysfunctional Families, can help family members and adults who grew up in unhealthy homes come to terms with their past and prepare for a happier future.

- For people with alcohol dependence and abuse, recovery is a lifelong process of change rather than a one-time treatment. Through therapy, education,

health **/ ONLINE**

The College Alcohol Study
http://www.hsph.harvard.edu/cas/test/index.shtml
The Harvard School of Public Health College Alcohol Study is an ongoing survey of more than 15,000 students at 140 colleges in 40 states. You can access the most recent survey results from this site.

Facts on Tap: Alcohol and Student Life
http://www.factsontap.org/collexp/Collexp.htm
This site provides statistics on campus alcohol use, tips to help cut down on or stop drinking, places to go for help, and more.

National Institute on Alcohol Abuse and Alcoholism
http://www.niaaa.nih.gov/
Answers frequently asked questions and provides online databases and publications on alcohol-related topics.

Please note that links are subject to change. If you find a broken link, use a search engine like http://www.yahoo.com *and search for the web site by typing in key words.*

 Campus Chat: How prevalent is binge drinking on your campus? Share your thoughts on our online discussion forum at **http://health.wadsworth.com**

Find It On InfoTrac: You can find additional readings related to alcohol via InfoTrac College Edition, an online library of more than 900 journals and publications. Follow the instructions for accessing InfoTrac that came packaged with your textbook; then search for articles using a key word search.

- **Suggested reading:** "A Summary of Alcohol Facts—Facts for Patients." *The Brown University Digest of Addiction Theory and Application,* March 1999, Vol. 18, Issue 3, p. S1.

  (1) List several ways that alcohol can adversely affect your brain and vision.

  (2) What is the only preventable cause of birth defects with accompanying mental retardation?

  (3) What percent of American families have to cope with alcohol-related problems?

For additional links, resources, and suggested readings on InfoTrac, visit our Health & Wellness Resource Center at **http://health.wadsworth.com**

and a reevaluation of what's meaningful in life, they can find hope for a better way of living. Relapses are so common that therapists believe they may be part of the process of recovery. Although painful, they may serve a purpose in developing the insight and motivation needed to break out of a self-destructive pattern once and for all.

Responsible drinking is a matter of you controlling your drinking, rather than the drinking controlling you. The Serenity Prayer, written by Protestant theologian Reinhold Niebuhr, summarizes the attitudes and values that can help people break free from their addictions and find purpose and meaning in life:

> *God grant me the Serenity*
> *To accept the things I cannot change;*
> *Courage to change the things I can; and*
> *Wisdom to know the difference.*

 Fighting Addiction. What is known about the chemistry of addiction?

Key Terms

The terms listed here are used within the chapter. Page numbers are included for each term. A definition of each term is given in the Glossary pages at the end of this book.

absorption 511	codependence 532	proof 510
alcohol abuse 525	delirium tremens (DTs) 530	relapse prevention 532
alcohol dependence 525	detoxification 530	
alcoholism 526	ethyl alcohol 510	
binge drinking 517	fetal alcohol effects (FAE) 524	
blood-alcohol concentration	fetal alcohol syndrome (FAS) 524	
(BAC) 510	intoxication 513	

Critical Thinking Questions

1. Driving home from his high school graduation party, 18-year-old Rick has had too much to drink. As he crosses the dividing line on the two-lane road, the driver of an oncoming car—a young mother with two young children in the backseat—swerves to avoid an accident. She hits a concrete wall and dies instantly; but her children survive. Rick has no record of drunk driving. Should he go to prison? Is he guilty of manslaughter? How would you feel if you were the victim's husband? if you were Rick's friend?

2. Some groups concerned about alcohol abuse advocate greater restrictions on availability, such as prohibiting the sale of alcoholic beverages in supermarkets, convenience stores, and gas stations. They would like to see a ban on advertisements, especially those aimed at young people. Opponents argue that laws have never been effective in controlling alcohol abuse. Do you think our society is too permissive in the way we allow alcohol to be promoted or sold? Would you support anti-alcohol laws? Why or why not?

3. What effects has alcohol use had in your life? Try making a list of the positive and negative effects your own alcohol use has had. Be specific. If you continue to drink at your current rate, what positive and negative effects do you think it will have on your future? What effects has other people's drinking had on your life? List family members and friends who drink regularly, and how their drinking has affected you.

References

1. Hales, Robert, et al. *American Psychiatric Press Textbook of Psychiatry.* 3rd ed. Washington, D.C.: American Psychiatric Press, 1999.

2. Renaud, Serge, et al. "Wine, Beer, and Mortality in Middle-aged Men From Eastern France." *Archives of Internal Medicine,* September 13, 1999.

3. Hoke, Franklin. "Alcohol Consumption Triggers Free-Radical Damage." University of Pennsylvania Medical Center Science News, September 11, 1999.

4. Koob, George. "Alcohol: The Chemistry of the Dark Side." Presentation, American Chemical Society, August 21, 1999.

5. Gronbaek, Morten, et al. "Alcohol and Mortality: Is There a U-Shaped Relation in Elderly People?" *Age and Ageing,* Vol. 27, Issue 6, November 1998.

6. Cullen, K. W., et al. "Gender Differences in Chronic Disease Risk Behaviors Through the Transition Out of High School," *American Journal of Preventive Medicine,* Vol. 17, No. 1, 1999.

7. Bradizza, Clara, et al. "Social and Coping Reasons for Drinking: Predicting Alcohol Misuse in Adolescents." *Journal of Studies on Alcohol,* Vol. 60, No. 4, July 1999.

8. Costa, Frances, et al. "Transition into Adolescent Problem Drinking: The Role of Psychosocial Risk and Protective Factors." *Journal of Studies on Alcohol,* Vol. 60, No. 4, July 1999.

9. Zoccolillo, Mark, et al. "Problem Drug and Alcohol Use in a Community Sample of Adolescents." *Journal of the American Academy of Child and Adolescent Psychiatry,* Vol. 38, Issue 7, July 1999.

10. "MADD, OJJDP Expand Program to Combat Underage Drinking." *Alcoholism & Drug Abuse Weekly,* Vol. 11, Issue 29, July 16, 1999.

11. Bradley, Ann. "Age of Drinking Onset Predicts Future Alcohol Abuse and Dependence." National Institute on Alcohol Abuse and Alcoholism, January 14, 1998.

12. Wechsler, Henry, et al. "College Alcohol Use: A Full or Empty Glass?" *Journal of American College Health,* Vol. 47, No. 6, May 1999.

13. Perkins, H., et al. "Misperceptions of the Norms for the Frequency of Alcohol and Other Drug Use on College Campuses." *Journal of American College Health,* Vol. 47, No. 6, May 1999.

14. Flaherty, Julie. "Ad Campaign Focuses on Binge-Drinking by College Students." *New York Times,* August 8, 1999. Reasons for Drinking: Predicting Alcohol Misuse in Adolescents." *Journal of Studies on Alcohol,* Vol. 60, Issue 4, July 1999.

15. Federal Office of Substance Abuse Prevention.

16. Staton, Michele, et al. "Risky Sex Behavior and Substance Use Among Young Adults." *Health and Social Work,* Vol. 24, Issue 2, May 1999.

17. Ullman, Sarah, et al. "Alcohol and Sexual Assault in a National Sample of College Women." *Journal of Interpersonal Violence,* Vol. 14, No. 6, June 1999.

18. Poulson, R. L., et al. "Alcohol Consumption, Strength of Religious Beliefs, and Risky Sexual Behavior in College Students." *Journal of American College Health,* Vol. 46, No. 5, March 1998.

19. Perkins, Wesley, "Stress-Motivated Drinking in Collegiate and Postcollegiate Young Adulthood: Life Course and Gender Patterns." *Journal of Studies on Alcohol,* Vol. 60, No. 2, March 1999.

20. Wechsler. "College Alcohol Use: A Full or Empty Glass?"

21. Opalka, Susie, and Yelena Spektor. "Fraternity, Sorority, Anything but Sobriety." GRIP Publications, 1999.

22. Brody, Jane. "Coping with Cold, Hard Facts on Teen-age Drinking." *New York Times,* April 6, 1999.

23. Hingson, Ralph. "College-Age Drinking Problems." *Journal of American College Health,* Vol. 47 No. 2, September 1998.

24. Keeling, Richard. "Drinking in College: The Politics of Research and Prevention." *Brown University Digest of Addiction Theory and Application,* Vol. 17, Issue 12, December 1998.

25. "Group of Boston Colleges Seeks Joint Strategy Against Campus Drinking." *Alcoholism & Drug Abuse Weekly,* Vol. 10, Issue 47, December 14, 1998.

26. National Institute on Alcohol and Alcohol Abuse.

27. Skaff, Marilyn, et al. "Gender Differences in Problem Drinking and Depression: Different Vulnerabilities." *American Journal of Community Psychology,* Vol. 27, Issue 1, February 1999.

28. Williams, Robert, and Lina Ricciardelli. "Gender Congruence in Confirmatory and Compensatory Drinking." *Journal of Psychology,* Vol. 133, Issue 3, May 1999.

29. Nolen-Hoeksema, Susan. "Women Think, Men Drink: The Link Between Gender, Depression and Alcohol." Presentation, American Psychological Association, Boston, August 1999.

30. Kirkpatrick, Jean. Personal interview.

31. National Highway Traffic Safety Administration.

32. Bruhnsen, Keith. Personal interview.

33. Hales. *American Psychiatric Press Textbook of Psychiatry.*

34. National Institute on Alcohol and Alcohol Abuse.

35. "Bibulous America."

36. Nixon, S., et al. "Cognitive Efficiency in Alcoholics and Polysubstance Abusers." *Alcoholism: Clinical and Experimental Research,* Vol. 22, No. 7, March 1999.

37. Swift, Robert. "Drug Therapy: Drug Therapy for Alcohol Dependence." *New England Journal of Medicine,* Vol. 340, No. 19, May 13, 1999.

38. Garbutt, James, et al. "Pharmacological Treatment of Alcohol Dependence: A Review of the Evidence." *Journal of the American Medical Association,* April 9, 1999.

39. Bruhnsen, Keith. Personal interview.

40. Burge, Sandra, and David Schneider, "Alcohol-Related Problems: Recognition and Intervention." *American Family Physician,* Vol. 59, No. 2. Jan. 15, 1999.

41. "Alcohol Researchers Prove Brief Intervention Successful in Older Problem Drinkers." National Institute on Alcohol Abuse and Alcoholism News Release, June 23, 1999.

42. "Alcohol Researchers Identify New Medication That Lessens Relapse Risk." National Institute on Alcohol Abuse and Alcoholism Press Office, August 30, 1999.

43. Soglin, Becky. "Parental Alcoholism Linked to Kids' Behavioral Problems." University of Iowa College of Medicine, August 21, 1999.

C H A P T E R

17

Tobacco Use, Misuse, and Abuse

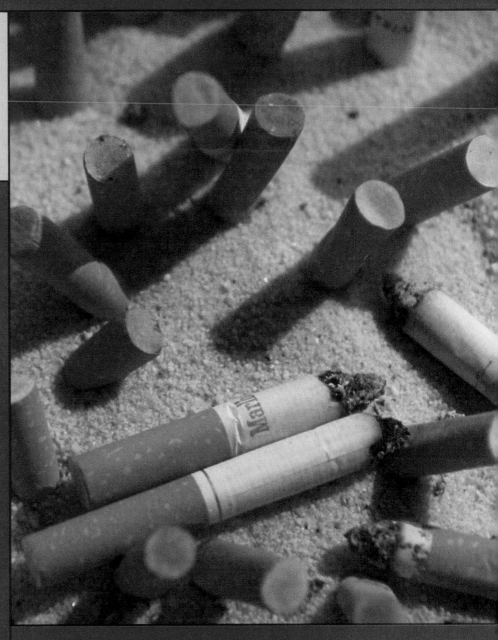

After studying the material in this chapter, you should be able to:

- **Describe** today's tobacco smokers and the common reasons why they smoke.
- **List** the health effects of smoking tobacco or using smokeless tobacco.
- **List** the health problems that can be prevented by quitting smoking.
- **Describe** the health effects of passive, or secondhand, tobacco smoke.
- **Discuss** several recommended ways to quit smoking.
- **Plan** a strategy for keeping your personal environment smoke-free.

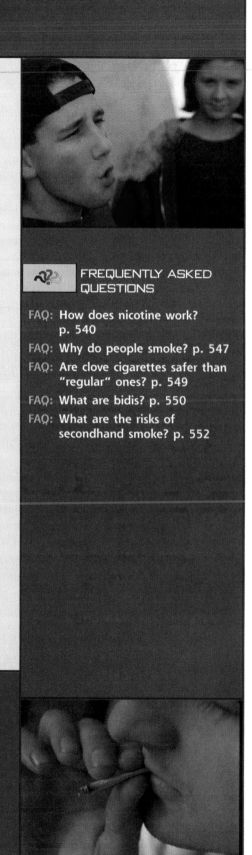

I magine living in a smoke-free society. No one would light up at the table next to yours at a restaurant. There wouldn't be clouds of smoke in airports, conference rooms, or theater lobbies. Parks and beaches wouldn't be littered with cigarette butts.

A generation ago the very idea would have seemed like a fantasy. Now in many places around the country, such scenes are a reality. Nationwide, nonsmokers now outnumber smokers by a ratio of two to one. The Food and Drug Administration (FDA), American Medical Association (AMA), and other health groups have targeted nicotine as a dangerous addictive drug and have launched an all-out campaign against this devastating killer.

Nevertheless, tobacco use remains the single leading preventable cause of death in the world. According to WHO statistics, tobacco products annually cause two million deaths in developed countries and one million in developing countries. The death toll is expected to rise to ten million a year by the 2020s, with 70 percent of these deaths in developed countries.[1]

In the United States, there also is reason for concern. Teen smoking rose throughout the nineties, with more youngsters lighting up at early ages. There also have been increases in the use of cigars and smokeless tobacco. If current trends continue, health officials fear a reversal in the progress that has been made and a rise in lung cancer and other tobacco-related ailments.

This chapter discusses the effects of tobacco on the body, smoking patterns, tobacco dependence, quitting smoking, smokeless tobacco, and passive smoking. The information it provides may help you to breathe easier today—and may help ensure cleaner air for others to breathe tomorrow. ❖

FREQUENTLY ASKED QUESTIONS

FAQ: **How does nicotine work?
p. 540**

FAQ: **Why do people smoke? p. 547**

FAQ: **Are clove cigarettes safer than
"regular" ones? p. 549**

FAQ: **What are bidis? p. 550**

FAQ: **What are the risks of
secondhand smoke? p. 552**

Tobacco and Its Effects

Tobacco, an herb that can be smoked or chewed, directly affects the brain. While its primary active ingredient is nicotine, there are almost 400 other compounds and chemicals in tobacco smoke, including gases, liquids, particles, tar, carbon monoxide, cadmium, pyridine, nitrogen dioxide, ammonia, benzene, phenol, acrolein, hydrogen cyanide, formaldehyde, and hydrogen sulfide. See Figure 17-1 for a summary of their physiological effects.

 ## How Does Nicotine Work?

A colorless, oily compound, **nicotine** is poisonous in concentrated amounts. If you inhale while smoking, 90 percent of the nicotine in the smoke is absorbed into your body. Even if you draw smoke only into your mouth and not into your lungs, you still absorb 25 to 30 percent of the nicotine. The FDA has concluded that nicotine is a dangerous, addictive drug that should be regulated. (See Figure 17-2.)

Nicotine stimulates the cerebral cortex, the outer layer of the brain that controls complex behavior and mental activity and enhances mood and alertness. Investigators have shown that nicotine may enhance smokers' performance on some tasks but leave other mental skills unchanged.[2] Nicotine also acts as a sedative. How often you smoke and how you smoke determine nicotine's effect on you. If you're a regular smoker, nicotine will generally stimulate you at first, then tranquilize you. Shallow puffs tend to increase alertness, because low doses of nicotine facilitate the release of the neurotransmitter *acetylcholine,* which makes one feel alert. Deep drags, on the other hand, relax the smoker, because high doses of nicotine block the flow of acetylcholine.

Nicotine stimulates the adrenal glands to produce adrenaline, a hormone that increases

blood pressure, speeds up the heart rate by 15 to 20 beats a minute, and constricts blood vessels (especially in the skin). Nicotine also inhibits the formation of urine, dampens hunger, irritates the membranes in the mouth and throat, and dulls the taste buds, so foods don't taste as good as they would otherwise. Nicotine is a major contributor to heart and respiratory diseases.

Tar

As it burns, tobacco produces **tar,** a thick, sticky dark fluid made up of several hundred different chemicals—many of them poisonous, some of them *carcinogenic* (enhancing the growth of cancerous cells). As you inhale tobacco smoke, tar and other particles settle in the forks of the branchlike bronchial tubes in your lungs, where precancerous changes are apt to occur. In addition, tar and smoke damage the mucus and the cilia in the bronchial tubes, which normally remove irritating foreign materials from your lungs.

Carbon Monoxide

Smoke from cigarettes, cigars, and pipes also contains **carbon monoxide,** the deadly gas that comes out of the exhaust pipes of cars, in levels 400 times those consid-

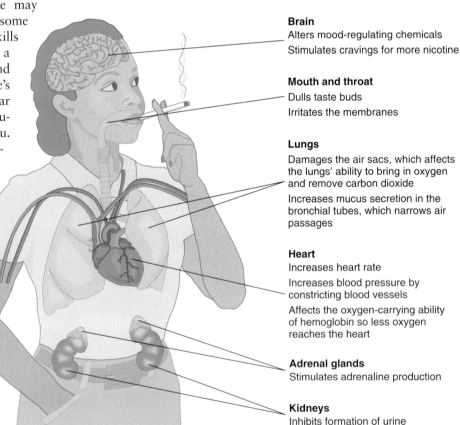

Brain
Alters mood-regulating chemicals
Stimulates cravings for more nicotine

Mouth and throat
Dulls taste buds
Irritates the membranes

Lungs
Damages the air sacs, which affects the lungs' ability to bring in oxygen and remove carbon dioxide
Increases mucus secretion in the bronchial tubes, which narrows air passages

Heart
Increases heart rate
Increases blood pressure by constricting blood vessels
Affects the oxygen-carrying ability of hemoglobin so less oxygen reaches the heart

Adrenal glands
Stimulates adrenaline production

Kidneys
Inhibits formation of urine

■ Figure 17-1 Some effects of smoking on the body.

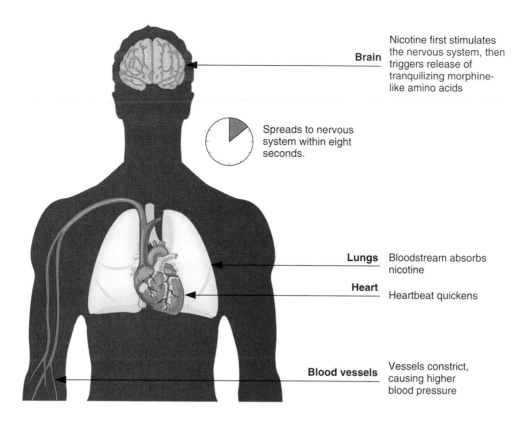

Brain Nicotine first stimulates the nervous system, then triggers release of tranquilizing morphine-like amino acids

Spreads to nervous system within eight seconds.

Lungs Bloodstream absorbs nicotine

Heart Heartbeat quickens

Blood vessels Vessels constrict, causing higher blood pressure

■ **Figure 17-2** The effects of nicotine, a fast-acting and potent drug, on the body.

ered safe in industry. Carbon monoxide interferes with the ability of the hemoglobin in the blood to carry oxygen, impairs normal functioning of the nervous system, and is at least partly responsible for the increased risk of heart attack and strokes in smokers.

The Impact of Tobacco

Smoking tobacco is the largest and most preventable cause of mortality in the United States, causing more than 400,000 deaths among smokers and another 50,000 deaths among nonsmokers exposed to environmental tobacco smoke. Nationally, smoking results in more than 5 million years of potential life lost each year.[3] Cigarette smoking is associated with elevated risk of mortality from all causes, several cardiovascular diseases, and cancer.[4]

Health Effects of Cigarette Smoking

If you're a smoker who inhales deeply and started smoking before the age of 15, you're trading a minute of future life for every minute you now spend smoking. Smoking not only eventually kills, it also ages you: Smokers get more wrinkles than nonsmokers. But the

effects of smoking are far more than skin-deep. A cigarette smoker is 10 times more likely to develop lung cancer than a nonsmoker and 20 times more likely to have a heart attack. Those who smoke two or more packs a day are 15 to 25 times more likely to die of lung cancer than are nonsmokers. Moreover, the danger of lung cancer skyrockets when smokers are also exposed to other carcinogens, such as asbestos. This double threat increases the risk of lung cancer to as much as 92 times that for nonsmokers not exposed to asbestos.

Heart Disease and Stroke

Although a great deal of publicity has been given to the link between cigarettes and lung cancer, heart attack is actually the leading cause of deaths for smokers. Smoking doubles the risk of heart disease, and smokers who suffer heart attacks have only a 50 percent chance of recovering. Smokers have a 70 percent higher death rate from heart disease than do nonsmokers, and those who smoke heavily have a 200 percent higher death rate.

The federal Office of the Surgeon General blames cigarettes for one out of every ten deaths attributable to heart disease. Smoking is more dangerous than are the two most notorious risk factors for heart disease: high blood pressure and high cholesterol. If smoking is combined with one of these, the chances of heart attack are four times greater. Women who smoke and use oral contraceptives have a ten times higher risk of suffering heart attacks than women who do neither.

Smoking also causes a condition called *cardiomyopathy*, which weakens the heart's ability to pump blood and results in the death of about 10,000 people a year. Although researchers don't know precisely how smoking poisons the heart muscle, they speculate that either nicotine or carbon monoxide has a direct toxic effect. Other coronary diseases may be associated with

Self-*Survey*   Are You Addicted to Nicotine?

Answer the following questions as honestly as you can by placing a check mark in the appropriate column:

	Yes	No
1. Do you smoke every day?	____	____
2. Do you smoke because of shyness and to build up self-confidence?	____	____
3. Do you smoke to escape from boredom and worries or while under pressure?	____	____
4. Have you ever burned a hole in your clothes, carpet, furniture, or car with a cigarette?	____	____
5. Have you ever had to go to the store late at night or at another inconvenient time because you were out of cigarettes?	____	____
6. Do you feel defensive or angry when people tell you that your smoke is bothering them?	____	____
7. Has a doctor or dentist ever suggested that you stop smoking?	____	____
8. Have you ever promised someone that you would stop smoking, then broken your promise?	____	____
9. Have you ever felt physical or emotional discomfort when trying to quit?	____	____
10. Have you ever successfully stopped smoking for a period of time, only to start again?	____	____
11. Do you buy extra supplies of tobacco to make sure you won't run out?	____	____
12. Do you find it difficult to imagine life without smoking?	____	____
13. Do you choose only those activities and entertainments during which you can smoke?	____	____
14. Do you prefer, seek out, or feel more comfortable in the company of smokers?	____	____
15. Do you inwardly despise or feel ashamed of yourself because of your smoking?	____	____
16. Do you ever find yourself lighting up without having consciously decided to?	____	____
17. Has your smoking ever caused trouble at home or in a relationship?	____	____

	Yes	No
18. Do you ever tell yourself that you can stop smoking whenever you want to?	____	____
19. Have you ever felt that your life would be better if you didn't smoke?	____	____
20. Do you continue to smoke even though you are aware of the health hazards posed by smoking?	____	____

If you answered Yes to one or two of these questions, there's a chance that you are addicted or are becoming addicted to nicotine. If you answered Yes to three or more of these questions, you are probably already addicted to nicotine.

Source: Nicotine Anonymous World Services, San Francisco.

Making Changes

Breaking the Habit

Here's a six-point program to help you or someone you love quit smoking. (*Caution:* Don't undertake the quit-smoking program until you have a two- to four-week period of relatively unstressful work and study schedules or social commitments.)

1. *Identify your smoking habits.* Keep a daily diary (a piece of paper wrapped around your cigarette pack with a rubber band will do) and record the time you smoke, the activity associated with smoking (after breakfast, in the car), and your urge for a cigarette (desperate, pleasant, or automatic). For the first week or two, don't bother trying to cut down; just use the diary to learn the conditions under which you smoke

2. *Get support.* It can be tough to go it alone. Phone your local chapter of the American Cancer Society, or otherwise get the names of some ex-smokers who can give you support.

3. *Begin by tapering off.* For a period of one to four weeks, aim at cutting down to, say, 12 or 15 cigarettes a day; or change to a lower-nicotine brand, and concentrate on not increasing the number of cigarettes you smoke. As indicated by your diary, begin by cutting out those cigarettes you smoke automatically. In addition, restrict the times you allow yourself to smoke. Throughout this period, stay in touch, once a day or every few days, with your ex-smoker friend(s) to discuss your problems.

4. *Set a quit date*. At some point during the tapering-off period, announce to everyone—friends, family, and ex-smokers—when you're going to quit. Do it with flair. Announce it to coincide with a significant date, such as your birthday or anniversary.

5. *Stop*. A week before Q-day, smoke only five cigarettes a day. Begin late in the day, say after 4:00 P.M. Smoke the first two cigarettes in close succession. Then, in the evening, smoke the last three, also in close succession, about 15 minutes apart. Focus on the negative aspects of cigarettes, such as the rawness in your throat and lungs. After seven days, quit

and give yourself a big reward on that day, such as a movie or a fantastic meal or new clothes.

6. *Follow up*. Stay in touch with your ex-smoker friend(s) during the following two weeks, particularly if anything stressful or tense occurs that might trigger a return to smoking. Think of the person you're becoming—the very person cigarette ads would have you believe smoking makes you. Now that you're quitting smoking, you're becoming healthier, sexier, more sophisticated, more mature, and better looking—and you've earned it!

Sources: American Cancer Society; National Cancer Institute.

---

smoking. *Aortic aneurysm* is a bulge in the aorta (the large artery attached to the heart) caused by a weakening of its walls. *Pulmonary heart disease* is a heart disorder caused by changes in blood vessels in the lungs. (See Chapter 13 for further discussion of heart disease.)

Even people who have smoked for decades can reduce their risk of heart attack if they quit smoking. However, recent studies indicate some irreversible damage to blood vessels. Progression of atherosclerosis—hardening of the arteries—among past smokers continues at a faster pace than among those who never smoked.[5]

In addition to contributing to heart attacks, cigarette smoking increases the risk of stroke two to three times in men and women, even after other risk factors are taken into account. According to one study of middle-aged men, giving up smoking leads to a considerable decrease in the risk of stroke within five years of quitting, particularly in smokers of less than 20 cigarettes a day. Those with hypertension show the greatest benefit. The risk for heavy smokers declines but never reverts back to that of men who never smoked.

Cancer

The American Cancer Society estimates that tobacco smoking is the cause of 28 percent of all deaths from cancer and the cause of more than 85 to 90 percent of all cases of lung cancer. The more people smoke, the longer they smoke, and the earlier they start smoking, the more likely they are to develop lung cancer.

Smokers of two or more packs a day have lung cancer mortality rates 15 to 25 times greater than nonsmokers. If smokers stop smoking before cancer has started, their lung tissue tends to repair itself, even if there were already precancerous changes. Former smokers who haven't smoked for 15 or more years have lung

cancer mortality rates only somewhat above those for nonsmokers.

Chemicals in cigarette smoke and other environmental pollutants switch on a particular gene in the lung cells of some individuals. This gene produces an enzyme that helps manufacture powerful carcinogens, which set the stage for cancer. The gene seems more likely to be activated in some people than others, and people with this gene are at much higher risk of developing lung cancer. However, smokers without the gene still remain at risk, because other chemicals and genes also may be involved in the development of lung cancer.

Smokers who are depressed are more likely to get cancer than nondepressed smokers. Although researchers don't know exactly how smoking and depression may work together to increase the risk of cancer, one possibility is that stress and depression cause biological changes that lower immunity, such as a decline in natural killer cells that fight off tumors.[6]

Among the new drugs that have improved the odds for survival of lung cancer patients is Taxotere (docetaxel), which, in one study, increased the one-year survival rate in patients from 19 to 32 percent.[7] Despite some advances in treating lung cancer, however, the prognosis for sufferers is not good. Even with vigorous therapy, fewer than 10 percent survive for five years after diagnosis. This is one of the lowest survival rates of any type of cancer. And if the cancer has spread from the lungs to other parts of the body, only 1 percent survive for five years after diagnosis. (See Chapter 14 for further discussion of cancer.)

Respiratory Diseases

Smoking quickly impairs the respiratory system. Even some teenaged smokers show signs of respiratory difficulty—breathlessness, chronic cough, excess phlegm production—when compared with nonsmokers of the same age. Cigarette smokers are up to 18 times more likely than are nonsmokers to die of noncancerous diseases of the lungs.

Cigarette smoking is the major cause of chronic obstructive lung disease (COLD), which includes emphysema and chronic bronchitis, in men and women. COLD is characterized by progressive limitation of the flow of air into and out of the lungs. In emphysema, the limitation of airflow is the result of disease changes in the lung tissue, affecting the bronchioles (the smallest air passages) and the walls of the alveoli (the tiny air sacs of the lung) (see Figure 17-3). Eventually, many of the air sacs are destroyed, and the lungs become much less able to bring in oxygen and remove carbon dioxide. As a result, the heart has to work harder to deliver oxygen to all organs of the body.

In chronic bronchitis, the bronchial tubes in the lungs become inflamed, thickening the walls of the bronchi, and the production of mucus increases. The result is a narrowing of the air passages. Smoking is more dangerous than any form of air pollution, at least for most Americans, but exposure to both air pollution and cigarettes is particularly harmful. Although each may cause bronchitis, together they have a synergistic effect—that is, their combined impact exceeds the sum of their separate effects.

Other Smoking-Related Problems

Smokers are more likely than nonsmokers to develop gum disease, and they lose significantly more teeth. Even those who quit have worse gum problems than people who never smoked at all. Smoking may also contribute to the loss of teeth and teeth supporting bone, even in individuals with good oral hygiene. (See Chapter 11 for more on oral health.)

Cigarette smoking is associated with stomach and duodenal ulcers; mouth, throat, and other types of cancer; and cirrhosis of the liver. Smoking may worsen the symptoms or complications of allergies, diabetes, hypertension, peptic ulcers, and disorders of the lungs or blood vessels. Some men who smoke ten cigarettes or more a day may experience sexual impotence. Cigarette smokers also tend to miss work one-third more often than do nonsmokers, primarily because of respiratory illnesses. In addition, each year cigarette-ignited fires claim thousands of lives.

Smoking and Medication

Smokers use more medications—aspirin, painkillers, sleeping pills, tranquilizers, antihistamines, cough medicines, stomach medicines, laxatives, diuretics, and antibiotics—than nonsmokers do. According to the American Pharmaceutical Association, nicotine and other tobacco ingredients speed up the process by which the body uses and eliminates drugs, so they may not be able to do what they're intended to do. As a result, smokers may have to take a medication more frequently than do nonsmokers. If you smoke, let your physician know so that he or she can adjust any prescriptions, if necessary.

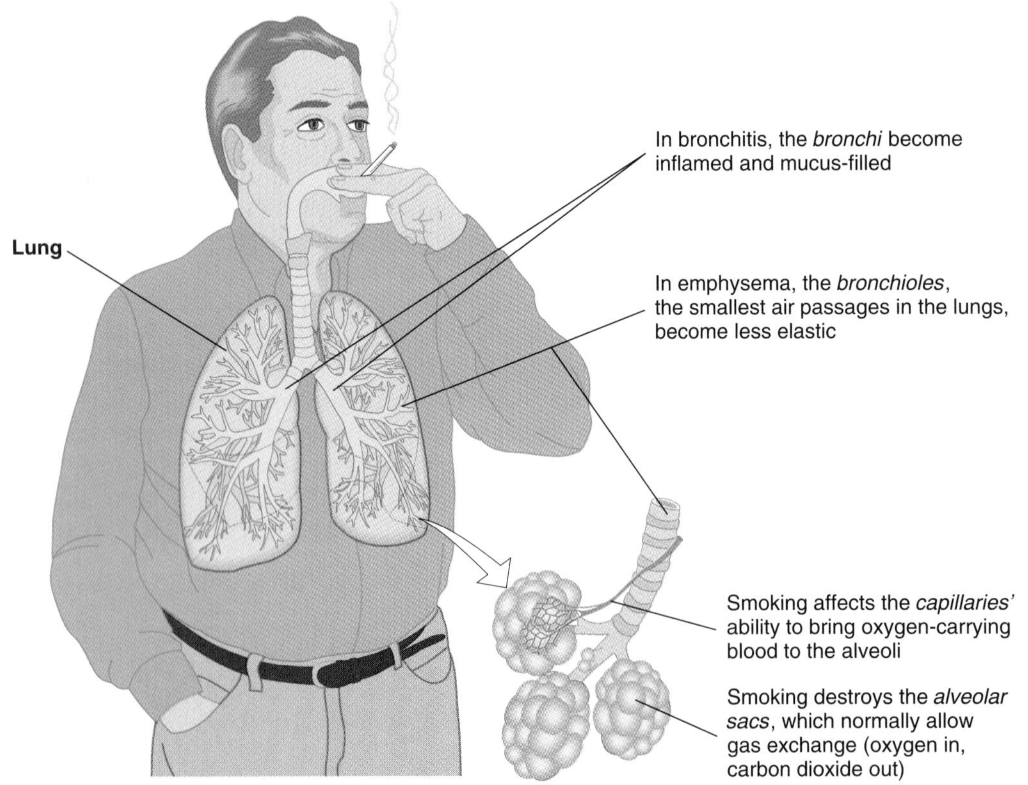

Lung

In bronchitis, the *bronchi* become inflamed and mucus-filled

In emphysema, the *bronchioles*, the smallest air passages in the lungs, become less elastic

Smoking affects the *capillaries'* ability to bring oxygen-carrying blood to the alveoli

Smoking destroys the *alveolar sacs*, which normally allow gas exchange (oxygen in, carbon dioxide out)

■ Figure 17-3 How smoking affects the lungs.

Among the drugs affected by smoking are antianxiety drugs (including Valium), painkillers (including Darvon), tricyclic antidepressants (including Elavil), anti-blood-clotting medications (such as heparin), antiasthmatic drugs (including theophylline), and the cardiovascular drugs known as beta blockers (such as propranolol).

The Financial Cost of Smoking

The total costs of cigarette smoking to American society include greater work absenteeism, higher insurance premiums, disability payments, and training costs to replace employees who die prematurely from smoking. In the course of a lifetime, the average smoker can expect to spend $10,000 to $20,000 on cigarettes—but that's only the beginning. The potential costs for medical services for a man between the ages of 35 and 39 who smokes heavily may be as high as $60,000. But the greatest toll—the pain and suffering of cancer victims and their loved ones—obviously cannot be measured in dollars and cents.

Smoking in America

Tobacco use remains the most serious and widespread addictive behavior in the world and the major cause of preventable deaths in our society. Although smoking by adults has declined, many young teenagers—particularly white girls—are smoking as much or more than they were ten years ago.

Strategies *for* Prevention

Why Not to Light Up

Before you start smoking—before you ever face the challenge of quitting—think of what you have to gain by *not* smoking:

✔ A significantly reduced risk of cancer of the larynx, mouth, esophagus, pancreas, and bladder.

✔ Half the risk of heart disease that smokers face.

✔ A lower risk of stroke, chronic obstructive lung disease (COLD), influenza, ulcers, and pneumonia.

✔ A lower risk of having a low-birth-weight baby.

✔ A longer life span.

✔ Potential savings of tens of thousands of dollars that you would otherwise spend on tobacco products and medical care.

Starting Early

Every day nearly 3,000 young people under the age of 18 become regular smokers.[8] More than 5 million children will die prematurely because they decide to start smoking. Eight percent of adults who currently smoke began to do so before the age of 18, at an average age of 12.5 years, and most were regular smokers by the age of 14. Among high school smokers who thought they wouldn't be smoking in five years, 73 percent still are.[9]

The earlier that smokers light up, the greater the dangers they face. Recent studies suggest that smoking in adolescence may trigger changes in DNA that put young people at higher risk for cancer even if they later quit. In studies of lung cancer patients, those with the worst genetic damage were not those who'd smoked the longest but those who started the youngest. And the earlier they started, the more severe the damage.[10]

Unfortunately, American children are starting to smoke at earlier ages. In 1999, the National Parents' Resource Institute for Drug Education reported that 4 percent of fourth graders, 7 percent of fifth graders, and nearly 15 percent of sixth graders had already smoked. More than three million teenagers are estimated to be smokers.[11]

It is no coincidence that so many people start to smoke early in life. The tobacco industry has deliberately targeted young teenagers by many means, including advertising in magazines with large youth readerships. Researchers estimate that the tobacco industry's promotional activities in the late 1990s will influence 17 percent of those who turn 17 years old each year to experiment with cigarettes.[12]

As Campus Focus: "Smoking by College Students" shows, most college students have tried cigarettes, and about one in five have smoked regularly.[13]

Smoking and Minorities

Cigarette smoking is a major cause of disease and death in all population groups. However, tobacco use varies within and among racial/ethnic minority groups. Among adults, American Indians and Alaska Natives have the highest rates of tobacco use. Nearly 40 percent of American Indian and Alaska Native adults smoke cigarettes, compared with 25 percent of adults in the overall U. S. population. They are more likely than any other racial/ethnic minority group to smoke tobacco or use smokeless tobacco. African-American and Southeast Asian men also have a high prevalence of smoking. Asian-American and Hispanic women have the lowest rates of smoking.[14]

Among adolescents, cigarette smoking prevalence increased in the 1990s among African Americans and

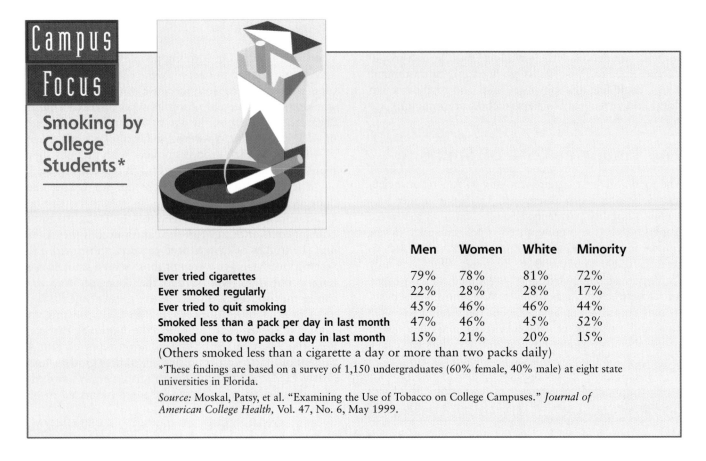

Campus Focus

Smoking by College Students*

	Men	Women	White	Minority
Ever tried cigarettes	79%	78%	81%	72%
Ever smoked regularly	22%	28%	28%	17%
Ever tried to quit smoking	45%	46%	46%	44%
Smoked less than a pack per day in last month	47%	46%	45%	52%
Smoked one to two packs a day in last month	15%	21%	20%	15%

(Others smoked less than a cigarette a day or more than two packs daily)

*These findings are based on a survey of 1,150 undergraduates (60% female, 40% male) at eight state universities in Florida.

Source: Moskal, Patsy, et al. "Examining the Use of Tobacco on College Campuses." *Journal of American College Health,* Vol. 47, No. 6, May 1999.

Hispanics after several years of substantial decline in all racial/ethnic minority groups. This increase was particularly striking among African American youths, who had shown the greatest decline of all minority groups during the 1970s and 1980s.

Tobacco has taken the greatest toll on the health of African Americans. Middle-aged and older African Americans are far more likely than their counterparts in other major racial/ethnic minority groups to die from coronary heart disease, stroke, or lung cancer. In the 1970s and 1980s, death rates from respiratory cancers (mainly lung cancer) increased among both African-American men and women. In the first half of the 1990s, these rates declined substantially among African-American men and leveled off in African-American women.

After increasing in the 1970s and 1980s, death rates from respiratory cancers decreased slightly among Hispanic men and women in the 1990s. In general, smoking rates among Mexican-American adults increase as they adopt the values, beliefs, and norms of American culture. Recent declines in the prevalence of smoking have been greater among Hispanic men with at least a high school education than among those with less education.

According to the U. S. Surgeon General, "adverse infant health outcomes," such as low-birth-weight babies, SIDS, and infant mortality, are especially high for African Americans, American Indians, and Alaska Natives who smoke. Cigarette smoking also increases these risks, especially for SIDS, among Asian Americans and Pacific Islanders and among Hispanics.

Smoking and Women

The World Health Organization (WHO) reports that 20 to 30 percent of women in wealthy nations smoke, compared with 2 to 10 percent of women in the developing nations. In the United States, 23 percent of women smoke, and more young women than men are starting the habit. This is a troubling trend because, once women start, they often find it difficult to quit, in part because they fear gaining weight.[15]

As noted in The X & Y Files: "Men, Women, and Tobacco," lung cancer now claims more women's lives than breast cancer. The risk of heart attack in women who smoke 25 or more cigarettes a day is more than 500 percent greater than the risk in women who don't smoke. Even smoking just one to four cigarettes a day doubles the risk. Women who smoke low nicotine cigarettes are four times more likely to have a first heart attack than women who don't smoke—the same risk as for those who smoke high-nicotine cigarettes.

Smoking directly affects women's reproductive organs and processes. Women who smoke are less fer-

The X&Y Files

Men, Women and Tobacco

For decades the rugged Marlboro man projected the popular image of smoking as a manly activity. Far more men than women smoked any form of tobacco—from cigarettes to pipes to cigars. In 1955, 57 percent of men smoked cigarettes, compared with 28 percent of women. By the 1960s the prevalence of smoking among men began to decrease, while more women started lighting up. In 1965, 52 percent of men and 34 percent of women smoked. From the 1960s to the 1980s the prevalence of smoking declined in both sexes, but more so among men than women. Since 1983, however, the decline has been comparable for both sexes.

According to the CDC, 28 percent of men and 22 percent of women in the United States smoke. However, the ways in which they use tobacco and the risks they face are not the same. Here are some key differences:

- **Types of tobacco.** Far more men than women smoke cigars or pipes or use any form of smokeless tobacco. As noted in this chapter, these forms of tobacco greatly increase their health risks. Women, especially African-American women, favor menthol cigarettes. Since smokers of these cigarettes tend to inhale more deeply with each drag, they potentially take in more nicotine than smokers of non-menthol cigarettes.

- **Lung cancer.** As male smoking has declined, so have lung cancer rates and deaths in men. The opposite has occurred with women. In the last 30 years, the lung cancer death rate among women has increased by more than 400 percent. An estimated 62,000 women die each year from lung cancer, which has surpassed breast cancer as the leading cause of cancer deaths among women.

- **Heart Disease.** Both men and women who smoke greatly increase their risk of heart attack and stroke. As discussed in Chapter 13, men tend to develop heart disease about a decade earlier than women. However, smoking cigarettes dramatically increases the risk of heart disease among premenopausal women who are also taking birth control pills.

- **Reproductive Health.** Smoking has been implicated as a culprit in male impotence. For women, smoking is associated with complications of pregnancy, early menopause, and reduced fertility. An estimated 18 to 20 percent of pregnant women smoke throughout their pregnancies. They face an increased risk of miscarriage, stillbirth, preterm delivery, and infant death. Their babies are more likely to have a low birth weight; their children have higher rates of asthma, ear infections, and violent behavior.

Sources: CDC's TIPS (Tobacco Information and Prevention Source). CDC. "Women Who Smoke Fact Sheet," 1999. Ward, Darrell. "Women Smoking Menthol Cigarettes Have Greater Nicotine Exposure." Ohio State University, March 31, 1999.

tile and experience menopause one or two years earlier than women who don't smoke. Smoking also boosts a woman's likelihood of developing cervical cancer and greatly increases the possible risks associated with taking oral contraceptives. Older women who smoke are weaker, have poorer balance, and are at greater risk of physical disability than nonsmokers.

Women who smoke also are more likely to develop osteoporosis, a bone-weakening disease. They tend to be thin, which is a risk factor for osteoporosis, and they enter menopause earlier, thus extending the period of jeopardy from estrogen loss.

Women who smoke during pregnancy increase their risk of miscarriage and pregnancy complications, including bleeding, premature delivery, and birth defects such as cleft lip or palate. Women who smoke are twice as likely to have an ectopic pregnancy (in which a fertilized egg develops in the fallopian tube rather than in the uterus) and to have babies of low birth weight as those who have never smoked. However, women who stop smoking before pregnancy reduce their risk of having a low-birth-weight baby to that of women who don't smoke. Even those who quit three or four months into the pregnancy have babies with higher birth weights than those who continue smoking throughout pregnancy. (See Chapter 10 for more information on the health risks associated with smoking during pregnancy.)

Why Do People Smoke?

Most Americans are aware that there is a health risk associated with smoking, but many don't know exactly what that risk is or how it might affect them. Other factors associated with the reasons for smoking are discussed in the following sections.

The two main factors linked with the onset of a smoking habit are age and education. The vast majority of white men (93 percent) with less than a high school education are current or former daily cigarette smokers. White women with similar educational backgrounds are also very likely to smoke or to have smoked every day. Latino men and women without a high school education are less likely to be or become daily smokers.

Heredity

Researchers speculate that genes may account for about 50 percent of smoking behavior, with environment playing an equally important role. Studies have shown that identical twins, who have the same genes, are more likely to have matching smoking profiles than fraternal twins. If one identical twin is a heavy smoker, the other is also likely to be; if one smokes only occasionally, so does the other.

Parental Role Models

Children who start smoking are 50 percent more likely than youngsters who don't smoke to have at least one smoker in their families. A mother who smokes seems a particularly strong influence on making smoking seem acceptable. The majority of youngsters who smoke say that their parents also smoke and are aware of their own tobacco use.

Adolescent Experimentation and Rebellion

Young people who are trying out various behaviors may take up smoking because they're curious or because they want to defy adults. Others simply want to appear grownup or cool. Increases in teen smoking are not inevitable, however. After a one-year anti-tobacco campaign in Florida, officials recorded the steepest drop in teen smoking in nearly two decades. Between 1998 and 1999, the number of middle school students who said they had smoked cigarettes in the past month dropped about 19 percent—from 18.5 percent of children smoking to 15 percent. Cigarette smoking among high school students fell about 8 percent, from 27.4 percent to 25.2 percent.[16]

In other research conducted by the CDC, about seven out of 10 high school students said they wanted to stop smoking, but only a small percentage were successful.

Teens often misjudge the addictive power of cigarettes. Many, sure that they'll be able to quit any time they want, figure that smoking for a year or two won't hurt them. But when they try to quit, they can't. Like older smokers, most young people who smoke have tried to quit at least once. The American Cancer Society has found that young smokers tend to become heavy smokers and that the longer anyone is exposed to smoke, the greater the health dangers.

Limited Education

People who have graduated from college are much less likely to smoke than are high school graduates; those with fewer than 12 years of education are most likely to smoke. An individual with 8 years or less of education is 11 times more likely to smoke than someone with postgraduate training.

Weight Control

Smokers burn up an extra 100 calories a day compared with nonsmokers—the equivalent of walking a mile—probably because nicotine increases metabolic rate. Once they start smoking, many individuals say they cannot quit because they fear they'll gain weight. The CDC estimates that women who stop smoking gain an average of eight pounds, while men put on an average of six pounds. One in eight women and one in ten men who stop smoking put on 29 pounds or more. The reasons for this weight gain include nicotine's effects on metabolism as well as emotional and behavioral factors, such as the habit of frequently putting something into one's mouth. Yet as a health risk, smoking a pack and a half to two packs a day is a greater danger than carrying 60 pounds in extra weight.

Weight gain for smokers who quit is not inevitable, however. Aerobic exercise helps increase metabolic rate; and limiting alcohol and foods high in sugar and fat can help smokers control their weight as they give up cigarettes.

Aggressive Marketing

Cigarette companies spend billions each year on advertisements and promotional campaigns, with manufacturers targeting ads especially at women, teens, minorities, and the poor. Most controversial are cigarette advertisements in magazines and media aimed at teenagers and even younger children. As part of a nationwide antismoking campaign, health and government officials have called for restrictions on cigarette ads, and manufacturers have agreed not to aim their sales efforts at children and teens.

Stress

In studies that have analyzed the impact of life stressors, depression, emotional support, marital status, and income, researchers have concluded that an individual with a high stress level is approximately 15 times as likely to be a smoker than a person with low stress. About half of smokers identify workplace stress as a key factor in their smoking behavior.

Why People Keep Smoking

Whatever the reasons for lighting up that first cigarette, very different factors keep cigarettes burning pack after pack, year after year. In national polls, four out of five smokers say that they want to quit but can't. The reason isn't a lack of willpower. Medical scientists have recognized tobacco dependence as an addictive disorder that may be more powerful than heroin dependence and that may affect more than 90 percent of all smokers.

Pleasure

According to the American Cancer Society, 87.5 percent of regular smokers find smoking pleasurable. Nicotine—the addictive ingredient in tobacco—is the reason. Researchers have shown that nicotine reinforces and strengthens the desire to smoke by acting on brain chemicals that influence feelings of well-being. This drug also can improve memory, help in performing certain tasks, reduce anxiety, dampen hunger, and increase pain tolerance.

Relief of Depression

Some people with depression use the mood-altering properties of nicotine to relieve depressive symptoms. People with a history of depression are significantly more likely to be smokers and to be diagnosed as nicotine-dependent. Smokers are more likely than nonsmokers to report depressive symptoms—and these symptoms may interfere with quitting. According to researchers, the likelihood of quitting smoking is about 40 percent lower among depressed than nondepressed smokers.

Dependence

Nicotine has a much more powerful hold on smokers than alcohol does on drinkers. Whereas about 10 percent of alcohol users lose control of their intake of alcohol and become alcoholics, as many as 80 percent of all heavy smokers have tried to cut down on or quit smoking but cannot overcome their dependence.

Nicotine causes dependence by at least three means:

- It provides a strong sensation of pleasure.
- It leads to fairly severe discomfort during withdrawal.

- It stimulates cravings long after obvious withdrawal symptoms have passed.

Few drugs act as quickly on the brain as nicotine does. It travels through the bloodstream to the brain in seven seconds—half the time it takes for heroin injected into a blood vessel to reach the brain. And a pack-a-day smoker gets 200 hits of nicotine a day—73,000 a year.

After a few years of smoking, the most powerful incentive for continuing to smoke is to avoid the discomfort of withdrawal. Generally, ten cigarettes a day will prevent withdrawal effects. For many who smoke heavily, signs of withdrawal, including changes in mood and performance, occur within two hours after smoking their last cigarette. Smokeless tobacco users also get constant doses of nicotine. However, absorption of nicotine by the lungs is more likely to lead to dependence than absorption through the linings of the nose and mouth. As with other drugs of abuse, continued nicotine intake results in tolerance (the need for more of a drug to maintain the same effect), which is why only 2 percent of all smokers smoke just a few cigarettes a day, or smoke only occasionally.

Use of Other Substances

Many smokers also drink or use drugs. According to the Addiction Research Foundation in Canada, tobacco smokers say cigarettes are harder to abandon than other drugs, even when they find them less pleasurable than their preferred drug of abuse. Individuals who drink excessively also find their cigarette habit a hard one to break.

Other Forms of Tobacco

Other ways of ingesting tobacco may be less deadly than smoking cigarettes, but all are dangerous. Smoking clove cigarettes, cigars, and pipes, and chewing or sucking on smokeless tobacco all put the user at risk of cancer of the lip, tongue, mouth, and throat—as well as other diseases and ailments.

 ### Are Clove Cigarettes Safer Than "Regular" Ones?

Sweeteners have long been mixed into tobacco, and clove, a spice, is the latest ingredient to be added to the recipe for cigarettes. Clove cigarettes typically contain two-thirds tobacco and one-third cloves. Consumers of these cigarettes are primarily teenagers and young adults.

Many users believe that clove cigarettes are safer than regular ones because they contain less tobacco, but this isn't necessarily the case. The CDC reports that people who smoke clove-containing cigarettes may be at risk of serious lung injury. Smoking clove cigarettes during a mild upper respiratory tract illness can lead to severe breathing difficulty. And clove cigarette smokers, like other cigarette smokers, can become addicted to the tobacco.

Clove cigarettes may actually be more harmful than conventional cigarettes. Puff for puff, they deliver twice as much nicotine, tar, and carbon monoxide as moderate-tar American brands. Moreover, eugenol, the active ingredient in cloves (which dentists have used as an anesthetic for years), deadens sensation in the throat, allowing smokers to inhale more deeply and hold smoke in their lungs for a longer time. Close chemical relatives of eugenol can produce the kind of damage to cells that may eventually lead to cancer.

 ## What Are Bidis?

Skinny, sweet-flavored cigarettes called **bidis** (pronounced "beedees") have become a smoking fad among teens and young adults. For centuries, bidis were popular in India, where they are known as the "poor man's cigarette" and sell for less than five cents a pack. Although they look strikingly like clove cigarettes or marijuana joints, bidis, available in flavors like grape, strawberry, and mandarin orange, are legal for adults and even minors in some states and are sold on the Internet as well as in stores. In one survey, 58 percent of high school students in San Francisco had tried bidis, and 31 percent smoke them at least once a month.[17] In another survey in inner city Boston, 40 percent of teens had tried a bidi, while nearly 16 percent currently smoked them, and nearly 8 percent said they were "heavy users" who had smoked more than 100.[18]

Although bidis contain less tobacco than regular cigarettes, their unprocessed tobacco is more potent. Smoke from bidis has about three times as much nicotine and carbon monoxide and five times as much tar as smoke from regular filtered cigarettes. Because bidis are wrapped in nonporous brownish leafs, they don't burn as easily as cigarettes, and smokers have to inhale harder and more often to keep them lit. In one study, smoking a single bidi required 28 puffs, compared to nine puffs for cigarettes.

Health authorities view bidis as "cigarettes with training wheels"—products that could lead to a lifetime of nicotine addiction because they are easy to buy and lack the health-warning labels required of cigarettes. Unlike regular cigarettes, which are smoked mostly by white youths, bidis also are popular among young Hispanics and blacks.[19]

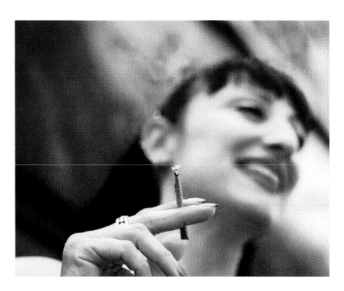

The smoke produced by bidis—skinny, flavored cigarettes—can contain higher concentrations of toxic chemicals than that in regular cigarettes.

Cigars

Cigar-smoking has become a widespread fad, particularly among men. Total cigar consumption in the United States totals approximately 4.5 billion cigars, and consumption of larger cigars increased by 50 percent from 1993 to 1997.[20] Although this trend may have started among adult men, it has spread to adolescents. In various state surveys, approximately 27 to 28 percent of high school students reported having smoked at least one cigar in the previous 30 days.[21] A national survey of high schoolers found that approximately 6 million students had smoked a cigar in the previous year. Although federal and state laws prohibit sale of cigars and other tobacco products to minors, many young people, including ninth graders, reported no difficulty in making such purchases.

Many cigar smokers of all ages assume that because they do not inhale the smoke, they are not at risk for heart disease or lung cancer. This is not the case. Recent research has found that cigar smoking boosts the risk of heart disease and of lung cancer. In an analysis of the medical records of 16,228 men who had never smoked cigarettes or cigars and another 1,546 who smoked only cigars, researchers found that, after adjusting for age and other risk factors, there was a direct link between sickness and the number of cigars smoked. Patients who smoked fewer than five cigars a day had a 34 percent greater risk of throat and oral cancers and a 57 percent greater risk of lung cancer than nonsmokers. Those who smoked five or more cigars a day had a 620 percent greater risk of throat and oral cancers and a 220 percent greater risk of lung cancer than nonsmokers. Those who did not inhale had lower rates of disease—though they were still significantly higher than those of nonsmokers. (See Figure 17-4.) Drinking three or more alcoholic drinks a day further raised their risk.[22]

Pipes

Many cigarette smokers switch to pipes to reduce their risk of health problems. But former cigarette smokers may continue to inhale, even though pipe smoke is more irritating to the respiratory system than cigarette smoke. People who have only smoked pipes and who do not inhale are much less likely to develop lung and heart disease than are cigarette smokers. However, they are as likely as cigarette smokers to develop—and die of—cancer of the mouth, larynx, throat, and esophagus.

Smokeless Tobacco

Other tobacco products may be taking the place of cigarettes in the mouths of Americans. The sale and consumption of smokeless tobacco products are rising, particularly among young males. These substances include snuff, finely ground tobacco that can be sniffed or placed inside the cheek and sucked, and chewing tobacco, which consists of tobacco leaves mixed with flavoring agents such as molasses. With both, nicotine is absorbed through the mucous membranes of the nose or mouth.

Although not as deadly as cigarette smoking, the use of smokeless tobacco is dangerous. It can cause cancer and noncancerous oral conditions and lead to nicotine addiction and dependence. Smokeless tobacco users are more likely than nonusers to become cigarette

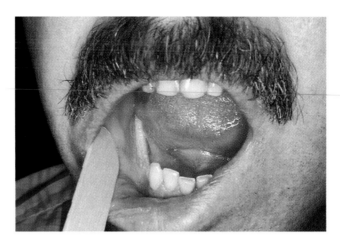

Chewing smokeless tobacco can damage the tissues of the mouth. In addition to causing oral cancer, the use of smokeless tobacco can lead to cancer of the larynx, esophagus, kidney, pancreas, and bladder.

smokers. Powerful carcinogens in smokeless tobacco include nitrosamines, polycyclic aromatic hydrocarbons, and radiation-emitting polonium. Its use can lead to the development of white patches on the mucous membranes of the mouth, particularly on the site where the tobacco is placed. Most lesions of the mouth lining that result from the use of smokeless tobacco dissipate six weeks after the use of tobacco products is stopped, according to a U. S. Air Force study. However, when first found, about 5 percent of leukoplakias are cancerous or exhibit changes that progress to cancer within ten years if not properly treated.[23] Cancers of the lip, pharynx, larynx, and esophagus have all been linked to smokeless tobacco.

An estimated 7 to 22 million people, many of them young, use snuff and chewing tobacco. In a national survey of 5,894 men and women from 72 colleges and universities, 22 percent of college men and 2 percent of college women used smokeless tobacco. The lowest percentage was in the Northeast, the highest, in the Southcentral region. In different regions, 8 to 36 percent of male high school students are regular users. Many are emulating professional baseball players who keep wads of tobacco jammed in their cheeks. Even when they spot lesions in their mouths, most do not seek medical help but continue to use smokeless tobacco.

In recent years, there has been a decline in chewing tobacco, but an increase in the use of moist snuff, a product that is higher in nicotine and potential cancer-causing chemicals. The use of snuff increases the likelihood of oral cancer by more than four times. Other effects include bad breath, discolored or missing teeth, cavities, gum disease, and nicotine addiction. In a study by the Oregon Research Institute, dental patients were three times more likely to quit snuff and chewing

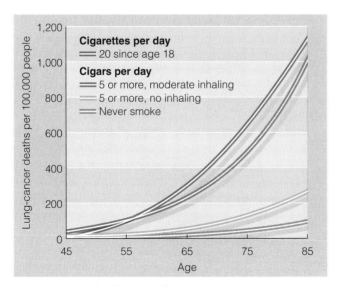

■ **Figure 17-4** The dangers of cigarettes versus cigars.

Sources: American Cancer Society, National Cancer Institute.

tobacco after hygienists taught them that smokeless tobacco was responsible for their mouth sores, bleeding gums, and receding gums.[24]

Environmental Tobacco Smoke

Maybe you don't smoke—never have, never will. That doesn't mean you don't have to worry about the dangers of smoking, especially if you live or work with people who smoke. **Environmental tobacco smoke,** or secondhand cigarette smoke, the most hazardous form of indoor air pollution, ranks behind cigarette smoking and alcohol as the third-leading preventable cause of death.

Mainstream and Sidestream Smoke

On the average, a smoker inhales what is known as **mainstream smoke** eight or nine times with each cigarette, for a total of about 24 seconds. However, the cigarette burns for about 12 minutes, and everyone in the room (including the smoker) breathes in what is known as **sidestream smoke.**

According to the American Lung Association, incomplete combustion from the lower temperatures of a smoldering cigarette makes sidestream smoke dirtier and chemically different from mainstream smoke. It has twice as much tar and nicotine, five times as much carbon monoxide, and 50 times as much ammonia. And because the particles in sidestream smoke are small, this

mixture of irritating gases and carcinogenic tar reaches deeper into the lungs. If you're a nonsmoker sitting next to someone smoking seven cigarettes an hour, even in a ventilated room, you'll take in almost twice the maximum amount of carbon monoxide set for air pollution in industry—and it will take hours for the carbon monoxide to leave your body.

What Are the Risks of Secondhand Smoke?

New research indicates that environmental tobacco smoke is even more dangerous than previously thought. According to the Centers for Disease Control and Prevention (CDC), every year environmental tobacco smoke causes 3,000 deaths from lung cancer. In a Harvard University study that tracked 10,000 healthy women who never smoked over ten years, regular exposure to other people's smoke at home or work almost doubled the risk of heart disease. On the basis of their findings, the researchers estimated that up to 50,000 Americans may die of heart attacks from environmental tobacco smoke every year, while 3,000 to 4,000 die of other forms of heart disease. As a cancer-causing agent, secondhand smoke may be twice as dangerous as radon gas and more than a hundred times more hazardous than outdoor pollutants regulated by federal law.

Families of Smokers: Living Dangerously

The most vulnerable nonsmokers are the spouses and children of smokers. Numerous epidemiological and

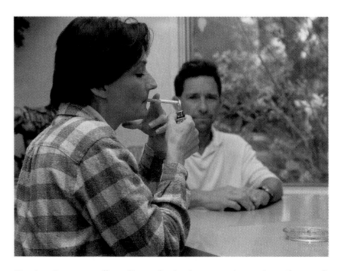

Passive (or secondhand) smoke is the most hazardous form of indoor air pollution.

autopsy studies have linked environmental tobacco smoke with lung cancer and other disorders. The nonsmoking spouses of smokers, for instance, are 30 percent more likely to die of heart disease than other nonsmokers.

Environmental tobacco smoke also poses great danger to young children. Those who breathe environmental tobacco smoke suffer from more asthma, wheezing, and bronchitis than children in smoke-free homes. Children regularly exposed to tobacco smoke also face increased risk of lung cancer, heart disease, and stroke.

Infants of parents who smoke are hospitalized for bronchitis and pneumonia more often than are youngsters in nonsmoking households. In addition, environmental tobacco smoke may increase the risk of sudden infant death syndrome (SIDS). Infants who died of SIDS were more likely to have been exposed to environmental tobacco smoke from their mothers, fathers, or care-providers. They also have more ear infections and asthma.[25]

Smoking during pregnancy has been associated with various behavioral and attention problems in childhood, including attention deficit-hyperactivity disorder and substance abuse. Researchers also have found an unexpected—and still unexplained—correlation between mothers who smoked during pregnancy and criminal violence in their sons. In a study of 4,000 Danish women, those who smoked a pack or more a day while pregnant were twice as likely to have boys who became violent. Some theorize that chemicals in smoke may somehow damage the developing brain.[26]

The negative effects of childhood exposure to environmental tobacco smoke persist even after youngsters leave home. In recent research at Ohio State University, college students who grew up in a smoking household had higher blood pressure and resting heart rates at rest and during psychological stress than those who grew up in smoke-free homes.[27]

The Politics of Tobacco

More than three decades after government health authorities began to warn of the dangers of cigarette smoking, tobacco remains a politically hot topic. After many years of difficult negotiations, the tobacco industry and attorneys general from nearly 40 states have reached a historic settlement. Major tobacco countries agreed to pay more than $200 billion to settle smoking-related lawsuits filed by states, to finance antismoking campaigns, to restrict marketing, to permit federal regulation of tobacco, and to pay fines if tobacco use by minors does not decline. In return, the industry would be protected against most tobacco-related lawsuits and the awarding of punitive damages.[28]

In the course of congressional hearings on this settlement, investigators discovered documents indicating that tobacco manufactures had been aware of nicotine's addictive potential and had deliberately directed advertising campaigns at adolescents and at African Americans, particularly those in inner cities.

Other groups are fighting smoking on different fronts. The federal government has launched a seven-year grass-roots antismoking coalition called Americans Stop Smoking Intervention Study (ASSIST) to combat cigarette smoking. Community leaders in some neighborhoods have whitewashed billboard ads for cigarettes. Some civic and consumer associations have proposed boycotting athletic events sponsored by tobacco companies. In some states, tough antismoking campaigns, financed by taxes on cigarettes, have led to impressive declines in cigarette sales.

The Fight for Clean Air

Nonsmokers, realizing that their health is being jeopardized by environmental tobacco smoke, have increasingly turned to legislative and administrative measures to clear the air and protect their rights. (See Figure 17-5.) Thousands of cities, towns, and counties now restrict smoking in public places or regulate the sale of tobacco to minors. Nationally, the airlines have banned smoking on domestic flights. Many institutions, including medical centers and some universities, no longer allow smoking on their premises. Some cities restrict smoking in bars, restaurants, and other public places.

Supporters of smoking restrictions argue that no one should be subjected involuntarily to the dangers of environmental tobacco smoke. They point out that other people's smoke can cause headaches or hoarseness, and may pose more serious health hazards. In addition, smokers jeopardize nonsmokers by increasing the danger of fire.

Opponents of smoking restrictions contend that banning smoking on the job might impair rather than enhance productivity, because employees would take more frequent breaks to go to lounges where smoking is permitted—or else would suffer the negative effects of nicotine withdrawal.

Quitting

Tobacco dependence may be the toughest addiction to overcome. One-third of smokers try to quit annually, but fewer than 10 percent succeed. Most people who eventually quit on their own have already tried other methods. Nicotine withdrawal symptoms can behave

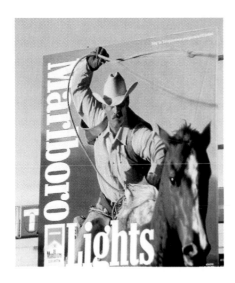
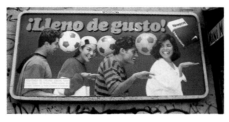
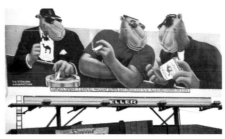

Tobacco advertising is aggressive, but tough antismoking campaigns have led to declines in cigarette sales.

like characters in a bad horror flick: Just when you think you've killed them, they're back with a vengeance. In recent studies, some people who tried to quit smoking reported a small improvement in withdrawal symptoms over two weeks, but then their symptoms leveled off and persisted. Others found that their symptoms intensified rather than lessened over time.[29]

According to therapists, quitting usually isn't a one-time event but a "dynamic process" that may take several years and four to ten attempts. The good news is that half of all living Americans who ever smoked have managed to quit. And thanks to new products and programs, it may be easier now than ever before to become an ex-smoker.

Quitting on Your Own

More than 90 percent of former smokers quit on their own—by throwing away all their cigarettes, by gradually cutting down, or by first switching to a less potent brand. One characteristic of successful quitters is that they see themselves as active participants in health maintenance and take personal responsibility for their own health. Often they experiment with a variety of strategies, such as learning relaxation techniques. In women, exercise has proven especially effective for quitting and avoiding weight gain.[30] Making a home a "smoke-free" zone also increases a smoker's likelihood of successful quitting.[31] (See Pulsepoints: "Ten Ways to

■ **Figure 17-5** Nonsmoker's bill of rights.

Nonsmoker's Bill of Rights

Nonsmokers Help Protect the Health, Comfort, and Safety of Everyone by Insisting on the Following Rights:

The Right to Breathe Clean Air
Nonsmokers have the right to breathe clean air, free from harmful and irritating tobacco smoke. This right supersedes the right to smoke when the two conflict.

The Right to Speak Out
Nonsmokers have the right to express — firmly but politely — their discomfort and adverse reactions to tobacco smoke. They have the right to voice their objections when smokers light up without asking permission.

The Right to Act
Nonsmokers have the right to take action through legislative means — as individuals or in groups — to prevent or discourage smokers from polluting the atmosphere and to seek the restriction of smoking in public places.

Consumer Health Watch

How Nonsmokers Can Clear the Air

- Let people know your feelings in advance by putting up "No Smoking" signs in your office, home, or car. If you're in a car and someone pulls out a cigarette, ask politely if the smoker can hold off until you reach your destination or stop for a break.
- When giving a party, designate a smoking room. Suggest that friends do the same for parties at their houses.
- If you're about to participate in a long meeting or class, suggest regular smoking breaks to avoid a smoke-filled room.

- At restaurants, always ask for a table in the nonsmoking section or, if there is none, one in a well-ventilated part of the restaurant.
- If someone's smoke is bothering you, speak up. Be polite, not pushy. Say something like, "Excuse me, but smoke bothers me."

Kick the Habit" for tips on how to smoke less—and less dangerously.)

Stop-Smoking Groups

Joining a support group doubles your chances of quitting for good. The American Cancer Society's FreshStart Program runs about 1,500 stop-smoking clinics, each with about 8 to 18 members meeting for eight 2-hour sessions over four weeks. Instructors explain the risks of smoking, encourage individuals to think about why they smoke, and suggest ways of unlearning their smoking habit. A quitting day is set for the third or fourth session.

The American Lung Association's Freedom from Smoking Program consists of eight 1- to 2-hour sessions over seven weeks. The approach is similar to the American Cancer Society's, but smokers keep diaries and team up with buddies. Ex-smokers serve as advisers on quitting day. Both groups estimate that 27 or 28 percent of their participants successfully stop smoking.

PULSE points

Ten Ways to Kick the Habit

1. **Use delaying tactics.** Have your first cigarette of the day 15 minutes later than usual, then 15 minutes later than that the next day, and so on.
2. **Distract yourself.** When you feel a craving for a cigarette, talk to someone, drink a glass of water, or get up and move around.
3. **Establish nonsmoking hours.** Instead of lighting up at the end of a meal, for instance, get up immediately, brush your teeth, wash your hands, or take a walk.
4. **Never smoke two packs of the same brand in a row.** Buy cigarettes only by the pack, not by the carton.

5. **Make it harder to get to your cigarettes.** Lock them in a drawer, wrap them in paper, or leave them in your coat or car.
6. **Change the way you smoke.** Smoke with the hand you don't usually use. Smoke only half of each cigarette.
7. **Keep daily records.** Chart your daily cigarette tally to see what progress you're making.
8. **Stop completely for just one day at a time.** Promise yourself 24 hours of freedom from cigarettes; when the day's over, make the same commitment for one more day. At the end of any 24-hour period, you can go back to smoking and not feel guilty.

9. **Spend more time in places where you can't smoke.** Take up bike-riding or swimming. Shower often. Go to movies or other places where smoking isn't allowed.
10. **Go cold turkey.** If you're a heavily addicted smoker, try a decisive and complete break. Smokers who quit completely are less likely to light up again than those who gradually decrease their daily cigarette consumption, switch to low-tar and low-nicotine brands, or use special filters and holders.

Stop-smoking classes are also available through health-science departments and student-heath services on many college campuses, as well as through community public health departments. The Seventh-Day Adventists sponsor a four-week Breathe Free Plan, in which smokers commit themselves to clean living (no smoking, alcohol, tea, or coffee, along with a balanced diet and regular exercise). Many businesses sponsor smoking-cessation programs for employees, which generally follow the approaches of professional groups. Motivation may be even higher in these programs than in programs outside the workplace, however, because some companies offer attractive incentives to participants, such as lower rates on their health insurance.

Some smoking-cessation programs rely primarily on **aversion therapy,** which provides a negative experience every time a smoker has a cigarette. This may involve taking drugs that make tobacco smoke taste unpleasant, undergoing electric shocks, having smoke blown at you, or rapid smoking (the inhaling of smoke every six seconds until you're dizzy or nauseated).

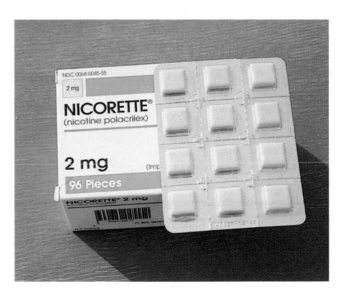

Nicorette gum, when chewed, gradually releases a nicotine resin and helps some smokers break their habit. Nicorette is now available without a prescription.

Nicotine Replacement Therapy

This approach uses a variety of products that supply low doses of nicotine in a way that allows smokers to taper off gradually over a period of months. They include nicotine gum (available in two doses) and slow-release skin patches. Although still experimental, a nasal spray also has shown promise.

In research studies, nicotine replacement is the only treatment for nicotine addiction that has proven clearly beneficial. When measured against a look-alike placebo treatment, nicotine gum and patches have doubled the initial quitting rate and the numbers of smokers who remain abstinent six months to one year later. However, even with these approaches, only about one smoker in four quits completely; about half of these remain abstinent over the long term.

Nicotine Gum

Nicotine gum, sold as Nicorette, contains a nicotine resin that's gradually released as the gum is chewed. Absorbed through the mucous membrane of the mouth, the nicotine doesn't produce the same rush as a deeply inhaled drag on a cigarette. However, the gum maintains enough nicotine in the blood to diminish withdrawal symptoms. A month's supply of Nicorette costs roughly $45.

Although this gum is lightly spiced to mask nicotine's bitterness, many users say that it takes several days to become accustomed to its unusual taste. Its side effects include mild indigestion, sore jaws, nausea,

heartburn, and stomachache. Also, because Nicorette is heavier than regular chewing gum, it may loosen fillings or cause problems with dentures. Drinking coffee or other beverages may block absorption of the nicotine in the gum; individuals trying to quit smoking shouldn't ingest any substance immediately before or while chewing nicotine gum.

Nicotine in any form is harmful, and nicotine gum should not be used during pregnancy or by people with heart disease. Most people use nicotine gum as a temporary crutch and gradually taper off it until they can stop chewing it relatively painlessly. However, 5 to 10 percent of users transfer their dependence from cigarettes to the gum. When they stop using Nicorette, they experience withdrawal symptoms, although the symptoms tend to be milder than those prompted by quitting cigarettes. Intensive counseling to teach smokers coping methods can greatly increase the success rates.

Nicotine Patches

Nicotine transdermal delivery system products, or patches, provide nicotine, their only active ingredient, via a patch attached to the skin by an adhesive. Like nicotine gum, the nicotine patch minimizes withdrawal symptoms, such as intense craving for cigarettes. Some insurance programs pay for patch therapy. Nicotine patches, which cost between $3.25 and $4 each, are replaced daily during therapy programs that run between 6 and 16 weeks. However, there is no evidence that continuing their use for more than eight weeks provides added benefit.

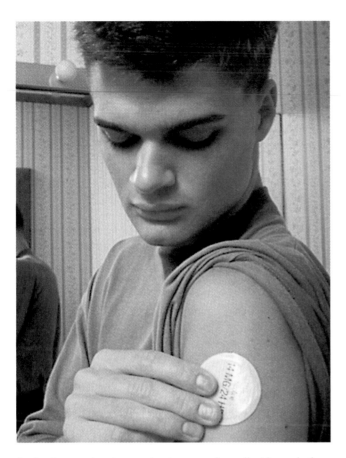

A nicotine patch releases nicotine transdermally (through the skin) in measured amounts, which are gradually decreased over time.

Some patches deliver nicotine around the clock and others for just 16 hours (during waking hours). Those most likely to benefit from nicotine patch therapy are people who smoke more than a pack a day, are highly motivated to quit, and participate in counseling programs. However, the nicotine patch is not a cure for a smoking habit. While using the patch, 37 to 77 percent of people are able to abstain from smoking. But the patch doesn't affect the psychological dependence that makes quitting smoking so hard. That's why the key to long-term success in quitting smoking is getting support. When combined with counseling, the patch can be about twice as effective as a placebo, enabling 26 percent of smokers to abstain for six months.

Because nicotine is a powerful, addictive substance, the use of nicotine patches for a prolonged period is not advised. Pregnant women and individuals with heart disease shouldn't use them. Patch wearers who smoke or use more than one patch at a time can experience a nicotine overdose; some users have even suffered heart attacks. Occasional side effects include redness, itching, or swelling at the site of the patch application; insomnia; dry mouth; and nervousness.

Bupropion (Zyban)

An alternative to the patch is **bupropion,** a drug initially developed to treat depression that is marketed in a slow-release form for nicotine addiction as Zyban. In studies that have combined Zyban with nicotine replacement and counseling, 40 to 60 percent of those treated have remained smoke-free for at least a year after completing the program.[32] This is much higher than the 10 to 26 percent success rates reported among smokers who try to quit using nicotine replacement alone. The combination of Zyban and nicotine replacement also prevented the initial weight gain that often accompanies quitting.[33]

Smoke-Free Days

Since 1976, a November day has been set aside in the United States for the annual Great American Smoke-Out, an idea promoted by the American Cancer Society to encourage smokers to give up cigarettes for 24 hours. As many as 36 percent of American smokers have given up cigarettes on Smoke-Out Day; about 5 to 6 percent have quit permanently; 15 percent reduced smoking for extended periods.[34] In addition, the World Health Organization has established World No-Tobacco Days in May to call on nations to urge tobacco users to abstain for at least one day and perhaps quit for good.

Other Ways to Quit

Hypnosis may help some people quit smoking. Hypnotherapists use their techniques to create an atmosphere of strict attention and give smokers in a mild trance positive suggestions for breaking their cigarette habit.

Acupuncture, in which a circular needle or staple is inserted in the flap in front of the opening to the ear, has also had some success. When smokers feel withdrawal symptoms, they gently move the needle or staple, which may increase the production of calming chemicals in the brain.

Making This Chapter Work for You

Clearing the Air

■ Many people have stopped smoking because of the health risks associated with tobacco use and because, as a social behavior, smoking has become unpopular. However, smoking is increasing among young white teens.

- Smokers may continue to smoke because they find smoking pleasurable or because the nicotine in cigarettes relieves feelings of depression. Most become dependent on nicotine, which is powerfully addictive. If they don't receive regular daily doses, smokers suffer withdrawal symptoms, such as irritability, anxiety, headache, and changes in performance.

- Nicotine affects mood, hunger, blood pressure, heart rate, and the performance of certain mental tasks. It also contributes to heart and respiratory diseases. The tar in cigarettes is carcinogenic and can damage the respiratory system.

- The incidence of heart attack and cardiomyopathy is high among smokers, possibly because of the effects of nicotine, which increases blood pressure and constricts blood vessels, and carbon monoxide, which diminishes oxygen received by the heart. In the United States, more people die of lung cancer, usually caused by smoking, than of any other type of cancer. Smoking also contributes to the development of other cancers, including cancer of the mouth and larynx, esophagus, bladder and kidney, and pancreas.

- Besides causing lung cancer, smoking can cause two types of chronic obstructive lung disease—emphysema and chronic bronchitis. Cigarette smoking is also associated with ulcers, liver disease, and gum disease and dental problems.

- Women who smoke face the additional risk of developing reproductive disorders such as cervical cancer. A pregnant woman who smokes has a high risk of miscarriage, ectopic pregnancy, or losing her baby shortly before, during, or after birth. Her baby may be born prematurely or underweight; with poor respiration, heart rate, muscle tone, or color; or with respiratory or heart disease.

health **/ ONLINE**

American Lung Association Tobacco Control
http://www.lungusa.org/tobacco/index.html
This site contains information about quitting smoking, smoking and pregnancy, tobacco control, smoking and targeted populations (minorities and teens), secondhand smoke, cigar smoking, and other tobacco topics.

CDC's TIPS: Tobacco Information and Prevention Source
http://www.cdc.gov/tobacco
Provides current tobacco-related news, Surgeon General's reports related to tobacco, tobacco research and data, guides on how to quit, educational materials, and other resources.

American Council on Science and Health: Tobacco
http://www.acsh.org/tobacco/index.html
Contains tobacco-related press releases, editorials, magazine articles, and additional links.

Please note that links are subject to change. If you find a broken link, use a search engine like http://www.yahoo.com *and search for the web site by typing in key words.*

 Campus Chat: Do actors and actresses who smoke onscreen influence people to smoke? Share your thoughts on our online discussion forum at **http://health.wadsworth.com**

Find It On InfoTrac: You can find additional readings related to tobacco via InfoTrac College Edition, an online library of more than 900 journals and publications. Follow the instructions for accessing InfoTrac that came packaged with your textbook; then search for articles using a key word search.

- **Suggested article:** "Making It Uncool: Ways to Prevent Teenage Smoking," by Robert Worth. *Washington Monthly,* March 1999, Vol. 31 Issue 3, p. 8.
  (1) What are the strategies used by the tobacco industry to encourage young people to smoke?
  (2) What strategies have been used by some states to curb smoking? How successful have they been?

For additional links, resources, and suggested readings on InfoTrac, visit our Health & Wellness Resource Center at http://health.wadsworth.com

■ Clove cigarettes may be more dangerous than conventional cigarettes because they contain more nicotine, tar, and carbon monoxide. Bidis, popular among the young, also may expose smokers to more harmful chemicals in smoke. People who chew tobacco or use snuff are at risk of nicotine addiction, teeth and gum conditions, and cancer of the mouth and throat.

■ Environmental, or secondhand, smoke is a dangerous carcinogen. Nonsmokers constantly exposed to cigarette smoke are at risk of many illnesses, including lung cancer and heart disease. The spouses and children of smokers are at greatest risk of developing lung cancer, heart disease, and other ailments.

■ Quitting cigarettes often requires four to ten attempts, but 90 percent of those who quit eventually succeed on their own. The health benefits of quitting smoking include longer life span and greatly reduced risk of heart disease, cancer, and other diseases. One approach to quitting smoking is gradually reducing the number of cigarettes smoked per day. Another is stopping all at once. People who need help to stop smoking can try stop-smoking groups or programs, aversion therapy, nicotine replacement (with gum or patches), medication, hypnosis, and acupuncture.

Learning to live without tobacco requires great commitment. If you smoke and want to stop, don't think of quitting as giving up something pleasant, but rather as beginning something even more pleasant. With every healthy breath you take, you're renewing yourself, becoming better—making a new you.

 The Smoking Gene. What brain chemical is affected by "the smoking gene"?

Key Terms

The terms listed here are used within the chapter. Page numbers are included for each term. A definition of each term is given in the Glossary pages at the end of this book.

aversion therapy 556	carbon monoxide 540	mainstream smoke 552
bidis 550	environmental tobacco smoke 552	sidestream smoke 552
bupropion 557	nicotine 540	tar 540

Critical Thinking Questions

1. Has smoking become unpopular among your friends or family? What social activities continue to be associated with smoking? Can you think of any situations in which smoking might be frowned upon?

2. How would you motivate someone you care about to stop smoking? What reasons would you give for them to stop? Describe your strategy.

3. According to the chapter, environmental tobacco smoke is even more dangerous than mainstream smoke. If you're a nonsmoker, how would you react to someone who's smoking in the same room as you? Define the rights of smokers and nonsmokers.

References

1. World Health Organization.
2. Heishman, Stephen. "Scientists Chart Nicotine Craving's Impact on Mental Skills." *Nicotine & Tobacco Research*, April 1999.
3. CDC's TIPS (Tobacco Information and Prevention Source). For latest data, check http://www.cdc.gov/nccdphp/osh/index.htm
4. Jacobs, David. "Cigarette Smoking and Mortality Risk: Twenty-Five-Year Follow-Up of the Seven Countries Study." *Archives of Internal Medicine*, Vol. 159:733–740, April 12, 1999.
5. Howard, George, et al. "Cigarette Smoking and Progression of Atherosclerosis." *Journal of the American Medical Association*, Vol. 279, No. 2, January 14, 1998.
6. Irwin, Michael. "Smoking and Depression Weakens the Immune System." *Psychosomatic Medicine*, May 1999.
7. Ertischek, Michelle. "Non-Small-Cell Lung Cancer Study Shows an Increased One-Year Survival Rate with Taxotere." University of Wisconsin, Madison News Bureau, June 3, 1999.

8. CDC's TIPS.

9. Ibid.

10. Gillyatt, Peta. "Younger Smokers May Face More Harm Than Late Starters." *Focus: News from Harvard Medical, Dental and Public Health Schools,* April 16, 1999.

11. Golden, Frederic. "Smoking Gun for the Young." *Time,* April 19, 1999.

12. Pierce, John, et al. "Tobacco Industry Promotion of Cigarettes and Adolescent Smoking." *Journal of the American Medical Association,* Vol. 279, No. 7, February 18, 1998.

13. Moskal, Patsy, et al. "Examining the Use of Tobacco on College Campuses." *Journal of American College Health,* Vol. 47, No. 6, May 1999.

14. Satcher, David. "Tobacco Use Among U.S. Racial/Ethnic Minority Groups—A Report of the Surgeon General." Centers for Disease Control and Prevention, 1998.

15. CDC. "Women Who Smoke Fact Sheet." 1999.

16. "Tobacco Use Among Middle and High School Students—Florida, 1998 and 1999 Fact Sheet." CDC TIPS. "Teen Smoking Drops for First Time." Centers for Disease Control and Prevention News Bureau, April 1, 1999.

17. "Psychedelic Smokes. (Indian Cigarettes Called Bidis Popular with Teenagers)." *Newsweek,* Vol. 133, No. 9, March 1, 1999.

18. Goldberg, Carey. "Study Details Smoking Fad Among Youth." *New York Times,* September 17, 1999.

19. Koch, Wendy. "Cheap, Flavored Smokes Are Latest Teen Fad." *USA Today,* August 5, 1999.

20. Satcher, David. "Cigars and Public Health." *New England Journal of Medicine,* Vol. 340, No. 23, June 10, 1999.

21. Morbidity and Mortality Weekly Report (MMWR). "Cigar Smoking Among Teenagers." *Journal of the American Medical Association,* Vol. 278, No. 1, July 2, 1997.

22. Iribarren, Carlos. "The Effect of Cigar Smoking on the Risk of Cardiovascular Disease, Chronic Obstructive Pulmonary Disease, and Cancer in Men." *New England Journal of Medicine,* June 10, 1999.

23. "Oral Lesions from Smokeless Tobacco Dissipate After Stopping." American Dental Association, July 15, 1999.

24. Severson, Herbert. "Tobacco Chewers Quit After Teachable Moment in Dental Chair." *Annals of Behavioral Medicine,* July 1999.

25. "Maternal Cigarette Smoking During Pregnancy Is an Independent Predictor for Symptoms of Middle Ear Disease at Five Years' Postdelivery." American Academy of Pediatrics, news release, August 2, 1999.

26. Weissman, Myrna, et al. "Maternal Smoking During Pregnancy and Psychopathology in Offspring Followed to Adulthood." *Journal of the American Academy of Child and Adolescent Psychiatry,* Vol. 38, No. 7, July 1999.

27. Frost, Pam. "Children of Smokers Suffer Negative Health Effects Later in Life." Ohio State University, April 1, 1999.

28. Meier, Eileen. "The Tobacco Settlement and 1999 Forecasts." *Nursing Economics,* Vol. 17, No. 1, January 1999.

29. Baker, Timothy. " Unrelenting Grip of Nicotine Withdrawal." Presentation, American Psychological Society, Denver, June 1999.

30. Turner, Scott. "Vigorous Exercise Helps Women Quit Smoking and Stay Smoke Free." Brown University News Bureau, June 13, 1999.

31. Pierce, John. "Smoke-Free Homes Increase Smokers' Chances to Quit." *Nicotine & Tobacco Research,* June 30, 1999.

32. Kirchner, Jeffrey. "Bupropion With or Without Patches for Smoking Cessation." *American Family Physician,* Vol. 59, No. 11, June, 1999.

33. "Study Finds Antismoking Drug Zyban Twice as Effective as Nicotine Patch." *Los Angeles Times,* March 4, 1999.

34. Morbidity and Mortality Weekly Report. "Impact of Promotion of the Great American Smokeout and Availability of Over-the-Counter Nicotine Medications." *Journal of the American Medical Association,* Vol. 278, No. 23, December 17, 1997.

VI

Health in Context

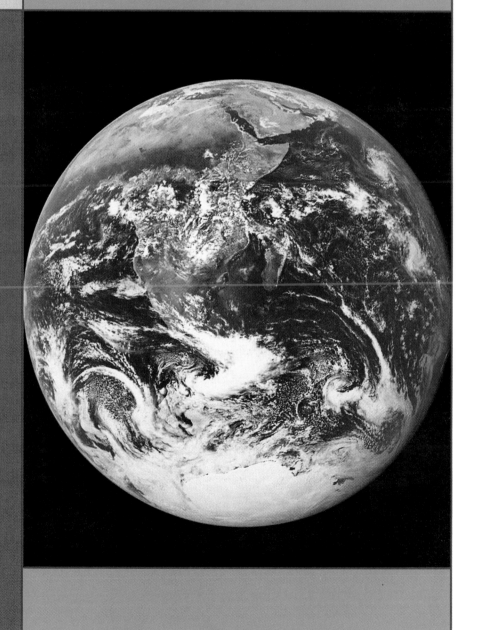

Personal health always involves more than a single individual. We are social beings, and we live our lives as part of a network of family, friends, acquaintances, colleagues, neighbors. Our actions affect others; others' behaviors have a significant impact on our wellbeing.

This is especially true of issues such as injury, violence, and sexual victimization, which are discussed in Chapter 18. For college students, staying safe is an essential part of staying healthy. Injury claims more lives of young Americans than illness. Threats such as violence and victimization are too serious and widespread for anyone to ignore.

Ultimately, all lives end in the same way. Death is as much a part of the real world as life itself. The quest to find meaning in dying is one of the challenges of living. All of us share something else: our planet. The problems of creating a healthy environment are many and complex. They too demand our attention and commitment.

18

Staying Safe: Preventing Injury, Violence, and Victimization

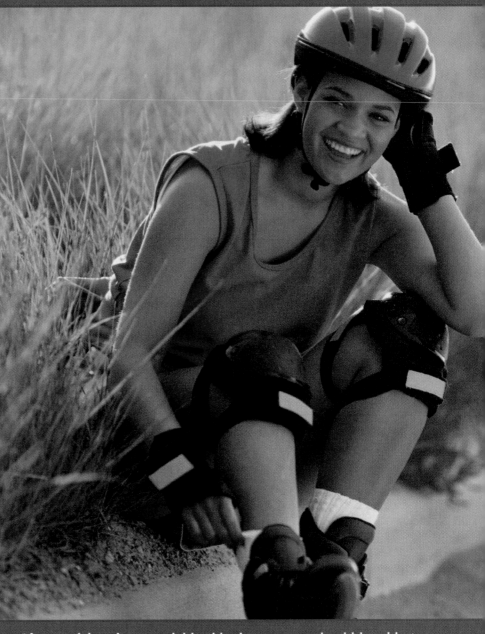

After studying the material in this chapter, you should be able to:

- **List** and **explain** factors that increase the likelihood of an accident.
- **Describe** safety procedures for road, residential, worksite, and outdoor safety.
- **Define** sexual victimization, sexual harassment, and sexual coercion, and **explain** how each can develop.
- **List** the different types of rape, and **describe** recommended actions for preventing rape.
- **Explain** the consequences of sexual violence.
- **Describe** the abuse pattern, and **explain** how it relates to child abuse and partner abuse.

The major threats to the well-being of most college students aren't illnesses but injuries. In all, injuries—intentional and unintentional—claim almost 150,000 lives a year.[1] Accidents, especially motor-vehicle crashes, kill more college-age men and women than all other causes combined; the greatest number of lives lost to accidents is among those 25 years of age. In recent years, another threat has claimed the lives of tens of thousands of Americans of all ages: violence. Each year more than 30,000 men, women, and children die and 100,000 are injured by firearms. Violent crime—murders, rapes, robberies, aggravated assaults—victimize more than four million Americans a year.[2]

Recognizing the threat of intentional and unintentional injury is the first step to ensuring your personal safety. You may think that the risk of something bad happening is simply a matter of chance, of being in the wrong place at the wrong time. That's not the case. Certain behaviors, such as using alcohol and drugs or not buckling your seat belt, greatly increase the risk of harm. Ultimately, you have more control over your safety than anyone or anything else in your life.

This chapter is a primer in self-protection that could help safeguard—perhaps even save—your life. Included are recommendations for commonsense safety on the road, at home, outdoors, and on the job. This chapter also explores other serious threats to personal safety in our society—violence, both public and domestic, and sexual victimization. ❖

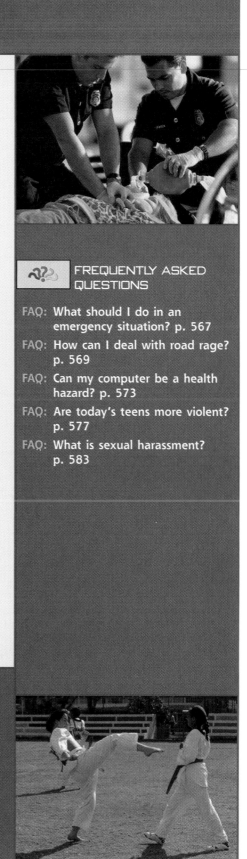

FREQUENTLY ASKED QUESTIONS

FAQ: **What should I do in an emergency situation?** p. 567

FAQ: **How can I deal with road rage?** p. 569

FAQ: **Can my computer be a health hazard?** p. 573

FAQ: **Are today's teens more violent?** p. 577

FAQ: **What is sexual harassment?** p. 583

Unintentional Injury: Why Accidents Happen

You may assume that most accidents happen without any warning. Yet often an accident is the unfortunate result of a series or combination of events. The more you know about the factors that increase the likelihood of an accident or injury, the more you can do to prevent it. (See Self-Survey: "Are You Doing Enough to Prevent Accidents?")

Unsafe Attitudes

Where do you feel safest? Chances are you'll answer by naming the places that are most familiar to you: your room, your home, your car. Yet that's where you're most likely to have an accident—often because you let your guard down. While listening to the morning news, you may forget to shut off a burner on the stove. Since there usually isn't much traffic on your street, you may back out of your driveway without looking both ways. Most of the time you, or someone with you, is able to correct such dangerous situations before a fire or collision occurs. But you can't count on always being so lucky.

Keep in mind that *feeling* safe is not the same as *being* safe. Away from home, unsafe attitudes can set the stage for unsafe behaviors. If you're overly confident in your driving skills, you may speed on a winding or wet road. If you're daydreaming, you may trip and fall as you hike. Keeping your wits about you is essential to keeping yourself safe.

Self-*Survey* — Are You Doing Enough to Prevent Accidents?

Accidents frequently result in serious injury, and a large number of deaths.

The following questions are designed to test how well you protect yourself and your family from accidental injury. The first group of questions concentrates on guarding against possible hazards in and around your house or apartment. The second group deals with safety measures that should be taken against accidents that might happen to you or your family on the road, whether in a vehicle or as pedestrians. The third group is concerned mainly with safety on vacations, when unfamiliar surroundings and activities present special hazards.

Group 1: Safety at Home
Answer Yes or No to the following questions:
1. Do you make it a point never to smoke in bed?
2. If you have fireplaces, do you keep screens around them?
3. When cooking, do you guard against accidental hot spills by positioning pan handles so that they don't extend outward?
4. Do you keep electrical cords out of the reach of children and avoid overloading electrical outlets?
5. Are you careful never to leave small children unsupervised in the kitchen or bathroom?
6. Are nightclothes and soft toys labeled to show that they're made of nonflammable materials?
7. Are medicines in your house kept in a secure place, out of children's reach and away from beds?
8. Are you careful never to store drugs or dangerous chemicals (bleach, paint-stripper, and so on) within children's reach or in incorrectly labeled containers?
9. If you own a gun, do you keep it unloaded, separate from the ammunition, and locked away?
10. Do you make a point of preventing your children from playing with objects small enough to be swallowed or inhaled?
11. Do you keep plastic bags away from your children?

12. When working around the house, do you wear safety glasses, earplugs, and protective clothing such as sturdy shoes?
13. Are your carpets firmly fixed, with no ragged spots or edges, and are loose rugs placed to minimize the risk of sliding or tripping?
14. Are your stairs, halls, and other passages lit brightly enough to read a newspaper?
15. Is it a rule in your house that nothing gets left on the stairs?
16. If you spill or drop something on the floor that might be slippery, do you always clean it up right away?
17. Do you keep nonslip mats both in and alongside the bath or shower?

Group 2: Safety on the Road
Answer Yes or No to the following questions:
18. Have you taught your children exactly how, when, and where to cross streets safely?
19. Have your children been taught the basic rules of the road to use when bicycling?
20. When walking in streets or open roads at twilight or in the dark, do all members of your family carry a flashlight, or wear a markedly visible outer garment, such as a white or luminous jacket?

21. Do you always drive within the speed limit and defensively?
22. Are you always careful not to drink if you're going to drive a car soon afterward?
23. Do you avoid driving when you feel unusually tired or ill, or if you're taking drugs (such as antihistamines) known to impair alertness?
24. Do you have your car fully serviced, including checking the lights, tires, windshield washer and wipers, brakes, and steering, either every 6,000 miles (10,000 km) or at least every six months?
25. Do you check at least once a week to make sure that your car windows, lights, mirrors, and reflectors are clean?
26. When driving, do you always try to keep a gap between your car and the one in front of you of at least a yard (or meter) for each mile-per-hour you're traveling?
27. Do you always make sure that you and all passengers in your car use available seatbelts?
28. Are any infants or toddlers riding in your car securely strapped into infant car seats?

Group 3: Safety on Vacations

Answer Yes or No to the following questions:
29. Are all members of your family able to swim or in the process of learning how to swim?
30. Do you test the depth of the water and go in feet first?
31. In a boat, does everyone always wear a life jacket?
32. If you do any skiing, hiking, or climbing, do you always go properly prepared with the right clothing and equipment?
33. When going on an excursion for a day or longer, do you tell someone what your route is and when you expect to return?
34. Do you and your family take full safety precautions and have the proper equipment when you engage in contact and other possibly dangerous sports?
35. Before taking up a new and potentially dangerous activity, such as hang gliding, do you make sure you get proper instruction?
36. During a vacation, do you make sure you get adequate rest and relaxation?

Evaluation

A No answer to any of the above questions indicates that you're not doing all you can to minimize your risk of accidents. You can and should take all the protective steps suggested by the questions.

Source: Kunz, Jeffrey, and Asher Finkel, eds. *The AMA Family Medical Guide.* New York: Random House, 1987.

Individual Risk Factors

Many factors influence an individual's risk of accident or injury, including those discussed in the following sections.

Age

The very young and the very old are the most susceptible to serious injury. Children may not recognize the danger of running into the street or jumping into a pool. In older people, a combination of factors—poor health, vision and hearing impairments, a faltering sense of balance, decreased agility, slower reflexes, and reduced resilience—make accidents a greater threat. Most victims of fatal accidents victims are males, often in their teens and twenties. Feeling full of life and energy, they may take dangerous risks because they think they're invulnerable. As noted in The X and Y Files: "Which Sex Is at Greater Risk of Personal Injury?" there also are sex differences in vulnerability to risk.

Alcohol and Drugs

An estimated 40 percent of Americans are involved in an alcohol-related accident sometime during their

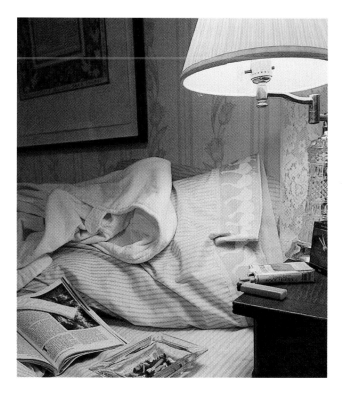

Home is a dangerous place. Many accidents happen at home—perhaps because we let down our guard there.

The X&Y Files

Which Sex Is at Greater Risk of Personal Injury?

Just like illness, injury doesn't discriminate against either sex. Both men and women can find themselves in harm's way—but for different reasons. Here are some sex differences in vulnerability:

- Men are ten times more likely to die of an occupational injury than women.

- Males are most often the victims and the perpetrators in homicides in the United States. In about 68 percent of cases reported by the Bureau of Justice Statistics, both the offender and the victim were male. In 22 percent, the offender was male, and the victim female. In 7.8 percent of all cases, the offender was female and the victim male, while in 2.3 percent both the offender and victim were female.

- Overall, men are 3.6 times more likely than women to be murdered and 9 times more likely to commit murder. Both men and women are more likely to kill or attempt to kill male victims than female victims.

- Women are the victims of three of every four murders of an intimate partner and about 85 percent of nonlethal intimate violence. Women between the ages of 16 and 24 experience the highest per capita rates of intimate violence.

- College men are nearly as likely as women to encounter unwanted sexual coercion. In a University of Washington study of nearly 300 students, 21 percent of the male participants and 28 percent of the female ones reported being recipients of one or more of five types of unwanted sexual contact. The men who experienced unwanted sexual contact reported more symptoms of depression than the other males in the study; there was no difference in depression symptoms for women who said they were sexually coerced and those who weren't. Women, however, were more likely to have had physical force used against them.

- According to the University of Washington survey, college men are more likely than women to report that they had unwanted sex or were pressured into having sex. In this study, 14 percent of the men and 8 percent of the women said they had unwanted sex; 8 percent of the men and 6 percent of the women said they had been pressured into having sex.

- Alcohol gets equal numbers of men and women—nearly half of those surveyed—into sexual situations that they later regret. Seventeen percent of the women and 9 percent of the men said someone had attempted to have intercourse with them when they didn't want to after giving them alcohol or drugs. And 6 percent of the women and 4 percent of the men said they had sex when they didn't want to after being given alcohol and drugs.

Sources: National Center for Health Statistics, Bureau of Justice Statistics. Schwarz, Joel . "College Men Nearly as Likely as Women to Report They Are Victims of Unwanted Sexual Coercion," University of Washington News Office, July 26, 1999.

---

lives. In nearly half of motor-vehicle deaths, either the driver or a pedestrian was intoxicated at the time of the crash. Other drugs also affect driving ability by impairing judgment and perceptions. (See Chapters 15 and 16.)

Stress

In times of tension and anxiety, we all pay less attention to what we're doing. We rush about; we don't take time to relax or rest. One common result is an increase in accidents during busy or stressful periods. If you find yourself having a series of small mishaps or "near-misses," it's important to do something to lower your stress level, rather than wait for something more harmful to happen. (See Chapter 2 on stress.)

Situational Factors

Some situations—such as driving on a curvy, wet road in a car with worn tires—are so inherently dangerous that they greatly increase the odds of an accident. But even when there's greater risk, you can lower the danger—for instance, you can't make the road dry, but you can make sure your tires and brakes are in good condition.

Thrill-Seeking

Some people crave the sensation of danger. To them, activities that others might find terrifying—such as sky-diving or parachute-jumping—are stimulating. The reason may be that they have lower than normal levels of the brain chemicals that regulate excitement. Because the stress of potentially hazardous sports may increase the levels of these chemicals, they feel pleasantly aroused rather than scared. However, their desire for this sensation could lead them to ignore safety precautions and jeopardize their safety.[3]

Left-Handedness

America's 33 million left-handed individuals, or "lefties," have nearly two accidents for every one suffered by right-handers. While left-handers are at greater risk in various situations and activities, driving seems especially dangerous for them. Left-handers are 85 percent more likely to have an accident-related injury when driving than are right-handers; the risk is greatest for left-handed men. According to Stanley Coren, author of *The Left-Hander Syndrome*, left-handers face more dangers because "the world was primarily designed by right-handers for the comfort and convenience of right-handers."

What Should I Do in an Emergency Situation?

Life-threatening situations rarely happen more than once or twice in any person's life. When they do, you must think and act quickly to prevent disastrous consequences.

- *Don't panic.* Your immediate response to an emergency may be overwhelming fear and anxiety. Take several deep breaths. Start by assessing the circumstances. Shout for help if you're in a public place. Look for any possible dangers to you or the victim, such as a live electrical wire or a fire. Seek medical assistance as quickly as possible. Don't attempt rescue techniques, such as cardiopulmonary resuscitation (CPR), unless you're trained. (For advice on

what to do in case of a heart attack, see the "Emergency!" section at the back of this book.)

- *Don't wait for symptoms to go away or get worse.* If you suspect that someone is having a heart attack or stroke, or has ingested something poisonous, *phone for help immediately.* A delay could jeopardize the person's life. Stay on the line long enough to give your name, address, and a brief description of the emergency.

- *Don't move a victim.* The person may have a broken neck or back, and attempting to move him or her could cause extensive damage or even death.

- *Don't drive.* Even if the hospital is just ten minutes away, you're better off waiting for a well-equipped ambulance with trained paramedics who can deliver emergency care on the spot. People rushing to emergency rooms are more likely to get into accidents themselves.

- *At home, keep a supply of basic first-aid items in a convenient place.* Make sure that emergency telephone numbers (ambulance service, police and fire departments, poison control center, your doctor and neighbors) are handy. If you can't find a number quickly, call the operator.

- *Don't do too much.* Often well-intentioned Good Samaritans make injuries worse by trying to tie tourniquets, wash cuts, or splint broken limbs. Also, don't give an injured person anything to eat or drink. (See "Emergency!" in the Hales Health Almanac at the back of this book for more on first-aid and emergency care.)

Safety on the Road

Every 14 seconds someone in America is injured in a traffic crash; every 12 minutes someone is killed. Motor vehicle accidents in the United States claim about 42,000 lives annually, more than any other form of unintentional injury. They are the leading cause of all deaths for people ages 6 to 27; only cancer and heart attacks claim more American lives. Far more people—more than 3.5 million annually—are injured in motor vehicle accidents. The economic toll of motor vehicle accidents also is high: an estimated total of $150 billion a year, including $17

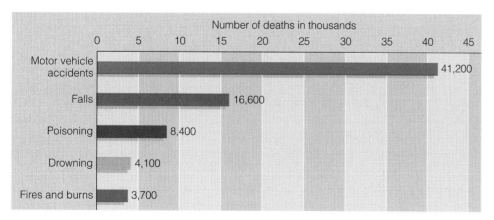

■ **Figure 18-1** Leading causes of fatal unintentional injuries in the United States, 1998.

Source: National Safety Council, **http://www.nsc.org/lrs/statinfo/99report.htm**

billion in medical and emergency expenses, lost productivity, and property loss.[4]

Safe Driving

Car crashes aren't accidents that just happen. Most are the result of unsafe vehicles, unsafe drivers, or unsafe driving techniques. Basic precautions can greatly increase your odds of reaching a destination alive. Vehicles equipped with seat belts, air bags, padded dashboards, safety glass windows, a steel frame, and side-impact beams all help protect against injury or death. The size and weight of a vehicle also matter. However, as sports utility vehicles (SUVs) and vans have become more popular, they've increased the risk to drivers of smaller cars, who are more likely to be injured in a collision with oversized vehicles.

According to a National Highway Traffic Safety Administration (NHTSA) telephone survey of drivers age 16 and older, most Americans want safer highways and more enforcement of traffic laws. Most called for more police monitoring of drivers on interstate highways and residential roads. Only a small percentage felt there was too much enforcement of speed limits, tailgating, and weaving in and out of traffic.[5]

Seat Belts and Air Bags

Seat belts have proven to be the most effective means of reducing fatalities and serious injuries when traffic crashes occur. They save an estimated 9,500 lives in America each year. When lap/shoulder belts are used properly, they reduce the risk of fatal injury to front seat passengers by 45 percent and the risk of moderate-to-critical injury by 50 percent. For light truck occupants, seat belts reduce the risk of fatal injury by 60 percent and moderate-to-critical injury by 65 percent.

Seat belts save lives in several ways. When a crash occurs, occupants continue to travel at the vehicle's original speed at the moment of impact. After the vehicle comes to a complete stop, unbelted occupants slam into the steering wheel, windshield, or into another part of the car. Seat belts reduce injuries from this second collision and also prevent ejection from the car. Three-quarters of the those ejected from passenger cars in a crash die.[6]

In national surveys, almost three-quarters of Americans say they are full-time seat belt users. However, of these, almost 10 percent acknowledge that they did not use their seat belts on at least one occasion during the preceding week. State laws that require motorists to "click it or ticket" make a difference, usually boosting seat belt use about 15 percentage points. However, even so, a significant percentage of drivers, including undergraduates do not use seat belts regularly. (See Campus Focus: "Are College Students Buckling Up?")

Typically, nonusers of seat belts also are high-risk drivers. They are more likely than others to drive after drinking and to be involved in a serious crash, yet they're the least likely to take responsibility for the social and economic consequences of their behavior. Although nonusers come from all segments of society, they are frequently male, younger than 30 years of age,

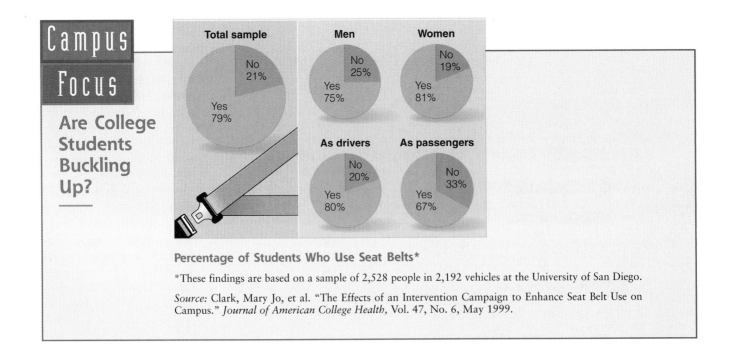

Campus Focus

Are College Students Buckling Up?

Percentage of Students Who Use Seat Belts*

*These findings are based on a sample of 2,528 people in 2,192 vehicles at the University of San Diego.

Source: Clark, Mary Jo, et al. "The Effects of an Intervention Campaign to Enhance Seat Belt Use on Campus." *Journal of American College Health,* Vol. 47, No. 6, May 1999.

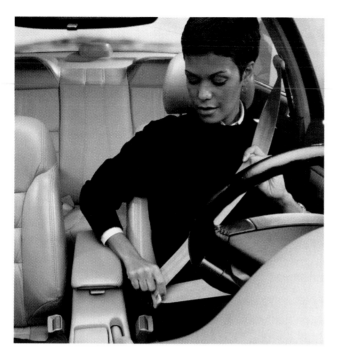

Buckling up is one of the simplest and most effective ways of protecting yourself from injury.

unmarried, have little or no post-secondary education, and often drive pickup trucks or sport utility vehicles. In NHTSA surveys, the female seat belt use rate is generally 10 percentage points higher than the male use rate. Overall seat belt use rates are highest in the suburbs, followed by cities, then rural areas.

Air bags also can save adult lives. Federal law requires that all cars manufactured since 1998 are equipped with air bags, but there is controversy over the potential hazard they pose to children. NHTSA has given automobile owners permission to deactivate air bags if a small child might be a front seat passenger. However, the American Academy of Pediatrics has argued that deactivation might pose an even greater risk by jeopardizing the safety of older children, teens, and adult passengers. It recommends that children be placed in the back seat, whether or not the car is equipped with a passenger air bag.

Unsafe Driving Behaviors

Drunk driving is the number one cause of serious motor-vehicle accidents. In recent years, there has been a decline in the number of fatalities caused by drunk driving, particularly among young people. The NHTSA attributes this decline to increases in the drinking age, to educational programs aimed at reducing nighttime driving by teens, to the formation of Students Against Driving Drunk (SADD) and similar groups, and to

changes in state laws that penalize drivers younger than age 21 for driving with even lower blood-alcohol concentration levels than were previously acceptable (from 0.01 to 0.05 percent). (See Chapter 16 for more information on blood-alcohol concentrations and drunk driving.)

Falling asleep at the wheel is second only to alcohol as a cause of serious motor-vehicle accidents. According to the National Commission on Sleep Disorders Research, each year 200,000 sleep-related motor-vehicle accidents claim more than 5,000 lives, cause hundreds of thousands of injuries, and lead to billions of dollars in indirect costs. Too little sleep, recent research suggests, may be as detrimental to driving skills as drinking too much. Individuals with sleep apnea, a nighttime breathing disruption, may be at particularly high risk of impaired response times on the road.[7]

Certain driving behaviors, such as speeding, tailgating, or running yellow lights, also increase the risk of an accident. According to a recent survey, more than half of Americans recognize that passing on the shoulder, failing to yield to merging traffic, and similar behaviors are dangerous, yet many still admit to doing so themselves. When asked about their driving in the past month, 62 percent of those surveyed said they had driven through yellow lights that were turning red, and 56 percent said they had driven 10 miles per hour over the speed limit.[8]

Cellular phones are helpful in alerting authorities to road hazards, congestion, or problem drivers, and they make it easier for motorists to summon help if they have a mechanical breakdown or another emergency. However, cell phones and other forms of wireless technology, such as on-board navigation systems, also create distractions that increase a driver's risk on the highways, according to an NHTSA report.[9] As many as 100 million Americans may be using cell phones in the coming years, and those who try to conduct business, check messages, or chat with friends as they drive could be putting themselves and others in danger. NHTSA research suggests that distraction or driver inattention is a primary or contributing factor in as many as 50 percent of all crashes. Actual accident reports cited by NHTSA document that drivers using cell phones have crashed into trees, struck stopped vehicles, and caused other cars to swerve out of control. Some communities have banned the use of cellular phones while driving.

 ## How Can I Deal with Road Rage?

According to the AAA Foundation for Traffic Safety, "violent aggressive driving"—a deliberate attempt to harm another driver after a traffic dispute—is rising by

7 percent per year. "The violent incidents that make the papers are still relatively rare," says Phil Berardelli, author of *The Driving Challenge*. "But what's equally horrible is the everyday climate of driving, the basic level of aggression that almost everyone participates in. The majority of drivers, women and men, drive more discourteously than they should."[10]

This habitual hostility can and often does erupt into the emotional outbursts known as road rage—a factor, says the National Highway Traffic Safety Administration, in as many as two-thirds of all fatal car crashes and one-third of nonfatal accidents.[11] Psychologist Arnold Nerenberg of Whittier, California, a specialist in motorway mayhem, estimates that there may be 1.78 billion episodes of road rage a year, resulting in more than 28,000 deaths and 1 million injuries.[12]

What transforms perfectly polite, well-mannered Joe and Jane Jekylls into hell-bent Mr. and Mrs. Hydes behind the wheel? Terror, says Stephanie Faulk of the AAA Foundation for Traffic Safety. "If someone darts in front of you, for a second you think you are going to die, and the fight or flight impulse kicks in. People are more likely to fight in a car because they're encased in a steel shell and they feel safe. And the other driver is anonymous. You can't see his face or hear his voice so you don't have any social cues to guide you. You think, 'I'll show him,' because the consequences seem remote." This isn't necessarily so. Road rage has led to deadly races, confrontations, and shootings.[13] Some strategies for reducing road rage include the following:

- *Lower the stress in your life.* Take a few moments to breathe deeply and relax your shoulders before putting the key in the ignition.

- *Consciously decide not to let other drivers get to you.* Decide that whatever happens, it's not going to make your blood pressure go up.

- *Slow down.* If you're going five or ten miles over the speed limit, you won't have the time you need to react to anything that happens.

- *Modify bad driving habits one at a time.* If you tend to tailgate slow drivers, spend a week driving at twice your usual following distance. If you're a habitual horn honker, silence yourself.

- *Be courteous—even if other drivers aren't.* Don't dawdle in the passing lane. Never tailgate or switch lanes without signaling. Don't use your horn or high beams unless absolutely necessary.

- *Never retaliate.* Whatever another driver does, keep your cool. Count to ten. Take a deep breath. If you yell or gesture at someone who's upset with you, the conflict may well escalate.

- *If you do something stupid, show that you're sorry.* On its web site, the AAA Foundation for Traffic

Strategies *for* Prevention

How to Drive Safely

✓ Don't drive while under the influence of alcohol or other drugs, including medications that may impair your reflexes, cause drowsiness, or affect your judgment. Never get into a car if you suspect the driver may be intoxicated or affected by a drug.

✓ Remain calm when dealing with drivers who are reckless or rude. Be alert and anticipate possible hazards. Don't let yourself be distracted by conversations, children's questions, arguments, food or drink, or scenic views. If you become exhausted, pull over and rest.

✓ Don't get too comfortable. Alertness matters. Use the rearview mirror often. Don't let passengers or packages obstruct your view. Use the turn signals when changing lanes or making a turn. If someone cuts you off, back off to a safe distance. When you can, drive so that you have enough space around you.

✓ Make sure small children are in safety seats. Unless pets are trained to ride quietly in a car, keep them in carrying cases.

✓ Drive more slowly if weather conditions are bad. Avoid driving at all during heavy rain, snow, or other conditions that affect visibility and road conditions. If you must drive in hazardous conditions, make sure that your car has the proper equipment, such as chains or snow tires, and that you know how to respond in case of a skid.

✓ Maintain your car properly, replacing windshield wipers, tires, and brakes when necessary. Keep flares and a fire extinguisher in your car for use in emergencies.

✓ To avoid a head-on collision, generally veer to the right—onto a shoulder, lawn, or open space. Steer your way to safety; avoid hitting the brakes hard once you leave the pavement. If you have to hit something stationary, look for a "soft" target— bushes, parked cars, woodframe buildings—as opposed to "hard" boulders, brick walls, trees, concrete abutments, and so on.

Safety solicited suggestions for automotive apologies. The most popular: slapping yourself on your forehead or the top of your head to indicate that you know you goofed. Such gestures can soothe a miffed motorist—and make the roads a slightly safer place for all of us to be.

Across the Lifespan: Seniors at the Wheel

About a third of all drivers are over age 55; their number will increase as the baby boom generation ages. Driving is very important to seniors, and most want to stay on the road as long as possible. While age alone is not an indicator of impairment, there are age-related changes that can affect driving ability. One is the ability of older drivers to safely maneuver through intersections.

About one-third of the fatalities of older drivers occur at intersections, and this figure jumps to more than half for drivers over the age of 80. Older drivers may have greater difficulties at intersections because of diminished capabilities, including deficits in vision, diminished spatial vision, and altered depth and motion perception. In a study of older drivers by the National Highway Traffic Safety Administration, one type of maneuvering error—infringing on others' right of way when changing lanes—occurred at a 90 percent rate on unfamiliar routes and 57 percent rate on familiar routes.[14]

Other studies have shown that, although half the people over age 85 meet motor vehicle bureau vision standards, many suffer weaknesses in other critical aspects of vision, such as recovery from glare. It takes up to two minutes for those over 85 to recover from glare, for instance, compared to 15 seconds for a person between ages 55 and 65. In one test of 900 volunteers over age 55, half couldn't pass a depth perception test; the ability of those over 85 to operate a vehicle when they had to divide their attention was half that of people under age 65.

As various regulatory agencies struggle with ways to evaluate the safety of older drivers, seniors can lower their risks by taking simple steps such as limiting night driving, avoiding freeways, driving during less crowded periods of the day, making practice runs of frequently traveled routes, and identifying and using alternate means of transportation.

Safe Cycling

Mile for mile, motorcycling is far more risky than automobile driving. The most common motorcycle injury is head trauma, which can lead to physical disability, including paralysis and general weakness, as well as problems reading and thinking. It can also cause personality changes and psychiatric problems, such as depression, anxiety, and uncontrollable mood swings and anger. Some improvement may occur naturally as swelling diminishes and the brain heals. However, complete recovery from head trauma can take four to six years, and the costs can be staggering. Head injury can also result in permanent disability, coma, and death. To prevent head trauma, motorcycle helmets are required in most states. Federal law dictates that a certain percentage of highway construction funds be reallocated for safety programs in states that don't require motorcycle helmets.

Approximately 80.6 million people ride bicycles. Each year, bicycle crashes kill about 900 of these individuals; about 200 of those killed are children under age 15. About 567,000 people go to hospital emergency departments annually with bicycle-related injuries; 350,000 of the injured are children under age 15. Of these children, about 130,000 suffer head injuries.

According to a national survey, 50 percent of all bicycle riders in the United States regularly wear bike helmets—43 percent every time they ride and 7 percent more than half the time. This represents a dramatic increase from 1991, when only 18 percent of bike riders reported wearing helmets. Safety is the primary reason that 98 percent of those surveyed gave for wearing a helmet, followed by the insistence of a parent or spouse. The reasons for not wearing a bike helmet included riding only a short distance, forgetting to put it on, or feeling that the helmet was uncomfortable.[15]

Consumer Health Watch

Buying a Bike Helmet

What should you look for in buying a helmet? Here are some basic guidelines:

- A government regulation requires all helmets produced after 1999 to meet the Consumer Product Safety Commission standard; look for a CPSC sticker inside the helmet. The Snell Memorial Foundation's B-90 standard and the ASTM standard are comparable to CPSC. The Snell B-95 standard is even better.

- Check the fit. The helmet should sit level on your head, touching all around, comfortably snug but not tight. The helmet should not move more than about an inch in any direction, regardless of how hard you tug at it.

- Pick a bright color for visibility. Avoid dark colors, thin straps, or a rigid visor that could snag in a fall.

- Look for a smooth plastic outer shell, not one with alternating strips of plastic and foam. Watch out for excessive vents, which put less protective foam in contact with your head in a crash. Mirrors should have a breakaway mount; the wire type mounted on eyeglasses can gouge an eye in a fall.

Most cyclists underestimate the annual number of bicycle-related deaths and emergency department injuries. For example, 72 percent of survey respondents believed there were 500 or fewer bicycle-related deaths every year. Similarly, 96 percent believed there were fewer than 50,000 bicycle-related injuries treated in hospital emergency departments every year. Safety helmets can reduce the risk of injury by 85 percent and could prevent one cyclist's death every day. (See Consumer Health Watch: "Buying a Bike Helmet.")

In addition to wearing helmets, cyclists should know and follow traffic rules: yield right-of-way appropriately, signal turns properly, obey stop signs, and so on. They should use bike lanes if they're available, and avoid weaving in and out of traffic or riding in the center of the street or against the flow of traffic. Bikes should have reflectors on the front, back, and both wheels, as well as taillights and headlights for night use.

Safety at Home

Every year home accidents claim more than 24,000 lives and cause nearly 25 million injuries. Poison poses the greatest threat, causing more than 17,000 deaths every year.[16] Half a million children swallow poisonous materials each year; 90 percent are under age 5. Adults may also be poisoned by mistakenly taking someone else's prescription drugs or taking medicines in the dark and swallowing the wrong one. In most cities, you can call a poison control center for advice. (See "Emergency!" in the Hales Health Almanac for first-aid advice for poisoning.)

Falls

Falls, the leading cause of fatal accidents at home, claim about 12,000 lives a year.[17] High heels or worn footgear, poor lighting, slippery or uneven walkways, broken stairs and handrails, loose or worn rugs, or objects left where people walk all increase the likelihood of a slip. Falls are an especially serious health risk for the elderly. Each year about one-third of all people 65 years of age or older who live at home fall; 6 to 10 percent of these falls result in injury, including fractures, muscle injuries, sprains, lacerations, and dislocations. Fearing another fall, older people may limit their activity, becoming less independent and fit.

Fires

You can prevent fires from occurring by making sure that the three ingredients of fire—fuel, a heat source,

Strategies *for* Prevention

Staying Safe at Home

✓ Wear gloves when using household cleaning products. Read labels carefully, and use the products only in well-ventilated rooms. Never combine cleaning products; doing so could produce a dangerous chemical reaction.

✓ Light stairways well. Remove clutter, cords, wires, and furniture from walking paths in living areas. Make sure carpets are attached firmly and area rugs are secure. Install nonskid mats in bathtubs and showers.

✓ Carry only loads you can see over. Clean up spills immediately, or mark the spill with a paper towel or wastebasket until you get a chance to clean it up. If you must walk over wet or slippery surfaces, take short steps to keep your center of balance beneath you. Slow down.

✓ To avoid shocks, be careful about anything involving electricity and water. Avoid using power tools in the rain; be careful with electrical heaters and other appliances, such as radios and hair dryers, in the bathroom; and use tools with nonconducting handles.

and oxygen—don't get a chance to mix. Almost anything can act as fuel for fire, including paper, wood, and, of course, flammable liquids such as oils, gasoline, and some paints. A heat source can be a spark from a

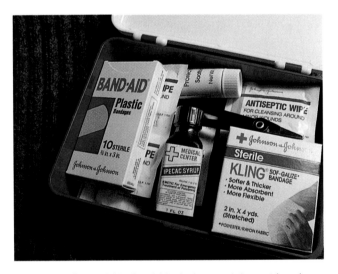

Your home first-aid kit should include (at minimum) bandages, sterile gauze pads, adhesive tape, scissors, cotton, antibiotic ointment, a needle, safety pins, calamine lotion, syrup of ipecac to induce vomiting, and a thermometer.

lighted match, pilot light, or an electrical wire. Oxygen is necessary for the chemical reaction between the fuel and heat source that causes combustion.

If a fire starts and it's small, you may be able to put it out with a portable fire extinguisher before it spreads. However, if the fire does get out of control, you might have only two to five minutes to get out of the house or building alive. A fire-escape plan can save time and lives. Sketch a plan of your house, apartment building, dormitory, or fraternity or sorority house. Identify two ways out of each room or apartment. Make sure everyone is familiar with these escape routes. Designate an area outside where all family members or dorm residents should meet after escaping from a fire.

If a fire breaks out in your dorm room, get out as quickly as possible, but don't run. Before opening a room door, place your hand on it. If it's hot, don't open it. If the door feels cool, open it slightly to check for smoke. If there's none, leave by your planned escape route. If you're on an upper floor and your escape routes are blocked, open a window (top and bottom, if possible) and wait or signal from the window for help. Never try to use an elevator in a fire.

If you can't leave your room safely during a fire, call for help and turn off the air-conditioning or heating systems. To block smoke, press sheets and towels (wet, if possible) around and under the door. Keep as close to the floor as possible (where there's likely to be more oxygen), and place a wet washcloth over your face to filter out smoke particles.

Strategies *for* Prevention

Staying Safe from Fires

✓ Keep gasoline, paint, oily rags, newspapers, plastics, glues, and lightweight materials away from pilot lights, heaters, and other sources of heat. Store flammables in metal cans. Clean up grease on stoves.

✓ Don't overload electrical circuits, use worn wiring, or use portable heaters that have no cutoff feature if they tip over.

✓ Check to see that at least one smoke detector has been installed on each floor of your dorm or home. Make sure that you have a multipurpose fire extinguisher available to put out small fires.

✓ Close bedroom doors when you sleep. Closed doors slow the spread of fire. Keep a flashlight by each bedside to light the way out at night.

On-the-Job Safety

The workplace is second only to the home as the most frequent site of accidents. More than 5,500 injury deaths occur on the job every year.[18] The industries with the highest fatality rates are mining; transportation, communication, and public utilities; construction; and agriculture, forestry, and fishing. Whatever your job, find out about potential hazards and learn the proper safety regulations. (Chapter 20 discusses some potential environmental hazards at work, including noise, toxic substances, and video display terminals.)

Can My Computer Be a Health Hazard?

As computers have become part of daily life for everyone from preschoolers to seniors, health professionals have learned a great deal about potential health problems, including repetitive motion injuries and vision-related difficulties.

Repetitive Motion Injuries

Repetitive motion injuries (RMI) have surpassed back and neck injuries as the number one claim for workers compensation injuries. Repeated motions—such as the hand and arm movements made while using a computer keyboard—all day, every day, can result in muscle and tendon strain and inflammation. About 20 percent of people with pain, tingling, or numbness in the hands may have carpal tunnel syndrome, an overuse injury caused by repetitive motions in the hands and wrists.[19] Symptoms include pain, swelling, and numbness and weakness in the hands or the arms. If these problems are identified early, permanent damage can generally be avoided by altering the work environment and allowing for more breaks during the day.

If you work at a computer, good posture and correct positioning of the computer screen and keyboard can help prevent repetitive motion injuries, eyestrain, and back strain (see Figure 18-2). Here are some additional tips:

• Place the keyboard so that your elbows are bent at a 90° angle and you don't have to bend your wrists to type.

• Use a chair that provides ample back support. Keep your thighs parallel to the floor and your feet on the floor. If your feet don't reach the floor, use a footrest.

• If you experience neck strain, place a document holder next to your screen so that you can view the materials you are typing more easily.

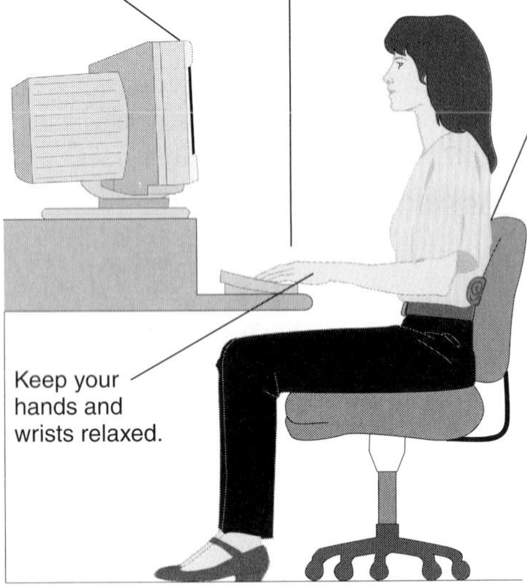

The screen should be at eye level (22–26 inches higher than your seat).

Position the keyboard so that your elbows are bent at a 90° angle and your hands and wrists are straight.

Sit straight in your chair; for extra back support, place a rolled-up towel behind you.

Keep your hands and wrists relaxed.

■ **Figure 18-2 Safe Computing**
By paying attention to your posture and your computer's position, you can help protect yourself from repetitive motion injury, back strain, and eyestrain.

• Every 15 minutes take a 30-second break, stretch your arms, and walk around the office. Take a 15-minute break at least once every two hours.

Vision Problems

Computer vision syndrome is a condition marked by tired and sore eyes, blurred vision, headaches and neck, shoulder, and back pain. The American Optometric Association estimates that it afflicts nearly 90 percent of workers who use computers, and it also is common among children and students of all ages.[20] The symptoms result from repeatedly stressing some aspect of the visual system, but they often disappear as soon as the person stops working at the computer.

The eye focuses on a computer image differently from the way it focuses on a printed one. The pixels that appear on a computer screen, unlike printed characters, are bright in the center and gradually fade away into the background color. This makes it difficult for the eye to sustain focus. Optometrists have developed a specific method, called a PRIO examination, that simulates how the eye responds to pixels on a VDT screen. It can determine the need and proper prescription for computer-only eyeglasses.

Working with Chemicals

Many different types of workers, from laboratory technicians to professional artists, must use dangerous chemicals to perform their jobs. Employers and manufacturers of these chemicals are required by federal law to inform workers about any potential hazards, as well as first-aid measures in case they're accidentally exposed.

Here are some safety guidelines to follow if you work with dangerous substances:

• Make sure your work space is adequately ventilated. This doesn't mean a fan, which just blows dust and fumes around, but the equivalent of a filtered vacuum cleaner at the source of the toxic material.

• Be careful with the storage and handling of flammable solvents. Label all toxic materials clearly and carefully. Store them in nonbreakable containers. Discard them according to the manufacturer's instructions.

• Wash yourself thoroughly with soap and water before taking a break. Don't sweep up: vacuum or wet mop.

• Do not eat or smoke when using toxic materials. Wear appropriate protective gear: air respirators, goggles, gloves, earplugs, and so on.

• If you're pregnant or planning to conceive, check with your doctor about any potential risks to an unborn child.

Recreational Safety

When you want to take a break, exercise, or simply enjoy yourself, you probably go outside. But if you aren't careful, even a simple stroll or swim can turn into a hazardous event. According to a study by the Johns Hopkins School of Public Health, every year 750,000 Americans are injured during recreational activities such as horseback riding, skiing, sledding, snowboarding, skating, and playground activities; 82,000 suffer head injuries requiring emergency room or hospital treatment. Two dangers on the increase are in-line skating (rollerblading) and skateboarding. Public health experts urge helmet use for sports such as rollerblading and skateboarding because such activities combine high speeds with exposure to traffic.

Handling Heat

Each year as many as 1,000 Americans die from heat-caused illnesses that are almost always preventable. Two common heat-related maladies are **heat cramps** and **heat stress.** Heat cramps are caused by hard work and heavy sweating in the heat. Heat stress may occur simultaneously or afterward, as the blood vessels try to keep body temperature down. **Heat exhaustion,** a third such malady, is the result of prolonged sweating with inadequate fluid replacement. (See Table 18-1.)

The first step in treating the above conditions is to stop exercising, move to a cool place, and drink plenty of water. Don't resume work or activity until all the symptoms have disappeared; see a doctor if you're suffering from heat exhaustion. **Heat stroke** is a life-threatening medical emergency caused by the breakdown of the body's mechanism for cooling itself. The treatment is to cool the body down: Move to a cooler environment; sponge down with cool water, and apply ice to the back of the neck, armpits, and groin. Immersion in cold water could cause shock. Get medical help immediately.

Coping with Cold

The tips of the toes, fingers, ears, nose, chin, and cheeks are most vulnerable to exposure to high wind speeds and low temperatures, which can result in **frostnip.** Because frostnip is painless, you may not even be aware of

---

Strategies *for* Prevention

Protecting Yourself from the Cold

✓ Dress appropriately. Choose several layers of loose clothing made of wool, cotton, down, or synthetic down. Make sure your head, feet, and hands are well protected. A pair of cotton socks inside a pair of wool socks will keep your feet warm.

✓ Don't go out in the cold after drinking. Alcohol can make you more susceptible to cold (see Chapter 16) and can impair your judgment and sense of time.

✓ When snowshoeing or cross-country skiing, always let a responsible person know where you're heading and when you expect to be back. Stick to marked trails. Don't eat snow; it could lower your body temperature.

✓ Carry an emergency kit that includes waterproof matches, a compass, a map, high-energy food, and water.

■ **Table 18-1** Heat Dangers

Illness	Symptoms	Treatment
Heat cramps	Muscle twitching or cramping; muscle spasms in arms, legs, and abdomen.	Stop exercising; cool off; drink water.
Heat stress	Fatigue, pale skin, blurred vision, dizziness, low blood pressure.	Stop exercising; cool off; drink water.
Heat exhaustion	Excessive thirst, fatigue, lack of coordination, increased sweating, elevated body temperature.	See a doctor.
Heat stroke	Lack of perspiration, high body temperature (over 105°F), dry skin, rapid breathing, coma, seizures, high pulse.	Cool the body; sponge; get medical help.

---

it occurring. Watch for a sudden blanching or lightening of your skin. The best early treatment is warming the area by firm, steady pressure with a warm hand; blowing on it with hot breath; holding it against your body; or immersing it in warm (not hot) water. As the skin thaws, it becomes red and starts to tingle. Be careful to protect it from further damage. Don't rub the skin vigorously or with snow, as you could damage the tissue.

More severe is **frostbite.** There are two types of frostbite, *superficial* and *deep.* Superficial frostbite, the freezing of the skin and tissues just below the skin, is characterized by a waxy look and firmness of the skin, although the tissue below is soft. Initial treatment should be to slowly rewarm the area. As the area thaws, it will be numb and bluish or purple, and blisters may form. Cover the area with a dry, sterile dressing, and protect the skin from further exposure to cold. See a doctor for further treatment. Deep frostbite, the freezing of skin, muscle, and even bone, requires medical treatment. It usually involves the tissues of the hands and feet, which appear pale and feel frozen. Keep the victim dry and as warm as possible on the way to a medical facility. Cover the frostbitten area with a dry, sterile dressing.

The gradual cooling of the center of the body may occur at temperatures above, as well as below, freezing—usually in wet, windy weather. When body temperature falls below 95°F, the body is incapable of rewarming itself because of the breakdown of the internal system that regulates its temperature. This state is known as **hypothermia.** The first sign of hypothermia is severe shivering. Then the victim becomes uncoordinated, drowsy, listless, confused, and is unable to speak properly. Symptoms become more severe as body temperature continues to drop, and coma or death can result.

Hypothermia requires emergency medical treatment. Try to prevent any further heat loss: Move the victim to a warm place, cover him or her with blankets, remove wet clothing, and replace it with dry garments. If the victim is conscious, administer warm liquids, not alcohol.

Drowning

Over the last few decades, deaths from drowning have declined. Possible reasons include less use of alcohol by swimmers and boaters, and an increase in body fat, which makes floating easier.[21] Toddlers under age 4 and teenage boys between 15 and 19 remain at greatest risk. Among young children, 90 percent of drownings occur in residential swimming pools.

The causes of drowning, in order of frequency, are becoming exhausted, being swept into deep water, losing support, becoming trapped or entangled, having a cramp or other attack, and striking an underwater object. Many drowning victims were strong swimmers. Most drownings occur at unorganized facilities, such as ponds or pools with no lifeguard present. Health officials believe that pool fencing alone, along with adequate gates and latches, could prevent as many as half of all drownings or near-drownings of children.

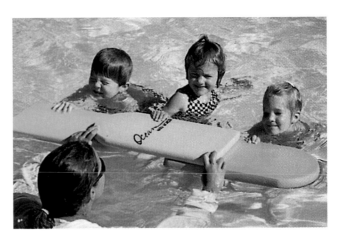

Water safety training can begin in early childhood. Swimming, treading water, and engaging in safe water practices are all important to preventing drownings.

Strategies *for* Prevention

How to Enjoy the Water Safely

✔ Learn "drownproofing," or ways of treading water or moving with minimal output of energy. Know your limits as a swimmer, and don't try to swim beyond your depth or capability.

✔ Don't swim after drinking. Don't swim in the dark, especially in the ocean. Find out about currents, undertows, or sharp underwater rocks before swimming in a strange place. Never dive before knowing the depth of the water below you.

✔ Always use a buddy system, even when swimming with a group. Even a strong swimmer can suffer a cramp or another problem that can jeopardize his or her ability to stay afloat.

✔ If thrown from a boat or canoe, stay with the craft and use it for support. Wear a personal flotation device whenever you're boating, rafting, or canoeing.

Intentional Injury

The scenes, for all their horror, have become familiar. A gunman bursts into an office building, a church, a school, a community center—places we think of as safe—and opens fire. Chaos erupts. People scream and run for cover. The wounded crumple in pain. Some die instantly. Within minutes an ordinary day in an ordinary place turns into a nightmare. As the news bulletins flash across television screens, there is a collective disbelief that such senseless slaughtering has happened yet again. When the shooters turn out to be children or teenagers gunning down their own classmates—as happened repeatedly in the late 1990s—the violence seems even more incomprehensible.

Is There an Epidemic of Violence in America?

What is happening in America? Legislators, teachers, doctors, law enforcement officials, parents, and citizens throughout the country are struggling to find an answer. The "epidemic" of violence—as health professionals describe it—began in the late 1980s and early 1990s. Despite a number of recent incidents, such as the Columbine High School shooting in 1999, the actual incidence of violent crime, including murder, has been declining.

According to the Bureau of Justice Statistics National Crime Victimization Survey, violent crime in the United States declined by almost 17 percent in the 1990s.[22] By the end of the 1990s, homicide rates had declined to levels last seen in the late 1960s, with the

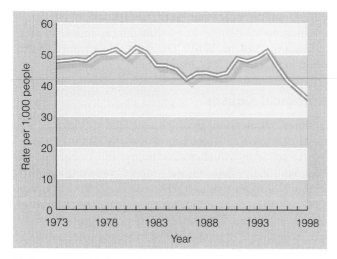

■ **Figure 18-3** Violent crime rates.

Source: Bureau of Justice Statistics:
http://www.ojp.usdoj.gov/bjs/glance/viort.htm

largest declines in the nation's biggest cities.[23] According to the Federal Bureau of Investigation's Uniform Crime Reports, the overall crime index rate has fallen almost 17 percent since 1991.[24]

Nevertheless, as an editorial in the *Journal of the American Medical Association* puts it, violence remains "widespread, long-lasting, and harmful to human health—in short, a major public health problem."[25] Increasingly, health professionals are speaking out against the threat of violence. The best approach to criminal violence, as to other public health problems, is prevention. They point to the successful campaigns that greatly reduced motor-vehicle injuries and deaths in the last decade and urge all Americans to employ similar strategies against violence.[26]

Victims of Violence: Who Is at Risk?

Statistics on violence tell only part of the story. Behind the numbers are real people: loving husbands, devoted mothers, talented workers, students dreaming of a future they would never live to see. No one is entirely safe from intentional injury, but some Americans are more vulnerable than others.

African Americans are disproportionately represented among both the victims and perpetrators of violent crimes. As noted in The X and Y Files: "Which Sex Is at Greater Risk of Personal Injury?" there also are gender differences. Men, for instance, are 3.6 times more likely than women to be murdered and 9 times more likely to commit murder. Young people are at much greater risk than older ones. One in 12 youths

between ages 12 and 15 are victimized in a violent crime every year, compared to one in 357 Americans over age 65. Young, black males are at highest risk. Even the very young become victims. The number of homicides of children under age 5 increased through most of the last two decades of the twentieth century but declined in the late 1990s.[27]

While many people assume that strangers present the greatest danger, this is not the case. Fewer than half of victims of nonfatal violence, such as robberies, do not know their assailant. Three in four sexual assaults are committed by someone the victim knows. In homicide cases, 45 percent of murder victims are related to or acquainted with their assailants, while only 15 percent are murdered by strangers; the others had an unknown relationship to their murderer.

Are Today's Teens More Violent?

A rash of multiple murders on school campuses has brought a new type of violent criminal into the public eye: a very angry, very young male who unleashes his rage through guns and firearms. However, overall, the amount of violence committed by teenagers—both in and out of school—has declined significantly since the early 1990s, according to a survey of 16,000 students in grades nine through twelve by the Centers for Disease Control and Prevention (CDC).[28]

The most dramatic decline in the CDC study involved teenagers carrying guns and other weapons: down from 26 percent in 1991 to 18 percent in 1997.

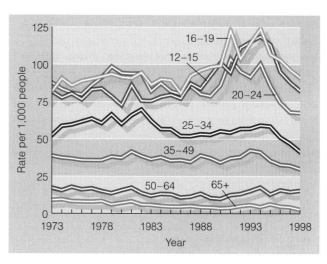

■ **Figure 18-4** Violent crime rates by age of victim.

Source: Bureau of Justice Statistics:
http://www.ojp.usdoj.gov/bjs/glance/rape.htm

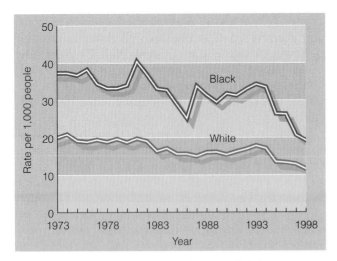

■ **Figure 18-5** Violent crime rates by race of victim.

Source: Bureau of Justice Statistics:
http://www.ojp.usdoj.gov/bjs/glance/race.htm

About 9 percent of students admitted carrying a weapon at school in 1997, down from almost 12 percent in 1993, the first year that question was asked. There was no statistically significant decrease, however, in the 12 percent of teenagers surveyed who had carried a weapon other than a gun in the previous month and no change in the proportion who said they had skipped school because they felt unsafe (4 percent), had been threatened or injured by a weapon at school (7 percent), or had had their property stolen or damaged at school (33 percent).

Various researchers credit the decline in teen violence to the nation's prospering economy, ebbing warfare between gangs that deal in crack cocaine, the shift to community policing, adoption of tougher school discipline policies and an expansion of violence prevention programs.[29] Despite these findings, many people perceive teenagers as increasingly dangerous. This widespread view has led lawmakers and prosecutors to crack down on juvenile offenders, often by trying more of them as adults.[30]

As discussed in the following section, mental health professionals have developed new insights into violent teens. Neuroimaging scans of the brain of a violent teen typically show several abnormalities that may reflect early head injuries, depression, and exposure to violence as a child.[31]

The Roots of Aggression and Violence

While anger is considered a normal, sometimes inevitable emotion, aggression—behavior with the intent to control or dominate—is a threat to individuals and to society. Angry people may want to push or punch someone; aggressive people carry through on such impulses and become violent. Why? The reasons, discussed in the following sections, are complex.

Biological Causes

Traumatic brain injury, which can lead to violent outbursts of explosive anger, is one of many medical factors associated with violence. As many as 70 percent of those who suffer head injuries report some degree of irritability or explosive rage. The use of alcohol or drugs before or after a head injury may increase the likelihood of such problems. Illnesses that affect the brain—stroke and neurologic diseases, brain tumors, infectious illnesses, epilepsy, metabolic disorders (such as hyperthyroidism or hypothyroidism), multiple sclerosis, and systemic lupus erythematosus—can also lead to aggressive behavior.[32]

Certain medications—painkillers, antianxiety agents, steroids, antidepressants, and over-the-counter sedatives (which may produce delirium)—can trigger aggression. Alcohol abuse, which lowers inhibitions against violent behavior and interferes with judgment, and many street drugs, including amphetamines, cocaine, and hallucinogens, are also associated with violence.

In searching for other biological abnormalities that may be linked with violence, neuroscientists have noted low levels of the neurotransmitter serotonin in men convicted of homicide. Serotonin is involved in the control of impulses, particularly toward violent or self-destructive acts. Other neurotransmitters also may play important roles in aggression, and the relations among these chemicals ultimately may prove more critical than the levels of any single one of them.

Sex chromosome abnormalities have been investigated but do not seem to lead to a greater tendency toward violence in, for example, men with an extra Y chromosome. The role of the male sex hormone testosterone also has been investigated. The highly competitive men most likely to dominate a situation or group—whether it's a seminar or a street gang—tend to have higher testosterone levels than other men. But testosterone in itself does not make men aggressive. Rather, scientists explain, it is only one of many contributing factors.

According to recent research, individuals with serious mental disorders may be somewhat more violent than the general population, especially immediately after discharge from the hospital.[33] Individuals with a serious mental illness (such as schizophrenia) report having been violent much more often than those with no mental disorder. However, alcohol and drug users are, as a group, more violent than individuals with serious mental illnesses.

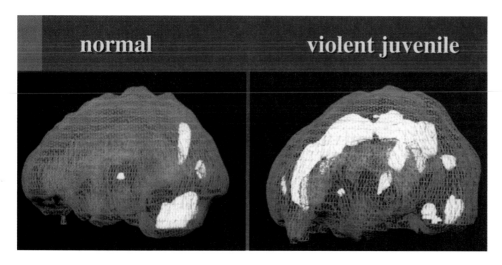

Scans of the brain of a 16-year-old who assaulted another teen show several abnormalities compared with a normal brain. They may reflect some combination of early head injuries, depression, and exposure to violence as a child.

Developmental Factors

Many developmental factors—childrearing practices, parental discipline, relations to peers, sex-role socialization, economic inequality, lack of opportunity, and media influences—contribute to violence. Parents who reject their youngsters, who are physically abusive, or who have a criminal history are most likely to have children with early signs of aggressive behavior. As discussed later in this chapter, violence in the home, especially when it is experienced at a young age, breeds more violence. Brutalized children learn to be brutal themselves. The reason for this may be that such children haven't learned effective ways to relate to others, or they may suffer from emotional and cognitive disorders.[34]

Hate Crimes

Recent years have seen the emergence of violent crimes motivated by hatred of a particular person's or group of persons' race, religion, sexual orientation, or political values. (See Figure 18-6.) They have included the dragging death of a young African-American man, the beating of a young gay man, the shooting of children and teachers at a Jewish community center in Los Angeles, and the killing of teens at a prayer service in Texas.[35] Politicians and government leaders have called for an expansion of hate-crime laws that would inflict especially severe sentences on those who commit violence on the basis of racism, sexism, homophobia, anti-Semitism, or other forms of prejudice.[36]

Hate may have been the motivation in some of the most baffling and disturbing of recent crimes: school shootings. The two young men who murdered class-mates, teachers, and themselves at Columbine High School in 1999 felt hated by others and eventually released their hatred and anger in a horrible shooting spree. Long after this tragedy, experts continue to try to pinpoint the influences that can fan hatred into violence, including inflammatory Internet web sites, violence in video games, television, and movies, and easy access to weapons.[37] Some school districts and national advocacy groups, such as the Seattle-based Committee for Children, are offering violence prevention programs to children as young as age 4, using techniques such as taking turns and dealing with angry feelings.[38]

Violence in the Media

The average American youth is exposed to 40,000 deaths and hundreds of thousands of incidents of other mayhem while growing up. Researchers estimate that, if television had never been invented, there would be 10,000 fewer murders, 70,000 fewer rapes, and 700,000 fewer assaults each year in the United States. Studies in the United States, Australia, Finland, Israel, and Poland have found that more aggressive children watch more television, prefer violent programs, identify with violent TV characters, and perceive violence as

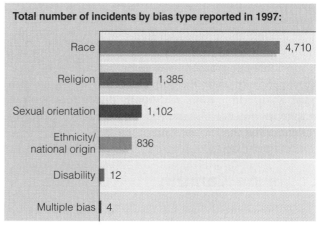

Total number of incidents by bias type reported in 1997:

Race	4,710
Religion	1,385
Sexual orientation	1,102
Ethnicity/national origin	836
Disability	12
Multiple bias	4

■ **Figure 18-6** Hate crimes by the numbers.

Source: Federal Bureau of Investigation.

more real than less aggressive youngsters. They also grow up to be more aggressive adults, with a higher likelihood of being convicted for serious crimes and for aggressive behavior in public and in their own homes. Experts now view the cumulative effects of violent entertainment as a "risk factor" that increases an individual's aggressiveness.[39]

Guns

Almost half of all homes in the United States contain at least one firearm, which may be kept for self-defense, hunting, target shooting, or collecting. Some 3 to 4 million handguns are circulating in the United States; an estimated 100,000 students carry a gun to school. In eight states, firearms kill more people than motor-vehicle accidents. Across the country, they are quickly becoming the leading cause of traumatic brain injury and traumatic death. For each fatal shooting, there are an estimated 2.6 injuries. The price tag for treating gun-related injuries has been estimated at $2.3 billion a year.[40]

Ease of access to a gun has consistently been found to increase homicide rates since, with a gun at hand, an assault, rape, robbery, or fight may well result in murder. It also increases the risk of suicide and accidental shootings by adults and children. Several states have passed Child Accident Prevention laws that make it a crime to leave a loaded firearm within easy reach of a child. However, gun control remains a highly controversial political issue, with intense debate between gun makers and owners and those working toward greater restrictions on gun ownership.

Social Factors

Extreme poverty, deprivation, unemployment, prejudice, discrimination, involvement with gangs, and repeated exposure to actual violence all contribute to aggressive and violent behavior. The risk of violence increases for those who can find few, if any, economic and social opportunities in mainstream society. Violence is most common among the poor, regardless of race. Most people of color, including those who grow up with poverty, discrimination, and family disruptions, do not engage in violence and are more likely to be victims of violent crime than white Americans.

Crime on Campus

Once considered havens from the meanness of America's streets, colleges and universities have seen a dramatic rise in crime in recent years. However, crime rates in these institutions are lower than in the general community.[41] Under the Federal Student Right to Know and Campus Security Act, all colleges and universities receiving federal funds must publish and make readily available the number of campus killings, assaults, sexual assaults, robberies, burglaries and other crimes, and their security policies.[42] (See discussions of sexual harassment and assault later in this chapter.)

Because of concerns about safety on campus, more schools are taking tougher stands on student behavior. Many have established codes of conduct barring the use of alcohol and drugs, fighting, and sexual harassment. Many also have instituted policies requiring suspension or expulsion for students who violate this code.[43]

Many campuses have set up public safety programs, which include late-night shuttle buses and escorts, student bicycle patrols, outdoor emergency phones, and increased numbers of police and security guards. Sexual-assaults services provide counseling, crisis intervention, and educational programs. Students are urged to walk in groups, lock doors and windows, and limit alcohol consumption. Freshman orientation often includes mandatory sessions on campus safety and sexual assault.

Family Violence

Violence doesn't stop at the front doors of America's homes. According to the Federal Bureau of Investigation, the most common and least-reported violent crimes are attacks in which the victim and the perpetrator knew each other at the time of or before the incident. One-third of all murders occur within families. Physical violence may occur in 20 to 30 percent of all American households. As with other forms of violent crime, there has been a decline in assaults and murders by intimates.[44]

Partner Abuse

During their lifetime, at least one of every five women will be assaulted by a partner or ex-partner. Domestic violence is the single most common cause of injury to women—more common than car accidents, muggings, and rapes combined—and accounts for 42 percent of female murders.

Battered women (who outnumber battered men ten to one) are victims of severe, deliberate, and repeated physical assaults, often accompanied by psychological abuse and threats on their lives. A significant proportion of women who visit emergency departments seek help for symptoms related to ongoing abuse, yet only 5 percent are identified as victims of domestic violence by the physicians who treat them.[45] A survey by the American Academy of Family Physicians found that most patients feel doctors should ask about domestic violence. In one study, 32 percent of women told physicians who inquired that they had been hit or hurt in their lifetime.[46]

The primary factors contributing to physical abuse are the degree of frustration and stress a man is under, his use of alcohol (involved in up to 60 percent of battering cases), and whether he was raised in an abusive home.[47] Only one in twenty men who beat their partners are violent outside the home; nine in ten refuse to admit that they have a problem. In homes where a wife is beaten, children also may be abused. The primary risk factors for domestic murder are poverty and household crowding; the lower a family's socioeconomic status—regardless of its racial or ethnic background—the greater the risk of deadly violence.[48]

Abused wives and children are often trapped in terror. Wives may stay with abusive husbands because of love, financial dependence, shame, guilt, fear of being pursued, harmed, or killed if they leave, or a sense of responsibility to their children. The incidence of alcoholism, substance abuse, depression, and suicide attempts is higher in battered women than others.

Child Abuse

Severe child abuse occurs an estimated 1.7 million times each year and claims the lives of as many as 5,000 children a year. However, many experts believe that the incidence of fatal child abuse is greatly underestimated.[49] Parents in every economic, social, educational, religious, and racial group abuse children, but poverty is a significant factor in abuse. Mistreatment is seven times more likely in families with incomes under $15,000.[50]

Abuse can take many forms: physical, psychological, or sexual. Physical abuse often leaves visible marks. However, emotional abuse—rejection, verbal cruelty such as constant berating and belittling, serious threats of harm, frequent tension in the home, and violent arguments among parents—can be just as devastating to a child.

Sexual abuse of children involves *any* sexual contact, whether it is sexually suggestive conversation, prolonged kissing, petting, oral sex, or intercourse, between an adult and child. Because children are not intellectually or emotionally mature enough to consent to sexual involvement, any such action is illegal and a violation of a child's rights.

Pedophilia, or child molestation, refers to abuse by individuals—teachers, babysitters, neighbors, and so on—who are not related to the child. **Incest** is sexual contact between two people who are closely related, including siblings as well as children and parents, grandparents, uncles, and aunts. Abuse—emotional, physical, or sexual—can affect every aspect of a child's life. Youngsters may develop physical symptoms, such as headaches, stomachaches, and sleep problems, and run

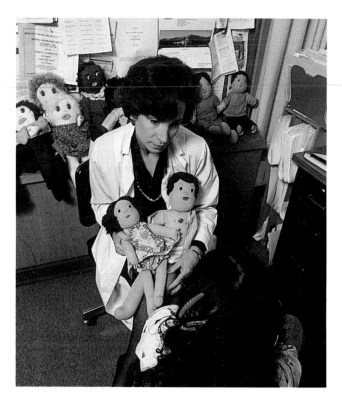

Child sexual abuse. Specialists in the field of child sexual abuse may use anatomically correct dolls to educate children about "okay" touches. These dolls may also be used in discussions with very young victims to clarify the nature of the abuse that has occurred.

into academic and social difficulties in school. Since children often blame themselves for whatever happened and assume they are responsible, they may develop a sense of hopelessness, shame, and pessimism. Some become clinically depressed or develop other mental or emotional problems that may continue into adolescence and adulthood, including more reports of headaches, depression, insomnia, obesity, and fatigue.

Abusing parents are not necessarily sick. Only 10 percent have mental disorders. Many other factors play a role: ignorance about childrearing, absence of role models, teenage parenthood, lack of a partner or supportive family network, and the stress of poverty. However, most abusive parents share a similar psychological history. As youngsters, they felt misunderstood, unrewarded, criticized, and denied the right to behave like children. Sometimes they were abused themselves, physically or psychologically, so they grew up feeling so worthless and unlovable that as adults they continue to search for mothering and love. Often such an individual will marry a person with problems similar to his or her own. When the new relationship cannot meet their psychological needs, they feel rejected. Their children may seem the last resort in obtaining the love they crave, and children who do not—cannot—live up to these unrealistic expectations in turn become the victims of abuse. In other cases, parents who cannot cope with daily stress may feel pushed beyond their ability to cope and end up abusing their children.

Many abusive families can be helped with appropriate treatment. Usually, this involves counseling for the entire family. Within the family structure, the abusive parent must learn to trust, to establish healthy intimate relationships, and to ask for help when it's needed. Parents must learn to view their children realistically; their children must realize that it's permissible to act like children.

The effects of any form of child abuse can be lifelong. Sexual abuse survivors suffer deep psychological wounds, including a profound sense of betrayal and loss. As adults, many find it hard to form intimate adult relationships and experience sexual difficulties. Other common problems include depression, feelings of guilt or shame, inability to trust, drug and alcohol abuse, and a vulnerability to other forms of victimization.

Helping the Victims of Violence

As their numbers have grown and their anguish has been recognized, the victims of violence have received greater attention. In the last decade, hundreds of shelters for battered wives and their children have been set up across the country. They offer physical and psychological treatment, and a haven where women can begin to rebuild their shattered self-esteem, as well as their daily lives. Rape counseling and crisis centers on college campuses and in the community provide various forms of assistance to victims of rape. In many cities, the telephone directory lists hot lines and resources. More than 400 victims' advocacy groups have been set up across the country to advise those hurt by crime. Support organizations help many survivors deal with the emotional aftermath of their experiences. (See "Your Health Directory" at the back of this book for listings.)

Sometimes well-intentioned friends and relatives add to the stress felt by the victims of violence. Here's how to offer comfort without implying criticism:

- Don't blame the victim. Even when no one doubts that the victim is completely innocent, individuals may be plagued by regrets and self-accusation: Why didn't I lock the windows? Why did I park on that dark street? Any second-guessing or implied criticism adds to this burden of blame and shame.
- Don't try to deny that it happened. Although it may be hard to talk about—or even listen to—what happened, the reality of the event must not be ignored. Denial makes victims doubt their own experience and question themselves at a time when they crave reassurance.

- Don't pressure the victim to talk—or not to talk. Some individuals need to go over every detail of what happened, again and again, until they work out their feelings of outrage and become ready to get on with their lives. Others find going into details too humiliating. Let the victim set the tone and limits for disclosure. Don't pry or prod.
- Don't try to rush the victim to leave the past behind and get on with his or her life. Recovery from any traumatic event takes time, and only the victim knows the appropriate pace. If, however, months pass without any lessening of symptoms or improvement in day-to-day functioning, family members and friends shouldn't hesitate to recommend that their loved one see a mental health professional.

Sexual Victimization and Violence

Sexual victimization refers to any situation in which a person is deprived of free choice and forced to comply with sexual acts. It is not only a woman's issue; in fact, men are also victimized. In recent years, researchers have come to view acts of sexual victimization along a continuum, ranging from behaviors such as street hassling, grabbing, and obscene telephone calls to rape, battering, and incest.

What Causes Sexual Victimization and Violence?

While obscene comments or calls may seem minor annoyances compared with acts of sexual violence, all forms of sexual victimization attack a person's integrity. The roots of this problem extend beyond individuals to our society and the beliefs and assumptions—many of them false—that it engenders:

- *Acceptance of myths about sexual conduct.* Our culture, consciously and unconsciously, teaches women not to make sexual advances and to limit sexual intimacy to love relationships. At the same time, men are encouraged to pursue sexual encounters with numerous partners and to view sex as an achievement. Men who accept these gender roles—particularly those who admit to using force or deception to obtain sex—may believe that women who say no really mean yes, and that women like to lead men on. They may also feel that coercion is legitimate in certain situations—for example, if a woman asks a man out or comes to his apartment or home.

• *Acceptance of male aggression.* Boys in our culture learn at early ages that "real men" are aggressive and powerful and are expected to make sexual conquests. Researchers have found that men who are predisposed to sexual violence typically want to avoid acting in any way that might be seen as feminine or sissy; strive for power, status, and control; act tough and unemotional; and tend to be aggressive and take risks. These collective attitudes, sometimes dubbed the "masculine mystique," are used to justify aggressive behavior by reducing women to sex objects.

• *The uncontrollable male sex drive.* Both men and women often believe—erroneously—that young men, once stimulated, cannot control their sexual appetites. Yet, as educators have pointed out, any college-age man would be able to stop immediately if his partner's parents walked into the room. A related myth is that stopping sexual activity is in some way harmful to a male; it isn't.

• *Blaming the victim.* Although victims of thefts, carjackings, and other crimes aren't blamed for what happened to them, women are often held responsible for "provoking" sexual attacks by wearing tight clothing, flirting, or going to a bar alone.

• *Trivializing.* Many acts of sexual victimization, such as the use of verbal slurs when talking about women's bodies, are treated as jokes or pranks rather than serious offenses. This makes such behaviors seem acceptable and denies the very real distress they cause.

• *Exposure to sexually violent material.* Repeated exposure to magazines, books, movies, and videos that link sex and violence may desensitize men to violence toward women so that they come to think of it as normal and acceptable. As they become more callous in their attitudes toward women, men are less inclined to view forced sexual activity, including rape, as wrong and are more likely to admit that they would commit rape if they could get away with it.

 ## What Is Sexual Harassment?

All forms of sexual harassment or unwanted sexual attention—from the display of pornographic photos to the use of sexual obscenities to a demand for sex by anyone in a position of power or authority—are illegal. (See Pulsepoints: "Ten Ways to Prevent Sexual Victimization.")

Sexual Harassment on the Job

The issue of sexual misconduct on the job exploded into the national consciousness at the confirmation hearings for Supreme Court Justice Clarence Thomas in 1991.

"Anita Hill's testimony [in which she described comments about pornographic movies and pubic hair on Coke bottles] sensitized women to things they didn't think about as sexual harassment before," says Barbara Gutek, Ph.D., author of *Sex and the Workplace* and a professor of psychology and business at the University of Arizona.[51] Various surveys have found rates of sexual harassment ranging from 42 to 66 percent. Overall, only 5 percent of sexual harassment victims are men— and their harassers are more likely to be other men than women. The incidence is not limited to low-paying jobs or any particular segment of the workforce. Several recent studies have revealed high rates of harassment in medical settings. In one survey of 133 physicians, 73 percent of the women and 22 percent of the men reported experiencing sexual harassment during their residency training.[52]

As defined by the Equal Employment Opportunity Commission, sexual harassment takes two basic forms: in **quid pro quo** harassment, a person in power or authority makes unwanted sexual advances as a condition for receiving a job, a promotion, or another type of favor; in harassment by means of a **hostile or offensive environment,** supervisors or coworkers engage in persistent inappropriate behaviors that make the workplace hostile, abusive, or otherwise unbearable.

"There's a spectrum of verbal, nonverbal and physical acts, ranging from making off-color remarks to grabbing someone's breast or buttocks," says consultant Susan L. Webb of Seattle, author of *Step Forward: Sexual Harassment in the Workplace.* "But sexual harassment always involves behavior that is related to or based on sex, that is deliberate or repeated, and that is not welcome, not asked for, and not returned."[53] Sexual comments, propositions, dirty jokes, suggestive looks or remarks, displays of pinups or pornography, "accidental" touches, pats, squeezes, pinches, fondling and ogling are all potentially offensive.[54]

"There isn't always a clear line," says Webb. "Each sexual harassment case has to be considered in its own context." The standard the courts use is whether a reasonable person would consider the behavior or environment abusive or hostile. Since most targets of sexual harassment are women, that usually translates into what a reasonable *woman* would think—which may be quite different from a man's view. Psychologist Gutek once asked 1,200 men and women how they would view a sexual proposition in the workplace. About 67 percent of the men said they would find it flattering, while 63 percent of the women said they would be insulted.[55]

Sexual harassment can affect employees in many ways—financially, psychologically, even physically. If they are fired because they refuse to endure sexual harassment, they may jeopardize their own and their family's economic security. Common psychological

PULSE *points*

Ten Ways to Prevent Sexual Victimization

1. **Challenge gender stereotypes.** Just because you're male doesn't mean you have to act in a macho, sexually aggressive way. Just because you're female doesn't mean you have to be passive and accepting of male behavior.

2. **Don't tolerate inappropriate language or behavior.** If you find someone's sexually crude language offensive, say so. If you don't like to be touched by casual acquaintances, back away, and keep your distance.

3. **Be careful of your sexual signals.** Men often assume that women who smile, make conversation, and flirt are signaling sexual availability. Women typically think they're just being friendly. Make sure you know the message you want to send—and don't assume you can tell what someone else is trying to signal.

4. **Choose safe settings.** If you're going out with someone you don't know well or have reservations about being alone with, suggest meeting in a public place or participating in a group activity.

5. **Think about your sexual expectations for a relationship.** What are you willing to do? How much sexual activity is enough? Where do you want to draw the line? Remember, your partner will be making decisions about the same things.

6. **Talk about sex.** Using the communication guidelines in Chapters 8 and 9, bring up the topic of sexual involvement. Let your date know from the beginning how you feel about sexual activity on first, second, third, or twentieth dates.

7. **Think ahead.** Rather than letting yourself get carried away by passion, anticipate what could happen if, for instance, you agree to go to your date's apartment for a drink or park in an isolated spot. State your feelings clearly.

8. **Say "no" clearly when you mean it, and accept "no" when you hear it.** If you're the one saying no, use a firm, even loud voice, and back up what you say with body language. If you're on the receiving end of a no, pay attention. A "no"—even if said quietly and shyly—still means no.

9. **Keep your wits about you.** Alcohol and other drugs can affect your judgment and inhibitions. You may become more sexually aggressive under their influence, or you may greatly increase your risk of being victimized.

10. **Call it like it is.** If you're the target of sexual taunts or unwanted propositions on campus or at work, say, "What you're doing is sexual harassment, and I'm going to report it." If a date or acquaintance won't respect your limits, one of the most effective defensive tactics is saying, "This is rape, and I'm calling the cops."

---

effects include crying spells, loss of self-esteem, anger, humiliation, shame, alienation, helplessness, and degradation. Many victims also suffer physical symptoms that stem directly from pressures associated with sexual harassment, including headache, stomach ailments, decreased appetite, weight loss, back and neck pain, decreased sleep, and other stress-related problems.

Workers who feel victimized by sexual harassment should document their complaints by writing down specific incidents (including dates, times, places, and what happened). It sometimes helps initially to confront the harasser, either in person or by writing a note, and state that you're not interested in his or her attention. Many companies have established grievance procedures for handling sexual harassment complaints. The courts have awarded substantial payments of both punitive and compensatory damage to victims of physical and verbal harassment and have held companies liable for failing to halt offensive actions.

Sexual Harassment on Campus

Sexual harassment starts early. In a survey conducted by the American Association of University Women, 81 percent of students in grades 9 through 11 said they had been harassed at least once. Of these, 76 percent of girls and 56 percent of boys reported that on at least one occasion they had been targets of sexual comments, jokes, or gestures; 65 percent of the girls and 42 percent of the boys said they had been touched, grabbed, or pinched in a sexual way. According to recent court rulings school districts can be sued if they know about and are "deliberately indifferent" to "severe, pervasive, and objectively offensive" student-to-student sexual harassment.[56]

As many as 30 to 40 percent of female undergraduates and 20 percent of male undergraduates have experienced some form of sexual harassment.[57] Professors or supervisors may pressure students into sexual involvement for the sake of a grade, recommendation, or special opportunity. If a student tries to end a sexual

Strategies *for* Change

Gender Etiquette on the Job

✓ Rely on courtesy rather than contact. Offer a handshake instead of a hug; an encouraging word, not a pat on the back.

✓ Use the same-sex standard. If you're not sure whether a comment is appropriate, think of what you would do with a colleague of the same sex.

✓ Give compliments on merit, not appearance or clothing.

✓ If you're a man, before making a comment or telling a joke, imagine how your mother, sister, or daughter would respond. If you're a woman, think of the impact your words might have on a father, brother, or son.

✓ Speak up. If you don't like your boss to rub your neck or you don't appreciate tasteless jokes on your e-mail, say, "I find your behavior offensive, and I'd appreciate your stopping it." Focus on the behavior, not the person, to take the emotion out of the interaction.

relationship, the professor or supervisor may threaten reprisals. Most harassment comes from male faculty members, but both men and women report having been harassed by either male or female faculty. In a recent University of Washington study, college men were almost as likely as women to report unwanted sexual contact and coercion. Overall, 21 percent of the men and 28 percent of the women said they had been recipients of at least one form of unwanted sexual contact.[58]

Sexual harassment can undermine students' well-being and academic performance. Its effects include diminished ambition and self-confidence, reduced ability to concentrate, sleeplessness, depression, physical aches, and ailments. Some students avoid classes or work with certain faculty members because of the risk of sexual advances. However, few file official grievances.

Because college administrations can be held legally responsible for allowing a hostile or offensive sexual environment, many schools have set up committees to handle such student reports and to take action against faculty members.[59] Universities also are discouraging and, in some cases, restricting consensual relationships between teachers and students, especially any dating of students by their academic professors or advisers. Although such relationships may seem consensual, in reality they may not be because of the power faculty members have to determine students' grades and futures. In some cases, students have sued their universi-

ties for failing to protect them from professors who pressured them into sexual liaisons.

If you encounter sexual harassment as a student, report it to the department chair or dean. If you don't feel that you're getting an adequate response to your complaint, talk with the campus representatives who handle matters involving affirmative action or civil rights. Federal guidelines prevent any discrimination against you in terms of grades or the loss of a job or scholarship if you report harassment. Schools that do not take measures to remedy harassment could lose federal funds.

Sexual Coercion and Rape

At a bar on a weekend night, a group of intoxicated young men grab a woman and squeeze her breasts as she struggles to get free. At a party, a man offers his date drugs and alcohol in the hope of lowering her resistance to sex. Although some people don't realize it, such actions are forms of sexual coercion (forced sexual activity), which is very common, on and off college campuses. In fact, about one in five college women report being forced to have sexual intercourse.

Sexual coercion can take many forms, including exerting peer pressure, taking advantage of one's desire for popularity, threatening an end to a relationship, getting someone intoxicated, stimulating a partner against his or her wishes, or insinuating an obligation based on the time or money one has expended. Men may feel that they need to live up to the sexual stereotype of taking advantage of every opportunity for sex. Women are far more likely than men to encounter physical force.[60]

Rape refers to sexual intercourse with an unconsenting partner under actual or threatened force. Sexual intercourse between a male over the age of 16 and a female under the "age of consent" (which ranges from 12 to 21 in different states) is called *statutory* rape. In *acquaintance* rape, or *date* rape, discussed in depth later in this chapter, the victim knows the rapist; in stranger rape, the rapist is an unknown assailant. Both stranger and acquaintance rapes are serious crimes that can have a devastating impact on their victims.

The motives of rapists vary. Those who attack strangers often have problems establishing intimate relationships, have poor self-esteem, feel inadequate, and may have been sexually abused as children. Some rapists report a long history of fantasizing about rape and violence, generally while masturbating. Others commit rape out of anger that they can't express toward a wife or girlfriend. The more sexually aggressive men have been, the more likely they are to see such aggression and violence as normal and to believe rape myths, such as that it's impossible to rape a woman who doesn't really want sex. Sexually violent and degrading

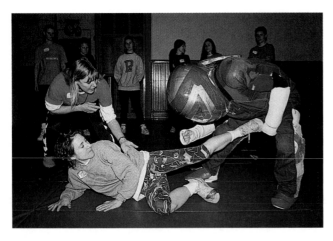

Model mugging courses train women to actively resist assault and rape.

photographs, films, books, magazines, and videos may contribute to some rapists' assaultive behaviors.[61] Hard-core pornography depicting violent rape has been strongly associated, not only with judging oneself capable of sexual coercion and aggression, but also with engaging in such acts.

Alcohol and drugs also play a major role. About 25 percent of both men and women report unwanted sexual experiences as a result of alcohol use. Many rapists drink prior to an assault, and alcohol may interfere with a victim's ability to avoid danger or resist attack.

For many years, the victims of rape were blamed for doing something to bring on the attack. Researchers have since shown that women are raped because they encounter sexually aggressive men, not because they look or act a certain way. However, while no woman is immune to attack, many rape victims are children or adolescents. In a recent survey, 54 percent of women who had been raped said the rape occurred before they were 18 years old. Twenty-two percent were under age 12; 32 percent were between the ages of 12 and 17.[62] Women who were sexually abused or raped as children are at greater risk than others. Scientists are exploring the reasons for this greater vulnerability.

Women who successfully escape rape attempts do so by resisting verbally and physically, usually by yelling and fleeing. Women who use forceful verbal or physical resistance (screaming, hitting, kicking, biting, running, and so on) are more likely to avoid rape than women who try pleading, crying, or offering no resistance.

Types of Rape

Although rape has long been viewed as an act of violence and domination, recent studies indicate that not all rapes fit into a single pattern. Within the broad category of rape are specific, but not mutually exclusive, subcate-

Strategies *for* Prevention

Reducing the Risk of Stranger Rape

Rape prevention consists primarily of making it as difficult as possible for a rapist to make you his victim:

✓ Don't advertise that you're a woman living alone. Use initials on your mailbox. Install and use secure locks on doors and windows, changing door locks after losing keys or moving into a new residence.

✓ Don't open your door to strangers. If a repairman or public official is at your door, ask him to identify himself and call his office to verify that he is a reputable person on legitimate business.

✓ Lock your car when it is parked, and drive with locked car doors. Should your car break down, attach a white cloth to the antenna and lock yourself in. If someone other than a uniformed officer stops to offer help, ask this person to call the police or a garage but do not open your locked car door.

✓ Avoid dark and deserted areas, and be aware of the surroundings where you're walking. Should a driver ask for directions when you're a pedestrian, avoid approaching his car. Instead, call out your reply from a safe distance.

✓ Have house or car keys in hand as you approach the door. Check the back seat before getting into your car.

✓ Carry a device for making a loud noise, like a whistle or, even better, a small pint-sized compressed air horn available in many sporting goods and boat supply stores. Sound the noise alarm at the first sign of danger.

✓ Take a self-defense class to learn techniques of physical resistance that can injure the attacker or distract him long enough for you to escape.

gories of the crime, including anger rape, power rape, sadistic rape, gang rape, and sexual gratification rape.[63]

Anger rape, usually on a total stranger, is motivated by hatred and a desire for revenge for the rejection the rapist feels he's suffered from women. Anger rapists often harbor long-standing hostility toward women, use far more physical violence than is needed for submission, and usually don't find the rape sexually gratifying.

Power rape is a generally premeditated attack motivated by a desire to dominate and control another person. Power rapists, unable to deal with stress and their sense of failure, may rape to regain a sense of power. They use only as much force as needed to make their victims submit and may find the rape sexually gratifying, even though that's not their primary motive.

Sadistic rape is a premeditated assault that often involves bondage, torture, or sexual abuse. Sadistic rapists find power and anger sexually arousing, and may subject victims to rituals of humiliation or torture. They're often preoccupied with violent pornography; their motives are more complex and difficult to understand than those of other types of rapists.

Gang rape involves three or more rapists. Men in close groups that drink and party together—such as fraternities or athletic teams—are more likely to participate in such assaults. The reasons may go beyond aggression and sexual gratification to the excitement and camaraderie the men feel while sharing the experience.

Sexual gratification rape is a usually impulsive attack by someone willing to use physical coercion for the sake of sex. These rapists generally use no more force than needed to get a partner to submit and may stop the attack if it becomes clear they'll have to use extreme violence to overcome resistance. Many acquaintance rapes fit into this category.

Acquaintance or Date Rape

Most rapes are committed by someone who is known to the victim. Both women and men report having been forced into sexual activity by someone they know. Many college students are in the age group most likely to face this threat: women aged 16 to 25 and men under 25. Women are most vulnerable and men are most likely to commit assaults during their senior year of high school and their first year of college. In several surveys of college students, 79.7 to 97.5 percent of the women and 62.1 to 93.5 percent of the men reported that they had been coerced into some unwanted sexual behavior.[64]

Often women who describe incidents of sexual coercion that meet the legal definition of rape don't label it as such. Often they have a preconceived notion that true "rape" consists of a blitzlike attack by a stranger. Or they may blame themselves for getting into a situation in which they couldn't escape, or they may feel some genuine concern for others who would be devastated if they knew the truth (for example, if the rapist were the brother of a good friend or the son of a neighbor). In studies of university students, both men and women who held less traditional gender roles tended to view rape scenarios involving acquaintances or spouses as more serious and were less likely to blame the victim.[65]

Men who admit to being sexually aggressive don't see themselves as would-be rapists. The reasons stem from our society's ambivalence about sexual violence and standards for "normal" interactions between potential sexual partners. According to various studies, 25 to 60 percent of college men have engaged in some

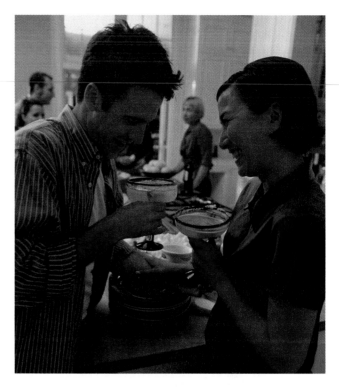

Acquaintance rape and alcohol use are very closely linked. Both men and women may find their judgment impaired or their communications unclear as a result of drinking.

form of sexual coercion. Most often these men simply ignored a woman when she said no or protested. In addition, many college men report engaging in sexual activity against their own wishes, most often because of male peer pressure or a desire to be popular.

The same factors that lead to other forms of sexual victimization can set the stage for date rape. Socialization into an aggressive role, acceptance of rape myths, and a view that force is justified in certain situations increase the likelihood of a man's committing date rape. Other factors can also play a role, including the following:

- *Personality and early sexual experiences.* Psychological studies haven't found that date rapists are more disturbed than other men. However, certain factors may predispose individuals to sexual aggression, including first sexual experience at a very young age, earlier and more frequent than usual childhood sexual experiences (both forced and voluntary), hostility toward women, irresponsibility, lack of social consciousness, and a need for dominance over sexual partners.

- *Situational variables (what happens during the date).* Men who initiate a date, pay all expenses, and provide transportation are more likely to be sexually aggressive, perhaps because they feel that they can call all the shots. For instance, a man may drive to an isolated area and park his car, setting the stage for a sexual assault.

- *Acceptance of sexual coercion.* Some social groups, such as fraternities or athletic teams, may encourage the use of alcohol; reinforce stereotypes about masculinity; and emphasize violence, force, and competition. The group's shared values, including an acceptance of sexual coercion, may keep individuals from questioning their behavior. In studies comparing self-admitted date rapists with college men who had not sexually victimized women, the rapists were more likely to have taken advantage of women—for example, by saying that they loved them—for the sake of sex. They also were much more likely to have friends who viewed rough sex and rape as justified—or even as something that would enhance their reputation among their peers.

- *Drinking.* Alcohol use is one of the strongest predictors of acquaintance rape. Men who've been drinking may not react to subtle signals, may misinterpret a woman's behavior as come-ons, and may feel more sexually aroused. At the same time, drinking may impair a woman's ability to communicate her wishes effectively and to cope with a man's aggressiveness. Alcohol also affects the way rape is perceived: Assailants suffer less blame when drunk than when sober, while victims may be considered more responsible for the rape if they were drunk.

- *Date rape drugs.* As discussed in Chapter 15, drugs such as Rohypnol (roofie, La Rocha, rope, Mexican Valium, Rib Roche, R-2), a tranquilizer used overseas, and gammahydroxybutrate of GHB (Liquid X), a depressant with potential benefits for people with narcolepsy, have been implicated in cases of acquaintance or date rape. Since both are odorless and tasteless, a woman has no way of knowing whether her drink has been tampered with. The subsequent loss of memory leaves her with no explanation for where she's been or what's happened in the hours before she regains consciousness. Women have reported waking up naked in college fraternity houses or in the apartments of dates or casual acquaintances with no recall of what happened.[66]

Rohypnol can cause impaired motor skills and judgment, lack of inhibitions, dizziness, confusion, lethargy, very low blood pressure, coma, and death. Its use has been outlawed in this country; rapists found guilty of giving this drug to one of their victims can get an additional 20 years tacked on to their prison sentences. Deaths also have been attributed to GHB overdoses.

- *Gender differences in interpreting sexual cues.* In research comparing college men and women, the men typically overestimated the woman's sexual availability and interest, seeing friendliness, revealing clothing, and attractiveness as deliberately seductive. In one study of date rapes, the men reported feeling "led on," in part because their female partners seemed to be dressed more suggestively than usual. They didn't define their behavior as rape, placed equal responsibility on their partners for what happened, and said that they'd behave similarly again. They also disagreed with their victims about the amount of force used and viewed the women's protests as token resistance.

Preventing Date Rape

For men:

- Remember that it's okay not to "score" on a date. Don't assume that a sexy dress or casual flirting is an invitation to sex.

- Be aware of your partner's actions. If she pulls away or tries to get up, understand that she's sending you a message—one you should acknowledge and respect.

- Restrict drinking, drug use, or other behaviors (such as hanging out with a group known to be sexually aggressive in certain situations) that could affect your judgment and ability to act responsibly.

- Think of the way you'd want your sister or a close woman friend to be treated by her date. Behave in the same manner.

For women:

- Be wary if the man calls all the shots (ordering for you at restaurants, planning what to do on your date); he may do the same when it comes to sex. If he pays for all expenses, he may think he's justified in using force to get "what he paid for." If you cover some of the costs, he may be less aggressive.

- Back away from a man who pressures you into other activities you don't want to engage in on a date, such as chugging beer or drag racing with his friends.

- Avoid misleading messages and avoid behavior that may be interpreted as sexual teasing. Don't tell him to stop touching you, talk for a few minutes, and then resume petting. If you know or feel at the onset of a relationship that you don't want to have sex with this person, say so.

- If, despite your clearly stated intentions, your date behaves in a sexually coercive manner, use a strategy of escalating forcefulness—direct refusal, vehement verbal refusal, and, if necessary, physical force.

- Avoid using alcohol or other drugs when you definitely do not wish to be sexually intimate with your date.

Male Rape

No one knows how common male rape is because men are less likely to report such assaults than women. In a recent survey in England, nearly 3 percent of men reported nonconsensual sexual experiences as adults.[67] Other researchers estimate that the victims in about 10 percent of acquaintance rape cases are men. These "hidden victims" often keep silent because of embarrassment, shame, or humiliation and their own feelings and fears about homosexuality and conforming to conventional sex roles.

Although many people think that men who rape other men are always homosexuals, most male rapists consider themselves to be heterosexual. Young boys aren't the only victims. The average age of male rape victims is 24. Rape is a serious problem in prison, where men may experience brutal assaults by men who usually resume sexual relations with women once they're released.

There have been reports of men forced by women to participate in sexual intercourse. Typically, these men feel very upset afterward because they functioned sexually in circumstances that they thought should have made it impossible to obtain an erection. They suffer a post-assault syndrome comparable to the rape trauma syndrome women experience, including psychological and sexual difficulties. Men raped by other men also suffer extreme emotional distress after an attack.

The Impact of Rape

Only a small percentage of college women who are raped report their assaults to the police; many don't even tell a close friend or relative about the assault. However, women who survive a rape can benefit from the support of others. If you are raped, call a friend or rape crisis center. Before you take a bath or shower, go to a doctor; you may later decide to report the rape. If you must go to a hospital, remember that you don't necessarily have to talk to the police. Talk to a counselor or health-care workers at the hospital about testing and antibiotics for sexually transmitted diseases and post-intercourse contraception (discussed in Chapter 10).

Sexual violence has both a physical and a psychological impact. Rape-related injuries include unexplained vaginal discharge, bleeding, infections, multiple bruises, and fractured ribs. Victims of sexual violence often develop chronic symptoms, such as headaches, backaches, high blood pressure, sleep disorders, pelvic pain, and sexual fertility problems.

The psychological scars of a sexual assault take a long time to heal. Therapists have linked sexual victimization with hopelessness, low self-esteem, high levels of self-criticism, and self-defeating relationships. Some

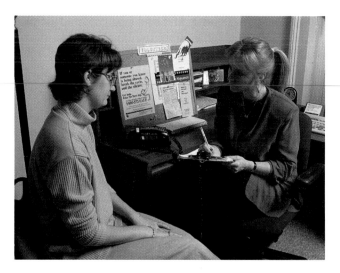

Counseling from a trained professional can help ease the trauma suffered by a rape victim.

have described a "rape trauma syndrome," similar to posttraumatic stress disorder, in which women suffer both acute symptoms, such as crying, shortly after the rape and long-term symptoms, which can persist for years and often include deeply disturbing flashbacks in which they "relive" the rape.

Acquaintance rape may cause fewer physical injuries but greater psychological torment. The victims of date rape are less likely to notify the police, in part because they fear that no one will believe their stories. Often too ashamed to tell anyone what happened, they may suffer alone, without skilled therapists or sympathetic friends to reassure them. Women raped by acquaintances blame themselves more, see themselves less positively, question their judgment, have greater difficulty trusting others, and have higher levels of psychological distress. Nightmares, anxiety, and flashbacks are common. The women may avoid others, become less capable of protecting themselves, and come to accept victimization as part of being a woman.

According to some researchers, victims of acquaintance rape rate themselves as less recovered than women raped by strangers for up to three years after the assault. Years after a rape, victims of date rape may still be struggling with rage against men and having problems establishing trusting relationships. Women who remain haunted by the sexual violence should seek professional help. A therapist can help them begin the slow process of healing.

What to Do in Case of Rape

If a woman has been raped, she will have to decide whether to report the attack to the police. Even an unsuccessful rape attempt should be reported because the information a woman may provide about the attack—the assaulter's physical characteristics, voice, clothes, car, even an unusual smell—may prevent another woman from being raped. A woman shouldn't bathe or change her clothes before calling the police. Semen, hair, and material under her fingernails or on her apparel all may be useful in identifying the man who raped her. Many rape victims find it very helpful to contact a rape crisis center, where qualified staff members assist in dealing with the trauma. Many colleges, universities, and large urban communities in the United States have such programs. Friends and family members should remember that many women will mistakenly blame themselves for the rape. However, the victim hasn't committed a crime—the man who raped her has.

Sexual Abuse of Children

Pedophilia, or child molestation, refers to abuse by individuals—teachers, babysitters, neighbors, and the like—who aren't related to the child. (Sexual abuse by family members is discussed earlier in this chapter.) Researchers find it difficult to make accurate estimates about the prevalence of child molestation. Many victims of childhood sexual abuse are under age 7 and may not realize that an adult's behavior is improper, or may not know how to distinguish between affection and inappropriate sexual contact. Older children may feel ashamed and not confide in their parents for fear of being punished. Even when they do inform them, the parents may not believe them, may be unable to handle the emotional trauma of finding out that some adult they love would "do that," or may not want to subject the child to the stress of a criminal investigation. Counseling can help the entire family.

Parents should explain to children at an early age the differences between okay touches, such as snuggles and hugs, and touches that are not okay (touches under clothes, touches to areas of the body that would be covered by a bathing suit, or any other touches that make a child feel uncomfortable or confused), and the differences between okay kisses and not-okay kisses (prolonged, tongue in mouth). Children also need to understand that they have rights, including the right to control their bodies and say no to being touched in a way that makes them uncomfortable. They should have a talk about strategies adults may use to get children to go along with their wishes, such as saying they're "teaching" them something that will make them feel good. Parents also should let children know that it's okay to scream, yell, run away, or get assistance from a trusted adult if they're in a situation that makes them feel uncomfortable. Youngsters should be encouraged to tell someone right away if an adult has touched them or done anything to make them feel uncomfortable. Stress that you will not be angry with them and that they will not get into trouble. Instruct them to tell anyone who tries to touch them that they will tell a responsible adult.

Halting Sexual Violence: Prevention Efforts

Sexual violence has its roots in social attitudes and beliefs that demean women and condone aggression. As colleges and universities have become more aware of the different forms of sexual danger, many have taken the lead in setting up primary prevention programs (including newspaper articles; seminars in dormitories, fraternities, and sororities; and lectures) to help students examine their attitudes and values, understand cultural influences, and develop skills for avoiding or escaping from dangerous situations. All men and women should understand the impact of socialization on their willingness to tolerate or participate in sexual victimization, recognize misleading rape myths, and develop effective ways of communicating to avoid misinterpretation of sexual cues. Students should also know where they can turn to learn more about and seek help for sexual victimization: counselors, campus police, deans of student affairs, fraternity or sorority representatives, campus ministers, and so on.

Discussion groups led by campus leaders and facilitated by students are very effective in producing positive peer pressure against rape and modeling alternatives to sexist male behaviors. Some campuses have found that all-male workshops are best at creating a safe environment in which men can talk with other men about gender-role expectations, expressing anger without violence, communication skills, and power and control issues.

In addition, practical institutional steps—such as providing adequate lighting, escort services, and clear policies against both violence and drug and alcohol abuse—can help. Some campuses offer self-defense classes, which teach women how to avoid becoming victims either by escaping or protecting themselves. Individuals who advocate such training believe that it can strengthen women's physical capacities and encourage them to be less passive in encounters with potential victimizers. Others, however, view self-defense behaviors as violent actions in themselves, and are concerned that they may lead to an increased risk of injury or death. Followup studies of college women have found that self-defense training increased their feelings of self-

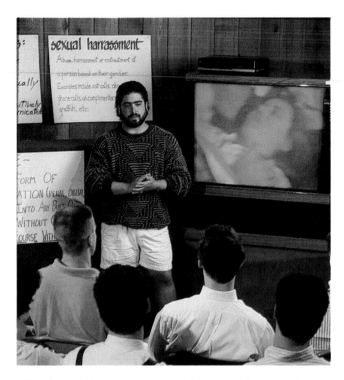

All-male workshops can generate discussion about gender roles, violence, and other societal ideas. These discussions may also provide positive pressure against rape and other forms of aggression against women.

improvement, a sense of control over their life, confidence, security, independence, and physical prowess.

Campuses are also providing "secondary prevention" by getting help to victims of sexual violence as soon as possible through rape crisis teams and emergency mental-health services; and "tertiary prevention" by working with victims to ameliorate the long-term effects of their experience through psychotherapy, educational services, and medical care.

Making This Chapter Work for You

Staying Alive and Healthy

- The major threats to the well-being of most college students are unintentional and intentional injuries. Accidents, especially motor-vehicle crashes, kill more college-age men and women than all other causes combined. Young people also are at risk of becoming victims of physical and sexual violence.

- The risk factors that increase the likelihood of accidents include unsafe attitudes and behaviors, alcohol and drug use, stress, age and gender, environmental conditions, and thrill-seeking.

- The most common causes of fatal accidents for Americans are motor-vehicle injuries. Using seat belts, practicing defensive driving, and being extra cautious and wearing a helmet when on a motorcycle or bicycle can increase your odds of staying safe on the road.

- The risk of accidents is greatest in the home. Falls are a common cause of injury, particularly for the elderly. Fires, another serious threat, can often be prevented by eliminating hazards, using caution with flammable materials, and knowing the proper way to use and maintain electrical appliances, including microwave ovens.

- Work-related risks range from obvious hazards, such as toxic chemicals, to more subtle dangers, such as trauma from repetitive motions like typing.

- Recreational safety demands common sense and proper planning. Anyone who exercises or spends a great deal of time outdoors should be aware of the early warning signs of problems related to temperature—whether they're caused by excess heat or extreme cold. Even strong swimmers are at risk of drowning, especially if they drink before diving into the water or ignore safety precautions.

- Health officials have declared violence a national emergency that threatens the well-being of all Americans. Homicide has become the tenth leading killer in the nation; among African-American youth, homicide is the most common cause of death. The costs to the economy total in the billions of dollars each year.

- Many factors contribute to aggression and violence: biological causes, such as traumatic brain injury, certain medications, and the abuse of drugs or alcohol; developmental factors, such as harsh parental discipline, relations to peers, sex-role socialization, economic inequality, and lack of opportunity; exposure to violence in the media; the widespread availability of guns; and social factors, such as extreme poverty, deprivation, unemployment, prejudice, discrimination, involvement with gangs, and repeated exposure to actual violence.

- Crime has increased on college and university campuses. Federal law requires disclosure of school crime statistics and security policies. Many campuses have set up safety programs, which include late-night shuttle buses and escorts, patrols, outdoor emergency phones, and increased numbers of guards.

- Physical violence may occur in 20 to 30 percent of all American households. Domestic violence is the single most common cause of injury to women—more common than car accidents, muggings, and rapes combined. Severe child abuse occurs an estimated 1.7 million times each year and claims the lives of as many as 5,000 children. Abusive partners or parents may have been abused themselves, and have low self-esteem and little sense of empathy. Abuse occurs within families of every racial, social, and economic group and takes many forms, including physical, sexual, and psychological abuse. All can cause long-term emotional distress.

■ Sexual victimization refers to any situation in which a person is deprived of free choice and is forced to comply with sexual acts. At its root are false beliefs and callous attitudes that stem from myths about sexual conduct, acceptance of male aggression, trivialization of the impact of sexual misconduct, blame of the victim, and exposure to sexually violent material.

■ Any unwanted sexual attention by a teacher, counselor, boss, coworker, or other authority figure constitutes sexual harassment and is illegal. The two basic forms are "quid pro quo" harassment, in which a person in power or authority makes unwanted sexual advances as a condition for receiving a job, a promotion, or another type of favor, and creation or tolerance of a "hostile or offensive environment," in which supervisors or coworkers engage in persistent inappropriate behaviors that make the workplace hostile, abusive, or otherwise unbearable.

■ Sexual coercion (forced sexual activity) is common on college campuses. Both men and women report that they have performed sexual acts because of peer pressure, a desire for popularity, a threatened end to

health **/ ONLINE**

National Safety Council
http://www.nsc.org/
This site provides resources and fact sheets on issues related to public safety, the environment, the community, and the workplace. Topics include auto safety, first aid, air quality, lead poisoning, sun safety, and disaster recovery.

National Center for Injury Prevention and Control
http://www.cdc.gov/ncipc/
Includes news, fact and data sheets, and publications concerning injury care, violence, and unintentional injuries.

U.S. Consumer Product Safety Commission
http://www.cpsc.gov/
This site spotlights consumer products that have been recalled, allows you to report unsafe products, and provides other resources related to product safety.

Please note that links are subject to change. If you find a broken link, use a search engine like http://www.yahoo.com *and search for the web site by typing in key words.*

 Campus Chat: In what environments do you feel the *least* safe, and why? (Examples: at work, at school, on the highway, in the city.) Share your thoughts on our online discussion forum at **http://health.wadsworth.com**

Find It On InfoTrac: You can find additional readings related to personal safety via InfoTrac College Edition, an online library of more than 900 journals and publications. Follow the instructions for accessing InfoTrac that came packaged with your textbook; then search for articles using a key word search.

• **Suggested reading:** "Bigger and Better Here: Road Rage Psychology of Drivers in the U.S.," by Andrew Stephen. *New Statesman,* April 2, 1999, Vol. 129, Issue 4430, p. 24.

  (1) What contributes to the phenomenon known as "road rage"?

  (2) What is the typical profile of an aggressive driver?

For additional links, resources, and suggested readings on InfoTrac, visit our Health & Wellness Resource Center at **http://health.wadsworth.com**

a relationship, intoxication, obligation, or unwanted physical stimulation.

■ Rape refers to sexual intercourse with an unconsenting partner, who may be a stranger or an acquaintance, under actual or threatened force. The different types of rape include anger rape, an unplanned violent physical attack, usually on a total stranger; power rape, a generally premeditated attack motivated by a desire to dominate and control; sadistic rape, which often involves bondage, torture, and sexual abuse; gang rape, involving three or more rapists; and sexual gratification rape, usually an impulsive attack by someone willing to use force to obtain sex.

■ Date or acquaintance rape, usually committed for the sake of sexual gratification, stems from the same factors that lead to other forms of sexual victimization, including male socialization into an aggressive role, widespread acceptance of rape myths, early sexual experiences (both forced and voluntary), the acceptance of sexual coercion, drinking, and gender differences in interpreting verbal and nonverbal sexual cues.

■ Sexual violence has both a physical and a psychological impact and can lead to chronic symptoms, such as pain in the head, stomach, back, or chest, as well as depression, low self-esteem, and self-defeating relationships. Victims of date rape, who may feel too ashamed to tell anyone what happened, may blame themselves more than those raped by strangers, see themselves less positively, question their judgment, have greater difficulty trusting others, and experience higher levels of psychological distress. Male rape victims, whether they're forced into sexual activity by a woman or another man, also suffer emotionally after an attack.

 Gun Violence. What should be done to prevent gun violence?

Key Terms

The terms listed here are used within the chapter. Page numbers are included for each term. A definition of each term is given in the Glossary pages at the end of this book.

computer vision syndrome 574	heat stress 575	pedophilia 581
frostbite 575	heat stroke 575	quid pro quo 583
frostnip 575	hostile or offensive environment 583	rape 585
heat cramps 574	hypothermia 575	repetitive motion injury (RMI) 573
heat exhaustion 575	incest 581	sexual coercion 585

Critical Thinking Questions

1. Can you name two risk factors in your daily life that might increase the likelihood of accidental injury? What actions have you taken to keep yourself safe? Are there any additional risk factors you haven't taken action to minimize or eliminate? What might you do about them?

2. A friend of yours, Eric, frequently makes crude or derogatory comments about women. When you finally call him on it, his response is, "I didn't say anything wrong. I like women." What might you say to him?

3. At one college, women raped by acquaintances or dates scrawled the names of their assailants on the walls of women's rest rooms on campus. Several young men whose names appeared on the list objected, protesting that they were innocent and were being unfairly accused. How do you feel about this method of fighting back against date rape? Do you think it violates the rights of men? How do you feel about naming women who've been raped in news reports? Are there circumstances in which a woman's identity should be revealed? Would fewer women report a rape if not assured of privacy?

References

1. National Center for Health Statistics (NCHS).
2. Bureau of Justice Statistics.
3. Greenfeld, Karl. "Life on the Edge." *Time,* September 6, 1999.
4. " People Saving People: Presidential Initiative for Increasing Seat Belt Use Nationwide." National Highway Traffic Safety Administration, available at http://www.nhtsa.dot.gov
5. Ibid.
6. Ibid.
7. Powell, Nelson, et al., "A Comparative Model: Reaction Time Performance in Sleep Disordered Breathing Versus Alcohol Impaired Controls." Presentation, American Academy of Otolaryngology Head and Neck Surgery, September 22, 1999.
8. "Views on Aggressive Driving Vary Across the U.S." Global Strategy Group news release, September 13, 1999.
9. "An Investigation of the Safety Implications of Wireless Communications in Vehicles." NHTSA Office of Public and Consumer Affairs, available at http://www.nhtsa.dot.gov
10. Berardelli, Phil. *The Driving Challenge.* McLean, VA: EPM Publishers, 1998.
11. AAA Foundation for Traffic Safety.
12. Nerenberg, Arnold. Personal interview.
13. Faulk, Stephanie. Personal interview.
14. "Older Drivers Have Some Problems Negotiating Intersections." *Traffic Tech,* No. 197, April 1999.
15. "National Survey Finds That Most People Want More Enforcement of Unsafe Driving." *Tech Transfer,* No. 187, January 1999.
16. National Center for Health Statistics (NCHS).
17. Ibid.
18. Ibid.
19. Atroshi, Isam, et al. "Prevalence of Carpal Tunnel Syndrome in a General Population." *JAMA,* Vol. 282, No. 2, July 14, 1999. "Detecting Carpal Tunnel Syndrome." *JAMA,* Vol. 282, No. 2, July 14, 1999.
20. Wojcik, Joanne. "Computer-Related Vision Woes Hard to See." *Business Insurance,* October 26, 1998.
21. Cummings, Peter, and Quan, Linda. "Trends in Unintentional Drowning: The Role of Alcohol and Medical Care." *JAMA,* Vol. 281, No. 23, June 16, 1999.
22. Bureau of Justice Statistics (available at www.ojp.usdoj.gov/bjs).
23. "Nation's Largest Cities Lead the Way as Homicides Fall to Lowest Rate in Three Decades." U.S. Department of Justice release, January 2, 1999.
24. Fox, James Alan. "Homicide Trends in the United States." Washington, D.C.: Federal Bureau of Investigation, 1999.
25. Cole, Thomas, and Annette Flanagin. "What Can We Do about Violence?" *JAMA,* Vol. 282, No. 5, August 4, 1999.
26. Wintemute, Garen. "Violence Prevention: Building on Success." *JAMA,* Vol. 282, No. 5, August 4, 1999.
27. Bureau of Justice Statistics (available at www.ojp.usdoj.gov/bjs).
28. Brener, Nancy, et al. "Recent Trends in Violence-Related Behaviors Among High School Students in the United States." *JAMA,* Vol. 282, No. 5, August 4, 1999.
29. Egan, Timothy. "Violence by Youths: Looking for Answers." *New York Times,* April 22, 1999.
30. Cooper, Kenneth. "Youth Violence Declines: CDC's National Study Defies Public Perceptions." *Washington Post,* August 4, 1999.
31. "Warning Signs of Teen Violence." American Psychological Association, April 22, 1999.
32. "Violence." American Psychological Association, 1999.
33. "Violence and Aggression in Psychiatric Patients." *Harvard Mental Health Letter,* Vol. 15, Issue 11, May 1999.
34. Begley, Sharon. "Why the Young Kill." *Newsweek,* May 3, 1999.
35. Sullivan, Andrew. "What's So Bad about Hate?" *New York Times Magazine,* September 25, 1999.
36. Levin, Brian, and Fein, Bruce. "Does America Need a Federal Hate-Crime Law?" *Insight on the News,* Vol. 14, No. 43, November 23, 1998.
37. Levy, Steven. "Loitering on the Dark Side." *Newsweek,* May 3, 1999.
38. Bronner, Ethan. "Experts Urge Swift Action to Fight Depression and Aggression." *New York Times,* April 22, 1999.
39. Mifflin, Lawrie. "Many Researchers Say Link Is Already Clear on Media and Youth Violence." *New York Times,* May 9, 1999.
40. Cook, Philip, et al. " The Medical Costs of Gunshot Injuries in the United States." *JAMA,* August 4, 1999.
41. Henson, Verna, and Stone, William. " Campus Crime: A Victimization Study." *Journal of Criminal Justice,* Vol. 27, No. 4, July–August, 1999.
42. Nicklin, Julie. "Colleges Differ Widely on How They Tally Incidents Under Crime-Reporting Law." *Chronicle of Higher Education,* Vol. 45, No. 38, May 28, 1999.
43. Agron, Joe. "Safe Havens: Preventing Violence and Crime in Schools." (Includes related article on security measures of University of California, Berkeley.) *American School & University,* Vol. 71, No. 6, February 1999.
44. Bureau of Justice Statistics (available at www.ojp.usdoj.gov/bjs).
45. Rodriguez, A., et al. "Screening and Intervention for Intimate Partner Abuse." *JAMA,* Vol. 282, No. 5, August 4, 1999.
46. "Patients Want Their Physicians to Ask About Family Conflict." *American Family Physician,* Feb. 15, 1999.
47. Leonard, Kenneth, and Quigley, Brian. "Drinking and Marital Aggression in Newlyweds: An Event-Based Analysis of Drinking and the Occurrence of Husband Marital Aggression." *Journal of Studies on Alcohol,* Vol. 60, Issue 4, July 1999.
48. Eisenstat, Stephanie, and Lundy Bancroft. "Primary Care: Domestic Violence." *New England Journal of Medicine,* Vol. 341, No. 12, September 16, 1999.
49. Herman-Giddens, E., et al. "Underascertainment of Child Abuse Mortality in the United States." *JAMA,* Vol. 282, No. 5, August 4, 1999.
50. "Protecting Our Children From Child Abuse." *JAMA,* August 4, 1999.
51. Gutek, Barbara. Personal interview.
52. Langelan, Martha. *Back Off? How to Confront and Stop Sexual Harassment and Harassers.* New York: Fireside, 1993.
53. Fisher, Anne. "After All This Time, Why Don't People Know What Sexual Harassment Means?" *Fortune,* Vol. 137, No. 1, January 12, 1998.
54. Susan Webb. Personal interview.
55. Gutek, Barbara.
56. Leo, John. "See Jane Sue Dick." *U.S. News & World Report,* Vol. 126, Issue 22, June 7, 1999.
57. Leitich, Keith. "Sexual Harassment in Higher Education." *Education,* Vol. 119, Issue 4, Summer 1999.
58. Schwarz, Joel. "College Men Nearly as Likely as Women to Report They Are Victims of Unwanted Sexual Coercion." University of Washington News Office, July 26, 1999.
59. Vickio, Craig, et al. "Combating Sexual Offenses on the College Campus: Keys to Success." *Journal of American College Health,* Vol. 47, No. 6, May 1999.
60. O'Sullivan, Lucia, et al. "A Comparison of Male and Female College Students' Experiences of Sexual Coercion." *Psychology of Women Quarterly,* Vol. 22, No. 2, June, 1998.

61. Crooks and Baur, 1999.
62. Reichert, Jennifer. "Many Rape Victims are Children and Adolescents, Survey Finds." *Trial,* Vol. 35, Issue 2, February 1999.
63. Crooks and Baur, 1999.
64. Ibid.
65. Simonson, Kelly, and Linda Subich. "Rape Perceptions as a Function of Gender-Role Traditionality and Victim-Perpetrator Association." *Sex Roles: A Journal of Research,* Vol. 40, Issue 7–8, April 1999.
66. Crooks and Baur, 1999.
67. Coxell, Adrian, et al. "Lifetime Prevalence, Characteristics, and Associated Problems of Non-Consensual Sex in Men: Cross Sectional Survey." *British Medical Journal,* Vol. 318, Issue 7187, March 27, 1999.

19

When Life Ends

After studying the material in this chapter, you should be able to:

- **Define** death and **explain** the stages of emotional reaction experienced in facing death.
- **Explain** the controversy surrounding the right to die, including the influence of culture on life-and-death decisions.
- **Describe** the impact of death on the grieving survivors.
- **List** and **explain** factors affecting the length and intensity of grief.
- **Explain** the purposes of a living will and a holographic will.

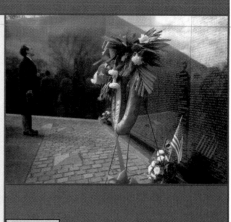

o one gets out of this life alive. Death is the natural completion of things, as much a part of the real world as life itself. If you're in your teens or twenties, death may seem remote, even unimaginable. That's normal: At all ages, we struggle to deny the reality of death. Yet we never escape it. We lose grandparents, aunts and uncles, parents, friends, coworkers, teachers, and neighbors. With every loss, part of us dies; yet each loss also reaffirms how precious life is.

The death that most fascinates and frightens us is our own. We hope that it won't come for a long, long time. We also hope that when it does come, we'll be able to face it with dignity and courage, and we wonder what, if anything, waits beyond death.

This chapter explores the meaning of death, describes the process of dying, provides practical information on medical and legal arrangements, and offers advice on comforting the dying and helping their survivors. ❖

 FREQUENTLY ASKED QUESTIONS

FAQ: **What are advance directives? p. 602**

FAQ: **What is a living will? p. 604**

FAQ: **What do we know about near-death experiences? p. 607**

FAQ: **Does grief affect health? p. 612**

FAQ: **How can survivors of a loss be helped? p. 612**

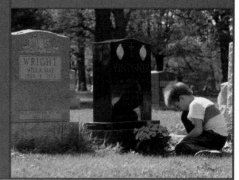

How We Die

In our society, death isn't a part of everyday life, as it once was. Because machines can now keep alive people who, in the past, would have died, the definition of death has become more complex. Death has been broken down into the following categories:

- *Functional death.* The end of all vital functions, such as heartbeat and respiration.
- *Cellular death.* The gradual death of body cells after the heart stops beating. If placed in a tissue culture or, as is the case with various organs, transplanted to another body, some cells can remain alive indefinitely.
- *Cardiac death.* The moment when the heart stops beating.
- *Brain death.* The end of all brain activity, indicated by an absence of electrical activity (confirmed by an *electroencephalogram, or EEG*) and a lack of reflexes. The notion of brain death is bound up with what we consider to be the actual person, or self. The destruction of a person's brain means that his or her personality no longer exists; the lower brain centers controlling respiration and circulation no longer function.
- *Spiritual death.* The moment when the soul, as defined by many religions, leaves the body.

When does a person actually die? The traditional legal definition of death is failure of the lungs or heart to function. However, because modern medicine is often able to maintain respiration and circulation by artificial means, most states have declared that an individual is considered dead only when the brain, including the brain stem, completely stops functioning. Brain-death laws prohibit a medical staff from "pulling the plug" if there is any hope of sustaining life.

The Meaning of Death

Death is not a mystery to those who have died. The living are the ones who struggle to find meaning in it. As far back as 60,000 years ago, prehistoric people observed special ceremonies when burying their dead. Many early cultures believed that people continued to exist after death and had the same needs that they did in life; hence they buried their loved ones with food, dishes, weapons, and jewels. Some religions, such as Christianity, believe that the dead will rise again; to them, the burial of the body is symbolic, like the planting of a seed in the earth to await rebirth.[1] Many Eastern religions share the belief that death marks the end only of physical existence and of the limited view of reality that human beings can grasp.

Death itself is a remote experience in most lives today, something that takes place off-stage in a hospital or nursing home. In earlier times, dying was a much more visible part of daily living. Families, friends, and other loved ones in a community would share in caring for those at the end of life. Our attitudes toward dying also have changed with the development of medical technology and the extension of the human life span. Some people will do anything to delay aging or defeat death itself through medical science or other means. Others see death as part of a natural biological process and work toward the goal of dying well, with dignity and without undue suffering.

Denial and Death

Most of us don't quite believe that we're going to die. A reasonable amount of denial helps us focus on the day-to-day realities of living. However, excessive denial can be life-threatening. Many drivers, for instance, refuse to buckle their seat belts, because they refuse to acknowledge that a drunk driver might collide with them. Similarly, cigarette smokers deny that lung cancer will ever strike them, and people who eat high-fat meals deny that they'll ever suffer a heart attack.

One important factor in denial is the nature of the threat. It's easy to believe that death is at hand when someone's pointing a gun at you; it's much harder to think that cigarette smoking might cause your death 20 or 30 years down the road. (See the Self-Survey: "How Do You Feel About Death?") Yet as Elisabeth Kübler-Ross, a psychiatrist who has extensively studied the process of dying, writes in *Death: The Final Stage of Growth:*

> It is the denial of death that is partially responsible for people living empty, purposeless lives; for when you live as if you'll live forever, it becomes too easy to postpone the things you know that you must do. You live your life in preparation for tomorrow or in the remembrance of yesterday,—and meanwhile, each today is lost. In contrast, when you fully understand that each day you awaken could be the last you have, you take the time that day to grow, to become more of who you really are, to reach out to other human beings.[2]

Emotional Responses to Death

Kübler-Ross has identified five typical stages of reaction that a person goes through when facing death (see Figure 19-1).

1. *Denial ("No, not me").* At first knowledge that death is coming, a terminally ill patient rejects the

Self-*Survey* How Do You Feel About Death?

This questionnaire isn't designed to test your knowledge. Instead, it should encourage you to think about your present attitudes toward death and how these attitudes may have developed. Answer the questions, to the best of your knowledge, by circling the appropriate letter.

1. Who died, in your first personal involvement with death?
   a. Grandparent or great-grandparent
   b. Parent
   c. Brother or sister
   d. Friend or acquaintance
   e. Stranger
   f. Public figure
   g. Animal
2. To the best of your memory, at what age were you first aware of death?
   a. Under 3 years
   b. 3–5 years
   c. 5–10 years
   d. 10 years or older
3. When you were a child, how was death talked about in your family?
   a. Openly
   b. With some sense of discomfort
   c. Only when necessary, and then with an attempt to exclude children
   d. As though it were a taboo subject
   e. Don't recall any discussion
4. Which of the following best describes your childhood conceptions of death?
   a. Heaven-and-hell concept
   b. Afterlife
   c. Death as sleep
   d. Cessation of all physical and mental activity
   e. Mysterious and unknowable
   f. Something other than the above
   g. No conception
   h. Can't remember
5. To what extent do you believe in a life after death?
   a. Strongly believe in it
   b. Tend to believe in it
   c. Uncertain
   d. Tend to doubt it
   e. Convinced it doesn't exist
6. Regardless of your belief about life after death, what is your wish about it?
   a. I strongly wish that there were a life after death.
   b. I am indifferent about life after death.
   c. I definitely prefer that there not be a life after death.
7. Has there been a time in your life when you wanted to die?
   a. Yes, mainly because of great physical pain
   b. Yes, mainly because of great emotional upset
   c. Yes, mainly to escape an intolerable social or interpersonal situation
   d. Yes, mainly because of great embarrassment
   e. Yes, for a reason other than one above
   f. No
8. What does death mean to you?
   a. The end, the final process of life
   b. The beginning of a life after death, a transition, a new beginning
   c. A joining of the spirit with a universal cosmic consciousness
   d. A kind of endless sleep, rest, and peace
   e. An interim period before being born again
   f. Termination of this life but survival of the spirit
   g. Don't know
   h. Other (specify)
9. What aspect of your own death is the most distasteful to you?
   a. I could no longer have any experiences.
   b. I'm afraid of what might happen to my body after death.
   c. I'm uncertain about what might happen to me if there is a life after death.
   d. I could no longer provide for my dependents.
   e. It would cause grief to my relatives and friends.
   f. All my plans and projects would come to an end.
   g. The process of dying might be painful.
   h. Other (specify)
10. How do you rate your present physical health?
    a. Excellent
    b. Very good
    c. Moderately good
    d. Moderately poor
    e. Extremely poor
11. How do you rate your present mental health?
    a. Excellent
    b. Very good
    c. Moderately good
    d. Moderately poor
    e. Extremely poor
12. Based on your present feelings, what is the probability of your taking your own life in the near future?
    a. Extremely high (feel very much like killing myself)
    b. Moderately high
    c. Between high and low
    d. Moderately low

e. Extremely low (very improbable that I would kill myself)

13. In your opinion, at what age are people most afraid of death?
    a. Up to 12 years
    b. 13–19 years
    c. 20–29 years
    d. 30–39 years
    e. 40–49 years
    f. 50–59 years
    g. 60–69 years
    h. 70 years and older

14. When you think of your own death (or when circumstances make you realize your own mortality), how do you feel?
    a. Fearful
    b. Discouraged
    c. Depressed
    d. Purposeless
    e. Resolved, in relation to life
    f. Pleasure, in being alive
    g. Other (specify)

15. What is your present orientation to your own death?
    a. Death-seeker
    b. Death-hastener
    c. Death-accepter
    d. Death-welcomer

e. Death-postponer
f. Death-fearer

16. If you were told that you had a terminal disease and a limited time to live, how would you want to spend your time until you died?
    a. I would make a marked change in my lifestyle to satisfy hedonistic needs (travel, sex, drugs, or other experiences).
    b. I would become more withdrawn—reading, contemplating, or praying.
    c. I would shift from my own needs to a concern for others (family and friends).
    d. I would attempt to complete projects, to tie up loose ends.
    e. I would make little or no change in my lifestyle.
    f. I would try to do one very important thing.
    g. I might consider committing suicide.
    h. I would do none of the above.

17. How do you feel about having an autopsy done on your body?
    a. Approve
    b. Don't care one way or the other
    c. Disapprove
    d. Strongly disapprove

Source: Shneidman, Edwin. "You and Death Questionnaire." *Psychology Today,* August 1970. Reprinted by permission of Sussex Publishers, Inc.

news. The denial overcomes the initial shock, and allows the person to begin to gather together his or her resources. Denial, at this point, is a healthy defense mechanism. It can become distressful, however, if it's reinforced by the relatives and friends of the dying patient.

2. *Anger ("Why me?").* In the second stage, the dying person begins to feel resentment and rage regarding imminent death. The anger may be directed at God or at the patient's family and caregivers, who can do little but try to endure any expressions of anger, provide comfort, and help the patient on to the next stage.

3. *Bargaining ("Yes, me, but . . .").* In this stage, a patient may try to bargain, usually with God, for a way to reverse, or at least postpone, dying. The patient may promise, in exchange for recovery, to do good works or to see family members more often. Alternatively, the patient may say, "Let me live long enough to see my grandchild born" or "to see the spring again."

4. *Depression ("Yes, it's me").* In the fourth stage, the patient gradually realizes the full consequences of his

or her condition. This may begin as grieving for health that has been lost, and then become anticipatory grieving for the loss that is to come of friends, loved ones, and life itself. This is perhaps the most difficult time: the dying person should not be left alone during this period. Neither should one try to cheer the patient, however, who must be allowed to grieve.

5. *Acceptance ("Yes, me; and I'm ready").* In this last stage, the person has accepted the reality of death: The moment looms as neither frightening nor painful, neither sad nor happy—only inevitable. The person who waits for the end of life may ask to see fewer visitors, to separate from other people, or perhaps to turn to just one person for support.

Several stages may occur at the same time and some may happen out of sequence. Each stage may take days or only hours or minutes. Throughout, denial may come back to assert itself unexpectedly—and hope for a medical breakthrough or a miraculous recovery is forever present.

Some experts dispute Kübler-Ross's basic five-stage theory as too simplistic, and argue that not all people go

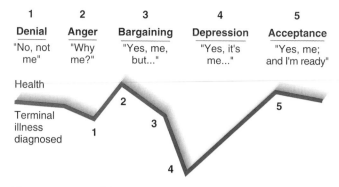

	1	2	3	4	5
	Denial	**Anger**	**Bargaining**	**Depression**	**Acceptance**
	"No, not me"	"Why me?"	"Yes, me, but..."	"Yes, it's me..."	"Yes, me; and I'm ready"

■ Figure 19-1 Kübler-Ross's five stages of adjustment to death.

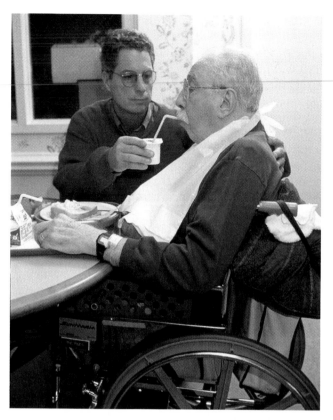

Humanitarian caregiving for both critically ill patients and their loved ones can help to take some of the fear out of death.

through such well-defined stages in the dying process. The way a person faces death is often a mirror of the way he or she has faced other major stresses in life: Those who have had the most trouble adjusting to other crises will have the most trouble adjusting to the news of their impending death.

An individual's will to live can postpone death for a while. In a study of elderly Chinese women, researchers found that their death rate decreased before and during a holiday during which the senior women in a household play a central role; it increased after the celebration. A similar temporary drop occurs among Jews at the time of Passover. However, different events may have different effects. In a study of 2,745,149 deaths, researchers at the University of California, San Diego, found that the prospect of an upcoming birthday postpones death in women but hastens it in men. The women were more likely to die in the week following their birthdays than in any other week during the year—and less likely in the week before. Among the men, however, mortality peaked shortly before their birthdays. The reason for this gender difference, the researchers speculated, may be that many people use birthdays to take stock of their ambitions versus their accomplishments. Men, who in our society often base their self-esteem on professional achievement, may be more likely to evaluate themselves in negative terms.[3] However, the will to live fluctuates greatly in terminal patients, varying along with depression, anxiety, shortness of breath, and sense of well-being.[4]

The family of a dying person experiences a spectrum of often wrenching emotions. Family members, too, may deny the verdict of death, rage at the doctors and nurses who can't do more to save their loved one, bargain with God to give up their own health if necessary, sink into helplessness and depression, and finally accept the reality of their anticipated loss.

One way of reducing the mystery and fear of death is to learn more about it. **Thanatology,** a term derived from the Greek god of death, Thanatos, refers to "the

discipline of humanitarian caregiving for critically ill patients and their grieving family members and friends." Such care, which may be provided by physicians, nurses, social workers, psychologists, and others, helps ensure that terminally ill patients receive the compassionate, respectful care they deserve. The more we all learn about the process of dying and about what can be done to help more people die more peacefully, the better we can understand, and offer support to, the terminally ill.

Ethical Dilemmas

Modern medicine can do more to delay or defy death than was once thought possible. However, the ability to sustain life in patients with no hope of recovery has created wrenching medical and moral dilemmas. Increasingly, lawyers, ethicists, and consumer advocates are arguing that health-care providers must recognize a fundamental right of patients: the right to die.

Health economists, noting that more than half of U. S. health-care dollars are spent in the last year of life, have questioned "heroic" measures to prolong the life of chronically ill elderly patients or those with fatal diseases. Policies on such aggressive measures vary from hospital to hospital and state to state; often medical staffs are not aware of patients' wishes. In one study of HMOs, a third of seniors had filed advance directives stating their end-of-life preferences, but only 15 percent had discussed them with a health-care professional.[5]

Some health-care facilities require that staff members try to resuscitate any patient whose heart stops unless a do-not-resuscitate (DNR) order has been written, usually with the family's permission. (DNR documents are discussed later in this chapter.) In other cases, physicians may decide against resuscitation despite the family's wishes if they think that treatment would be futile and that the family's objections are not based on the patient's values or best interests.

Another major ethical concern is the fate of an estimated 5,000 to 10,000 unconscious Americans who are being kept alive by artificial means. Some are in a **coma**, a state of total unconsciousness. They may have no sense of where they are, no memory, and no experience of pain. Others are in a **persistent vegetative state**, in which they're awake and yet unaware. They open their eyes; their brain waves show the characteristic patterns of waking and sleep. They can usually breathe on their own after a few weeks on artificial respiration; they can cough; the pupils of their eyes respond to light; but they do not respond to pain. The questions of when to use and when to discontinue artificial means of life support remain among the most challenging ethical dilemmas facing health-care workers and the families of critically ill patients.[6]

Preparing for Death

Throughout this book we have stressed the ways in which you can determine how well and how long you live. You can also make decisions about the end of your life, particularly its impact on other people. In order to clarify your thinking on this difficult subject, ask yourself the following questions:

- Would I prefer to receive or not to receive any specific treatments if I were unconscious or incapable of voicing my opinion?

- Would I like my bodily systems to be kept functioning by extraordinary life-sustaining measures, even though my natural systems had failed? If I could not survive without mechanical assistance, would I want to be kept alive or resuscitated if my heart were to stop?

- Would I like the state to decide how to distribute my property or provide for my children (if any), or my family to decide how to handle my funeral arrangements?

- Would I care to give someone else, by donating my organs, the same possibilities for life that I have had?

You can assure that your wishes are heeded by several means, including advance directives, such as health-care proxies and living wills; a holographic will; and an organ donation card.

What Are Advance Directives?

Every state and the District of Columbia have laws authorizing the use of **advance directives** to specify the kind of medical treatment individuals want in case of a medical crisis. However, very few Americans, including only 4 to 24 percent of men and women have any type of advance directive. These documents are important because, without clear indications of a person's preferences, hospitals and other institutions often make decisions on an individual's behalf, particularly if family members are not available or disagree.

According to the Patient Self-Determination Act, health-care facilities that receive Medicare or Medicaid reimbursements must advise patients of their rights to sign advance directives for health-care decisions, such as whether they want to be kept alive by artificial means. These statements allow medical professionals to know and follow an individual's wishes, or the wishes of a person to whom the patient has given authority to make decisions on his or her behalf. However, as mentioned earlier, they often are ignored by physicians and other hospital workers committed to sustaining life at all costs.[7]

A *health-care proxy* is an advance directive that gives someone else the power to make decisions on your behalf. (See Figure 19-2.) People typically name a relative or close friend as their agent. Let family and friends know your thoughts about treatments and life-support. You also should let your primary physician know about the type of care you would or wouldn't want to receive in various circumstances, such as an accident that results in an irreversible coma, but you should not designate your doctor as your agent. Many states prohibit this. Even when allowed, it is not a good idea because your doctor's primary responsibility is to administer care.

It also is possible to sign an advance directive specifying that you do not want to be resuscitated in case your heart stops beating or that you want to be allowed to die naturally.[8] **Do-not-resuscitate (DNR)** orders apply mainly to hospitalized, terminally ill patients. However, in some states, it is possible to complete a "nonhospital DNR" form that specifies an individual's wish not to be resuscitated at home. Patients in the final stages of advanced cancer or AIDS may choose to use

Except in California, where they must be renewed every five years, living wills are effective until they're revoked. Still, it's considered a good idea to initial and date your living will every few years to show that it still expresses your wishes.

"Imminent" is used on many living wills to express the inevitability and timing of death, but it's open to varying interpretations. A recent Virgina court decision found that it doesn't necessarily mean "immediately, at once, within a few days," and that a comatose person who's within a few months of death falls within the definition.

Except in California, Idaho, and Oregon, living wills have a space to specify treatment you do or don't want. Ask your physician what to include here. You can:
- Ask for or prohibit use of artificial feeding tubes, cardiopulmonary resuscitation, antibiotics, dialysis, and respirators.
- Ask for pain medication to keep you comfortable.
- State whether you would prefer to die in the hospital or at home.
- Designate a proxy—someone to make decisions about your treatment when you're unable.
- Donate organs or other body parts.

If your directions are contrary to state law, they'll be ignored, but the rest of the document will stand.

DIRECTIVE TO PHYSICIANS

Directive made this _____ day of _____ (month, year). I, _____ being of sound mind, willfully and voluntarily make known my desire that my life shall not be artificially prolonged under the circumstances set forth below, and do hereby declare:

If at any time I should have an incurable condition caused by injury, disease, or illness certified to be a terminal condition by two physicians, and where the application of life-sustaining procedures would serve only to artificially prolong the moment of death and where my attending physician determines that my death is imminent whether or not life-sustaining procedures are utilized, I direct that such procedures be withheld or withdrawn, and that I be permitted to die naturally.

In the absence of my ability to give directions regarding the use of such life-sustaining procedures, it is my intention that this directive shall be honored by my family and physicians as the final expression of my legal right to refuse medical or surgical treatment and accept the consequences from such refusal.

If I have been diagnosed as pregnant and that diagnosis is known to my physician, this directive shall have no force or effect during the course of my pregnancy.

Other directions:
This directive shall be in effect until it is revoked. I understand the full import of this directive, and I am emotionally and mentally competent to make this directive. I understand that I may revoke this directive at any time.

Signed _____

City, County, and State of Residence _____

The declarant has been personally known to me and I believe him/her to be of sound mind. I am not related to the declarant by blood or marriage, nor would I be entitled to any portion of the declarant's estate on his/her decease, nor am I the attending physician of the declarant or an employee of the attending physician or a health facility in which the declarant is a patient, or a patient in the health care facility in which the declarant is a patient, or any person who has a claim against any portion of the estate of the declarant upon his/her decease.

Witness _____   Witness _____

"Life-sustaining procedures" are those that only prolong the process of dying. Most states include feeding and hydration tubes in this definition.

In some states a physician who will not carry out a patient's wishes must make a "good faith effort" to locate a doctor who will; other states require the physician to actually find someone and specify penalties—in some cases, jail terms—for failure to do so.

In some states the living will is valid for pregnant women. Others exclude women during all or part of their pregnancy, although that has been challenged on the grounds that a woman's right to privacy doesn't end when she becomes pregnant.

You can revoke or amend your living will at any time simply by making a statement to a physician, nurse, or other health care worker.

Several states provide for the appointment of a proxy. In others decisions may be delegated through a document called a Durable Power of Attorney.

In some states, your signature must be notarized. Elsewhere, the signature of the witnesses is adequate although if you're in a hospital or nursing home in some states you may need as an additional witness the chief of staff or medical director.

■ Figure 19-2 Preparing a physician's directive.

Source: Reprinted by permission of Health Publishing Group.

such forms to protect their rights in case paramedics are called to their home.

Whereas a health-care proxy allows you to name someone to make health-care decisions for you, a power of attorney designates someone to make financial decisions on your behalf. An aging parent might give a son or daughter the power to file tax returns, pay bills, or handle other financial matters. One partner might give similar authorization to another. Power-of-attorney forms are sold at many large stationery or office supply stores. Some experts advise consulting with an attorney to make sure your power of attorney is "durable"— meaning that it remains in effect even if you should become mentally incapacitated.

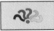 ## What Is a Living Will?

Living wills aren't just for people who don't want to be kept alive by artificial means. Individuals can also use these advance directives to indicate that they want all possible medical treatments and technology used to prolong their lives. Most states recognize living wills as legally binding, and a growing number of health-care professionals and facilities are offering patients help in drafting living wills. You can obtain state-specific forms for living wills and health-care proxies free from an organization called Choice in Dying (1-800-989-WILL). Computer software for preparing such documents also is available. (See Figure 19-3.)

Once the forms are completed, make copies of your living will and other advance directives and give them to anyone who might have input in decisions on your behalf. Also give copies to your physician or health-care organization, and ask that they be made part of your medical record.

The Holographic Will

Perhaps you think that only wealthy or older people need to write wills. However, if you're married, have children, or own property, you should either hire a lawyer to draw up a will, or write a **holographic will** yourself, specifying who you wish to raise your children or who should have your property. If you die *intestate* (without a will), the state will make these decisions for you. Even a modest estate can be tied up in court for a long period of time, depriving family members of money when they need it most.

Many states will recognize a handwritten (not typed) statement by you, through which you can accomplish the following:

- Name a family member or friend as the executor, the person who sees that your wishes are carried out.
- List the things you own and to whom you want them to go; include addresses and telephone numbers, if possible.
- Select a guardian for your children (if any), presumably someone whose ideas about raising children are similar to your own. Be sure that they are willing and able to accept this responsibility before writing them into your will.
- Specify any funeral arrangements.
- Be sure to keep the will in a safe place, where your executor, family members, or closest beneficiary can get to it quickly and easily; tell them where it is.

The Gift of Life

If you're at least 18 years old, you can fill out a donor card (see Figure 19-4), agreeing to designate, in the event of your death, any organs or tissues needed for transplantation. Corneas may help a blind person see, for example. Kidneys, or even a heart, may be transplanted. The donation takes effect upon your death and is a generous way of giving others the possibilities for life that you have had yourself. The card should be filled out and signed; some must be signed in the presence of two witnesses. Attach the donor card to the back of your driver's license or I.D. card. (Whole-body donations may require other arrangements.)

The Process of Dying

Most people who have a fatal or **terminal illness** prefer to know the truth about their health and chances for recovery. (See Table 19-1.) Even when they're not officially informed by a doctor or relative, most fatally ill people know or strongly suspect that they're dying. Dying people usually make it clear whether they want to talk about death and to what extent. The most frequent concern is how much time is left. Usually physicians can give only a rough estimate, such as "several weeks or months."

Once death was a taboo topic even between doctors and patients. Filled with a zeal to heal, physicians viewed death as the enemy; it caused a sense of medical impotence and failure that often led them to pull away from dying patients. However, surveys of physicians show changes in the last two decades. Today's doctors are much more open to communicating with dying patients and their families on issues concerning death.[9]

A LIVING WILL

To My Family, Doctors, and All Those Concerned with My Care:

I, _____, being of sound mind, make this statement as a directive to be followed if I become unable to participate in decisions regarding my medical care.

If I should have an incurable or irreversible mental or physical condition with no reasonable expectation of recovery. I direct my attending physician to withhold or withdraw treatment that merely prolongs my dying. I further direct that treatment be limited to measures to keep me comfortable and to relieve pain.

> This declaration sets forth your directions regarding medical treatment.

These directions express my legal right to refuse treatment. Therefore, I expect my family, doctors, and everyone concerned with my care to regard themselves as legally and morally bound to act in accord with my wishes, and in so doing to be free of any legal liability for having followed my directions.

> You have the right to refuse treatment you do not want, and you may request the care you do want.

I especially do not want _____
_____
_____
_____
_____
_____
_____

> You may list specific treatment you do not want (for example, cardiac resuscitation, mechanical respiration, artificial feeding/fluids by tube); otherwise, your general statement, top left, will stand for your wishes.

Other instructions/comments: _____
_____
_____
_____

> You may want to add instructions or care you do want—for example, pain medication, or that you prefer to die at home if possible.

Proxy Designation Clause: Should I become unable to communicate my instructions as stated above, I designate the following person to act on my behalf:

Name _____

Address _____

If the person I have named above is unable to act on my behalf, I authorize the following person to do so:

Name_____

Address_____

> If you want, you can name someone to see that your wishes are carried out, but you do not have to do this.

This living will declaration expresses my personal treatment preferences. The fact that I may have also executed a document in the form recommended by state law should not be construed to limit or contradict this living will declaration, which is an expression of my common-law and constitutional rights.

Signed: _____ Date: _____

Witness:_____ Witness:_____

Address:_____ Address:_____

> Sign and date here in the presence of two adult witnesses, who should also sign.

Keep the assigned original with your personal papers at home. Give signed copies to doctors, family, and proxy. Review your declaration from time to time: initial and date it to show it still expresses your intent.

■ **Figure 19-3** A sample form for a living will.

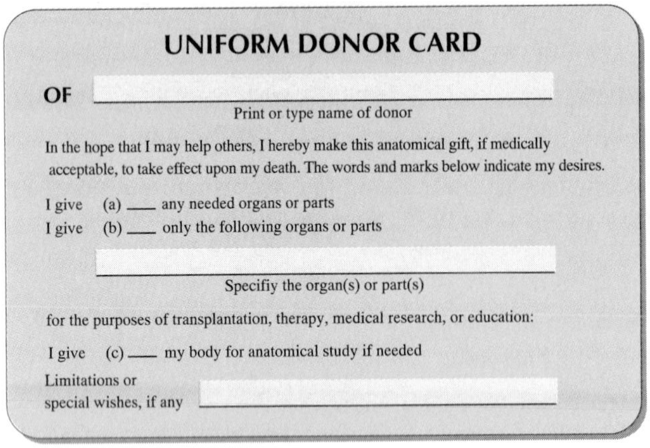

UNIFORM DONOR CARD

OF ______________________

Print or type name of donor

In the hope that I may help others, I hereby make this anatomical gift, if medically acceptable, to take effect upon my death. The words and marks below indicate my desires.

I give (a) ___ any needed organs or parts

I give (b) ___ only the following organs or parts

____

Specifiy the organ(s) or part(s)

for the purposes of transplantation, therapy, medical research, or education:

I give (c) ___ my body for anatomical study if needed

Limitations or special wishes, if any ______________________

■ **Figure 19-4** Example of a uniform donor card.

They, too, benefit from open, honest conversations with their patients.[10]

Patients also are letting doctors know what they want and need when dealing with a fatal illness. As one woman with terminal lung cancer put it, "Beyond pain control, the three elements we most need are feeling cared about, being respected, and enjoying a sense of continuity, be it in relationships or in terms of spiritual awareness." The greatest gift, she notes, is simply being there and listening. "Just as there is no 'right' way for a person to die, there is no right way to be with the dying. The willingness to extend to the patient with freshness, innocence, and sincere concern far outweighs any technique or expertise."[11]

Living While Dying

As life expectancy has increased and high technology interventions have multiplied, many health-care professionals as well as citizens and social organizations have begun to demand a better way of caring for those who are dying. The Center to Improve Care of the Dying in Washington, D.C., has set goals for reintegrating dying within living, thus enhancing the prospect for growth at the end of life. These experts talk of "dying well," "living while dying," and "physician-assisted living." They aim to change our way of thinking about dying so that we view the end of life as a time of love and reconciliation, and transcendence of suffering.[12]

As discussed later in this chapter, physicians who care for the dying are being urged to do all that they can to eliminate pain. They are encouraged not to withhold opioid drugs, such as morphine, simply out of fear of addiction.[13] More efforts are being made for patients to be taken care of at home, with appropriate support and well-informed guidance.[14]

In fact, most older Americans do spend their last days at home and die peacefully. According to a study of nearly 4,000 individuals over age 65 who died, more than half were in good to excellent health a year before death. About a fourth were still in good health a month before they died. Eighty percent were mentally alert; 60 percent were mobile. More than half died in their sleep.

Older people frequently have several serious health problems, rather than any single condition that leads to their demise. In one report, 20 variables—including age, sex, income, cardiovascular abnormalities, smoking, lack of exercise, and impaired cognitive function—contributed to mortality. But, as medical experts emphasize, what is less important than the predictors of death is the quality of life before death.

Pain Relief

Pain remains a major problem for the terminally ill. In a survey of 170 advanced cancer patients, 86 percent of caregivers indicated that their patients experienced pain; 70 percent rated the pain as severe. The researchers speculated that various factors might get in the way of adequate pain relief for the dying, including medical care providers' hesitancy to prescribe opioid medications, family members who have concerns about these drugs, and patients who either don't report pain or fear medication.[15]

■ **Table 19-1** Attitudes Toward the Dying

Percent of Ethnic Group Who Believe:	Korean Americans	Mexican Americans	African Americans	European Americans
A patient should be told diagnosis of metastatic cancer.	47%	65%	89%	87%
A patient should be told of terminal prognosis.	35	48	63	69
A patient should decide about the use of life support.	28	41	60	65

Source: The University of Southern California

However, a painful death is not inevitable, even for patients with advanced cancer. The World Health Organization has developed pain relief guidelines that would provide effective pain relief for most terminal cancer patients in their own homes. The guidelines include several medications, including nonopioid pain relievers, anti-ulcer drugs, anti-nausea drugs, and, if needed, opioids. In addition to standard pain medication, researchers have also experimented with such restricted drugs as marijuana (for the relief of nausea in cancer patients undergoing chemotherapy) and heroin (as a painkiller for people who don't respond well to other narcotics).

Hospice: Caring When Curing Isn't Possible

A **hospice** is a homelike health-care facility or program that helps dying men and women who can afford such care to live their final days to the fullest, as free as possible from disabling pain and mental anguish. Hospice workers generally work in teams, usually consisting of a nurse, physician, social worker, chaplain, and trained volunteers. Other professionals, such as a physical therapist, may join the team when needed. These workers provide the comfort, support, and care dying patients need until they do die.

Hospice programs offer a combination of medical and emotional care that involves not only the patient but also the family members or others concerned with caring for the patient. Most hospice patients have life expectancies of six months or less, and are no longer receiving treatments aimed at curing their diseases. When someone is available to provide care, patients remain in their own homes. Hospice nurses regularly visit all home patients and are available around the clock.

For patients requiring care that the family cannot provide, round-the-clock care is available at the hospice facility. Unlike a traditional hospital, where the focus is on diagnosis, cure, and treatment, a hospice works to make what is left of life pain-free and comfortable. Visiting hours for relatives and friends are flexible, with no restrictions on visits by children and grandchildren. Hospice services are covered, in full or in part, by most major insurance companies.[16]

 ## What Do We Know About Near-Death Experiences?

In recent years, the number of reports of **near-death experiences** has grown, thanks largely to advances in

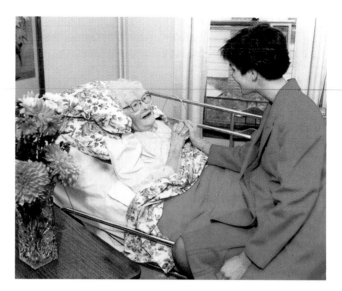

A hospice provides care and support and helps people die with comfort and dignity.

emergency medical care. Most such experiences are remarkably similar, whether they occur in children or adults, whether they're the result of accidents or illnesses, even whether the individuals actually are near death or only think they are. Some individuals who have survived a close brush with death report **autoscopy** (watching, from several feet in the air, resuscitation attempts on their own bodies) or **transcendence** (the sense of passing into a foreign region or dimension). Some see light, often at the end of a tunnel. Their vision seems clearer; their hearing, sharper. Some recall scenes from their lives or feel the presence of loved ones who have died. Many report profound feelings of joy, calm, and peace. Fewer than 1 percent of those who've reported near-death experiences described them as frightening or distressing, although a larger number recall transitory feelings of fear or confusion.[17]

Many near-death experiences occur in individuals who've been sedated or given other medications; however, many others do not. Several studies have shown that individuals who received medication or anesthesia were actually less likely to remember near-death experiences than those who hadn't had any drugs. Some scientists have speculated that lack of oxygen, changes in blood gases, altered brain functioning, or the release of neurotransmitters (messenger chemicals in the brain) may play a role in near-death experiences. However, there's little solid evidence that physiological events are responsible. There's also no proof that wishful thinking, cultural conditioning, post-traumatic stress, or other psychological mechanisms may be at work. For now, the most that scientists can say for sure about this medical mystery is that it needs further study.

The X&Y Files

Who Cares for the Dying?

D eath is the fate of all humans, male and female, but when someone becomes terminally ill, a woman—usually the patient's wife, daughter, or sister—is most likely to provide most of the day-to-day care. A recent study of 988 patients of both sexes whose doctors expected them to die within six months and who lived in five cities and one rural county in the United States found that family members provide primary care in 96 percent of cases. Of the caregivers, 72 percent were women. Among the services they provided were complex nursing tasks, such as changing feeding tubes and giving intravenous medication. However, when women themselves are dying, they—unlike most men—typically must rely on paid assistance for more than half of the types of care that they need.

The psychological toll that caregiving takes on women may depend on whether they are caring for a parent or a spouse. According to a Stanford University School of Medicine study involving 81 women ages 50 to 85, daughters who serve as the primary caregivers for an ailing parent display more cardiovascular stress than wives who care for ailing husbands. However, wives show more stress than daughters when merely talking about the unpleasant side of taking care of their husbands. When talking about the negative aspects of caregiving, the wives' blood pressure rose to a greater extent than the daughters did.

Sources: Emanuel, Ezekiel, et al. "Assistance from Family Members, Friends, Paid Care Givers, and Volunteers in the Care of Terminally Ill Patients." *New England Journal of Medicine,* Vol. 341, No. 13, September 23, 1999. "Heart-Rending Situation." *American Fitness,* Vol 7, No. 11, January 1999.

Suicide

Suicide is among the ten leading causes of death in the United States; each year 25,000 to 55,000 people kill themselves. And for every completed suicide, there are 10 to 40 unsuccessful attempts. (Chapter 4 presents a detailed discussion of the risk factors and warning signs of suicide.)

One of the main factors leading to suicide is illness, especially terminal illness. Approximately three-fourths of those who commit suicide consult a physician, most with medical complaints, within the six-month period prior to their deaths. Disease, medication, and the fear of pain or of being a burden to one's family can breed depression, a primary factor among those who attempt suicide. Treatment can make a difference. Only 10 to 14 percent of those who survive a suicide attempt take their lives in the next ten years.[18] Fatally ill individuals who talk about suicide should be taken seriously; family physicians can arrange for them to talk with psychotherapists. (Physician-assisted suicide is discussed below.)

"Rational" Suicide

An elderly widow suffering from advanced cancer takes a lethal overdose of sleeping pills. A young man with several AIDS-related illnesses shoots himself. A woman in her fifties, diagnosed as having Alzheimer's disease, asks a doctor to help her end her life. Are these suicides "rational" because these individuals used logical reasoning in deciding to end their lives?

The question is intensely controversial. Advocates of the right to "self-deliverance" argue that individuals in great pain or faced with the prospect of a debilitating, hopeless battle against an incurable disease can and should be able to decide to end their lives. As legislatures and the legal system tackle the thorny questions of an individual's right to die, mental health professionals worry that, even in those with fatal diseases, suicidal wishes often stem from undiagnosed depression.

In one classic study of 44 terminally ill individuals, 34 had never been suicidal or wished for death. The remaining ten (seven who did desire early death and three who specifically considered suicide) all had severe depression. Their despair and preoccupation with dying may well have contributed to their willingness to consider suicide. Numerous studies have indicated that most patients with painful, progressive or terminal illnesses do not want to kill themselves. The percentage of those who report thinking about suicide ranges from 5 to 20 percent; most of these have major depressions. Many mental health professionals argue that what makes patients with severe illnesses suicidal is depression, not their physical condition.

Because depression may indeed warp the ability to make a rational decision about suicide, mental health professionals urge physicians and family members to make sure individuals with chronic or fatal illnesses are evaluated for depression and given medication, psychotherapy, or both. It is also important for everyone to allow enough time—an average of three to eight weeks—

to see if treatment for depression will make a difference in their desire to keep living.

Physician-Assisted Suicide

If patients have a right to die, should doctors help them end their lives? Physicians have been willing to stop any extraordinary efforts to sustain life (for example, by withholding oxygen or ending intravenous feedings); such actions are referred to as passive **euthanasia,** or **dyathanasia.** Euthanasia, the active form of so-called mercy killing, has generally been viewed as illegal and unethical. Euthanasia has been tolerated for years in the Netherlands, but it is not technically legal there.

In 1994, Oregon passed the "Death with Dignity" act and became the first state to legalize physician-assisted suicide for terminally ill patients. Despite numerous legal challenges, the act became law in 1997. However, the law bars suicide assistance for anyone whose judgment may be impaired by a mental disorder.[19]

Jack Kevorkian, M.D., a Michigan pathologist, has stirred public debate by using a "suicide machine" to help end the life (at their request) of dozens of people suffering from chronic, but not necessarily fatal, illnesses. He has been found guilty of murder charges. The Michigan Supreme Court has since ruled physician-assisted suicide a "common law felony." Some medical groups, such as the American Medical Association, oppose as unethical any physician's involvement in euthanasia.[20] Others argue that individuals have the right to end their own lives and that physicians who provide prescriptions for lethal doses of certain drugs are acting out of compassion. The debate, which has reached the U. S. Congress, continues to stir passion and controversy.[21]

The Practicalities of Death

At a time of great emotional pain, grieving family members must cope with medical, legal, and practical concerns, including obtaining a medical certificate of the cause of death, registering the death, and making funeral arrangements. They may also want to arrange for organ donations and, in some circumstances, an autopsy.

Funeral Arrangements

A burial is typically the third most expensive purchase of a lifetime, behind the cost of a house and car.[22] The average national costs range as high as $6,000, although they vary considerably. (See Consumer Health

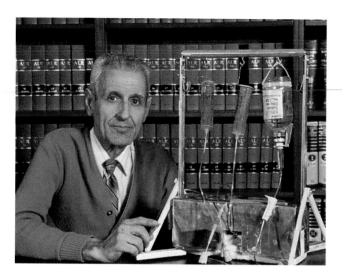

Dr. Jack Kevorkian designed this suicide machine to enable patients with fatal or incurable diseases to take their own lives.

Watch: "What You Should Know About Funeral Costs.") Memorial societies are voluntary groups that help people plan in advance for death. They obtain services at moderate cost, keep the arrangements simple and dignified, and—most importantly, perhaps—ease the emotional and financial burden on the rest of the family when death finally does come.

A body can be either buried or cremated. Burial requires the purchase of a cemetery plot, which many families do decades before death. If the body is to be cremated, you must comply with some additional formalities, with which the funeral director can help you. After a cremation (incineration of the remains), you can either collect the ashes to keep, bury, or scatter yourself, or ask the crematorium to dispose of them.

The tradition of a funeral may help survivors come to terms with the death, enabling them both to mourn their loss and to celebrate the dead person's life. Alternatively, the body may be disposed of immediately, through burial, cremation, or bequeathal to a medical school, and a memorial service held later.

Funerals are usually held two to four days after the death. Many have two parts: a religious ceremony at a church or funeral home, and a burial ceremony at the grave site. In a memorial service, the body is not present, which may change the focus of the service from the person's death to his or her life.

Autopsies

An autopsy is a detailed examination of a body after death, also called a postmortem exam. There are two types:

Consumer Health Watch

What You Should Know About Funeral Costs

About half the people responsible for making or for overseeing final arrangements report that, before meeting with a funeral director, they had no idea of how much a funeral might cost. Survivors are usually not only grieving and emotionally distressed but also pressed for time when it comes to making final arrangements. One local cemeterian estimated that there are more than 70 tasks to be completed after a family death. It would be wise to review the following information before you need it:

- Have an idea of what your final costs are likely to be before meeting with the funeral director. This puts you and other family members in a better position to understand the options, to serve as your own advocate, and to make an informed purchase.

- Final costs may vary considerably depending on which funeral home you choose, and whether you choose burial or cremation. In a study of 62 funeral homes in the Kansas City area, the median cost of staff and equipment for a graveside service was $200, with prices ranging from $65 to $3,440. Always ask about all the options.

- The Federal Trade Commission requires that all funeral homes provide a "General Price List" to anyone who requests it in person. Check with the local chapter of the Funeral and Memorial Society (if available) for additional information.

- The American Association of Retired Persons (AARP) is an excellent source of consumer-oriented information on final arrangements. Other community agencies may also sponsor talks and seminars on the subject.

Source: Bern-Klug, Mercedes, et al. "What Families Know About Funeral-Related Costs: Implications for Social Work Practice." *Health and Social Work*, Vol. 24, No. 2, May, 1999.

---

1. *Medicolegal.* This is an autopsy performed to establish the cause of death and to gather information about the death for use as evidence in any legal proceedings. It is done to detect any crimes and to help identify the proper person for prosecution, to investigate possible industrial hazards or contagious diseases that may endanger the public health, or to establish the cause of death for insurance purposes.

2. *Medical/educational.* This is an autopsy performed, usually in the hospital where the person died, to increase medical knowledge and to determine a more exact cause of death. It may be requested by the attending physician or the family, but it cannot be performed without the family's permission.

Autopsies can be extremely valuable in establishing an accurate cause of death, revealing a different diagnosis that might have led to a change in therapy and prolonged survival in about 10 percent of cases. Thirty years ago about 50 percent of patients who died in hospitals were autopsied. However, the autopsy rate in the United States has been steadily declining, and today about 10 to 20 percent of deaths in teaching hospitals are autopsied. Physicians are arguing for an increase in autopsies as the best method for establishing the cause of death, helping to spot infectious diseases, aiding medical education, and helping assure the high quality of medical practice.

Grief

An estimated 8 million Americans lose a member of their immediate families each year. The death of a loved one may be the single most upsetting and feared event in a person's life.

The death of a family member produces a wide range of reactions, including anxiety, guilt, anger, and financial concern. Many see the death of an old person as less tragic (usually) than the death of a child or young person. A sudden death is more of a shock than one following a long illness. A suicide can be particularly devastating, because family members may wonder whether they could have done anything to prevent it. The cause of death can also affect the reactions of friends and acquaintances. Some people express less sympathy and support when individuals are murdered or take their own lives.

Encountering death can make us feel alone and vulnerable. The most common and one of the most painful experiences is the death of a parent. When both parents die, individuals may feel like orphaned children. They mourn, not just for the father and mother who are gone, but for their lost role of being someone's child.

The death of a child can be even more devastating. Grieving may continue for many years. Eventually par-

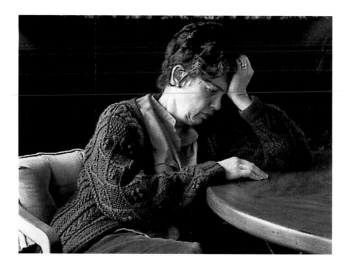

Grief can take an enormous physical and psychological toll on family members and loved ones.

ents may be able to resolve their grief and accept the death as "God's will" or as "something that happens." Time erases their pain, and they feel a desire to get on with their lives, consciously putting the loss behind them. Others deal with their grief by keeping busy, or by substituting other problems or situations to take their minds off their loss. Yet many parents who lose a child continue to grieve for many years. Although the pain of their loss diminishes with time, they view it as part of themselves and describe an emptiness inside—

even though most have rich, meaningful, and happy daily lives.

The loss of a mate can also have a profound impact, although men's and women's responses to the death—and their subsequent health risks—may depend on how their spouses died. Men whose wives die suddenly face a much greater risk of dying themselves than those whose wives die after a long illness. On the other hand, women whose husbands die after a long illness face greater risk than other widows. The reason may be that men whose wives were chronically ill learned how to cope with the loss of their nurturers, while women who spend a long time caring for an ill husband may be at greater risk because of the combined burdens of caregiving and loss of financial support.

All grieving people continue to need support for many months. The anniversary of a death or the first several holidays spent alone can be particularly difficult. (See Pulsepoints: "Ten Ways to Cope with Grief.") For individuals who remain intensely distressed, or whose grief does not ease over time, therapy and medication may be enormously helpful—and potentially life-saving. Grieving parents, partners, or adult children are at increased risk of serious physical and mental illness, suicide, and premature death. The family members of a suicide victim are especially likely to need, and benefit from, professional help in sorting out their feelings of failure, anger, and sorrow.

PULSE*points*

Ten Ways to Cope with Grief

1. **Accept your feelings**—sorrow, fear, emptiness, whatever—as normal.

2. **Don't try to deny emotions** such as anger, guilt, despair, or relief.

3. **Let others help you**—by bringing you food, by taking care of daily necessities, by providing companionship and comfort. (It will make them feel better, too.)

4. **Express your feelings**—through tears, recollections, and talking with others—so that you can accept the loss.

5. **Don't feel that you must be strong and brave and silent,** though you have every right to keep your grief private.

6. **Face each day as it comes.** Let yourself live in the here-and-now until you're ready to face the future.

7. **Give yourself time**—perhaps more than you ever imagined—for the pain to ebb, the scars to heal, and your life to move on.

8. **Commemorate.** A funeral or memorial service can help you come to terms with a loved one's death and provides an opportunity to celebrate the dead person's life.

9. **Don't think there's a right or wrong way to grieve.** Mourning takes many forms, and there's no set timetable for working through the various stages of grief.

10. **Seek professional counseling** if you remain intensely distressed for more than six months or your grief does not ease over time. Therapy can be enormously helpful—and can help prevent potentially serious physical and psychological problems.

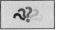 ## Does Grief Affect Health?

Men and women who lose partners, parents, or children endure so much stress that they're at increased risk of serious physical and mental illness, and even of premature death. Studies of the health effects of grief have found the following:

- Grief produces changes in the respiratory, hormonal, and central nervous systems, and may affect functions of the heart, blood, and immune systems.

- Grieving adults may experience mood swings between sadness and anger, guilt and anxiety. They may feel physically sick, lose their appetites, sleep poorly, or fear that they're going crazy because they "see" the deceased person in different places.

- Friends and remarriage offer the greatest protection against health problems.

- Some widows may have increased rates of depression, suicide, and death from cirrhosis of the liver. The greatest risk factors are poor previous mental and physical health, and a lack of social support.

Methods of Mourning

Grief is a psychological necessity, not self-indulgence. Psychotherapists refer to grief as work, and it is—slow, tedious, and painful. Yet only by working through grief, by dealing with feelings of anger and despair, and adjusting emotionally and intellectually to the loss, can bereaved individuals make their way back to the living world of hope and love.

Some widows and widowers move through the grieving process without experiencing extreme distress. Others stop somewhere in the midst of normal grieving and become clinging and overreliant, continue to pine for the deceased, or show signs of denial, avoidance, or anxiety. Individuals who lose children or spouses in car accidents are particularly likely to remain depressed and anxious years later. One of the most devastating losses is the death of a child killed by a drunk driver. Many years afterward parents often cannot find any "meaning" in what happened.

 ## How Can Survivors of a Loss Be Helped?

Although we grieve for the dead, the living are the ones who need our help. Bereavement is such an intense state that survivors may be too numb or too stunned to ask for help. Family and friends must take the initiative and

spend time with them, even if that means sitting together silently. Offer empathy and support, and let the grieving person know with verbal and nonverbal expressions that you care and wish to help. Simply being there is enough to let your friend know you care.

You may also wish to write a simple note expressing your sympathy. A phrase, such as "I want to let you know I'm thinking of you and praying for you," can mean a great deal. A small gift, such as a book or plant, is also thoughtful. Or you can invite your friend to do something with you. Choose something you know your friend might enjoy—a walk in the country or a concert. And don't just give your help over the first few days or weeks and then withdraw. Grieving people continue to need support for many months. The first anniversary of a death or the first holiday spent alone can be particularly difficult.

Most bereaved people don't need professional psychological counseling. In most instances, sharing their feelings with friends is all that's needed. However, you should urge a friend or relative to seek help if he or she shows no sign of grieving, or exhibits as much distress a year after the loss as during the first months. The family members of a suicide victim are those most likely to need, and benefit from, professional help in sorting out their feelings of failure, anger, and sorrow.

Making This Chapter Work for You

Understanding the Meaning of Death

- Many states define death as the end of all functioning of the brain, including those parts of the brain that control breathing and circulation. But while death itself is an end, dying can be a long, complex process.

- Individuals with fatal illnesses may go through various emotional stages: denial, anger, bargaining, depression, and acceptance.

- The ability to sustain life by artificial means has created agonizing dilemmas for health-care professionals and the families of individuals in vegetative states. The courts have upheld an individual's right to refuse treatment and have allowed patients with no hope of recovery to be removed from ventilators and feeding tubes.

- You can assure that your wishes concerning heroic treatments are heeded by several means, including "advance directives," such as health-care proxies and living wills. They allow individuals to state their wishes for treatment options and to designate a friend or relative to make decisions for them.

- In many states, a handwritten holographic will is considered a legal document.

- People over 18 years of age can designate that in the event of their death, their organs are to be donated to others.

- Dying patients often share common physical and mental symptoms, whether they die in a hospital or at home.

- Hospice care provides comfort, support, and needed treatment for the terminally ill in a home or home-like setting.

- Many individuals with deadly or severe illnesses may consider suicide. Often they are suffering from untreated depression.

- Euthanasia involves active participation in ending a dying person's life. Dyathanasia refers to passive willingness to withhold or stop any extraordinary measures to sustain life.

- Some lawmakers and patient advocates no longer believe that it's unethical for doctors to aid in the suicide of a rational patient, but physician-assisted suicide has raised many thorny legal and ethical issues.

- When a loved one dies, individuals must deal with many practical matters, including funeral and burial arrangements. They may be asked their approval for an autopsy to determine the cause of death or to advance medical knowledge or training.

- Grief encompasses many feelings, including sadness, anger, guilt, despair, confusion, relief, and fear, and has profound effects on the body. Various individuals

health **/ ONLINE**

Before I Die: Medical Care and Personal Choices
http://www.wnet.org/archive/bid/
This PBS web site explores some of the medical, ethical, and social issues surrounding end-of-life care in America today via six real-life stories. It also includes numerous articles on topics like hospices, living wills, advance directives, and paying for long-term care.

Last Rights
http://www.last-rights.com/main.html
Provides information on how to talk about death, how to ensure that one's wishes are carried out after death, how to draft a living will, and more.

Bereavement Self-Help Resources Guide
http://www.inforamp.net/~bfo/guide/index.html
This site provides online resources for those who have lost a loved one, including information about support groups and dealing with grief.

Please note that links are subject to change. If you find a broken link, use a search engine like http://www.yahoo.com *and search for the web site by typing in key words.*

Campus Chat: Are you for or against physician-assisted suicide? Explain your position and share your thoughts on our online discussion forum at **http://health.wadsworth.com**

 Find It On InfoTrac: You can find additional readings related to topics discussed in this chapter via InfoTrac College Edition, an online library of more than 900 journals and publications. Follow the instructions for accessing InfoTrac that came packaged with your textbook; then search for articles using a key word search.

- **Suggested reading:** "The Dying Adult: Coping With Loss," by Colin Murray Parkes. *British Medical Journal*, April 25, 1998, Vol. 316, No. 7140, p. 1313.

  (1) What are two common problems that arise when people come close to death?

  (2) What are the five stages of death acceptance described by Elizabeth Kübler-Ross? Why have these stages been criticized?

For additional links, resources, and suggested readings on InfoTrac, visit our Health & Wellness Resource Center at http://health.wadsworth.com

mourn in different ways, depending on the cause of the death, the age and health of the person who died, and the survivor's age and life circumstances.

Thinking about death can be difficult. It can also be peaceful, depending on how we envision what is beyond. Realizing that life won't go on forever can be a frightening thought. However, the realization that our lives have limits is what makes every day, every minute, of living so very precious.

Key Terms

The terms listed here are used within the chapter. Page numbers are included for each term. A definition of each term is given in the Glossary pages at the end of this book.

advance directives   602
autoscopy   607
coma   602
do-not-resuscitate (DNR)   602
dyathanasia   609

euthanasia   609
holographic will   604
hospice   607
living wills   604
near-death experiences   607

persistent vegetative state   602
terminal illness   604
thanatology   601
transcendence   607

Critical Thinking Questions

1. Do you think that coming to terms with mortality allows an individual to live each day to its fullest, rather than putting off what he or she would like to do until tomorrow? How does this concept affect your own life? Explain. Do you believe in a next life or a greater reality? If so, how does this affect your view of life and death?

2. In 20 cases over the last 50 years, family members accused of mercy killings of fatally ill relatives have gone to trial. One was a father who held off hospital workers with a pistol while he unplugged his baby's respirator. Another was a man who suffocated his wife, who had Alzheimer's disease, with a pillow. Only three of the defendants were sentenced to jail. Do you think these individuals should have been put on trial?

Should all have been punished? Are there circumstances that would make mercy killing a crime in some cases but not in others?

3. As many as 10,000 people in this country are chronically unconscious, kept alive by artificial respirators and feeding tubes. What if you were in an accident that left you in a vegetative state? Would you want doctors to do everything possible to fight for your life? Would you want to spend months or even years totally unaware of your surroundings? Should health-care professionals have the right to declare that anyone is too old, too ill, or too frail to try to save? Should they have the right to insist that someone live on even if that person isn't experiencing much of a "life"?

References

1. Jones, L. Gregory. "Shaped by Lament and Hope." *The Christian Century,* Vol. 116, Issue 12, April 14, 1999.
2. Kübler-Ross, Elisabeth. *Death: The Final Stage of Growth.* Englewood Cliffs, NJ: Prentice-Hall, 1975.
3. Phillips, David, et al. "The Birthday: Lifeline or Deathline?" *Psychosomatic Medicine,* September–October 1992.
4. Chochinov, Harvey Max, et al. "Will to Live in the Terminally Ill." *Lancet,* Vol. 354, No. 9181, September 4, 1999.
5. Gordon, Nancy, and Shade, Starley. "Advance Directives Are More Likely Among Seniors Asked About End-of-Life Care Preferences." *Archives of Internal Medicine,* April 12, 1999.
6. "Heart-Rending Situation." *American Fitness,* Vol. 17, Issue 1, January 1999.
7. Parkman, Cynthia, and Barbara Calfee. "Advance Directives: Honoring Your Patient's End-of-Life Wishes." *Nursing,* Vol. 27, No. 4, April 1997.

8. Thomas, William, et al. "Advance Directives in the Perioperative Setting." *AORN Journal,* Vol. 66, No. 4, October 1997.
9. Dickinson, George, et al. "Twenty Years Beyond Medical School." *Archives of Internal Medicine,* August 9, 1999.
10. Mirando, Sally. "Doctors Can Benefit from Spending Time with Their Dying Patients." *British Medical Journal,* Vol. 318, No. 7200, June 26, 1999.
11. Fahnestock, Deborah. "Partnership for Good Dying." *JAMA,* Vol. 282, No. 7, August 18, 1999.
12. Khan, Mark. "Our Duty Lasts Until the End of Life." *British Medical Journal,* Vol. 219, Issue 7206, August 7, 1999.
13. "Clinical Practice Guidelines, No. 9, Management of Cancer Pain." Agency for Health Care Policy and Research; available on the Internet at http://www.ahcpr.gov
14. Reichel, William. "End-of-Life Care and Family Practice." *American Family Physician,* Vol. 59, Issue 6, March 15, 1999.

15. Lindgren, Maryclaire. "Cancer Patients Die Painfully." *Cancer Weekly Plus,* April 19, 1999.

16. Friedrich, M. "Hospice Care in the United States." *JAMA,* May 12, 1999.

17. Wrenn, Robert. "The Near Death Experience," *Omega—The Journal of Death and Dying,* Vol. 35, No. 4, December 1997.

18. Chochinov. "Will to Live in the Terminally Ill."

19. Fenn, Darien, and Ganzini, Linda. "Attitudes of Oregon Psychologists Toward Physician-Assisted Suicide and the Oregon Death with Dignity Act." *Professional Psychology: Research and Practice,* Vol. 30, No. 3, June 1999.

20. Baron, Charles. "Assisted Dying." *Trial,* Vol. 35, No. 7, July, 1999.

21. Salem, Tania. "Physician-Assisted Suicide." *Hastings Center Report,* Vol. 29, No. 3, May 1999.

22. Bern-Klug, Mercedes, et al. "What Families Know About Funeral-Related Costs: Implications for Social Practice." *Health and Social Work,* Vol. 24, No. 2, May, 1999.

20

Working Toward a Healthy Environment

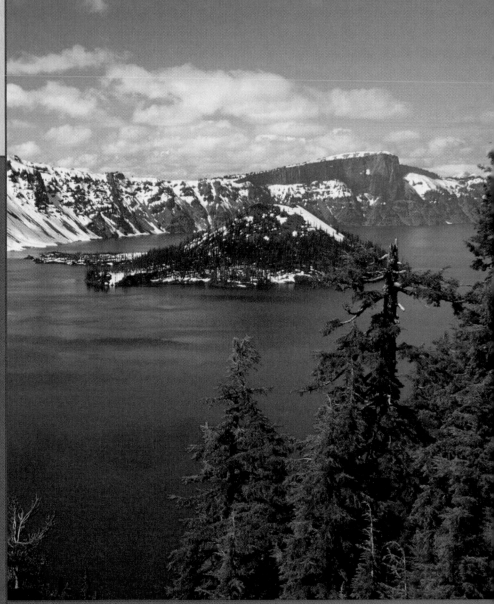

After studying the material in this chapter, you should be able to:

- **List** and **explain** the major hazards to the survival of our planet.
- **List** and **explain** the major types of indoor pollution.
- **Explain** the hazardous impact of chemicals on air, land, and water.
- **Describe** ways to protect your ears from noise-induced hearing loss.
- **Define** *electromagnetic fields*, and **describe** the recommended procedures to protect yourself from their dangers.
- **Explain** the risks of radiation.

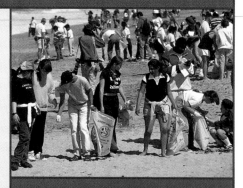

I n some ways, this is both the best and the worst of times for the planet we call home. Never before has global attention focused so sharply on the fate of the world. Never before have scientists known so much about the complexities of life on earth. Yet, at the same time, the threats to our planet have never seemed so great nor the quest for solutions so challenging.

The World Health Organization (WHO) has stated that "a healthy environment is not only a need, it is also a right," a right that everyone—governments, businesses, research institutions, communities, and individuals—is responsible for upholding. If you, as a citizen of the world, don't become part of the solution, you end up as part of the problem. And, the fact is, you *can* help find solutions. The first step is realizing that you have a personal responsibility for safeguarding the health of your environment and, thereby, your own well-being.

This chapter explores the complex interrelationships between your world and your well-being. It discusses the major threats to the environment—including overpopulation; atmospheric changes; depletion of resources; air, water, and noise pollution; chemical risks; and radiation—and provides specific guidance on what you can do about them. ❖

 FREQUENTLY ASKED QUESTIONS

FAQ: **How big is the world's population? p. 619**

FAQ: **What is global warming? p. 621**

FAQ: **What is acid rain? p. 626**

FAQ: **Is bottled water better? p. 630**

FAQ: **What health risks are caused by pesticides? p. 631**

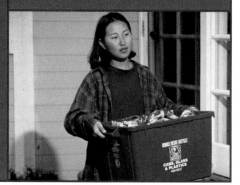

The State of the Environment

The planet earth—once taken for granted as a ball of rock and water that existed for our use for all time—now is seen as a single, fragile **ecosystem** (a community of organisms that share a physical and chemical environment). Our environment is a closed ecosystem, powered by the sun. The materials needed for the survival of this planet must be recycled over and over again. Increasingly, we're realizing just how important the health of this ecosystem is to our own well-being and survival. However, as shown in Campus Focus: "Do Students Care about the Environment?" the majority of undergraduates do not share this concern.

At the beginning of the twenty-first century, environmental experts predict new dangers to human life and health.[1] These include acts of biological or chemical terrorism, natural disasters, contamination of water supplies, and hazardous waste disposal.[2] One of the greatest challenges is the creation of a shared vision of a global society that is fair and equitable to all people today and for generations to come.[3] This will require a different type of health decision-making—one that takes into account both individual and societal risks and that may lead to recommended action, such as bans on potential toxins, before definitive scientific knowledge is available.[4]

Our Planet, Our Health

Our environment affects our well-being both directly and indirectly. Changes in temperature and rainfall patterns disturb ecological processes in ways that can be hazardous to health.[5] For instance, patterns of infectious disease change as insects like mosquitoes and ticks, influenced by temperature variations, travel in new directions, breed in new places, and transmit illness to new groups of people. The deterioration of the environment has already contributed to the emergence of several diseases that affect the brain and nervous system, including transmissible spongiform encephalopathy and Creutzfeldt-Jakob disease.[6] Warmer weather—a consequence of changes in atmospheric gases and climate discussed later in this chapter—worsens urban-industrial air pollution and, if the air also is moist, increases concentrations of allergenic pollens and fungal spores. Not all climactic changes are harmful, however. Warmer winters, as an example, might mean fewer illnesses and lower cold-weather mortality.[7]

No individual is immune to environmental health threats. Depletion of the ozone layer has already been implicated in the increase in skin cancers and cataracts. Global warming, according to some theorists, might lead to change in one-third to one-half of the world's vegetation types and to the extinction of many plant and animal species. A warmer world is expected to produce more severe flooding in some places and more severe droughts in others, jeopardizing natural resources and the safety of our water supply. These are truly problems without borders.[8]

For good or for ill, we cannot separate our individual health from that of the environment in which we live. The air we breathe, the water we drink, the chemicals we use all have an impact on the quality of our lives. At the same time, the lifestyle choices we make, the products we use, the efforts we undertake to clean up a beach or save wetlands affect the quality of our environment.

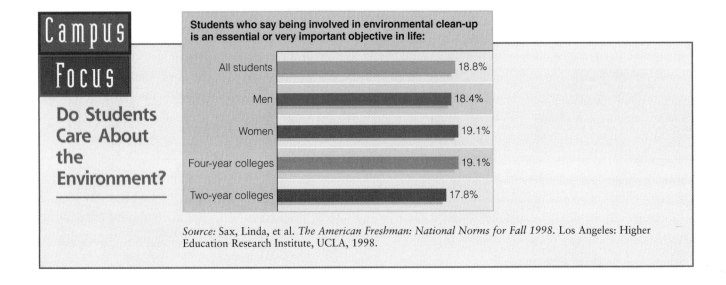

Campus Focus

Do Students Care About the Environment?

Students who say being involved in environmental clean-up is an essential or very important objective in life:

All students	18.8%
Men	18.4%
Women	19.1%
Four-year colleges	19.1%
Two-year colleges	17.8%

Source: Sax, Linda, et al. *The American Freshman: National Norms for Fall 1998.* Los Angeles: Higher Education Research Institute, UCLA, 1998.

Multiple Chemical Sensitivity

The proliferation of chemicals in modern society has led to an entirely new disease, **multiple chemical sensitivity (MCS)**, also called environmentally triggered illness, twentieth-century disease, universal allergy, or chemical AIDS. MCS was first described almost a half century ago when a Chicago allergist treated a number of patients who reported becoming ill after being exposed to various petrochemicals. Since that time, many more cases of MCS have been reported, yet there is no agreed-upon definition for the condition, no medical test that can diagnose it, and no proven treatment.[9]

According to medical theory, people become chemically sensitive in a two-step process: First, they experience a "major" exposure to a chemical, such as a pesticide, a solvent, or a combustion product. The sensitized person then begins to react to low-level chemical exposures from ordinary substances, such as perfumes and tobacco smoke. In other words, these low-level exposures trigger a physiological response. Over time, chemically unrelated substances may induce symptoms such as chest pain, depression, difficulty remembering, dizziness, fatigue, headache, inability to concentrate, nausea, and aches and pains in muscles and joints.[10]

Individuals who may be at risk of MCS include Persian Gulf veterans, industrial workers, occupants of "sick buildings" with high levels of indoor pollutants, and people who live near contaminated sites. Because of the variety of racial, ethnic, and socioeconomic groups affected, an increasing number of medical professionals have become convinced that MCS is a real and serious health problem that requires extensive investigation.

The Fight to Save the Earth

Concern over the future of our environment has brought the nations of the world together in a search for solutions. One problem is the great chasm between rich countries, concentrated in the northern hemisphere, and poor nations, mainly in the south. Affluent nations have more cars, more heavy industry, and higher energy consumption. For instance, the United States, with only 5 percent of the world's population, uses a much greater percentage of the earth's resources than any other region of the world. Poor countries tend to blame the industrialized nations for environmental problems, whereas the rich nations fear that the high birthrates and rapid industrialization of developing nations may jeopardize the progress that has been made in limiting pollution and protecting the environment.

Increasingly, all nations are recognizing the need to abandon destructive practices in favor of "sustainable" development—that is, economic growth that doesn't

cause irreparable damage to the environment. Ever since the United Nations Conference on Environment and Development, also called the Earth Summit, in 1992 the International Conference on Population and Development in Cairo in 1994, and the Kyoto Conference on Global Warming in 1997, some 150 countries have been working toward both economic and political solutions to environmental woes. For instance, they've agreed that polluters ought to bear the cost of the damage they cause to the environment, that family planning should be promoted, that special priority should be given to the needs of developing countries, and that emissions of certain dangerous gases should be cut back.

Formed in 1970 and often under fire for being too lax or too tough, the Environmental Protection Agency (EPA) has helped enforce laws to ensure clean air and water; manage solid waste; and control toxic substances, pesticides, radiation, and other potential dangers. In addition, many private groups, such as Friends of the Earth and the Audubon Society, have been working to preserve and restore natural resources. Although no one denies that the environment is in peril, there is also great promise in working together at community, corporate, national, and international levels to overcome the threats to the planet.

 ## How Big Is the World's Population?

In the year 1800, about 1 billion people lived on earth. The world's population grew to 2 billion in the next 130

Strategies *for* Change

How to Slow Population Growth

Policymakers suggest that social and political changes are critical in preventing global overpopulation:

✔ Improve the quality of reproductive services and family planning services around the globe.

✔ Meet current needs for contraception. This alone could cut the population projections for the year 2100 by nearly 2 billion.

✔ Increase access to education for girls and opportunities for women. Educated women with recognized status—whether because of paid jobs or positions of respect with-in the community—have fewer and healthier children.

✔ Involve men. Men who share equally in childrearing take more responsibility for family planning.

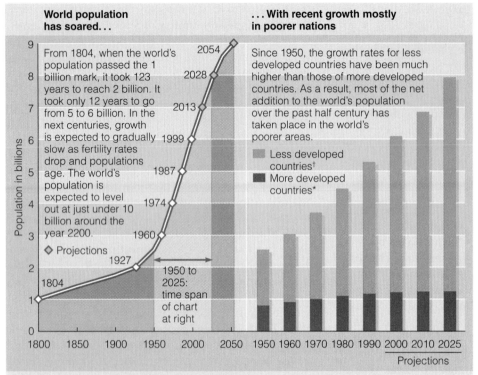

World population has soared...

From 1804, when the world's population passed the 1 billion mark, it took 123 years to reach 2 billion. It took only 12 years to go from 5 to 6 billion. In the next centuries, growth is expected to gradually slow as fertility rates drop and populations age. The world's population is expected to level out at just under 10 billion around the year 2200.

◇ Projections

1804
1927
1960
1974
1987
1999
2013
2028
2054

1950 to 2025: time span of chart at right

Population in billions

1800 1850 1900 1950 2000 2050

...With recent growth mostly in poorer nations

Since 1950, the growth rates for less developed countries have been much higher than those of more developed countries. As a result, most of the net addition to the world's population over the past half century has taken place in the world's poorer areas.

☐ Less developed countries†
☐ More developed countries*

1950 1960 1970 1980 1990 2000 2010 2025
Projections

* "More developed" countries and areas include North America, Europe, Japan, Australia and New Zealand. †"Less developed" countries include all of Africa, all of Asia except Japan, the Transcaucasian and Central Asian countries of the former Soviet Union, all of Latin America and the Caribbean, and all of Oceania except Australia and New Zealand.

■ Figure 20-1 The growing world population.

Source: New York Times, Sunday, September 19, 1999. Reprinted by permission.

years (1930); to 3 billion in 30 years (1960); to 4 billion in 15 years (1975); to 5 billion in 12 years (1987): In 1999 it reached 6 billion. The world population, which is now growing more slowly, could stabilize at 8 billion by the year 2025. (The point at which the number of births equals the numbers of deaths is called **zero population growth.**) However, the population crisis is far from over. Just ten countries, led by China and India, account for 60 percent of the world's population increase. At least 74 countries—including Ethiopia, El Salvador, Nigeria, Iran, Iraq, and Syria—are expected to double their populations in the next 30 years.[11] (See Figure 20-1.)

Birth control has become a critical public health issue, as well as a personal concern, around the world. Yet according to the Alan Guttmacher Institute, a nonprofit research and public education agency, approximately one in six women of reproductive age—nearly 230 million in all—do not have access to effective, reversible contraception and voluntary sterilization. More than one in four of the 190 million pregnancies to women worldwide every year end in abortion; many women say their last birth was unwanted or mistimed.

In most countries, there is a gap between the number of children women want and the number they have. Around the world, women spend half to three-quarters of their childbearing years trying to avoid pregnancy. No matter where she lives in the world, a woman must use some form of effective contraception for at least 20 years of her life if she wants to limit her family size to two children.

Pollution

Any change in the air, water, or soil that could reduce its ability to support life is a form of **pollution.** Natural events, such as smoke from fires triggered by lightning, can cause pollution. The effects of pollution depend on the concentration (amount per unit of air, water, or soil) of the **pollutant,** how long it remains in the environment, and its chemical nature. An *acute effect* is a severe immediate reaction, usually after a single, large exposure. For example, pesticide poisoning can cause nausea and dizziness, even death. A *chronic effect* may take years to develop or may be a recurrent or continuous reaction, usually after repeated exposures. The development of cancer after repeated exposure to a pollutant such as asbestos is an example of a chronic effect.

Environmental agents that trigger changes, or **mutations,** in the genetic material, the DNA, of living cells are called **mutagens.** The changes that result can lead to the development of cancer. As previously discussed, a substance or agent that causes cancer is a *carcinogen:* all carcinogens are mutagens; most mutagens are carcinogens (see Chapter 14). Furthermore, when a mutagen affects an egg or a sperm cell, its effects can be passed on to future generations. Agents that can cross the placenta of a pregnant woman and cause a spontaneous abortion or birth defects in the fetus are called **teratogens.**

Pollution is a hazard to all who breathe. Those with respiratory illnesses are at greatest risk during days when smog or allergen counts are high. However, even healthy joggers are affected; carbon monoxide has been shown to impair their exercise performance. The effects of carbon monoxide are much worse in smokers, who already have higher levels of the gas in their blood.[12]

Toxic substances in polluted air can enter the human body in three ways: (1) through the skin, (2) through the digestive system, and (3) through the lungs. The combined interaction of two or more hazards can produce an effect greater than that of either one alone. Pollutants can affect an organ or organ system directly or indirectly.

Among the health problems that have been linked with pollution are the following:

- Headaches and dizziness.
- Eye irritation and impaired vision.
- Nasal discharge.
- Cough, shortness of breath, and sore throat.
- Constricted airways.
- Chest pains and aggravation of the symptoms of colds, pneumonia, bronchial asthma, emphysema, chronic bronchitis, lung cancer, and other respiratory problems.
- Birth defects and reproductive problems.
- Nausea, vomiting, and stomach cancer.

Changes in the Atmosphere

According to one still-controversial theory, the use of carbon (fossil) **fuels** such as oil and gas, the burning of tropical forests, and methane emissions (produced mainly by cattle and the cultivation of rice) have led to a buildup of the so-called *greenhouse gases* (principally, carbon dioxide, methane, and nitrous dioxide). The **greenhouse effect**—an environmental phenomenon in which the buildup of greenhouse gases leads to warming of the planet—has already led to record warmth. In the future it may increase global temperatures by 33.8°F within 30 years and by 37.4°F within 100 years. (See the following section on global warming.)

The **ozone layer** is a region of the upper atmosphere where ozone, created by the energy of sunlight acting on ordinary oxygen, repels the most dangerous ultraviolet radiation from the sun. *Chlorofluorocarbons (CFCs)*, which are gases used in fire extinguishers, refrigerators, air-conditioning units, and styrofoam, rise into the atmosphere and damage this protective layer. In the past, products in aerosol cans contained high levels of CFCs, but all aerosols now sold in the United States must not exceed legal limits for CFC levels. However, because these products can still contribute to the destruction of the ozone layer, consumers are advised to switch to nonaerosol sprays.

One result of the shrinking of the ozone cover has been a dramatic increase in skin cancer, particularly its deadliest form: malignant melanoma (see also Chapter 14). In 1930 the average person's risk of melanoma was one in 1,500; it is now one in 75. Most of the world's industrialized nations have agreed to cut their production and use of ozone-destroying chemicals and to provide funds to help developing countries obtain alternatives to these substances. In the future, developing countries will be crucial to planetary well-being. Although Asia now produces only 17 percent of greenhouse gases, its carbon dioxide emissions are rising at four times the world average. (See Figure 20-2.)

 ## What Is Global Warming?

The earth's surface temperature has been rising steadily over the last twenty years, according to the World Meteorological Organization.[13] Over the past 100 years, the global average temperature has risen by about one degree centigrade, although this warming has not been uniform. More of the warming has occurred over land than over water, more at night than during the day, and more in winter than in summer.[14] No one can predict exactly what effects a continuing temperature rise may have, but some experts have predicted severe drought and a rise in ocean levels of 2 to 20 feet—conditions that will affect everyone on earth. Ways to prevent these consequences include increasing the globe's tree cover (which accelerates carbon dioxide removal) and reducing fossil fuel combustion.

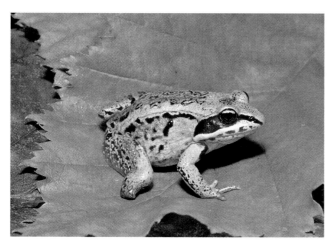

Environmental factors may be to blame for a rise in the number of deformed frogs, toads, and salamanders that have been discovered in recent years.

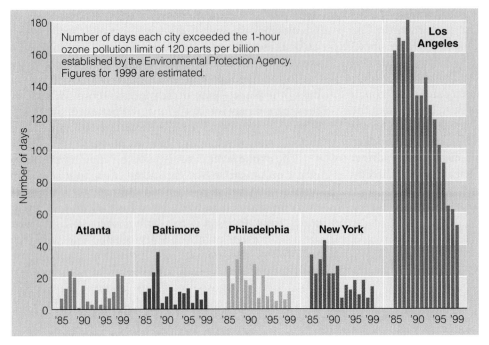

■ Figure 20-2 Ozone pollution.

Source: Environmental Protection Agency. Reprinted by permission of *The New York Times.*

Why is our planet getting warmer? Scientists and policy makers have been heatedly debating this question for years. Global warming may have many causes, including natural processes like volcanic activity and solar radiation and human activities that have resulted in atmospheric changes. (See Figure 20-3.) Some scientists argue that the mean surface temperatures of the last 100 years are not unusual, but the extremely rapid warming since 1975 cannot be explained by natural forces alone.[15]

The consequences of global warming are many and include even planetary motion. According to French scientists, higher temperatures may be slowing earth's daily spin by around half a millisecond every century.[16] A more visible consequence is the melting of the Antarctic ice shelves, flat expanses of ice up to 1,000 feet thick, which extend into the ocean from opposite sides of the Antarctic Peninsula. Satellite imagery shows that chunks of ice, some the size of aircraft carriers, are breaking off the shelves and drifting into the sea. The shelves themselves will probably disappear within a few years, but most scientists do not now think they will raise sea levels since they are already displacing ocean water in their frozen state.[17] Within the next century, though, if global warming continues, the sea level will probably creep up more modestly, by about a foot or two, enough to endanger beachfront property and cost billions of dollars of damage.[18]

Rising temperature during the summer on the arctic tundra may increase both snowfall and the emission of

carbon dioxide. This may further contribute to atmospheric changes. However, farms, forests, and grasslands—if protected from development—may help counterbalance this trend. According to scientists' calculations, agricultural lands could remove from 40 to 80 billion metric tons of carbon from the atmosphere over the next 50 to 100 years and store it in the soil.[19]

For the last ten years, world leaders have been focusing on global warming and its potential consequences. Politicians and scientific experts continue to debate which measures—if any—should be taken to slow or stop global warming. Meanwhile, emissions of greenhouse gases are rising faster than expected, and it seems unlikely that any of the international goals for reducing emissions early in the twenty-first century will be met.[20]

Depletion of the Earth's Resources

A major concern is the loss of tropical rainforests, which play a vital role in regulating climate. As tropical rainforests shrink, their capacity to absorb carbon dioxide declines, hastening the onset and increasing the extent of global warming. Each year 40 to 50 million acres of trees worldwide—an area the size of the state of Washington—are cut up for timber or to clear land for agriculture and other development.

The decrease in rainforests has led to the extinction of many species of plants and wildlife. But the loss of life forms isn't confined to rainforests. As development continues in the next half-century, about 25 percent of the estimated 250,000 known plant species may become extinct. Three-fourths of the world's bird species are declining or facing extinction, as are a third of North America's freshwater fish and two-thirds of the world's 150 primate species.

The world's oceans are also threatened. Many U.S. coastal fishing grounds are contaminated with *polychlorinated biphenyls (PCBs)* from insulation and electronics manufacturing. These chemicals can cause cancer in fish, and the birds who eat them may be

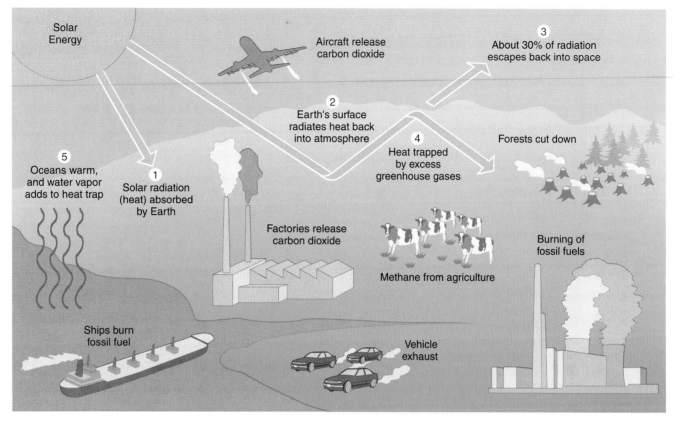

■ Figure 20-3 **Why the World is Heating Up**
The buildup of carbon dioxide and other greenhouse gases in the atmosphere could result in the greatest climatic change in human history. A combination of factors, including the burning of fossil fuels and deforestation, is causing the atmosphere to retain heat. Scientists estimate that the world will be as much as 37.4°F warmer within a hundred years—the hottest it's been in two million years.

unable to reproduce or may produce damaged eggshells. (See the further discussion of PCBs later in this chapter.)

What You Can Do to Protect the Planet

By the choices you make and the actions you take, you can improve the state of the world. No one expects you to sacrifice every comfort or spend great amounts of money. However, for almost everyone, there's plenty of room for improvement. If enough people make small individual changes, they can have an enormous impact. (See the Self-Survey: "Are You Doing Your Part for the Planet?")

Going "Green"

As a consumer, you have a great deal of influence on manufacturers and distributors. When making purchases, consider their environmental impact. A simple switch—from plastic wrap to wax paper, for example—can make a difference. However, it can be difficult to know which choice is best for the environment. For years, for example, environmental and consumer groups have differed about disposable versus cloth diapers. Disposable diapers, though convenient, don't break down; cloth diapers can be reused, but laundering them requires energy and produces wastewater and air pollution. One compromise that suits some parents is using cloth diapers at home and disposable diapers when out. (See Pulsepoints: "Ten Ways to Protect the Planet" for other practical suggestions for protecting the planet.)

Precycling and Recycling

One basic principle of buying green is **precycling**: buying products packaged in recycled materials. According to Earthworks, a consumer group, packaging makes up a third of what Americans throw away. When you precycle, you consider how you're going to dispose of a product and the packaging materials before purchasing it. For example, you might choose eggs in recyclable

Self-*Survey*   Are You Doing Your Part for the Planet?

You may think that there is little you can do, as an individual, to save the earth. But everyday acts can add up and make a difference in helping or harming the planet on which we live.

	Almost Never	Sometimes	Always
1. Do you walk, cycle, car pool, or use public transportation as much as possible to get around?	_____	_____	_____
2. Do you recycle?	_____	_____	_____
3. Do you reuse plastic and paper bags?	_____	_____	_____
4. Do you try to conserve water by not running the tap as you shampoo or brush your teeth?	_____	_____	_____
5. Do you use products made of recycled materials?	_____	_____	_____
6. Do you drive a car that gets good fuel mileage and has up-to-date emission control equipment?	_____	_____	_____
7. Do you turn off lights, televisions, and appliances when you're not using them?	_____	_____	_____
8. Do you avoid buying products that are elaborately packaged?	_____	_____	_____
9. Do you use glass jars and waxed paper rather than plastic wrap for storing food?	_____	_____	_____
10. Do you take brief showers rather than baths?	_____	_____	_____
11. Do you use cloth towels and napkins rather than paper products?	_____	_____	_____
12. When listening to music, do you keep the volume low?	_____	_____	_____
13. Do you try to avoid any potential carcinogens, such as asbestos, mercury, or benzene?	_____	_____	_____
14. Are you careful to dispose of hazardous materials (such as automobile oil or antifreeze) at appropriate sites?	_____	_____	_____
15. Do you follow environmental issues in your community and write your state or federal representative to support "green" legislation?	_____	_____	_____

Making Changes

Count the number of items you've checked in each column. If you've circled 10 or more in the "always" column, you're definitely helping to make a difference. If you've circled 10 or more in the "never" column, read this chapter carefully, particularly the "Strategies for Change" to find out how and why you should make some changes. If you've mainly circled "sometimes," you're moving in the right direction, but you need to be more consistent and more conscientious.

cardboard packages rather than plastic ones and look for refillable bottles.

Recycling—collecting, reprocessing, marketing, and using materials once considered trash—has become a necessity for several reasons. We've run out of space for all the garbage we produce, waste sites are often health and safety hazards, recycling is cheaper than landfill storage or incineration (which is a major source of air pollution), and recycling helps save energy and natural resources. Different communities take different approaches to recycling. Many provide regular curbside pickup of recyclables, which is so convenient that a majority of those eligible for such services participate.

Most programs pick up bottles, cans, and newspapers—either separated or mixed together. Other communities have drop-off centers where consumers can leave recyclables. Conveniently located and sponsored by community organizations (such as charities or schools), these centers accept beverage containers, newspapers, cardboard, metals, and other items.

Buy-back centers, usually run by private companies, pay for recyclables. Many centers specialize in aluminum cans, which offer the most profit. Some operate in supermarket parking lots; other centers have regular hours and staff members who carefully weigh and evaluate recyclables. In some places, "reverse vending machines"

PULSE *points*

Ten Ways to Protect the Planet

1. **Plant a tree.** Even a single tree helps absorb carbon dioxide and produces cooling that can reduce the need for air-conditioning.

2. **Look for simply packaged items.** Whenever possible, choose items packed in recycled materials or something recyclable.

3. **Bring your own bag.** Whenever possible, avoid using plastic or paper bags for items you could carry in a cloth or string carry all.

4. **Hit the switch.** Turn off all electrical appliances (TVs, CD players, radios, lights) when you're not in the room or paying attention to them.

5. **Avoid disposables.** Use a mug instead of a paper or Styrofoam cup, a sponge instead of a paper towel, a cloth napkin instead of a paper one.

6. **Be water wise.** Turn off the tap while you shave or brush your teeth. Install water-efficient faucets and shower heads. Wash clothes in cold water.

7. **Cancel junk mail.** It consumes 100 million trees a year. To get off mailing lists, write: Direct Mail Association, Mail Preference Service, P.O. Box 9008, Farmingdale, NY 11735-9008

8. **Spare the seas.** If you live near the coast or are picnicking or hiking near the ocean, don't use plastic bags (which are often blown into the water) or plastic six-pack holders (which can get caught around the necks of sea birds).

9. **Don't buy products made of endangered substances.** Examples include coral, ivory, tortoise shell, or wood from endangered forests (teak, mahogany, ebony, rosewood).

10. **Speak out.** Write to your senators and congressional representatives, who vote on pollution controls, budgets for the enforcement of safety regulations, and the preservation of forests and wildlife. Identify the particular bill or issue you're addressing. Be as specific, brief, and to the point as possible, and make sure you have the correct addresses:

Hon. [Your District's Congressperson]
United States House of Representatives
Washington, DC 20515

or

Senator [Your State's Senator]
United States Senate
Washington, DC 20510

---

accept returned beverage containers and provide deposit refunds, in the form of either cash or vouchers. Enthusiasm and support for recycling has grown, and, thanks to these efforts along with new manufacturing techniques and other technological advances, Americans are consuming some natural materials, such as aluminum and steel, at lower rates.

With composting—which some people describe as nature's way of recycling—the benefits can be seen as close as your backyard. Organic products, such as leftover food and vegetable peels, are mixed with straw or other dry material and kept damp. Bacteria eat the organic material and turn it into a rich soil. Some people keep a compost pile (which should be stirred every few days) in their backyards; others take their organic garbage (including mowed grass and dead leaves) to community gardens or municipal composting sites.

Clearing the Air

The good news is that, in most places in the United States, you can breathe easier today than you might have a quarter-century ago (see Figure 20-2). Smog has declined by about a third, although there are now 85 percent more vehicles being driven 105 percent more miles a year. In Los Angeles, smog has decreased by almost 50 percent, even though the city's vehicle population has risen 65 percent. Several urban areas, such as Detroit and Kansas City, have been removed from the federal smog watch list, and none has been added.[21] Current model automobiles emit an average of 80 percent less pollution per mile than was emitted by new cars in 1970, and the fuel efficiency of new cars has reduced the typical car's average annual gasoline consumption by around 300 gallons—more than enough fuel to take the average driver across the United States and back again.

The bad news is that air quality still is far from optimal in many places. According to the Harvard School of Public Health, living in a city with even moderately sooty air may shorten your life span by about a year. In fact, air pollution can be as harmful to breathing capacity as smoking. Residents of polluted cities are exposed to some of the same toxic gases, such as nitrogen oxide and carbon monoxide, found in cigarettes.

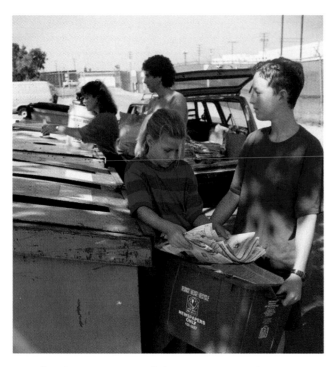

Recycling is an easy way to help save energy and conserve resources.

Air pollution of any sort can cause numerous ill effects. As pollutants destroy the hairlike cilia that remove irritants from the lungs, individuals may suffer chronic bronchitis, characterized by excessive mucus flow and continuous coughing. Emphysema may develop or worsen, as pollutants constrict the bronchial tubes and destroy the air sacs in the lungs, making breathing more difficult. In addition to respiratory diseases, air pollution also contributes to heart disease, cancer, and weakened immunity. For the elderly and people with asthma or heart disease, polluted air can be life-threatening. Even

Strategies *for* Change

Doing Your Part for Cleaner Air

✓ Drive a car that gets high gas mileage and produces low emissions. Keep your speed at or below the speed limit.

✓ Keep your tires inflated and your engine tuned. Recycle old batteries and tires. (Most stores that sell new ones will take back old ones.)

✓ Turn off your engine if you're going to be stopped for more than a minute.

✓ Collect all fluids that you drain from your car (motor oil, antifreeze) and recycle or dispose of them properly.

healthy individuals can be affected, particularly if they exercise outdoors during high-pollution periods.

Smog

A combination of smoke or gases and fog, **smog** is made up of chemical vapors from auto exhaust and industrial and commercial pollutants that react with sunlight, including volatile organic compounds, carbon monoxide, nitrogen oxides, sulfur oxides, particulate, and ozone. The most obvious sources of these pollutants are motor vehicles, industrial factories, electric utilities plants, and wood-burning stoves.

Gray-air, or *sulfur-dioxide,* smog, often seen in Europe and much of the eastern United States, is produced by burning oil of high sulfur content. Among the cities that must deal with gray-air smog are Chicago, Baltimore, Detroit, and Philadelphia. Like cigarette smoke, gray-air smog affects the cilia in the respiratory passages; the lungs are unable to expel particulate, such as soot, ash, and dust, which remain and irritate the tissues. This condition is hazardous to people with the chronic respiratory problems described in Chapter 14.

Brown-air, or *photochemical,* smog is found in large traffic centers such as Los Angeles, Salt Lake City, Denver, Mexico City, and Tokyo. This type of smog results principally from nitric oxide in car exhaust reacting with oxygen in the air, forming nitrogen dioxide, which produces a brownish haze and, when exposed to sunlight, other pollutants.

One of these, *ozone,* the most widespread pollutant, can impair the body's immune system and cause long-term lung damage. (Ozone in the upper atmosphere protects us by repelling harmful ultraviolet radiation from the sun; but ozone in the lower atmosphere is itself a harmful component of air pollution.) As seen in Figure 20-2, ozone pollution has decreased since 1985. Automobiles also produce carbon monoxide, a colorless and odorless gas that diminishes the ability of red blood cells to carry oxygen. The resulting oxygen deficiency can affect breathing, hearing, and vision.

 ## What Is Acid Rain?

The burning of fossil fuels, such as oil and gas, and the smelting of certain ores, such as copper and nickel, can produce **acid rain**—rain, sleet, snow, mist, fog, and clouds containing sulfuric acid and nitric acid. These pollutants are carried through the atmosphere long distances from their sources and fan to earth when it rains. Acid rain, which is believed to be declining in some regions, has damaged buildings, monuments, and other structures.[22]

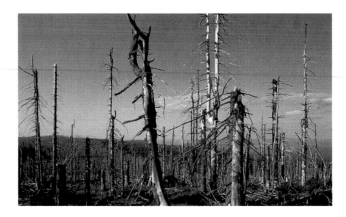

The effects of acid rain on a forest.

Indoor Pollutants

Because people in industrialized nations spend more than 90 percent of their time in buildings, the quality of the air they breathe inside can have an even greater impact on their well-being than outdoor pollution. The most hazardous form of indoor air pollution is cigarette smoke. Passive smoking—inhaling others' cigarette smoke—may rank behind active smoking and alcohol use as the third-leading preventable cause of death. Each year secondhand cigarette smoke kills 53,000 nonsmokers. (See Chapter 17 for a complete discussion of smoke's harmful effects.)

Formaldehyde

Unlike outdoor contaminants from exhaust pipes or smokestacks, indoor pollutants come from the very materials the buildings are made of and from the appliances inside them. For instance, formaldehyde, commonly used in building materials, carpet backing, furniture, foam insulation, plywood, and particle board, can cause nausea, dizziness, headaches, heart palpitations, stinging eyes, and burning lungs. Formaldehyde has been shown to cause cancer in animals. Most manufacturers have voluntarily quit using it, but many homes already contain materials made with urea-formaldehyde, which can seep into the air. To avoid formaldehyde exposure, buy solid wood or nonwood products whenever possible; and ask about the formaldehyde content of building products, cabinets, and furniture before purchasing them.

Asbestos

Asbestos, a mineral widely used for building insulation, has been linked to lung and gastrointestinal cancer among asbestos workers and their families, although it may take 20 to 30 years for such cancer to develop. If fibers from asbestos home insulation or fireproofing become airborne, they can cause progressive and deadly lung diseases, including cancer. More than 200,000 lawsuits have been filed for asbestos-related injuries, and as many as 300,000 American workers may have died from asbestos-linked diseases, including lung cancer.[23] The danger may be greatest for those who smoke and are also exposed to asbestos.[24]

If you're concerned about asbestos in your home, don't waste money searching for asbestos in the air. The results of such tests are meaningless. To check a building material for asbestos, put three small pieces in a film canister and send it to an EPA-approved laboratory. The cost for testing is usually $25 to $75 per sample. If you find asbestos in your house, sealing it may be safer than removing it. Contact your state or city health department for advice. If asbestos must be removed, have it done by professionals.[25]

Lead

A danger both inside and outside our homes is lead, which lurks in some 57 million American homes, most built before 1960, with walls, windows, doors, and banisters coated with more than 3 million metric tons of lead paint.[26] One out of every six youngsters—as many as 4 million American boys and girls—may have toxic levels of lead in their bodies; millions more are at risk of poisoning from lead in the air they breathe or the water they drink. "In terms of the number of children affected, the number at risk and the dire effects of exposure, lead is the number-one environmental threat to

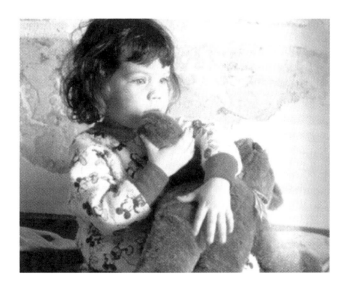

Lead-based paint poses a hazard, especially to young children, who can be poisoned even by ingesting small amounts of paint chips.

our youngsters," says pediatrician John Rosen, M.D., chairman of the advisory committee on childhood lead poisoning for the CDC.

Fetuses and children under age 7 are particularly vulnerable to lead because their nervous systems are still developing and because their body mass is so small that they ingest and absorb more lead per pound than adults.[27] Even 10 micrograms (millionths of a gram) of lead per deciliter of blood—the CDC standard for lead poisoning—can kill a child's brain cells and cause poor concentration, reduced short-term memory, slower reaction times, and learning disabilities.

Adults exposed to low levels of lead (which once were thought to be safe) may develop headaches, high blood pressure, irritability, tremors, and insomnia.[28] Health effects increase with exposure to higher levels and include anemia, stomach pain, vomiting, diarrhea, and constipation. Long-term exposure can impair fertility and damage the kidneys.[29] Workers exposed to lead may become sterile or suffer irreversible kidney disease, damage to their central nervous system, stillbirths, or miscarriages.

The CDC and the American Academy of Pediatrics recommend annual testing of blood levels of lead in all children from age 9 months to 6 years, regardless of where they live. High-risk youngsters—those who live or play in older housing (especially if a building is in poor condition or undergoing renovation); those who live with someone who uses lead for a job or hobby; and those who live near a lead smelter, a processing plant, or a heavily traveled road or highway—should be screened every two or three months until age 3 and every six months until age 6. High levels of ascorbic acid (vitamin C) have been associated with a lower rate of elevated blood lead levels.[30]

Mercury

While free of lead, some popular, easy-to-use latex paints may contain potentially hazardous mercury, which manufacturers routinely added until a 1990 ban to prevent the growth of mold and mildew. The threat of mercury poisoning is greatest during painting and immediately after. Even mercury in medical devices, such as sphygmomanometers that measure blood pressure, can be a hazard.[31] Symptoms of mercury poisoning include a racing heartbeat, sweating, aching limbs, kidney problems, hand tremors, peeling skin, and emotional problems.

Carbon Monoxide and Nitrogen Dioxide

Carbon monoxide (CO) gas, which is tasteless, odorless, colorless, and nonirritating, can be deadly. Produced by the incomplete combustion of fuel in space heaters, furnaces, water heaters, and engines, it reduces the delivery of oxygen in the blood. Every year an estimated 10,000 Americans seek treatment for CO inhalation; at least 250 die because of this silent killer. Those most at risk are the chronically ill, the elderly, pregnant women, and infants. Typical symptoms of CO poisoning are headache, nausea, vomiting, fatigue, and dizziness. A blood test can measure CO levels; inhaling pure oxygen speeds removal of the gas from the body. Most people who don't lose consciousness as a result of CO poisoning recover completely.

Another dangerous gas, nitrogen dioxide, can reach very high levels if you use a natural gas or propane stove in a poorly ventilated kitchen. This gas may lead to respiratory illnesses. Pilot lights are a steady source of nitrogen dioxide; to reduce exposure, switch to spark ignition.

Radon

Radioactive radon—which diffuses from rock, brick, and concrete building materials and natural soil deposits under some homes—produces charged decay products that cling to dust particles, which often lodge in the lungs. Once trapped inside, radon can reach levels that may increase the risk of lung cancer. EPA estimates that the inhalation of indoor radon is responsible for approximately 14,000 lung cancer deaths per year. Radon levels tend to be highest in areas with granite and black shale topped with porous soil. If you live in a high-radon area, don't panic. Your hypothetical risk of dying from radon-caused lung cancer is about equal to the known risk of dying in a home fire or fall. Check with the geology department at the nearest university or with your state health department to find out if they've performed radon tests in your area. If there may be danger, you can buy a radon detector. In most homes, the readings turn out to be low. If not, your state health department can provide guidelines for bringing them down.

Protecting Yourself from Indoor Air Pollution

- If you live in a formaldehyde-insulated home, keep heat and humidity down, because formaldehyde vapors increase in hot, humid weather. Air conditioning and dehumidifiers reduce such emissions. An air-to-air heat exchanger can increase the circulation of outside air without sharply increasing heating costs. Treatment with specially formulated sealants can cut formaldehyde emissions from wood products to 1 percent of their original level.

- Before renovating your home, inspect pipe and furnace coverings and insulation in attics and crawlspaces for signs of cracking, flaking, or loose asbestos.

- To minimize lead exposure, watch out for peeling or chipping lead paint, particularly from window sills and frames, which can release dust contaminated with lead. Watch out when scraping or sanding lead-based paint. Water flowing through lead pipes, brass faucets, or pipes connected with lead solder can contain lead. Imported products sold in cans may contain lead that leaches in from the solder. (Most domestic cans do not use lead solder.) Lead in the glaze used for ceramic dishes or cookware can leach into food.

- To prevent carbon monoxide poisoning, provide adequate ventilation when using wood stoves, space heaters, and fireplaces. Make sure that your furnace has adequate air intake. Don't use ovens or gas ranges to heat your home, or operate gasoline-powered engines in confined spaces. Never burn charcoal inside a home, recreational vehicle, or tent. The Consumer Product Safety Commission recommends installing at least one CO detector, which sounds an alarm before the gas reaches hazardous levels, in all homes.

- Limit your use of cleaners and aerosols that fill the air with chemicals, and ventilate your house immediately after their use. Air your house daily or as often as possible—particularly in the winter, when pollutants build up inside.

Protecting Your Hearing

Loudness, or the intensity of a sound, is measured in **decibels (dB)**. A whisper is 20 decibels; a conversation in a living room is about 50 decibels. On this scale, 50 isn't two and a half times louder than 20, but 1,000 times louder: Each 10-dB rise in the scale represents a tenfold increase in the intensity of the sound.

Sounds under 75 dBs don't seem harmful. However, prolonged exposure to any sound over 85 dBs (the equivalent of a power mower or food blender) or brief exposure to louder sounds can harm hearing. The noise level at rock concerts can reach 110–140 dBs—about as loud as an air raid siren. Personal sound systems (boom boxes) can blast sounds of up to 115 dBs. Cars with extremely loud music systems, known as boom cars, can produce an earsplitting 145 dBs—louder than a jet engine or thunderclap.

Most hearing loss occurs on the job. The people at highest risk are firefighters, police, military personnel, construction and factory workers, musicians, farmers, and truck drivers. Other sources of danger include live or recorded high-volume music, recreational vehicles, airplanes, lawn-care equipment, woodworking tools, some appliances, and chain saws (see Figure 20-4).[32]

The Effects of Noise

The healthy human ear can hear sounds within a wide range of frequencies (measured in **hertz**), from the low-frequency rumble of thunder at 50 hertz to the high-frequency overtones of a piccolo at nearly 20,000 hertz. High-frequency noise damages the delicate hair cells that serve as sound receptors in the inner ear. Damage first begins as a diminished sensitivity to frequencies around 4,000 hertz—the highest notes of a piano. Early symptoms of hearing loss include difficulty understanding speech and tinnitus (ringing in the ears). Brief, very loud sounds, such as an explosion or gunfire, can produce immediate, severe, and permanent hearing loss. Longer exposure to less intense but still hazardous sounds, such as those common at work or in public places, can impair hearing gradually, often without the individual's awareness.

Conductive hearing loss, often caused by ear infections, cuts down on perception of low-pitched sounds. Sensorineural loss involves damage or destruction of the sensory cells in the inner ear that convert sound waves to nerve signals.

Noise can harm more than our ears: High-volume sound has been linked to high blood pressure and other stress-related problems that can lead to heart disease, insomnia, anxiety, headaches, colitis, and ulcers. Noise frays the nerves; people tend to be more

Strategies *for* Prevention

Protecting Your Ears

✓ If you must live or work in a noisy area, wear hearing protectors to prevent exposure to blasts of very loud noise. Don't think cotton or facial tissue stuck in your ears can protect you; foam or soft plastic earplugs are more effective. Wear them when operating lawn mowers, weed trimmers, or power tools.

✓ Soundproof your home by using draperies, carpets, and bulky furniture. Put rubber mats under washing machines, blenders, and other noisy appliances. Seal cracks around windows and doors.

✓ When you hear a sudden loud noise, press your fingers against your ears. Limit your exposure to loud noise. Several brief periods of noise seem less damaging than one long exposure.

✓ Be careful if you wear Walkman-type stereos. The volume is too high if you can feel the vibrations.

✓ Beware of large doses of aspirin. Researchers have found that eight aspirins a day can aggravate the damage caused by loud noise; twelve aspirins daily can cause ringing in the ears (tinnitus).

✓ Don't drink in noisy environments. Alcohol intensifies the impact of noise and increases the risk of lifelong hearing damage.

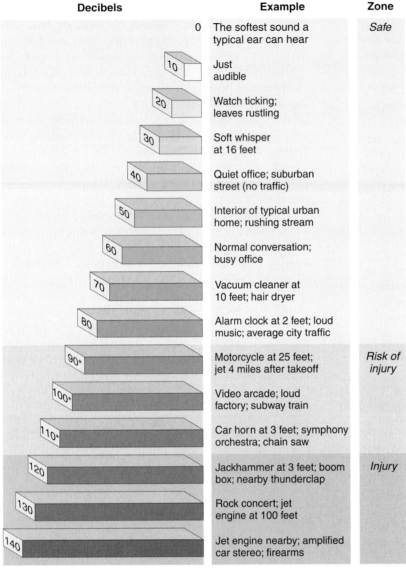

Decibels	Example	Zone
0	The softest sound a typical ear can hear	Safe
10	Just audible	
20	Watch ticking; leaves rustling	
30	Soft whisper at 16 feet	
40	Quiet office; suburban street (no traffic)	
50	Interior of typical urban home; rushing stream	
60	Normal conversation; busy office	
70	Vacuum cleaner at 10 feet; hair dryer	
80	Alarm clock at 2 feet; loud music; average city traffic	
90*	Motorcycle at 25 feet; jet 4 miles after takeoff	Risk of injury
100*	Video arcade; loud factory; subway train	
110*	Car horn at 3 feet; symphony orchestra; chain saw	
120	Jackhammer at 3 feet; boom box; nearby thunderclap	Injury
130	Rock concert; jet engine at 100 feet	
140	Jet engine nearby; amplified car stereo; firearms	

*Note: The maximum exposure allowed on the job by federal law, in hours per day, is as follows: 90 decibels—8 hours; 100 decibels—2 hours; 110 decibels—1/2 hour.

■ **Figure 20-4** Loud and louder. The human ear perceives a 10-decibel increase as a doubling of loudness. Thus, the 100 decibels of a subway train sounds much more than twice as loud as the 50 decibels of a rushing stream.

able and possibly dangerous quantities of man-made chemicals. Some make water look or taste funny. Others have lethal effects at very high concentrations. Some contaminants enter the water as a result of natural processes, such as the decay of vegetation. Others are the result of urban development, industrial activity, and agricultural runoff.[33]

Many toxic chemicals and heavy metals—including lead, mercury, cadmium, and chromium that can cause kidney and nervous system damage and birth defects—accumulate in fish and shellfish, which can pass them on to humans. Several states have had to ban fishing in specific areas because the contamination level posed a significant risk of cancer or other health effects.[34]

Each year the CDC reports an average of 7,400 cases of illness related to the water people drink. (See Chapter 12 on infectious diseases.) The most common culprits include parasites, bacteria, viruses, chemicals, and lead. Health officials suggest having your water tested if you live near a hazardous waste dump or industrial park, if the pipes in your house are made of lead or joined together with lead solder, if your water comes from a well, or if you purchase it from a private company. Check to see if your state health department or local water supplier will provide free testing. If not, use a state-certified laboratory that tests water in accordance with EPA standards.

anxious, irritable, and angry when their ears are constantly barraged with sound. Even unborn babies respond to sounds; some researchers speculate that noise, particularly if it stresses the mother, may be hazardous to the fetus.

Is Your Water Safe to Drink?

According to various EPA reports, as many as 37 percent of public water-supply systems contains measur-

Is Bottled Water Better?

Is bottled water better? That's what consumers have often assumed. Yet in the past, the Food and Drug Administration (FDA) simply defined bottled water as "sealed in bottles or other containers and intended for human consumption." Bottled water wasn't required to be "pure" or even to be tested for toxic chemicals. However, the FDA has called for federal monitoring of the purity of bottled water. Some states, including California and New York, have their own bottled-water safety standards to ensure that bottled water is at least as safe as drinking water. In cases where public drinking water has been contaminated (for instance, by a toxic spill) and health authorities advise using bottled waters, check the label to make sure that the brand you purchase has been tested or undergone purification treatment.

Fluoride

About half (53 percent) of Americans drink water containing fluoride, an additive to water and toothpaste that helps teeth resist decay. According to the American Dental Association (ADA), tooth decay is 50 to 70 percent lower in areas with fluoridated water. However, laboratory rats given fluoridated water have shown a high rate of bone cancer. The more fluoride they drank in their water, the more likely they were to develop this cancer. But this type of cancer is extremely rare in humans, and the estimated lifetime risk to any individual from drinking fluoridated water is less than one in 5,000.

Federal health officials have found no evidence that fluoride causes cancer in humans and have concluded that its benefits far outweigh any risks. However, excessive fluoride can increase bone loss and fractures in pre- and postmenopausal women. Health professionals advise consumers to use only small amounts of fluoridated toothpastes, rinse thoroughly after brushing, and use fluoride supplements only when the home water supply is known to be deficient.

Chlorine

Three-quarters of the American population drinks water treated with chlorine to kill disease-causing bacteria. The Council on Environmental Quality has warned that people drinking chlorinated water have a 53 percent greater risk of getting colon and bladder cancer and a 13 to 93 percent greater risk of getting rectal cancer than those not drinking chlorinated water. There may even be a link between soft water and a higher rate of cardiovascular disease, perhaps because soft water in some areas tends to have more sodium in it.

Lead

Long recognized as a hazard in paint and dust, lead can also leach from pipes into the drinking supply. The highest risk exists in cities with older housing and lead pipes or water lines.

Chemical Risks

Each year, a thousand new chemicals join the 50,000–75,000 already in common use. Workers exposed to chemicals on the job may be at highest risk.[35] In most cases, little is known about their potential ill effects.

No relationship has been found between fertility, as measured by time to pregnancy (that is, the time taken for a couple to conceive once they decide they want to), and male exposure to pesticides.[36] Exposure to pesticides may, however, pose a risk to pregnant women and their unborn children.

An estimated 50,000–70,000 U.S. workers die each year of chronic diseases related to past exposure to toxic substances, including lung cancer, bladder cancer, leukemia, lymphoma, chronic bronchitis, and disorders of the nervous system. "**Endocrine disruptors**," chemicals that act as or interfere with human hormones, particularly estrogen, may pose a different threat. Scientists are investigating their impact on fertility, falling sperm counts, and cancers of the reproductive organs.[37]

 ## What Health Risks Are Caused by Pesticides?

The chemical agents used to destroy unwanted insects, plants, and fungi save billions of dollars of valuable crops from pests; at the same time, they may endanger human health and life. **Chlorinated hydrocarbons** include several high-risk substances—such as DDT, kepone, and chlordane—that have been restricted or

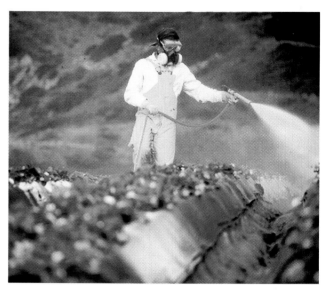

Pesticides protect crops from harmful insects, plants, and fungi but may endanger human health.

banned because they may cause cancer, birth defects, neurological disorders, and damage to wildlife and the environment. They are extremely resistant to breakdown.

Organic phosphates, including chemicals such as malathion, break down more rapidly than do the chlorinated hydrocarbons. Most chlorinated hydrocarbons are highly toxic, causing cramps, confusion, diarrhea, vomiting, headaches, and breathing difficulties. Higher levels in the blood can lead to convulsions, paralysis, coma, and death. Farm workers and those in the surrounding communities are at greatest risk for pesticide exposure. However, even city dwellers aren't out of range. About half (52 percent) of Americans use insect repellents, including some made with potent insecticides.[38]

Toxic Chemicals, Metals, and Wastes

The family of 75 chemicals called **dioxins** can linger in the body for years. In sunlight, dioxins break down fairly quickly into less toxic compounds. However, when they get into the upper layers of the soil, they retain their original structure. Long-term exposure to dioxin—a chemical linked to birth defects, tumors, and skin problems—may damage the body's immune system and may increase the risk of infections or possibly cancer.

Polychlorinated biphenyls (PCBs) belong to a family of 209 chemical compounds that are widely used as coolants and lubricants in electrical equipment; in insulating fluids; and in the manufacture of common products such as plastics, adhesives, paints, and varnishes. PCBs made their way into the environment when industries discharged PCB-laden wastes into rivers and streams, or disposed of them in open landfills. A possible human carcinogen, PCB is no longer commercially produced in the United States, but high levels of PCB remain in certain parts of the country, and in eggs, poultry, and fish.[39]

In the United States, exposure to the heavy metal cadmium results mainly from inhaling cigarette smoke or city air. Cadmium may be linked to high blood pressure and heart disease. The use of beryllium, a metal with many industrial uses (fluorescent bulb manufacture, for example), has increased 500 percent over the past 25 years. According to the EPA, beryllium can cause severe respiratory problems, including bronchitis and lung cancer.

Before the environmental laws of the last two decades, industry dumped most of its waste into open pits, abandoned mines, or nearby rivers. The EPA has identified thousands of potentially dangerous dumps, pits, ponds, and landfills across the nation (Figure 20-5). Many of these are designated industrial-waste sites, but even the local landfill can be a danger.

The burning of garbage and industrial waste in the country's toxic-waste incinerators has created a new problem: emissions containing dangerous pollutants, such as lead, which can damage children's central nervous systems, and cancer-causing dioxins.[40] Toxic waste dumps often end up near low-income areas, placing those populations at greatest risk. Other sources of pollution are the 2 million or more storage tanks containing gasoline, petroleum, and other chemicals, which are buried underground at gas stations, factories, and other sites around the country. The EPA estimates that 10 to 30 percent of these may be leaking their contents

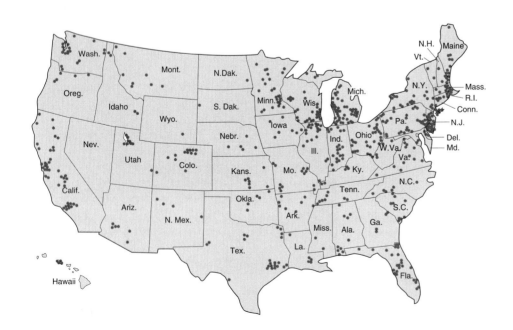

■ Figure 20-5 **Hazardous Waste Dumps**
Each dot represents a hazardous waste dump that poses a serious threat to life. These are sites on the EPA's priority list for cleanup, but there are many other dangerous waste dumps in the United States.

into the water supply. New laws are requiring the replacement of some tanks.

Invisible Dangers

Among the unseen threats to health are various forms of radiation.

Electromagnetic Fields

Any electrically charged conductor generates two kinds of invisible fields: electric and magnetic. Together they're called **electromagnetic fields (EMFs)**. For years, these fields, produced by household appliances, home wiring, lighting fixtures, electric blankets, and overhead power lines, were considered harmless. However, epidemiological studies revealed a link between exposure to high-voltage lines and cancer (especially leukemia, a blood cancer) in electrical workers and children.

Laboratory studies on animals have shown that alternating current, which changes strength and direction 60 times a second (and electrifies most of North America), emits fields that may interfere with the normal functioning of human cell membranes, which have their own electromagnetic fields. The result may be mood disorders, changes in circadian rhythms (our inner sense of time), miscarriage, developmental problems, or cancer. Researchers have documented an increase in breast cancer deaths in women who worked as electrical engineers, electricians, or in other high-exposure jobs and a link between EMF exposure and an increased risk of leukemia and possibly brain cancer.[41]

In 1999 after six years of congressionally mandated research, the National Institute of Environmental Health Sciences concluded that the evidence of a risk of cancer and other human disease from the electric and magnetic fields around power lines is "weak." This finding applies to the extremely low frequency electric and magnetic fields surrounding both the big power lines that distribute power and the smaller but closer electric lines in homes and appliances. However, the researchers also noted that EMF exposure "cannot be recognized as entirely safe."[42]

The strongest evidence for health effects came from statistical associations of childhood leukemia and chronic lymphocytic leukemia in adults exposed to EMFs on the job, such as electric utility workers, machinists, and welders. "While the support from individual studies is weak," according to the report, "these epidemiological studies demonstrate, for some methods of measuring exposure, a fairly consistent pattern of a small, increased risk." Laboratory studies and investigations of basic biological function do not support these epidemiological associations.[43]

Appliances that are used only briefly, such as hair dryers, are probably less dangerous than electric blankets, which people sleep under for an entire night. Expectant mothers who often use electric blankets or heated water beds during winter have a higher miscarriage rate than nonusers; babies conceived in the winter by electric blanket-users grow more slowly in the womb and tend to have a lower birth weight than others. Federal officials urge "prudent avoidance" of electric blankets for women who are pregnant or hoping to conceive.

Strategies *for* Prevention

Protecting Yourself from Electromagnetic Fields

✓ Sit at least 3 feet from a 19-inch television screen, and even farther from a larger screen. Sit at least 13 inches from the computer screen. Install a special screen on your computer that can block out some of the radiation.

✓ If you use a plug-in electric alarm clock, which produces strong magnetic fields, keep it at least 3 feet away from your head at night. Some experts suggest switching to a battery-powered or wind-up clock.

✓ Use electric blankets only to warm the bed. Unplug the blanket or remove it before climbing under the covers. Children and pregnant women should avoid using them entirely.

Video Display Terminals (VDTs)

Chances are there's a **video display terminal (VDT)** in your life—at the school library, at the office where you work, or maybe in your home. Is it a health hazard? The answer is a definite maybe. Although VDTs have been blamed for increases in reproductive problems. miscarriages, low infant birthweights, and cataracts, repeated measurements of radiation from VDTs have shown that leakage is well below present standards for safe occupational exposure. However, VDTs emit electromagnetic fields from all sides, not just the screen, and the strongest emissions are from the sides, backs, and tops of monitors. At least in theory, working next to someone using a computer may be more hazardous than using one yourself. Scientists are continuing to investigate possible links between VDT use and health hazards.

Microwaves

Microwaves (extremely high frequency electromagnetic waves) increase the rate at which molecules vibrate; this vibration generates heat. There's no evidence that existing levels of microwave radiation encountered in the environment pose a health risk to people, and all home microwave ovens must meet safety standards for leakage.

Another concern about the safety of microwave ovens stems from the chemicals in plastic wrapping and containers used for them, which may leak into food. Some, such as DEHA, a chemical that makes plastic more pliable, can cause cancer in mice in high concentrations. Consumers should be cautious about using clingy plastic wrap when reheating leftovers, and plastic-encased metal "heat susceptors" included in convenience foods such as popcorn and pizza. Although these materials seem safe when tested in conventional ovens at temperatures of 300°F–350°F, microwave ovens can boost temperatures to 500°F.

Ionizing Radiation

Radiation that possesses enough energy to separate electrons from their atoms, leaving charged ions, is called **ionizing radiation.** Its effects on health depend on many factors, including the amount, length of exposure, type, part of the body exposed, and the health and age of the individual.

We're surrounded by low-level ionizing radiation every day. Most comes from cosmic rays and radioactive minerals, which vary according to geography. (Denver has more than Atlanta, for instance, because of its altitude.) Man-made sources, including medical and dental X rays, account for approximately 18 percent of the average person's lifetime exposure.

Radiation exposure in humans is measured in units called rads and rems. A *rad (radiation absorbed dose)* is a measure of the energy deposited by ionizing radiation when it's absorbed by an object. A *rem (roentgen equivalent man)* is a measure of the biological effect of ionizing radiation. Different types of radiation cause different amounts of damage. The rem measurement takes this into account. For X rays, rads and rems are equivalent. A quantity of 1 rad or 1 rem is a substantial dose of radiation. Smaller doses are measured in *millirads (thousandths of a rad)* or *millirems (thousandths of a rem).* The average annual radiation exposure for a person in the United States is about one-tenth of a rem.

Although high levels of radiation are most dangerous, even low-level radiation can be harmful to health. According to the National Research Council, the risk of getting cancer from small amounts of radiation is four times more than had been previously estimated, and there's much greater danger of mental retardation among babies exposed to radiation in the womb from eight to fifteen weeks after conception.

Diagnostic X Rays

The EPA estimates that 30 to 50 percent of the 700 million X rays taken every year in the United States are unnecessary. However, doctors sometimes prescribe X rays or newer imaging techniques involving radiation, such as CT scans, to protect themselves from malpractice suits, and hospitals benefit financially from the heavy use of X-ray equipment.

Dental X rays involve little radiation, but many people receive so many so often that they're second only to chest examinations in frequency. Dentists typically obtain radiographs of all the teeth at the beginning of a patient's care, and again every three to five years. However, you can cut down on total X rays by bringing previous films with you or having your dentist forward copies when you switch dentists.

Always ask why an X ray is being ordered. Don't give your consent unless there's a clear need. Keep a record of the date and location of every X-ray exam. Some of these X rays may someday provide information that would make more X rays unnecessary. Ask the radiologist to explain specifically how much radiation you'll be exposed to, and be sure to wear a protective leaded apron. There's no sense in refusing a needed medical X ray just because you're afraid of the radiation exposure. Under certain circumstances, the benefits far outweigh the risks.

Radioactivity

The emission of nuclear radiation by radioactive materials is called radioactivity. The degree of damage it causes depends on the particular type of radioactivity, as well as the dosage. The following are the three major kinds of radioactivity:

1. *Alpha particles.* The slowest and least penetrating; cannot pass through the skin and are not a health hazard unless the emitting material is ingested or inhaled.

2. *Beta particles.* Can penetrate slightly into the body; if the emitting material is ingested, can affect the bones and thyroid.

3. *Gamma rays.* Similar to X rays and the most hazardous; can pass right through the human body.

Irradiated Foods

The use of radiation on food, from either radioactive substances or devices that produce X rays, is known as **irradiation.** It doesn't make the food radioactive; its primary benefit is to prolong the food's useful life. Like the heat in canning, irradiation can kill all the microorganisms that might grow in a food; the sterilized food can then be stored for years in sealed containers at room temperature without spoiling. In addition, low-dose irradiation can inhibit the sprouting of vegetables such as potatoes and onions, and delay the ripening of some fruits, such as bananas, mangoes, tomatoes, pears, and avocados—cost-saving benefits of great appeal to the food industry.

Irradiated foods are believed to be safe to eat, and the federal government has approved their distribution. Most research has focused on low-dose irradiation to delay ripening and destroy insects. Nutritional studies have shown no significant decreases in the quality of the foods, but high-dose treatments may cause vitamin losses similar to those that occur during canning. It's also possible that the ionizing effect of radiation creates new compounds in foods that may be mutagenic/carcinogenic.

Nuclear Reactors and Radioactive Wastes

In the United States, nuclear power hasn't become a major energy source. One reason is the fear of a possibly catastrophic accident, such as those that occurred at Three Mile Island in Pennsylvania in 1979 and at Chernobyl in the former Soviet Union in 1986. Even if no accidents occur, a nuclear plant is expected to be safe for only about 30 years. After that, parts of the reactor mechanism are so weakened by radioactivity that they must be removed and the plant shut down.

More than 23,000 tons of highly radioactive waste materials—sometimes called *radwaste*—have accumulated around the 111 operating nuclear power plants in the United States. Each year the world produces about 1 million cubic feet of intermediate and high-level waste—that's equal to a cube about 100 feet on each side. Researchers have documented higher than normal rates of cancer among those who live near nuclear facilities.

Most nuclear wastes haven't found a permanent home. Military radwaste—some 380,000 cubic meters' worth, equivalent to a giant cube 240 feet wide—is scattered across the nation, in liquid vats or underwater barrels. The U.S. Congress has allocated $3 billion to the cleanup of hazardous wastes surrounding weapons stores, plants, and bases. Some radioactive byproducts must be stored for periods of 10 to 20 times their half-lives (the time it takes the radioactivity to reduce to one-half its original amount). This means that it will be tens of thousands of years before the radioactivity of these byproducts reaches safe levels.

Making This Chapter Work for You

Creating a Healthier World

- The term *environment* refers to the conditions under which you live—including the air you breathe, the water you drink, the sounds you hear. Decisions you make every day—about what you buy, use, and throw away—have an impact on the environment. Your health depends on the interaction between the environment's impact on your well-being and your impact on your environment.

- The earth is a closed ecosystem or community of organisms sharing a physical and chemical environment that depends on materials that must be recycled over and over again.

- Threats to the environment include overpopulation, atmospheric changes, and the depletion of resources. In recent decades, both the United States and other nations have joined together to take steps to protect planetary well-being.

- As the world's population continues to soar, family planning has become a global public health issue. The critical steps to slowing population growth include improving the quality of reproductive and family planning services, meeting current needs for contraception, increasing access to education for girls, and involving men in family planning.

- Pollution—any change in the air, water, or soil that could reduce its ability to support life—can have acute, or immediate, effects as well as chronic, or long-term, ones. Pollutants that trigger changes, or mutations, in the genetic material, the DNA, of living cells are called mutagens.

- Atmospheric changes, such as the warming of the planet because of a buildup of gases and the depletion of the protective ozone layer, can have an impact on the well-being of everyone on earth. Most of the world's industrialized nations have agreed to take steps to stop or limit environmentally destructive practices.

- Other environmental concerns include the widening gap between rich and poor in and among nations, poverty, homelessness, and hunger.

- Individuals can make environmentally responsible decisions by precycling, recycling, and choosing products that do not harm the environment.

■ In most places in the United States, air quality has improved in the last 25 years. However, it remains less than optimal in many places, and living in a city with even moderately sooty air may shorten your life span by about a year.

■ Indoor air pollutants include environmental tobacco smoke, formaldehyde, asbestos, lead, carbon monoxide gas, nitrogen dioxide, and radioactive radon.

■ The most widespread form of environmental pollution is invisible: noise. Sounds above 85 decibels can damage sound receptors in the inner ear, resulting in hearing problems. Rock concerts and powerful stereos can produce sounds as loud as—and sometimes louder than—jackhammers and jet planes.

■ Air pollution may be caused by natural events, such as dust storms or forest fires; or it may be man made, as is smog, which may cause or worsen emphysema, chronic bronchitis, lung and stomach cancer, and heart disease.

■ The water that we drink may also be dangerous because of additives such as fluoride and chlorine, and contamination by toxic chemicals.

■ Chemical threats to health include industrial wastes, pesticides, lead, dioxin, PCBs, and heavy metals, such as cadmium and beryllium.

■ Electromagnetic fields produced by appliances, electrical wires, televisions, and VDTs may cause biological changes in body tissues in humans and animals.

■ Sources of potentially harmful ionizing radiation include X rays, food irradiation, radioactive wastes, and nuclear power plants. Even low levels of radiation can damage the genetic material in the body's cells and result in cancer and birth defects.

health / ONLINE

Environmental Protection Agency
http://www.epa.gov/
A comprehensive, general resource site for information on environmental topics. Includes news, publications, databases, software, and laws and regulations related to environmental protection.

National Library for the Environment
http://www.cnie.org/nle/
This site is a gateway to population and environment news from hundreds of online sources.

CDC: Environmental Health
http://www.cdc.gov/health/environm.htm
This site provides basic information about several environmental health topics, including air pollution, carbon monoxide poisoning, earthquakes, floods, hurricanes, lead poisoning, and tornadoes.

Please note that links are subject to change. If you find a broken link, use a search engine like
http://www.yahoo.com *and search for the web site by typing in key words.*

 Campus Chat: Is our society doing enough to protect the environment? Share your thoughts on our online discussion forum at **http://health.wadsworth.com**

Find It On InfoTrac: You can find additional readings related to health and the environment via InfoTrac College Edition, an online library of more than 900 journals and publications. Follow the instructions for accessing InfoTrac that came packaged with your textbook; then search for articles using a key word search.

• **Suggested reading:** "Flowers that Fight Pollution," by Dan Johnson. *The Futurist*, April 1999, Vol. 33, Issue 4, p. 6.
  (1) What is phytoremediation, and how can it fight pollution?
  (2) What are some of the disadvantages of phytoremediation?

For additional links, resources, and suggested readings on InfoTrac, visit our Health & Wellness Resource Center at
http://health.wadsworth.com

Environmental problems can seem so complex that you may think there's little you can do about them. That's not the case. This world can be made better instead of worse. The job isn't easy, and all of us have to do our part. Just as many diseases of the previous century have been eradicated, so, in time, we may be able to remove or reduce many environmental threats. Your future—and our planet's future—may depend on it.

 6 Billion and Counting. What problems are caused by a growing population?

Key Terms

The terms listed here are used within the chapter. Page numbers are included for each term. A definition of each term is given in the Glossary pages at the end of this book.

acid rain   626
chlorinated hydrocarbons   631
decibel (dB)   629
dioxins   632
ecosystem   618
electromagnetic fields (EMFs)   633
endocrine disruptors   631
fuels   621
greenhouse effect   621
hertz   629

ionizing radiation   634
irradiation   635
microwaves   634
multiple chemical sensitivity
   (MCS)   619
mutagen   620
mutation   620
organic phosphates   632
ozone layer   621
pollutant   620

pollution   620
polychlorinated biphenyls
   (PCBs)   632
precycling   623
recycling   624
smog   626
teratogen   620
video display terminal (VDT)   633
zero population growth (ZPG)   619

Critical Thinking Questions

1. How do you personally contribute to environmental pollution? How might you change your practices to protect the environment instead?

2. In the past few years, we've witnessed the end of the Cold War era in which nuclear war was often considered the ultimate health threat. Do you feel that nuclear war is still the number-one threat to health, or have other issues replaced it? What, in your opinion, is the number-one health threat?

3. In one Harris poll, 84 percent of Americans said that, given a choice between a high standard of living (but with hazardous air and water pollution and the depletion of natural resources) and a lower standard of living (but with clean air and drinking water), they would prefer clean air and drinking water and a lower standard of living. What about you? What exactly would you be willing to give up: air conditioning, convenience packaging and products, driving in your own car rather than using public transportation? Do you think that most people are willing to change their lifestyles to preserve the environment?

References

1. Costanza, Robert. "Four Visions of the Century Ahead: Will It Be Star Trek, Ecotopia, Big Government, or Mad Max?" *Futurist*, Vol. 33, No. 2, February 1999.

2. Coleman, Gary. "Challenges Enough for a Century." *Journal of Environmental Health*, Vol. 62, No. 1, July–August 1999.

3. Tong, Shilu, and Lu, Ying. "Major Issues in the Environmental Health Decision-Making Process." *Journal of Environmental Health*, Vol. 62, No. 1, July–August 1999.

4. Briley, Richard, et al. "Hindsight is 20/20." *Journal of Environmental Health*, Vol. 62, No. 1, July–August 1999.

5. Obassi, G. "Can Global Health Weather Global Climate?" *U. N. Chronicle*, Vol. 36, No. 1, Spring 1999.

6. Hartmann, Thom. "No Place to Escape." *Tikkun*, Vol. 14, No. 3, May–June 1999.

7. "Environmental Health." *JAMA*, Vol. 282, No. 2, July 14, 1999.

8. Krieger, D. J., and Hoehn, J. P. "The Economic Value of Reducing Environmental Health Risks." *Journal of Environmental Management*, May 1999.

9. "All-Around Health." *Sierra*, Vol. 84, No. 4, July 1999.

10. Gist, Ginger. "Multiple Chemical Sensitivity—The Role of Environmental Health Professionals." *Journal of Environmental Health*, Vol. 61, No. 6, January–February 1999.

11. Wiant, Chris. "Which Came First—The Carrot or the Stick?" *Journal of Environmental Health*, Vol. 61, No. 10, June, 1999.

12. Baxter, Jamie, and Eyles, John. "The Utility of In-Depth Interviews for Studying the Meaning of Environmental Risk." *Professional Geographer*, Vol. 51, No. 2, May, 1999.

13. Goch, Lynna. "It's Getting Hot Down Here." *Best's Review-Property-Casualty Insurance Edition*, Vol. 100, No. 4, August 1999. Nash, Madeleine. "The Case for a Shifting Climate is Heating Up." *Time*, Vol. 154, No. 6, August 9, 1999.

14. Tangley, Laura. " A Hot, Dry, Puzzling Summer." *U. S. News & World Report*, Vol. 127, No. 6, August 9, 1999.

15. Karlen, Wibjorn, et al. "Man-Made Versus Natural Climate Change." *Ambio*, Vol. 28, No. 4, June 1999.

16. Matthews, Robert. "Days Just Drag: We Knew Earth Was Getting Hotter . . . Now It's Slower, Too." *New Scientist*, Vol. 162, No. 2193, July 3, 1999.

17. Laber, Emily. "Meltdown." *Sciences*, Vol. 39, No. 4, July, 1999.

18. Kulash, Damian. "Facing Up to Global Climate Challenge." *Transportation Quarterly*, Vol. 53, No. 3, Summer 1999.

19. "New Weapons Help Fight Global Warming." *Engineering & Technology for a Sustainable World*, Vol. 6, No. 7, July 1999.

20. Visco, Ignazio. "Policy Challenges Arising from Climate Change." *OECD Economic Outlook*, No. 65, June 1998.

21. Wald, Matthew. "A Bad Year but Not a Hideous Year for Smog." *New York Times*, September 10, 1999.

22. Schindler, David. "From Acid Rain to Toxic Snow." *Ambio*, Vol. 28, No. 4, June 1999.

23. Mullenix, Linda. "Court Nixes Latest Settlement Class; Court Strikes Down 'Limited Fund' Settlement Class but Leaves Issues Unanswered." *National Law Journal*, Vol. 21, No. 51, August 16, 1999).

24. Taylor, Stuart, Jr. "Why Congress Should Fix the Asbestos Litigation Mess." *National Journal*, Vol. 31, No. 28, July 10, 1999.

25. Savage, David. "Another Asbestos Deal Undone; Justices Urge Legislative Solution to Liability Mess." *ABA Journal*, Vol. 85, August, 1999.

26. Morrison, Dorothy. "Lead-based Paint Hazards: Funding Opportunities Provide Control." *Public Management*, Vol. 80, No. 1, January 1998.

27. Rothenberg, Stephen, et al. "Maternal Blood Lead Level During Pregnancy in South Central Los Angeles." *Archives of Environmental Health*, Vol. 54, No. 3, May, 1999.

28. Elreedy, Salma, et al. "Relations Between Individual and Neighborhood-Based Measures of Socioeconomic Position and Bone Lead Concentrations Among Community-Exposed Men: The Normative Aging Study." *American Journal of Epidemiology*, Vol. 150, No. 2, July 15, 1999.

29. Fletcher, Alicia, et al. "Reasons for Testing and Exposure Sources Among Women of Childbearing Age with Moderate Blood Lead Levels." *Journal of Community Health*, Vol. 24, No. 3, June 1999.

30. Simon, Joel, and Hudes, Esther. "Relationship of Ascorbic Acid to Blood Lead Levels." *JAMA*, Vol. 281, No. 24, June 23, 1999.

31. Rennie, A. C., et al. "Mercury Poisoning After Spillage at Home from a Sphygmomanometer on Loan from Hospital." *British Medical Journal*, Vol. 319, No. 7206, August 7, 1999.

32. Staples, Susan, et al. "Noise Disturbance from a Developing Airport: Perceived Risk or General Annoyance?" *Environment and Behavior*, Vol. 31, No. 5, September 1999.

33. Barzilay, Joshua, et al. *The Water We Drink: Water Quality and Its Effects on Health*. New Brunswick, N.J.: Rutgers University Press, 1999.

34. Copley, Jon. "Smoke on the Water." *New Scientist*, Vol. 163, No. 2200, August 21, 1999.

35. Harrington, J. M. "Safety, Health and Environmental Hazards at the Workplace." *British Medical Journal*, Vol. 318, No. 7189, April 10, 1999.

36. Abell, A., et al. "Effects of Pesticide Exposure on Time to Pregnancy: Results of a Multicenter Study in France and Denmark." *American Journal of Epidemiology*, Vol. 150, No. 2, July 15, 1999.

37. "Endocrine Disruptors: A Scientific Perspective." American Council on Science and Health, July 12, 1999. Available at http://www.acsh.org

38. Weiss, Michael. "Keeping Bugs at Bay." *American Demographics*, July 1999.

39. Young, Frank. "Environmental Quality in the U. S. States." *Social Indicators Research*, Vol. 46, No. 2, February 1999.

40. Pearch, Fred. "Errors of Emission." *New Scientist*, Vol. 155, No. 2102, October 4, 1997.

41. Rutter, Terri. "Electromagnetic Fields May Be Carcinogenic." *British Medical Journal*, Vol. 317, No. 7150, July 4, 1998.

42. "Environmental Health Institute Report Concludes Evidence Is 'Weak' that Electric and Magnetic Fields Cause Cancer." National Institute of Environmental Health Sciences press release, June 15, 1999.

43. "EMFs—Doubts Linger over Possible Risks." *Science News*, Vol. 156, No. 1, July 3, 1999.

Hales Health

Almanac

Health Information on the Internet ■

Emergency ■

A Consumer's Guide to Medical Tests ■

Counting Your Calories and Fat ■

Your Health Directory ■

Health Information on the Internet

Using the Internet

The Internet: A Gateway to Health Information

What are the very latest statistics on the incidence of AIDS? Are any new drugs in the works for the treatment of diabetes? How can I get in touch with others who suffer from asthma? Is it possible to make a low-fat chocolate cake? These are the kinds of questions you can answer from your home or computer lab, with the help of the Internet. The Internet is a gold mine of information for the student of health. It can help you with research for your schoolwork, and also with personal questions and concerns about your own health. But the Internet is not comprehensively catalogued, and finding the information you need can be daunting. This guide will introduce you to health resources on the Internet and how to find them.

When you first start to explore the world of the Internet, it can seem overwhelming. What are the practical uses of the Internet for the student of health and the health care consumer?

- *Educational resources.* Most colleges and universities now have Internet hosts and World Wide Web sites. Faculty often post course information and syllabi on line, and some courses are even offered entirely on line. Some instructors require students to do tutorials or other projects on the Internet, or to do research using the Internet. In addition, you may be able to get general information about your school, its policies, programs, graduation requirements, and faculty on the Net.

- *Research.* The Internet is a repository for many health journals, government statistics, archives, and other sources of scholarly information. In addition, subscribing to a mailing list or posting to a newsgroup in an area of interest can yield new sources of information that would be hard to get elsewhere.

- *Graduate school and career information.* The Internet is a great resource for those interested a career in a health-related field. Most graduate schools have web sites that list their programs, entrance requirements, faculty profiles, and other information of interest to prospective students. And once you get that degree you can consult online listings of jobs available in many areas of health care.

- *Self-help and support.* The Internet is a good way of providing information and support to people who might not otherwise have access to it. There are dozens of newsgroups and mailing lists that offer support and advice for people dealing with all kinds of health-related issues, from Alzheimer's caregivers to people with eating disorders to athletes comparing training programs.

- *Goods and services.* As many people have discovered, the web can serve as an electronic shopping mall. For people with concerns about health it can be a place to order books, software, or journals of interest, sign up for classes or conferences, or even get online professional consultations (though we're not recommending that).

The World Wide Web

The World Wide Web is an information retrieval system designed to offer a user-friendly graphical interface with the Internet. You can surf the web using any one of a number of different programs called browsers, such as Netscape or Microsoft Explorer. Many web sites now offer exciting capabilities, such as audio, video, animation clips, and interactivity. Each web site has its own unique address, or URL. URLs often begin with the characters http://. To go to a web site, you can either type its URL into the box at the top of your browser, or click on a hyperlink from another page that will take you to the new site. Hyperlinks often appear as color or underlined text, and offer links to other web sites that may be of interest.

There are thousands of sites related to health and wellness on the World Wide Web. As a starting point, you can try using any of the sources listed in the Health Online boxes in this book, or at this book's web site at http://health. wadsworth.com. Or you can try to look for specific information by doing a web search.

Bookmarks

When you find a web site you will want to return to again in the future, you can "bookmark" it. To bookmark a site, go to that site and choose "bookmark" from your menu bar. Your browser will record the address of that site in your bookmark folder. Anytime you want to return to that site, you simply open the bookmark folder and click on the title of that web site.

Tips for Using the World Wide Web

- *Be patient.* Accessing a web site can take time depending on how elaborate the site is, how fast your modem can download the information, and what time of day you are surfing. You can speed things up a bit by turning off the "auto load image" option in your browser.

- *Keep in mind that glitches can occur in the transfer process.* Sometimes the server of the web site you are trying to reach may be down, there may be a lot of activity on that site, or there may be line noise. Just try again to load the web site, or try again later.

- *Because the Web is so dynamic, sites and links change every day.* You might find some links on web pages that go nowhere, if the link has moved their pages to a new server or address.

- *Remember that while the web is a great source of information, not everything on it is true.* It is up to you to evaluate the information you get from the web; see the section on Thinking Critically about Health Information on the Internet.

Searching the Web

How do you go about finding web sites that might interest you? One way is to use one of the popular directories on the web called search engines. A search engine allows you to type in keywords on the topic that you are interested in, and it will retrieve sites that contain those words. Some of the larger and more popular search engines are:

- **Yahoo!**
  http://www.yahoo.com

- **Alta Vista**
  http://altavista.digital.com

- **Excite**
  http://www.excite.com

- **Hot Bot**
  http://www.hotbot.com

- **Lycos**
  http://www.lycos.com

- **Infoseek**
  http://www.infoseek.com

- **WebCrawler**
  http://webcrawler.com

To use a search engine, type in one of the URLs listed above. When the home page for the site comes up you will notice a "search" box in which you can type one or more key words or phrases. The engine will then search all the sites in its index and return a list to you, with hyperlinks and sometimes short descriptions, of those that contain your keywords.

There is no single search engine that contains all the contents of the Internet. After connecting to a search engine for the first time, it is a good idea to read the tool's description, search options, and rules and restrictions. Each engine offers a different "view" of the web and you'll want to tailor your query to make the best use of that system. Some search engines contain indexes to huge amounts of online information, so it pays to make precise queries so you don't get thousands of sites returned to you. It is also possible to make queries that are too precise and retrieve no results.

The key to an effective search is picking the right keywords. Commonly used words make poor search keywords; try to find distinctive words or combinations of words. If you use several keywords, separate them with one of these three operators: AND, OR, and NOT. Using the word AND actually narrows the results you obtain in a search. For example, if you search for "pregnancy AND teen," you will get back only sites that contain both these keywords. The word "OR" broadens the search results. You may try searching "pregnancy AND teen OR adolescent," to find sites that refer to teen or adolescent pregnancy. To limit your results, you can use the word NOT. Searching for "pregnancy AND teen NOT United States" might help you find sites that deal with teen pregnancy in other countries.

Now that you have done your search, you may end up with hundreds or even thousands of results—or only a few. If you have more results than you can handle, try making the keywords in your search more precise. See if you can think of words that uniquely identify what you are looking for, and use several relevant keywords. If you have too few results, try another search engine, using synonyms or variations on your keywords, or be less specific in your query.

News Groups

News groups are a way of discussing topics over the Internet with other people who share the same interests or concerns. They are a popular way to establish an online community, share information, and give and receive support. For example, a person suffering from a relatively rare disorder may not know anyone else with the same problems and concerns on campus or in town, but he or she can frequent a news group specifically for people with that disorder to learn about other peoples' experiences, the latest treatments, and just to commiserate. Or a person who is trying to quit smoking can participate in a newsgroup to share frustrations, tips, and successes. But, as always, be aware that not everything posted to a news group is necessarily true; you must be a critical thinker.

Many commercial online services offer members-only news groups to their subscribers, but there are many other news groups available to anyone. To find a news group on a topic of interest to you, try looking on the Deja News web page, http://www.dejanews.com, which lists hundreds of news groups. Some health-related news groups are listed in the Resources section of this appendix.

News group addresses are grouped into several broad categories called hierarchies. Listed below are some of the standard hierarchies that relate to health.

- **alt**
  groups generally alternative in nature (i.e., alt.sex)

- **bionet**
  groups discussing biology and biological sciences (i.e., bionet.immunology)

- **misc**
  groups that don't fit into other categories (i.e., misc.fitness)

- **rec**
  groups discussing hobbies, sports, music, and art (i.e., rec.food)

- **sci**
  groups discussing subjects related to the science and scientific research (i.e., sci.epidemiology)

- **soc**
  groups discussing social issues including politics, social programs, etc. (i.e., soc.college)

• **talk**
public debating forums on controversial issues (i.e., talk.abortion)

Before you make a posting to a news group, you may want to "lurk" for awhile, that is, read the discussion without contributing your own posting. Lurking will give you a sense of the kinds of postings that are appropriate for that news group and what the news group culture is like. It is also a good idea to read the news group's "FAQ," or list of answers to frequently asked questions.

Postings to many news groups are updated frequently, so if an item is of interest to you, you should print it or save it to your computer since it may be gone the next day. After lurking for awhile, you can join in the discussion by posting a message to the news group. You may also want to reply only to the originator of a certain message. You may want to join in on the discussion of an already-existing topic, or start your own "thread."

Mailing Lists

Mailing lists (or listservs) are groups of people who "get together" via e-mail to discuss a specific topic. Mailing lists offer a way to participate in lively discussions, stay up on current research, or find out answers to burning questions. There are mailing lists on nearly every topic imaginable. Mailing lists are similar to news groups in that they are forums for discussion, but the messages are delivered to your e-mail account instead of to a public bulletin board. Here's how it works:

• First, find a mailing list dealing with a subject you are interested in discussing with others (i.e., attention deficit disorder).

• In order to get involved in a discussion group, you have to subscribe to it. To subscribe, send an e-mail to that mailing list's "subscribe" address with the word "subscribe" in the subject line and in the main body of the text. Also include your e-mail address.

• Usually, the listserv will then subscribe you to the list and send you instructions on how to "post" to the group. "Posting" means that you send out a comment to the entire mailing list that you have subscribed to.

• Every time any member posts to the listserv, all the subscribers get that posting as an e-mail message in their mailbox.

• Once you have subscribed you will begin to receive e-mail messages from the mailing list. Be careful though: some discussion groups have a large following and you may find your mailbox filling up faster than you can read the messages.

• Again, evaluate carefully any information you get from a mailing list to make sure it is accurate.

Thinking Critically About Health Information on the Internet

Unlike information in most books and journals, anyone can post information or advice on the Internet. Some of this information can be misleading or downright harmful, so it is important to use your best critical thinking skills to evaluate health information you find on the Internet. When evaluating information on the Net, ask yourself the following questions.

• *Who is the author or sponsor of the information?* The author of the site is usually listed at the top or bottom of a site's home page. Be very wary of any anonymous site. Sites that are maintained by established schools or universities, government agencies, professional organizations, or other established organizations like the American Cancer Society are probably trustworthy. Sites created by individuals or other groups may or may not contain valid information; see if you can verify their information in other places. And keep in mind that many sites contain links to other pages which may be maintained by other less (or more) reliable sources.

• *Is it current?* Many sites post the date of their most recent modification. Look for sites where you can determine when the information was created or modified; many of the best sites are updated weekly or even daily.

• *What is the purpose of the site?* The hidden purpose of some health web sites is to sell products or act as a vehicle for advertisements. Be wary of any site that tries to sell you things or get your money. Also beware of sites that seem to be trying to persuade you of things, promote "miracle cures" or anything that seems too good to be true. There are also people who use news groups and other chat forums to sell or persuade. Be skeptical and use your common sense.

• *Who is the intended audience?* Some Internet information is intended for doctors and other health care professionals; although the information may be accurate, it may be too difficult for a layperson to interpret on their own. Other web sites or Internet forums are targeted toward people with specific problems or disorders, students, or the general public.

• *Is the information verifiable?* To get a better perspective on information from the Internet, see if you can verify it with other sources. Before you follow any health advice you get from the Net, check it out with your physician.

Health Resources on the Internet

Hundreds of health-related Internet addresses can be found at http://health.wadsworth.com Also see "Your Health Directory" near the back of this Almanac—it contains web site adresses for several health-related organizations.

Emergency!

By definition, an emergency is a situation in which you have to think and act fast. Start by assessing the circumstances. Shout for help if you're in a public place. Look for any possible dangers to you or the victim, such as a live electrical wire or a fire. Seek medical assistance as quickly as possible. Dial 911, the operator, or a local emergency phone number, and keep it near every phone in your house. Don't attempt rescue techniques, such as cardiopulmonary resuscitation (CPR), unless you are trained. If you have a car, be sure you know the shortest route from your home to the nearest 24-hour hospital emergency department.

Supplies

Every home should have a kit of basic first aid supplies kept in a convenient location out of the reach of children. Stock it with the following:

- Bandages
- Sterile gauze pads and bandages
- Adhesive tape
- Scissors
- Cotton balls or absorbent cotton
- Cotton swabs
- Thermometer
- Syrup of ipecac to induce vomiting
- Antibiotic ointments
- Sharp needle
- Safety pins
- Calamine lotion

Keep a similar kit in your car or boat. You might want to add some extra items from your home, such as a flashlight, soap, blanket, paper cups, and any special equipment that a family member with a chronic illness may need.

Bleeding

Blood loss is frightening and dangerous. Direct pressure stops external bleeding. Since internal bleeding can also be life-threatening, you must be aware of the warning signs.

For an Open Wound

1. Apply direct pressure over the site of the wound. Cover the entire wound.
2. Use sterile gauze, a sanitary napkin, a clean towel, sheet, or handkerchief or, if necessary, your washed bare hand.

Ice or cold water in a pad will help stop bleeding and decrease swelling.

3. Apply firm, steady pressure for five to fifteen minutes. Most wounds stop bleeding within a few minutes.
4. If the wound is on a foot, hand, leg, or arm, use gravity to help slow the flow of blood. Elevate the limb so that it is higher than the victim's heart.
5. If the bleeding doesn't stop, press harder.
6. Seek medical attention if the bleeding was caused by a serious injury, if stitches will be needed to keep the wound closed, or if the victim has not had a tetanus booster within the last ten years.

For Internal Bleeding

1. Suspect internal bleeding if a person coughs up blood, vomits red or brown material that looks like coffee grounds, passes blood in urine or stool, or has black, tar-like bowel movements.
2. Do not let the victim take any medication or fluids by mouth until seen by a doctor, because surgery may be necessary.
3. Have the victim lie flat. Cover him or her lightly.
4. Seek immediate medical attention.

For a Bloody Nose

1. Have the victim sit down, leaning slightly forward so the blood does not run down his or her throat. The person should spit out any blood in his or her mouth.
2. Use the thumb and forefingers to pinch the nose. If the victim can do the pinching, apply a cold compress to the nose and surrounding area.
3. Apply pressure for ten minutes without interruption.
4. If pinching does not work, gently pack the nostril with gauze or a clean strip of cloth. Do not use absorbent cotton, which will stick. Let the ends hang out so you can remove the packing easily later. Pinch the nose, with the packing in place, for five minutes.
5. If a foreign object is in the nose, do not attempt to remove it. Ask the person to blow gently. If that does not work, seek medical attention.
6. The nose should not be blown or irritated for several hours after a nosebleed stops.

Breathing Problems

If a person appears to be unconscious, approach carefully. The victim may be in contact with electrical current. If so, make sure the electricity is shut off before touching the victim. The first function you should check is respiration. Tap or shake the victim's shoulder gently, shouting, "Are you all right?" Look for any signs of breathing: Can you hear breath sounds? Can you feel breath on your cheek? If the person is breathing, do not perform mouth-to-mouth resuscitation.

If you aren't certain if the victim is breathing, or if there are no signs of breath, follow these steps:

1. Lay the person on his or her back on the floor or ground. Roll the victim over if necessary, being careful to turn the head with the remainder of the body as a unit to avoid possible neck injury. Loosen any tight clothing around the neck or chest.

2. Check for any foreign material in the mouth or throat and remove it quickly.

3. Open the airway by tilting the head back and lifting the chin up.

4. Pinch the nostrils shut with your thumb and index finger.

5. Take a deep breath, open your mouth wide and place it securely over the victim's, and give two slow breaths, each lasting 1 to 10 seconds. Remove your mouth, turn your head, and check to see if the victim's chest rises and falls. If you hear air escaping from the victim's mouth and see the chest fall, you know that you are getting air into the lungs.

6. Repeat once every five seconds (twelve breaths per minute) until professional help takes over, or the victim begins breathing on his or her own. It may take several hours to revive someone. If you stop, the victim may not be able to breathe on his or her own. Once the person does begin to breathe independently, always get professional help.

7. If air doesn't seem to be entering the chest, or the chest doesn't fall between breaths, tilt the head further back. If that doesn't work, follow the directions for choking emergencies later in this section.

8. If the victim is a child, do not pinch the nose shut. Cover both the mouth and nose with your mouth, and place your free hand very lightly on the child's chest. Use small puffs of air rather than big breaths. Feel the chest inflate as you blow, and listen for exhaled air. Repeat once every three seconds (twenty breaths per minute).

Broken Bones

If you suspect that a person has broken a leg, do not move him or her unless there is immediate danger.

1. Check for signs of breathing. If there is none or breathing is very weak, administer mouth-to-mouth resuscitation.

2. If the person is bleeding, apply direct pressure on the site of the wound.

3. Try to keep the victim warm and calm.

4. Do not try to push a broken bone back into place if it is sticking out of the skin. You can apply a moist dressing to prevent it from drying out.

5. Do not try to straighten out a fracture.

6. Do not allow the victim to walk.

7. Splint unstable fractures to prevent painful motion.

Burns

1. If fire caused the burn, cool the affected area with water to stop the burning process.

2. Remove the victim's garments and jewelry and cover him or her with clean sheets or towels.

3. Call for help immediately.

4. If chemicals caused the burn, wash the affected area with cool water for at least twenty minutes. Chemical burns of the eye require immediate medical attention after flushing with water for twenty minutes.

Choking

A person with anything stuck in the throat and blocking the airway can stop breathing, lose consciousness, and die within four to six minutes. A universal signal of distress because of choking is clasping the throat with one or both hands. Other signs are an inability to talk and noisy, difficult breathing. You need to take immediate action, but *NEVER* slap the victim's back. This could make the obstruction worse.

If the victim can speak, cough, or breathe, do not interfere. Coughing alone may dislodge the foreign object. If the choking continues without lessening, call for medical help.

If the victim cannot speak, cough, or breathe but is conscious, use the Heimlich maneuver, as follows

1. Stand behind the victim (who may be seated or standing) and wrap your arms around his or her waist.

2. Make a fist with one hand and place the thumb side of your fist against the victim's abdomen, just above the navel. Grasp your fist with your other hand and press into his or her abdomen with a quick, upward thrust. Do not exert any pressure against the rib cage with your forearms.

3. Repeat this procedure until the victim is no longer choking or loses consciousness.

4. If the person is lying facedown, roll the victim over. Facing the person, kneel with your legs astride his or her hips. Put the heel of one hand below the rib cage and place your other hand on top. Press into the abdomen with a quick, upward thrust. Repeat thrusts as needed.

5. If you start choking when you're by yourself, place your fist below your rib cage and above your navel. Grasp this fist with your other hand and press into your abdomen with a quick, upward thrust. You also can lean over a fixed, horizontal object, such as a table edge or chair back, and press your upper abdomen against it with a quick, upward thrust. Repeat as needed until you dislodge the object.

If the Victim Is Unconscious

1. Place him or her on the ground and give mouth-to-mouth resuscitation as described earlier.

2. If the victim does not start breathing and air does not seem to be going into his or her lungs, roll the victim onto his or her back and give one or more manual thrusts: Place one of your hands on top of the other with the heel of the bottom hand in the middle of the abdomen, slightly above the

navel and below the rib cage. Press into the abdomen with a quick, upward thrust. Do not push to either side. Repeat 6 to 10 times as needed.

3. Clear the airway. Hold the victim's mouth open with one hand and use your thumb to depress the tongue. Make a hook with the index finger of your other hand and, using a gentle, sweeping motion, reach into the victim's throat and feel for a swallowed foreign object in the airway.

4. Repeat the following steps in this sequence:
   - Six to ten abdominal thrusts
   - Probe in mouth
   - Try to inflate lungs
   - Repeat

5. If the victim suddenly seems okay, but no foreign material has been removed, take him or her directly to the hospital. A foreign object, such as a fish or chicken bone or other jagged object, could do internal damage as it passes through the victim's system.

If the Victim Is a Child

1. If the child is coughing, do nothing. The coughing alone may dislodge the object.

2. If the airway is blocked and the child is panicky and fighting for breath, do *NOT* probe the airway with your fingers to clear an unseen foreign object. You might push the material back into the airway, worsening the obstruction.

3. For an infant younger than a year, hang the child over your arm so that the head is lower than the trunk. Using the heel of your hand, administer four firm blows high on the back between the shoulder blades. For a bigger child, follow the same procedure, but invert the child over your knee rather than your arm.

4. After four back blows, perform four chest thrusts (the Heimlich maneuver as described above).

Drowning

A person can die of drowning four to six minutes after breathing stops. Although prevention is the wisest course, follow these steps in case of a drowning emergency:

1. Get the victim out of the water fast. Be extremely cautious, because a drowning person may panic and grasp at a rescuer, endangering that individual as well. If possible, push a branch or pole within the victim's reach.

2. If the victim is unconscious, use a flotation device if at all possible. Carefully place the person on the device. Once out of the water, place the victim on his or her back.

3. If the victim is not breathing, start mouth-to-mouth resuscitation. Continue until the person can breathe unassisted or help arrives. (Note that it may take an hour or two for a drowning victim to resume independent breathing.) Do not leave the victim alone for any reason.

4. Once the person is breathing without assistance, even if he or she is still coughing, you need only stay nearby until professional help arrives.

Electrical Shock

1. If you suspect that an electrical shock has knocked a person unconscious, approach very carefully. Do not touch the victim unless the electricity has been turned off.

2. Shut off the power at the plug, circuit breaker, or fuse box. Simply shutting off an appliance does not remove the shock hazard. Use a dry stick to move a wire or downed power line from the victim. Keep in mind that you also are in danger until the power is off.

3. If the person's breathing is weak or has stopped, follow the steps for mouth-to-mouth resuscitation.

4. Even if the victim returns to consciousness, call for medical help. While waiting, cover the victim with a blanket or coat to keep him or her warm. Place a blanket underneath the body if the surface is cold. Be sure the person lies flat if conscious, with legs raised. If the victim is unconscious, place him or her on one side, with a pillow supporting the head. Do not give the victim anything to eat or drink.

5. Electrical burns can extend deep into the tissue, even when they appear minor. Do not put butter, household remedies, or sprays on burns without a doctor's instruction. Do not use ice or cold water on an electrical burn that is more than two inches across.

Heart Attack

Chest pain can be caused by indigestion, strained muscles, or lung infections. The warning signs of a heart attack are:

- Intense pain that lasts for more than two minutes, produces a tight or crushing feeling, is centered in the chest, or spreads to the neck, jaw, shoulder, or arm
- Shortness of breath that is worse when the person lies flat and improves when the person sits
- Heavy sweating
- Nausea or vomiting
- Irregular pulse
- Pale or bluish skin or lips
- Weakness
- Severe anxiety, feeling of doom

If an individual develops these symptoms:

1. Call for emergency medical help immediately.

2. Have the person sit up or lie in a semi-reclining position. Loosen tight clothing. Keep him or her comfortably warm.

3. If the person loses consciousness, turn on his or her back and check for breathing and pulse. If vomiting occurs, turn the victim's head to one side and clean the mouth.

4. If the person has medicine for angina pectoris (chest pain) and is conscious, help him or her take it.

5. If the person is unconscious, and you are trained to perform cardiopulmonary resuscitation (CPR), check for a pulse at the wrist or neck. If there is none, begin CPR in conjunction with mouth-to-mouth resuscitation. Do not

attempt CPR unless you are trained. It is not a technique you can learn from a book.

Poisoning

Many common household substances, including glue, aspirin, bleaches, and paint, can be poisonous. Make sure you know the emergency numbers for the Poison Control Center and Fire Department Rescue Squad. Keep them near your telephone. Be prepared to provide the following information:

- The kind of substance swallowed and how much was swallowed

- If a child or adult swallowed the substance

- Symptoms

- Whether or not vomiting has occurred

- Whether you gave the person anything to drink

- How much time it will take to get to an emergency room

The Poison Control Center or rescue team will tell you whether or not to induce vomiting or neutralize a swallowed poison. Here are some additional guidelines:

1. Always assume the worst if a small child has swallowed or might have swallowed something poisonous. Call the local Poison Control Center or emergency number (911 in many areas). Keep the suspected item or container with you to answer questions.

2. Do not give any medications unless a physical or the Poison Control Center instructs you to do so.

3. Do not follow the directions for neutralizing poisons on the container unless a doctor or the Poison Control Center confirms that they are appropriate measures to take.

4. If the child is conscious, give moderate doses of water to dilute the poison.

5. If a poisoning victim is unconscious, make sure he or she is breathing. If not, give mouth-to-mouth resuscitation. Do not give anything by mouth or attempt to simulate the person. Call for emergency help immediately.

6. If the person is vomiting, make sure he or she is in a position in which he or she cannot choke on what is brought up.

7. While vomiting is the fastest way to expel swallowed poisons from the body, never try to induce vomiting if the person has swallowed any acid or alkaline substance, which can cause burns of the face, mouth, and throat (examples include ammonia, bleach, dishwasher detergent, drain and toilet cleaners, lye, oven cleaners, or rust removers), or petroleum-like products, which produce dangerous fumes that can be inhaled during vomiting (examples include floor polish, furniture wax, gasoline, kerosene, lighter fluid, turpentine, and paint thinner).

A Consumer's Guide to Medical Tests

✓ **What They Tell the Doctor**
✓ **How Often You Need Them**
✓ **What to Do About Abnormal Results**

D o you wonder what the doctor sees when he looks into your eyes with that little light, or what it means when your blood or urine test is normal? In this section we cover some of the most common tests your doctor does, what they tell, and how often they should be done.

General Information

- Always ask your doctor what tests are being done, why they are being ordered, what they involve, and what the results mean.
- No test is foolproof. If a result is unexpected, whether normal or abnormal, your doctor should repeat the test before making any decisions.
- Modern X-ray machines expose you to a minuscule amount of radiation. Nevertheless, be sure to tell the physician or X-ray technician if there is even a chance you may be pregnant.
- Often a doctor orders a test because that is the only way to prove you do *not* have a disease.

Allergy Skin Testing

- Skin testing is still the most reliable method.
- The physician either pricks your skin twenty to forty or more times to introduce a tiny bit of potentially allergic material or injects a small amount.
- Children who are frightened by multiple needle sticks and are unlikely to sit still for as long as necessary may have blood (RAST) tests instead.

What results mean

If you develop redness or a hivelike bump around an area, you are probably allergic to the injected substance. Sometimes you can avoid the offending material, but things like pollen and dust are everywhere. Your allergist may recommend desensitizing shots to reduce your reaction. Note that the results of skin tests won't be reliable if you take antihistamines within 48 hours of the test.

How often to be tested

Skin tests are necessary only if you cannot get allergy relief from other measures such as over-the-counter medications, reducing mold and dust in the house, and staying away from animals.

Blood Pressure Reading

- High blood pressure, a major cause of stroke and heart attacks, usually causes no symptoms.
- The upper number in a reading—the systolic—refers to peak amount of pressure generated when your heart pumps blood, the lower number—the diastolic—measures the least amount of pressure.

What results mean

Most doctors today think the lower the pressure the better, which means a reading of 120/80 or less. Because the mere anxiety of having your blood pressure taken can cause a mild elevation, your doctor will want to repeat an abnormal test, ideally on a different day, before diagnosing high blood pressure.

How often to be tested

Everyone—no matter how healthy—should have a blood-pressure reading taken at least once a year, more often if you have high blood pressure.

Blood Tests

- Blood may be taken from either a finger prick or, more commonly, a vein in your arm.
- See below for information on cholesterol testing, which is also done from a blood sample.

Complete Blood Count (CBC)

This is the most commonly performed of all blood tests.

What results mean

A *low red-cell count,* called anemia, can be caused by something as simple as too little iron in your diet, as complex as an abnormality in your digestion, or as serious as a bone marrow problem or silent bleeding. Iron deficiency is the most frequent cause, with women who menstruate and limit their intake of red meat at the greatest risk. If your doctor diagnoses this problem, ask about making dietary changes as well as taking iron supplements.

A high white-cell count, a measure of the body's defenses against infection, usually indicates some kind of infection. Depending on the type of cell that predominates, your doctor may be able to identify whether you have a bacterial or viral infection.

Platelets, the first participants in blood clotting, may be decreased because of a viral infection, abnormal bleeding, or for no identifiable reason.

Chemistry Panels (Chem 12 or 18, SMA 12 or 24)

Kidney, bone, liver, pancreas, prostate, and some glandular functions are screened by these tests.

What results mean

An abnormality may signal a problem that needs treatment. Because accuracy decreases when many tests are run together, any specific abnormal test should be repeated, especially if unexpected.

CAT (Computerized Axial Tomography) Scan

- A CAT scan is 100 times more sensitive than an X ray.
- You lie as motionless as possible in a large tube while an X-ray beam travels 360 degrees around you. The test takes about an hour.

What results mean

The test can help diagnose such conditions as tumors, blood clots, cysts, and bleeding in the brain as well as in various other organs.

Cholesterol Test

- Anyone can have a high cholesterol level, but you are more apt to be at risk if there is a family history of early heart attacks, strokes, or high cholesterol tests.
- Your doctor will look at not only total cholesterol but also the levels of high-density lipoprotein (HUL), the "good" cholesterol that prevents cholesterol from sticking to your blood vessels, and low-density lipoprotein (LDL), the "bad" cholesterol that does the reverse.

What results mean

Experts today think optimum cholesterol levels are below 200 mg/ml of blood. The following chart shows the risk by age of various cholesterol levels.

Cholesterol Risk Chart

Age	Moderate Risk	High Risk
20–29	200–220 mg/ml	Over 220
30–39	220–240	Over 240
Over 40	240–260	Over 260

Persistently high cholesterol values will prompt your doctor to advise dietary and lifestyle changes—less fat intake, more exercise—and perhaps medication. This will particularly be the case if LDL levels also are high (less than 130 mg/ml is considered desirable, 130–159 is borderline risk, and over 160 is high risk).

How often to be tested

If your cholesterol level is under 200 and your LDL level is under 130, repeat the test every five years. If your test is borderline, repeat it annually. (Note that the test should be taken when you have not eaten for at least twelve hours.)

If you have a family history of cholesterol problems, have your children tested annually from age 2; if you don't, have them tested around age 10 and every few years thereafter. Children under 2 should not be given a low-cholesterol diet; they need extra fat to make brain tissue and hormones for growth.

Fundoscopy

- The doctor looks into your eye with a little light.

What results mean

The beginnings of cataracts may be visible, as well as irregularities in the blood vessels that indicate damage from high cholesterol (fatty deposits in the blood vessels), high blood pressure (narrowing and notching), diabetes, or other diseases. If the optic nerve is swollen, there may be excess pressure inside your skull.

What your doctor *cannot* see are the early signs of glaucoma, which can lead to blindness if not treated. Over age 20, have a pressure check for glaucoma from an opthalmologist or optometrist every three years—or every year if you have a family history of glaucoma.

Heart Tests

- The following tests are listed from the simplest through the most complicated.
- Also see listings for blood pressure readings, cholesterol tests, and pulse.

Electrocardiogram (EKG, ECG)

- A machine amplifies the electrical signals from your heart and records them on paper.

What results mean

An EKG can detect such things as an enlarged heart, abnormal levels of potassium or calcium, disease of the small vessels of the heart, and where an abnormal heart rhythm originates. It is a nonspecific test, however, and more advanced studies should be done if serious disease is suspected.

Echocardiogram

This is a painless test in which sound waves are used to produce a picture of the heart in action on a TV-type screen.

What results mean

The test investigates the size of the heart chambers, the thickness of the walls, how the four heart valves are working, and the condition of the membrane surrounding the heart. Mitral valve prolapse, a common minor abnormality, often shows up on this test, as well as more serious problems.

Stress Test

Your heart rate, blood pressure, and EKG are constantly monitored as you exercise on a treadmill that goes faster and faster with a steeper and steeper incline. This test—also called an exercise tolerance test or treadmill test—should be performed in the presence of a cardiologist and in or near a hospital in case the strain causes heart problems that need emergency treatment. The test should be stopped immediately if you experience any lightheadedness, chest pain, nausea, or palpitations.

What results mean

The changes that an increasing strain on the heart causes can tell your doctor if you are at risk of a heart attack. This is because a blockage in the coronary arteries—the blood vessels that feed your heart muscle—may show up only during exercise.

Angiography

A dye is injected into various arteries, and X rays are taken.

What results mean

The doctor can detect blockages in the blood vessels that can lead to heart attack or stroke, as well as aneurysms (weakened spots in the blood-vessel walls). The test carries some risk of causing stroke.

Kidney Tests

- The tests noted here involve taking X rays. In addition, ultrasound (similar to an echocardiogram) can be used to outline the kidneys.

Intravenous Pyelogram (IVP)

After an iodine-containing substance is injected into a vein, X rays are taken at five-minute intervals to show the outlines of the kidney, ureter, and bladder.

What results mean

Tumors, kidney stones, and swelling of the kidney tissue can be seen, as well as blockage to urine flow or a mass that may be pressing on the kidney. A kidney that is not functioning will not appear on the X ray, and one in an abnormal position can be found.

Voiding Cystourethrogram (VCUG)

A technician will fill your bladder with a dye injected through a catheter and take X rays while you urinate.

What results mean

If you have recurrent urinary-tract infections, the test will show if there is a significant backup of urine from the bladder into the ureter, in which case daily antibiotics may be needed to prevent infection. Investigating recurrent urinary tract infections is particularly important for children.

Magnetic Resonance Imaging (MRI)

- MRI uses no radiation but produces pictures of the brain that are much more detailed than those of a CAT scan.

What results mean

In addition to locating bleeding or tumors, as a CAT scan does, the test picks up subtle signs such as those of Parkinson's disease and multiple sclerosis in the brain or a herniated disc in the spinal column.

Mammography

- Only a small amount of radiation is used to take the mammogram. You usually stand up and put your breast on a photographic plate where it is compressed with a plastic shield or balloonlike device. It shouldn't hurt. If your breasts are tender at certain times in your menstrual cycle, schedule your mammogram when they are least sensitive.

- Mammograms can detect breast abnormalities at easily treated stages before you can feel them, but they are not foolproof. Examine your breasts monthly.

What results mean

Mammograms can detect cysts, abscesses, and tumors. Whether a mass is benign or malignant is hard to tell in the early stages, so abnormalities usually need to be biopsied or removed totally to determine treatment.

How often to be tested

Although there is controversy over the benefits of mammography for women under 50, many experts still recommend having a first mammogram between ages 35 and 40, followed by one every two years between 40 and 50, and yearly thereafter. If your mother or sister has had breast cancer, consult your doctor for an appropriate schedule. And if you have a lump, pain, or nipple discharge, have a mammogram right away, no matter what your age.

You also should have a breast examination by a doctor at least every three years between ages 20 and 40, and every year after 40.

Pap Smear

- A routine part of every gynecological examination.

- Your doctor takes a painless swab from the cervix and vaginal walls and sends it to a lab for analysis.

What results mean

Pap smears can detect not only cervical cancer but also inflammation and many infections, minor and more serious; they also provide important information about the state of your female hormones. A normal test is termed class 1, and abnormal results are graded by degree into four classifications, with only the most severe—a class V test—signifying outright cancer. Treatment depends on the diagnosis and may range from doing nothing for a minor inflammation to, in rare cases, a hysterectomy for cancer. Because the error rate of Pap smears is high, the doctor should always repeat an abnormal test.

How often to be tested

Women who are on birth control pills and are sexually active should have a Pap smear every six months; other women should be checked every year.

Physical Examination

- The routine physical exam generally includes a pulse and blood-pressure reading, measure of height and weight, blood tests (including a cholesterol test), fundoscopy, and sometimes other tests as well, such as a stool test for blood.

What results mean

A physical exam serves as a general measure of health and sometimes picks up early signs of disease.

How often to have a physical exam

Most doctors no longer recommend yearly physicals for everybody. A good schedule to follow instead is to have a complete checkup every four or five years under age 40, every three years between 40 and 50, every two years between 50 and 60, and every year after that. At any age, you should have more frequent examinations if you have chronic medical problems such as diabetes or high blood pressure, are obese, or smoke cigarettes.

Pulse

- To take your own pulse, press two fingertips over the artery in your wrist, just below the base of the thumb. Count the beats in 20 seconds, then multiply by 3.

What results mean

The normal pulse rate—the speed at which your heart pumps blood—is 60–80 beats a minute; it should be regular, without skipped or extra beats. Abnormal rates can be due to thyroid problems (too high causes a fast rate, too low a slow one), heart problems, anxiety (even the stress of a physical exam), or weakness from an illness such as the flu or other problems.

    The character of your pulse is also important. A discrepancy between the strength of the pulse on one side of the neck and the other may mean you are in danger of a stroke. A pulse that is abnormally strong and bounding can signal a problem with a heart valve. If the pulse is weak, you may have blockages in your blood vessels from diabetes, atherosclerosis (hardening of the arteries), or a variety of other disorders.

Stomach and Intestinal Tests

- Though most of these tests are uncomfortable, they generally are not painful.

Barium Enema

Barium, a radioactive material, is instilled in your large intestine through a tube inserted into your anus. Because barium is constipating, drink fluids afterward. Don't be alarmed if you have white stools for a day or two.

What results mean

The doctor will be able to see tumors or polyps, any obstructions, and other abnormalities.

Gastroscopy and Proctoscopy

In gastroscopy, for which you will be sedated, the doctor looks into the stomach with a flexible tube that goes through your mouth. The procedure is essentially the same for proctoscopy, except that the doctor looks into your large intestine through a tube inserted into your anus.

What results mean

Your doctor can see where bleeding comes from, remove a polyp, or biopsy a mass.

Upper GI Series

You will be asked to down a drink of barium so that X rays can be taken of the esophagus, stomach, duodenum, and sometimes the small intestine.

What results mean

Your doctor can diagnose swallowing disorders, hiatus hernias, ulcers, tumors, and some inflammations of the stomach and small bowel.

Stool Test for Occult Blood

A small sample of stool that remains on the doctor's glove after a rectal exam or that is collected by you at home is tested for blood that is invisible to the eye.

What results mean

This test is done routinely as part of a regular checkup to detect the earliest sign of cancer of the colon. It is also part of an investigation of anemia or abdominal pain. If your test is positive, tell your doctor if you recently ate radishes, turnips, or red meat, took large doses of vitamin C or iron pills, or had a nosebleed. All of these things can produce misleading results.

Urinalaysis

- Urine can tell about the health not only of the kidneys but also of other organ systems.

What results mean

Specific gravity is the degree to which your urine is concentrated or diluted. If it is persistently too dilute, your doctor may ask for a first morning sample to see how well your kidneys concentrate your urine overnight. Urine that is too concentrated may indicate poor fluid intake, decreased kidney function, or dehydration from vomiting and diarrhea.

    pH or acidity or alkalinity is useful information when there is a history or possibility of kidney stones, urinary-tract infection, or kidney disease.

    Glucose or sugar in the urine may mean you have diabetes. You will need a blood test to confirm the diagnosis, as some families filter sugar easily through their kidneys but do not have any disease. Inflammation of the pancreas and thyroid problems also may cause sugar in the urine.

    Blood in the urine may mean infection, a stone, or an inflammation of the kidney. Excessive exertion such as running sometimes causes some blood to leak into the urine; this usually disappears after resting.

Protein molecules are large and under normal conditions should not filter into the urine. However, they may appear in small amounts in the urine after strenuous exercise or an illness, especially one with a fever. In large amounts, protein in the urine warrants a search for an underlying kidney problem.

Nitrites, substances produced when bacteria multiply, may be the earliest or only sign of an infection.

White blood cells may be present because of a urinary-tract or vaginal infection.

X Ray

- The simple X ray is a nonspecific test that is being replaced more and more by CAT scans, magnetic resonance imaging, and other tests.

What results mean

An X ray can detect such things as an enlarged heart, a broken bone, a sinus infection, or pneumonia.

Counting Your Calories and Fat

T otal calorie values for each item in this table were rounded to the nearest 5 calories (calories from fat and fat grams were not). The portion sizes are given in common household units and in grams. The portion size shown may not be the amount that you eat. If you choose larger or smaller portions than listed, increase or decrease the calorie and fat counts accordingly. Check nutrition labels on foods for additional information, including saturated fat, cholesterol, and sodium content.

Breads, Cereals, and Other Grain Products

BREADS	Calories	Fat grams	Calories from fat
Bagel			
plain, 1, 3-1/2 inch diameter	195	1	10
oat bran, 1, 3-1/2 inch	180	1	8
poppy seed, 1, Sara Lee	190	1	9
Cracked-wheat bread, 1, 25g slice	65	1	9
French bread, 1, 25g slice	70	1	7
Pita bread			
white, 1, 6-1/2 inch diameter	165		6
whole wheat, 1, 6-1/2 inch diameter	170		15
Pumpernickel, 1, 32g slice	80	1	9
Raisin, 1, 26g slice	70	1	10
Rye, 1, 32g slice	85	1	10
White			
regular, 1, 25g slice	65	1	8
Wonder bread light, 2 slices, 45g	80	1	9
Whole wheat			
regular, 1, 25g slice	70	1	11
Wonder bread, 2 slices, 45g	80	<1	14

Rolls

	Calories	Fat grams	Calories from fat
Croissant, prepared w/butter, 1, 57g	230	12	108
Dinner, 1, 28g	85	2	19
Frankfurter or hamburger, 1, 43g	125	2	20
French, 1, 38g	105	2	15
Hard, 1 3-1/2 inch, 57g	165	2	22

Quick breads, Biscuits, Muffins, Breakfast Pastries

	Calories	Fat grams	Calories from fat
Biscuit			
plain, 2-1/2 in diameter, 60g	210	10	88
from dry mix, 3 inch diameter, 57g	190	7	62
from refrig. dough, 2-1/2 diam., 27g	95	4	36
Banana bread, 1 slice, 60g	195	57	
Coffee cake			
cinnamon w/crumb topping, 63g	265	15	132
butter streusel, Sara Lee, 41g	160	7	63
Danish			
cheese, Sara Lee, individual, 36g	130	8	72
cheese-filled, Entenmann's, fat-free 54g	130	0	0
Doughnuts			
plain cake, 1, 47g	200	11	97
glazed, 1, 45g	190	10	93
English muffin, plain, 1, 57g	135	1	9

Muffin	Calories	Fat grams	Calories from fat
blueberry, 2-1/2 inch, 1, 57g	160	4	33
bran w/raisins, Dunkin' Donuts 1, 104g	310	9	81
Pancake			
plain, from dry mix, 1, 56g	200	1	9
plain, frozen Aunt Jemima, 3, 114g	185	2	22
Waffle			
plain, 7 inch diameter, 75g	220	11	95
blueberry, frozen, Eggo, 2, 78g	220	8	72

Breakfast Cereal

	Calories	Fat grams	Calories from fat
All-Bran, 1/2 cup, 30g	80	1	9
Bran flakes, 3/4 cup, 28g	100	1	9
Cheerios, 1-1/4 cup, 28g	110	2	18
Corn flakes, 1 cup, 30g	110	0	0
Cream of Wheat			
regular or instant, cooked, 2/3 cup, 168g	100	0	0
instant, cooked, 2/3 cup, 161g	100	<1	0
mix'n eat, 1 pkg., 28g	100	0	0
Frosted Flakes, 3/4 cup, 30g	120	0	0
Frosted Mini-Wheats, 1 cup, 55g	190	1	9
Grape-Nut Flakes, 1 cup, 28g	100	1	9
Granola, date nut, Erewhon, 1/4 cup, 28g	130	6	50
Oatmeal			
reg., quick, or instant, cooked, 1 cup, 234g	145	2	21
cinnamon & spice, Instant , 1 pkg., 46g	170	2	18
Raisin bran, 1 cup, 55g	170	1	9
Rice Chex, 1 cup, 31g	120	0	0
Rice Krispies, 1-1/4 cup, 30g	110	0	0
Shredded wheat, Quaker	220	2	14
Special K, 1 cup, 30g	110	0	0
Total, 1 cup, 28g	100	1	9
Wheaties, 1 cup, 28g	100	1	9

Pasta and Rice

	Calories	Fat grams	Calories from fat
Macaroni			
cooked, plain, 1/2 cup, 65g	95	<1	3
spinach, cooked, Ronzoni, 1/2 cup, 67g	105	<1	4
Pasta			
fresh, cooked, plain, 1 cup, 170g	225	2	16
homemade w/egg, cooked, 1 cup, 170g	220	3	27
Ravioli, cheese, cooked, Contadina, 1/3 container, 190g	270	11	99
Rice, cooked, 1/2 cup			
Brown, medium grain, 98g	110	1	7
White, glutinous, 120g	115	<1	2
White, long grain instant, 82g	80	<1	1
White, medium grain, 93g	120	<1	2
Wild rice, 82g	85	<1	3
Spaghetti, cooked, plain, 1 cup, 140g	155	<1	4

Crackers

	Calories	Fat grams	Calories from fat
Cheez-it, Sunshine, 24 crackers, 32g	140	8	72
Finn-Crisp dark, 3 crackers, 15g	60	0	0
Matzo, plain, 1 (28g)	110	<1	4
Ritz, Nabisco, 4 crackers, 14g	70	4	36
Saltine, 10 crackers, 28g	120	4	36
Soup or oyster, 4 crackers, 14g	70	4	36
Triscuit, Nabisco, 6 crackers, 28g	120	4	36

Fruits

	Calories	Fat grams	Calories from fat

Fruits
(calories in cooked and canned
fruit include both fruit and liquid)

	Calories	Fat grams	Calories from fat
Apple, raw, sliced, 1/2 cup, 55g	30	<1	2
Applesauce, 1/2 cup			
sweetened, 128g	95	<1	2
unsweetened, 122g	50	<1	1
Apricots			
canned, heavy syrup, 3 halves, 85g	70	<1	1
canned, light syrup pack, 3 halves, 85g	55	<1	0
dried, cooked without sugar, 1/2 cup, 125g	105	<1	2
raw, 4 halves, 78g	35	<1	3
Avocados			
California, 3 inch, 1/2, 86g	155	15	135
Florida, 3-5/8 inch, 1/2, 152g	170	13	121
Banana, medium, 114g	105	1	5
Blueberries, 1/2 cup			
frozen, unsweetened, 78g	40	<1	4
frozen, sweetened, 115g	95	1	5
raw, 72g	40	<1	3
Cherries, 1/2 cup			
raw, sweet, 72g	50	1	6
sweet, frozen, sweetened, 130g	115	<1	2
sour red, frozen, unsweetened, 78g	35	<1	3
Cranberry sauce, sweetened, 1/4 cup, 70g	110	0	0
Dates, dried, 10, 83g	230	<1	3
Fruit cocktail, canned, 1/2 cup			
juice pack, 124g	55	<1	0
heavy syrup, 128g	95	<1	1
Grapefruit, raw, 3-3/4 inch, 1/2, 118g	40	<1	1
Melon, honeydew, cubed, 1/2 cup, 85g	30	<1	1
Oranges, 1/2 cup			
mandarin, canned, light syrup, 122g	80	0	0
raw, sections, 90g	40	<1	1
Peaches			
canned, in juice, 1/2 cup, 77g	55	0	0
canned, in light syrup, 1/2 cup, 77g	70	<1	1
Pears			
canned, in light syrup, 1 half, 77g	35	<1	1
dried, without added sugar, 1/2 cup, 128g	165	<1	4
Pineapple			
canned, juice pack, 1/2 cup, 125g	75	<1	1
raw, diced, 1/2 cup, 78g	40	<1	3
Plums			
canned, juice pack, 3, 95g	55	<1	0
raw, 2-1/8 inch diameter, 66g	35	<1	4
Prunes			
dried, cooked, without sugar, 1/2 cup, 106g	115	<1	2
dried, uncooked, 10, 84g	200	<1	4
Raisins, seedless, 1/4 cup, 41g	125	<1	2
Raspberries, 1/2 cup			
frozen, unsweetened, 125g	61	1	6
raw, 62g	30	<1	3
Rhubarb, cooked, sweetened, 1/2 cup, 120g	140	<1	1
Tangerines, sections, 1/2 cup, 98g	45	<1	2
Watermelon, 10 inches x 1 inch, 480g	155	2	19

Juices

	Calories	Fat grams	Calories from fat
Apple juice or cider, 1 cup, 249g	120	0	0
Apricot nectar, canned, 3/4 cup, 188g	105	<1	2
Cranberry juice cocktail, 3/4 cup, 190g	110	<1	2
Grape juice			
bottled, 3/4 cup, 188g	110	0	0
from frozen concentrate, 3/4 cup, 188g	96	<1	2
Grapefruit			
Lemonade, 3/4 cup			
homemade, prepared w/sugar, 186g	90	0	0
from frozen concentrate, 186g	75	<1	0
Orange juice, 3/4 cup			
fresh, 186g	85	<1	3
from frozen concentrate, 187g	85	<1	1
Pineapple juice, canned, 3/4 cup, 188g	105	<1	1
Prune juice, canned, 3/4 cup, 192g	135	<1	1
Snapple, 1 bottle			
Dixie Peach, 295g	140	0	0
Lemonade, 240g	110	0	0
Passion Supreme, 309g	160	0	0
Pink Grapefruit Cocktail, 249g	120	0	0
V-8 juice, canned, 3/4 cup, 182g	35	0	0

Vegetables

	Calories	Fat grams	Calories from fat
Alfalfa sprouts, raw, 1 cup, 33g	10	<1	2
Artichoke, cooked, medium, 120g	60	<1	2
Asparagus, 1/2 cup			
canned, drained, 120g	25	1	7
cooked, drained, 90g	20	<1	3
Bean sprouts, Mung, raw, 1/2 cup, 52g	15	<1	1
Beet greens, cooked, drained, 1/2 cup, 72g	20	<1	1
Beets, 1/2 cup			
canned, sliced, drained, 85g	25	<1	1
cooked, sliced, drained, 85g	35	<1	1
Broccoli, 1/2 cup			
frozen florets, cooked, 71g	20	0	0
raw, chopped, 44g	10	<1	1
Brussels sprouts, cooked, drained, 1/2 cup, 78g	30	<1	4
Cabbage, 1/2 cup			
Chinese bok-choy, shredded, raw, 35g	5	<1	1
shredded, raw, 35g	10	<1	1
shredded, cooked, drained, 75g	15	<1	3
Carrots			
frozen, sliced, cooked, drained, 1/2 cup, 73g	25	<1	1
raw, 7-1/2 inches x 1-1/8 inch, 72g	30	<1	1
Cauliflower, 1/2 cup			
frozen, cooked, drained, 90g	15	<1	2
raw, 1 inch pieces, 50g	10	<1	1
Celery, raw			
cooked, drained, 1/2 cup, 75g	15	<1	1
raw, 7-1/2 in x 1-1/4 inch, 40g	5	<1	1
Corn, cooked			
canned, yellow, cream style, 1/2 cup, 128g	90	1	5
canned, solids & liquid, 1/2 cup, 128g	80	1	5
frozen, white, cooked, drained, 1/2 cup, 82g	65	<1	1
on the cob, drained, 1 ear, 140g	85	1	9
Cucumber, raw, sliced, 1/2 cup, 52g	10	<1	1
Eggplant			
cooked, drained, 1 inch pieces, 1/2 cup, 48g	15	<1	1
in tomato sauce, 1 cup, 231g	75	<1	3
Green beans, 1/2 cup			
canned, drained, 68g	25	0	0
cooked, drained, 62g	20	<1	2
frozen, French style 85g	25	0	0
raw, snap, 55g	15	<1	1
Kale, cooked, drained, 1/2 cup, 65g	20	<1	2
Lettuce			
iceberg, 1/4 of a 6-inch head, 135g	20	<1	2
looseleaf, shredded, 1/2 cup, 28g	5	<1	1
romaine, shredded, 1/2 cup, 28g	5	<1	4
Lima beans, cooked, drained, 1/2 cup, 85g	105	<1	2
Mushrooms			
canned, pieces, drained, 1/2 cup, 78g	20	<1	2
raw, whole, 1, 18g	5	<1	1
shiitake, cooked, 1/2 cup, 73g	40	<1	1

Onions	Calories	Fat grams	Calories from fat
canned, solids & liquid, 1 inch, 63g	10	<1	1
raw, chopped, 1/2 cup, 80g	30	<1	1
Peas, green, 1/2 cup			
frozen, cooked, drained, 80g	60	<1	2
raw, 72g	50	<1	3
Peppers, sweet, red or green, 1/2 cup			
cooked, drained, 68g	20	<1	1
raw, 50g	15	<1	1
Potatoes			
baked, w/skin, 4-3/4 inch x 2-1/3 inch, 156g	220	<1	2
boiled, no skin, 2-1/2 inch diameter, 135g	115	<1	1
hash browns, Ore-Ida frozen, 1 patty, 85g	70	<1	0
mashed, w/whole milk, 1/2 cup, 105g	80	1	6
scalloped, frozen, Stouffer's, 1/2 pkg., 165g	135	6	52
Tater Tots, frozen, Ore-Ida, 1-1/4 cup, 85g	160	7	63
Spinach, 1/2 cup			
frozen, cooked, drained, 95g	25	<1	2
raw, chopped, 28g	5	<1	1
Squash, 1/2 cup			
summer, cooked, drained, 90g	20	<1	3
winter, baked cubes, 102g	40	1	6
Sweet potatoes			
baked in skin, 5 inches x 2 inches, 114g	115	<1	1
canned, mashed, 128g	130	<1	2
Tomato sauce, canned, 1/2 cup, 112g	35	<1	2
Tomatoes, 1/2 cup			
canned, stewed, 103	35	0	0
raw, chopped, 90g	20	<1	3
Turnip greens, cooked, drained, 1/2 cup, 72g	15	<1	2
Turnips, cooked, mashed, 1/2 cup, 115g	20	<1	1

Meat, Poultry, Fish, and Alternates

(Serving sizes are cooked, edible parts.)

Beef

	Calories	Fat grams	Calories from fat
Beef liver, 3 oz, 85g			
braised	135	4	37
pan-fried	185	7	61
Corned beef, canned, 1 oz, 28g	70	4	38
Ground beef, broiled, medium, 3 oz, 85g			
extra lean	220	14	125
ground chuck	230	16	141
regular	245	18	158
Roast beef, 3 oz, 85g			
bottom round, lean & fat	160	6	56
eye of round, lean & fat	195	11	98
pot roast, lean & fat	280	20	182
rib, lean & fat	300	24	216
tip round, lean & fat	160	7	60
Sirloin, broiled, lean & fat, 30 oz, 85g	165	6	55
Veal, loin, lean only, roasted, 30 oz, 85g	150	6	53

Lamb

Ground lamb, broiled, 3 oz, 85g	240	17	150
Leg of lamb, lean & fat roasted, 3 oz, 85g	250	18	158
Shoulder chop, lean & fat, braised, 3 oz, 85g	295	20	185

Pork

Bacon, thick, broiled, 1 slice, 10g	55	4	40
Bacon, Canadian, grilled, 1 slice, 23g	45	2	18
Ham			
center slice, 3 oz, 85g	170	11	99
canned, lean, 3 oz, 85g	100	4	35
canned, regular, 30 oz, 85g	190	13	116

	Calories	Fat grams	Calories from fat
Pork chop, loin, broiled, 3 oz, 85g	205	11	100
Pork loin ribs, braised, 3 oz, 85g	250	18	165
Pork roast, center loin, 3 oz, 85g	200	11	103
Pork roast, sirloin, 3 oz, 85g	175	8	72
Pork shoulder, roasted, 3 oz, 85g	245	20	180

Sausage and Luncheon Meats

Bologna, 1 slice, 28g			
beef & pork	90	8	72
turkey	55	4	40
Braunschweiger, 1 slice, 18g	65	6	52
Chicken breast			
Oscar Mayer, roasted, 1 slice, 28g	25	<1	3
Healthy Choice, roasted, 3 slices, 28g	30	<1	4
Ham, boiled, 1 slice, 21g	20	1	9
Salami			
beef, 1 slice, 23g	60	5	43
turkey, 10% fat, 1 oz, 28g	45	3	24
Sausage, summer, beef, 1 slice, 23g	70	6	54
Turkey			
Oscar Mayer, roasted, 1 slice, 28g	25	1	7
Oscar Mayer, fat free, smoked, 4 slices, 52g	40	<1	3

Poultry

Chicken breast, 1/2 breast			
boneless, w/out skin, roasted, 86g	140	3	28
boneless, w/skin, flour fried, 98g	220	9	78
Chicken drumstick, 1			
w/out skin, roasted, 72g	75	2	22
w/skin, roasted, 81g	110	6	52
Chicken liver, simmered, 1/2 cup, 70g	110	4	34
Chicken, thigh, 1			
w/out skin, roasted, 71g	110	6	51
w/skin, roasted, 81g	155	10	86
Turkey, ground, cooked, 1 patty, 82g	195	11	97
Turkey, roasted			
dark meat w/out skin, diced, 1/2 cup, 64g	120	5	42
dark meat w/skin, 3 oz, 85g	190	10	88
light meat w/out skin diced, 1/2 cup, 64g	100	2	19
light meat w/skin, 3 oz, 85g	170	7	64
Turkey liver, simmered, 1/2 cup, 70g	120	4	38

Fish and Shellfish

Anchovies, canned in oil, drained, 5, 20g	45	2	17
Clams, canned, drained, 1/2 cup, 80g	120	2	14
Fish fillets			
breaded, frozen, 2, 99g	280	19	171
breaded, Healthy Choice, 1, 99g	160	5	45
Flounder, cooked, dry heat, 3 oz, 85g	100	1	12
Halibut, cooked, dry heat, 3 oz, 85g	120	2	22
Salmon 3 oz, 85g			
Chinook, cooked, dry heat	195	11	102
Chum, cooked, dry heat	130	4	37
Coho, cooked, moist heat	155	6	57
Sardines, Atlantic, canned in oil, drained solids, 2, 24g	50	3	25
Sea Bass, cooked, dry heat, 3 oz, 85g	105	2	20
Shrimp, cooked			
breaded & fried, 4, 30g	75	4	33
moist heat, large, 4 22g	20	<1	2
Tuna, light, canned in water, 1/2 cup, 74g	85	1	5

Eggs

Fried, whole, 1, 46g	90	7	62
Hard-cooked, whole, 1, 50g	80	5	48
Poached, 1 whole, , 50g	75	5	45
Scrambled, w/marg. & whole milk, 1, 64g	105	8	7

	Calories	Fat grams	Calories from fat
Soft-boiled, whole, 1, 50g	80	6	50
Whites, raw, 1, 33g	15	0	0

Beans and Peas

	Calories	Fat grams	Calories from fat
Baked beans, canned			
pork & beans, tomato sauce, 1/2 cup, 114g	100	1	13
w/pork, molasses & sugar, 1/2 cup, 126g	190	6	58
Black-eyed peas, 1/2 cup			
canned, solids & liquid, 120g	90	1	6
cooked, drained, 1/2 cup, 82g	80	<1	3
Chick-peas (garbanzos), canned, 1/2 cup, 120g	145	1	12
Black beans, cooked, 1/2 cup, 86g	115	<1	4
Kidney beans, cooked, 1/2 cup, 88g	110	<1	4
Lima beans, cooked, drained, 1/2 cup, 85g	105	<1	2
Navy beans, cooked, 1/2 cup, 91g	130	1	5
Refried beans, canned, 1/2 cup, 126g	135	1	12

Nuts and Seeds

	Calories	Fat grams	Calories from fat
Almonds, unblanched			
dried, 3 Tbs., 28g	165	15	133
dry roasted, 3 Tbs., 26g	150	13	119
Cashews, dry roasted, 3 Tbs., 28g	165	13	118
Coconut, dried, sweetened, flaked, 2 Tbs., 9g	45	3	27
Peanut butter, 2 Tbs., 32g	190	14	126
Peanuts, roasted			
dry roasted, 3 Tbs., 28g	165	14	125
honey roasted, 3 Tbs., 28g	170	14	126
Pecans, dried, 1/2 cup, 28g	190	19	173
Pine nuts, dried, 1 Tbs., 10g	50	5	46
Pistachios, dry roasted, 3 Tbs., 28g	170	15	135
Sesame seeds			
Tahini, raw kernels, 1 Tbs., 15g	85	7	65
dried, kernels, 1 Tbs., 8g	45	4	39
Sunflower seeds, dry roasted, 3 Tbs., 28g	165	14	127
Walnuts, dried, 1/4 cup, 28g	180	18	158

Meat Substitutes

	Calories	Fat grams	Calories from fat
Burger, vegetarian			
Vege burger, Natural Touch, 1, 64g	140	6	54
Veggie Sizzler, nonfat, Soy Boy, 1, 85g	90	0	0
Hot dog, Not Dogs, 1, 43g	105	5	45
Tofu			
fried, 2-3/4 x 1 x 1/2 inch, 29g	80	6	53
regular, 1/2 cup, 124g	95	6	53

Dairy Products

Cheese

	Calories	Fat grams	Calories from fat
American, light, 1 slice, 28g	70	4	36
Blue, crumbled (not packed) 1/4 cup, 34g	120	10	87
Brie, 1 oz, 28g	95	8	70
Cheddar			
1-inch cube, 17g	70	6	51
light, 1 slice, 28g	70	4	36
Colby, 10 oz, 28g	110	9	79
Cottage cheese, 1/2 cup			
creamed, large curd, 113g	115	5	46
dry curd, 73g	60	<1	3
lowfat, 1% fat, 113g	80	1	10
Cream cheese, 2 Tbs.			
light, Philadelphia brand, 28g	60	5	45
regular, 30g	105	10	94
whipped, Philadelphia brand, 28g	100	10	90

	Calories	Fat grams	Calories from fat
Feta, 1 oz, 28g	75	6	54
Mozzarella, 1 oz, 28g			
regular	80	6	54
part skim	70	4	40
Parmesan, grated, 1 Tbs., 5g	25	2	14
Swiss			
1-inch cube, 15g	55	4	37
light, 1 slice, 28g	70	3	27

Cream

	Calories	Fat grams	Calories from fat
Half & half, 1 Tbs., 15g	20	2	16
Heavy, whipping, 1 Tbs., 15g	50	6	48
Sour cream			
cultured, 2 Tbs., 24g	50	5	45
light, 50% less fat, 2 Tbs., 30g	40	2	22
Whipped cream, pressurized, 1 Tbs., 3g	10	1	6

Imitation Cream Products

	Calories	Fat grams	Calories from fat
Coffee creamers			
non-dairy, liquid, Coffee Rich, 1 Tbs., 14g	25	1	13
non-dairy, liquid, Int'l Delight, 1 Tbs., 15g	45	2	14
Sour cream			
imitation, cultured, nondairy, 2 Tbs., 28g	60	5	49
imitation, non-butterfat, 2 Tbs., 24g	45	4	36
powdered, Coffee-Mate, 1 tsp., 2g	10	1	6
Whipped topping			
non-dairy, pressurized, 2 Tbs., 9g	25	2	19
non-dairy, frozen, Cool Whip, 1 Tbs., 4g	10	1	7

Milk

	Calories	Fat grams	Calories from fat
Buttermilk, 1% fat, 1 cup, 245g	100	2	19
Chocolate milk, 1 cup, 250g			
lowfat, 1% fat	160	2	22
whole	210	8	76
Condensed, sweetened, 2 Tbs., 38g	125	3	30
Evaporated, canned, 2 Tbs., 32g			
lowfat	30	1	5
skim	25	<1	1
whole	40	2	21
Lowfat, 1% fat, 1 cup, 244g	100	3	23
Skim, 1 cup, 245g	85	<1	4
Whole, 3.3% fat, 1 cup, 244g	150	8	73

Yogurt

	Calories	Fat grams	Calories from fat
Fruit flavors, custard, Yoplait, 1 cont., 170g	190	4	36
Fruit-on-the-bottom, lowfat, 1 cont., 226g	230	3	27
Plain, 1 cont., 226g			
lowfat	145	4	32
nonfat	125	<1	4

Soups

Canned Soups

(Canned, condensed soups are prepared with water, unless otherwise noted.)

	Calories	Fat grams	Calories from fat
Bean & ham, Healthy Choice, 1/2 can, 228g	220	4	36
Beef broth, ready-to-serve, 1 cup, 240g	15	1	5
Black bean, Healthy Valley, 1 cup, 240g	110	0	0
Chicken broth, ready-to-serve, 1/2 can, 249g	30	3	27
Chicken noodle, Campbell's, 1 cup, 226g	60	2	18
Chicken rice, 1 cup, 241g	60	2	17
Clam chowder, New England			
frozen, Stouffer's 1 cup, 227g	180	9	81
prepared w/skim milk, 1 cup, 233g	100	2	18
prepared w/water, Campbell's, 1 cup, 224g	80	2	20
Cream of Chicken, 1 cup, 244g	110	7	62
Cream of mushroom, 1 cup			

	Calories	Fat grams	Calories from fat
prepared w/water, 244g	130	9	81
prepared w/whole milk, 248g	205	14	122
Minestrone			
prepared w/water, 1 cup, 241g	80	3	23
ready-to-serve, Hain, 1/2 can, 270g	160	3	27
Tomato, 1 cup			
prepared w/water, 244g	85	2	17
prepared w/whole milk, 248g	160	6	54
Vegetable			
prepared w/water, 1 cup, 241g	90	1	9
ready-to-serve, Pritikin, 1/2 can, 209g	70	0	0

Dried or Dehydrated Soups

	Calories	Fat grams	Calories from fat
Black bean, Nile Spice, 1 container, 309g	180	1	5
Chicken vegetable, 1 cup, 251g	50	1	7
Cream of chicken, 1 cup, 261g	105	5	48
Mushroom, 1 cup, 253g	95	1	44
Onion, 1 pkg., 7g	20	<1	4
Split pea, 1 cup, 271g	135	2	14
Tomato, 1 cup, 265g	105	2	22

Desserts, Snack Foods, and Candy

Cakes

	Calories	Fat grams	Calories from fat
Angel food, 1/12 of 10 inch tube, 50g	130	<1	1
Boston Cream Pie, 1/6 of 20 oz, 92g	230	8	70
Carrot cake, Sara Lee, snack size, 1, 52g	180	7	63
Cheesecake, plain, 1/6 of 17 oz, 80g	255	18	160
Cupcake, 1			
chocolate, Hostess, 46g	170	5	45
yellow, w/icing, 36g	130	4	34
Devil's food, w/icing, 1/6 of 9 inch, 69g	235	8	72
Fruitcake, 1 slice, 34g	140	4	35
Pound cake, Sara Lee, 1/10 of cake, 30g	130	7	63
Yellow cake, w/icing, 1/8 of 8 oz, 64g	240	9	84

Cookies and Bars

	Calories	Fat grams	Calories from fat
Brownies, chocolate			
frozen, Weight-Watchers, 1, 36g	100	3	27
from mix, 2 inch square, 33g	140	7	59
Chocolate chip			
Chips Ahoy!, 3, 32g	160	8	72
refrigerated, Pillsbury, 2, 31g	140	7	59
Creme sandwich, Nabisco, 2, 28g	140	6	54
Fig bar, 2, 31g	110	2	21
Gingersnaps, Sunshine, 6, 28g	120	4	36
Graham crackers, 4, 1-1/2 squares, 28g	120	2	18
Oatmeal raisin, Barbara's, 2, 38g	160	7	63
Oreo, Nabisco, 2, 28g	100	4	36
Shortbread, 1-5/8 inch square, 4, 32g	160	8	69
Vanilla wafers, Nabisco, 7, 28g	120	4	36

Pies

	Calories	Fat grams	Calories from fat
Apple, 1/8 of 9 inch pie, 155g	410	19	175
Blueberry, 1/8 of 9 inch, 147g	360	17	157
Cherry, 1/8 of 9 inch pie, 180g	485	22	198
Chocolate cream, 1/8 of 9 inch, 142g	400	23	206
Custard, 1/8 of 9 inch, 127g	260	11	102
Lemon meringue, 1/8 of 9 inch, 127g	360	16	147
Pumpkin, 1/8 of 9 inch, 155g	315	14	130

Other Desserts

	Calories	Fat grams	Calories from fat
Custard, baked, 1/2 cup, 141g	150	7	60

	Calories	Fat grams	Calories from fat
Frozen yogurt, vanilla, 1/2 cup			
Haagen-Dazs, 98g	160	2	22
Yoplait, soft, 72g	90	3	27
Gelatin, Jell-O, 1/2 cup, 140g	80	0	0
Ice cream, vanilla, 1/2 cup			
regular, 10% fat, 66g	135	7	65
Haagen-Dazs, 106g	260	17	153
Ice cream, chocolate, 1/2 cup			
regular, 10% fat, 66g	145	7	65
Haagen-Dazs, 106g	270	17	153
Ice milk sandwich, Weight Watchers, 78g	160	4	36
Juice bars			
Strawberry, Fruit'n Juice, Dole, 74g	70	0	0
Strawberry, Welch's, 85g	80	0	0
Puddings, from mix, prepared w/2% milk			
butterscotch, 1/2 cup, 148g	150	2	20
chocolate, 1/2 cup, 147g	150	2	20
tapioca, 1/2 cup, 141g	145	2	22
vanilla, 1/2 cup, 144g	140	2	20
Sherbet, 1/2 cup, 87g	135	2	17

Snack Foods

	Calories	Fat grams	Calories from fat
Corn chips, 3/4 cup, 28g	155	9	85
Crackers (see Crackers)			
Nuts (see Nuts and Seeds)			
Popcorn			
air-popped, 1 cup, 8g	30	<1	3
microwave, natural flavor, 1 cup, 8g	35	2	18
Potato chips, 1 cup, 28g	150	10	90
Pretzels			
Dutch, twisted, 2-3/4 inch, 2, 32g	120	1	10
Sticks, 2-1/2 x 1/8 inch, 60, 30g	115	1	9
Twists, thin, Rold Gold, 10, 28g	110	1	9

Candy

	Calories	Fat grams	Calories from fat
Caramel, plain, 3/4 inch, 8g	30	1	6
Fudge, chocolate, 1 cu inch, 17g	65	1	13
Gum drops, 8, 28g	110	0	0
Hard candy, 5, 28g	105	0	0
Jellybeans, 10 large or 26 small, 28g	105	<1	1
Hershey's Kisses, 6, 28g	150	9	81
Lollipops, 1, 28g	110	0	0

Beverages

(Milk and juices are in Dairy Products and Fruits sections.)

Carbonated Sodas

	Calories	Fat grams	Calories from fat
Cola, 1-1/2 cup, 370g	150	<1	0
Diet cola, w/aspartame, 1-1/2 cup, 355g	4	0	0
Gingerale, 1-1/2 cup, 366g	125	0	0
Grape soda, 1-1/2 cup, 372g	160	0	0
Lemon-lime, 1-1/2 cup, 368g	145	0	0
Orange soda, 1-1/2 cup, 372g	180	0	0
Root beer, 1-1/2 cup, 370g	150	0	0

Coffee and Tea

	Calories	Fat grams	Calories from fat
Coffee			
brewed, 1 cup, 235g	5	<1	0
brewed, decaffeinated, 1 cup, 240g	3	0	0
instant, 1 cup, 240g	5	0	0
Tea, brewed, 1 cup 237g	2	<1	0
Tea, brewed herb, unflavored, 1 cup, 236g	2	<1	0
Tea, iced, instant, lemon flavored			
sweetened w/aspartame, 1 cup, 259g	2	0	0
sweetened w/sugar, made w/4 tsp., 23g	85	<1	0

	Calories	Fat grams	Calories from fat

Alcoholic Beverages

	Calories	Fat grams	Calories from fat
Beer, 1-1/2 cup, 355g			
light	100	0	0
regular	145	0	0
nonalcoholic	50	0	0
Gin, Rum, Whiskey, or Vodka,			
80-proof, 1 jigger, 42g	95	0	0
Wine, 1 glass			
red, 147g	105	0	0
white, 147g	100	0	0
Wine cooler, 1 glass, 360g	175	< 1	0
Wine, dessert, 1 glass			
dry, 59g	75	0	0
sweet, 59g	90	0	0

Fats, Oils, and Condiments

Fats and Oils

	Calories	Fat grams	Calories from fat
Butter			
regular or unsalted, 1 tsp., 5g	35	4	37
whipped, 1 Tbs., 11g	80	9	80
Margarine			
spread, tub, 1 Tbs., 14g	75	9	75
stick, 1 Tbs., 14g	100	11	100
Oil			
corn, 1 Tbs., 14g	120	14	122
olive, 1 Tbs., 14g	120	14	122
vegetable spray, 1-1/4 seconds, 1g	5	1	5
Salad dressing			
blue cheese, 1 Tbs., 15g	75	8	72
French 1 Tbs., 16g	65	6	57
French, low calorie, 1 Tbs., 16g	20	1	9
Italian, 1 Tbs., 15g	70	7	64
Italian, low calorie, 1 Tbs., 16g	15	1	12
mayonnaise-like, 1 Tbs., 15g	55	5	43
thousand island, 1 Tbs., 16g	60	6	50

Condiments

	Calories	Fat grams	Calories from fat
Barbecue sauce, 1 Tbs., 15g	15	< 1	3
Catsup, 1 Tbs., 15g	15	< 1	0
Gravy, canned			
au jus, 1/4 cup, 60g	10	< 1	1
beef, 1/4 cup, 58g	30	1	12
chicken, 1/4 cup, 60g	45	3	30
turkey, 1/4 cup, 60g	30	1	11
Horseradish, prepared, 1 tsp., 5g	2	< 1	0
Mustard, prepared, 1 tsp., 5g	4	< 1	2
Olives			
black, canned, small, 3, 10g	10	1	9
green, medium, 4, 13g	15	2	14
green, stuffed, 10, 34g	35	4	34
Pickles			
dill, kosher spears, 1, 28g	5	0	0
sweet, gherkins, small, 2-1/2 inches, 2, 30g	40	< 1	0
Relish, sweet pickle, 2 Tbs., 30g	40	< 1	1
Soy sauce, tamari, 1 Tbs., 18g	10	< 1	0
Tartar sauce, 1 Tbs., 14g	75	8	68

Sugar, Jams, and Jellies

	Calories	Fat grams	Calories from fat
Chocolate syrup			
fudge-type, 2 Tbs., 42g	145	6	51
thin-type, 2 Tbs., 38g	82	< 1	3
Honey, 1 Tbs., 21g	65	0	0
Jams and preserves, 1 Tbs., 20g	50	< 1	0
Jellies, 1 Tbs., 19g	50	< 1	0
Maple syrup, 2 Tbs., 40g	105	< 1	1
Sugar			
brown, unpacked, 1 cup, 145g	545	0	0
white, granulated, 1 tsp., 4g	15	0	0

Fast Foods

Burgers and Sandwiches

	Calories	Fat grams	Calories from fat
Burger King			
Big Fish	700	41	370
Broiler Chicken	550	29	260
Double Cheeseburger with Bacon	640	39	350
Hamburger	330	15	140
Whopper	640	39	350
McDonald's			
Big Mac	530	28	250
Filet-O-Fish	360	16	150
Hamburger	270	10	90
MacLean Deluxe	350	12	110
McChicken	570	30	270
McGrilled Chicken	510	30	270
Wendy's			
Big Bacon Classic	610	33	290
Chicken Club	500	23	200
Grilled Chicken Sandwich	310	8	70
Hamburger, with everything	420	20	180

Salads, Fries, and Miscellaneous

(Salad values are given for salads without dressing.)

	Calories	Fat grams	Calories from fat
Burger King			
Broiled Chicken Salad	200	10	90
French fries, medium	370	20	180
Garden Salad	100	5	45
Salad dressing, 30g, thousand island	140	12	110
Salad dressing, 30g, ranch	180	19	170
Salad dressing, 30g, reduced calorie Italian	15	< 1	5
McDonald's			
Chef Salad	210	11	100
Fajita Chicken Salad	160	6	60
French fries, large	450	22	200
French fries, small	210	10	90
Salad dressing, 1 pkg., blue cheese	190	17	150
Salad dressing, 1 pkg., lite vinaigrette	50	2	20
Salad dressing, 1 pkg., ranch	180	19	170
Pizza Hut			
Breadsticks, 5	770	25	223
Buffalo wings, 12	565	35	310
Cheese pizza, 1/8 of med., thin crust	205	8	75
Cheese pizza, 1/8 of med., pan pizza	260	11	98
Pepperoni pizza, 1/8 of med., thin crust	215	10	69
Veggie Lover's, 1/8 of med., thin crust	185	7	61
Wendy's			
Baked potato, plain	310	0	0
Baked potato w/chili and cheese	620	24	220
Baked potato w/sour cream and chives	380	6	60
Deluxe Garden Salad	110	6	50
Salad dressing, 2 Tbs., blue cheese	170	19	170
Salad dressing, 2 Tbs., fat-free French	30	0	0
Salad dressing, 2 Tbs., ranch	90	10	90

Desserts

	Calories	Fat grams	Calories from fat
Burger King			
Dutch apple pie	300	15	140
McDonald's			
Baked apple pie	260	13	120
Cookies	260	9	80
Pizza Hut			
Dessert pizza, 1/8 of med.	245	5	46
Wendy's			
Chocolate chip cookies, 1, 57g	270	11	100

Your Health Directory

In *An Invitation to Health*, I emphasize that you shoulder a great deal of responsibility for your health and the quality of your life. Given the complexity of our minds and bodies and the many social and environmental factors that affect us, this responsibility can be a very heavy burden. But your load can be made lighter if you know where to turn for health information, services, and support.

In this directory, you will find more than 100 health-related topics and about 250 resources, including addresses, phone numbers, and web sites for government agencies, community organizations, professional associations, recovery groups, and Internet sources. Many of these organizations and groups have toll-free 800 or 888 phone numbers, and an increasing number of them have web sites (one caution: as you may have experienced, web site addresses—like street addresses and phone numbers—do change on occasion). Much of the material available from these groups is free.

Also included in Your Health Directory are clearinghouses and information centers that are especially rich sources of health knowledge. Their main purpose is to collect, help manage, and disseminate information. Clearinghouses often perform other services as well, such as creating original publications and providing tailored responses to individual requests. These organizations also may provide referrals to other groups that can help you.

Many of the groups listed here have local offices or chapters. You can call, write, or visit the web sites of these organizations to find out if there is a branch in your vicinity, or you can check your local telephone directory.

The purpose of this directory is to help you be in control of your health. If you know where to turn for answers to your questions and if you know what choices you have, you may find that you have more control over your life.

General Information Resources

Agency for Health Care Policy Research

2101 E. Jefferson Street
Suite 501
Rockville, MD 20852
(301) 594-1360
http://www.ahcpr.gov/

Go Ask Alice

http://www.goaskalice.columbia.edu

Internet Grateful Med

National Library of Medicine (offers assisted searching in online databases of the NLM)
8600 Rockville Pike
Bethesda, MD 20894
(808) 638-8480
(301) 402-1076
http://igm.nim.nih.gov

National Center for Health Statistics (NCHS)

(produces vital statistics and health statistics for the United States)
Division of Data Services
6525 Belcrest Road, Room 1064
Hyattsville, MD 20782-2003
(301) 458-4636
http://www.cdc.gov/nchswww/index.htm

ODPHP National Health Information Center

P.O. Box 1133
Washington, D.C. 20013-1133
(301) 565-4167
(800) 336-4797

National Institutes of Health (NIH)

9000 Rockville Pike
Bethesda, MD 20892
(301) 496-4000
http://www.nih.gov

New York Online Access to Health

http://www.noah.cuny.edu

Tel-Med Health Information Service

(provides taped messages on health concerns) See white pages of telephone directory for listing

Yahoo Health Directory

http://www.yahoo.com/health

Resources By Topic

▶ Abortion

National Abortion Federation

(provides information about abortion and referral for abortion services)
1755 Massachusetts Ave., N.W.
Suite #600
Washington, DC 20036
(202) 667-5881
(800) 772-9100
http://www.prochoice.org

▶ Accident Prevention

Centers for Disease Control and Prevention

1600 Clifton Road N.E.
Atlanta, GA 30333
(404) 639-3311
http://www.cdc.gov

National Safety Council

1121 Spring Lake Drive
Itasca, IL 60143-3201
(630) 285-1121
(800) 621-7619
http://www.nsc.org

▶ Adoption

Adoptees' Liberty Movement Association (ALMA) Society

(provides assistance for adopted children to locate natural parents and for natural parents to locate relinquished children)
P.O. Box 727
Radio City Station
New York, NY 10101-0727
(212) 581-1568
http://www.almanet.com

AASK (Adopt a Special Kid)

(provides assistance to families who adopt older and handicapped children)
1025 N. Reynolds Road
Toledo, OH 43615
(419) 534-3350
http://www.adoptamerica.org

▶ Aging

American Association of Retired Persons

601 E Street, N.W.
Washington, DC 20049
(800) 424-3410
(202) 434-2277
http://www.aarp.org

Gray Panthers

733 15th Street, N.W., Suite 437
Washington, DC 20005
(800) 280-5362
(202) 737-6637
http://graypanthers.org

▶ AIDS (Acquired Immunodeficiency Syndrome)

Gay Men's Health Crisis

119 West 24th Street
New York, NY 10011
(212) 807-6664
http://www.gmhc.org

National AIDS Hotline

(800) 342-2437

San Francisco AIDS Foundation

995 Market St.
San Francisco, CA 94103
(415) 487-3000
http://www.sfaf.org

▶ Alcohol Abuse and Alcoholism

Al-Anon and Alateen

(support groups for friends and relatives of alcoholics)
281 Independence Blvd.
Virginia Beach, VA 23462
(757) 499-1443
http://www.al-anon-alateen.org

See also white pages of telephone directory for listing of local chapter

Alcohol Hotline

(800) ALCOHOL

Alcoholics Anonymous

307 Seventh Ave., 2nd Floor
New York, NY 10001
(212) 647-1680
http://www.alcoholics-anonymous.org

See also white pages of telephone directory for listing of local chapter

National Association of Children of Alcoholics

11426 Rockville Pike, Suite 100
Rockville, MD 20852
(888) 55-4COAS
(301) 468-0985
http://www.health.org/nacoa

National Clearinghouse for Alcohol and Drug Information

P.O. Box 2345
Rockville, MD 20847-2345
(800) 729-6686
(301) 468-2600
http://www.health.org/index.htm

National Institute on Alcohol Abuse and Alcoholism

6000 Executive Boulevard
Willco Building
Bethesda, MD 20892-7003
(301) 443-3860
http://www.niaaa.nih.gov

Women for Sobriety, Inc.

(support group for women with drinking problems)
P.O. Box 618
Quakertown, PA 18951-0618
(800) 333-1606
(215) 536-8026
http://www.mediapulse.com/wfs/

See also Drug Abuse; Drunk Driving Groups

▶ Alternative Medicine

National Center for Complementary and Alternative Medicine (NCCAM)
(888) 644-6226
http://altmed.od.nih.gov/nccam

▶ Alzheimer's Disease

Alzheimer's Association National Office

919 N. Michigan Avenue, Suite 1000
Chicago, IL 60611-1676
(800) 272-3900
(312) 335-8700
www.alz.org

▶ Arthritis

Arthritis Foundation

1330 West Peachtree Street
Atlanta, GA 30309
(800) 283-7800
(404) 872-7100
http://www.arthritis.org

▶ Asthma

Asthma and Allergy Foundation of America

1233 Twentieth St., N.W., Suite 402
Washington, DC 20036
(800) 7-ASTHMA
(202) 466-7643
http://www.aafa.org/home.html

Lung Line

National Jewish Center for Immunology and Respiratory Medicine
(information and referral service)
1400 Jackson Street
Denver, CO 80206
(800) 222-5864
(303) 388-4461
http://www.njc.org/Markethtml/Lungline.html

▶ Attention Deficit Disorder

National Attention Deficit Disorder Association (National ADDA)

1788 Second Street, Suite 200
Highland Park, IL 60035
(847) 432-ADDA
http://www.add.org

Children and Adults with Attention Deficit Disorder (CHADD)

8181 Professional Place, Suite 201
Landover, MD 20785
(301) 306-7070
http://chadd.org/

Learning Disabilities Association (LDA)

4156 Library Road
Pittsburgh, PA 15234-1349
(412) 341-1515
http://www.ldanatl.org

▶ Automobile Safety

American Automobile Association (AAA)

1000 AAA Drive #28
Heathrow, FL 32746-5080
(407) 444-4240
http://www.aaa.com

See also white or yellow pages of telephone directory for listing of local chapter

Insurance Institute for Highway Safety

1005 North Glebe Road, Suite 800
Arlington, VA 22201
(703) 247-1500
www.highwaysafety.org/

National Highway Traffic Safety Association

Office of Publications
400 7th Street, S.W.
Room 6123
Washington, DC 20590
(202) 366-2587
http://www.nhtsa.dot.gov

Auto Safety Hotline

(for consumer complaints about auto safety and child safety seats, and requests for information on recalls)
(800) 424-9393

▶ Birth Control and Family Planning

Advocates for Youth

(offers programs aimed at reducing teenage pregnancy)
1025 Vermont Avenue, N.W., Suite 200
Washington, D.C. 20005
(202) 347-5700
http://www.advocatesforyouth.org

American College of Obstetricians and Gynecologists

(provides literature and contraceptive information)
409 12th Street, S.W., P.O. Box 96920
Washington, DC 20090-6920
(202) 638-5577
http://www.acog.com

Association for Voluntary Surgical Contraception (AVSC)

(provides information and referrals to individuals considering tubal ligation or vasectomy)
440 Ninth Ave.
New York, NY 10001
(212) 561-8000

Planned Parenthood Federation of America (PPFA)

810 Seventh Avenue
New York, NY 10019
(212) 541-7800
http://www.plannedparenthood.org

See also white or yellow pages of telephone directory for listing of local chapter

▌ Birth Defects

Cystic Fibrosis Foundation (CFF)

6931 Arlington Road
Bethesda, MD 20814
(800) FIGHT-CF
(301) 951-4422
http://www.cff.org

March of Dimes Birth Defects Foundation

1275 Mamaroneck Avenue
White Plains, NY 10605
(888) 663-4637
(914) 428-7100
http://www.modimes.org

▌ Blindness

American Foundation for the Blind

11 Penn Plaza, Suite 300
New York, NY 10001
(800) AFB-LINE
(212) 502-7661
http://www.afb.org

National Federation for the Blind

1800 Johnson Street
Baltimore, MD 21230
(800) 638-7518
(410) 659-9314
http://www.nfb.org

National Library Service for the Blind and Physically Handicapped

Library of Congress
1291 Taylor Street, N.W.
Washington, DC 20542
(800) 424-8567
(202) 707-5100
http://www.loc.gov/nls

▌ Blood Banks

American Red Cross

11th Floor
1621 N. Kent Street
Arlington, VA 22209
(703) 248-4222
http://www.redcross.org

See also white or yellow pages of telephone directory for listing of local chapter

▌ Breast Cancer

Reach to Recovery

(support program for women who have undergone mastectomies as a result of breast cancer)
American Cancer Society
2200 Lake Blvd.
Atlanta, GA 30319
(800) ACS-2345
(404) 816-7800
www2.cancer.org/state/ga/index.html

▌ Burn Injuries

National Burn Victim Foundation

246-A Madisonville Road
P.O. Box 409
Basking Ridge, NJ 07920
(201) 676-7700
http://www.nbvf.org

Phoenix Society for Burn Victims

(self-help organization for burn victims and their families)
11 Rust Hill Road
Levittown, PA 19056
(800) 888-BURN
(215) 946-BURN
http://www.firealert.com/phoenix.htm

▌ Cancer

American Cancer Society

2200 Lake Blvd.
Atlanta, GA 30319
(800) 227-2345
(404) 816-7800
http://www.cancer.org

Cancer Information Service

National Cancer Institute
31 Center Dr., MSC 2580
Building 31, Room 10A03
Bethesda, MD 20892-2580
(800) 4-CANCER
(301) 435-3848
http://www.nci.nih.gov/hpage/cis.htm

Leukemia Society of America, Inc.

600 Third Avenue
New York, NY 10016
(800) 955-4LSA
(212) 573-8484
http://www.leukemia.org

National Coalition for Cancer Survivorship

1010 Wayne Avenue, Suite 505
Silver Springs, MD 20910-5600
(877) 622-7937
http://www.cansearch.org

National Council on Independent Living

2111 Wilson Boulevard, Suite 405
Arlington, VA 22201
(703) 525-3406
www.arcat.com/arcatcos

R. A. Bloch Cancer Foundation (Cancer Connection)

(support group that matches cancer patients with volunteers who are cured, in remission, or being treated for same type of cancer)
4435 Main Street, Suite 500
Kansas City, MO 64111
(800) 433-0464
(816) 932-8453
http:www.blochcancer.org

▌ Child Abuse

National Center for Assault Prevention

(provides services to children, adolescents, mentally retarded adults, and elderly)
606 Delsea Drive
Sewell, NJ 08080
(800) 258-3189
(609) 582-7000
http://www.ncap.org

National Child Abuse Hotline

(800) 422-4453

National Committee for the Prevention of Child Abuse

(provides literature on child abuse prevention programs)
200 S. Michigan Avenue
17th Floor
Chicago, IL 60604-2404
(312) 663-3520
http://www.preventchildabuse.org

Parents Anonymous

(self-help group for abusive parents)
675 W. Foothill Blvd., Suite 220
Claremont, CA 91711-3475
(909) 621-6184
http://www.parentsanonymous-natl.org

▌ Childbirth

American College of Nurse-Midwives

(RNs who provide services through the maternity cycle)
818 Connecticut Avenue, N.W.
Suite 900
Washington, D.C. 20006
(202) 728-9860
www.midwife.org/

American College of Obstetricians and Gynecologists

409 12th Street, S.W.
P.O. Box 96920
Washington, D.C. 20090-6920
(202) 638-5577
http://www.acog.com

Lamaze International

1200 19th Street, N.W.
Suite 300
Washington, D.C. 20036-2422
(800) 368-4404
(202) 857-1128
http://www.lamaze-childbirth.com

International Childbirth Education Association

P.O. Box 20048
Minneapolis, MN 55420
(612) 854-8660
http://www.icea.org

▶ Child Health and Development

National Center for Education in Maternal and Child Health

2000 15th Street, N.
Suite 701
Arlington, VA 22201
(703) 524-7802

National Institute of Child Health and Human Development

31 Center Drive, MSC-2425
Building 31/2A32
Bethesda, MD 20892-2425
(301) 496-5133
www.nichd.nih.gov/

▶ Chiropractic

American Chiropractic Association

1701 Clarendon Boulevard
Arlington, VA 22209
(800) 986-INFO
(703) 276-8800
http://www.amerchiro.org

▶ Consumer Information

Consumer Information Center

(catalog of publications developed by federal agencies for consumers)
Department WWW
Pueblo, CO 81009
(888) 878-3256
http://www.pueblo.gsa.gov

Consumer Product Safety Commission

Office of Information Services
4330 East-West Highway
Bethesda, MD 20814-4408
(800) 638-2772

(301) 504-0990
http://www.cpsc.gov

Consumers Union of United States

(tests quality and safety of consumer products; publishes *Consumer Reports* magazine)
101 Truman Avenue
Yonkers, NY 10703
(914) 378-2000
http://www.consumerreports.org

Council of Better Business Bureaus (CBBB)

4200 Wilson Boulevard, Suite 800
Arlington, VA 22203-1804
(703) 276-0100
http://www.bbb.org

See also white or yellow pages of telephone directory for listing of local chapter

Food and Drug Administration (FDA)

Office of Consumer Affairs
Consumer Inquiries
5600 Fishers Lane (HFE-88)
Rockville, MD 20857
(888) INFO-FDA
(463-6332)
http://www.fda.gov

▶ Crime Victims

Crisis Prevention Institute, Inc.

(offers programs on non-violent physical crisis interventions)
3315-K N. 124th Street
Brookfield, WI 53005
(800) 558-8976
(262) 783-5787
www.crisisprevention.com

National Association for Crime Victims Rights (NACVR)

P.O. Box 16161
Portland, OR 97292
(503) 252-9012

▶ Death and Grieving

Share

(support group for parents who have suffered loss of newborn baby)
c/o St. John's Hospital
800 E. Carpenter Street
Springfield, IL 62769
(217) 544-6464

▶ Dental Health

American Dental Association (ADA)

211 E. Chicago Avenue
Chicago, IL 60611
(312) 440-2500
http://www.ada.org

National Institute of Dental Research

Office of Communication
9000 Rockville Pike
Building 31, Room 2C35

Bethesda, MD 20892-2190
(301) 496-4261
http://www.nidr.nih.gov

▶ Depressive Disorders

National Depressive and Manic Depressive Association (NDMDA)

730 N. Franklin, Suite 501
Chicago, IL 60610-3526
(312) 642-0049
(800) 826-3632
http://www.ndmda.org

▶ DES (Diethylstibestrol)

DES Action, USA

(support group for persons exposed to DES)
1615 Broadway
Suite 510
Oakland, CA 94612
(510) 465-4011
http://www.desaction.org

▶ Diabetes

American Diabetes Association

National Center
1701 North Beauregard St.
Alexandria, VA 22311
(800) DIABETES (342-2383)
(703) 549-1500
http://www.diabetes.org

Juvenile Diabetes Foundation International (JDFI)

120 Wall Street
New York, NY 10005-4001
(800) JDF-CURE
(212) 785-9500
http://www.jdfcure.org

National Diabetes Information Clearinghouse

31 Center Dr., MSC 2560
Bethesda, MD 20892-2560
(301) 654-3327
http://www.niddk.nih.gov

▶ Digestive Diseases

National Digestive Diseases Information

Clearinghouse (NDDIC)
Box NDDIC
2 Information Way
Bethesda, MD 20892-3570
(301) 654-3810
www.niddk.nih.gov

▶ Domestic Violence

Batterers Anonymous

(self-help group designed to rehabilitate men who abuse women)
1850 N. Riverside Avenue
Suite 220

Rialto, CA 92376
(909) 355-1100

National Coalition Against Domestic Violence (NCADV)

P.O. Box 18749
Denver, CO 80218
(303) 839-1852
www.ncadv.org/

National Domestic Violence Hotline

(800) 799-SAFE

National Network to End Domestic Violence

701 Pennsylvania, N.W., Suite 900
Washington, D.C. 20004
(202) 347-9520

▶ **Down Syndrome**

National Association for Down Syndrome (NADS)

P.O. Box 4542
Oak Brook, IL 60522-4542
(630) 325-9112
http://www.nads.org

National Down Syndrome Society (NDSS)

666 Broadway, 8th Floor
New York, NY 10012-2317
(800) 221-4602
(212) 460-9330
http://www.ndss.org

▶ **Drug Abuse**

Cocaine Anonymous World Services

P.O. Box 2000
Los Angeles, CA 90049-8000
(800) 347-8998
(310) 559-5833
http://www.ca.org

Narcotics Anonymous (NA)

(support group for recovering recent narcotics addicts)
P.O. Box 9999
Van Nuys, CA 91409
(818) 773-9999
http://www.wsoinc.com

See also white or yellow pages of telephone directory for listing of local chapter

National Cocaine Hotline

(800) COCAINE

National Institute on Drug Abuse Helpline

(800) 662-4357
http://nida.nih.gov

National Parents Resource Institute for Drug Education (PRIDE)

3610 Dekalb Technology Parkway, Suite 105
Atlanta, GA 30340

(770) 458-9900
http://www.prideusa.org

Substance Abuse Prevention

Alcohol, Drug Abuse, and Mental Health Administration
5600 Fishers Lane
Rockwall 2 Building
Rockville, MD 20857
(301) 443-0365

▶ **Drunk Driving Groups**

Mothers Against Drunk Driving

P.O. Box 541688
Dallas, TX 75354-1688
(800) GET-MADD
http://www.madd.org

See also white pages of telephone directory for listing of local chapter

Remove Intoxicated Drivers (RID)

P.O. Box 520
Schenectady, NY 12301
(518) 372-0034
(518) 393-HELP
www.crisny.org/not-for-profit/ridusal

Students Against Drunk Driving (SADD)

P.O. Box 800
Marlboro, MA 01752
(508) 481-3568
www.saddonline.com

▶ **Eating Disorders**

American Anorexia/Bulimia Association (AA/BA)

(self-help group that provides information and referrals to physicians and therapists)
165 West 46th Street, #1108
New York, NY 10036
(212) 575-6200
www.aabainc.org

Anorexia Nervosa and Related Eating Disorders (ANRED)

(provides information and referrals for people with eating disorders)
P.O. Box 5102
Eugene, OR 97405
(800) 931-2237
(541) 344-1144
http://www.anred.com

▶ **Environment**

Environmental Protection Agency (EPA)

Public Information Center
PM 211-B
401 M Street, S.W.
Washington, D.C. 20460
(202) 260-2080
http://www.epa.gov

Greenpeace, USA

1436 U Street, N.W.
Washington, D.C. 20009
(800) 326-0959
(202) 462-1177
http://www.greenpeaceusa.org

Natural Resources Defense Council

40 West 20th Street
New York, NY 10011
(212) 727-2700
http://www.nrdc.org

Sierra Club

85 2nd Street, 2nd Floor
San Francisco, CA 94105-3441
(415) 977-5500
http://www.sierraclub.org

World Wildlife Fund

1250 24th Street, N.W.
P.O. Box 97180
Washington, D.C. 20077-7180
(800) CALL-WWF
(202) 293-4800
http://www.wwfus.org

▶ **Epilepsy**

Epilepsy Foundation of America

4351 Garden City Drive
Landover, MD 20785-2267
(800) EFA-1000
(301) 459-3700
http://www.efa.org

▶ **Gay and Lesbian Organizations and Services**

Human Rights Campaign

919 18th St.
Washington, D.C. 20006
(202) 628-4160
http://www.hrc.org

National Gay and Lesbian Task Force (NGLTF)

1700 Kalorama Rd., N.W.
Washington, D.C. 20009-2624
(202) 332-6483
http://www.ngltf.org

Parents, Family, and Friends of Lesbians and Gays (P-FLAG)

1101 14th Street, N.W, Suite 1030
Washington, D.C. 20005
(202) 638-4200
http://www.pflag.org

▶ **Handicapped and Disabled**

American Alliance for Health, Physical Education, Recreation, and Dance (AAHPERD)

(provides information about recreation and fitness opportunities for the handicapped)
1900 Association Drive

Reston, VA 20191
(703) 476-3400
http://www.aahperd.org

National Council on Independent Living

2111 Wilson Boulevard
Suite 405
Arlington, VA 22201
(703) 525-3406
www.arcat.com/arcatcos

National Library Service for the Blind and Physically Handicapped

Library of Congress
1291 Taylor Street, N.W.
Washington, D.C. 20542
(800) 424-8567
(202) 707-5100
http://www.loc.gov/nls

Special Olympics International (SOI)

1325 G Street, N.W.
Suite 500
Washington, D.C. 20005
(202) 628-3630
http://www.specialolympics.org

▌ Hazardous Waste

Environmental Protection Agency (EPA)

Public Information Center
PM 211-B
401 M Street, S.W.
Washington, D.C. 20460
(202) 260-2080
http://www.epa.gov

Hazardous Waste Hotline Information

(800) 424-9346

▌ Health Care

American Association for Therapeutic Humor (AATH)

(publishes a newsletter and sponsors seminars for people in the helping professions)
222 S. Merimac Street, Suite 303
St. Louis, MO 63105
(314) 863-6232
http://aath.org

American Medical Association

515 N. State Street
Chicago, IL 60610
(312) 464-5000
http://www.ama-assn.org

American Nurses Association

600 Maryland Avenue, S.W.
Suite 100 West
Washington, D.C. 20024-2571
(800) 274-4ANA
(202) 651-7000
http://www.nursingworld.org

Medical Self-Care Magazine

P.O. Box 717
Inverness, CA 94937

▌ Health Education

Center for Health Promotion and Education

Centers for Disease Control and Prevention
Mail Stop A34
1600 Clifton Road, N.E.
Atlanta, GA 30333
(404) 639-3534
(800) 311-3435
www.cdc.gov/

▌ Hearing Impairment

American Society for Deaf Children

(resource group for parents of hard of hearing and deaf children)
1820 Tribute Rd., Suite A
Sacramento, CA 95815
(800) 942-ASDC
(916) 641-6084
www.deafchildren.org/

Better Hearing Institute (BHI)

(provides educational and resource materials on deafness)
Box 1840
Washington, D.C. 20013
(800) EAR-WELL
(703) 684-3391
http://www.betterhearing.org

▌ Heart Disease

American Heart Association (AHA)

7272 Greenville Avenue
Dallas, TX 75231
(800) 242-8721
(214) 373-6300
http://www.americanheart.org

National Heart, Lung, and Blood Institute

(provides information on cardiovascular risk factors and disease)
4733 Bethesda Avenue, Suite 530
Bethesda, MD 20814
(800) 575-9355
http://www.nhlbi.nih.gov/index.htm

▌ Holistic Medicine

American Holistic Medical Association (NHMA)

6728 Old McLean Village Drive
McLean, VA 22101
(703) 556-8729—fax
http://www.ahmaholistic.com

▌ Homeopathy

National Center for Homeopathy (NCH)

801 N. Fairfax Street, Suite 306

Alexandria, VA 22314
(703) 548-7790
http://www.healthworld.com/nch

▌ Hospice

National Hospice Organization

1700 Diagchal Rd., Suite 300
Arlington, VA 22314
(703) 243-5900
http://nho.org

▌ Immunization

National Center for Prevention Services

Centers for Disease Control
1600 Clifton Road, N.E.
Atlanta, GA 30333
(404) 639-3311
(800) 311-3435

▌ Infant Care

American Red Cross

1621 N. Kent Street, 11th Floor
Arlington, VA 22209
(703) 248-4222
http://www.redcross.org

LaLeche League International

(provides information and support to women interested in breast-feeding)
1400 N. Meacham Road
Schaumburg, IL 60173-4048
(800) LA-LECHE
(847) 519-7730
http://www.lalecheleague.org

▌ Infectious Diseases

Centers for Disease Control and Prevention

1600 Clifton Road, N.E.
Atlanta, GA 30333
(404) 639-3534
http://www.cdc.gov

▌ Infertility

Resolve, Inc.

(offers counseling, information, and support to people with problems of infertility)
1310 Broadway
Somerville, MA 02144-1779
(617) 623-0744
http://www.resolve.org

▌ Inherited Diseases

Alliance of Genetic Support Groups

(provides information about inherited diseases; publishes a directory of genetic counseling services)
35 Wisconsin Circle, Suite 440
Chevy Chase, MD 20815
(800) 336-GENE
www.research.mdacc.tmc.edu

▶ Kidney Disease

American Kidney Fund (AKF)

(provides information on financial aid to patients, organ transplants, and kidney-related diseases)
6110 Executive Boulevard, Suite 1010
Rockville, MD 20852
(800) 638-8299
(301) 881-3052
http://www.akfinc.org

American Association of Kidney Patients (AAKP)

100 S. Ashley Dr., Suite 280
Tampa, FL 33602-5346
(800) 749-2257
http://www.aakp.org

National Kidney Foundation (NKF)

30 East 33rd Street, Suite 1100
New York, NY 10016
(800) 622-9010
(212) 889-2210
http://www.kidney.org

Learning Disorders

Learning Disabilities Association of
America (LDA)
4156 Library Road
Pittsburgh, PA 15234-1349
(412) 341-1515
www.npin.org/reswork/workorgs/
ldaa.html

▶ Liver Disease

American Liver Foundation (ALF)

75 Maiden, Suite 603
New York, NY 10038
(800) 465-4837
www.liverfoundation.org/

▶ Lung Disease

American Lung Association (ALA)

432 Park Ave. South, 8th Floor
New York, NY 10016
(800) LUNG-USA
(212) 889-3370
http://www.lungusa.org

NHLBI Educational Program Information Center

(provides information on cardiovascular risk factors)
P.O. Box 30105
Bethesda, MD 20824
(301) 951-3260
www.nhlbi.nih.gov/

National Jewish Center for Immunology and Respiratory Medicine

899 Logan St., Suite 600
Denver, CO 80203
(303) 860-6600
www.weitz.com/colorado/national_
jewish.asp

▶ Lupus Erythematosus

Lupus Foundation of America (LPA)

1300 Piccard Drive, Suite 200
Rockville, MD 20850-4303
(301) 670-9292
(800) 558-0121
http://www.lupus.org/lupus/index.html

▶ Marriage and Family

Women Work! The National Network for Women's Employment

(national advocacy group for women over 35 who have lost their primary means of support through death, divorce, or disabling of spouse)
1625 K Street N.W., Suite 300
Washington, D.C. 20006
(202) 467-6346

Alliance for Children & Families

1701 K Street, N.W., Suite 200
Washington, D. C. 20006
(202) 223-3447
http://www.alliance1.org

Stepfamily Association of America

(provides information and publishes quarterly newsletter)
650 J Street, Suite 205
Lincoln, NE 68508
(402) 477-7837
(800) 735-0329
http://www.stepfam.org

▶ Medical Information

Medic Alert Foundation

(provides those with medical problems bracelets or neck chains with special emblems to alert medical or law enforcement personnel)
P.O. Box 819008
Turlock, CA 95381-1009
(800) 344-3226
(209) 668-3333
www.aoa.dhhs.gov/AOA/dir/121.html

▶ Medications (Prescriptions and Over-the-Counter)

Food and Drug Administration (FDA)

Office of Consumer Affairs Public
Inquiries
5600 Fishers Lane (HFE-88)
Rockville, MD 20857
(888) 463-6332 (INFO-FDA)
http://www.fda.gov

▶ Mental Health

American Psychiatric Association

1400 K Street, N.W.
Washington, D.C. 20005
(202) 682-6000
http://www.psych.org

American Psychological Association

750 First Street, N.E.
Washington, D.C. 20002-4242
(202) 336-5500
http://www.apa.org

National Alliance for the Mentally Ill (NAMI)

(self-help advocacy organization for persons with schizophrenia and depressive disorders and their families)
200 N. Glebe Road, Suite 1015
Arlington, VA 22203-3754
(800) 950-NAMI
(703) 524-7600
www.nami.org/

National Institute of Mental Health

Information Resources and Inquiries
Branch
6001 Executive Blvd., Rm 8184 MSC
9663
Bethesda, MD 20892-9663
(301) 443-4513
www.nimh.nih.gov/

National Mental Health Association (NMHA)

1021 Prince Street
Alexandria, VA 22314-2971
(800) 969-NMHA
(703) 684-7722
http://www.nmha.org

Recovery, Inc.

(self-help group for former mental patients)
Association of Nervous and Former
Mental Patients
802 N. Dearborn Street
Chicago, IL 60610
(312) 337-5661

▶ Mental Retardation

Association for Retarded Citizens (ARC)

1010 Wayne Ave., Suite 650
Silver Spring, MD 20910
(301) 565-3842
http://www.thearc.org

▶ Missing and Runaway Children

Child Find of America

(800) I-AM-LOST

National Center for Missing and Exploited Children (NCMEC)

699 Prince St., Suite 550
Alexandria, VA 22314
(800) 843-5678
http://www.missingkids.org

Runaway Hotline

(800) 621-4000

▶ Neurological Disorders

National Institute of Neurological and Communicative Disorders and Stroke

National Institutes of Health
P.O. Box 5801
Bethesda, MD 20824
(301) 496-4000
www.ninds.nih.gov/

▶ Nutrition

American Dietetic Association

216 West Jackson Boulevard
Chicago, IL 60606-6995
(312) 899-0040
http://www.eatright.org

American Society for Nutritional Sciences (AIN)

9650 Rockville Pike
Bethesda, MD 20814-3990
(301) 530-7050
www.faseb.org/ain

Food and Drug Administration (FDA)

Office of Consumer Affairs
Public Inquiries
5600 Fishers Land (HFE-88)
Rockville, MD 20857
(888) 463-6332 (INFO-FDA)
http://www.fda.gov

Food and Nutrition Board

Institute of Medicine
2101 Constitution Avenue, N.W.
Washington, D.C. 20418
(202) 334-2383
www4.nas.edu/IOM/IOMHeme.nsf

Food and Nutrition Information Center

National Agricultural Library
Room 304
10301 Baltimore Avenue
Beltsville, MD 20705-2351
(301) 504-5719
http://www.nalusda.gov/fnic/

▶ Occupational Safety and Health

Occupational Safety and Health Administration

U.S. Dept. of Labor
Office of Public Affairs—Room N3647
200 Constitution Ave.
Washington, D.C. 20210
(202) 693-1999

▶ Organ Donations

The Living Bank (TLB)

(provides information and acts as registry and referral service for people wanting to donate organs for research or transplantation)
P.O. Box 6725

Houston, TX 77265
(800) 528-2971

▶ Osteopathic Medicine

American Osteopathic Association (AOA)

142 East Ontario Street
Chicago, IL 60611
(800) 621-1773
http://www.am-osteo-assn.org

▶ Parent Support Groups

National Organization of Mothers with Twin Clubs (NOMOTC)

P.O. Box 438
Thompson Station, TN 37179-0438
(615) 595-0936 & (877) 540-2200
www.nomotc.org

Parents Anonymous

(self-help group for abusive parents)
675 W. Foothill Boulevard, Suite 220
Claremont, CA 91711-3475
(909) 621-6184
www.parentsanonymous_natl.org

Parents Without Partners, Inc.

1650 South Dixie Highway, Suite 510
Boca Raton, FL 33432
(561) 391-8833
http://www.parentswithoutpartners.org

▶ Pesticides

National Pesticides Telecommunications Network

Agricultural Chemistry Extension
Oregon State University
333 Weniger Hall
Corvallis, OR 97331
(800) 858-7378

▶ Phobias

Anxiety Disorders Association of America (ADAA)

(provides information about phobias and referrals to therapists and support groups)
11900 Parklawn Drive, Suite 100
Rockville, MD 20852
(301) 231-9350
http://www.adaa.org

TERRAP Programs

(headquarters for national network of treatment clinics for agoraphobia)
932 Evelyn Street
Menlo Park, CA 94025
(415) 327-1312
(800) 2-PHOBIA
www.terrap.com/default.htm

▶ Physical Fitness
See local yellow and white pages of telephone directory for listing of local health clubs and YMCAs, YWCAs, and Jewish Community Centers

Cooper Institute for Aerobics Research

12330 Preston Road
Dallas, TX 75230
www.cooperinst.org/

President's Council on Physical Fitness and Sports

200 Independence Ave., S.W.
Humphrey Bldg., Room 738 H
Washington, D.C. 20201
(202) 690-9000

Women's Sports Foundation

Eisenhower Park
East Meadow, NY 11554
(516) 542-4700
(800) 227-3988
http://www.lifetimetv.com/WoSport/

▶ Poisoning
See emergency numbers listed in the front of your local phone directory

National Poison Hotline

(800) 962-1253

▶ Pregnancy

National Center for Education in Maternal and Child Health

2000 15th Street N., Suite 701
Arlington, VA 22201-2617
(703) 524-7802

▶ Product Safety

Consumer Product Safety Commission

4330 East-West Highway
Bethesda, MD 20814-4408
(800) 638-CPSC
http://www.cpsc.gov

▶ Radiation Control and Safety

Center for Devices and Radiological Health

Office of Consumer Affairs
5600 Fishers Lane HFC-210
Rockville, MD 20857
http://www.fda.gov/cdrh/index.html

National Institute of Environmental Health Sciences

P.O. Box 12233
Research Triangle Park, NC 27709
(919) 541-3345
http://www.niehs.nih.gov

▶ Rape
See white pages of telephone directory for listing of local rape crisis and counseling centers

National Clearinghouse on Marital and Date Rape

(for-profit referral service)

2325 Oak Street
Berkeley, CA 94708
(510) 524-1582
http://members.aol.com/ncmdr/
  index.html

National Coalition Against Sexual Assault

912 N. 2nd Street
Harrisburg, PA 17102
(717) 232-6745

▶ Reye's Syndrome

National Reye's Syndrome Foundation

426 North Lewis
P.O. Box 829
Bryan, OH 43506
(419) 636-2679
(800) 233-7393
www.bright.net/ ~ reyessyn

▶ Self-Care/Self-Help

National Self-Help Clearinghouse (NSHC)

(provides information about self-help groups)
25 West 43rd Street, Room 620
New York, NY 10036
(212) 354-8525
http://selfhelpweb.org/

United Way of America

701 N. Fairfax Street
Alexandria, VA 22314-2045
(703) 836-7100
http://www.unitedway.org

▶ Sex Education

American Association of Sex Educators, Counselors, and Therapists (AASECT)

P.O. Box 238
Mount Vernon, IA 52314
(319) 895-6203
http://www.aasect.org

Advocates for Youth

(develops programs and material to educate youth on sex and sexual responsibility)
1025 Vermont Avenue, N.W.
Suite 200
Washington, D.C. 20005
(202) 347-5700
www.advocatesforyouth.org/

Planned Parenthood Federation of America (PPFA)

810 Seventh Avenue
New York, NY 10019
(212) 541-7800
http://www.plannedparenthood.org

Sex Information and Education Council of the U.S. (SIECUS)

(maintains an information clearinghouse on all aspects of human sexuality)
130 West 42nd Street, Suite 350
New York, NY 10036
(212) 819-9770
http://www.siecus.org

▶ Sexual Abuse and Assault

National Center for Assault Prevention

(provides services to children, adolescents, mentally regarded adults, and elderly)
606 Delsea Drive
Sewell, NJ 08080
(856) 582-7000
(800) 258-3189

National Committee for Prevention of Child Abuse

200 S. Michigan Avenue, Suite 1700
Chicago, IL 60604
(312) 663-3520

Parents United International

(support group for individuals—and their families—who have experienced molestation as children)
615 15th Street
Modesto, CA 95354-2510
(209) 572-3446

▶ Sexually Transmitted Diseases

Centers for Disease Control and Prevention

1600 Clifton Road, N.E.
Atlanta, GA 30333
(404) 639-3311
http://www.cdc.gov

Herpes Resource Center

American Social Health Association
P.O. Box 13827
Research Triangle Park, NC 27709-3827
(919) 361-8488
http://www.ashastd.org/herpes/
  hrc.html

National STD Hotline

(800) 227-8922

▶ Sickle Cell Disease

Center for Sickle Cell Disease

Howard University
2121 Georgia Avenue, N.W.
Washington, D.C. 20059
(202) 806-7930

Sickle Cell Disease Association of America

200 Corporate Pointe, Suite 495
Culver City, CA 90230-7633

(310) 216-6363
(800) 421-8453

▶ Skin Disease

National Psoriasis Foundation

6600 S.W. 92nd Avenue, Suite 300
Portland, OR 97223
(503) 244-7404
http://www.psoriasis.org

▶ Sleep and Sleep Disorders

American Narcolepsy Association

1255 Post Street, Suite 404
San Francisco, CA 94109

American Sleep Disorders Association

200 First Street, S.W.
Rochester, MN 55905
(507) 266-8900
http://www.asda.org

Better Sleep Council

501 Wythe St.
Alexandria, VA 22314
(703) 683-8371
www.bettersleep.org/

▶ Smoking and Tobacco

Action on Smoking and Health (ASH)

(provides information on non-smokers' rights and related subjects)
2013 H Street, N.W.
Washington, D.C. 20006
(202) 659-4310
http://ash.org

American Cancer Society

(provides information about quitting smoking and smoking cessation programs)
2200 Lake Blvd.
Atlanta, GA 30319
(800) 227-2345
http://www.cancer.org

American Heart Association

(provides information about quitting smoking and smoking cessation programs)
7272 Greenville Avenue
Dallas, TX 75231
(800) 242-8721
(214) 373-6300
http://www.americanheart.org

American Lung Association

(provides information about quitting smoking and smoking cessation programs)
432 Park Ave. South, 8th Floor
New York, NY 10016
(800) LUNG-USA
(212) 889-3370
http://www.lungusa.org

Americans for Nonsmokers' Rights

2530 San Pablo Avenue, Suite J
Berkeley, CA 94702
(510) 841-3032
http://www.no-smoke.org

▶ Stress Reduction

Association for Applied Psychophysiology and Biofeedback (AABP)

10200 W. 44th Avenue, Suite 304
Wheat Ridge, CO 80033
www.aabp.org

▶ Stroke

Council on Stroke

American Heart Association
7272 Greenville Avenue
Dallas, TX 75321
(214) 373-6300
www.americanheart.org

National Institute of Neurological and Communicative Disorders and Stroke

National Institutes of Health
P.O. Box 5801
Bethesda, MD 20824
(301) 496-4000
www.ninds.nih.gov/

▶ Stuttering

National Center for Stuttering

200 East 33rd Street
New York, NY 10016
(800) 221-2483
(212) 532-1460
http://www.stuttering.com

▶ Sudden Infant Death Syndrome (SIDS)

SIDS Alliance

(provides information and referrals for families who have lost an infant because of SIDS)
1314 Bedford Avenue, Suite 210
Baltimore, MD 21208

(800) 221-7437
(410) 653-8226
www.sidsalliance.org/

▶ Suicide Prevention

American Association of Suicidology (AAS)

1636 Connecticut Avenue, N.W.
2nd Floor
Washington, D.C. 20009
(202) 667-6363
http://www.cyberpsych.org/index.html

National Runaway Switchboard

3080 N. Lincoln Avenue
Chicago, IL 60657
(800) 621-4000
(773) 880-9860
http://nrs.crisisline.org/about.htm

▶ Terminal Illness

Choices in Dying—The National Council for the Right to Die (CID)

(promotes research on death and dying and works for the right of terminally ill persons to refuse extraordinary life-prolonging measures)
200 Varick Street, 10th Floor
New York, NY 10014-4810

Make-a-Wish Foundation of America (MAWFA)

(dedicated to granting the special wishes of terminally ill children)
100 W. Clarendon Avenue
Suite 2200
Phoenix, AZ 85013
(800) 722-9474
(602) 279-9474
http://www.wish.org

Make Today Count (MTC)

(self-help group for persons with terminal illness)
1235 E. Cherokee Street
Springfield, MO 65804
(800) 432-2273
(417) 885-3324
www.userpages.itis.com/lemoll/
index2.html#site

▶ Weight Control

Overeaters Anonymous (OA)

7133-B
Darby Ave.
Reseda, CA 91335
(818) 881-4776

Take Off Pounds Sensibly (TOPS)

P.O. Box 07360
4575 S. Fifth Street
Milwaukee, WI 53207-0360
(800) 932-8677
(414) 482-4620
www.tops.org

Weight Watchers International

175 Crossways Park West
Woodbury, NY 11797
(516) 390-1657
http://www.weight-watchers.com

▶ Wellness

Wellness Associates

(publishes The Wellness Inventory)
706 West Junior Terrace
Chicago, IL 60613
(773) 935-6377
www.wellness-associates.com

▶ Women's Health

Boston Women's Health Book Collective

(authors of The New Our Bodies, Ourselves, a well-known book on women's health)
240A Elm Street
Somerville, MA 02144
(617) 625-0271
www.ourbodiesourselves.org

National Women's Health Network (NWHN)

514 10th Street N.W., Suite 400
Washington, D.C. 20004
(202) 347-1140
www.womenshealthnetwork.org

Photography Credits

Glossary

abscess A localized accumulation of pus and disintegrating tissue.

absorption The passage of substances into or across membranes or tissues.

abstinence Voluntary refrainment from sexual intercourse.

acid rain Rain with a high concentration of acids produced by air pollutants emitted during the combustion of fossil fuels and the smelting of ores; damages plant and animal life and buildings.

acquired immunodeficiency syndrome (AIDS) The final stages of HIV infection, characterized by a variety of severe illnesses and decreased levels of certain immune cells.

acupuncture A Chinese medical practice of puncturing the body with needles inserted at specific points to relieve pain or cure disease.

acute injuries Physical injuries, such as sprains, bruises, and pulled muscles, which result from sudden traumas, such as falls or collisions.

adaptive response The body's attempt to reestablish homeostasis or stability.

addiction A behavioral pattern characterized by compulsion, loss of control, and continued repetition of a behavior or activity in spite of adverse consequences.

additive Characterized by a combined effect that is equal to the sum of the individual effects.

additives Substances added to foods to enhance certain qualities, such as appearance, taste, or freshness.

adjustment disorder An extraordinary response to a stressful event or situation.

adoption The legal process for becoming the parent to a child of other biological parents.

advance directives Documents that specify individual's preferences regarding treatment in a medical crisis.

aerobic circuit training Combining aerobic and strength exercises to build both cardiovascular fitness and muscular strength and endurance.

aerobic exercise Physical activity in which sufficient or excess oxygen is continually supplied to the body.

after-intercourse methods Treatments, such as large doses of oral contraceptives,

menstrual extraction, or dilation and curettage, given after unprotected intercourse to prevent pregnancy.

ageism A form of discrimination based on myths about aging and the elderly.

aging The characteristic pattern of normal life changes that occur as an individual gets older.

alcohol abuse Continued use of alcohol despite awareness of social, occupational, psychological, or physical problems related to its use, or use of alcohol in dangerous ways or situations, such as before driving.

alcohol dependence Development of a strong craving for alcohol due to the pleasurable feelings or relief of stress or anxiety produced by drinking.

alcoholism A chronic, progressive, potentially fatal disease characterized by impaired control of drinking, a preoccupation with alcohol, continued use of alcohol despite adverse consequences, and distorted thinking, most notably denial.

allergy A hypersensitivity to a particular substance in one's environment or diet.

allopathic medicine Conventional or orthodox Western medicine.

allostasis The body's ability to adapt to constantly changing environments.

altruism Acts of helping or giving to others without thought of self-benefit.

Alzheimer's disease A progressive deterioration of intellectual powers due to physiological changes within the brain; symptoms include diminishing ability to concentrate and reason, disorientation, depression, apathy, and paranoia.

amenorrhea The absence or suppression of menstruation.

amino acids Organic compounds containing nitrogen, carbon, hydrogen, and oxygen; the essential building blocks of proteins.

amnion The innermost membrane of the sac enclosing the embryo or fetus.

amphetamine Any of a class of stimulants that trigger the release of epinephrine, which stimulates the central nervous system; users experience a state of hyperalertness and energy, followed by a crash as the drug wears off.

anabolic steroids Drugs derived from testosterone and approved for medical use,

but often used by athletes to increase their musculature and weight.

anaerobic exercise Physical activity in which the body develops an oxygen deficit.

androgynous Not tied to traditional gender roles, as in a marriage.

androgyny The expression of both masculine and feminine traits.

anemia A condition characterized by a marked reduction in the number of circulating red blood cells or in hemoglobin, the oxygen-carrying component of red blood cells.

angina pectoris A severe, suffocating chest pain caused by a brief lack of oxygen to the heart.

angioplasty Surgical repair of an obstructed artery by passing a balloon catheter through the blood vessel to the area of disease and then inflating the catheter to compress the plaque against the vessel wall.

anorexia nervosa A psychological disorder in which refusal to eat and/or an extreme loss of appetite leads to malnutrition, severe weight loss, and possibly death.

antagonistic Opposing or counteracting.

antibiotics Substances produced by microorganisms, or synthetic agents, that are toxic to other types of microorganisms; in dilute solutions, used to treat infectious diseases.

antidepressant A drug used primarily to treat symptoms of depression.

antioxidants Substances that prevent the damaging effects of oxidation in cells.

antiviral drug A substance that decreases the severity and duration of a viral infection if taken prior to or soon after onset of the infection.

anxiety A feeling of apprehension and dread, with or without a known cause; may range from mild to severe and may be accompanied by physical symptoms.

anxiety disorders A group of psychological disorders involving episodes of apprehension, tension, or uneasiness, stemming from the anticipation of danger and sometimes accompanied by physical symptoms, which cause significant distress and impairment to an individual.

aorta The main artery of the body, arising from the left ventricle of the heart.

appetite A desire for food, stimulated by anticipated hunger, physiological changes within the brain and body, the availability of food, and other environmental and psychological factors.

arrhythmia Any irregularity in the rhythm of the heartbeat.

arteriosclerosis Any of a number of chronic diseases characterized by degeneration of the arteries and hardening and thickening of arterial walls.

arthritis Inflammation of the joints.

artificial insemination The introduction of viable sperm into the vagina by artificial means for the purpose of inducing conception.

assertive Behaving in a confident manner to make your needs and desires clear to others in a nonhostile way.

asthma A disease or allergic response characterized by bronchial spasms and difficult breathing.

atherosclerosis A form of arteriosclerosis in which fatty substances (plaque) are deposited on the inner walls of arteries.

atrial fibrillation A condition characterized by an irregular, abnormally rapid heartbeat.

atrium (plural atria) Either of the two upper chambers of the heart, which receive blood from the veins.

attention deficit/hyperactivity disorder (ADHD) A spectrum of difficulties in controlling motion and sustaining attention, including hyperactivity, impulsivity, and distractibility.

autoimmune Resulting from the attack on body tissue by an immune system that fails to recognize the tissue as self.

autonomy The ability to draw on internal resources; independence from familial and societal influences.

autoscopy The sensation of one's self being outside its body, often experienced by individuals in near-death medical crises.

aversion therapy A treatment that attempts to help a person overcome a dependence or bad habit by making the person feel disgusted or repulsed by that habit.

axon The long fiber that conducts impulses from the neurons nucleus to its dendrites.

axon terminal The ending of an axon, from which impulses are transmitted to a dendrite of another neuron.

ayurveda A traditional Indian medical treatment involving meditation, exercise, herbal medications, and nutrition.

bacteria (singular, bacterium) One-celled microscopic organisms; the most plentiful pathogens.

bacterial vaginosis A vaginal infection caused by overgrowth and depletion of various microorganisms living in the vagina, resulting in a malodorous white or gray vaginal discharge.

barbiturates Antianxiety drugs that depress the central nervous system, reduce activity and induce relaxation, drowsiness, or sleep; often prescribed to relieve tension and treat epileptic seizures or as a general anesthetic.

barrier contraceptives Birth-control devices that block the meeting of egg and sperm, either by physical barriers, such as condoms, diaphragms, or cervical caps, or by chemical barriers, such as spermicide, or both.

basal body temperature The body temperature upon waking, before any activity.

basal metabolic rate (BMR) The number of calories required to sustain the body at rest.

behavior therapy Psychotherapy that emphasizes application of the principles of learning to substitute desirable responses and behavior patterns for undesirable ones.

benign hypertrophy Enlargement of the prostate gland, resulting in a pinching of the urethra.

benzodiazepines Antianxiety drugs that depress the central nervous system, reduce activity and induce relaxation, drowsiness, or sleep; often prescribed to relieve tension, muscular strain, sleep problems, anxiety, and panic attacks; also used as an anesthetic and in the treatment of alcohol withdrawal.

bidis Skinny, sweet-flavored cigarettes.

binge drinking For a man, having five or more alcoholic drinks at a single sitting; for a woman, having four drinks or more at a single sitting.

binge eating The rapid consumption of an abnormally large amount of food in a relatively short time.

biofeedback A technique of becoming aware, with the aid of external monitoring devices, of internal physiological activities in order to develop the capability of altering them.

bipolar disorder Severe depression alternating with periods of manic activity and elation.

bisexual Sexually oriented toward both sexes.

blended family A family formed when one or both of the partners bring children from a previous union to the new marriage.

blood-alcohol concentration (BAC) The amount of alcohol in the blood, expressed as a percentage.

body mass index (BMI) The percentage of fat in ones body.

bone-marrow transplantation A cancer treatment involving high doses of radiation or chemotherapy during which the marrow is destroyed and then replaced with healthy bone marrow.

botulism Possibly fatal food poisoning, caused by a type of bacterium, which grows and produces its toxin in the absence of air and is found in improperly canned food.

bradycardia An abnormally slow heart rate, under 60 beats per minute.

breech birth A birth in which the infant's buttocks or feet pass through the birth canal first.

bulimia nervosa Episodic binge eating, often followed by forced vomiting or laxative abuse, and accompanied by a persistent preoccupation with body shape and weight.

bupropion A drug, also known as Zyban, for treating nicotine addiction that is an alternative to the nicotine patch.

burnout A state of physical, emotional, and mental exhaustion resulting from constant or repeated emotional pressure.

caesarean delivery The surgical procedure in which an infant is delivered through an incision made in the abdominal wall and uterus.

calorie The amount of energy required to raise the temperature of 1 gram of water by 1 Celsius. In everyday usage related to the energy content of foods and the energy expended in activities, a calorie is actually the equivalent of a thousand such calories, or a kilocalorie.

candidiasis An infection of the yeast Candida albicans, commonly occurring in the vagina, vulva, penis, and mouth and causing burning, itching, and a whitish discharge.

capillary A minute blood vessel that connects an artery to a vein.

carbohydrates Organic compounds, such as starches, sugars, and glycogen, that are composed of carbon, hydrogen, and oxygen, and are sources of bodily energy.

carbon monoxide A colorless, odorless gas produced by the burning of gasoline or tobacco; displaces oxygen in the hemoglobin molecules of red blood cells.

carcinogen A substance that produces cancerous cells or enhances their development and growth.

cardiopulmonary resuscitation (CPR) A method of artificial stimulation of the heart and lungs; a combination of mouth-to-mouth breathing and chest compression.

cardiovascular fitness The ability of the heart and blood vessels to circulate blood through the body efficiently.

celibacy Abstention from sexual activity; can be partial or complete, permanent or temporary.

cell-mediated The portion of the immune response that protects against parasites, fungi, cancer cells, and foreign tissue, primarily by means of T cells, or lymphocytes.

certified social worker A person who has completed a two-year graduate program in counseling people with mental problems.

cervical cap A thimble-sized rubber or plastic cap that is inserted into the vagina to fit over the cervix and prevent the passage of sperm into the uterus during sexual intercourse; used with a spermicidal foam or jelly, it serves as both a chemical and a physical barrier to sperm.

cervix The narrow, lower end of the uterus that opens into the vagina.

chanchroid A soft, painful sore or localized infection usually acquired through sexual contact.

chemoprevention The use of natural or synthetic substances to reduce the risk of developing cancer.

chiropractic A method of treating disease, primarily through manipulating the bones and joints to restore normal nerve function.

chlamydial infections A sexually transmitted disease caused by the bacterium Chlamydia trachomatis, often asymptomatic in women, but sometimes characterized by urinary pain; if undetected and untreated, may result in pelvic inflammatory disease (PID).

chlorinated hydrocarbons Highly toxic pesticides, such as DDT and chlordane, that are extremely resistant to breakdown; may cause cancer, birth defects, neurological disorders, and damage to wildlife and the environment.

cholesterol An organic substance found in animal fats; linked to cardiovascular disease, particularly atherosclerosis.

chronic fatigue syndrome (CFS) A cluster of symptoms whose cause is not yet known; a primary symptom is debilitating fatigue.

chronic obstructive lung disease (COLD) Any one of several lung diseases characterized by obstruction of breathing, including emphysema and chronic bronchitis.

circumcision The surgical removal of the foreskin of the penis.

cirrhosis A chronic disease, especially of the liver, characterized by a degeneration of cells and excessive scarring.

clinical practice guidelines Recommendations used by physicians to determine appropriate health care for specific conditions.

clitoris A small erectile structure on the female, corresponding to the penis on the male.

cocaine A white crystalline powder extracted from the leaves of the coca plant which stimulates the central nervous system and produces a brief period of euphoria followed by a depression.

codependence An emotional and psychological behavioral pattern in which the spouses, partners, parents, children, and friends of individuals with addictive behaviors allow or enable their loved ones to continue their self-destructive habits.

cognitive therapy A technique used to identify an individual's beliefs and attitudes, recognize negative thought patterns, and educate in alternative ways of thinking.

cohabitation Two people living together as a couple, without official ties such as marriage.

coitus interruptus The removal of the penis from the vagina before ejaculation.

colpotomy Surgical sterilization by cutting or blocking the fallopian tubes through an incision made in the wall of the vagina.

coma A state of total unconsciousness.

companion-oriented marriage A marital relationship in which the partners share interests, activities, and domestic responsibilities.

complementary medicine and alternative medicine (CAM) A term used to apply to all health care approaches, practices, and treatments not widely taught in medical schools, not generally used in hospitals, and not usually reimbursed by medical insurance companies.

complementary proteins Incomplete proteins that, when combined, provide all the amino acids essential for protein synthesis.

complete proteins Proteins that contain all the amino acids needed by the body for growth and maintenance.

complex carbohydrates Starches, including cereals, fruits, and vegetables.

conception The merging of a sperm and an ovum.

computer vision syndrome A condition caused by computer use marked by tired and sore eyes, blurred vision, headaches, and neck, shoulder, and back pain.

conditioning The gradual building up of the body to enhance one or more of the three main components of physical fitness: flexibility, cardiovascular or aerobic fitness, and muscular strength and endurance.

condom A latex sheath worn over the penis during sexual acts to prevent conception and/or the transmission of disease; some condoms contain a spermicidal lubricant.

congestive heart failure Inability of the heart to pump at normal capacity, resulting in decreased blood flow throughout the body, collection of blood fluids in the lungs, and pulmonary congestion.

constant-dose combination pill An oral contraceptive that releases synthetic estrogen and progestin at constant levels throughout the menstrual cycle.

contraception The prevention of conception; birth control.

coping mechanism Any of several conscious and unconscious mental processes that enable a person to cope with a difficult situation or problem; usually healthier, more mature, and more effective than a defense mechanism.

coronary angiography A diagnostic test in which a thin tube is threaded through the blood vessels of the heart, a dye is injected, and X rays are taken to detect blockage of the arteries.

coronary bypass Surgical correction of a blockage in a coronary artery by grafting an artery from the patients leg or chest wall onto the damaged artery to detour blood around the blockage.

corpus luteum A yellowish mass of tissue that is formed, immediately after ovulation, from the remaining cells of the follicle; it secretes estrogen and progesterone for the remainder of the menstrual cycle.

Cowpers glands Two small glands that discharge into the male urethra; also called bulbourethral glands.

crib death The unexplained death of an apparently healthy baby under one year of age during sleep; also called sudden infant death syndrome (SIDS).

cross-training Alternating two or more different types of fitness activities.

crucifers Plants, including broccoli, cabbage, and cauliflower, that contain large amounts of fiber, proteins, and indoles.

culture The set of shared attitudes, values, goals, and practices of a group that are internalized by an individual within the group.

cunnilingus Sexual stimulation of a woman's genitals by means of oral manipulation.

cystitis Inflammation of the urinary bladder.

decibel (dB) A unit for measuring the intensity of sounds.

deleriants Chemicals, such as solvents, aerosols, glue, cleaning fluids, petroleum products, and some anesthetics, that produce vapors with psychoactive effects when inhaled.

delirium tremens (DTs) The delusions, hallucinations, and agitated behavior following withdrawal from long-term chronic alcohol abuse.

dementia Deterioration of mental capability.

dendrites Branching fibers of a neuron that receive impulses from axon terminals of other neurons and conduct these impulses toward the nucleus.

depression In general, feelings of unhappiness and despair; as a mental illness, also characterized by an inability to function normally

depressive disorders A group of psychological disorders involving pervasive and sustained depression.

dermatitis Any inflammation of the skin.

designer drugs Illegally manufactured psychoactive drugs that have dangerous physical and psychological effects.

detoxification The supervised removal of a poisonous or harmful substance (such as a drug) from the body; a therapy for alcoholics in which they are denied alcohol in a controlled environment.

diabetes mellitus A disease in which the inadequate production of insulin leads to failure of the body tissues to break down carbohydrates at a normal rate.

diagnostic-related group (DRG) A category of conditions requiring hospitalization for which the cost of care has been determined prior to a client's hospitalization.

diaphragm A bowl-like rubber cup with a flexible rim that is inserted into the vagina to cover the cervix and prevent the passage of sperm into the uterus during sexual intercourse; used with a spermicidal foam or jelly, it serves as both a chemical and a physical barrier to sperm.

diastole The period between contractions in the cardiac cycle, during which the heart relaxes and dilates as it fills with blood.

digestion The process of chemically and mechanically breaking down foods into compounds capable of being absorbed by body cells.

dilation and evacuation (D and E) A medical procedure in which the contents of the uterus are removed through the use of instruments.

dioxins A family of chemicals used in industry; some forms are believed to be extremely toxic.

distress A negative stress stage that may result in illness.

do-not-resuscitate (DNR) A directive expressing an individual's preference that resuscitation efforts not be made during a medical crisis.

drug Any substance, other than food, that when taken, affects bodily functions and structures.

drug abuse The excessive use of a drug in a manner inconsistent with accepted medical practice.

drug misuse The use of a drug for a purpose (or person) other than that for which it was medically intended.

dyathanasia The act of permitting death by the removal or ending of any extraordinary efforts to sustain life; passive euthanasia.

dysfunctional Characterized by negative and destructive patterns of behavior between partners or between parents and children.

dysmenorrhea Painful menstruation.

dyspareunia A sexual difficulty in which a woman experiences pain during sexual intercourse.

dysthymia Frequent, prolonged mild depression.

eating disorders Bizarre, often dangerous patterns of food consumption, including anorexia nervosa, bulimia nervosa, and bulimarexia.

e coli (Escherichia coli) a bacteria often spread through undercooked or inadequately washed foods.

ecosystem A community of organisms sharing a physical and chemical environment and interacting with each other.

ectopic pregnancy A pregnancy in which the fertilized egg has implanted itself outside the uterine cavity, usually in the fallopian tube.

ejaculation The expulsion of semen from the penis.

ejaculatory duct The canal connecting the seminal vesicles and vas deferens.

electrocardiogram (ECG, EKG) A graphic record of the electric current associated with heartbeats.

electromagnetic fields (EMFs) The invisible electric and magnetic fields generated by an electrically charged conductor.

embryo An organism in its early stage of development; in humans, the embryonic period lasts from about the second to the eighth week of pregnancy.

emotional health The ability to express and acknowledge one's feelings and moods.

emotional intelligence A term used by some psychologists to evaluate the capacity of people to understand themselves and relate well with others.

enabling To unwittingly contribute to a person's addictive or abusive behavior. Components of enabling include shielding or covering up for an abuser/addict; controlling them; taking over responsibilities; rationalizing addictive behavior; or cooperating with them.

endocrine disruptors Synthetic chemicals that interfere with the ways that hormones work in humans and wildlife.

endocrine system The group of ductless glands that produce hormones and secrete them directly into the blood for transport to target organs.

endometrium The mucous membrane lining the uterus.

endorphins Mood-elevating, pain-killing chemicals produced by the brain.

endurance The ability to withstand the stress of continued physical exertion.

enkephalins Naturally occurring opioids that the body uses to relieve pain and stress.

environmental tobacco smoke Secondhand cigarette smoke; the third leading preventable cause of death.

epididymis That portion of the male duct system in which sperm mature.

epidural block An injection of anesthesia into the membrane surrounding the spinal cord to numb the lower body during labor and childbirth.

epilepsy A variety of neurological disorders characterized by sudden attacks (seizures) of violent muscle contractions and unconsciousness.

ergogenic aids Dietary supplements that purport to boost strength and enhance athletic performance, such as androstenedione and creatine.

erogenous Sexually sensitive.

estrogen The female sex hormone that stimulates female secondary sex characteristics.

ethyl alcohol The intoxicating agent in alcoholic beverages; also called ethanol.

eustress Positive stress, which stimulates a person to function properly.

euthanasia Any method of painlessly causing death for a terminally ill person.

failure rate The number of pregnancies that occur per year for every 100 women using a particular method of birth control.

fallopian tubes The pair of channels that transport ova from the ovaries to the uterus; the usual site of fertilization.

false negative A diagnostic test result that falsely indicates the absence of a particular condition.

false positive A diagnostic test result that falsely indicates the presence of a particular condition.

family A group of people united by marriage, blood, or adoption, residing in the same household, maintaining a common culture, and interacting with one another on the basis of their roles within the group.

fat-soluble vitamins Vitamins absorbed through the intestinal membranes, with the aid of fats in the diet or bile from the liver, and stored in the body.

fellatio Sexual stimulation of a man's genitals by means of oral manipulation.

fertilization The fusion of the sperm and egg nuclei.

fetal alcohol effects (FAE) Milder forms of FAS, including low birth weight, irritability as newborns, and permanent mental impairment as a result of the mother's alcohol consumption during pregnancy.

fetal alcohol syndrome (FAS) A cluster of physical and mental defects in the newborn, including low birth weight, smaller-than-normal head circumference, intrauterine growth retardation, and permanent mental impairment caused by the mother's alcohol consumption during pregnancy.

fetus The human organism developing in the uterus from the ninth week until birth.

fiber Indigestible materials in food that lower blood cholesterol or facilitate digestion and elimination.

flap surgery Surgical removal of diseased tissue and bone from under the gums of the teeth.

flexibility The range of motion allowed by one's joints; determined by the length of muscles, tendons, and ligaments attached to the joints.

food allergies Hypersensitivities to particular foods.

food toxicologists Specialists who detect toxins in food and treat the conditions toxins produce.

frostbite The freezing or partial freezing of skin and tissue just below the skin, or even muscle and bone; more severe than frostnip.

frostnip Sudden blanching or lightening of the skin on hands, feet, and face, resulting from exposure to high wind speeds and low temperatures.

fungi (singular, fungus) Organisms that reproduce by means of spores.

gallstones Clumps of solid material, usually cholesterol, that form in bile stored in the gallbladder.

gamma butyrolactone (GBL) The main ingredient in gamma hydroxybutyrate (GHB), also known as the "date rape drug"; once ingested, GBL converts to GHB and can cause the ingestor to lose consciousness.

gamma globulin The antibody-containing portion of the blood fluid (plasma).

gamma hydroxybutyrate (GHB) A brain messenger chemical that stimulates the release of human growth hormone; commonly abused for its high and its alleged ability to trim fat and build muscles. Also known as "blue nitro" or the "date rape drug."

gender Maleness or femaleness, as determined by a combination of anatomical and physiological factors, psychological factors, and learned behaviors.

gene therapy A cancer treatment involving the insertion of genes into a patient.

general adaptation syndrome (GAS) The sequenced physiological response to a stressful situation; consists of three stages: alarm, resistance, and exhaustion.

generalized anxiety disorder (GAD) An anxiety disorder characterized as chronic distress.

generic Refers to products without trade names that are equivalent to other products protected by trademark registration.

gerontologist A specialist in the interdisciplinary field that studies aging.

gingivitis Inflammation of the gums.

glia Support cells for neurons in the brain and spinal cord that separate the brain from the bloodstream, assist in the growth of neurons, speed transmission of nerve impulses, and eliminate damaged neurons.

gonadotropins Gonad-stimulating hormones produced by the pituitary gland.

gonads The primary reproductive organs in a man (testes) or woman (ovaries).

gonorrhea A sexually transmitted disease caused by the bacterium Neisseria gonorrhoeae; symptoms include discharge from the penis; women are generally asymptomatic.

greenhouse effect An environmental phenomenon in which the buildup of carbon dioxide and other greenhouse gases leads to warming of the planet.

guided imagery An approach to stress control, self-healing, or motivating life changes by means of visualizing oneself in the state of calmness, wellness, or change.

gum disease Inflammation of the gum and bones that hold teeth in place.

hallucinogen A drug that causes hallucinations.

hashish A concentrated form of a drug, derived from the cannabis plant, containing the psychoactive ingredient TCH, which causes a sense of euphoria when inhaled or eaten.

health A state of complete well-being, including physical, psychological, spiritual, social, intellectual, and environmental components.

health maintenance organization (HMO) An organization that provides health services on a fixed-contract basis.

health promotion An educational and informational process in which people are helped to change attitudes and behaviors in an effort to improve their health.

heat cramps Painful muscle spasms caused by vigorous exercise accompanied by heavy sweating in the heat.

heat exhaustion Faintness, rapid heart beat, low blood pressure, an ashen appearance, cold and clammy skin, and nausea, resulting from prolonged sweating with inadequate fluid replacement.

heat stress Physical response to prolonged exposure to high temperature; occurs simultaneously with or after heat cramps.

heat stroke A medical emergency consisting of a fever of at least 105°F, hot dry skin, rapid heart-beat, rapid and shallow breathing, and elevated or lowered blood pressure, caused by the breakdown of the body's cooling mechanism.

helminth A parasitic roundworm or flatworm.

hemoglobin The oxygen-transporting component of red blood cells; composed of heme and globin.

hepatitis An inflammation and/or infection of the liver caused by a virus, often accompanied by jaundice.

herbal medicine An ancient form of medical treatment using substances derived from trees, flowers, ferns, seaweeds, and lichens to treat disease.

herbology The practice of herbal medicine.

hernia The abnormal protrusion of an organ or body part through the tissues of the walls containing it.

herpes simplex A condition caused by one of the herpes viruses and characterized by lesions of the skin or mucous membranes; herpes virus type 2 is sexually transmitted, and causes genital blisters or sores.

hertz A unit for measuring the frequency of sound waves.

heterosexual Primary sexual orientation toward members of the other sex.

holistic An approach to medicine that takes into account body, mind, emotions, and spirit.

holographic will A will wholly in the handwriting of its author.

home health care Provision of medical services and equipment to patients in the home to restore or maintain comfort, function, and health.

homeopathy A system of medical practice that treats a disease by administering dosages of substances that would in healthy persons produce symptoms similar to those of the disease.

homeostasis The body's natural state of balance or stability.

homosexual Primary sexual orientation toward members of the same sex.

hormones Substances released in the blood that regulate specific bodily functions.

hormone replacement therapy (HRT) The use of supplemental hormones during and after menopause.

hospice A homelike health-care facility or program committed to supportive care for terminally ill people.

host A person or population that contracts one or more pathogenic agents in an environment.

hostile or offensive environment A workplace made hostile, abusive, or unbearable by persistent inappropriate behaviors of coworkers or supervisors.

human immunodeficiency virus (HIV) A type of virus that causes a spectrum of health problems, ranging from a symptomless infection to changes in the immune system, to the development of life-threatening diseases because of impaired immunity.

human papilloma virus (HPV) A pathogen that causes genital warts and increases the risk of cervical cancer.

humoral A portion of the immune response that provides lifelong protection against bacterial or viral infections, such as mumps, by means of antibodies whose production is triggered by the release of antigens upon first exposure to the infectious agent.

hunger The physiological drive to consume food.

hydrostatic weighing The weighing of a person in water to distinguish buoyant fat from denser muscle.

hypertension High blood pressure occurring when the blood exerts excessive pressure against the arterial walls.

hypothermia An abnormally low body temperature; if not treated appropriately, coma or death could result.

hysterectomy The surgical removal of the uterus.

hysterotomy A procedure in which the uterus is surgically opened and the fetus inside it removed.

immune deficiency Partial or complete inability of the immune system to respond to pathogens.

immunity Protection from infectious diseases.

immunotherapy A series of injections of small but increasing doses of an allergen, used to treating allergies.

implantation The embedding of the fertilized ovum in the uterine lining.

impotence A sexual difficulty in which a man is unable to achieve or maintain an erection.

incest Sexual relations between two individuals too closely related to contract a legal marriage.

incomplete proteins Proteins that lack one or more of the amino acids essential for protein synthesis.

incubation period The time between when a pathogen enters the body and the first symptom.

indemnity A form of insurance that pays a major portion of medical expenses after a deductible amount is paid by the insured person.

indoles Naturally occurring chemicals found in foods such as winter squash, carrots, and crucifers; may help lower cancer risk.

induced abortion A procedure to remove the uterine contents after pregnancy has occurred.

infertility The inability to conceive a child.

infiltration A gradual penetration or invasion.

inflammation A localized response by the body to tissue injury, characterized by swelling and the dilation of the blood vessels.

inflammatory bowel disease (IBD) A digestive disease that causes frequent and intense diarrhea, abdominal pain, gas, fever, and rectal bleeding. Crohn's disease is an inflammation anywhere in the digestive tract, and ulcerative colitis causes severe ulcers in the inner lining of the colon and rectum.

informed consent Permission (to undergo or receive a medical procedure or treatment) given voluntarily, with full knowledge and understanding of the procedure or treatment and its consequences.

influenza Any number of a type of fairly common, highly contagious viral diseases.

inhalants Substances that produce vapors having psychoactive effects when sniffed.

integrative medicine An approach that combines traditional medicine with alternative/complementary therapies.

intercourse Sexual stimulation by means of entry of the penis into the vagina; coitus.

interpersonal therapy (IPT) A technique used to develop communication skills and relationships.

intimacy A state of closeness between two people, characterized by the desire and ability to share one's innermost thoughts and feelings with each other either verbally or nonverbally.

intoxication Maladaptive behavioral, psychological, and physiologic changes that occur as a result of substance abuse.

intramuscular Into or within a muscle.

intrauterine device (IUD) A device inserted into the uterus through the cervix to prevent pregnancy by interfering with implantation.

intravenous Into a vein.

ionizing radiation A form of energy emitted from atoms as they undergo internal change.

irradiation Exposure to or treatment by some form of radiation.

irritable bowel syndrome A digestive disease caused by intestinal spasms, resulting in frequent need to defecate, nausea, cramping, pain, gas, and a continual sensation of rectal fullness.

isokinetic Having the same force; exercise with specialized equipment that provides resistance equal to the force applied by the user throughout the entire range of motion.

isometric Of the same length; exercise in which muscles increase their tension without shortening in length, such as when pushing an immovable object.

isotonic Having the same tension or tone; exercise requiring the repetition of an action that creates tension, such as weight lifting or calisthenics.

kidney stones Formations of calcium salts or minerals that form in the kidneys; may be passed out of the body in urine, surgically removed, or decomposed by high-frequency sound waves.

labia majora The fleshy outer folds that border the female genital area.

labia minora The fleshy inner folds that border the female genital area.

labor The process leading up to birth: effacement and dilation of the cervix; the movement of the baby into and through the birth canal, accompanied by strong contractions; and contraction of the uterus and expulsion of the placenta after the birth.

lacto-vegetarians People who eat dairy products as well as fruits and vegetables (but not meat, poultry, or fish).

Lamaze method A method of childbirth preparation taught to expectant parents to help the woman cope with the discomfort of labor; combines breathing and psychological techniques.

laparoscopy A surgical sterilization procedure in which the fallopian tubes are observed with a laparoscope inserted through a small incision, and then cut or blocked.

laparotomy A surgical sterilization procedure in which the fallopian tubes are cut or blocked through an incision made in the abdomen.

licensed clinical social worker (LCSW). See certified social worker.

lifestyle An individual's way of life, as indicated and expressed by one's daily practices, interests, possessions, and so on.

lipoprotein A compound in blood that is made up of proteins and fat; a high-density lipoprotein (HDL) picks up excess cholesterol in the blood; a low-density lipoprotein (LDL) carries more cholesterol and deposits it on the walls of arteries.

listeria A bacteria commonly found in deli meats, hot dogs, and soft cheeses that can cause an infection called listeriosis.

living will A written statement providing instructions for the use of life-sustaining procedures in the event of terminal illness or injury.

lochia The vaginal discharge of blood, mucus, and uterine tissue that occurs after birth.

locus of control An individual's belief about the source of power and influence over one's life.

lumpectomy The surgical removal of a breast tumor and its surrounding tissue.

Lyme disease A disease caused by a bacterium carried by a tick; it may cause heart arrhythmias, neurological problems, and arthritis symptoms.

lymph nodes Small tissue masses in which some immune cells are stored.

mainstream smoke The smoke inhaled directly by smoking a cigarette.

mainstreaming The placement of disabled students into regular school classes with specialized attention given in the classroom or in separate sessions.

major depression Sadness that does not end.

male pattern baldness The loss of hair at the vertex, or top, of the head.

malpractice The failure of a doctor or other health-care professionals to provide appropriate and skillful medical or surgical treatment.

mammography A diagnostic X-ray exam used to detect breast cancer.

managed care Health-care services and reimbursement predetermined by third-party insurers.

marijuana The drug derived from the cannabis plant, containing the psychoactive ingredient THC, which causes a mild sense of euphoria when inhaled or eaten.

marriage and family therapist A psychiatrist, psychologist, or social worker who specializes in marriage and family counseling.

mastectomy The surgical removal of an entire breast.

masturbation Manual (or nonmanual) self-stimulation of the genitals, often resulting in orgasm.

medical history The health-related information collected during the interview of a client by a health-care professional.

meditation A group of approaches that use quiet sitting, breathing techniques, and/or chanting to relax, improve concentration, and become attuned to one's inner self.

menarche The onset of menstruation at puberty.

menopause The complete cessation of ovulation and menstruation for twelve consecutive months.

menstruation Discharge of blood from the vagina as a result of the shedding of the uterine lining at the end of the menstrual cycle.

mental disorder Behavioral or psychological syndrome associated with distress or disability or with a significantly increased risk of suffering death, pain, disability, or loss of freedom.

mental health The ability to perceive reality as it is, to respond to its challenges, and to develop rational strategies for living.

meta-analysis Summarization and review of research in a particular area to evaluate the results of several large clinical trials in a uniform manner.

metastasize To spread to other parts of the body via the bloodstream or lymphatic system.

microwaves Extremely high frequency electro-magnetic waves that increase the rate at which molecules vibrate, thereby generating heat.

migraine headache Severe headache resulting from the constriction, then dilation of blood vessels within the brain; sometimes accompanied by vomiting and nausea.

mindfulness A method of stress reduction that involves experiencing the physical and mental sensations of the present moment.

minerals Naturally occurring inorganic substances, small amounts of some being essential in metabolism and nutrition.

minilaparotomy A surgical sterilization procedure in which the fallopian tubes are cut or sealed by electrical coagulation through a small incision just above the pubic hairline.

minipill An oral contraceptive containing a small amount of progestin and no estrogen, which prevents contraception by making the mucus in the cervix so thick that sperm cannot enter the uterus.

miscarriage A pregnancy that terminates before the twentieth week of gestation; also called spontaneous abortion.

mitral valve prolapse A condition in which a valve in the heart is abnormally long and floppy, which can cause heart murmurs.

mononucleosis An infectious viral disease characterized by an excess of white blood cells in the blood, fever, bodily discomfort, a sore throat, and kidney and liver complications.

mons pubis The rounded, fleshy area over the junction of the female pubic bones.

mood A sustained emotional state that colors one's view of the world for hours or days.

moral The internal standard of right and wrong by which one makes judgments and decisions.

multiphasic pill An oral contraceptive that releases different levels of estrogen and progestin to mimic the hormonal fluctuations of the natural menstrual cycle.

multiple chemical sensitivity (MCS) A sensitivity to low-level chemical exposures from ordinary substances, such as perfumes and tobacco smoke, that results in physiological responses like chest pain, depression, dizziness, fatigue, and nausea. Also known as environmentally triggered illness.

mutagen An agent that causes alterations in the genetic material of living cells.

mutation A change in the genetic material of a cell or cells that is brought about by radiation, chemicals, or natural causes.

myocardial infarction (MI) A condition characterized by the dying of tissue areas in the myocardium, caused by interruption of the blood supply to those areas; the medical name for a heart attack.

near-death experiences See autoscopy.

negligence The failure to act in a way that a reasonable person would act.

neoplasm Any tumor, whether benign or malignant.

nephrosis A cluster of symptoms indicating chronic damage to the kidneys.

neuron The basic working unit of the brain, which transmits information from the senses to the brain and from the brain to specific body parts; each nerve cell consists of an axon, an axon terminal, and dendrites.

neuropsychiatry The study of the brain and mind.

neurotransmitters Chemicals released by neurons that stimulate or inhibit the action of other neurons.

nicotine The addictive substance in tobacco; one of the most toxic of all poisons.

nocturnal emissions Ejaculations while dreaming; wet dreams.

non-exercise activity thermogenesis (NEAT) The process of burning calories through non-volitional activities such as walking and gardening,

noncompliance Failure to take a prescription drug according to the doctor's instructions.

nongonococcal urethritis (NGU) Inflammation of the urethra caused by organisms other than the gonococcus bacterium.

nonopioids Chemically synthesized drugs that have sleep-inducing and pain-relieving properties similar to those of opium and its derivatives.

norms The unwritten rules regarding behavior and conduct expected or accepted by a group.

nucleus The central part of a cell, contained in the cell body of a neuron.

nutrients Elements in food that the body cannot produce on its own, which are essential for growth, repair, and energy.

nutrition The science devoted to the study of dietary needs for food and the effects of food on organisms.

obesity The excessive accumulation of fat in the body; a condition of being 20% or more above the ideal weight for a person of that height and gender.

obsessive-compulsive disorder (OCD) An anxiety disorder characterized by obsessions and/or compulsions that impair one's ability to function and form relationships.

oncogene A gene that, when activated by radiation or a virus, may cause a normal cell to become cancerous.

opioids Drugs that have sleep-inducing and pain-relieving properties, including opium and its derivatives and nonopioid, synthetic drugs.

optimism The tendency to seek out, remember, and expect pleasurable experiences.

oral contraceptives Preparations of synthetic hormones that inhibit ovulation; also referred to as birth control pills or simply the pill.

organic phosphates Toxic pesticides that may cause cancer, birth defects, neurological disorders, and damage to wildlife and the environment.

organic Term designating food produced with, or production based on the use of, fertilizer originating from plants or animals, without the use of pesticides or chemically formulated fertilizers.

orgasm A series of contractions of the pelvic muscles occurring at the peak of sexual arousal.

osteopathy The manipulation of the spine and other structural parts of the body to treat disorders.

osteoporosis A condition common in older people in which the bones become increasingly soft and porous, making them susceptible to injury.

outcomes The ultimate impacts of particular treatments or absence of treatment.

ovary The female sex organ that produces egg cells, estrogen, and progesterone.

over-the-counter (OTC) drugs Medications that can be obtained legally without a prescription from a medical professional.

overloading Method of physical training involving increasing the number of repetitions or the amount of resistance gradually to work the muscle to temporary fatigue.

overtrain Working muscles too intensely or too frequently, resulting in persistent muscle soreness, injuries, unintended weight loss, nervousness, and an inability to relax.

overuse injuries Physical injuries to joints or muscles, such as strains, fractures, and tendinitis, which result from overdoing a repetitive activity.

ovo-lacto-vegetarians People who eat eggs, dairy products, and fruits and vegetables (but not meat, poultry, or fish).

ovulation The release of a mature ovum from an ovary approximately 14 days prior to the onset of menstruation.

ovulation method A method of birth control based on the observation of changes in the consistency of the mucus in the vagina to predict ovulation.

ovum (plural, ova) The female gamete (egg cell).

oxytocin A hormone that has been linked to one's ability to bond with others; also plays a key role in inducing labor during childbirth.

ozone layer An upper layer of the earth's atmosphere that protects the earth from harmful ultra-violet radiation from the sun.

panic attack A short episode characterized by physical sensations of light-headedness, dizziness, hyperventilation, and numbness of extremities, accompanied by an inexplicable terror, usually of a physical disaster such as death.

panic disorder An anxiety disorder in which the apprehension or experience of recurring panic attacks is so intense that normal functioning is impaired.

Pap smear A test in which cells removed from the cervix are examined under a microscope for signs of cancer; also called a Pap test.

pathogen A microorganism that produces disease.

PCP (phencyclidine) A synthetic psychoactive substance that produces effects similar to other psychoactive drugs when swallowed, smoked, sniffed, or injected, but may also trigger unpredictable behavioral changes.

pedophilia Sexual contact between an adult and an unrelated child.

pelvic inflammatory disease (PID) An inflammation of the internal female genital tract, characterized by abdominal pain, fever, and tenderness of the cervix.

penis The male organ of sex and urination.

percutaneous transluminal coronary angioplasty (PTCA) A procedure for unclogging arteries; also called balloon angioplasty.

perimenopause The period from a woman's first irregular cycles to her last menstruation.

perinatology The medical specialty concerned with the diagnosis and treatment of pregnant women with high-risk conditions and their fetuses.

perineum The area between the anus and vagina in the female and between the anus and scrotum in the male.

periodentitis Severe gum disease in which the tooth root becomes infected.

persistent vegetative state A state of being awake and capable of reacting to physical stimuli, such as light, while being unaware of pain or other environmental stimuli.

personality disorder An inflexible, maladaptive pattern of behavior that impairs an individuals ability to function.

phobia An anxiety disorder marked by an inordinate fear of an object, a class of objects, or a situation, resulting in extreme avoidance behaviors.

physical dependence The physiological attachment to, and need for, a drug.

physical fitness The ability to respond to routine physical demands, with enough reserve energy to cope with a sudden challenge.

phytochemicals Chemicals such as indoles, coumarins, and capsaicin, which exist naturally in plants and have disease-fighting properties.

placenta An organ that develops after implantation and to which the embryo attaches, via the umbilical cord, for nourishment and waste removal.

plaque The sludgelike substance that builds up on the inner walls of arteries.

pneumonia An inflammation of the lungs caused by infection or irritants.

pollutant A substance or agent in the environment, usually the by-product of human industry or activity, that is injurious to human, animal, or plant life.

pollution The presence of pollutants in the environment.

polyabuse The misuse or abuse of more than one drug.

polychlorinated biphenyls (PCBs) A family of chemical compounds, ranging from light, oily fluids to greasy or waxy substances, that have been widely used as industrial coolants and lubricants and in the manufacture of plastics, paints, and varnishes; a possible human carcinogen.

positive psychology An approach that emphasizes building one's personal strengths rather than treating weaknesses.

postpartum depression The emotional downswing that occurs after having a baby due to hormonal changes, physical exhaustion, and psychological pressures.

posttraumatic stress disorder (PTSD) The repeated reliving of a trauma through nightmares or recollection.

potentiating Making more effective or powerful.

preconception care Health care to prepare for pregnancy.

precycling The use of products that are packaged in recycled or recyclable material.

preferred provider organization (PPO) A group of physicians contracted to provide health care to members at a discounted price.

premature ejaculation A sexual difficulty in which a man ejaculates so rapidly that his partner's satisfaction is impaired.

premature labor Labor that occurs after the twentieth week but before the thirty-seventh week of pregnancy.

premenstrual dysphoric disorder (PMDD) A disorder that causes symptoms of psychological depression during the last week of the menstrual cycle.

premenstrual syndrome (PMS) A disorder that causes physical discomfort and psychological distress prior to a woman's menstrual period.

prevention Information and support offered to help healthy people identify their health risks, reduce stressors, prevent potential medical problems, and enhance their well-being.

primary care Ambulatory or outpatient care provided by a physician in an office, emergency room, or clinic.

progesterone The female sex hormone that stimulates the uterus, preparing it for the arrival of a fertilized egg.

progestin-only pill See minipill.

progressive relaxation A method of reducing muscle tension by contracting, then relaxing certain areas of the body.

promotion The process of enabling people to improve and increase control over their health in order to achieve a state of optimal health.

proof The alcoholic strength of a distilled spirit, expressed as twice the percentage of alcohol present.

prostate gland A structure surrounding the male urethra that produces a secretion that helps liquefy the semen from the testes.

prostatitis Inflammation of the prostate gland.

protection Measures that an individual can take when participating in risky behavior to prevent injury or unwanted risks.

protein A substance that is basically a compound of amino acids; one of the essential nutrients.

protozoa Microscopic animals made up of one cell or a group of similar cells.

psoriasis A chronic skin disorder caused by stress, skin damage, or illness and resulting in scaly, deep-pink, raised patches on the skin.

psychiatric drugs Medications that regulate a person's mental, emotional, and physical functions to facilitate normal functioning.

psychiatric nurse A nurse with special training and experience in mental health care.

psychiatrists Licensed medical doctors with additional training in psychotherapy, psychopharmacology, and treatment of mental disorders.

psychoactive Mood-altering.

psychodynamic Interpreting behaviors in terms of early experiences and unconscious influences.

psychological dependence The emotional or mental attachment to the use of a drug.

psychologists Mental health care professionals who have completed doctoral or graduate programs in psychology and are trained in a variety of psychotherapeutic techniques, but who are not medically trained and do not prescribe medications.

psychoneuroimmunology A scientific field that explores the relationships between and among the mind, the central nervous system, and the immune system.

psychoprophylaxis See Lamaze method.

psychotherapy Treatment designed to produce a response by psychological rather than physical means, such as suggestion, persuasion, reassurance, and support.

psychotropic Mind-affecting.

pyelonephritis Inflammation of the kidney.

quackery Medical fakery; unproven practices claiming to cure diseases or solve health problems.

quadrantectomy The surgical removal of a large portion of the breast and surrounding lymph glands.

quid pro quo A form of harassment in which a person in power or authority makes unwanted sexual advances as a condition for receiving a job, promotion, or favor.

rape Sexual penetration of a female or a male by means of intimidation, force, or fraud.

rapid-eye-movement (REM) sleep Regularly occurring periods of sleep during which the most active dreaming takes place.

receptors Molecules on the surface of neurons on which neurotransmitters bind after their release from other neurons.

recycling The processing or reuse of manufactured materials to reduce consumption of raw materials.

reflexology A treatment based on the theory that massaging certain points on the foot or hand relieves stress or pain in corresponding parts of the body.

refractory period The period of time following orgasm during which the male cannot experience another orgasm.

rehabilitation medicine The use of surgical procedures, medication, and physical therapy to improve the condition of patients with disabling conditions such as blindness, deafness, and arthritis.

relative risk The risk of developing cancer in persons with a certain exposure or trait compared to the risk in persons who do not have the same exposure or trait.

reinforcements Rewards or punishments for a behavior that will increase or decrease one's likelihood of repeating the behaviors.

relapse prevention An alcohol recovery treatment method that focuses on social skills training to develop ways of preventing or minimizing a relapse.

rep (or repetition) In weight training, a single performance of a movement or exercise.

repetitive motion injury (RMI) Inflammation of or damage to a part of the body due to repetition of the same movements.

rescue marriage A marital relationship in which one partner has had a traumatic childhood and views marriage as a way of healing the past.

resting heart rate The number of heartbeats per minute during inactivity.

reuptake Reabsorption by the originating cell of neurotransmitters that have not connected with receptors and have been left in synapses.

rhythm method A birth-control method in which sexual intercourse is avoided during those days of the menstrual cycle in which fertilization is most likely to occur.

romantic marriage A marital relationship in which sexual passion never fades.

rubella An infectious disease that may cause birth defects if contracted by a pregnant woman; also called German measles.

satiety A feeling of fullness after eating.

saturated fat A chemical term indicating that a fat molecule contains as many hydrogen atoms as its carbon skeleton can hold. These fats are normally solid at room temperature.

schizophrenia A general term for a group of mental disorders with characteristic psychotic symptoms, such as delusions, hallucinations, and disordered thought patterns during the active phase of the illness, and a duration of at least six months.

scrotum The external sac or pouch that holds the testes.

seasonal affective disorder (SAD) An annual rhythm of depression that appears to be linked to seasonal variations in light.

secondary sex characteristics Physical changes associated with maleness or femaleness, induced by the sex hormones.

self-actualization A state of wellness and fulfillment that can be achieved once certain human needs are satisfied; living to one's full potential.

self-efficacy Belief in one's ability to accomplish a goal or change a behavior.

self-esteem Confidence and satisfaction in oneself.

self-talk Repetition of positive messages about one's self-worth to learn more optimistic patterns of thought, feeling, and behavior.

semen The viscous whitish fluid that is the complete male ejaculate; a combination of sperm and secretions from the prostate gland, seminal vesicles, and other glands.

seminal vesicles Glands in the male reproductive system that produce the major portion of the fluid of semen.

set A person's expectations or preconceptions about a situation or experience; mind-set.

set-point theory The proposition that every person has an unconscious control system for keeping body fat (and therefore weight) at a pre-determined level, or set point.

sets In weight training, the number of repetitions of the same movement or exercise.

sex Maleness or femaleness, resulting from genetic, structural, and functional factors.

sexual addiction A preoccupation with sex so intense and chronic that an individual cannot have a normal sexual relationship with a spouse or lover; sexual compulsion.

sexual coercion Sexual activity forced upon a person by the exertion of psychological pressure by another person.

sexual compulsion See sexual addiction.

sexual dysfunction The inability to react emotionally and/or physically to sexual stimulation in a way expected of the average healthy person or according to one's own standards.

sexual health The integration of the physical, emotional, intellectual, and social aspects of sexual being in ways that are positively enriching and that enhance personality, communication, and love.

sexuality The behaviors, instincts, and attitudes associated with being sexual.

sexually transmitted diseases (STDs) Any of a number of diseases that are acquired through sexual contact.

sexual orientation Sexual attraction to (and behavior with) individuals of one's own sex, the other sex, or both.

sidestream smoke The smoke emitted by a burning cigarette and breathed by everyone in a closed room, including the smoker; contains more tar and nicotine than mainstream smoke.

simple carbohydrates Sugars; like all carbohydrates, they provide the body with glucose.

skin calipers An instrument used to pinch skin folds at the arms, waist, and back to determine the percentage of body fat.

smog A grayish or brownish fog caused by the presence of smoke and/or chemical pollutants in the air.

social isolation A feeling of unconnectedness with others caused by and reinforced by infrequency of social contacts.

social phobia A severe form of social anxiety marked by extreme fears and avoidance of social situations.

sperm The male gamete produced by the testes and transported outside the body through ejaculation.

spermatogenesis The process by which sperm cells are produced.

spinal block An injection of anesthesia directly into the spinal cord to numb the lower body during labor and childbirth.

spiritual health The ability to identify one's basic purpose in life and to achieve one's full potential; the sense of connectedness to a greater power.

spiritual intelligence The capacity to sense, understand, and tap into ourselves, others, and the world around us.

sterilization A surgical procedure to end a person's reproductive capability.

stimulant An agent, such as a drug, that temporarily relieves drowsiness, helps in the performance of repetitive tasks, and improves capacity for work.

strength Physical power; the maximum weight one can lift, push, or press in one effort.

stress The nonspecific response of the body to any demands made upon it; may be characterized by muscle tension and acute anxiety, or may be a positive force for action.

stressor Specific or nonspecific agents or situations that cause the stress response in a body.

stroke A cerebrovascular event in which the blood supply to a portion of the brain is blocked.

subcutaneous Under the skin.

suction curettage A procedure in which the contents of the uterus are removed by means of suction and scraping.

sudden infant death syndrome (SIDS) See crib death.

synapse A specialized site at which electrical impulses are transmitted from the axon terminal of one neuron to a dendrite of another.

synergistic Characterized by a combined effect that is greater than the sum of the individual effects.

syphilis A sexually transmitted disease caused by the bacterium Treponema pallidum, and characterized by early sores, a latent period, and a final period of life-threatening symptoms including brain damage and heart failure.

systemic disease A pathologic condition that spreads throughout the body.

systole The contraction phase of the cardiac cycle.

tachycardia An abnormally rapid heart rate, over 100 beats per minute.

tamoxifen An estrogen-based medication that can help reduce the likelihood of developing cancer.

tar A thick, sticky dark fluid produced by the burning of tobacco, made up of several hundred different chemicals, many of them poisonous, some of them carcinogenic.

target heart rate Sixty to eighty-five percent of the maximum heart rate; the heart rate at which one derives maximum cardiovascular benefit from aerobic exercise.

teratogen Any agent that causes spontaneous abortion or defects or malformations in a fetus.

terminal illness An illness in which death is inevitable.

testes (singular, testis) The male sex organs that produce sperm and testosterone.

testosterone The male sex hormone that stimulates male secondary sex characteristics.

thallium scintigraphy A diagnostic test in which radioactive isotopes are injected into the bloodstream, and images of the rays emitted by the isotopes are captured and then translated into images of the heart as it pumps.

thanatology The discipline of humanitarian care-giving for critically ill patients and their grieving family members and friends.

toxicity Poisonousness; the dosage level at which a drug becomes poisonous to the body, causing either temporary or permanent damage.

toxic shock syndrome (TSS) A disease characterized by fever, vomiting, diarrhea, and often shock, caused by a bacteria that releases toxic waste products into the bloodstream.

traditional marriage A marital relationship in which the roles of the partners are distinct; defined by gender-based cultural norms and expectations.

transcendence The sense of passing into a foreign region or dimension, often experienced by a person near death.

trans fats Fats formed when liquid vegetable oils are processed to make table spreads or cooking fats, and also found in dairy and beef products; considered to be especially dangerous dietary fats.

transgendered Having a gender identity opposite one's biological sex; transsexual.

transient ischemic attack (TIA) A cerebrovascular event in which the blood supply to a portion of the brain is blocked temporarily; repeated attacks are predictors of more severe strokes.

trichomoniasis An infection of the protozoa Trichomonas vaginalis; females experience vaginal burning, itching, and discharge, but male carriers may be asymptomatic.

triglyceride A blood fat that flows through the blood after meals and is linked to increased risk of coronary artery disease.

tubal ligation The suturing or tying shut of the fallopian tubes to prevent pregnancy.

tubal occlusion The blocking of the fallopian tubes to prevent pregnancy.

tuberculosis A highly infectious bacterial disease that primarily affects the lungs and is often fatal.

tumor suppressor genes Genes that normally control cell growth. Many cancers are linked to defects in a tumor suppressor gene.

twelve-step programs Self-help group programs based on the principles of Alcoholics Anonymous.

ulcer A lesion in, or an erosion of, the mucous membrane of an organ.

unsaturated fat A chemical term indicating that a fat molecule contains fewer hydrogen atoms than its carbon skeleton can hold. These fats are normally liquid at room temperature.

urethra The canal through which urine from the bladder leaves the body; in the male, also serves as the channel for seminal fluid.

urethral opening The outer opening of the thin tube that carries urine from the bladder.

urethritis Infection of the urethra.

uterus The female organ that houses the developing fetus until birth.

vagina The canal leading from the exterior opening in the female genital area to the uterus.

vaginal contraceptive film (VCF) A small dissolvable sheet saturated with spermicide that can be inserted into the vagina and placed over the cervix.

vaginal spermicide A substance that kills or neutralizes sperm, inserted into the vagina in the form of a foam, cream, jelly, or suppository.

vaginismus A sexual difficulty in which a woman experiences painful spasms of the vagina during sexual intercourse.

values The criteria by which one makes choices about one's thoughts and actions and goals and ideals.

vas deferens Two tubes that carry sperm from the epididymis into the urethra.

vasectomy A surgical sterilization procedure in which each vas deferens is cut and tied shut to stop the passage of sperm to the urethra for ejaculation.

vector A biological or physical vehicle that carries the agent of infection to the host.

vegans People who eat only plant foods.

ventricle Either of the two lower chambers of the heart, which pump blood out of the heart and into the arteries.

video display terminal (VDT) A screen or monitor that emits electromagnetic fields from all sides; these fields may lead to increased reproductive problems, miscarriages, low birth weights, and cataracts.

virus A submicroscopic infectious agent; the most primitive form of life.

visualization An approach to stress control, self-healing, or motivating life changes by means of guided, or directed, imagery.

vital signs Measurements of physiological functioning; specifically, temperature, blood pressure, pulse rate, and respiration rate.

vitamins Organic substances that are needed in very small amounts by the body and carry out a variety of functions in metabolism and nutrition.

waist-to-hip ratio The proportion of one's waist circumference to one's hip circumference.

wellness A state of optimal health.

withdrawal Development of symptoms that cause significant psychological and physical distress when an individual reduces or stops drug use.

zero population growth (ZPG) The state at which the number of births equals the number of deaths.

zygote A fertilized egg.

Index

health and, 16, 20
health care and, 343
job etiquette and, 585
life expectancy and, 19
loneliness and, 87
physical fitness and, 130, 131
sexual attraction and, 264
smoking and, 546–547
stress and, 45
stroke and, 436
Gender identity, 250
General adaptation syndrome (GAS), 40, 41
Generalized anxiety disorder (GAD), 103
General Social Survey (GSS), 256
Generic drugs, 480
Gene therapy
  for cancer, 461
  for cardiovascular disease, 434
Genetically engineered foods, 186
Genetic disorders, 324. See also Heredity
Genetic testing, 30–31
Genital warts, 391, 399–400
German measles
  immunization against, 378
  pregnancy and, 320
Gestational diabetes, 462
Gestational surrogacy, 326
GHB (gamma hydroxybutyrate), 140, 500, 588
Giardiasis, 371
GIFT (gamete intrafallopian transfer), 326
Gingivitis, 339
Gingko biloba, 115
Global health, 21. See also Environment
  contraception and, 290
Global warming, 621–622, 623
Glycerol, 141
GnRH (gonadotropin–releasing hormone), 250, 256
Goals
  identity and, 75
  realistic, 26
Goleman, Daniel, 69–70
Gonadotropin-releasing hormone (GnRH), 250
  menstrual cycle and, 256
Gonadotropins, 250
Gonads, 250
Gonorrhea, 390, 396–397
Gordon, James, 14
Gorman, Jack, 479
Government, health financing by, 363
Grafenberg spot (G spot), 276
Grains, 155
Grand, mal seizures, 463
Great American Smoke-Out, 557
"Green" (phencyclidine), 498
Greenhouse effect, 621
Grief, 610–612
Group B streptococcus, 385
Growth, puberty and, 251–252
G spot, 276
GSS (General Social Survey), 256

Guided imagery, 57
Gum disease, 339–340
  smoking and, 544
Guns
  suicide and, 108–109
  violence and, 580
Gyms, 146–147

H

Hall, Judith, 223
Hallucinogens, 487, 488, 494–495
  driving and, 490
Happiness, 78–81
Hashish, 491
Hate crimes, 579
Hazelden Recovery Center, 502
HCG (human chorionic gonadotropin), 254
HDL (high-density lipoprotein), 157, 159, 419
Headache, stress-related, 44
Healing rituals, religious, 18
Health. See also Wellness
  changes for improvement of, 15
  of college students, 23
  components of, 14
  definition of, 14
  diversity and, 21–23
  environmental, 19
  global, 21
  grief and, 612
  holistic approach to, 14
  intellectual, 19
  physical, 14
  prevention and, 29–30
  promotion of, 31–32
  psychological, 14, 16, 67–91
  sexual, 252–263
  social, 17–19
  spiritual, 16–17, 18
  stress effects on, 41–44. See also Stress
Health behavior, 23–26
  decisions and, 26
  enabling factors in, 26
  goal setting for, 26
  habits and, 27
  high-risk, 31
  predisposing factors in, 24–25
  reinforcing factors in, 26
  successful change in, 27–29
Health care, 335–366
  access to, 341–347
  dental, 339–340
  elective treatments and, 346–347
  home, 360
  medical research and, 339
  medical rights and, 347–350
  news and, 338
  online medical advice and, 336–338
  payment for, 360–363
  practitioners of, 357–358
  self-care, 336, 337
  treatment plan and, 346
Health-care facilities, 358–360

Health-care proxy, 602–604
Health-care system, 357–360
Health-change contract, 27, 28
Health claims, of products, 25
Health clubs, 146–147
Health education, 29–34
Health maintenance organizations (HMOs), 362–363
Health promotion, 18–19
Health protection, 30–31
  in elderly, 33–34, 147
Health risks. See Risks
Health span, life span and, 32–34
Healthy People 2000, 19–21
Healthy People 2010, 21
Hearing, protection of, 629–630
Heart. See also Cardiovascular disease
  function of, 414
  gender and, 16
  stress effects on, 42–43
Heart attack, 429–431
Heart rate, 336
  abnormalities in, 431
  target, 132–133
Heat
  exercise and, 144–145
  illness related to, 574–575
  pregnancy and, 318
Heat cramps, 574–575
Heat exhaustion, 575
Heat stress, 575
Heat stroke, 575
Helicobacter pylori, ulcers and, 466
Helmets, bike, 571
Helminths, 371–372
Hemoglobin, iron and, 166
Hemophilus influenza type B (HIB)
  infection, immunization against, 379
Hemorrhagic stroke, 435
Hepatitis A, 382–383
  food-borne, 187
Hepatitis B, 382–383, 391
  immunization against, 379
Hepatitis C, 383
Hepatitis D, 383
Herbal ecstasy, 501–502
Herbal medicine, 353–354. See also
  Complementary and alternative medicine (CAM)
  for mental disorders, 115
Heredity, 30–31, 324
  cancer and, 448–449
  cardiovascular disease and, 420
  smoking and, 548
Hernia, 467
Heroin, 487, 488
Heroine, 496
Herpes, 390, 398–399
Heterosexuality, 269
HGH (human growth hormone), 140
HIB (Hemophilus influenza type B)
  infection, immunization against, 379
High-density lipoprotein (HDL), 157, 159, 419